Biomedical
Ethics

Biomedical Ethics

THIRD EDITION

Thomas A. Mappes
Frostburg State University

Jane S. Zembaty
University of Dayton

McGraw-Hill, Inc.
New York St. Louis San Francisco Auckland Bogotá
Caracas Lisbon London Madrid Mexico Milan
Montreal New Delhi Paris San Juan Singapore
Sydney Tokyo Toronto

Biomedical Ethics

Copyright © 1991, 1986, 1981 by McGraw-Hill, Inc. All
rights reserved. Printed in the United States of America.
Except as permitted under the United States Copyright Act
of 1976, no part of this publication may be reproduced or
distributed in any form or by any means, or stored in a data
base or retrieval system, without the prior written permission of the publisher.

3 4 5 6 7 8 9 0   HAL   HAL   9 5 4 3 2

ISBN 0-07-040126-8

This book was set in Plantin by the College Composition Unit
in cooperation with Waldman Graphics, Inc.
The editors were Cynthia Ward and David Dunham;
the production supervisor was Kathryn Porzio.
The cover was designed by Marie-Christine Lawrence.
Arcata Graphics/Halliday was printer and binder.

Library of Congress Cataloging-in-Publication Data

Biomedical ethics / [edited by] Thomas A. Mappes, Jane S. Zembaty.—
    3rd ed.
        p.   cm.
    Reprinted from various sources.
    Includes bibliographical references.
    ISBN 0-07-040126-8
    1. Medical Ethics.   2. Bioethics.   I. Mappes, Thomas A.
    II. Zembaty, Jane S.
    [DNLM: 1. Bioethics—collected works.   2. Ethics, Medical-
collected works.   W 50 B6153]
R724.B49   1991
174.2—dc20
DNLM/DLC
for Library of Congress   90-6069

CONTENTS

v

PREFACE

The third edition of *Biomedical Ethics*, like its predecessors, is designed to provide an effective teaching instrument for courses in biomedical ethics. Although the basic character of the book remains unchanged, it has been substantially revised and updated. Virtually 50 percent of the book's readings are new to the third edition, and a number of new chapter subsections have been developed. For example, there is now material on such topics as AIDS and the duty of physicians to treat (Chapter 2), hospital ethics committees (Chapter 3), treatment decisions for incompetent adults (Chapter 6), maternal/fetal conflicts (Chapter 8), and age-based health-care rationing (Chapter 10).

In this third edition we have retained all the structural features that made earlier editions of the book effective teaching instruments. Thus we have maintained the comprehensive character of the text, once again organized the subject matter so that it unfolds in an efficient and natural fashion, and retained a number of helpful editorial features, such as the argument sketches that precede each selection and the annotated bibliographies at the end of each chapter. We have also retained (and updated) the appendix of case studies. Finally, inasmuch as the value of any textbook anthology is largely dependent upon the quality of its readings, we have once again assembled a set of readings characterized by high-quality analysis and, to the greatest extent possible, clarity of writing style. As in the past, we have also taken care to choose readings that reflect diverse viewpoints with regard to the leading issues in biomedical ethics. Although many of the selections are written by philosophers, the collection also includes writings by lawyers, physicians, scientists, and theologians, as well as relevant judicial opinions and official codes. Such a distribution reflects the interdisciplinary nature of biomedical ethics.

As the table of contents makes clear, this book is extremely comprehensive. We have placed a premium on comprehensiveness in order to allow individual instructors wide latitude regarding the choice of subject matter. In aiming at comprehensiveness, we have been especially concerned to widen the discussion of the professional-patient relationship (Chapters 2 and 3) so that it does not focus exclusively on the physician-patient relationship but also reflects the significant role of nurses in medical care. As for the overall organization and development of subject matter, subsection by subsection, chapter by chapter, we are confident that it unfolds in an efficient and natural fashion. We believe that our organization forestalls some of the perplexities and confusions that students often experience in biomedical ethics. For example, it seems important to us that students consider the concept of mental illness before they discuss involuntary civil commitment (Chapter 5). Similarly, it seems important that students discuss the morality of suicide and the refusal of life-sustaining treatment (Chapter 6) before they discuss the morality of euthanasia (Chapter 7), and so on. Still, we wish to emphasize the relative detachability of our various subsections and chapters. The issues of biomedical ethics are in many ways intertwined and overlapping. Thus there may be many reasons why an individual instructor would prefer to rearrange the order of presentation of our subsections and chapters.

The introductions to each chapter of this book provide one of its most important editorial features. In the introductions we explicitly identify the central issues in each chapter and scan the various positions on these issues together with their supporting argumentation. Whenever possible, we draw out the relationship between the arguments that appear in a certain chapter and the ethical theories, concepts, and principles discussed in our introductory chapter. Whenever necessary, we also provide conceptual and factual information. In this vein, as a matter of course, we explicate the meaning of technical biomedical terms and introduce relevant biomedical information. The purpose of the chapter introductions is to enhance the effectiveness of the book as a teaching instrument. This same central purpose is shared by the book's other editorial features, which include biographical as well as argument sketches preceding each selection and annotated bibliographies at the end of each chapter. The annotated bibliographies provide substantial guidance for further reading and research. The various entries in the bibliographies, like the various readings in each chapter, reflect diverse viewpoints.

We wish to thank the University of Dayton Department of Philosophy and Frostburg State University for their support of this project. We are indebted to the Kennedy Institute, Georgetown University, whose bioethics library has been a significant ally in our research efforts. We are also indebted to the reference librarians at both the University of Dayton and Frostburg State University, and to the following professors who provided Cynthia Elmas of McGraw-Hill with useful review information: Kathleen Barlow, Ball State University; Melvin Brandon, Spring Hill College; Patrick Coffey, Marquette University; Judith Erlen, University of Pittsburgh; Robert Martin, St. Leo College; Gerald Matross, Merrimack College; Thomas Miller, Ball State University; James Moran, Daemen College; Terrence McConnell, University of North Carolina, Greensboro; James Tubbs, Mercy College; Mary Williams, University of Delaware; Richard Wright, University of Toledo; and Thomas Young, Mansfield University of Pennsylvania. We are especially grateful to Lawrence P. Ulrich, University of Dayton, and Joy Kroeger Mappes, Frostburg State University, for their valuable criticisms and advice. Lawrence P. Ulrich also provided much of the material in our original set of case studies. Finally, we must express our thanks to Sky Cappucci for her exemplary work as a research assistant, to Ami Shuster and Shelley Drees for their valuable help with manuscript preparation, and to Vera Mappes and Matt Walls for their assistance in proofreading.

Thomas A. Mappes
Jane S. Zembaty

CHAPTER 1

BIOMEDICAL ETHICS AND ETHICAL THEORY

A number of ethical issues (or problem areas) may be identified as associated with the practice of medicine and/or the pursuit of biomedical research. This set of ethical issues constitutes the subject matter of biomedical ethics. The proper task of biomedical ethics is to advance reasoned analysis in an effort to clarify and resolve such issues. What we term "biomedical ethics" is also commonly termed "bioethics." Although both terms have some measure of currency, we prefer "biomedical ethics" in order to make explicit the concern with issues associated with the practice of medicine.

THE NATURE OF BIOMEDICAL ETHICS

In order to properly situate biomedical ethics as a subdiscipline within the more general discipline of ethics, it is necessary to briefly discuss the nature of ethics as a philosophical discipline. Ethics, understood as a philosophical discipline, can be conveniently defined as the *philosophical* study of morality. As such, it must be immediately distinguished from the *scientific* study of morality, often called "descriptive ethics." The goal of descriptive ethics is to attain empirical knowledge about morality. The practitioner of descriptive ethics is dedicated to describing actually existing moral views and, subsequently, explaining such views by advancing an account of their causal origin. Moral views, no less than other aspects of human experience, provide behavioral and social scientists a range of phenomena that stand in need of explanation. For example, why does a certain individual have such a Victorian view of sexual morality? A Freudian psychologist may attempt an explanation in terms of basic Freudian categories and early childhood experience. Why does a particular group of people manifest such a high incidence of moral opposition to abortion? A sociologist may attempt an explanation in terms of relevant socialization factors. If most of the members of the group were raised as Roman Catholics, this fact is probably relevant to the desired explanation.

Ethics as a philosophical discipline stands in contrast to descriptive ethics. (Hereafter, the expression "ethics" will be used to designate the philosophical discipline, as distinct from descriptive ethics.) Philosophers commonly subdivide ethics into (1) normative ethics and (2) metaethics (analytic ethics), although the precise relationship of these two branches is a matter of some dispute. In normative ethics, philosophers attempt to establish what is morally right and what is morally wrong with regard to human action. In metaethics, philosophers are said to be concerned with an analysis of both moral concepts (e.g., the concept of duty or the concept of a right) and moral reasoning. It seems plausible to maintain that deliberations in normative ethics are to some extent dependent upon and cannot be completely detached from metaethical considerations. But whatever the precise relationship between normative ethics and metaethics, it is important to see that *normative ethics* is logically distinct from *descriptive ethics*. Whereas descriptive ethics attempts to describe (and explain) those moral views which in fact *are accepted*, normative ethics attempts to establish which moral views are *justifiable* and thus *ought to be accepted*. In *general* normative ethics, the task is to advance and provide a reasoned justification of an overall theory of moral obligation, thereby establishing an ethical theory that provides a general answer to the question: What is morally right and what is morally wrong? In *applied* normative ethics, as opposed to general normative ethics, the task is to resolve particular moral problems—for example: Is abortion morally justifiable?

In light of the distinctions just made, it is now possible to identify biomedical ethics as one branch of applied (normative) ethics. The task of biomedical ethics is to resolve ethical problems associated with the practice of medicine and/or the pursuit of biomedical research. Clearly, since there are ethical problems associated with other aspects of life, there are other branches of applied ethics. Business ethics, for example, is concerned with the ethical problems associated with the transaction of business. Importantly, in all branches of applied ethics, the particular issues under discussion are *normative* in character. Is this particular practice right or wrong? Is it morally justifiable? In applied ethics, the concern is not to establish which moral views people do in fact have. That is a descriptive matter. The concern in applied ethics, as in general normative ethics, is to establish which moral views people *ought* to have.

The following questions are typically raised in biomedical ethics. Is a physician morally obligated to tell a terminally ill patient that he or she is dying? Are breaches of medical confidentiality ever morally justifiable? Is abortion morally justifiable? Is euthanasia morally justifiable? Normative ethical questions such as these are concerned with the morality of certain practices. Other questions in biomedical ethics focus on the ethical justifiability of laws. It is one thing to discuss the morality of suicide but quite another thing (although related) to discuss the justifiability of laws that would permit suicide intervention. Is society justified in enacting laws that would restrict the availability of abortion? Is society justified in enacting laws that would allow others to commit an individual, against his or her will, to a mental institution? The appearance of questions of this latter type signifies that biomedical ethics must rely not only on the theories of general normative ethics but also on the theories of social-political philosophy and philosophy of law. In these latter disciplines, a central theoretical question concerns the justifiable limits of law. Strictly speaking, if biomedical ethics is a type of applied ethics, ethics must be broadly understood as encompassing social-political philosophy and the philosophy of law.

Although many of the ethical issues falling within the scope of biomedical ethics have historical roots, especially insofar as they are related to various codes of medical ethics, biomedical ethics did not crystallize into a full-fledged discipline until very recently. Only since about 1970 have the various trappings of a relatively autonomous discipline become manifest. Centers for research in biomedical ethics have emerged, most notably The Hastings Center (now located in Briarcliff Manor, New York) and the Kennedy Institute, Center for Bioethics, Georgetown University (Washington, D.C.). Journals such as the *Hastings Center Report* and the *Journal of Medicine and Philosophy* have sprung into existence. Bibliographies have been produced, conferences abound, and the field has its own encyclopedia, *The Encyclopedia of*

Bioethics (1978). An increasing number of philosophers, as well as theologians, now identify biomedical ethics as an area of specialization.

If, as is clear, many of the ethical issues falling within the scope of biomedical ethics are not historically unprecedented, why is it that biomedical ethics has emerged as a vigorous and highly visible discipline only recently? Two cultural developments are at the root of the contemporary prominence of biomedical ethics: (1) the awesome advance of biomedical research as attended by the resultant development of biomedical technology; and (2) the practice of medicine in an increasingly complicated institutional setting.

Consider first the impact of recent biomedical research. It has been responsible not only for the creation of historically unprecedented ethical problems but also for adding new dimensions to old problems and making the solving of those old problems a matter of greater urgency. Some developments—for example, those associated with reproductive technologies such as *in vitro* fertilization—seem to present us with ethical problems that are genuinely unprecedented. More commonly, however, the advance of biomedical research has simply added complexity to old problems and created a sense of urgency with regard to their solution. Euthanasia is not a new problem; but our ability to save the lives of severely impaired newborns who would have died in the past and our ability to sustain the biological processes of irreversibly comatose individuals have added new dimensions and, surely, a new urgency. Abortion is not a new problem, but the development of various techniques of prenatal diagnosis has created the new possibility of genetic abortion. Indeed, the many successes of biomedical research in our own time, as manifested in the associated technological developments, call attention to the value of systematic biomedical research on human subjects and thus occasion reexamination of ethical limitations with regard to human experimentation.

The practice of medicine in an increasingly complicated institutional setting is, along with the advance of biomedical research, largely responsible for the contemporary prominence of biomedical ethics. In the past, the practice of medicine was largely confined within the bounds of the physician-patient relationship. Now, however, hospitals and other medical institutions are intimately intertwined with physicians and allied personnel in the delivery of medical care. Moreover, we have become increasingly conscious of issues of social justice. We hear talk of a right to health care and are confronted with numerous problems of allocation.

It is frequently said that biomedical ethics is an interdisciplinary field, and some explication of its interdisciplinary character might prove helpful. There is a sense in which biomedical ethics is interdisciplinary within philosophy itself, that is, inasmuch as it applies the theories of social-political philosophy and philosophy of law as well as those of ethics narrowly defined. There is also a sense in which biomedical ethics is interdisciplinary precisely because the issues under discussion are frequently approached not only from the vantage point of moral philosophy (the dominant vantage point in the collection of readings in this text), but also from the vantage point of moral theology. Whereas philosophical analysis proceeds on the basis of *reason alone*, theological analysis proceeds on the basis of *faith*, within a framework of "revealed truth." There is yet a third sense in which biomedical ethics is said to be interdisciplinary. In this sense, the most prominent one, biomedical ethics is interdisciplinary in that it necessarily requires the input of medicine and biology. (It also utilizes, where relevant, the empirical findings of the social sciences.) Medical and biological facts are an essential part of the grist for the mill of ethical evaluation. But it is also important to recognize that the *experience* of medical personnel and researchers is often essential to ensure that ethical discussions retain firm contact with the concrete realities that permeate the practice of medicine and the pursuit of biomedical research.

Although the issues of biomedical ethics are essentially normative, they are often intertwined with both conceptual issues and factual (i.e., empirical) issues. For example, suppose we are concerned with the ethical acceptability of intervention for the sake of preventing a person from committing suicide. Our basic concern is with a normative question; however, we must face the problem of clarifying the nature of suicide, a conceptual issue. For example, if a Jehovah's Witness, on the basis of religious principle, refuses a lifesaving blood transfusion, is the resultant death to be classified as a suicide? In addition to facing conceptual perplexities, we are also faced with an important factual question. Do those who typically attempt suicide really want to die? Presumably psychologists and sociologists have important things to tell us on this score. In the end, of course, we want to apply relevant ethical principles to the issue of the ethical acceptability of intervention for the sake of preventing a person from committing suicide. But ethical principles are applied in the light of conceptual structures and factual beliefs. In the case of some issues in biomedical ethics, underlying factual issues are especially prominent. For example, in addressing the normative question of whether it is ever morally permissible to use children as research subjects, it is important to consider a factual question. To what extent can therapeutic techniques be developed for children in the absence of research employing children as research subjects? In the case of other issues in biomedical ethics, associated conceptual issues command special attention. For example, one could hardly discuss the normative issue of whether the involuntary civil commitment of the mentally ill is a justifiable social practice without closely examining the concept of mental illness. To give a second example, in considering the morality of euthanasia, the distinction between active and passive euthanasia invites conceptual clarification.

It is helpful to approach the literature of biomedical ethics with an eye toward distinguishing conceptual, factual, and normative issues. Furthermore, with regard to normative issues, the central issues of biomedical ethics, one cannot hope to properly situate argumentation in biomedical ethics without some awareness of the various types of ethical theory developed in general normative ethics. Such theories provide the frameworks within which many of the arguments in biomedical ethics are formulated.

ETHICAL THEORIES

An ethical theory provides an ordered set of moral standards (in some cases, simply one *ultimate* moral principle) that is to be used in assessing what is morally right and what is morally wrong regarding human action in general. An ethical theory, in this sense, is a theory of moral obligation. A proponent of any such theory puts it forth as a framework within which a person can correctly determine, on any given occasion, what he or she (morally) ought to do.

The Critical Assessment of Competing Ethical Theories

Since a number of competing ethical theories may be identified, the question immediately arises, what criteria are relevant to an assessment of these competing theories? There is no easy way to answer this very fundamental and very controversial question, but let us start with those considerations whose relevance is unlikely to be disputed. Any theory in any field is rightly expected to be internally consistent. Thus a theory can be faulted on the basis of lack of coherence. In a similar vein, any theory is surely flawed to the extent that it is either unclear and/or incomplete. It might also be claimed that lack of simplicity should count against a theory, but the relevance of this consideration is somewhat more problematic. Perhaps simplicity should be understood as a subsidiary criterion, one whose relevance is limited to the case of deciding between two theories otherwise judged to be equally defensible. Surely a theory that exhibits simplicity is more elegant, more aesthetically pleasing, than one that does not. But if the latter theory is otherwise more adequate, it would seem to retain a superiority over the former.

If the above considerations are relevant to a critical assessment of theories in any field, we must yet identify considerations relevant to our particular concern, the critical assessment of (normative) ethical theories. Responsive to this task, it is suggested that the following criteria should be identified as embodying the two most important considerations. (1) The implications of an ethical theory must be reconcilable with our experience of the moral life. (2) An ethical theory must provide effective guidance where it is most needed, that is, in those situations where substantive moral considerations can be advanced on both sides of an issue. Although many philosophers would endorse the relevance of these two criteria, perhaps not so many would be willing to assign them the exclusive prominence suggested here. Nevertheless, in support of identifying (1) and (2) as the principal criteria relevant to a critical assessment of competing ethical theories, it can be pointed out that analogous considerations are clearly relevant (and prominent) in the critical assessment of empirical (i.e., scientific) theories. When competing empirical theories are under critical examination, it is surely relevant to ask which of the competitors gives a better account of the facts. It is also relevant to ask which of the competitors is superior in terms of heuristic value, that is, which can function to guide future research most effectively. In embracing the priority of (1) and (2), we are saying that an adequate ethical theory must achieve two major goals, analogous to the goals that must be achieved by an adequate empirical theory. An adequate ethical theory must accord with the "facts" of the moral life as we experience it, and it must function heuristically by guiding us when we are confronted with moral perplexity. An ethical theory should, on one hand, make sense out of the moral life by exhibiting the structure underlying our ordinary moral thinking. On the other hand, it should illuminate our moral judgment precisely where it is experienced to falter—in the face of moral dilemmas.

There is certainly no suggestion here that the standards embodied in (1) and (2) can be applied in some mechanical-like fashion to assess the relative adequacy of a proposed ethical theory. Intellectual judgments on these matters are necessarily complex and subtle. In saying, for example, that an adequate ethical theory must accord with our experience of the moral life, we certainly do not want to insist that each and every divergence from the verdict of "commonsense morality" must be interpreted as counting against an ethical theory. Perhaps we would be better advised to revise our moral judgment in light of the theory. (In empirical science, fact-theory mismatches are sometimes resolved not by modifying the theory but by reinterpreting the facts in the light of the theory.) In embracing (1), we undoubtedly commit ourselves to a point of view incompatible with the acceptance of an ethical theory that is revisionary in some wholesale sense, but we do not commit ourselves to the view that "commonsense morality" is sacrosanct. If an ethical theory successfully captures the underlying structure of our ordinary moral thinking, it will of course be true that its implications in large measure accord with our ordinary moral thinking. If the theory, however, cannot be reconciled with a relatively smaller range of our ordinary moral judgments, we may decide to interpret this disharmony as the product of inconsistency in "commonsense morality" rather than as an inadequacy in the proposed theory.

Teleological versus Deontological Theories

With the introduction of criteria (1) and (2), we are now prepared to undertake a survey of alternative ethical theories. Our immediate concern is the identification, articulation, and critical consideration of those ethical theories that are at once both prominent in general normative ethics and frequently reflected in argumentation advanced in biomedical ethics.

In contemporary discussions, ethical theories are frequently grouped into two basic, and mutually exclusive, classes—*teleological* and *deontological*. Any ethical theory that claims the rightness and wrongness of human action is *exclusively* a function of the goodness and badness of the consequences resulting directly or indirectly from that action is a teleological theory. Consequences are all-important here. A deontological theory maintains, in contrast, that the rightness and wrongness of human action is *not exclusively* (in the extreme case, not at all) a function of the goodness and badness of consequences. In accordance with this specification, a theory is deontological (rather than teleological) if it places limits on the relevance of teleological considerations. Thus an ethical theory in which the moral rightness and wrongness of human action is construed as totally independent of the goodness and badness of consequences would be only one kind, albeit the strongest or most extreme kind of deontological theory.

The most prominent teleological ethical theory is the theory known as "utilitarianism." The adequacy of utilitarianism and the issue of its proper explication continue to be dominant concerns in contemporary discussions of ethical theory. For this reason, and especially because much argumentation in biomedical ethics is based on utilitarian reasoning, utilitarianism warrants our detailed attention. However, it should first be noted that utilitarianism is not the only ethical theory that is rightly categorized as teleological. One other notable teleological theory is the theory known as "ethical egoism." The basic principle of ethical egoism can be phrased as follows: *A person ought to act so as to promote his or her own self-interest.* An action is morally right if, when compared to possible alternatives, its consequences are such as to generate the greatest balance of good over evil *for the agent.* (The impact of action on other people is irrelevant except as it may indirectly affect the agent.) Ethical egoism is a teleological theory precisely because, by the terms of the theory, the rightness and wrongness of human action is exclusively a function of the goodness and badness of consequences.

Ethical egoism is an enormously problematic theory, a theory whose implications seem to be intensely at odds with our ordinary moral thinking. Under certain conditions, ethical egoism leads us to the conclusion that it is a person's moral obligation to perform an action that is flagrantly antisocial in nature. Consider this example. Mr. *A* loves to set buildings on fire; nothing makes him happier than watching a building burn down. He recognizes that arson destroys property and subjects human life to serious risk, but he happens to be a thoroughly unsympathetic person, one whose well-being is not negatively affected by the misfortune of others. Of course, it would not be in *A*'s best self-interest (and thus would not be *A*'s moral obligation) to burn down a building if there is a good chance that he will be caught. (The punishment for arson is severe.) But if *A* is very clever, and it is virtually certain that he will not be caught, ethical egoism seems to imply that arson is the morally right thing for him to do.

Another problematic feature of ethical egoism is that it cannot be publicly advocated without inconsistency. Suppose that Ms. *B* embraces ethical egoism. Accordingly, she considers it her moral obligation always to act in such a way as to promote her individual self-interest. Can she now publicly advocate ethical egoism, that is, encourage others to adopt the view that each person's moral obligation is to act in such a way as to promote his or her individual self-interest? No. Since it is to *her* advantage that others *not* act egoistically, it follows that it would be immoral for her to publicly advocate ethical egoism.

In reducing morality to considerations of personal prudence, it can be argued, ethical egoism destroys the very sense behind morality. Morality, it would seem, functions (at least in part) to restrict the pursuit of personal self-interest. It is not that morality prohibits the pursuit of personal self-interest; rather it functions to place limits on this pursuit. In "collapsing" morality into prudence, ethical egoism does not accord with a commonly experienced phenomenon of the moral life, the tension between self-interest and morality, between "what would be best for me" and "what is the morally right thing."

In fairness to ethical egoism, it must be noted that its proponents have sometimes devised ingenious arguments in an attempt to minimize the sort of difficulties just discussed. However, ethical egoism is not widely defended in contemporary discussions of ethical theory, and it surely plays an insignificant role in discussions of biomedical ethics. It has been introduced primarily as a notable instance of a teleological yet nonutilitarian theory. Attention will now be focused on utilitarianism.

In its classical formulation, utilitarianism is found most prominently in the works of two English philosophers, Jeremy Bentham (1748–1832) and John Stuart Mill (1806–1873). In contemporary discussions, a distinction is made between two kinds of utilitarianism—*act-utilitarianism* and *rule-utilitarianism*. Although it is somewhat controversial whether a significant distinction can be maintained between these two versions of utilitarianism, it will be presumed for the sake of exposition that two distinct utilitarian ethical theories can indeed be articulated.

Act-Utilitarianism

Human action typically takes place within the fabric of our social existence. Thus an action performed by one person often impacts not only on the agent but on the lives of many others. Consider a man who refuses to stop smoking even though he suffers from emphysema. He will not be the only one to suffer the consequences; certainly those who care about him will also. His refusal to give up smoking, since it has the effect of further damaging his health, also produces a higher level of anxiety among the members of his family. Among the other detrimental consequences of his continuing to smoke is the negative impact, although small, on the productivity of those around him when he smokes. But the various consequences of a single action are seldom uniformly good or uniformly bad. In addition to the bad consequences already indicated, there are also a number of good consequences that result from the refusal to stop smoking. Most notably, the emphysema patient continues to derive the satisfaction associated with cigarette smoking. In addition, it is likely that his continuing to smoke will make him less irritable around others. When the various consequences of a single action are fully analyzed, more often than not we find ourselves confronted with a mixture of good and bad. If a person throws a late-night party, it is true that those in attendance may derive a great deal of pleasure, but it is also true that the neighbors may lose out on some much-needed sleep.

The basic principle of act-utilitarianism can be stated as follows: *A person ought to act so as to produce the greatest balance of good over evil, everyone considered.* Act-utilitarianism stands in vivid contrast to ethical egoism, which directs a person always to act so as to produce the greatest balance of good over evil *for oneself* (i.e., the agent). The act-utilitarian is committed to the proposition that the interests of everyone affected by an action are to be weighed in the balance along with the interests of the agent. Everyone's interests are entitled to an impartial consideration. According to the act-utilitarian, an action is morally right if, when compared to possible alternatives, its likely consequences are such as to generate the greatest balance of good over evil, everyone considered. If we refer to the net balance of good over evil (everyone considered) that is likely to be produced by a certain action as its (overall) *utility*, then we can say that act-utilitarianism directs a person always to choose that alternative which has the greatest utility. Thus we can express the basic principle of act-utilitarianism as follows: A person ought to act so as to maximize utility.

For the act-utilitarian, calculation is a paramount element in the moral assessment of action. The question is always, what is the utility of each of my alternatives in this particular set of circumstances? But any system of utilitarian calculation must ultimately be anchored in some conception of "intrinsic value" (i.e., that which is good or desirable in and of itself). The act that will maximize utility (by our definition) is the act that is likely to produce the greatest balance of good over evil, everyone considered. But what is to count as "good" and what as "evil" in our calculations? The answers provided within the framework of classical utilitarianism reflect a so-called "hedonistic" theory of intrinsic value. According to Bentham, only pleasure (understood broadly to include any type of satisfaction or enjoyment) has intrinsic value; only pain (understood broadly to include any dissatisfaction, frustration, or displeasure) has intrinsic disvalue. According to Mill, only happiness has intrinsic value; only unhappiness has intrinsic disvalue. To what extent there is substantive disagreement between Bentham and Mill on this matter is a complex question that cannot be dealt with here. It should be mentioned, however, that many contemporary utilitarian thinkers have embraced more elaborate and nonhedonistic theories of intrinsic value. Nevertheless, for the sake of exposition, we shall presume that a hedonistic theory of intrinsic value, in the spirit of Bentham and Mill, underlies utilitarian calculation.

In the spirit of act-utilitarianism, in order to determine what I should do in a certain situation, I must first attempt to delineate alternative paths of action. Next I attempt to foresee the consequences (sometimes numerous and far-reaching) of each alternative action. Then I attempt, in each case, to evaluate the consequences and to weigh the good against the bad, considering the impact of my action on everyone whom it is likely to affect. Such a reckoning will reveal the act that is likely to produce the greatest balance of good over evil, and this act is the morally right act for me in my particular circumstances. (If it appears likely that two competing actions would produce the same balance of good over evil, then either action will qualify as the morally correct action.) In some situations, it is true, no matter what I do, more evil (pain or unhappiness) will come into the world than good (pleasure or happiness). In such unfortunate situations, according to the act-utilitarian, the morally right act is that one which will bring the least amount of evil into the world.

Act-utilitarianism can rightly be understood as a form of "situation ethics." The act-utilitarian has no sympathy for the notion that certain kinds of actions are intrinsically wrong, that is, wrong by their very nature. Rather, a certain kind of action (e.g., lying) may be wrong in one set of circumstances, yet right in a different set of circumstances. The circumstances in which an action is to be performed are relevant to its morality (i.e., its rightness or wrongness) because the consequences of the action will vary depending on the circumstances. Thus the morality of action is a function of the situation confronting the agent—"situation ethics."

The situational character of act-utilitarianism is reflected in the act-utilitarian attitude toward moral rules. Among the "commonsense rules of morality" are the following: "do not kill," "do not injure," "do not steal," "do not lie," "do not break promises," and so forth. According to the act-utilitarian, these rules are to be understood merely as rules of thumb. They are, for the most part, reliable guides for human action, especially relevant when time constraints undermine the possibility of careful calculation. In most circumstances, acting in accordance with a moral rule is the way to maximize utility, but in some cases this is not so. In these latter cases, whenever there is good reason to believe that breaking a moral rule will produce a greater balance of good over evil (everyone considered), the right thing to do is to break it. In such a case, it would be wrong to follow the rule. Lying is usually wrong, breaking promises is usually wrong, killing is usually wrong, but whenever circumstances are such that there is good reason to believe that breaking a certain moral rule will maximize utility, the rule should be broken. Of course, the act-utilitarian insists, one must be cautious in concluding that any given exception to a moral rule is indeed justified. One must be wary of rationalization and not allow one's own interests to weigh more heavily than the interests of others in the utilitarian calculation. And most importantly, one must not be simple-minded in a consideration of the likely consequences of breaking a moral rule. Indirect and long-term consequences must be considered as well as direct and short-term consequences. Lying on a certain occasion may seem to promote most effectively the interests of those immediately involved, but perhaps the lie will provide a bad example for less reflective people, or perhaps it will contribute to a general breakdown of trust among human beings. In this same vein, one prominent contemporary act-utilitarian emphasizes the significance of the long-term, indirect consequences of promise breaking, while at the same time exhibiting the underlying act-utilitarian attitude toward moral rules:

> The rightness or wrongness of keeping a promise on a particular occasion depends only on the goodness or badness of the consequences of keeping or of breaking the promise on that particular occasion. Of course part of the consequences of breaking the promise, and a part to which we will normally ascribe decisive importance, will be the weakening of faith in the institution of promising. However, if the goodness of the consequences of breaking the rule is *in toto* greater than the goodness of the consequences of keeping it, then we must break the rule....[1]

Act-utilitarianism has often been criticized on the grounds that, due to the extensive sort of calculations it seems to demand, it cannot function as a useful guide for human action. In the spirit of this criticism, the following questions are asked: How can I possibly predict all the consequences of my actions? How am I to assign weights to the various kinds of human satisfactions—for example, the pleasure of eating a cheeseburger versus the aesthetic enjoyment of the ballet? How am I to weigh the anxiety of one person against the inconvenience of another? And besides, how am I supposed to have time to do these extensive calculations? Act-utilitarians, in response to such questions, usually appeal rather directly to "common sense." They say, typically: There is no escape from a consideration of probabilities in rational decision making; predict as best you can, weigh as best you can, considering the time you have available for deliberation. All that can be expected is that you come to grips with the likely consequences of your alternatives in a serious-minded, sensible way, and then act accordingly.

Examples of Act-Utilitarian Reasoning in a Biomedical Context   The following examples are provided in an effort to exhibit act-utilitarian reasoning as it might arise in a biomedical context. It is not claimed that an act-utilitarian must necessarily reach the conclusion suggested in each case. It is only claimed that an act-utilitarian might plausibly reach the stated conclusion. In fact, an act-utilitarian can always assert that some likely consequence, either overlooked or insufficiently emphasized in a particular case, is the decisive one.

(1) A severely impaired newborn, believed to have no realistic chance of surviving more than a few weeks, has contracted pneumonia. (The treatment of impaired newborns is discussed in Chapter 7.) A physician, in conjunction with the parents of the infant, must decide whether to fight off the pneumonia with antibiotics, thereby prolonging the life of the infant. The alternative is simply to allow the infant to die. It seems clear that the interests of all those immediately involved are best served by deciding not to treat the pneumonia. Surely the infant has nothing to gain, and something to lose, by a slight extension of a pain-filled life. The parents, whose suffering cannot be eradicated whatever action is taken, nevertheless will find some relief knowing that their child's suffering has ended. In addition, hospital resources can be better utilized than to prolong the dying process of an infant who cannot benefit from further treatment. But there may be decisive consequences of an indirect, long-term nature. Perhaps allowing this infant to die will contribute to a breakdown of protective attitudes toward infants in general. No, the risk of this untoward consequence seems minimal. Withholding antibiotics, thereby allowing the infant to die, is the right thing to do in this particular case.

(2) A biomedical researcher, on the basis of animal studies she has conducted, believes that a certain drug therapy has great promise for the treatment of a particular kind of cancer in human beings. At present, however, her primary concern is to establish an appropriate dosage level for human beings; there have been several troublesome side effects exhibited by the an-

imals who received large doses of the drug. Over the years, the researcher has found that students at her university are very willing to volunteer themselves as research subjects in experiments that can be identified as presenting only minimal risks to themselves. They are, however, understandably reluctant to volunteer for experiments that seem to present more substantial risks. The researcher in this particular case cannot honestly say that there are no substantial risks for research subjects. She expects, in particular, that perhaps 30 to 40 percent of the research subjects will have to contend with very prolonged nausea. But, if she is honest in conveying this information to potential research subjects, it is unlikely that they will volunteer in sufficient numbers. (The ethics of experimentation on human subjects is discussed in Chapter 4.) Perhaps, she reasons, it is justifiable in this particular case to withhold information about the risk of very prolonged nausea. After all, it is very likely that numerous people will eventually derive great benefit from the therapeutic technique under study. Surely this likely benefit far outweighs the short-term discomfort of a much smaller number. But suppose the deception comes to light. If those who routinely volunteer as research subjects are given a reason to distrust those conducting the experiments, the overall research effort will be impaired, and human welfare will be damaged greatly. This seems to be a decisive consideration. In this particular case, then, deception would be wrong. (If there were no realistic chance of the deception being discovered, it seems that the conclusion would be different.)

(3) In the 1960s when kidney dialysis machines were scarce, it was not possible for all who needed them to be accorded access. A hospital administrator or perhaps a committee has been charged with the responsibility of deciding, in essence, whose lives will be saved. (Such "microallocation decisions" are discussed in Chapter 10.) On a particular occasion, when there is room for one more patient, there are two candidates in great need. One of the candidates, a civic-minded woman of 40, is married and the mother of four children. The other candidate, an unmarried man of the same age, is known to be a drifter and an alcoholic. It seems clear, at first glance, that the consequences of saving the woman's life are far superior to those of saving the man's life. Her husband, her children, and the community in general would be negatively affected in very substantial ways by her death. But is it not problematic to accord a person access to a scarce medical resource on the basis of his or her social role? If a precedent of this sort is set, will not those whose lives are less "socially useful" become somewhat anxious and fearful? On the other hand, perhaps this negative consequence will be balanced by a positive consequence, that is, people will be more inclined to become "socially useful." It still seems clear that the woman in this case should have priority over the man.

Critical Assessment of Act-Utilitarianism   Act-utilitarianism seems to fare poorly when measured against a previously identified standard: The implications of an ethical theory must be reconcilable with our experience of the moral life. In a number of ways, it can be argued, act-utilitarianism clashes with our experience of the moral life. This failure to accord with our ordinary moral thinking is reflected in the following well-known objections to act-utilitarianism.

(1) *Act-Utilitarianism Confronts Individuals with an Overly Demanding Moral Standard.* We are accustomed to thinking that at least some of our decisions are matters of "mere prudence," rightly decided on the basis of "what is best for me." Which major a college student should choose is a good example of a choice that we are inclined to consider essentially a nonmoral matter, a matter of "mere prudence." According to the act-utilitarian, however, a person is continually under a moral obligation to produce the greatest balance of good over evil, everyone considered. Whereas ethical egoism seems to wrongly "collapse" morality into prudence, it would seem that act-utilitarianism "expands" morality so as to destroy the realm of prudence. No aspect of a person's life can be considered merely a matter of prudence. Every decision is a moral decision, to be made on the basis of utilitarian calculation. But, however noble

it might be for a college student to decide his or her major on the basis of a utilitarian calculation, it would seem that one is certainly not under an obligation to proceed in this manner. Doing so, we would ordinarily say, is not one's duty but, rather, is something "above and beyond the call of duty." Act-utilitarianism, in directing a person always to act so as to maximize utility, seems problematically to imply that it is one's duty to act in a way that we ordinarily consider "above and beyond the call of duty."

(2) *Act-Utilitarianism Does Not Accord with Our Experience of Particular, Morally Significant Relationships.* In our experience of the moral life, we are continually aware of highly particular, morally significant relationships that exist between ourselves and others. We are related to particular individuals in a host of morally significant ways, such as spouse to spouse, parent to child, creditor to debtor, promiser to promisee, employer to employee, teacher to student, physician or nurse to patient. In view of such relationships, it is ordinarily thought, we have special obligations—obligations that function to restrict the effort to maximize utility. Parents, we are strongly inclined to say, are obligated to care for their children even if there is good reason to think that the time and energy necessary for this task would maximize utility if redirected to some other task. In the same way, by virtue of the special relationship that exists between a physician and a patient, would it not be wrong for a physician to make decisions regarding patient treatment in the manner of an act-utilitarian? For a physician to damage the interests of an individual patient in an effort to maximize utility surely seems wrong. W. D. Ross, who has vigorously pressed this overall line of criticism against act-utilitarianism, asserts that the "essential defect of the...theory is that it ignores, or at least does not do full justice to, the highly personal character of duty."[2]

(3) *Act-Utilitarianism Does Not Accord with Our Conviction That Individuals Have Rights.* The notion of rights plays an important part in our ordinary moral thinking, but act-utilitarianism seems incapable of accommodating this notion. Moreover, in certain circumstances, the action that would maximize utility (and thus the right action according to the act-utilitarian) is one that we are inclined to consider seriously immoral precisely because it entails the violation of some person's right. For example, it seems that act-utilitarianism would allow an innocent person to be unjustly punished, as long as circumstances were such as to make this line of action the one that would generate the greatest balance of good over evil. Suppose extreme social unrest has been created by a wave of unsolved crimes. The enraged crowd will violently erupt, bringing massive evil into the world, unless the authorities punish someone (anyone) in an effort to appease the appetite for vengeance. So act-utilitarianism seems to allow the unjust treatment of a person as a scapegoat, as a mere means to a social end. But surely an innocent person has a right not to be punished, and it is by reference to this right that the wrongness of "scapegoating" is most naturally understood. Similarly, "the common moral opinion that painless undetected murders of old unhappy people are wicked, no matter what benefits result"[3] can be thought to rest on the contention that people, however old and unhappy, nevertheless have a *right* to life. It is often asserted against act-utilitarianism that it is a defective theory because it allows "the end to justify the means." At least part of the sense behind this charge can be made out in reference to the notion of rights. Certain means of achieving a desirable social end are simply wrongful because they entail the violation of a person's right. Contra act-utilitarianism, such means cannot be justified by the end.

Act-utilitarians have responded in two different ways to the overall claim that the theory cannot be reconciled with our ordinary moral thinking. Some say, in essence, "so much the worse for our ordinary moral thinking." In their view, we must simply overhaul our collective moral consciousness and embrace the mind-set of the act-utilitarian. Most act-utilitarians, however, do not adopt this revisionary stance. Rather, they seek to demonstrate that the clash between act-utilitarianism and our ordinary moral thinking is not nearly so severe as the above criticisms suggest. They argue that, when act-utilitarianism is properly applied, when all the significant long-term, indirect consequences are taken into account, the theory does not give rise to conclusions that seem so patently objectionable. It is very doubtful, however, that this strategy of argument can completely rescue act-utilitarianism from its difficulties.

Perhaps act-utilitarianism fares better when measured against the second of our previously identified standards: An ethical theory must provide effective guidance where it is most needed. At the very least, it must be said in favor of act-utilitarianism that it provides a reasonably clear decision procedure, a sense of direction, for the resolution of moral dilemmas. In the face of moral considerations that incline our judgment in conflicting ways, act-utilitarianism counsels us to analyze the likely consequences of alternative actions, in order to determine the alternative that will maximize utility. Still, however well act-utilitarianism might be thought to fare with regard to our second standard, it seems to be a seriously defective theory as measured against our first standard. Indeed, in contemporary times, most utilitarian thinkers have rejected act-utilitarianism in favor of a theory known as rule-utilitarianism.[4]

Rule-Utilitarianism

The basic principle of act-utilitarianism has previously been formulated as follows: A person ought to act so as to produce the greatest balance of good over evil, everyone considered. In contrast, the basic principle of rule-utilitarianism can be formulated as follows: *A person ought to act in accordance with the rule that, if generally followed, would produce the greatest balance of good over evil, everyone considered.* If the demand to produce the greatest balance of good over evil, everyone considered, is referred to as the principle (standard) of utility, then the principle of utility is the basic ethical principle in both the act-utilitarian and the rule-utilitarian systems. However, in the act-utilitarian system, determining the morally correct action is a matter of assessing alternative actions directly against the standard of utility; whereas in the rule-utilitarian system, determining the morally correct action involves an *indirect* appeal to the principle of utility. In the spirit of rule-utilitarianism, a moral code is first established by reference to the principle of utility. That is, a set of valid moral rules is established by determining which rules (as opposed to conceivable alternatives), if generally followed, would produce the greatest balance of good over evil. In rule-utilitarianism, individual actions are morally right if they are in accord with those rules.

The difference between act-utilitarian reasoning and rule-utilitarian reasoning can be represented schematically as follows:

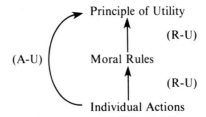

Act-utilitarian reasoning embodies a single-stage procedure, rule-utilitarian reasoning a two-stage procedure. Because the act-utilitarian is committed to assessing individual actions strictly on the basis of utilitarian considerations, act-utilitarianism is often referred to as "extreme" or "unrestricted" utilitarianism. Because the rule-utilitarian is committed to developing a moral code (a set of moral rules) on the basis of utilitarian considerations and then assessing individual actions not on the basis of utilitarian considerations but on the basis of accordance with the moral rules that have been established, rule-utilitarianism is often referred to as "restricted" utilitarianism.

For the act-utilitarian, moral rules have a very subordinate status. They are merely "rules of thumb," providing some measure of practical guidance. For the rule-utilitarian, moral rules assume a much more fundamental status, indeed a theoretical primacy. Only in reference to established moral rules can the moral assessment of individual actions be carried out. Thus the first and most crucial step for the rule-utilitarian is the articulation of a set of moral rules, themselves justified on the basis of utilitarian considerations. Underlying this task is the question of which rules (as opposed to conceivable alternatives), if generally followed, would produce the greatest balance of good over evil, everyone considered. That is, which rules, if adopted or recognized in our moral code, would maximize utility?

As a first approximation of a set of moral rules that could be justified on the basis of utilitarian considerations, consider the "commonsense rules of morality," rules such as "do not kill," "do not steal," "do not lie," "do not break promises." It is not difficult to visualize such rules as resting upon a utilitarian foundation. Surely the consequences of the adoption of the rule "do not kill" are dramatically better than the consequences of the adoption of the rule "kill whenever you want." If the latter rule were generally followed, society would be reduced to a profoundly uncivilized level. Similarly, the consequences of the adoption of the rule "do not steal" are dramatically better than the consequences of the adoption of the rule "steal whenever you want." If the former rule is generally followed, individuals will enjoy an important measure of personal security. If the latter rule were adopted by a society, anxiety and tension would dominate social existence. As for lying and promise breaking, if people felt free to engage in such behavior, the numerous advantages that derive from human trust and cooperation would evaporate. But the rules thus far exhibited as having a utilitarian foundation are essentially prohibitions. Are there not also rules of a more positive sort that could also be justified on the basis of utilitarian considerations? It would seem so. Consider rules such as "come to the aid of people in distress" and "prevent innocent people from being harmed." It surely seems that human welfare would be enhanced by the adoption of such rules as part of the overall fabric of our moral code.

According to the rule-utilitarian, an individual action is morally right when it accords with the rules or moral code established on a utilitarian basis. But the account of moral rules thus far presented is too simplistic. In order to be plausible, the rules that constitute the moral code must be understood as incorporating certain exceptions. The need to recognize justified exceptions is perhaps most apparent when we remember that moral rules, if stated unconditionally, can easily come into conflict with each other. When an obviously agitated person waves a gun and inquires as to the whereabouts of a third party, it may not be possible to act in accordance with both the rule "do not lie" and the rule "prevent innocent people from being harmed." Indeed, it is precisely this sort of situation that inclines us to consider incorporating an exception into our rule against lying. Suppose we say, "Do not lie *except* when necessary to prevent an innocent person from being harmed." When the possibility of a justified exception is raised, the rule-utilitarian employs the following decision procedure. The question is posed, Would the adoption of the rule with the exception have better consequences than the adoption of the rule without the exception? If so, the exception is a justified one; the rule incorporating the exception has greater utility than the rule without the exception. In the face of our proposed exception to the rule against lying, the rule-utilitarian would probably conclude that it does constitute a justified exception. The adoption of the rule "do not lie *except* when necessary to protect an innocent person from being harmed" would seem to preserve essentially all the social benefits provided by the adoption of the rule "do not lie," while at the same time bringing about an additional social benefit, an increased measure of personal security for potential victims of assault.

Examples of Rule-Utilitarian Reasoning in a Biomedical Context   (1) A substantive problem in biomedical ethics (discussed in Chapter 2) has to do with the morality of a physician's lying to a patient, in particular, whether it is right for a physician to lie to a patient, saying that the patient's illness is not terminal when it is believed to be so. The rule-utilitarian would conceptualize this issue as raising the possibility of a justified exception to the rule against lying. (Notice that an act-utilitarian, in contrast, would insist on assessing every individual case on its own utilitarian merits.) Suppose we consider incorporating into the rule against lying an exception to this effect: "*except* when in the judgment of a physician it would be better for a patient that he or she not know that his or her illness is believed to be terminal." Would the adoption of the rule incorporating this exception have better consequences than the adoption of the rule without the exception? The correct answer to this question is perhaps arguable, but it would seem that the rule-utilitarian would conclude that the proposed exception is an unjustified one. It is perhaps true that adoption of a rule incorporating the proposed exception would result in many patients being spared (at least temporarily) the distress that accompanies knowledge of one's impending death. On the other hand, it seems that this gain would be dwarfed by the distress and anxiety that would emerge from the erosion of trust within the confines of the physician-patient relationship. Whether a more limited exception could be formulated to a rule-utilitarian's satisfaction remains an open question.

(2) Another substantive problem in biomedical ethics (discussed in Chapter 7) has to do with the morality of mercy killing. Suppose a terminally ill patient, in great pain, requests that a physician terminate his or her life by administering a lethal dose of a drug. Such a case can be said to raise the issue of voluntary (active) euthanasia. The rule-utilitarian would conceptualize this issue (and other issues such as suicide and abortion) as raising the possibility of a justified exception to our rule against killing. Notice that at least one exception to our rule against killing is relatively uncontroversial. Killing in self-defense is justifiable, according to the rule-utilitarian, because although the adoption of the rule "do not kill" has dramatically better consequences than the adoption of the rule "kill whenever you want," adoption of the rule "do not kill *except* in self-defense" has still better consequences. As for voluntary (active) euthanasia, perhaps we should say that strong rule-utilitarian arguments can be advanced on both sides of the issue. Rule-utilitarian proponents of voluntary (active) euthanasia emphasize that social acceptance of this practice would result in great benefits—the primary one being that many dying people would be able to escape an extension of an anguished dying process. On the other side of the issue, however, we find, among a number of important concerns, insistence that availability of the lethal dose would create a climate of fear and anxiety among the elderly. Will dying people not come to feel that their families, to whom they have become a burden, expect them to ask for the lethal dose?

(3) A final illustration of rule-utilitarian reasoning in a biomedical context can be presented in reference to the principle of medical confidentiality (discussed in Chapter 3). This principle, which has an obvious basis in a rule-utilitarian structure, demands that information revealed within the context of a therapeutic relationship be held confidential. If patients could not rely on this expectation, they would be reluctant to communicate information that is essential to their proper treatment. Still, are there not justifiable exceptions to the principle of medical confidentiality? Suppose, for example, a patient reveals to his or her psychiatrist an intention to kill or injure a third party. Is it not incumbent upon the psychiatrist to break medical confidentiality in an effort to ensure protection for the third party? The situation just described is the basis of the *Tarasoff* case considered in Chapter 3, and rule-utilitarian arguments on both sides of the issue can be found in the judicial opinions presented. There is an obvious benefit associated with the recognition of an exception to medical confidentiality based on the interests of innocent third parties. Namely, threatened people will sometimes be saved from injury and death. On the other hand, it is argued, emotionally disturbed patients are

likely to become more inhibited in communicating with psychiatrists; thus their cures will be inhibited, and a greater incidence of violence against innocent people will result.

Critical Assessment of Rule-Utilitarianism   Rule-utilitarianism, it would seem, goes a long way toward alleviating the perceived difficulties of act-utilitarianism. Although act-utilitarians have charged rule-utilitarians with "superstitious rule-worship,"[5] it is act-utilitarianism rather than rule-utilitarianism that seems to clash with our ordinary moral thinking on this score. Indeed, rule-utilitarianism, in somewhat vivid contrast to act-utilitarianism, seems to fare reasonably well when measured against the standard that the implications of an ethical theory must be reconcilable with our experience of the moral life.

Whereas act-utilitarianism seems to confront individuals with an overly demanding moral standard, placing each of us under a continuing obligation to maximize utility with each of our actions, rule-utilitarianism is far less demanding of individuals. It requires only that individuals conform their actions to the rules that constitute a utilitarian-based moral code, and this requirement accords well with our ordinary moral thinking. Rule-utilitarianism also seems to accord reasonably well with our experience of particular, morally significant relationships. We commonly perceive ourselves as having special obligations arising out of our various morally significant relationships, and we think of these obligations as incompatible with functioning in the manner of an act-utilitarian. Parents have a special obligation to care for their children, physicians have a special obligation to act in the interests of their patients, and so forth. But such special obligations can be understood as having a rule-utilitarian foundation, as deriving from rules that, if generally followed, would maximize utility. Thus rule-utilitarianism seems to remedy another perceived difficulty of act-utilitarianism.

It is less clear that rule-utilitarianism is capable of providing a complete remedy for another perceived difficulty of act-utilitarianism, that is, its inability to provide an adequate theoretical foundation for individual rights. Surely rule-utilitarianism does not lead us so easily as does act-utilitarianism to conclusions that are incompatible with our ordinary moral thinking about the rights of individuals. For example, in suggesting that the painless murder of an old, unhappy person is the right thing as long as it can be done in complete secrecy, act-utilitarianism seems to clash violently with our conviction that such an action is patently objectionable, inasmuch as it constitutes a violation of a person's right to life. Rule-utilitarianism, in contrast, would never lead us to the conclusion that this sort of killing is morally legitimate. Surely the consequences of adopting the rule "do not kill *except* in the case of old, unhappy people who can be killed in complete secrecy" are dramatically worse than the consequences of adopting the rule without such an exception. If the rule with the exception were adopted, the lives of elderly people would be filled with anxiety and fear. In addition to rescuing utilitarian thinking from such obvious clashes with our ordinary moral thinking, rule-utilitarianism does suggest a way of accommodating the notion of individual rights. Just as our special obligations can be understood as deriving from rules in a utilitarian-based moral code, so too can an individual's rights be understood in this fashion. A person's right to life, for example, can be understood as a correlate of our utilitarian-based rule against killing. Of course, whatever exceptions are properly incorporated into our rule against killing will factor out as limitations on a person's right to life. Whether rule-utilitarianism in this manner can provide an adequate theoretical foundation for individual rights is a very controversial matter. Its critics charge that it cannot.

Closely related to the claim that rule-utilitarianism does not provide an adequate theoretical foundation for individual rights is the somewhat broader claim that rule-utilitarianism fails to provide an adequate theoretical grounding for what we take to be the obligations of justice. This broader criticism, which is also vigorously advanced against act-utilitarianism, is surely the principal residual difficulty confronting rule-utilitarianism. Critics of rule-utilitarianism allege, for example, that the theory is compatible with the blatant injustice of enslaving one segment of a society's population or at least discriminating against this segment. The idea is that social rules discriminating against an explicitly identified minority group might function to maximize utility by bringing about more happiness in the advantaged majority than unhappiness in the disadvantaged minority. Rule-utilitarians are inclined to argue in response to this line of criticism that when the consequences of adopting "unjust rules" are completely analyzed, it is never true that their adoption can be justified on utilitarian grounds. Rather, the rule-utilitarian contends, "the rules of justice" rest on a secure utilitarian foundation. Whether rule-utilitarianism, in this manner, can adequately be reconciled with the perceived obligations of justice is a matter of contemporary debate.

Rule-utilitarianism also seems to fare reasonably well when measured against the second of our suggested standards: An ethical theory must provide effective guidance where it is most needed. In the dilemma situation, where one moral rule, or principle, inclines us one way, another moral rule, or principle, inclines us another way, the rule-utilitarian instructs us to establish relative priority by considering the consequences of incorporating appropriate exceptions into the rules that are in conflict. The dilemma is to be resolved by adoption of a rule that will maximize utility. Although this decision procedure sometimes entails very complex factual analysis and deliberation, it does seem to provide us a substantial measure of explicit guidance. Since rule-utilitarianism also seems to be reasonably harmonious with our ordinary moral thinking, it is an ethical theory that cannot easily be dismissed.

Kantian Deontology

The most prominent of the classical deontological theories is that developed by the German philosopher Immanuel Kant (1724–1804). Kantian deontology continues to command substantial attention in contemporary discussions of ethical theory and, importantly, is the underlying framework of much argumentation in biomedical ethics. In both of these respects, Kantian deontology is similar to utilitarianism and, like utilitarianism, warrants our detailed attention.

Kant sees utilitarianism as embodying a radically wrong approach in ethical theory. He emphasizes the need to avoid the "serpent-windings" of utilitarian thinking and refers to the Principle of Utility as "a wavering and uncertain standard." There is indeed a single, fundamental principle that is the basis of all moral obligation, but this fundamental principle is *not* the Principle of Utility. The "supreme principle of morality," the principle from which all of our various duties derive, is called by Kant the "Categorical Imperative."

Our present objective is an exposition of Kantian deontology. But the enormous complexity of Kant's moral philosophy is a formidable obstacle to any concise exposition of the structure of Kant's ethical system. In particular, we are faced with the problem that Kant formulated the basic principle of his system, the Categorical Imperative, in a number of different ways. Although Kant insists that his various formulations are all equivalent, this contention is explicitly denied by many of his expositors and critics. Thus, if we are to provide a coherent account of Kantian deontology, mindful of the need to provide an account that is especially useful in dealing with issues in biomedical ethics, it seems advisable to settle on a favored formulation of the Categorical Imperative. Since two of Kant's formulations of the Categorical Imperative are especially prominent, it will suffice for our purposes to choose a favored formulation from these two.

According to what we will call the "first formulation," the Categorical Imperative tells us: "Act only on that maxim through which you can at the same time will that it should become a universal law."[6] According to what we will call the "second formulation," the Categorical Imperative tells us: "Act in such a way that you always treat humanity, whether in your own person or in the person of any other, never simply as a means, but always at the same time as an end."[7] The first formulation of the Categorical Imperative has often been compared with the Golden Rule ("do unto others as you would have them do unto you"), and it may be true that both of these principles, when suitably interpreted, have roughly the same implications. At any rate, it is apparently the case that Kant considered the first formulation to be the most basic of all his formulations. Yet, despite this fact, and despite the fact that ethical theorists have tended to pay more attention to the first formulation than the second, it is the second formulation that we take to have greater promise for the task at hand. Two major reasons can be advanced for choosing to exhibit the structure of Kant's ethical system in reference to the second formulation of the Categorical Imperative. First, the second formulation embodies a central notion—respect for persons—that is somewhat easier to grasp and apply than the more formalistic notion of universalizability, which is the core element of the first formulation. Second, when argumentation in biomedical ethics reflects a Kantian viewpoint, it is almost always couched in terms of the second formulation rather than the first.

Kantian deontology is an ethics of respect for persons. In Kant's view, every person, by virtue of his or her humanity (i.e., rational nature) has an inherent dignity. All persons, as rational creatures, are entitled to respect, not only from others but from themselves as well. Thus the Categorical Imperative directs each of us to "act in such a way that you always treat humanity, whether in your own person or in the person of any other, never simply as a means, but always at the same time as an end." From this fundamental principle, according to Kant, a host of particular duties can be derived. The resultant system of duties includes duties to self as well as duties to others. And in each of these cases, "perfect duties" must be distinguished from "imperfect duties," thus generating a fourfold classification of duties: (1) perfect duties to self, (2) imperfect duties to self, (3) perfect duties to others, (4) imperfect duties to others. Although the distinction between perfect and imperfect duties is not a transparent one, its structural importance in the Kantian system is hard to overemphasize. Perfect duties require of us that we do or abstain from certain acts. *There are no legitimate exceptions to a perfect duty.* Such duties are binding in all circumstances, because certain kinds of action are simply incompatible with respect for persons, hence strictly impermissible. Imperfect duties, by contrast, require of us, in some overall sense, that we pursue or promote certain goals (e.g., the welfare of others). However, action in the name of these goals must never be at the expense of a perfect duty. One of Kant's most prominent commentators relates the distinction between perfect and imperfect duties to the Categorical Imperative in the following way: "We transgress perfect duties by treating any person *merely* as a means. We transgress imperfect duties by failing to treat a person as an end, even though we do not actively treat him as a means."[8]

Our discussion of Kant's fourfold classification of duties will begin with a consideration of perfect duties to others. A transgression in this category of duty occurs whenever one person treats another person merely as a means. It is strictly impermissible for person *A* to treat person *B* merely as a means because such treatment is incompatible with respect for *B* as a person. Notice that Kant does not claim that it is morally wrong for one person to use another as a means. His claim is that it is morally wrong for one person to use another *merely* as a means. In the ordinary course of life, it is surely unavoidable (and morally unproblematic) that each of us in numerous ways uses others as means to achieve our various ends. A college teacher uses students as a means to achieve his or her livelihood. A college student uses instructors as a means of gaining knowledge and skills. Such human interactions, presumably based on the voluntary participation of the respective parties, are quite compatible with a principle of respect for persons. But respect for persons entails that each of us recognize the rightful authority of other persons (as rational beings) to conduct their individual lives as they see fit. We may legitimately recruit others to participate in the satisfaction of our personal ends, but they are used merely as a means whenever we undermine the voluntary or informed character of their consent to interact with us in some desired way. Person A coerces person B at knifepoint to hand over $200. A uses B merely as a means. If A had requested of B a gift of $200, leaving B free to determine whether or not to make the gift, A would have proceeded in a manner compatible with respect for B as a person. Person C deceptively rolls back the odometer of a car and thereby manipulates person D's decision to buy the car. C uses D merely as a means. C has acted in a way that is strictly incompatible with respect for D as a person.

In the Kantian system, among the most notable of our perfect duties to others are: (1) the duty not to kill an innocent person, (2) the duty not to lie, and (3) the duty to keep promises. Murder (the killing of an innocent person), lying, and promise breaking are actions that are intrinsically wrong. However beneficial the consequences of such an action might be in a given circumstance, the action is strictly impermissible. (Notice the anti-utilitarian character of Kant's thinking.) The murderer exhibits obvious disrespect for the person of the victim. The liar, in misinforming another person, violates the respect due to that person as a rational creature with a fundamental interest in the truth. A person who makes a promise issues a guarantee upon which the recipient of the promise is entitled to rely in his or her future planning. The promise breaker shows disrespect for a person in undermining the effort to conduct the affairs of one's life. By murdering, lying, or promise breaking, an agent uses another person merely as a means to the agent's own ends.

According to Kant, each person has not only perfect duties to others but also perfect duties to self. The Categorical Imperative demands that no person (including oneself) be treated merely as a means. It is no more permissible to manifest disrespect for one's own person than to do so for the person of another. Kant insists, for example, that each person has a perfect duty to self to avoid drunkenness. Since drunkenness undermines a person's rational capacities, it is incompatible with respect for oneself as a rational creature. Kant believes that individuals debase themselves in the effort to achieve pleasure via inebriation. Inebriates treat themselves merely as a means (to the end of pleasure). But surely the foremost example of a perfect duty to self in the Kantian system is the duty not to commit suicide. To terminate one's own life, Kant insists, is strictly incompatible with respect for oneself as a person. In eradicating one's very existence as a rational creature, a person treats oneself merely as a means (ordinarily to the end of avoiding discomfort or distress). Suicide is an action that is intrinsically wrong, and there are no circumstances in which it is morally permissible.

In addition to the notion of perfect duties (both to self and others), the Kantian system also incorporates the notion of imperfect duties. Whereas perfect duties require, in essence, strict abstention from those actions that involve using a person merely as a means, imperfect duties have a very different underlying sense. Imperfect duties require the promotion of certain goals. In broad terms, there are two such goals—an agent's personal perfection (i.e., development) and the happiness or welfare of others. Respect for oneself as a person requires commitment to the development of one's capacities as a rational being. Thus Kant spoke of an imperfect duty to self to develop one's talents. The sense of this duty is that, by and large, it is up to each individual to decide which talents to cultivate and which to deemphasize. But a person is not free to abandon the goal of personal development. Although the duty to develop one's talents requires no *specific* actions, it does require each individual to formulate a plan of life that embodies a commitment to the goal of personal development.

Before discussing Kant's final category of duty, imperfect duty to others, it will prove helpful to introduce the notion of *beneficence*.[9] If one acts in such a way as to further the happiness or welfare of another, then one acts beneficently. (A benevolent person is one who is inclined to act beneficently.) Beneficence may be contrasted with *nonmaleficence*, which is ordinarily understood as the noninfliction of harm on others. One who harms ("does evil" to) another acts in a maleficent fashion. One who *refrains* from harming others acts in a nonmaleficent fashion. One who acts, in a more positive way, to contribute to the welfare of others acts in a beneficent fashion. Beneficence is a generic notion that can best be understood as including the following types of activity: (1) preventing evil or harm from befalling someone; (2) removing an evil that is presently afflicting someone; (3) providing benefits ("doing good") for someone. Although it is sometimes difficult to decide which of these categories is the most appropriate classification for a particular beneficent action, the following examples seem relatively straightforward. Pushing someone out of the path of an oncoming car is an example of (1). Curing a patient's disease is an example of (2). Giving someone a $100 gift is an example of (3).

According to Kant, respect for other persons requires not only that we avoid using them merely as a means (by the observance of our perfect duties to others) but also that we commit ourselves in some general way to furthering their happiness or welfare. Thus Kant considers what we will call the "duty of beneficence" to be an imperfect duty to others. As with the duty to develop our talents, an imperfect duty to self, the duty of beneficence requires no *specific* actions. One does not violate the duty of beneficence by refusing to act beneficently in any individual case where the opportunity arises. What is required instead of specific actions is that each person incorporate in his or her life plan a commitment to promoting the well-being of others. Individuals are free to choose the sorts of actions they will embrace in an effort to further the well-being of others (e.g., contributing to the relief of famine victims); they are not free to abandon the general goal of furthering the well-being of others.

Since the duty of beneficence is an imperfect duty in the Kantian system, action in the name of beneficence must never be taken at the expense of a perfect duty. For example, it is impermissible to lie or break a promise in an effort to save a third party from harm. The same is true with regard to the imperfect duty to develop one's talents. For example, if one has resolved (quite properly) to develop one's creative powers, it is nevertheless impermissible to do so by "creatively" defrauding others.

The Kantian Framework in a Biomedical Context   With our exposition of Kantian deontology now complete, we are in a position to exhibit some of the more important applications of this ethical theory in the realm of biomedical ethics. To begin with, the theory has an obvious relevance to the much-discussed problem of whether or not a physician may justifiably lie to a patient (an issue discussed in Chapter 2). Since every person has a perfect duty to others not to lie, a straightforward implication of Kantian deontology is that a physician may *never* lie to a patient. If a patient, diagnosed as terminally ill by a physician, inquires about his or her prognosis, the physician may be much inclined to lie, motivated by a desire to protect the patient from the psychological turmoil that would accompany knowledge of his or her true condition; but action in the name of beneficence (an imperfect duty) may never be at the expense of a perfect duty. This same analysis is applicable to the use of placebos by physicians. Sometimes a patient becomes psychologically dependent on a certain medication. When the medication is discontinued, because the physician is convinced it is no longer needed and because its continued use represents a threat to health, the patient complains of the reemergence of symptoms. If such a patient is given a placebo, that is, a therapeutically inert but harmless substance, misrepresented as a medication, the patient may feel fine. Nevertheless, despite the fact that placebos may be capable of enhancing patient welfare, their employment entails lying and thus is morally impermissible.

Kantian deontology has some very important and very direct implications for the ethics of experimentation with human subjects (the topic of Chapter 4). Since it is morally wrong for any person to use any other person merely as a means, it follows that it is morally wrong for a biomedical researcher to use a human research subject merely as a means. And from this consideration it is but a short step to the requirement of voluntary informed consent as a basic principle of research ethics. If a researcher is engaged in a study that involves human subjects, we may presume that the immediate "end" being sought by the researcher is the successful completion of the study. But notice that the researcher may desire this particular end for any number of reasons: the speculative understanding it will provide; the technology it will make possible; the eventual benefit of humankind; personal recognition in the eyes of the scientific community; a raise in pay; and so forth. This mixture of self-centered and benevolent motivations may be considered the researcher's less immediate ends. Now, if researchers are to avoid using their research subjects merely as means (to the ends of the researchers), surely they must refrain from coercing the participation of their subjects and, in addition, provide information about the research project (most notably, risks to the subjects) sufficient for the subjects to make a rational decision with regard to their personal participation. Thus respect for persons demands that researchers honor the requirement of voluntary informed consent.

Suppose a researcher explains to a potential research subject how important it is that he or she consent to participate. There is no question but that the research project at issue, if brought to a successful conclusion, will provide substantial benefit to humankind. Does the potential subject have a moral obligation to participate? Surely not. Within the framework of Kantian deontology, the duty of beneficence is an imperfect duty. A person must on occasion act beneficently, but there is no obligation to perform any *specific* beneficent action. Interestingly enough, the same line of thought would seem to apply to the question, does a physician have a moral obligation to come to the aid of a seriously injured person (not by prior agreement the physician's patient) in an emergency situation?

Critical Assessment of Kantian Deontology   Are the implications of Kantian deontology reconcilable with our experience of the moral life? Can this theory function to provide effective guidance in the face of perceived moral dilemmas? These two questions reflect the criteria suggested earlier as most central to the assessment of the relative adequacy of an ethical theory.

Before indicating some of the ways in which Kantian deontology can be thought to be at odds with our ordinary moral thinking, it is important to emphasize that the theory does successfully account for crucial aspects of our experience of the moral life. To begin with, Kantian deontology provides an obvious foundation for the "commonsense rules of morality." The wrongfulness of actions that fly in the face of these rules—actions such as killing, injuring, stealing, lying, breaking promises—can very plausibly be understood as flowing from the Categorical Imperative. The Kantian deontologist maintains that these actions are wrong because they involve treating another person merely as a means, and there is something very compelling about the notion of respect for persons as the core notion of morality.

Kantian deontology also seems to provide a secure foundation for the notion of individual rights, a notion that is very prominent in our ordinary moral thinking. Individual rights, in the Kantian system, are to be understood as the correlates of our perfect duties to others. (Imperfect duties, in contrast, do not generate rights.) For example, each of us has a perfect *duty* not to kill an innocent person; thus every innocent person has a *right* not to be killed. More generally, every person has a right not to be used by another merely as a means. An innocent person has a right not to be punished, no matter how socially desirable the consequences might be in a certain set of circumstances. A potential research subject has a right not to be coerced or deceived into participation, even if the satisfactory completion of the study promises great benefit for humankind. In its insistence that individual rights cannot be overridden by "utilitarian" considerations, Kantian deontology achieves accord with our firmly entrenched (if somewhat vague) conviction that the "end does not justify the means."

Yet, there are aspects of Kantian deontology that cannot be easily reconciled with our experience of the moral life. One very prominent difficulty has to do with the Kantian contention that keeping promises and not lying are both duties of perfect obligation. We are quite at home, in our ordinary moral thinking, with both a duty to keep promises and a duty not to lie, but it is the exceptionless character of these duties in the Kantian system that we find troublesome. Surely in extreme cases, we are inclined to say, these duties must yield to more weighty moral considerations. For example, if a person breaks a rather trivial promise (say, to return a book at a certain time) in order to respond to the needs of a person in serious distress, surely he or she has not acted immorally. Or again, if a person lies to a would-be murderer about the whereabouts of the intended victim, surely the liar has not (all things considered) acted immorally. The Kantian deontologist sees in such examples a clash between a perfect duty and the imperfect duty of beneficence, and the Kantian teaching is that the former may never yield to the latter. But it would seem that a theory with such implausible implications stands in need of revision. Perhaps the problem is not only that Kantian deontology overstates the significance of certain "perfect" duties but that it understates the significance of the duty of beneficence, at least that aspect of beneficence that has to do with preventing serious harm from befalling another or alleviating the serious distress of another.

In our everyday existence as moral agents, we are accustomed to the idea that we have a number of important duties to others. It is less clear that the Kantian notion of duties to self can be reconciled with our experience of the moral life. This is difficult territory. For one thing, the issue of suicide (discussed in Chapter 6) seems to confound our moral "common sense" in a way that blatant wrongs such as murder, rape, and slavery do not. Still, despite significant disagreement, suicide is widely held to be morally wrong. But the issue is this: Do those who consider suicide morally wrong experience the duty not to commit suicide as a duty to self? It seems more likely that this duty is experienced as a duty to others (who may be negatively affected by one's suicide) or, in the case of religious believers, as a duty to God. A similar argument could be made with regard to the imperfect duty to develop one's talents.

It cannot be denied that Kantian deontology, to a substantial degree, is reconcilable with our experience of the moral life. On the other hand, it appears that the theory is attended with some significant and unresolved difficulties. How does Kantian deontology fare when measured against the second of our standards, the requirement that an ethical theory provide effective guidance in the face of moral dilemmas? Once again, it seems, the verdict is somewhat mixed.

It might be argued that Kantian deontology, by sorting our various duties into the categories of perfect and imperfect and assigning priority to perfect duties, provides us with a structure in terms of which moral dilemmas can be resolved. And this is perhaps true to the extent that our perplexity can be analyzed in terms of perfect duties marshaled against imperfect duties, but even here it is difficult to overlook the fact that the priority of perfect over imperfect duties is itself a somewhat problematic feature of Kantian deontology. One is tempted to say that even if the theory provides reasonably *clear* guidance, it fails to provide *correct* guidance. And what is one to do when confronted with a perfect duty in conflict with another perfect duty? Kantian deontology does not even seem to recognize the possibility of such conflicts, but consider the following example. Suppose a patient discusses a certain sensitive matter (e.g., euthanasia) with a nurse, who promises not to tell the patient's family that the matter was discussed. The next day a family member directly asks the nurse if this matter was discussed. Thus the perfect duty to tell the truth seems to come into direct conflict with the perfect duty to keep a promise. Is it possible that the guiding idea of respect for persons could somehow resolve the question of which of these duties must be preferred? Or must one resort, perhaps in utilitarian fashion, to a consideration of consequences?

W. D. Ross's Theory of Prima Facie Duties

In a book entitled *The Right and the Good* (1930), the English philosopher W. D. Ross proposed a deontological theory that has received considerable attention among ethical theorists.

The point of departure for the development of Ross's theory is his concern to provide a defensible account of "cases of conscience," that is, situations that confront us with a conflict of duties. One perceived line of obligation pulls us in one direction, another perceived line of obligation pulls us in a contrary direction. We find ourselves unsettled and uncertain, but cannot avoid a choice. Which duty takes precedence over the other? The parent of a young child has promised to attend a community meeting, but the child seems to need special attention. Since our social existence is complex, conflict-of-duty situations are a recurrent feature of our daily life. In the biomedical context, such situations are pervasive.

For understandable reasons, Ross maintains that neither the Kantian nor the utilitarian can provide an account of conflict-of-duty situations that harmonizes with what he calls "ordinary moral consciousness." We have recently considered the relevant deficiency in the Kantian approach. It is implausible to maintain that the duty of beneficence can never take precedence over the duty to keep promises or the duty not to lie. As for the utilitarian approach, and here it is clear that Ross has act-utilitarianism in mind, this theory's insistence that in reality we have only the one duty of maximizing utility clashes with our conviction that we have distinct lines of obligation to distinct people. In order to provide an adequate account of conflict-of-duty situations, Ross maintains, it is essential to introduce the notion of "prima facie duty." The Latin phrase "prima facie," now commonplace in moral philosophy, literally means "at first glance." But the word "conditional" best expresses the sense of the phrase as Ross intends it. A prima facie duty is a conditional duty. A prima facie duty (as opposed to an absolute duty) can be overridden by a more stringent duty.

According to Ross, there are no absolute, or unconditional, duties, only prima facie duties. But what is the basis of our prima facie duties? Both the utilitarian and the Kantian assert that our various duties have a unitary basis in a fundamental principle of morality. The utilitarian believes that our various duties can be derived from the Principle of Utility. The Kantian believes that our various duties can be derived from the Categorical Imperative. Ross, in vivid contrast, maintains that our various prima facie duties have no unitary basis. Rather, they emerge out of our numerous "morally significant relations," relations such as promisee to promiser, creditor to debtor, spouse to spouse, child to parent, friend to friend, citizen to the state, fellow human being to fellow human being. "Each of these relations is the foundation of a *prima facie* duty, which is more or less incumbent on me according to the circumstances of the case."[10]

In unproblematic circumstances, where we are bound by only one prima facie duty, this particular prima facie duty is our *actual* duty. In conflict-of-duty situations, where two (or more) prima facie duties compete for priority, only one of these duties, the more stringent one in the circumstances, can be our actual duty. We have, for example, both a prima facie duty to keep promises and a prima facie duty to assist those who are in need. According to Ross, when these two duties come into conflict, it is clear (in terms of our "ordinary moral consciousness") that the duty to keep promises is usually more incumbent upon us than the duty to assist those who are in need. But if the promise is relatively trivial and the need of another is compelling— a matter of serious distress—then it is equally clear that the priority is reversed. In the difficult cases, Ross maintains, there is in principle no hard and fast rule to apply. In his view, the best anyone can do is to make a reflective, "considered decision" as to which of the competing prima facie duties has the priority in any given situation.

According to Ross, "there is nothing arbitrary about [our] *prima facie* duties. Each rests on a definite circumstance which cannot seriously be held to be without moral significance."[11] Accordingly, he proposes the following division of our prima facie duties.

(1) *Duties of fidelity* include keeping promises, honoring contracts and agreements, and telling the truth. Duties in this class rest on a person's previous acts. In giving one's word to do something, a person creates the duty to do so. (Ross thinks that by entering a conversation,

a person implicitly agrees to tell the truth.) Notice that a person's so-called role responsibilities can be identified as an important subclass of duties of fidelity. A teacher has certain responsibilities as a teacher, a physician certain responsibilities as a physician, a nurse certain responsibilities as a nurse. In taking on a certain social role, a person brings into existence various duties of fidelity. In addition, further duties of fidelity arise out of agreements (both explicit and implicit) that a person enters into while functioning in a professional capacity.

(2) *Duties of reparation* also rest on a person's previous acts. Any person, by wrongfully treating someone else, creates the duty to rectify the wrong that has been perpetrated. For example, if *A* steals a certain amount of money from *B*, *A* thereby brings into existence the duty to repay this amount. (3) *Duties of gratitude* rest on previous acts of other persons, that is, beneficial services provided by them. If *A* has provided a good service for *B* when *B* was in need, *B* thereby stands under a duty to provide a good service for *A* when *A* is in need.

(4) *Duties of beneficence* "rest on the mere fact that there are other beings in the world whose condition we can make better."[12] (5) *Duties of nonmaleficence* rest on the complementary fact that we can also make the condition of our fellow human beings worse. The duties in this category, which Ross recognizes as especially stringent, can be summed up under the heading of "not injuring others." The duty not to kill and the duty not to steal are obvious examples.

(6) *Duties of justice* "rest on the fact or possibility of a distribution of pleasure or happiness (or of the means thereto) which is not in accordance with the merit of the persons concerned."[13] Benefits are to be distributed in accordance with personal merit, and existing unjust patterns of distribution are to be rectified. (7) *Duties of self-improvement* "rest on the fact that we can improve our own condition."[14]

Prima Facie Duties in a Biomedical Context   Ross's framework of prima facie duties is helpful for conceptualizing many of the moral dilemmas that arise in a biomedical context. In analyzing such dilemmas as they arise from the point of view of health-care professionals, the category of duties of fidelity is especially important. Consider, for example, the physician-patient relationship (a topic under discussion in Chapter 2). The social understanding or implicit agreement that underlies this relationship undoubtedly includes a number of important provisions. Among these are the provision that the physician is to act in the best medical interest of the patient and the provision that the physician is to keep confidential any personal information that comes to light within the context of the physician-patient relationship. In the very act of accepting a patient for treatment, a physician thereby incurs a number of important prima facie duties of fidelity.

Suppose a physician is convinced that lying to a patient is in the best medical interest of the patient. In Ross's scheme, the prima facie duty not to lie, itself a duty of fidelity, comes into conflict with another duty of fidelity, the prima facie duty to act in the best medical interest of the patient. Since neither duty is unconditional, in one case the duty not to lie might be more incumbent upon the physician, whereas in another case the duty to act in the best interest of the patient might be the more stringent duty. Suppose, in a different case, a physician is treating a patient suffering from a condition that renders the patient in his or her occupation a danger to others. The patient, for example, is a bus driver subject to blackouts. The patient is desperate to keep his or her job and refuses to divulge the problem to his or her employer. Should the physician break medical confidentiality and notify the patient's employer, in an effort to ensure the public safety? In this case, the prima facie duty of beneficence comes into conflict with a duty of fidelity, the prima facie duty to keep medical confidentiality. (Justifiable exceptions to the duty to keep medical confidentiality are discussed in Chapter 3.)

Among the explicit role responsibilities of a typical hospital nurse is the obligation to follow a physician's orders in the treatment of patients. By the simple act of accepting employment in the hospital setting, a nurse thereby incurs, among other numerous duties of fidelity, the prima facie duty to obey a physician's orders. But an important moral dilemma for the hospital nurse arises when, in the judgment of the nurse, following a physician's order would be detrimental to the patient. (This dilemma is discussed in Chapter 3.) Thinking in terms of Ross's theory, we can structure the dilemma as follows. The prima facie duty to follow a physician's orders comes into conflict with two other prima facie duties. First there is a relevant duty of nonmaleficence. A nurse should not act in a way that would, in effect, injure another person. Second, there is another relevant duty of fidelity, deriving from the fact that a nurse has an implicit contract or agreement with the patient to act in his or her best medical interest. Is the collective force of these two prima facie duties more incumbent upon the nurse than the prima facie duty to follow a physician's orders? Since the duty of nonmaleficence is recognized by Ross (and "ordinary moral consciousness") as especially stringent, it seems that in most cases, at least where the potential harm to patients is significant, the nurse must conclude that it would be wrong to follow the physician's order.

Abstracting from any relevant role responsibilities on the part of health-care professionals, the issue of the moral justifiability of mercy killing (discussed in Chapter 7) might be conceptualized, in accordance with Ross's scheme, as a moral dilemma involving the conflict between a duty of beneficence and a duty of nonmaleficence. A terminally ill person suffering unbearable pain, it would seem, would benefit from an immediate and painless death. Thus we have on one hand a duty of beneficence—the prima facie duty to come to the assistance of a person in serious distress—and on the other hand we have a duty of nonmaleficence—the prima facie duty not to kill.

Critical Assessment of Ross's Theory   Since Ross developed his theory of prima facie duties explicitly in reference to the promptings of "ordinary moral consciousness," it would be surprising if his theory could not be reconciled with our experience of the moral life. Indeed, let us put aside whatever worries might be expressed on this score, for there is a much more obvious deficiency in Ross's theory. Recall that we have asked not only that an ethical theory be reconcilable with our experience of the moral life but also that it provide us with effective guidance where it is most needed, in the face of moral dilemmas. And despite the fact that Ross's theory provides us with a helpful framework for conceptualizing our moral dilemmas, it provides us with virtually no substantive guidance for resolving them.

In the difficult cases, where two prima facie duties come into strong conflict, Ross holds that there are no principles we can appeal to in an effort to make an appropriate decision. The most we can do, in his view, is render a "considered decision" as to which duty is more incumbent upon us in a certain situation. Although it is fine to be told to make a considered decision, what exactly is worthy of consideration in reaching a decision? Can we resist, however vaguely, falling back on some sort of utilitarian standard? A rule-utilitarian, in particular, might argue that Ross's entire system of prima facie duties could be exhibited on the basis of a rule-utilitarian foundation. And in this way, the advantages of thinking in terms of prima facie duties could be combined with a utilitarian methodology for mediating among conflicting duties.

RELEVANT CONCEPTS AND PRINCIPLES

The foregoing examination of some major normative ethical theories provides the groundwork for a brief exploration of several important concepts in biomedical ethics. The most central of these concepts are autonomy, paternalism, and rights. Closely associated with these concepts is a set of principles, called "liberty-limiting principles," which are often invoked in order to justify limitations on individual liberty. This section provides a brief examination of these relevant concepts and principles.

Autonomy

Many discussions in biomedical ethics presume the importance of individual autonomy, stressing the right of autonomous decision makers to determine for themselves what will be done to their bodies. This "right of self-determination" is said to limit what physicians, nurses, and other professionals can justifiably do to patients. In fact, this right is often taken so seriously that professionals who act against their patients' wishes, even to save their patients' lives, are condemned as morally blameworthy and leave themselves open to charges of battery. In view of all this, it is useful to discuss the following questions, the first a conceptual question, the second an ethical one. (1) What sense of autonomy is operative in the widespread presumption that individual autonomy is an important value? and (2) What is the ethical basis for the value accorded to individual autonomy?

The Concept of Autonomy   In discussions of ethics, autonomy is typically defined as self-governance or self-determination. Individuals are said to act autonomously when they, and not others, make the decisions that affect their lives and act on the basis of their decisions. This general characterization needs to be explicated, however, since autonomy is a complex notion. Writers in biomedical ethics often conceptually distinguish several senses of autonomy in order to clarify some of the issues raised when questions are asked about justified infringements or limitations of individual autonomy: (1) autonomy as liberty of action; (2) autonomy as freedom of choice; and (3) autonomy as effective deliberation.[15] A brief consideration of these three senses of autonomy will also serve to emphasize the various ways in which an individual's action, thought, or choice may be less than fully autonomous.

1 Autonomy as Liberty of Action   Think of a would-be physician, Mark, who sits under a tree waiting for medical knowledge to permeate his being. No one is forcing Mark to sit under the tree. He is free to leave anytime he chooses. His action results from his conscious intention to sit under the tree. (He does not mistakenly believe, for example, that he is sitting in medical school.) His action is also voluntary in the sense that it is not the result of coercion or duress. If autonomy is treated simply as a synonym for "liberty of action," then Mark is acting autonomously insofar as his action is intentional and voluntary. Mark's autonomy would be violated, however, if he were physically forced to sit under the tree or if someone were to coerce him into sitting there by threatening him with harm.

When autonomy is identified with liberty of action, the primary contrast drawn is between autonomy and coercion. Coercion always involves the deliberate use of force or the threat of harm. The coercer's purpose is to get the person being coerced to do something he or she would not otherwise be willing to do. "Occurrent" coercion involves the use of physical force. "Dispositional" coercion involves the threat of harm.[16] An unscrupulous medical researcher, for example, might literally force individuals to participate as research subjects, as was done in Nazi Germany. This is occurrent coercion. But the researcher might also bring about the desired participation by threatening reluctant patients with some harm, such as the withdrawal of care essential for the patient's recovery. This is dispositional coercion. Moreover, with regard to the threat of harm, human beings can coerce other human beings either directly or by enacting laws that threaten them with harm. So laws as well as individuals can be coercive. For example, a physician is constrained from performing some late abortions by laws that threaten harm (in the form of punishment) to those who perform such operations.

2 Autonomy as Freedom of Choice   Suppose that a pregnant woman decides, after carefully weighing all the alternatives, that abortion is the best alternative in her situation. If she is very poor and public funds to pay for the abortion are not forthcoming, she is not free to act on her decision. Note that her lack of freedom is not due to coercion. Nevertheless, her autonomy is limited because her range of choices is narrowed. The same might be true of a weak, terminally ill patient who wants to speed the dying process but may be unable to do so because physical weakness makes any act, such as jumping out of a window, impossible. If others are unwilling to help hasten the patient's death, the patient's freedom of choice is limited. Or consider the patient who does not want to go through the process of choosing between alternative forms of treatment (surgery versus chemotherapy, for example) and asks the physician to make the choice without giving the patient any details about the risks and benefits of each. If the physician does not accede to the request and insists upon giving the patient the requisite information, the patient's liberty of action is not being constrained by coercion. Nonetheless, the patient's freedom of choice is narrowed insofar as the way he or she is treated is not in accordance with the preferred choice.

3 Autonomy as Effective Deliberation   The accounts of limitations on autonomy provided in the discussions of autonomy as liberty of action and autonomy as freedom of choice focus on factors external to the agent which limit his or her autonomy. The first focuses on the coercion exerted on the agent by others, either directly or indirectly. The second focuses on the unavailability of options which the agent might have chosen. By contrast, autonomy as effective deliberation focuses on the agent's internal states and on related internal constraints.

In most discussions in biomedical ethics, autonomy is closely allied with rationality. An autonomous individual is characterized as one who is capable of making *rational* and *unconstrained* decisions and acting accordingly. An individual *exercises* autonomy in this sense when he or she acts without constraint on the basis of rational and unconstrained decisions. The criteria of rationality and constraint are central here. Under what conditions are individuals and their decisions and actions unconstrained? We have already discussed some of the constraints on an individual's actions. Our present discussion focuses on autonomy and constraints in relation to the agent's decision-making process. This requires distinguishing between two senses of rationality.

According to the first sense of rationality, individuals are properly described as rational when they are capable of choosing the best means to some chosen end. In this sense of rationality, someone in our society who wants to be a physician and attends medical school in order to attain this end is acting rationally. Someone with the same desire who, like Mark in our earlier example, sits under a tree and meditates for twelve hours a day, waiting for medical knowledge to "permeate his being," is acting irrationally. To be rational in this sense entails being capable of reasoning well on the basis of good evidence about the best means to achieve some end. Someone in our society, for example, who does not use contraceptives during intercourse because she believes that an amulet she wears will keep her from getting pregnant is acting irrationally. To be rational in this sense also entails being able to postpone immediate gratification when such postponement is necessary to achieve chosen goals. Would-be physicians in medical school who party every night because they desire the pleasures of partying, even though this seriously jeopardizes their chances of succeeding in school, are acting irrationally.

A second sense of rationality involves choosing ends rather than means to those ends. All thinking beings have goals or ends they believe are in their interest to pursue. Being able to select and identify appropriate goals or interests is an important aspect of rationality. In this sense of rationality, an individual is properly described as rational if he or she is capable of choosing appropriate ends, although what counts as an appropriate end is a notorious matter of dispute. One who chooses unprofitable or self-destructive ends, for example, may be characterized as irrational. Would-be suicides are often described as irrational in this sense, as are masochists. Would-be suicides might sometimes be rational in the first sense, that is, capable of choosing the most efficient and painless way to end their lives. However, those who hold that the choice of death as an end is always inappropriate would consider all would-be suicides irrational in the second sense.

If rational acts must be based on decisions concerning the best means to maximize appropriately chosen ends, a fully rational person will have to have a number of abilities:

1. The ability to formulate appropriate goals, especially long-term goals.

2. The ability to establish priorities among these goals.

3. The ability to determine the best means to achieve chosen goals.

4. The ability to act effectively to realize these goals.

5. The ability to either abandon the chosen goals or modify them if the consequences of using the available means are undesirable or if the means are inadequate.

To sum up the discussion of autonomy as effective deliberation thus far, an individual is autonomous in this sense only if he or she possesses the abilities requisite for effective reasoning and the disposition to exercise those abilities. But these abilities can be limited in many ways. When they are, decisions and actions may be less than fully rational. First, some individuals may not have sufficiently developed the necessary abilities or may even be incapable of sufficiently developing them. Second, even individuals who have the requisite abilities may be unable to *exercise* them on a particular occasion due to various internal factors. Emotions such as fear may make the impartial weighing of information impossible. Laziness may keep an individual from learning all the pertinent information. The presence of pain or the use of drugs may also affect the exercise of reasoning abilities. It may be best, therefore, to speak of *degrees* of rationality and irrationality since many factors can make decisions and actions less than fully rational without pushing them to the irrational end of the spectrum.

Furthermore, autonomy as effective deliberation may be constrained in ways that do not affect the "rationality" of the decision. A lack of appropriate information, lies, and deception can all limit the effective exercise of the abilities required for rational deliberation. Physicians, for example, can constrain their patients' decision-making processes by deliberately withholding information. A patient who is told about only one possible kind of therapy and lacks information about alternatives cannot weigh the relative risks and benefits of all possible therapies in relation to long-term ends. In that situation a patient's "choice" of the therapy recommended by the physician is less than fully autonomous. Yet the choice might be rational both because the patient's deliberative process has been logical and because it may actually be in the latter's best interests in light of long-term goals. But to the extent that the patient's decision-making processes are constrained by the lack of information, the patient is not free to effectively exercise his or her autonomy.

In summary, to be completely autonomous or self-determining, an individual must possess the characteristics necessary for effective deliberation, be free of internal constraints in the exercise of those abilities, and be neither coerced by others nor have his or her range of options narrowed by them. A person's autonomy can be infringed upon, limited, or usurped by others in many ways including coercion, deception, lying, failing to supply necessary information, and narrowing the individual's range of options, for example, by refusing to act in accordance with his or her expressed desires. It can also be diminished by internal factors, such as strong emotions, the lack of appropriate capacities, fever, compulsion, and severe pain. To respect others' autonomy or right of self-determination is to treat them as individuals having the abilities required to be rational decision makers, capable of identifying their own interests and making their own reflective choices about the best means to advance these. An individual (A) fails to respect a person's (B's) autonomy if A imposes constraints on B's deliberative process or liberty of action or if A narrows B's range of choices. In each of these cases, A interferes in some way with the effective exercise of B's autonomy, and this is prohibited by the principle of respect for autonomy.

Autonomous Decisions and Appropriate Ends   Concern is often expressed in biomedical ethics about the ends or values appropriate for human beings to pursue. This concern was mentioned in the discussion of autonomy as effective deliberation. The principle of respect for persons requires noninterference with others' autonomy and exercise of autonomy. But when an individual chooses ends that seem inappropriate or irrational or makes a decision whose implementation is likely to bring about such ends, others question the competency of the decision maker and thus his or her autonomy (in the third sense). What does the principle of respect for autonomy require of medical personnel when a patient's expressed choices are inconsistent with the professionals' conceptions of appropriate human goals?

One way of approaching the issue is to distinguish between actions and choices that are in keeping with an individual's usual choices and those that are not. Individuals have a history of choices and decision making. The values that shape some lives may be considered irrational and inappropriate by others and yet be firmly held and carefully thought out. For example, a Jehovah's Witness on religious grounds risks his life by refusing blood transfusions deemed essential by his physician. This refusal is consistent with the values and beliefs that govern his life. There are no good grounds for questioning the rationality of the refusal when it is understood in the context of his ultimate values. And there are no good grounds for rejecting those ultimate values as inconsistent with the choices of an autonomous agent. In another case a 22-year-old patient who has no history of strong religious belief is in severe pain and has a temperature of 103°. When told she needs surgery and possibly blood transfusions, she refuses both, saying she wants to die so she can go to heaven where there is no pain. This case is clearly different from the Jehovah's Witness case. First, her physical condition provides good grounds for questioning the rationality and, therefore, autonomy of her decision. Second, her statement is not in accordance with her past history of decisions and values. If prior to the illness, she had expressed strong religious beliefs that made her present "decision" intelligible, her present physical condition might not provide sufficient grounds for questioning her autonomy. If there is good reason to believe that her new goal was "chosen" when her abilities for effective deliberation were severely constrained by her physical condition, however, then we have grounds for questioning the rationality of that goal in her case. Here, the principle of respect for autonomy does not seem to require treating her expressed wishes as those of an autonomous agent. But suppose she remained in pain for a prolonged period and her temperature fluctuated and was often normal. Suppose that knowing the prognosis and the future pain she would be experiencing, she has gone through a long reflective process culminating in the adoption of religious beliefs that give her great hope of an afterlife. In light of this hope and an evaluation of a very negative prognosis provided by medical professionals, she decides not to have the surgery. Here, her decision may not be in keeping with her history of decisions since she has chosen new ultimate values. Nonetheless, there may be good reason to hold that her decisions are autonomous ones, which should be respected in keeping with the principle of respect for persons.

One way of rephrasing the issue is as follows. Under what conditions are the ultimate ends or values that guide a patient's decisions to be accepted as those of an autonomous decision maker by medical professionals and accorded the respect that is required by the principle of autonomy? A possible answer is that either (1) the values must be firmly and consistently held over a long period of time; or (2) if there is a change in ultimate ends or values, there must be good grounds for thinking that the change is the result of a reflective reassessment of ends and values.

The Value of Autonomy   What is the basis for the moral value accorded to individual autonomy? The strongest claims regarding its moral primacy come from Kant and from certain other deontologists. In Kant's view, persons, unlike things, must always be accorded respect as self-determining subjects. They must be treated as ends in themselves and never merely as objects. For Kant, the fundamental principle of morality, respect for persons as moral agents, entails respect for personal autonomy. Such respect is due them as a right—autonomous agents are entitled to respect. If persons were not taken to be autonomous agents, there would be no basis for the moral responsibility we have toward other human beings, which precludes our using them, as we do cattle, chickens, rocks, land, and trees, simply to serve our own ends. But how does Kant understand autonomy?

Kant's primary focus is on the autonomy of the will. For Kant, "Autonomy of the will is the property the will has of being a law to itself."[17] What Kant calls the "dignity of man as a rational creature" is due to human beings possessing just that property that enables them to govern their own actions in accordance with rules of their own choosing. Putting aside many complexities in Kant's own thinking, a Kantian position central in biomedical ethics describes autonomy in terms of self-control, self-direction, or self-governance. The individual capable of acting on the basis of effective deliberation, guided by reason, and neither driven by emotions or compulsions nor manipulated or coerced by others, is, on a Kantian position, the model of autonomy.

For utilitarians, autonomy is an important value. John Stuart Mill, who speaks of individuality rather than autonomy, argues, for example, that liberty of action and thought is essential in developing both the intellectual and character traits necessary for truly human happiness:

> The human faculties of perception, judgment, discriminative feeling, mental activity, and even moral preference, are exercised only in making a choice. He who does anything because it is the custom makes no choice. He gains no practice either in discerning or in desiring what is best. The mental and moral, like the muscular powers, are improved by being used....
>
> He who lets the world, or his own portion of it, choose his plan of life for him, has no need of any other faculty than the ape-like one of imitation. He who chooses his plan for himself employs all his faculties. He must use observation to see, reasoning and judgment to foresee, activity to gather materials for decision, discrimination to decide, and when he has decided, firmness and self-control to hold to his deliberate decision....
>
> Where, not the person's own character, but the traditions or customs of other people are the rule of conduct, there is wanting one of the principal ingredients of human happiness.[18]

For Mill, persons possessing "individuality" are autonomous in a very strong sense, reflectively choosing their own plans of life, making their own decisions without manipulation by others, and exercising firmness and self-control in acting on their decisions.

Despite the high value placed on autonomy by utilitarians, their interest in autonomy differs from the Kantian one. On a Kantian view, respect for the personal autonomy of rational agents is entailed by the fundamental principle of morality, which serves as a limiting criterion for all moral conduct. That is, it places limits on what one individual can do to another human being without acting immorally. As noted earlier, one person can never use another as a subject in a medical experiment without his or her consent, no matter what potential good consequences for society as a whole might result. For a utilitarian such as Mill, respect for individual autonomy has utility value. A society that fosters respect for persons as autonomous agents will be a more progressive and, on balance, a happier society because its citizens will have the opportunities to develop their capacities to act as rational, responsible moral agents. If it could be shown that respect for individual autonomy does not have sufficient utility value, the utilitarian might have no good grounds for objecting to practices that infringe upon that autonomy.

Liberty-Limiting Principles

Since autonomy is accorded such great moral significance, a moral justification must be given for any infringement on or limitation or usurpation of autonomy. Many of the discussions in biomedical ethics explore such *proposed* justifications. The following exposition will center on the most general kinds of reasons advanced in these discussions.

Six suggested general reasons, most frequently considered when limitations of liberty (one aspect of autonomy) are at issue, are embodied in six principles, often called "liberty-limiting principles," stated below.[19] It is important to note at the outset that while some writers advance these principles as legitimate liberty-limiting principles, others argue against the legitimacy of many, or even most, of them.

1. A person's liberty is justifiably restricted to prevent that person from harming others (the harm principle).

2. A person's liberty is justifiably restricted to prevent that person from offending others (the offense principle).

3. A person's liberty is justifiably restricted to prevent that person from harming himself or herself (the principle of paternalism).

4. A person's liberty is justifiably restricted to benefit that person (the principle of extreme paternalism).

5. A person's liberty is justifiably restricted to prevent that person from acting immorally (the principle of legal moralism).

6. A person's liberty is justifiably restricted to benefit others (the social welfare principle).

These liberty-limiting principles are most frequently discussed when questions are raised about the justification of coercive laws, such as laws limiting access to hallucinogenic drugs. But the considerations they embody are also pertinent when applied to individual acts and practices that infringe upon or limit others' *autonomy*. It should also be noted that more than one of these principles might be advanced to justify a proposed limitation or infringement.

The harm principle is the most widely accepted liberty-limiting principle. Few will dispute that the law is within its proper bounds when it constrains individuals from performing acts that will seriously harm other persons or will seriously impair important institutional practices. Laws that threaten thieves, murderers, and the like with punishment, for example, are usually perceived as a necessary part of any social system. Individual acts of coercion whose intent is to prevent individuals from harming others are also usually considered morally permissible. A bystander, for example, who prevents a terrorist from killing or wounding someone, is praised and not blamed for interfering with the terrorist's action. Aside from the harm principle, however, the moral legitimacy of the liberty-limiting principles under discussion here is a matter of dispute.

According to the offense principle, the law may justifiably be invoked to prevent offensive behavior in public. "Offensive" behavior is understood as behavior that causes shame, embarrassment, or discomfort to onlookers. In the leading example of the relevance of the offense principle to biomedical ethics, individuals who behave offensively in public are sometimes involuntarily committed to mental institutions, even though their behavior poses no serious threat of harm to themselves or others. If individuals are committed to mental institutions simply because their behavior is considered offensively eccentric, then the offense principle is being invoked, at least implicitly. Attacks on the use of such grounds to deprive individuals of much of their autonomy are attacks on the legitimacy of the offense principle.

According to the principle of legal moralism, liberty may justifiably be limited to prevent immoral behavior or, as it is often expressed, to "enforce morals." Acts such as kidnapping, murder, and fraud are undoubtedly immoral, but the principle of legal moralism does not have to be invoked to justify laws against them. An appeal to the harm principle already provides a widely accepted independent justification. The principle of legal moralism usually comes to the fore only when so-called victimless crimes are at issue. Is it justifiable to legislate against homosexual acts, gambling, or prostitution simply on the grounds that such activities are thought to be morally unacceptable? In biomedical ethics, the principle of legal moralism is sometimes invoked, at least implicitly, when it is argued that suicide is an immoral act and that, therefore, it is justifiable to act to prevent suicide, even if the decision to commit it is the result of careful deliberation. Many do not accept the principle of legal moralism as a legitimate liberty-limiting principle, however. Mill holds, for example, that to accept the principle is tantamount to permitting a "tyranny of the majority."

The social welfare principle also has some relevance in biomedical ethics. According to this principle, individual autonomy can justifiably be restricted to benefit others. Such justifications are sometimes attempted in discussions of biomedical and behavioral research. It is argued, for example, that using human beings as research subjects without informing them (thus bypassing their consent) is morally justified if the research project promises some potentially great benefit to others in society. Those who find such justifications questionable may be wary about accepting the social welfare principle as a legitimate liberty-limiting principle.

The liberty-limiting principles that are most prominent in the literature of biomedical ethics are the paternalistic principles. Disagreements about the legitimacy of paternalistic justifications affect the resolution of a number of important issues in biomedical ethics. Physicians or nurses, for example, who lie to patients in order to spare them pain are often accused of acting on questionable (i.e., paternalistic) grounds. The paternalistic justifications offered for certain laws that are of special concern in biomedical ethics are also frequently attacked. Among such laws are those that allow courts to commit individuals to mental institutions either in order to keep them from harming themselves or in order to force them to receive treatment. Because of the centrality of paternalism in biomedical ethics, it is essential to examine the concept of paternalism as well as some of the arguments offered both for and against paternalistic actions and practices.

Paternalism

The definition of paternalism most widely cited is Gerald Dworkin's:

> [Paternalism is] the interference with a person's liberty of action justified by reasons referring exclusively to the welfare, good, happiness, needs, interests, or values of the person being coerced.[20]

When paternalism in the legal system is at issue, this definition is acceptable since laws, backed by force or the threat of harm, are by nature coercive. However, many of the actions considered paternalistic in biomedical ethics do not fit this definition. Consider the following examples, which are similar to some discussed in our earlier presentation of autonomy.

1. A physician decides not to tell a patient that he has Alzheimer's disease. The patient had frequently asserted that if he were ever to receive such a diagnosis, he would immediately proceed to commit suicide as efficiently and painlessly as possible because the life of an Alzheimer's disease victim was antithetical to everything he valued. The physician, who believes that the patient will commit suicide if informed of his condition, considers deliberate premature death a morally unacceptable harm to the patient and, therefore, withholds the information.

2. A physician refuses to perform an abortion on a woman who lives in a small, isolated town with no other physicians. They both know that the woman cannot afford to travel elsewhere to have the abortion. The physician refuses to perform the abortion because she believes that the woman will eventually regret the decision and become seriously depressed about it.

3. A patient asks a physician not to give him information about relevant alternative treatments, but to make the choice for him. The physician insists upon giving the patient the information because the physician believes the patient will be better off if he makes his own decision.

Note that none of these cases involve coercion; yet they can all be correctly described as paternalistic interferences, limitations, or infringements on autonomy. In each of the cases, a physician has in one way or another infringed upon or limited a patient's autonomy. In both the second and third cases, a physician has narrowed a patient's range of choices to exclude the preferred choices, ostensibly for the patient's own good. In the first case, a physician has denied a patient information vital to effective deliberation about the balance of his life, again for his own good (i.e., to keep him from harming himself). In the first and second cases physicians have treated patients as individuals incapable of making the correct judgments about their own best interests. In all three cases, a physician has effectively usurped a patient's decision-making power, substituting his or her judgment for the patient's. While it is difficult to capture this sense of paternalism in a precise definition, a rough definition can be given as follows:

Paternalism is the interference with, limitation of, or usurpation of individual autonomy justified by reasons referring exclusively to the welfare or needs of the person whose autonomy is being interfered with, limited, or usurped.

Is such paternalistic behavior ever morally justified? If yes, under what conditions do paternalistic grounds constitute good reasons, either for coercion or for effectively taking decisions out of the individuals' hands for their own good? In considering the justifiability of paternalistic actions, keep in mind the difference between the principle of paternalism and the principle of extreme paternalism. The latter would apply to paternalistic actions whose intent is to benefit individuals; whereas the former would apply to paternalistic actions whose intent is to keep individuals from harm.

In the framework of Kantian ethical theory, the moral fundamentality of individual autonomy seems to prohibit any paternalistic actions when the individuals affected are capable of self-governance or self-determination. It would always be morally wrong, for example, for physicians to withhold information about surgical procedures from patients simply because the physicians believed that their patients would refuse to undergo potentially beneficial procedures if informed of all the risks. Charles Fried, a contemporary ethicist who adopts a Kantian approach to paternalism in the medical context, maintains that patients must never be denied relevant information. By withholding it, physicians fail to treat patients as ends in themselves. In Fried's view, patients can never be treated simply as means to ends, even when the ends in question are their own ends (e.g., their restored health).[21]

John Stuart Mill provides the classical utilitarian statement on the illegitimacy of paternalistic actions. This statement is frequently cited in court opinions concerning the right of self-determination in medical matters. Mill argues:

> [O]ne very simple principle [is] entitled to govern absolutely the dealings of society with the individual in the way of compulsion and control, whether the means used be physical force in the form of legal penalties, or the moral coercion of public opinion. That principle is, that the sole end for which mankind are warranted, individually or collectively, in interfering with the liberty of action of any of their number, is self-protection. That the only purpose for which power can be rightfully exercised over any member of a civilized community, against his will, is to prevent harm to others. His own good, either physical or moral, is not sufficient warrant. He cannot rightfully be compelled to do or forbear because it will be better for him to do so, because it will make him happier, because, in the opinions of others, to do so would be wise, or even right.[22]

In this statement, Mill asserts that while prevention of harm to others is sometimes sufficient justification for interfering with another's autonomy, the individual's own good never is. Mill rejects paternalistic interventions because of the high utility value that he assigns to individual autonomy. In assigning it this value, Mill assumes that individuals are, on the whole, better judges of their own interests than anyone else, so that minimizing paternalistic interventions will maximize human happiness. Mill himself qualified his strong rejection of paternalism, stating:

> [T]his doctrine is meant to apply only to human beings in the maturity of their faculties. We are not speaking of children, or of young persons below the age which the law may fix as that of manhood or womanhood. Those who are still in a state to require being taken care of by others, must be protected against their own actions as well as external injury.[23]

In the kinds of cases he cites, Mill assumes that people are justified in acting paternalistically because they are better judges of an individual's interests than is the individual himself or herself. Arguing in this way, Mill seems to open the door for the justification of paternalism in the case of individuals who may not be able to correctly identify and advance their own interests because they lack the required level of ability for effective deliberation. Such individuals, often described as having "diminished autonomy" insofar as they lack the necessary abilities or capacities for self-determination, include infants, young children, and the severely mentally retarded. It is important to see that the paternalistic restrictions Mill allows may limit autonomy as liberty of action since they may involve coercion. They may also limit autonomy in the second sense discussed earlier since they narrow the range of available choices. But they do not limit autonomy in the sense central to Mill's, as well as Kant's, moral position since those with diminished autonomy lack what is essential for an appropriate level of effective rational deliberation.

Many contemporary attempts to justify *some* paternalistic actions adopt an approach similar to Mill's, stressing the apparently diminished autonomy of those who are treated paternalistically. If they were fully autonomous, the argument runs, they would want the benefits involved and would want to avoid the harms. Those who argue in this way must deal with an underlying conceptual issue. They must identify the criteria that should be used in determining whether a person's autonomy is sufficiently diminished to justify paternalism. In light of our earlier discussion of rationality, constraint, and autonomy, it seems plausible to hold the following view regarding diminished autonomy. When a person's autonomy (in the third sense) is *severely* constrained by intellectual lacks (e.g., lack of reasoning ability or ignorance of relevant facts), and when acting on decisions made under such constraints will probably result in some serious, irrevocable harm, the individual's autonomy would seem to be sufficiently impaired to justify paternalistic acts. Two examples may be helpful here. People under the influence of hallucinogenic drugs who decide to leap from twentieth-floor windows in order to get home more quickly, believing that they (like Superman) can fly, are hardly acting in an autonomous manner. Their decisions are grossly inconsistent with the best inductive evidence we possess regarding what happens to human beings who leap out of windows. Severely retarded individuals who decide to go out alone in a busy city but are incapable of understanding traffic signals would also seem to be acting in a much less than fully autonomous way. They are unaware of the kind of risk they would be running by going out alone. In both cases, there is good reason to assume that the individuals are incapable, whether temporarily or permanently, of the level of reasoning required for sufficiently autonomous decision making. Paternalistic interventions seem to be justified here in light of the high value placed on life and the permanent or temporary inability of the individuals involved to understand that acting on their decisions could be fatal.

Does the fact that a decision will result in death or some other serious, irrevocable harm *always* provide sufficient grounds for the claim that autonomy is so severely diminished that paternalism is justified? Some especially problematic cases involve decisions to commit suicide. Many suicide attempts are the result of temporary disorientation associated with drugs, alcohol, or extreme, but temporary, depression. In accordance with our earlier discussion of rationality and autonomy, decisions to commit suicide in these cases are far from fully rational and autonomous. Cases involving individuals who are so severely constrained in their reasoning that they are temporarily or permanently incapable of correctly assessing the probable severely harmful results of their acts would seem to provide clear instances of sufficiently diminished autonomy. As already noted, however, some decisions to end or risk life may be based on carefully thought-out reasons and may be either consistent with the person's own long-term conception of a satisfying or meaningful life or the result of a new but reflective reassessment of ultimate values and goals. It would beg the question to call these latter decisions irrational and, therefore, nonautonomous, in order to justify paternalistic interventions, simply on the grounds that the person's intended act will probably result in serious self-harm. It may be that in the case of those ends that are usually considered highly undesirable (e.g., death or the possibility of severe injury), it should be presumed that the individual's choice is not rational and, therefore, not an autonomous one. This presumption would justify, at best, temporarily constraining someone from certain acts in order to establish the rationality of the choice. In summary, paternalistic actions are justified when they are necessary either (1) to keep persons with severely diminished autonomy from doing themselves serious, irrevocable harm or (2) to temporarily constrain persons from acting to bring about *presumably* irrational self-harming ends until it can be determined whether the individuals are acting autonomously. This kind of paternalism, often called "weak paternalism," is consistent with the position of those who agree with Mill's criticism of paternalism. The interventions do not show a lack of respect for individual autonomy. Rather, they are attempts either to prevent individuals from seriously harming themselves when they are acting non-autonomously or to prevent them from harming themselves until it can be determined whether their acts are indeed autonomous ones. Such weak paternalism stands in contrast to strong paternalism, which maintains that paternalistic treatment is sometimes justified even when (1) and (2) do not apply.

Note that the distinction between weak and strong paternalism is not the same as the distinction between paternalism and extreme paternalism (as reflected in the statement of liberty-limiting principles). Discussions of the distinction between weak and strong paternalism usually focus on actions and practices whose intention is to prevent harm and thus on the principle of paternalism rather than the principle of extreme paternalism. However, a similar distinction can be made in regard to extreme paternalism. A weak form of extreme paternalism would allow paternalistic interferences intended to benefit those whose autonomy is severely diminished. This would stand in contrast to a strong form of extreme paternalism, which would allow beneficial paternalistic interferences even in the case of persons whose autonomy is not severely diminished.

The severely or even mildly mentally retarded may pose special problems when questions of justified paternalism are raised, precisely because they *may* lack the abilities necessary for autonomy as effective deliberation. Whether the mildly retarded lack such abilities is a matter of dispute, however. Many people classified as mildly mentally retarded are capable of effective deliberation if they are given appropriate training and information. In the case of mentally retarded individuals who are capable of effective deliberation, paternalistic treatment would seem to be justified only if strong paternalism is justified. But if strong paternalism is not justified in the case of the nonmentally retarded, then it would also not be justified in the case of mildly mentally retarded individuals capable of effective deliberation. On the other hand, in the case of mentally retarded individuals whose autonomy is diminished to the point that paternalistic interferences in their lives would be instances of weak paternalism, paternalistic actions whose intent is to benefit these individuals could be as justifiable as those whose intent is to keep them from harm.

Is strong paternalism ever justified? One defense of strong paternalism rests on a prudential argument that itself appeals to the importance of autonomy. We are aware that we often act in ignorance and that we are often tempted to act in ways incompatible with what we see as our long-term interests. Acting in ignorance, or too weak-willed to resist temptation, we may do ourselves serious irreversible harm of a sort that would severely diminish our autonomy. We are also aware that accidents, illnesses, diseases, and emotional pressures may diminish our rational capacities and thus our autonomy. We should be willing, therefore, to accept those paternalistic acts, laws, and practices whose intent is either to protect individual autonomy from being severely diminished or, if it has already been diminished, to restore it. This argument is advanced in order to justify the following kinds of laws: (1) laws, such as those against the sale of laetrile, that protect us against our own ignorance; (2) laws, such as those against the sale of hallucinogenic drugs (without prescription), that protect us against our own weaknesses of the will and/or ignorance; and (3) laws that allow courts and psychiatrists to commit the "mentally ill" to institutions against their will in order to cure them (restore their autonomy) or to keep them from the kind of self-harm that might further reduce their autonomy. The same sort of prudential argument is sometimes invoked to justify paternalistic acts by physicians when these acts are performed to prevent some serious deterioration of the patient's autonomy. However, some of the constraining interventions that would seem to be justified by this line of argument are very problematic. Some individuals, for example, might prefer to give in to temptations, weighing the pleasures of using hallucinogenic drugs more highly than its dangers or risks. Others might want to have access to laetrile, hoping that it will help and willing to risk the possibility that it might not. The involuntary civil commitment of the mentally ill for their own good is perhaps even more questionable, as some of the readings in Chapter 5 bring out.

A radically different defense of paternalism on the part of the state is offered by critics of the liberal individualist tradition, which is associated with both natural right theorists such as John Locke and utilitarians such as Mill. These critics question the need to justify laws and government practices whose intent is to benefit or keep from self-harm the members of society being constrained. In this view, a need to justify the state's interference with individual autonomy arises from a social-political theory that misunderstands the relation between the state and the individual and mistakenly stresses the primacy of individual interests rather than the interests of the social whole. The ideal of the liberal-individualist tradition in social-political theory is a society with a minimal amount of state interference with individual autonomy. Critics of this social-political ideal reject the justifications that are offered in defense of the primacy accorded individual autonomy as simply expressions of an ideological commitment to "Western liberal thought." The ideology of the critics stresses the primacy of the interests of society as a whole. A social-political system committed to the latter ideal perceives all individual acts as significant for society at large and government regulation of any of those acts as part of the state's legitimate role. Any final assessment of such a defense of state paternalism, of course, is intimately intertwined with the resolution of fundamental questions about the relation between the individual and the state.

In a totally different vein, indirect support for opposition to paternalism comes from certain sociologists, psychologists, and other social theorists who offer analyses to explain the recent emphasis on antipaternalism in American society. They attribute much of the recent stress on antipaternalism to a growing awareness of both the class differences in our society and the fact that those who perform paternalistic acts (e.g., psychiatrists, judges, physicians, and the administrators and staffs of mental institutions) are usually members of the upper-middle class, while those who are treated paternalistically are usually members of the poorer, less-privileged classes. An awareness of this class difference, and of the related differences in interests and values, gives rise to serious doubts about both the ability and the willingness of those wielding paternalistic authority to act in the interests of those whom they typically constrain. On this analysis, it is not the moral legitimacy of the principle of paternalism that is really at issue when paternalistic acts and practices are increasingly rejected. Rather, what is at issue are the abuses resulting from so-called paternalistic acts that do not in fact serve to benefit (or keep from harm) the individuals constrained, but do serve the ends of the members of the professions wielding paternalistic authority. This line of argument is intended to point out that the current antipaternalistic stress is probably not the result of conscious deliberation about the legitimacy of central ethical principles but a rejection of what passes as justified paternalism in a class society in which the "constrainers" are neither knowledgeable nor altruistic enough to perceive correctly the interests of those they constrain. However, the factual claims, if correct, tend to support a Mill-like claim that unless the interests and values of constrainers and constrainees coincide, individual self-interest is better served in the long run if paternalism is rejected rather than accepted.

The Language of Rights

Many discussions in biomedical ethics, including discussions of autonomy and paternalism, are couched in the language of rights. People are said, for example, to have rights to health, privacy, or life. It is also said that our most fundamental right is the right to self-determination. Paternalistic medical practices are described as "infringements" on this fundamental right. Those who defend the legalization of euthanasia appeal to a "right to death with dignity," antiabortionists to a "fetus's right to life," and advocates of national health insurance to a "right to health care." Such appeals may sometimes invoke constitutional or legal rights, but more often they appeal to purported *moral* rights which, it is said, *must* be acknowledged by all moral agents and by society, and which ought, sometimes, to be guaranteed by being enacted as legal rights. One example of a document that invokes the language of rights is the "UN Declaration of Human Rights." This document announces that all persons have a right to medical treatment as well as to many other things, such as a decent standard of living. "Human rights" here may be understood as one species of moral rights. The rights asserted by the UN Declaration are certainly not legal ones since there is no international system of laws that recognizes and guarantees them for all human beings. A citizen of the United States, for example, cannot walk into a hospital, demand and receive treatment simply on the basis of the claim that the UN Declaration proclaims his or her right to such care. Those who argue that the United States should have a national health insurance system do, however, often claim that there is a "moral" right to adequate health care that our society must recognize and guarantee through its legal system.

Although talk of moral rights is commonplace in biomedical ethics, some ethicists argue that using the language of rights may hinder rather than help us in our attempts to develop an understanding of the moral issues that arise in the biomedical context. Rights talk, it is said, often engenders confusions that result, at least in part, from a lack of agreement regarding answers to the following types of questions about moral rights: (1) How do we determine what kinds of entities have rights and what kinds do not? Do fetuses have rights? Animals? Children? The mentally retarded? (2) When there is a conflict of rights, how should we resolve the conflict? Do the rights of the fetus take precedence over the rights of the woman bearing it? (3) When there is a disagreement about the existence of a specific right, how do we determine whether such a right exists? Is there, for example, a right to health care?

Conflicting claims using the language of rights cannot be resolved in a rational way unless these types of questions are answered. If legal or constitutional rights are at issue, we can answer such questions by examining the laws and constitutional decisions bearing on the rights in question. If moral rights are at issue, however, answering them requires agreement about the system of moral rules and principles that should be used as a basis for determining what moral rights must be recognized by all moral individuals and societies. In the absence of such agreement, disagreements over conflicting claims using the language of rights would seem to be disguised and confused disagreements about the more fundamental issues discussed earlier in this introduction—issues centering on the correctness of competing ethical theories, principles, and values. Suppose two individuals disagree about the existence of a moral right to death with dignity, for example. That dispute, it seems, can be resolved only if both individuals lay out the reasons supporting their claims. These reasons must include statements of the ethical principles and rules that support the conflicting views about rights. In attempting to determine which of the claimants is correct, we will have to examine the merits of any competing principles and rules and choose among them. If a choice cannot be made, it seems that the debate about rights cannot be settled.

Rights talk is also often criticized for very different reasons than those just discussed. An overemphasis on establishing legal rights, such as the right to adequate medical care, for example, is said to obscure the "emptiness" of many such rights in practice. Critics of some of the mainstream articles in biomedical ethics sometimes argue that the emphasis on rights ignores the social-cultural reality that makes the exercise of many rights problematic for the poor, the uneducated, and the otherwise disadvantaged members of our society. What is needed, they argue, is not a proliferation of government-backed rights but a radical reorganization of the existing institutions and social structures that are responsible for many of the moral dilemmas discussed in biomedical ethics.

Given the problems mentioned above, it might seem more useful to avoid the language of rights in our disputes and phrase our problems in terms of conflicting ethical theories, principles, rules, and values. However, since so many disputes in biomedical ethics invoke the language of rights, a brief examination of the concept of a right is a necessary prerequisite to understanding and evaluating many of the arguments in this text.

What is involved in the claim that someone has a right to X? Several theses, which are not all mutually compatible, are prominent in contemporary philosophical discussions.

(1) *The Correlativity Thesis: Any right entails a correlative obligation on others either not to interfere with one's liberty or to provide something.* On this thesis, A has a right to X only if others have a correlative obligation to provide A with X or to not interfere with A's pursuit of X. A has a right to health care, for example, only if others (individuals or groups) have a correlative obligation to provide A with health care. A has a right to privacy only if others have a correlative obligation not to interfere with A's privacy. The rights in question may be legal ones (those recognized and guaranteed by some system of laws) or moral ones (those required by a system of moral principles and rules).

(*a*) *The Correlativity Thesis and Positive Rights.* When the rights at issue carry correlative obligations to provide the rights holder with some benefit, good, opportunity, or service, they are often called "positive rights," or sometimes, "welfare rights." If A has a positive right to a minimum income, for example, then someone has a correlative obligation to provide it. Note that on the correlativity view, if A has a right to be provided with X, the bearer of the correlative obligation must be specifiable. If A has a right to health care, it would be useless to claim simply that someone somewhere has an obligation to provide that care. On the correlativity thesis, there must be some definite person or group who must acknowledge A's right and provide the necessary care on demand. If the state recognizes such a right through appropriate legislation, then a legal right is established, and the state through its legitimate agencies and representatives takes on the legal obligations involved. If the rights in question are only moral rights, however, then on the correlativity thesis, a full-fledged account of rights (given perhaps from a Kantian or utilitarian perspective) would involve specifying the individuals or groups who are morally obligated to fulfill the requisite obligations.

(*b*) *The Correlativity Thesis and Negative Rights.* When the rights at issue carry correlative obligations of noninterference, they are often called "negative rights," or sometimes, "liberty rights." If A has a negative right to X, no one should prevent A from pursuing X. Here again there is a correlation between rights and obligations. For example, if A has negative rights to privacy, then others have an obligation to refrain from interfering with A's privacy. Here there is no correlative obligation to provide some benefit but only an obligation, incumbent on all, not to interfere with the exercise of some rights. As in the case of positive rights, rights of noninterference may be either legal or moral or both. Negative rights are the kinds of rights that were proclaimed and defended in the seventeenth and eighteenth centuries by upholders of natural rights, such as John Locke. They asserted natural rights to life, liberty, and property, for example. Holders of this view perceived the natural negative rights they asserted as moral rights belonging to all rational agents independently of any legal system. In contrast, twentieth-century defenders of moral rights have often been concerned primarily with positive rights, such as the right to health care. In biomedical ethics, both negative and positive rights are invoked. When considering claims about rights, it is sometimes important to ask whether the writer is treating a right as a negative or a positive right. A right to life, for example, may be read as a negative right if it is understood as asserting that others have an obligation not to interfere with an individual by taking his life. A right to life is sometimes asserted as a positive right, however. Here the claim is that others have an obligation to provide the rights holder with the necessities needed to maintain life.

(2) *The Only Rights That Exist Are Legal Rights.* A has a right to X if and only if it is specifically granted by law. In this view, all other rights talk is simply rhetorical. As Jeremy Bentham, a noted utilitarian, argued in the nineteenth century, "Right...is the child of law: from *real* laws come *real* rights; but from *imaginary* laws, from laws of nature,...come *imaginary* rights."[24] Upholders of this view often argue that appeals to any rights other than legal or constitutional rights are simply disguised appeals to *values.* Rights exist only where there are correlative obligations assigned to specific individuals or groups and where there is a system of codified rules—a system that includes rules regarding both the enforcement of obligations and

the provision of redress for persons whose rights are infringed. Assertions of rights, such as natural rights or the human rights asserted in the UN Declaration, that are not recognized and guaranteed by some legal system are simply assertions of values and are binding on no one. Sometimes a value held by a particular society is used as the basis for establishing a legal right in that society. If it is, the value and the right (a legal right) coincide; but if it is not, the value in question is mistakenly described if it is characterized as a right. (If, for example, enough value is placed on the health of all our citizens, we may eventually enact the legislation that will guarantee all Americans a legal right to equal access to medical care. It would simply be rhetorical, however, to claim that such a legal right *must* be established because all human beings have a "moral right" to health care.) If this position on rights is correct, all appeals to moral rights to bolster claims in biomedical ethics would be pointless except as rhetorical devices used to underscore the moral importance of the values being asserted.

(3) *Legal Rights Are Not the Only Kinds of Rights, but Not All Rights Entail Correlative Duties.* Declarations of human rights, such as the one proclaimed by the United Nations, are statements of moral ideals that all societies should strive to realize. These moral ideals do not entail correlative duties. Recently, for example, a resolution introduced in Congress asserted a "right to food" for all human beings. A protester, understanding rights in sense 1(*a*), argued that guaranteeing food for everyone in the world would severely lower American living standards. The sponsoring congressman, understanding rights in sense 3, responded that the resolution would impose *no* correlative obligations on the United States to guarantee food to everyone either at home or abroad. It would merely provide a guideline for future policy—a goal toward which to strive. This concept of a right is one possible interpretation of the language of human rights. To the extent that such ideals are acknowledged and guaranteed by a legal system, of course, they become legal rights entailing correlative duties and, therefore, fall under either 1(*a*) or 1(*b*).

The charge is sometimes made that only a deontological ethical theory is capable of providing a theory of moral rights that will include a theory of correlative obligations binding on all moral agents. A utilitarian theory, it is said, can at best provide only a theory of values and goals. This is debatable, and many rule-utilitarians would not agree. It is not surprising, however, that utilitarians often advocate the second and third positions on moral rights, whereas deontologists usually support the correlativity view, at least in the case of those rights considered most fundamental, such as the right of self-determination.

THE RESOLUTION OF MORAL DISAGREEMENTS

Moral issues in biomedical ethics have generated a great deal of controversy. Disagreements are common; moral consensus, relatively rare. Sometimes, in regard to the use of age as a criterion in the distribution of health-care resources, for example, the relevant questions are just beginning to be asked, and the relevant issues are just beginning to be explored. However, in other cases (e.g., abortion) the issues have been explored in depth. Various writers have presented positions, others have responded, and more carefully thought-out views have emerged through dialectical exchange. Anyone approaching biomedical ethics for the first time by using this text, presented with opposing positions strongly defended by their upholders, cannot help but wonder whether any moral agreement on the issues is possible. When there is so much disagreement, can we hope to resolve moral controversies? If yes, what procedures should we use? On what principles can we rely? Several ways of approaching moral disagreements, presented below, may facilitate the resolution of controversies or, at the very least, clarify the nature of the disagreements.

(1) *Getting Clear about the Relevant Facts.* Many times, moral disagreements can be traced to disagreements about relevant facts. People may disagree, for example, about whether cancer patients should be told the truth about their condition. Sometimes, discussion may show that the disputants agree on the principle that the truth should always be given to patients who want it and can handle it appropriately. In such cases, the disagreement may be due to a radical difference in the disputants' beliefs about the effect of such information on patients' psychological states or about patients' desires to be told the truth. Sissela Bok's article in Chapter 2 gets to the heart of this *factual* disagreement. She presents the results of relevant factual studies in order to challenge physicians who claim that many cancer patients do not want the truth and that truthful information often harms patients. A lack of appropriate factual information or a disagreement about the facts is often present in other controversies as well. Utilitarians may disagree about the possible good and bad effects that establishing a right to health care or legalizing euthanasia may have on society. Critics of medical paternalism may overestimate the ability of the seriously ill to effectively deliberate about their care. It is useful, therefore, in thinking about issues in biomedical ethics, to examine the possibility that factual considerations may have to be explored and relevant information acquired. This is not an easy task since in many instances it will require a knowledge of psychology, sociology, and, even, economics. But a recognition of the nature of the problem—that the problem is a factual one and not a disagreement on moral principles—is a first step toward a resolution.

(2) *Conceptual Clarification.* Controversies can sometimes be settled or clarified if the disputants can agree about the meaning of a relevant concept (e.g., paternalism or autonomy). In our earlier discussion of rights, for example, the dispute between the congressman advocating a right to food and his opponent was due in part to a very different understanding of rights. Disagreements in regard to abortion are sometimes disagreements about just what is involved in the concept of person. The disputants might agree that there are some things it is never acceptable to do to persons but, given their different conceptions of personhood, disagree about whether the fetus is a person. In the case of euthanasia, conceptual clarification is essential since many of the pro and con arguments are unclear to the disputing parties when expressions such as "euthanasia," "passive euthanasia," and "active euthanasia" are understood differently. Conceptual clarification will not resolve a disagreement when the conceptual differences are effectively the result of differences in moral beliefs, but, even then, such clarification can help to bring out the nature of the disagreement more clearly.

(3) *Agreement on Ethical Theory, Moral Principles, or Values.* If the disputants can agree on a moral theory or a set of moral principles or the centrality of certain values, many disputes can be resolved. For example, if individuals can agree that the offense principle is *not* an acceptable liberty-limiting principle, then they would agree that committing those diagnosed as mentally ill to institutions *solely* on the grounds that their behavior is offensive to others is not morally permissible. Or if they can agree that rule-utilitarianism is the strongest ethical theory, then they can approach all moral issues from that standpoint. It is important to see, however, that even without agreement on the best ethical theory, it is possible to agree on the correctness of crucial moral principles, such as the principle of respect for persons, or the centrality of certain values. The President's Commission for the Study of Ethical Problems in Medicine and Biomedical and Behavioral Research, for example, recently completed the task of determining just what values ought to guide decision making in the provider-patient relationship. Commission members agreed that two values were central: promotion of a patient's well-being and respect for a person's self-determination. Having reached this agreement, they were able to proceed to explore the relevant concepts and develop more specific recommendations about moral decision making in the health-care context. (Chapter 2 contains a selection from their report.)

It is important to see, however, that even when there is agreement on some principles, rules, or values, disagreements can still arise in a particular context. Different values, rules, or principles may conflict, for example. Our earlier discussion of W. D. Ross illustrates the kinds of conflicts that can arise among prima facie duties. Thus individuals might agree on the correctness of rules asserting that both beneficence and nonmaleficence are prima facie duties, and yet they may disagree about which takes precedence in a particular context, when acting in accordance with one duty means violating the other. When this occurs, further discussion is necessary to determine whether agreement can be secured on which value, rule, or principle should have priority in a given context. Disagreement can also arise about whether a principle or rule applies in a particular case. As noted earlier, for example, there is a general agreement that the harm principle is a legitimate liberty-limiting principle. Invoking the harm principle, then, two individuals might agree that persons who pose a serious threat of harm should be committed to institutions. Yet they might hold opposing views on the question of whether the majority of those diagnosed as mentally ill should be committed to hospitals without their consent. The reason for this difference of opinion might be due to very different beliefs regarding the extent of potential harm to others posed by the majority of those diagnosed as mentally ill. If they pose no serious threat of harm to others, then the harm principle does not apply, and their commitment cannot be justified on such grounds. Thus resolution of the controversy here hinges on the evaluation of relevant factual material in order to determine whether the harm principle can be legitimately applied to justify commitment.

As the articles in this text demonstrate, attempts at factual and conceptual clarification play an important role in the ongoing exploration of issues in biomedical ethics. They also demonstrate the importance of agreeing on ethical principles, rules, and fundamental values. Also worth noting are some typical philosophical methods writers use both to show the inadequacies of an opposing position and to explore possible problems in a position they themselves are developing. One such method involves using examples and opposing counterexamples to show that a proposed conceptual account is inadequate because it is either too narrow or too broad. For example, suppose paternalism is defined in such a way that coercion is a necessary component of any paternalistic action. The inadequacies of this definition can be shown by providing examples of actions appropriately characterized as paternalistic that do not involve coercion. In contrast, suppose a paternalistic act is defined as any act that benefits someone. That definition can be shown to be too broad by providing examples of actions satisfying the definition that would not be considered paternalistic. In a simple business transaction, for example, Jones buys a chair from Smith rather than Caldwell, simply because Smith has a better product at a fair price. Smith benefits from the transaction by making a profit. But there is no reason to consider Jones's action paternalistic. Other methods used by philosophers include pointing out either the inconsistencies in a position or the, perhaps unexpected, consequences following from a line of argument. It was pointed out to Mary Anne Warren, whose article on abortion is reprinted in Chapter 8, for example, that the arguments she offers in defense of abortion would also justify infanticide. Warren was faced with the need to either (1) rethink her original line of argument; (2) accept the morality of infanticide; or (3) develop a new argument that would enable her to maintain that abortion is moral but infanticide is not. Her postscript, also reprinted in Chapter 8, is Warren's response to this line of criticism. In conclusion, when reading the articles in this text, it is useful both to recognize the stratagems the authors employ in their arguments and to use the stratagems just discussed to evaluate and criticize the arguments they advance.

T.A.M. and J.S.Z.

NOTES

1 J. J. C. Smart, "Extreme and Restricted Utilitarianism," in Michael D. Bayles, ed., *Contemporary Utilitarianism* (New York: Doubleday, 1968), p. 100.
2 W. D. Ross, *The Right and the Good* (Oxford: The Clarendon Press, 1930), p. 22.

3 Alan Donagan, "Is There a Credible Form of Utilitarianism?" in *Contemporary Utilitarianism*, p. 189. Donagan's point is that act-utilitarianism is "monstrous" and "incredible" because it seems to recommend such murders.

4 The distinction between act-utilitarianism and rule-utilitarianism is a distinction that has become prominent only in contemporary times. Accordingly, the writings of Bentham and Mill are somewhat ambiguous with regard to these categories. Although Bentham is probably rightly understood as an act-utilitarian, a very strong case can be made for interpreting Mill as a rule-utilitarian. See, for example, J. O. Urmson, "The Interpretation of the Moral Philosophy of J. S. Mill," in *Contemporary Utilitarianism*, pp. 13–24.

5 Smart, "Extreme and Restricted Utilitarianism," p. 107.

6 Immanuel Kant, *Groundwork of the Metaphysic of Morals*, trans. H. J. Paton (New York: Harper & Row, 1964), p. 88.

7 *Ibid.*, p. 96.

8 H. J. Paton, *The Categorical Imperative: A Study in Kant's Moral Philosophy* (Chicago: University of Chicago Press, 1948), p. 172.

9 The account of beneficence suggested here follows an analysis presented by Tom L. Beauchamp and James F. Childress in chapters 4 and 5 of *Principles of Biomedical Ethics*, 2d ed. (New York: Oxford University Press, 1983).

10 Ross, *The Right and the Good*, p. 19.

11 *Ibid.*, p. 20.

12 *Ibid.*, p. 21.

13 *Ibid.*

14 *Ibid.*

15 Writers in biomedical ethics and social philosophy characterize autonomy differently. Bruce L. Miller, for example, distinguishes four senses of autonomy, including: autonomy as liberty of action, autonomy as authenticity, autonomy as effective deliberation, and autonomy as moral reflection. (The discussion in this chapter follows Miller to some extent, but diverges in important ways.) Gerald Dworkin prefers to distinguish between liberty and freedom on the one hand and autonomy on the other, using "autonomy" much more narrowly than Miller. See Bruce L. Miller, "Autonomy and the Refusal of Lifesaving Treatment," *Hastings Center Report* 11 (August 1981), pp. 25–28; and Gerald Dworkin, "Autonomy and Informed Consent," in President's Commission: *Making Health Care Decisions*, Appendix G (1982), pp. 63–81.

16 The distinction between occurrent and dispositional coercion is made by Michael D. Bayles in "A Concept of Coercion," in J. Roland Pennock and John D. Chapman, eds., *Coercion: Nomos XIV* (Chicago: Aldine-Atherton, 1972), pp. 16–29.

17 Kant, *Groundwork*, p. 108.

18 John Stuart Mill, *Utilitarianism, On Liberty, Essay on Bentham*, ed. Mary Warnock (New York: New American Library, 1962), pp. 187, 185. All quotations in this chapter are from *On Liberty* in this edition.

19 Joel Feinberg's discussion of such principles served as a guide for the formulations adopted here. See Joel Feinberg, *Social Philosophy* (Englewood Cliffs, N.J.: Prentice-Hall, 1973), chapter 2.

20 Gerald Dworkin, "Paternalism," *The Monist* 56 (January 1972), p. 65.

21 Charles Fried, *Medical Experimentation: Personal Integrity and Social Policy* (New York: American Elsevier, 1974), p. 101.

22 Mill, *On Liberty*, p. 135.

23 *Ibid.*

24 Jeremy Bentham, *Anarchical Fallacies*, ed. John Bowring, Vol. 2 (New York: Russell and Russell, 1962; as reproduced from the 1843 edition), p. 220.

ANNOTATED BIBLIOGRAPHY: CHAPTER 1

Bayles, Michael D., ed.: *Contemporary Utilitarianism* (New York: Doubleday, 1968). This volume includes ten articles by contemporary philosophers. Various points of view on the nature and justifiability of utilitarian theory are represented.

Callahan, Daniel: "Bioethics as a Discipline," *Hastings Center Studies* 1 (no. 1, 1973), pp. 66–73. Callahan specifies three tasks for the bioethicist: (1) identifying ethical issues, (2) providing a systematic means of thinking through these issues, and (3) helping physicians and scientists make correct decisions. He calls for the development of a unique methodology for bioethics and emphasizes that the discipline must serve the needs of physicians and scientists, "at whatever cost to disciplinary elegance."

Caplan, Arthur L.: "Ethical Engineers Need Not Apply: The State of Applied Ethics Today," *Science, Technology, & Human Values* 6 (Fall 1980), pp. 24–32. Caplan presents criticisms of what he calls the "engineering model" of applied ethics. According to this model, applied ethics is only a technical process whereby existing theory is used to solve particular moral problems.

Childress, James F.: *Who Should Decide?: Paternalism in Health Care* (New York: Oxford, 1982). In this extended discussion of paternalism, Childress examines the metaphors and principles underlying the disputes about professional paternalism in health care.

Clouser, K. Danner: "Bioethics," *Encyclopedia of Bioethics* (1978), vol. 1, pp. 115–127. In this article, written for those who are "seeking a conceptual grasp of the field itself," Clouser situates medical ethics within the broader field of bioethics. Against those who contend that bioethics will have to develop new ethical principles, he argues that it simply involves "ordinary morality applied to new areas of concern."

Donagan, Alan: *The Theory of Morality* (Chicago: University of Chicago, 1977). In this book, Donagan provides a theory of morality whose philosophical basis is Kant's "second formulation" of the Categorical Imperative.

Dworkin, Gerald: *The Theory and Practice of Autonomy* (Cambridge: Cambridge University Press, 1988). In Part 1, Dworkin examines the nature and value of autonomy. In Part 2, he applies the general framework developed in Part 1 to various moral questions.

Feinberg, Joel: *Social Philosophy* (Englewood Cliffs, N.J.: Prentice-Hall, 1973). Feinberg gives a detailed account of legal and moral rights and of liberty-limiting principles.

Gorovitz, Samuel: "Bioethics and Social Responsibility," *The Monist* 60 (January 1977), pp. 3–15. Calling attention to a number of philosophical topics that cut across a variety of bioethical issues, Gorovitz contends that philosophers have a unique and essential role to play in bioethics. He also attempts to identify some of the genuinely new ethical problems that have arisen out of recent developments in biomedical research.

Kant, Immanuel: *Groundwork of the Metaphysic of Morals*, translated and analyzed by H. J. Paton (New York: Harper & Row, 1964). In this work, a basic reference point, Kant offers an overall statement and defense of his ethical theory.

Lindley, Richard: *Autonomy* (Atlantic Highlands, N.J.: Humanities Press, 1986). After examining various conceptions of autonomy and some related principles, Lindley discusses several specific practical problems regarding autonomy, including social practices in regard to those who are mentally handicapped or mentally ill.

Macklin, Ruth: "Moral Concerns and Appeals to Rights and Duties: Grounding Claims in a Theory of Justice," *Hastings Center Report* 6 (October 1976), pp. 31–38. Macklin criticizes contemporary appeals to rights in debates in biomedical ethics, arguing that we cannot settle disputes about rights until we work out a theory of rights.

Mill, John Stuart: *Utilitarianism, On Liberty, Essay on Bentham*, edited by Mary Warnock (New York: New American Library, 1962). In his famous essay *Utilitarianism*, Mill offers a classic statement of the utilitarian position. In his equally well-known essay *On Liberty*, he defends the classic libertarian position rejecting strong paternalism and all liberty-limiting principles other than the harm principle.

Sartorius, Rolf, ed.: *Paternalism* (Minneapolis: University of Minnesota Press, 1983). The papers in this two-part collection of articles were all written by participants in a conference on paternalism held in 1980. The papers in the first part were all published previously and include, for example, Gerald Dworkin's frequently reprinted article "Paternalism." The second part contains papers prepared for the conference.

Taylor, Paul W.: *Principles of Ethics: An Introduction* (Encino, Calif.: Dickenson, 1975). Chapter 4 of this book provides a very valuable discussion of utilitarianism. Also helpful is the exposition of ethical egoism in Chapter 3 and the exposition of Kant's ethical system in Chapter 5.

APPENDIX: SELECTED REFERENCE SOURCES IN BIOMEDICAL ETHICS

Lineback, Richard H., ed.: *The Philosopher's Index* (Bowling Green, Ohio: Philosophy Documentation Center, Bowling Green State University). This reference source, issued quarterly, is "an international index to philosophical periodicals and books." Both a subject index and an author index are provided. The subject index identifies useful material on virtually any topic of importance in biomedical ethics.

Reich, Warren T., ed. in chief: *Encyclopedia of Bioethics* (New York: Macmillan, 1978). This four-volume set, though somewhat dated, remains a valuable reference in biomedical ethics. The set contains 314 articles, and each article is followed by a selected bibliography.

Walters, LeRoy, and Tamar Joy Kahn, eds.: *Bibliography of Bioethics* (Washington, D.C.: Kennedy Institute of Ethics, Georgetown University). This bibliography, whose volumes are issued annually, is the most comprehensive source available. Its cumulated contents are also available from BIOETHICSLINE, an on-line data base of the National Library of Medicine. (The data base is updated bimonthly.)

CHAPTER 2

PHYSICIANS' OBLIGATIONS AND PATIENTS' RIGHTS

INTRODUCTION

What moral rules should govern physicians in dealing with patients? Are physicians ever morally justified in acting paternalistically to their patients? Are they ever morally justified in withholding information from patients, lying to them, or treating them without their consent? This chapter deals with such questions as it examines some of the fundamental moral issues associated with the physician-patient relationship and, consequently, with many of the other issues in this book.

Codes of Medical Ethics

The "Hippocratic Oath," reprinted in this chapter, reflects the traditional paternalism of the medical profession. The oath requires physicians to act so as to "benefit" the sick and "keep them from harm," but says nothing about patients' rights. Most of the medical codes of ethics developed through the years by the American Medical Association exemplify a similar approach. They state the standards that should guide physicians in their professional relationships with patients and others but remain silent on patients' rights. According to the 1957 AMA code, for example, the objective of the medical profession is to use its scientifically based expertise to "render service to humanity."[1] Physicians are expected to promote the well-being of their patients, but nothing is said about any patient right to participate knowledgeably in making the decisions that define that "well-being." In contrast, the discussions that have taken place over the last twenty years in biomedical ethics have frequently emphasized patients' rights, especially their right of self-determination. This emphasis reflects a growing change in lay attitudes toward health-care professionals, especially physicians.

For a long time physicians were viewed as dedicated, hardworking, selfless individuals who could be expected to do everything in their power to benefit their patients. Patients, on the other hand, were viewed as dependent individuals having an obligation to trust their physicians, who were assumed to be personally concerned with their patients' well-being. It was often taken for granted that doctors, because of their purported wisdom, objectivity, benevolence, and skill were in the best position to decide what was in their patients' best interests. Professional codes of medical ethics reflected this view of the physician-patient relationship, affirming that physicians would act to benefit their patients and would not exploit the often vulnerable patients over whom they frequently held great influence and power.

Current attitudes toward physicians are very different, due to many factors including the following. First, the physician-patient relationship has become increasingly impersonal as the growth of medical knowledge and technology has made modern medicine more complex. Growing complexity has led to an increase in specialization and the growth of large, depersonalized medical institutions. Second, the rise of "iatrogenic illnesses," illnesses resulting from medical interventions, has sometimes raised doubts about the skills of physicians. Publicity about medical mistakes and questionable medical practices has further eroded some of the lay trust in the judgments of physicians and in their selfless dedication to their patients' well-being. Third, a growing awareness of the economic and educational differences between physicians and many of their patients has resulted in doubts about the capacity of physicians to perceive the best interests of their patients and to act accordingly.

In keeping with such changes in lay attitudes toward physicians, many recent discussions of medical ethics, including Robert M. Veatch's in this chapter, have attempted first to make explicit and then to criticize the paternalism implicit in traditional codes of medical ethics. Veatch and others reject as morally unacceptable professional codes that seem to sanction using paternalistic reasons to justify medical practices (e.g., lying or withholding relevant information for a "patient's own good") that violate a patient's right of self-determination. In its 1980 statement, "Principles of Medical Ethics," reprinted in this chapter, the American Medical Association takes account of some of these criticisms, and for the first time, explicitly affirms the physician's commitment to "dealing honestly with patients" and respecting their rights.

Paternalism and Respect for Patient Autonomy

A question must be raised: Is acting in accordance with the traditional commitment to fostering a patient's well-being always compatible with acting in accordance with the principle of respect for patient autonomy? In one of this chapter's readings, Tom L. Beauchamp and Laurence B. McCullough maintain that the two goals are not always compatible as they develop two models of the physician-patient relationship. The first model, rooted in the Hippocratic tradition, gives centrality to the principle of beneficence, which requires one to help others further their important and legitimate interests, and to abstain from injuring them. In the medical context, the principle of beneficence is sometimes encapsulated in the comment that health-care professionals have an obligation to promote their patients' best interests. Beauchamp and McCullough contrast the beneficence model with the autonomy model, which assigns centrality to the principle of respect for patient autonomy. They maintain that neither model alone can provide a sufficient basis for physicians' responsibilities but that both are necessary to a full-fledged account of physicians' obligations. According to Beauchamp and McCullough, just as the principles of beneficence and respect for autonomy are prima facie principles generating prima facie obligations, so, too, with the models. Each generates prima facie obligations that may conflict—a conflict that Beauchamp and McCullough see as an inescapable dimension of medical practice. Rejecting the view that the obligations generated by the principle of autonomy are always overriding, Beauchamp and McCullough hold that which obligations are overriding in a particular medical context depends on the circumstances of the case. Since to give precedence to the principle of beneficence when it conflicts with the principle of autonomy is to act paternalistically, Beauchamp and McCullough would maintain that medical paternalism is sometimes justified.

As presented in Chapter 1, paternalism is the interference with, limitation of, or usurpation of individual autonomy justified by reasons referring exclusively to the welfare or needs of the person whose autonomy is being interfered with, limited, or usurped. In acting paternalistically, physicians in effect act as if they, and not their patients, are best able to identify what is in their patients' best interests as well as the best means to advance those interests. Veatch, who in this chapter discusses four possible models of the physician-patient relationship, sees the paternalistic (or "priestly") model as incompatible with the values of individual freedom and individual dignity, or, to use the language of Chapter 1, as incompatible with the principle of respect for another's autonomy or right of self-determination. Terrence F. Ackerman, however, argues in this chapter that real respect for patient autonomy may require physicians to engage in paternalistic practices in order to assist patients in regaining some of the autonomy lost because of the constraining effects of illness. While affirming the importance of honesty and respect for patients' rights, Ackerman criticizes the above mentioned "Principles of Medical Ethics," questioning their adequacy as a moral framework designed to guide physician-patient interaction. To understand his concern, it is helpful to discuss two kinds of cases in which the values perceived as fundamental in physician-patient interactions—promotion of a patient's medical well-being and respect for patient autonomy—appear to conflict.

First, a patient's abilities for any effective deliberation may be so severely constrained by illness (e.g., high fever, delirium) that autonomous decisions are virtually impossible and "apparent" decisions may not even be in accordance with the patient's history of decisions and values. In such cases, the promotion of a patient's well-being may require acting against his or her expressed wishes. This would appear to violate the principle of respect for autonomy. But the conflict between the two values may not be real. If the patient's autonomy as effective deliberation is so severely diminished and the desires expressed are also inconsistent with the patient's history and values, the principle of respect for autonomy would not even seem to apply. When there are compelling reasons for believing that a patient's decisions are not autonomous and that as a result the patient cannot exercise the right of self-determination, no paternalistic usurpation of that right is involved when decisions are made for the patient.

Second, the patient and physician may disagree about just what constitutes a patient's well-being. A physician, for example, might insist on continuing aggressive treatment in the case of a cancer patient, even though past treatment has brought no positive results. The patient might have a strong desire to discontinue the therapy advocated by the physician and to let life end without the additional discomforts caused by the therapy. To foster the patients' well-being then, the physician might think it necessary to resort to paternalistic practices intended to circumvent the patient's decision. Here the physician may see a conflict between two obligations—an obligation to promote the patient's well-being, as understood from some objective medical standpoint, and an obligation to respect the patient's right of self-determination. The physician may believe that any chance of prolonging life, no matter how slight, justifies continuing treatment. However, although the beneficence model as Beauchamp and McCullough present it does include the prolongation of life as a good and its premature termination as a harm, the model itself does not commit one to the prolongation of life irrespective of the harms arising to the patient in the process of prolongation. Thus the physician's belief that this life must be prolonged, whatever the discomfort to the patient and no matter how brief the resulting prolongation, may be due to the physician's subjective values rather than to some unquestionably objective medical values. The patient, however, may believe that a few extra days or weeks of uncomfortable in-hospital life, with an infinitely small chance of prolonging life further, are not worth the price. If the patient's decision is the result of reflection and in keeping with the patient's history of decisions and values, respect for autonomy would seem to require the physician to act in accordance with the *patient's* perception of his or her well-being. If the patient's decision is not in accordance with the patient's history of decisions and values but *is* the result of a careful reflective reevaluation of those values, respect for autonomy would again seem to require the physician to act in accordance with the patient's choices. The conflict here is not between an obligation to respect autonomy and an obligation to promote a patient's well-being but between two different conceptions of "well-being." The physician is not faced with having to choose to violate either the principle of respect for a patient's autonomy or the obligation to promote the patient's well-being; rather, he or she is faced with having to accept the patient's conception of what constitutes the patient's well-being and acting accordingly. The problem arises because whether something promotes an individual's well-being is to some extent a subjective judgment. That this is as true in health-care as in other areas of human life is emphasized by the President's Commission for the Study of Ethical Problems in Medicine and Biomedical and Behavioral Research in one of the readings in this chapter. The Commission notes that frequently when health-care decisions are made that are intended to promote a patient's well-being, no objective medical criteria necessitate one particular decision.

The problematic cases that concern Ackerman arise because of the constraining effects illness has on autonomy. In relation to the first kind of case, for example, it is sometimes difficult to judge whether a patient's capacity for effective deliberation is sufficiently undermined by illness so that the question of an infringement of the right of self-determination does not arise. In the face of such uncertainty, does the physician's obligation to promote the patient's well-being entail an obligation to act so as to "restore the patient's autonomy" to the greatest extent possible, given the nature of the patient's illness, even if this involves some measure of paternalism? Ackerman holds that the physician's obligation is to act to restore autonomy. He gives examples intended to show how psychological states, such as depression, or social factors, such as family influence, can constrain a patient's decision making. Ackerman argues that physicians' obligations include the obligation to act in ways that will offset the effects of these constraints in order to make the patient more autonomous. It is not clear that all of Ackerman's examples involve paternalism, since they do not all involve the usurpation of patients' decision making. However, physicians who act as Ackerman recommends run the danger exemplified by the second kind of case when they fail to see that a disagreement with a patient about some course of treatment may not be due to the constraining effects of illness on autonomy but to a disagreement about values.

Truth-Telling

As noted above, traditional codes of medical ethics have little to say about deception, lying, or truth-telling. Yet some of the most widely disputed issues in biomedical ethics center on the physician's obligation to be truthful with the patient and on the patient's right to know the truth. Until recently, it was not unusual for physicians to lie to seriously ill patients about their illnesses for paternalistic reasons. Nor was it unusual for physicians to prescribe alternating injections of sterilized water with injections of pain-killing drugs for patients who were told that all the injections contained some opiate. In the first kind of case, physicians often argued that patients did not want to know the truth or that the truth would harm the patient. In the second kind of case, they often argued that the deceptive practices were justified because water does have a psychotherapeutic effect and yet is much less dangerous to the patient than too-frequent injections of opiates. This latter view is succinctly expressed in a letter written to *The Lancet*:

> Whenever pain can be relieved with a ml of saline, why should we inject an opiate? Do anxieties or discomforts that are allayed with starch capsules require administration of a barbiturate, diazepam, or propoxyphene?[2]

In one of the readings in this chapter, Mack Lipkin defends paternalistically motivated deception and withholding of information. Is Lipkin correct? Are physicians ever morally justified in such lies and deceptive practices? If yes, under what conditions are their lies and deceptions justified?

One way to approach these questions is to begin with the more general questions: Is it always morally wrong to lie? Is it always morally correct to tell the truth? In answering these questions, of course, we must give reasons to justify the position taken. If it is *always* wrong to lie or to intentionally deceive others, then it is wrong for anyone, including physicians, to do so. If lies and intentional deception are *sometimes* morally acceptable, then it is necessary to specify the conditions that make them acceptable. Once these conditions are determined, we can then explore the particular physician-patient situation to see if it satisfies them.

Rule-utilitarians, for example, faced with deciding under what conditions, if any, lies and intentionally deceptive practices are justified, would have to consider the possible consequences of adopting and following a particular rule. In the medical context, for example, they would ask, "What would be the effect on the physician-patient relationship if physicians followed the rule, 'Lie to your patients whenever you believe that doing so is in the patient's best interests'?" In weighing the potential consequences of following such a rule, they would have to take account of the erosive effect that following it would have on patients' trust in the veracity of physicians.

How would the rule-utilitarian respond to a physician who argued as follows: Physicians ought to lie to patients because (1) most patients do not want to know the truth, and (2) the truth can be harmful to patients. Thus moral rules that forbid lying to patients are not in keeping with the Principle of Utility. First the utilitarian would have to examine the two factual claims underpinning this view, a task carried out by Sissela Bok in this chapter. Bok argues that (1) many patients do want to know the truth, and (2) physicians tend to overestimate the possible harmful consequences of telling patients the truth and to underestimate the possible good ones. The rule-utilitarian who agreed with Bok's analysis would still be faced with determining whether exceptions should be built into a rule prohibiting lying to patients. These exceptions would be designed to cover cases where there is very strong evidence to show that a patient does not want to know or would be seriously harmed by knowing. The rule-utilitarian would then have to determine whether the harm done to these patients would be outweighed by the balance of good consequences generated by adopting and following a rule that prohibits all lying in the physician-patient relationship.

Deontologists, of course, take a different approach. Immanuel Kant, whose deontological position is discussed in Chapter 1, is usually read as defending an "absolutist" position: All lies, including those done out of altruistic motives, are wrong. Not all deontologists agree with this absolutist position. As noted in Chapter 1, W. D. Ross maintains, for example, that there is a prima facie obligation not to lie or intentionally deceive but that this obligation can sometimes be overridden by some other prima facie obligation. In the physician-patient relationship, the overriding obligation might sometimes be the physician's obligation to promote the patient's medical well-being. Contrary to Ross, Joseph S. Ellin, in this chapter, takes an absolutist position in his prohibition of all lying in the physician-patient relationship. Ellin argues that it is always wrong for the physician to lie to patients but that the physician does not have even a prima facie obligation not to deceive. He bases his argument on his conception of the physician-patient relationship, seeing it as a fiduciary relationship. A "fiduciary relationship" is one of trust, often between unequals, where one party (e.g., the physician) is committed to promoting the well-being of the dependent party (e.g., the patient). Since trust is an essential element in a fiduciary relationship and lying seriously undermines trust, all lying is morally unacceptable. But, Ellin argues, this is not true of deceptive practices such as the use of placebos. In the medical context, deceptive practices may be simply one tool used by physicians to achieve the aims of the fiduciary relationship.

Informed Consent

Discussions about truth-telling and lying in medical ethics frequently arise in conjunction with discussions of the requirement of informed consent. It is now widely accepted that both law and morality require that no medical interventions be performed on competent adults without their informed and voluntary consent. But lying to patients or even withholding information from them can seriously undermine their ability to make informed decisions and, therefore, to give informed consent. In order to be able to give such consent, and thereby to exercise their right of self-determination, patients must have access to the necessary relevant information, and physicians are usually the only ones in a position to supply it. Judge Spotswood W. Robinson III affirms this point in a judicial opinion reprinted in this chapter, when he argues that physicians have a duty to "satisfy the vital informational needs of the patient."

The informed consent requirement is a relatively recent addition to the ethical constraints governing the physician-patient relationship. Traditional codes of medical ethics have nothing to say about any physician obligation to inform patients about the risks and benefits of alternative diagnostic and treatment techniques. The doctrine of informed consent was first introduced into case law in 1956. Since then, however, it has received a great deal of attention in biomedical ethics as both a legal and an ethical requirement. In 1982, for example, Congress assigned the task of determining the ethical and legal implications of the informed consent requirement to the aforementioned President's Commission. In its report, the Commission describes ethically valid consent "as an ethical obligation that involves a process of shared decisionmaking based upon the mutual respect and participation [of patients and health professionals]"[3] and identifies two values as providing the ethical foundation of the requirement: respect for the patient's autonomy, or the right of self-determination, and the promotion of the patient's well-being.

Much of the literature on informed consent focuses on several difficulties that affect the application of the requirement: (1) Who is *competent* to give consent? (2) When is consent *informed* consent? That is, how much information must a patient receive and understand before his or her consent is informed rather than partially informed or uninformed? (3) When is consent *voluntary* consent? Each of these questions will be briefly examined in order to show some of the difficulties that affect the application of the requirement. It is important to note that the problems here are both conceptual and empirical. The meaning of the concepts "informed," "competent," and "voluntary" must be explicated so that it can be determined just what counts as voluntary and informed consent. Then in a particular case, it must be determined whether the individual in question is capable of giving voluntary and informed consent.

(1) Who is competent to give consent? The patient who is sick enough to be in a hospital or institution may not be functioning normally enough to be a rational decision maker. Patients who are under great emotional stress, who are frightened or in severe pain, are often considered to be less than competent decision makers. In a burn center in California, for example, the following procedure is used when a patient with burns over 60 percent of his or her body is admitted. During the first two hours after the patient is severely burned there is no pain since the nerve endings are anesthetized. Patients during this time are given a choice. They can opt either to start a course of treatment, which will be prolonged and excruciatingly painful but may save their lives, or to simply receive pain-killing medication and care until they die. Can a patient in such circumstances, even if free from pain, be considered rational enough to weigh these alternatives? Recent work on the topic of competency stresses that it is not "all or nothing." The Commission's report, for example, maintains that individuals should be judged to be incapable of decision making only when they lack the ability to make decisions that promote their well-being in keeping with their own previously expressed values and preferences. James Drane in this chapter suggests a sliding-scale model for competency; different standards of competence apply depending on the kinds of medical decisions being made.

(2) How much information must patients be given before their consent is informed? Suppose a patient suffering from breast cancer agrees to have a radical mastectomy. She is not told that studies indicate that this radical surgery is no more effective than much less radical surgery. Has the patient been given sufficient information to guarantee that her decision is a fully informed one? What criteria must the physician use in determining when sufficient information has been given? Is more information better than less? Studies have shown that patients receiving long, detailed explanations of the risks and purposes of a procedure may comprehend and retain very little of the significant information. In contrast, those who are given less detailed information may be able to comprehend and retain more of the important facts.[4] It is sometimes argued that lay persons, unlike medical professionals, cannot understand enough about the procedures, the risks, and other factors to ever give fully informed consent. In many cases, it is asserted, the most that can be hoped for is that the patient will *assent* to the procedure. (A parallel point is developed in the context of experimentation in Chapter 4 by Franz J. Ingelfinger.) An additional complication here is that physicians often make their own decisions in conditions of uncertainty. They cannot give patients information that they themselves do not possess.

(3) When is consent really voluntary? It is often argued that it is very easy to manipulate even highly competent patients into giving consent when the request is made by someone in a position of authority. For example, it has been shown that physicians, whose patients sometimes see them as "god" figures, and psychiatrists, whose judgments patients trust, find it very easy to get the consent they request. When patients are influenced in this way, is their consent sufficiently voluntary?

Recent work on informed consent, such as that of the President's Commission, stresses the importance of the process of communication and of the patient's cognitive-information processing. Studies have been undertaken to both understand and improve the procedures used to get "informed consent."[5] If the goal is informed consent, it seems insufficient to simply hand over information to patients via a form or a short conversation listing possible risks and alternatives; rather, it is necessary to determine how much the patient has understood and, perhaps, even some of the other factors that may be affecting the patient's decision, such as concern about a physician's reaction to a refusal. Take the example of a terminally ill, diabetic, cancer-ridden patient who, after repeatedly rejecting amputation of his gangrenous left foot, suddenly assented. His consent appeared to be both voluntary and informed. However, given his past history and the staff's knowledge of his values, a decision was made to call in an ethical counselor to determine the reasons for the patient's change of mind. After a long conversation with the patient, the counselor learned that the patient had consented to the amputation only because he erroneously believed that without his consent the physician and the hospital would refuse to continue their care. Once he understood that his belief was incorrect, he withdrew his assent to the amputation. The staff members' knowledge of this patient's character and values as well as their concern that the consent be truly informed and voluntary may not be the norm, but this case illustrates that informed consent requires something more than forms and cursory rituals. It also shows the need for medical professionals to better understand the communication processes they use to achieve informed consent.

In one of this chapter's readings, Charles W. Lidz, Paul S. Appelbaum, and Alan Meisel present two models of informed consent. The first, called the "event model," sees the obtainment of informed consent as an event that occurs at a single point in time. The second, called the "process model," stresses the ongoing nature of the communication process taking place between physicians and patients and the need to integrate the information required by patients into an ongoing exchange. On the process model, the obtainment of informed consent is not a single event but a continuous part of the treatment process.

Some Other Issues Regarding Physicians' Obligations

Do physicians have an obligation, stemming from their professional roles, to provide health care even when doing so puts them at risk? For example, do physicians have an obligation to take care of individuals who either have AIDS or who are infected with the human immunodeficiency virus (HIV)? The latter, while not exhibiting symptoms of AIDS, nevertheless can transmit the virus. In two of this chapter's readings, Edmund D. Pellegrino and John D. Arras address both the general question of physicians' obligations to provide care even when doing so puts them at personal risk and questions dealing specifically with physicians' obligations toward those with AIDS or those who are infected with HIV. In the concluding reading in this chapter, Pellegrino together with David C. Thomasma addresses another troubling question regarding conflicts of interest: What should physicians do when serving their patients' interests conflicts with their own self-interest or the interests of the institutions (e.g., hospitals) with which they are associated?

J.S.Z.

NOTES

1 American Medical Association, "Principles of Medical Ethics," *Journal of the American Medical Association*, vol. 164, no. 10 (July 6, 1957), p. 1119.

2 J. Sice, "Letter to the Editor," *The Lancet* 2 (1972), p. 651.

3 President's Commission for the Study of Ethical Problems in Medicine and Biomedical and Behavioral Research, *Making Health Care Decisions*, vol. 1, p. 2.

4 On this point, see Ralph J. Alfidi, "Controversy, Alternatives, and Decisions in Complying with the Legal Doctrine of Informed Consent," *Radiology* 114 (January 1975), pp. 231–234.

5 Barrie R. Cassileth, et al., "Informed Consent—Why Are Its Goals Imperfectly Realized?" *New England Journal of Medicine* 302 (1980), pp. 896–900; and T. M. Grundner, "On the Readability of Surgical Consent Forms," *ibid.*, pp. 900–902.

Medical Codes of Ethics

The Hippocratic Oath

Little is known about the life of Hippocrates, a Greek physician born about 460 B.C. We know that he was a widely sought, well-known, and influential healer who is said to have lived 85, 90, 104, or 109 years. A collection of documents known as the *Hippocratic Writings* (largely written from the fifth to the fourth century, B.C.) is believed to represent the remains of the Hippocratic school of medicine. Some of the works in this collection are credited to Hippocrates. The oath reprinted here, however, is believed to have been written by a philosophical sect known as the Pythagoreans in the latter part of the fourth century, B.C.

For the Middle Ages and later centuries, the Hippocratic Oath embodied the highest aspirations of the physician. It sets forth two sets of duties: (1) duties to the patient and (2) duties to the other members of the guild (profession) of medicine. In regard to the patient, it includes a set of absolute prohibitions (e.g., against abortion and euthanasia) as well as a statement of the physician's obligation to help and not to harm the patient.

I swear by Apollo Physician and Asclepius and Hygieia and Panaceia and all the gods and goddesses, making them my witnesses, that I will fulfil according to my ability and judgment this oath and this covenant:

To hold him who has taught me this art as equal to my parents and to live my life in partnership with him, and if he is in need of money to give him a share of mine, and to regard his offspring as equal to my brothers in male lineage and to teach them this art—if they desire to learn it—without fee and covenant; to give a share of precepts and oral instruction and all the other learning to my sons and to the sons of him who has instructed me and to pupils who have signed the covenant and have taken an oath according to the medical law, but to no one else.

I will apply dietetic measures for the benefit of the sick according to my ability and judgment; I will keep them from harm and injustice.

I will neither give a deadly drug to anybody if asked for it, nor will I make a suggestion to this effect. Similarly I will not give to a woman an abortive remedy. In purity and holiness I will guard my life and my art.

I will not use the knife, not even on sufferers from stone, but will withdraw in favor of such men as are engaged in this work.

Whatever houses I may visit, I will come for the benefit of the sick, remaining free of all intentional injustice, of all mischief and in particular of sexual relations with both female and male persons, be they free or slaves.

What I may see or hear in the course of the treatment or even outside of the treatment in regard to the life of men, which on no account one must spread abroad, I will keep to myself holding such things shameful to be spoken about.

If I fulfill this oath and do not violate it, may it be granted to me to enjoy life and art, being honored with fame among all men for all time to come; if I transgress it and swear falsely, may the opposite of all this be my lot.

Principles of Medical Ethics (1980)
American Medical Association

This 1980 version of the ethical code of the American Medical Association states the standards that should guide physicians in their relationships with (1) patients, (2) colleagues, (3) members of allied health professions, and (4) society. Unlike the Hippocratic Oath, it does not expressly assert the physician's obligation to help patients and keep them from harm. Rather, it asserts that a physician "shall be dedicated to providing competent medical service with compassion and respect for human dignity." Unlike earlier codes it explicitly calls for both honesty in dealing with patients and colleagues and respect for patients' rights.

PREAMBLE

The medical profession has long subscribed to a body of ethical statements developed primarily for the benefit of the patient. As a member of this profession, a physician must recognize responsibility not only to patients, but also to society, to other health professionals, and to self. The following Principles adopted by the American Medical Association are not laws, but standards of conduct which define the essentials of honorable behavior for the physician.

PRINCIPLES

I. A physician shall be dedicated to providing competent medical service with compassion and respect for human dignity.

II. A physician shall deal honestly with patients and colleagues, and strive to expose those physicians deficient in character or competence, or who engage in fraud or deception.

Reprinted with permission of the publisher from *American Medical News*, August 1/8, 1980, p. 9.

III. A physician shall respect the law and also recognize a responsibility to seek changes in those requirements which are contrary to the best interests of the patient.

IV. A physician shall respect the rights of patients, of colleagues, and of other health professionals, and shall safeguard patient confidences within the constraints of the law.

V. A physician shall continue to study, apply and advance scientific knowledge, make relevant information available to patients, colleagues, and the public, obtain consultation, and use the talents of other health professionals when indicated.

VI. A physician shall, in the provision of appropriate patient care, except in emergencies, be free to choose whom to serve, with whom to associate, and the environment in which to provide medical services.

VII. A physician shall recognize a responsibility to participate in activities contributing to an improved community.

Models for Ethical Medicine in a Revolutionary Age
Robert M. Veatch

Robert M. Veatch is director of the Kennedy Institute of Ethics, Georgetown University, and adjunct professor at Georgetown Medical School. He has a Ph.D. in medical ethics as well as an M.S. in pharmacology. Veatch's edited books include *Medical Ethics* (1989) and *Cross Cultural Perspectives in Medical Ethics: Readings* (1989). He is the author of numerous books including *A Theory of Medical Ethics* (1981), *The Foundations of Justice: Why the Retarded and the Rest of Us Have Claims to Equality* (1986), and *The Patient as Partner: A Theory of Human-Experimentation Ethics* (1987).

Veatch presents four possible models for the moral relationship between the physician and the patient: (1) *The Engineering Model*: The physician is an applied scientist who presents the facts to the lay person but leaves all the decisions to the latter; (2) *The Priestly Model*: The physician, guided by the principle "Benefit and do no harm," plays a paternalistic role in relation to the patient; (3) *The Collegial Model*: The physician and lay person are seen as equal colleagues sharing common interests and striving for a common goal; and (4) *The Contractual Model*: The physician and lay person are not perceived as equals but as having some mutual interests and sharing ethical authority and responsibility. Veatch draws out the ethical implications of these different models.

Most of the ethical problems in the practice of medicine come up in cases where the medical condition or desired procedure itself presents no moral problem. Most day-to-day patient contacts are just not cases which are ethically exotic. For the woman who spends five hours in the clinic waiting room with two screaming children waiting to be seen for the flu, the flu is not a special moral problem; her wait is. When medical students practice drawing blood from clinic patients in the cardiac care unit—when teaching material is treated as material—the moral problem is not really related to the patient's heart in the way it might be in a more exotic heart transplant. Many more blood samples are drawn, however, than hearts transplanted. It is only by moving beyond the specific issues to more basic underlying ethical themes that the real ethical problems in medicine can be dealt with.

Most fundamental of the underlying themes of the new medical ethics is that health care must be a human right, no longer a privilege limited to those who can afford it. It has not always been that way, and, of course, is not

Reprinted with permission of the author and the publisher from *Hastings Center Report*, vol. 2 (June 1972), pp. 5–7.

anything near that in practice today. But the norm, the moral claim, is becoming increasingly recognized. Both of the twin revolutions have made their contribution to this change. Until this century health care could be treated as a luxury, no matter how offensive this might be now. The amount of real healing that went on was minimal anyway. But now, with the biological revolution, health care really is essential to "life, liberty, and the pursuit of happiness." And health care is a right for everyone because of the social revolution which is really a revolution in our conception of justice. If the obscure phrase "all men are created equal" means anything in the medical context where biologically it is clear that they are not equal, it means that they are equal in the legitimacy of their moral claim. They must be treated equally in what is essential to their humanity: dignity, freedom, individuality. The sign in front of the prestigious, modern hospital, "Methadone patients use side door," is morally offensive even if it means nothing more than that the Methadone Unit is located near that door. It is strikingly similar to "Coloreds to the back of the bus." With this affirmation of the right to health care, what are the models of professional-lay relationships which permit this and other basic ethical themes to be conveyed?

1 *The Engineering Model* One of the impacts of the biological revolution is to make the physician scientific. All too often he behaves like an applied scientist. The rhetoric of the scientific tradition in the modern world is that the scientist must be "pure." He must be factual, divorcing himself from all considerations of value. It has taken atomic bombs and Nazi medical research to let us see the foolishness and danger of such a stance. In the first place the scientist, and certainly the applied scientist, just cannot logically be value-free. Choices must be made daily—in research design, in significance levels of statistical tests, and in perception of the "significant" observations from an infinite perceptual field, and each of these choices requires a frame of values on which it is based. Even more so in an applied science like medicine choices based upon what is "significant," what is "valuable," must be made constantly. The physician who thinks he can just present all the facts and let the patient make the choices is fooling himself even if it is morally sound and responsible to do this at all the critical points where decisive choices are to be made. Furthermore, even if the physician logically could eliminate all ethical and other value considerations from his decision-making and even if he could in practice conform to the impossible value-free ideal, it would be morally outrageous for him to do so. It would make him an engineer, a plumber making repairs, connecting tubes and flushing out clogged systems, with no questions asked. Even though I strongly favor abortion reform, I am deeply troubled by a physician who really believes abortion is murder *in the full sense* if he agrees to either perform one or refer to another physician. Hopefully no physician would do so when confronted with a request for technical advice about murdering a post-natal human.

2 *The Priestly Model* In proper moral revulsion to the model which makes the physician into a plumber for whom his own ethical judgments are completely excluded, some move to the opposite extreme, making the physician a new priest. Establishment sociologist of medicine Robert N. Wilson describes the physician-patient relationship as religious. "The doctor's office or the hospital room, for example," he says, "have somewhat the aura of a sanctuary,... the patient must view his doctor in a manner far removed from the prosaic and the mundane."

The priestly model leads to what I call the "As-a syndrome." The symptoms are verbal, but the disease is moral. The chief diagnostic sign is the phrase "speaking-as-a...." In counseling a pregnant woman who has taken Thalidomide, a physician says, "The odds are against a normal baby and 'speaking-as-a-physician' that is a risk you shouldn't take." One must ask what it is about medical training that lets this be said "as-a-physician" rather than as a friend or as a moral man or as a priest. The problem is one of generalization of expertise: transferring of expertise in the technical aspects of a subject to expertise in moral advice.

The main ethical principle which summarizes this priestly tradition is "Benefit and do no harm to the patient." Now attacking the principle of doing no harm to the patient is a bit like attacking fatherhood. (Motherhood has not dominated the profession in the Western tradition.) But Fatherhood has long been an alternative symbol for the priestly model; "Father" has traditionally been a personalistic metaphor for God and for the priest. Likewise, the classical medical sociology literature (the same literature using the religious images) always uses the parent-child image as an analogy for the physician-patient relationship. It is this paternalism in the realm of values which is represented in the moral slogan "Benefit and do no harm to the patient." It takes the locus of decision-making away from the patient and places it in the hands of the professional. In doing so it destroys or at least minimizes the other moral themes essential to a more balanced ethical system. While a professional group may affirm this principle as adequate for a professional ethic, it is clear that society, more generally, has a much broader set of ethical norms. If the professional group is affirming one norm while society affirms another for the same circumstances, then the physician is placed in the uncomfortable position of having to decide whether his loyalty is to the norms of his professional group or to those of the broader society. What would this larger set of norms include?

a *Producing Good and Not Harm* Outside of the narrowest Kantian tradition, no one excludes the moral duty of producing good and avoiding harm entirely. Let this be said from the start. Some separate producing good and avoiding evil into two different principles placing greater moral weight on the latter, but this is also true within the tradition of professional medical ethics. The real difference is that in a set of ethical norms used more universally in the broader society producing good and avoiding harm is set in a much broader context and becomes just one of a much larger set of moral obligations.

b *Protecting Individual Freedom* Personal freedom is a fundamental value in society. It is essential to being truly human. Individual freedom for both physician and patient must be protected even if it looks like some harm is going to be done in the process. This is why legally competent patients are permitted by society to refuse blood transfusions or other types of medical care even when to the vast majority of us the price seems to be one of great harm. Authority about what constitutes harm and what constitutes good (as opposed to procedures required to obtain a particular predetermined good or harm) cannot be vested in any one particular group of individuals. To do so would be to make the error of generalizing expertise.

c *Preserving Individual Dignity* Equality of moral significance of all persons means that each is given fundamental dignity. Individual freedom of choice and control over one's own life and body contribute to that dignity. We might say that this more universal, societal ethic of freedom and dignity is one which moves beyond B. F. Skinner.

Many of the steps in the hospitalization, care, and maintenance of the patient, particularly seriously ill patients, are currently an assault on that dignity. The emaciated, senile man connected to life by IV tubes, tracheotomy, and colostomy has difficulty retaining his sense of dignity. Small wonder that many prefer to return to their own homes to die. It is there on their own turf that they have a sense of power and dignity.

d *Truth-Telling and Promise-Keeping* As traditional as they sound, the ethical obligations of truth-telling and promise-keeping have retained their place in ethics because they are seen as essential to the quality of human relationships. It is disturbing to see these fundamental elements of human interaction compromised, minimized, and even eliminated supposedly in order to keep from harming the patient. This is a much broader problem than the issue of what to tell the terminal carcinoma patient or the patient for whom there has been an unanticipated discovery of an XYY chromosome pattern when doing an amniocentesis for mongol-

ism. It arises when the young boy getting his measles shot is told "Now this won't hurt a bit" and when a medical student is introduced on the hospital floor as "Doctor." And these all may be defended as ways of keeping from harming the patient. It is clear that in each case, also, especially if one takes into account the long-range threat to trust and confidence, that in the long run these violations of truth-telling and promise-keeping may do more harm than good. Both the young boy getting the shot and the medical student are being taught what to expect from the medical profession in the future. But even if that were not the case, each is an assault on patient dignity and freedom and humanity. Such actions may be justifiable sometimes, but the case must be awfully strong.

e *Maintaining and Restoring Justice* Another way in which the ethical norms of the broader society move beyond concern for helping and not harming the patient is by insisting on a fair distribution of health services. What we have been calling the social revolution, as prefigurative as it may be, has heightened our concern for equality in the distribution of basic health services. If health care is a right then it is a right for all. It is not enough to produce individual cases of good health or even the best aggregate health statistics. Even if the United States had the best health statistics in the world (which it does not have), if this were attained at the expense of inferior health care for certain groups within the society it would be ethically unacceptable.

At this point in history with our current record of discriminatory delivery of health services there is a special concern for restoring justice. Justice must also be compensatory. The health of those who have been discriminated against must be maintained and restored as a special priority.

3 *The Collegial Model* With the engineering model the physician becomes a plumber without any moral integrity. With the priestly model his moral authority so dominates the patient that the patient's freedom and dignity are extinguished. In the effort to develop a more proper balance which would permit the other fundamental values and obligations to be preserved, some have suggested that the physician and the patient should see themselves as colleagues pursuing the common goal of eliminating the illness and preserving the health of the patient. The physician is the patient's "pal." It is in the collegial model that the themes of trust and confidence play the most crucial role. When two individuals or groups are truly committed to common goals then trust and confidence are justified and the collegial model is appropriate. It is a very pleasant, harmonious way to interact with one's fellow human beings. There is an equality of dignity and respect, an equality of value contributions, lacking in the earlier models.

But social realism makes us ask the embarrassing question. Is there, in fact, any real basis for the assumption of mutual loyalty and goals, of common interest which would permit the unregulated community of colleagues model to apply to the physician-patient relationship?

There is some proleptic sign of a community of real common interests in some elements of the radical health movement and free clinics, but for the most part we have to admit that ethnic, class, economic, and value differences make the assumption of common interest which is necessary for the collegial model to function a mere pipedream. What is needed is a more provisional model which permits equality in the realm of moral significance between patient and physician without making the utopian assumption of collegiality.

4 *The Contractual Model* The model of social relationship which fits these conditions is that of the contract or covenant. The notion of contract should not be loaded with legalistic implications, but taken in its more symbolic form as in the traditional religious or marriage "contract" or "covenant." Here two individuals or groups are interacting in a way where there are obligations and expected benefits for both parties. The obligations and benefits are limited in scope, though, even if they are expressed in somewhat vague terms. The basic norms of freedom, dignity, truth-telling, promise-keeping, and justice are essential to a contractual relationship. The premise is trust and confidence even though it is recognized that there is not a full mutuality of interests. Social sanctions institutionalize and stand behind the relationship, in case there is a violation of the contract, but for the most part the assumption is that there will be a faithful fulfillment of the obligations.

Only in the contractual model can there be a true sharing of ethical authority and responsibility. This avoids the moral abdication on the part of the physi-cian in the engineering model and the moral abdication on the part of the patient in the priestly model. It also avoids the uncontrolled and false sense of equality in the collegial model. With the contractual relationship there is a sharing in which the physician recognizes that the patient must maintain freedom of control over his own life and destiny when significant choices are to be made. Should the physician not be able to live with his conscience under those terms the contract is not made or is broken. This means that there will have to be relatively greater open discussion of the moral premises hiding in medical decisions before and as they are made.

With the contractual model there is a sharing in which the patient has legitimate grounds for trusting that once the basic value framework for medical decision-making is established on the basis of the patient's own values, the myriads of minute medical decisions which must be made day in and day out in the care of the patient will be made by the physician within that frame of reference.

In the contractual model, then, there is a real sharing of decision-making in a way that there is realistic assurance that both patient and physician will retain their moral integrity. In this contractual context patient control of decision-making on the individual level is assured without the necessity of insisting that the patient participate in every trivial decision. On the social level community control of health care is made possible in the same way. The lay community is given and should be given the status of contractor. The locus of decision-making is thus in the lay community, but the day-to-day medical decisions can, with trust and confidence, rest with the medical community. If trust and confidence are broken the contract is broken.

Medical ethics in the midst of the biological and social revolutions is dealing with a great number of new and difficult ethical cases: in vitro fertilization, psychosurgery, happiness pills, brain death, and the military use of medical technology. But the real day-to-day ethical crises may not be nearly so exotic. Whether the issue is in an exotic context or one which is nothing more complicated medically than a routine physical exam, the ethos of ethical responsibility established by the appropriate selection of a model for the moral relationship between the professional and the lay communities will be decisive. This is the real framework for medical ethics in a revolutionary age.

Two Models of Moral Responsibility in Medicine
Tom L. Beauchamp and Laurence B. McCullough

Tom L. Beauchamp is professor of philosophy at Georgetown University, specializing in ethics, bioethics, and applied philosophy. He is also senior research scholar at the Center for Bioethics of the Kennedy Institute of Ethics at Georgetown. Widely published, Beauchamp is the author of *Philosophical Ethics* (1982) as well as the coauthor of *A History and Theory of Informed Consent* (1986) and *Principles of Biomedical Ethics* (3d ed., 1989). Laurence B. McCullough is professor of medicine and community medicine and is affiliated with the Center for Ethics, Medicine, and Public Issues at Baylor College of Medicine. He is the coauthor of *Health Care: Its Psychosocial Dimensions* (1981) and "Respect for Autonomy and Medical Paternalism Reconsidered." Beauchamp and McCullough are coauthors of *Medical Ethics: The Moral Responsibilities of Physicians*, from which this selection is excerpted.

Beauchamp and McCullough explore two models of physician moral responsibility. The *beneficence model* gives primacy to the principle of beneficence, whereas the *autonomy model* gives primacy to the principle of respect for autonomy. Beauchamp and McCullough bring out some of the historical and philosophical sources of each model and identify four interconnected elements in each. On their analysis, each model includes (1) a conception of the general moral end of medicine (in each case the end is the same—the promotion of the patient's best interests); (2) a fundamental moral principle that provides the perspective from which the patient's best interests will be perceived; (3) a set of obligations (or duties) deriving from this principle; and (4) a set of virtues deriving from this principle. Beauchamp and McCullough conclude by claiming that the conflict generated by the two models is an inescapable dimension of medical practice.

In this [article] we examine two broad models of moral responsibility that...share a common origin in the moral purpose of promoting the best interests of the patient. Each model is developed in terms of two fundamental perspectives from which those interests can be interpreted.

The first model understands the patient's best interests exclusively from the perspective of medicine. By medicine we mean the repository of tested knowledge, skills, and experience constituting the science and art of the cure, alleviation, and prevention of disease and injury. Medicine in this sense establishes the main sources for discovering and corroborating hypotheses about health and disease, which, in turn, form the basis for diagnosis, treatment, and prognosis. So understood, medicine provides what we designate an *objective* perspective on the patient's best interests. "Objective" means sim-

ply that the perspective transcends the particular and sometimes idiosyncratic beliefs or approach of the individual physician. The goals of the medical enterprise, as well as the duties and virtues of the physician, are expressed in terms of both goods that should be sought on behalf of patients and harms to be avoided. Because the principle of beneficence expresses the moral significance of seeking the greater balance of good over harm for another, we call this the *beneficence model* of moral responsibility in medicine.

The second model interprets the best interests of the patient exclusively from the perspective of the patient, as he or she understands them. This perspective may sometimes be starkly different from that of medicine. The physician's respect for the patient's values and beliefs is the source of the duties and virtues appropriate to the second model. Because the principle of respect for autonomy expresses the moral significance of respecting another's values and beliefs, we call this the *autonomy model* of moral responsibility in medicine.

Models based in the utterly different commitments of the principles of beneficence and autonomy might at first glance seem to be in hopeless opposition, forcing the physician to choose one to the exclusion of the other. On closer examination this conclusion proves to be unwarranted. Each model is best viewed as capturing a valid but *partial* perspective on the responsibilities of physicians. Just as a theory of the moral life would be impoverished if it contained but a single principle, such as beneficence or respect for autonomy, so would a theory of the moral responsibilities of physicians be impoverished if but one model were accepted as the exclusive authority.[1] Medicine is enhanced and dignified by both, although, like moral principles, the two models can come into frustrating conflict.

We use the language of *models* (rather than *principles*) to convey the idea of a complex pattern that shows the arrangement of its parts—like, for example, an architect's model. The verb "to model" can also mean "to give shape to" and "to make a tool of." In developing these models we are giving shape to what is only inchoate and unsystematically formed in medical practice, as well as in the history of medical ethics. We are simultaneously forming a tool useful in clinical practice. A mere abstract theoretical model would scarcely serve our practical objectives.[2]

Each model embraces four interconnected elements:

1. The general *moral end* of medicine: to promote the patient's best interests;

2. A *principle* that provides the moral significance of distinct perspectives on the patient's best interests;

3. *Obligations* (or duties) that derive from this principle; and

4. *Virtues* that derive from this principle.

THE BENEFICENCE MODEL

The word "beneficence" is broadly used in English. Its meanings include the doing of good, the active promotion of good, kindness, and charity. However, any principle specifying the duty of beneficence will have a narrower meaning. In its most general form, a broadly formulated principle of beneficence requires that one help others further important and legitimate interests and abstain from injuring them....[3]

The central question for beneficence within the patient-physician relationship is "What does it mean for the physician to seek the greater balance of good over harm in the care of patients?" The beneficence model answers this question in terms of the perspective that medicine takes on the patient's best interests. That perspective gives the principle of beneficence specific clinically oriented meanings that define the goods and harms to be balanced. Because this perspective cannot be adequately understood if torn from its historical roots, we rely on historical writings and practices as a major source for the elements of the beneficence model.

Ancient Sources of the Model

The earliest expression of the beneficence model of moral responsibility in medicine is found in the influential Hippocratic writings,[4] whose distinctive features are influential to the present day.[5] The Hippocratic Oath[6] characterizes medical practitioners as a group of committed men (women were excluded from medicine in Greek society) set apart from and above others in society. Ludwig Edelstein's scholarly studies of the Oath and other Hippocratic writings have shown that this and other peculiar features of the Oath—e.g., its prohibitions against surgery, against the pharmacological inducement of abortion, and against the giving of "deadly drugs"—have their roots in the ancient Greek religious sect known as Pythagoreanism.[7] Influence from the main lines of Greek philosophical ethics seems absent, and the Oath fails to address what we would today consider fundamental ethical issues in the patient-physician relationship. Veracity and informed consent, for example, are nowhere mentioned, and most of the subjects addressed in contemporary medical ethics are not given even passing notice.

Because of its sources in the religious traditions of Pythagoreanism and its lack of a philosophical justification, the Hippocratic Oath is clearly not a philosophical document. Nonetheless, the Oath sets out some of the basic features of the beneficence model. Like oaths in general it is a solemn promise witnessed by others (in the case of ancient Greek physicians, first by a portion and then by the full panoply of the Greek gods and goddesses). By taking the Oath, one becomes committed to a distinctive moral goal or purpose of medicine as the basis of one's medical practice. Unlike descriptive or declarative statements that merely assert something, swearing an oath is a performative utterance: By subscribing to it, one is committed to live in accordance with that purpose and its implications for professional practice.

The preprofessional person is transformed into the professional at least in part by the commitment ritualized in the taking of an oath. An oath, of course, is ceremonial by comparison to the commitment, which has been in formation as the young apprentice grows into the profession—i.e., is trained professionally and comes to understand and live by the obligations and virtues established in the profession.

The moral purpose of medicine appears in a central passage from the Oath: "I will apply dietetic measures to the benefit of the sick according to my ability and judgment; I will keep them from harm and injustice."[8] This statement acknowledges the physician's special knowledge and skills and his or her commitment to principles requiring the use of those skills in order to benefit patients. This, according to the Oath, is the proper moral end of medicine, and commitment to that end makes one a physician.

By itself the Hippocratic Oath is a bare skeleton of the beneficence model of moral responsibility; it sheds scant light on the concepts that define what it means to "benefit the sick," while avoiding "harm and injustice." We must turn to other portions of the Hippocratic writings for a fuller account of the perspective from which acting in the patient's best interests is to be understood. Consider the following passage from *The Art*: "I will define what I conceive medicine to be. In general terms, it is to do away with the sufferings of the sick, to lessen the violence of their diseases, and to refuse to treat those who are overmastered by their diseases, realizing that in such cases medicine is powerless."[9]

Medicine is here conceived to have limited purposes. Its purpose is not, for example, to preserve life above all else—a distinctly modern notion.[10] Medical interventions to limit pain and suffering or to attempt curative therapy must hold out some reasonable prospect for success. This view of medicine keenly appreciates the discipline's limits. It also provides the context for the later remark in the *Epidemics*: "Declare the past, diagnose the present, foretell the future; practice these acts. As to disease, make a habit of two things—*to help, or at least to do no harm*."[11] This text does *not* say "first (or 'above all') do no harm" (*primum non nocere*, to use a later Latin formulation).

The basic roles and concepts that give substance to the principle of beneficence in medicine are as follows: The positive benefit the physician is obligated to seek is the cure of disease and injury if there is a reasonable hope of cure; the harms to be avoided, prevented, or removed are the pain and suffering of injury and disease. In addition, the physician is enjoined from *doing* harm.

This consideration, too, must be included in the beneficence model because physician interventions themselves can inflict unnecessary pain and suffering on patients. The Hippocratic texts hold that inflicting pain and suffering is permissible in those cases in which the physician is attempting to reverse a threat to health—e.g., administering an emetic[12] after the accidental ingestion of a poison. Inflicting such pain and suffering on a patient in order to eliminate a deadly substance from the body is justified because the patient is on balance benefited. When the patient cannot be benefited by further intervention, the inflicted pain and suffering is unnecessary and to be avoided. Thus, in its first formulation in Western medical ethics, the beneficence model of moral responsibility adapts the principle of beneficence to patient care by providing a medically oriented account of how to balance goods over harms.

A number of elements of the beneficence model emerge from ancient Greek medical ethics. First, the model builds its account of the moral responsibilities of the physician in terms of the moral purpose or end of medicine: promoting the patient's best interests as understood from medicine's perspective. Second, on this basis, it provides meanings for the key concepts in the principle of beneficence—"good" and "harm"—that are specific to medicine. In this way, the abstract principle of beneficence is adapted to the medical context. Third, it employs this principle to show that the primary, though prima facie, obligation of the physician is to benefit the patient, with prevention of unnecessary harm serving as the limiting condition....

The Elements of the Model

This model is built on a conception of goods and harms that underlie applications of the principle of beneficence in the model, and our construction of the model must begin with these goods and harms as medicine understands them. We believe that the following list expresses what medicine is to seek and avoid.[13]

Goods	Harms
Health	Illness
Prevention, elimination, or control of disease (morbidity) and injury	Disease (morbidity) and injury
Relief from unnecessary pain and suffering	Unnecessary pain and suffering

Amelioration of handi-	Handicapping condi-
capping conditions	tions
Prolonged life	Premature death

The goods and harms accepted by the beneficence model are rarely discussed in modern medicine as *values*, perhaps because they are such deeply embedded presuppositions in clinical practice and training. Increasingly, however, physicians are becoming aware of how these basic values, and many judgments derived from them, shape clinical decisionmaking. Even in highly quantified clinical decisionmaking, value judgments may be at work. Subtle tradeoffs, for example, between different levels of medically induced (iatrogenic) morbidity may be under constant evaluation.[14] Some specific examples will illustrate how such reasoning plays a role in medicine.

Consider the prophylactic use of drugs to reduce the risk of coronary and cerebrovascular disease in individuals at risk for such disease. Dr. Michael Oliver has argued that for patients who are otherwise healthy, a balance must be struck between maintaining health and risking illness caused by the use of these drugs. He calls for a change in current practice by limiting the use of prophylactic treatment to only those cases where there is good evidence, and not mere supposition, to believe that the benefits outweigh the risks.[15]

Drs. James Reuler and Donald Girard have identified how considerations about pain and its relief should figure in the primary physician's management of elderly patients with cancer.[16] They first distinguish benign forms of chronic pain in patients without cancer and argue that addicting drugs, with the morbidity and suffering they cause, should not be used for such pain. The presence of cancer in an elderly patient, however, leads them to change their balancing of these goods and harms. In these cases, the physician should be concerned not only about the relief of pain but about the patient's anxiety that medication will not be administered unless or until the pain renews its onslaught. Such anxiety can be a significant form of suffering for such patients. Hence, they argue that pain medications, including those with addictive potential, should be administered to cancer patients as required....

In addressing the surgical management of deformities of the lower extremities of patients with cerebral palsy, Dr. Robert Samilson argues that the general goal of such surgical treatment is increased function.[17] At the same time, the burdens of surgery should not be imposed in every case of the loss of function in the lower extremities. Surgery is acceptable only when the handicap to be corrected or ameliorated promotes the patient's overall well-being, e.g., enabling the patient to sit erect or to flex the knee.

Finally, Dr. Paul Brown identifies similar judgments that must be made in cases of orthopedic surgery where the alternatives are surgical amputation involving the upper extremities and an attempt to reattach, for example, a severed finger. In language remarkably similar to Dr. Gregory's, Dr. Brown develops the duties and virtues that characterize the beneficence model.[18] After a review of the literature, together with a discussion of clinical experience, Dr. Brown concludes that the relevant goods and harms are not simply those of having or not having one's finger remain part of one's body. The good of the reattachment of one's finger must be weighed against the possibility that it may be nonfunctional or only partly functional or even aesthetically displeasing to the patient. In some cases, he concludes, amputation may be more consistent with the patient's best interests than reattachment.

As these examples indicate, in applications of the principle of beneficence in medicine, goods of medical intervention must constantly be weighed against risks of harms presented by disease and handicaps, as well as by the medical interventions themselves. Beneficence includes the obligation to balance benefits against harms, benefits against alternative benefits, and harms against alternative harms. It also requires that the physician maintain the professional skills required to properly weigh and balance the alternatives. (Here, "Know your business" becomes a moral imperative ingredient in the model itself.) If this balancing leads a physician to conceive his or her obligations to patients differently from patients' assessments, the beneficence model simply dictates that the physician act in accordance with the ends of medicine. Therefore, the physician cannot kill, assist suicide, administer drugs with no hope of a medically indicated effect, and the like. However, the model has no power to show that the physician's medical judgment must *always* override the patient's. The model simply frames the physician's obligations in terms of medically specific ways of providing benefits and avoiding harms.

The elements of the beneficence model build on each other to provide an integrated account of the moral dimensions of the physician's role—its moral end, its moral principle, its moral obligations, and its moral virtues. In schematic form, these elements are as follows:

1. *The Moral End of Medicine*: The end of medicine is the promotion of the patient's best interest, as understood from the perspective of medicine.

2. *Basic Moral Principle*: The principle of beneficence is the sole fundamental principle. It requires the physician to promote goods for patients, as medicine sees those goods, and to avoid harms, as medicine sees those harms.

3. *Derivative Moral Obligations*: From the principle of beneficence the physician's role-related obligations are derived: honest communication, confidentiality, fidelity, and the like.

4. *Derivative Moral Virtues*: From the principle of beneficence the physician's role-related virtues are also derived: truthfulness, trustworthiness, faithfulness, and the like.

THE AUTONOMY MODEL

In contrast to the beneficence model, the autonomy model takes the *values and beliefs of the patient* to be the primary moral consideration in determining the physician's moral responsibilities in patient care: If the patient's values directly conflict with medicine's values, the fundamental responsibility of physicians is to respect and to facilitate a patient's self-determination in making decisions about his or her medical fate. The obligations and virtues of the physician thus flow from the principle of respect for autonomy. This model is not without support in the history of medical ethics, but has its major sources in the histories of law and philosophy.

Legal Sources of the Model

A key feature of the principle of respect for autonomy has been developed in legal contexts, where "self-determination" has a venerable history and is taken to be synonymous with what we are calling autonomy—that is, the ability to understand one's situation and pursue personal goals free of governing constraints. The principle of self-determination means that one has sovereignty over one's life—a sovereignty that protects privacy as well as rights to control what happens to one's person and property. In its original development in the law, the intrinsic worth of the individual, including the right to personal sovereignty, was advanced primarily as a check

or limit on the authority of the state or another person. For example, the Bill of Rights and the "due process" amendments to the United States Constitution were so fashioned. The central theme is that a person's sovereignty limits the sphere into which others may legitimately intrude.

Individual sovereignty needs protection for two reasons. First, there is a danger of imbalance in power between the individual and the state (or other parties) in favor of the latter. Individual rights provide a corrective to this imbalance by insuring that individuals as individuals will be given due consideration and respect. Second, conflicts arise between an individual's perception of his or her best interests and another's perception of those interests. Rights of individual sovereignty protect an individual's freedom to choose his or her best interests. The legal principle of respect for self-determination is applied to questions concerning the physician's responsibility because patients and physicians are unequal in their possession of information and their power to control the circumstances under which they meet. Typically, one party is fit and medically knowledgeable, the other sick and medically ignorant.[19] Legal rights are a way of limiting the physician's power and of protecting the patient from unwarranted intrusions—such as surgery without consent, involuntary commitment to a mental institution, and public disclosure of information contained in hospital records....

The relationship between patients and physicians is seen by the law in contractual and fiduciary terms. The implications for the responsibilities of the physician are clear and forceful. The physician is not to assume that, simply because an individual is under the physician's care, the physician is therefore free (as the *fiduciary*) to pursue the best interests of the patient as medicine might conceive them. To do so would be to deny the "equal standing" ingredient in the contractual dimension of the patient-physician relationship. The physician's responsibility cannot be sharply divorced from the patient's self-determined choices and decisions, including best interests as defined by the patient....

Philosophical Sources of the Model

Like the Hippocratic Oath, the word "autonomy" is a legacy from ancient Greece. The Greek *autos* (self) and *nomos* (rule or law) first combined to refer to self-governance in the Greek city-state. The most general idea of personal autonomy in moral philosophy is still self-governance: forming one's own self by adequate knowledge and understanding, free from controlling interferences by others or by personal limitations. The general idea of autonomy is linked in philosophical literature to several allied concepts, such as the freedom to choose, the creation of a personal moral position, and accepting responsibility for one's actions. There is near uniform agreement in this literature that a person lacking critical internal capacities for self-rule—and not mere freedom from external controls or constraints—lacks something integral to self-governance. Thus the autonomous person is both free of external control and in control of his or her affairs. One is autonomous in this sense only if one is capable of controlled deliberation and free action.

While a more precise analysis of autonomy remains a matter of philosophical controversy, we define an autonomous decision as follows: A person's decision is autonomous if it derives from the person's own values and beliefs, is based on adequate information and understanding, and is not determined by internal or external constraints that compel the decision. A person's autonomy is reduced if some of these conditions are unsatisfied or only weakly satisfied....

A *principle* of respect for autonomy requires that persons be enabled to order their values and beliefs and to choose and act free from the controlling interventions of others. Even if risk that to others may appear foolhardy is involved, this principle demands noninterference and respect as the proper responses to the autonomous choices of persons. For example, autonomous, informed patients have the right to decide that medical intervention to prevent death is unacceptable; these patients have the right to refuse further treatment, even in the face of certain death.[20] However, such rights do not always have overriding authority, and hence the burden of proof for an intervention can in principle be met....

The philosophical roots of this principle of respect for autonomy are not as easily traceable to ancient Greece as are the Hippocratic roots of the beneficence model. Indeed, their most prominent formulations are found in the philosophical ethics of the seventeenth and eighteenth centuries. In particular, the work of the British philosopher John Locke[21] and the German philosopher Immanuel Kant[22] have proven to be of monumental historical influence. Locke was concerned about the power of the state and the protection of individual rights. He delineated both a sphere of individual autonomy that any morally just state must respect and a doctrine of basic entitlements to noninterference that every individual possesses prior to the formation of a political order. There are four such rights in Locke's system: the rights to life, liberty, health, and possessions. The state cannot interfere with these rights without a valid authorization from the individual. Like the legal principle of respect for self-determination, Locke's rights protect against intervention without consent.

There is, however, more to the principle of respect for autonomy in the history of philosophy than Locke's orientation. Philosophers after Locke generally de-emphasized the relationship between the citizen and the state. Kant's theory is especially noteworthy. He was interested in the conditions for the establishment of a moral community whose defining mark would be mutual respect. A requirement that we treat one another as free to choose is fundamental for him. We thus should not treat others as means to our own ends (i.e., just as we please) without their consent. To do so would involve disrespect for their autonomous determinations, and so would disrespect them as autonomous agents. Thus, in evaluating the decisions and actions of others, we have a duty to accord them the same right to their judgments that we possess, and they in turn must treat us in the same way.

Following the courses charted by Locke and Kant, subsequent moral philosophy has generally supported the following interpretation of the principle of respect for autonomy: Autonomous decisions and actions should not be constrained by others. Two observations are in order about this principle: (1) As formulated, this broad principle has no exceptions built into it that express valid conditions or interventions that allow us to limit autonomy. However, respect for autonomy is a prima facie principle, and so can be overridden by other moral principles that permit constraints on autonomy. (2) All persons who do not have informational or related mental deficiencies or some form of internal or external governing constraints on their will are autonomous and can make autonomous decisions. All persons of this description fall under the scope of this principle. However, the principle of respect for autonomy must not be interpreted as applying to all individuals. Some individuals fail to act autonomously because they are incapacitated or coerced. Someone with reduced autonomy is highly dependent on others and in at least some respect incapable of making choices based on controlled deliberations. For example, young children, drug addicts, senile individuals, and many institutionalized populations, such as the mentally retarded, may suffer from reduced autonomy. For such persons the principle of respect for autonomy may be inapplicable. . . .

The Elements of the Model

Like the beneficence model, the autonomy model takes its beginning in the moral injunction to promote the patient's best interests. The distinctive feature of the autonomy model is its insistence that the individual patient's perspective on and interpretation of his or her best interests is fundamental.

No independent, objective list of medical goods and harms can be developed that is comparable to the list in the beneficence model because the individual's perspective is vastly more individualistic than the objective medical perspective that defines goods and harms in the beneficence model. . . .

The autonomy model insists on respect for the patient's decisions in matters of care. From this point of view, the physician's obligations are not to interfere with the patient's autonomous choices but to assist in their implementation insofar as professional skills and knowledge permit. Like those of the beneficence model, the elements of the autonomy model build on each other to form an interwoven pattern of the moral dimensions of the physician's role—its moral end, its principles, its obligations, and its virtues. These can be represented schematically as follows:

1. *The Moral End of Medicine*: The end of medicine is the promotion of the patient's best interests, as determined by the individual patient's autonomous decisions.

2. *Basic Moral Principle*: The principle of respect for autonomy is the sole fundamental principle. It requires the physician to respect the patient's autonomous decisions and actions regarding medical care.

3. *Derivative Moral Obligations*: From the principle of respect for autonomy the physician's role-related moral obligations are derived: disclosure of medical information, confidentiality, fidelity, and the like.

4. *Derivative Moral Virtues*: From the principle of respect for autonomy the physician's role-related virtues are derived: truthfulness, equanimity, faithfulness, and the like. . . .

The conflict generated by the two models is an inescapable dimension of medical practice: a conflict between the patient's best interests understood from the perspective of medicine and the patient's best interests understood from the perspective of the patient. That conflict is not, as is sometimes thought, an artifact of malpractice suits and contemporary philosophical ethics. Quite the opposite is the case: This conflict is the inevitable result of the histories, traditions, beliefs, and practices in medicine, law, and philosophy that we have traced in this [article]. (However, to say the conflict is inevitable is only to acknowledge its inevitability in *our* social system. That social systems in China, Japan, Bangladesh, and Saudi Arabia may have largely escaped such conflicts is neither a refutation of the claim nor a demonstration that some alternative social system is in some respect preferable to our own and for that reason to be emulated. . . .

Medicine as known in the West has inherited a complex history, and physicians presently must determine their responsibility to their patients in terms of both models. This is a basic demand in medical ethics because adopting one model *exclusively* will result in the sacrifice of significant values. To use the beneficence model as a trump to override the demands of the autonomy model may result in failure to respect the moral integrity of patients; and to use the autonomy model as a trump to override the demands of the beneficence model may require physicians to act contrary to some of the most basic values of medicine. . . .

NOTES

1 Allan Crimm and Raymond Greenberg, both physicians, criticize the single model approach in their "Reflections on the Doctor-Patient Relationship," in *Ethical Dimensions of Clinical Medicine*, ed. Dennis A. Robbins and Allen R. Dyer (Springfield, Ill.: Charles C Thomas, Publisher, 1981), pp. 104–10. See also David C. Thomasma, "Limitations of the Autonomy Model for the Doctor-Patient Relationship," *The Pharos* (Spring 1983): 2–5.

2 For accounts of other pertinent models in the medical ethics literature, see John Arras and Robert Hunt, eds., *Ethical Issues in Modern Medicine*, 2d ed. (Palo Alto, Calif.: Mayfield Publishing Co., 1983), Part One, Section I, which includes Robert M. Veatch's influential essay, "Models for Ethical Med-

icine in a Revolutionary Age," *Hastings Center Report* 2 (1972): 5–7; President's Commission for the Study of Ethical Problems in Medicine and Biomedical and Behavioral Research, *Making Health Care Decisions* (Washington, D.C.: U.S. Government Printing Office, 1982), pp. 36–39; Gregory Pence, *Ethical Options in Medicine* (Oradell, N.J.: Medical Economics Company, Book Division, 1980), pp. 185–221; and Albert R. Jonsen, Mark Siegler, and William Winslade, *Clinical Ethics* (New York: Macmillan Publishing Company, 1982), pp. 11–50.

3 See Earl Shelp, "To Benefit and Respect Persons: A Challenge for Beneficence in Health Care," in *Beneficence and Health Care*, ed. Earl Shelp (Dordrecht, Holland: D. Reidel Publishing Co., 1982), pp. 200–204; and Tom L. Beauchamp and James Childress, *Principles of Biomedical Ethics*, 2d ed. (New York: Oxford University Press, 1983), Chapters 4–5.

4 W. H. S. Jones, trans. *Hippocrates* (Cambridge: Harvard University Press, the Loeb Classical Library, 1923).

5 For an analysis of these features, see Ludwig Edelstein, *Ancient Medicine: Selected Papers of Ludwig Edelstein*, ed. Owsei Temkin and C. Lilian Temkin (Baltimore: The Johns Hopkins University Press, 1967).

6 See "Oath of Hippocrates," in Ludwig Edelstein, "The Hippocratic Oath: Text, Translation, and Interpretation," *Bulletin of the History of Medicine*, Supplement 1 (Baltimore: The Johns Hopkins University Press, 1943), p. 3.

7 See Edelstein, *Ancient Medicine*, passim.

8 "Oath of Hippocrates," p. 3.

9 Hippocrates, "The Art," in *Hippocrates*, trans. Jones, Vol. II, p. 193.

10 Darrel Amundsen, "The Physician's Obligation to Prolong Life: A Medical Duty without Classical Roots," *Hastings Center Report* 8 (August 1978): 23–30.

11 Hippocrates, "Epidemics," in *Hippocrates*, trans. Jones, Vol. I, p. 165 (emphasis added).

12 An emetic is a substance that induces vomiting.

13 We draw this list of medical goods and harms from both historical and contemporary sources. See also Eric Cassell, "The Nature of Suffering and the Goals of Medicine," *New England Journal of Medicine* 306 (18 March 1982): 639. This list of goods and harms does not differ significantly from that offered by, for example, Albert R. Jonsen et al. in *Clinical Ethics*, pp. 13–14. We view educating and counseling patients (their #5) as a *means* to securing the goods on their list.

14 Allan S. Brett, "Hidden Ethical Issues in Clinical Decision Analysis," *New England Journal of Medicine* 305 (5 November 1981): 1150–52.

15 Michael F. Oliver, "Risks of Correcting the Risks of Coronary Disease and Stroke with Drugs," *New England Journal of Medicine* 306 (4 February 1982): 297–98.

16 James B. Reuler and Donald E. Girard, "The Primary Care Physician's Role in Cancer Management," *Geriatrics* 36 (November 1981): 41–50.

17 Robert L. Samilson, "Current Concepts of Surgical Management of Deformities of the Lower Extremities in Cerebral Palsy," *Clinical Orthopedics* 158 (July–August 1981): 99–107.

18 Paul W. Brown, "The Rational Selection of Treatment for Upper Extremity Amputations," *Orthopedic Clinics of North America* 12 (October 1981): 843–48.

19 Drummond Rennie, "Informed Consent by 'Well-Nigh Abject' Adults," *New England Journal of Medicine* 302 (17 April 1980): 917.

20 President's Commission for the Study of Ethical Problems in Medicine and Biomedical and Behavioral Research, *Deciding to Forego Life-Sustaining Treatment* (Washington, D.C.: U.S. Government Printing Office, 1983), p. 244ff; and (for the theoretical grounding of this claim in autonomy) *Making Health Care Decisions* (Washington, D.C.: U.S. Government Printing Office, 1982), p. 44ff., esp. p. 47.

21 John Locke, *Two Treatises of Government*, ed. Peter Laslett (Cambridge: Cambridge University Press, 1960).

22 Immanuel Kant, *Groundwork of the Metaphysic of Morals*, trans. H. J. Paton (New York: Harper & Row, 1964).

Why Doctors Should Intervene
Terrence F. Ackerman

Terrence F. Ackerman is chair of the department of human values and ethics at the University of Tennessee and an adjunct member in medical ethics at St. Jude Children's Hospital. He is the author of "Medical Ethics and the Two Dogmas of Liberalism" and "Experimentation in Bioethics Research," and he is coeditor of *Clinical Medical Ethics: Exploration and Assessment* (1987).

Ackerman criticizes the notion of respect for autonomy that identifies it with noninterference. He argues that noninterference fails to respect patient autonomy because it does not take account of the transforming effects of illness. Ackerman's major contention is that the autonomy of those who are ill is limited by all kinds of constraints—physical, cognitive, emotional, and social. Ackerman argues in favor of medical paternalism, where appropriate, maintaining that real respect for the autonomy of patients requires physicians to actively attempt to neutralize the impediments that interfere with patients' choices, helping them to restore control over their lives.

Patient autonomy has become a watchword of the medical profession. According to the revised 1980 AMA Principles of Medical Ethics,[1] no longer is it permissible for a doctor to withhold information from a patient, even on grounds that it may be harmful. Instead the physician is expected to "deal honestly with patients" at all times. Physicians also have a duty to respect the confidentiality of the doctor-patient relationship. Even when disclosure to a third party may be in the patient's interests, the doctor is instructed to release information only when required by law. Respect for the autonomy of patients has given rise to many specific patient rights—among them the right to refuse treatment, the right to give informed consent, the right to privacy, and the right to competent medical care provided with "respect for human dignity."

While requirements of honesty, confidentiality, and patients' rights are all important, the underlying moral vision that places exclusive emphasis upon these factors is more troublesome. The profession's notion of respect for autonomy makes noninterference its essential feature. As the Belmont Report has described it, there is an obligation to "give weight to autonomous persons' considered opinions and choices while refraining from ob-

Reprinted with permission of the author and the publisher from *Hastings Center Report*, vol. 12 (August 1982), pp. 14–17.

structing their actions unless they are clearly detrimental to others."[2] Or, as Tom Beauchamp and James Childress have suggested, "To respect autonomous agents is to recognize with due appreciation their own considered value judgments and outlooks even when it is believed that their judgments are mistaken." They argue that people "are entitled to autonomous determination without limitation on their liberty being imposed by others."[3]

When respect for personal autonomy is understood as noninterference, the physician's role is dramatically simplified. The doctor need be only an honest and good technician, providing relevant information and dispensing professionally competent care. Does noninterference really respect patient autonomy? I maintain that it does not, because it fails to take account of the transforming effects of illness.

"Autonomy," typically defined as self-governance, has two key features. First, autonomous behavior is governed by plans of action that have been formulated through deliberation or reflection. This deliberative activity involves processes of both information gathering and priority setting. Second, autonomous behavior issues, intentionally and voluntarily, from choices people make based upon their own life plans.

But various kinds of constraints can impede autonomous behavior. There are physical constraints—confinement in prison is an example—where internal or external circumstances bodily prevent a person from deliberating adequately or acting on life plans. Cognitive constraints derive from either a lack of information or an inability to understand that information. A consumer's ignorance regarding the merits or defects of a particular product fits the description. Psychological constraints, such as anxiety or depression, also inhibit adequate deliberation. Finally, there are social constraints—such as institutionalized roles and expectations ("a woman's place is in the home," "the doctor knows best") that block considered choices.

Edmund Pellegrino suggests several ways in which autonomy is specifically compromised by illness:

> In illness, the body is interposed between us and reality—it impedes our choices and actions and is no longer fully responsive.... Illness forces a reappraisal and that poses a threat to the old image; it opens up all the old anxieties and imposes new ones—often including the real threat of death or drastic alterations in life-style. This ontological assault is aggravated by the loss of... freedoms we identify as peculiarly human. The patient... lacks the knowledge and skills necessary to cure himself or gain relief of pain and suffering.... The state of being ill is therefore a state of "wounded humanity," of a person compromised in his fundamental capacity to deal with his vulnerability.[4]

The most obvious impediment is that illness "interposes" the body or mind between the patient and reality, obstructing attempts to act upon cherished plans. An illness may not only temporarily obstruct long-range goals; it may necessitate permanent and drastic revision in the patient's major activities, such as working habits. Patients may also need to set limited goals regarding control of pain, alteration in diet and physical activity, and rehabilitation of functional impairments. They face considerable difficulties in identifying realistic and productive aims.

The crisis is aggravated by a cognitive constraint—the lack of "knowledge and skills" to overcome their physical or mental impediment. Without adequate medical understanding, the patient cannot assess his or her condition accurately. Thus the choice of goals is seriously hampered and subsequent decisions by the patient are not well founded.

Pellegrino mentions the anxieties created by illness, but psychological constraints may also include denial, depression, guilt, and fear. I recently visited an eighteen-year-old boy who was dying of a cancer that had metas-tasized extensively throughout his abdomen. The doctor wanted to administer further chemotherapy that might extend the patient's life a few months. But the patient's nutritional status was poor, and he would need intravenous feedings prior to chemotherapy. Since the nutritional therapy might also encourage tumor growth, leading to a blockage of the gastrointestinal tract, the physician carefully explained the options and the risks and benefits several times, each time at greater length. But after each explanation, the young man would say only that he wished to do whatever was necessary to get better. Denial prevented him from exploring the alternatives.

Similarly, depression can lead patients to make choices that are not in harmony with their life plans. Recently, a middle-aged woman with a history of ovarian cancer in remission returned to the hospital for the biopsy of a possible pulmonary metastasis. Complications ensued and she required the use of an artificial respirator for several days. She became severely depressed and soon refused further treatment. The behavior was entirely out of character with her previous full commitment to treatment. Fully supporting her overt wishes might have robbed her of many months of relatively comfortable life in the midst of a very supportive family around which her activities centered. The medical staff stalled for time. Fortunately, her condition improved.

Fear may also cripple the ability of patients to choose. Another patient, diagnosed as having a cerebral tumor that was probably malignant, refused life-saving surgery because he feared the cosmetic effects of neurosurgery and the possibility of neurological damage. After he became comatose and new evidence suggested that the tumor might be benign, his family agreed to surgery and a benign tumor was removed. But he later died of complications related to the unfortunate delay in surgery. Although while competent he had agreed to chemotherapy, his fears (not uncommon among candidates for neurosurgery) prevented him from accepting the medical intervention that might have secured him the health he desired.

Social constraints may also prevent patients from acting upon their considered choices. A recent case involved a twelve-year-old boy whose rhabdomyosarcoma had metastasized extensively. Since all therapeutic interventions had failed, the only remaining option was to involve him in a phase 1 clinical trial. (A phase 1 clinical trial is the initial testing of a drug in human subjects. Its primary purpose is to identify toxicities rather than to evaluate therapeutic effectiveness.) The patient's course had been very stormy, and he privately expressed to the staff his desire to quit further therapy and return home. However, his parents denied the hopelessness of his condition, remaining steadfast in their belief that God would save their child. With deep regard for his parents' wishes, he refused to openly object to their desires and the therapy was administered. No antitumor effect occurred and the patient soon died.

Various social and cultural expectations also take their toll. According to Talcott Parsons, one feature of the sick role is that the ill person is obligated " . . . to seek *technically competent* help, namely, in the most usual case, that of a physician and to *cooperate* with him in the process of trying to get well."[5] Parsons does not describe in detail the elements of this cooperation. But clinical observation suggests that many patients relinquish their opportunity to deliberate and make choices regarding treatment in deference to the physician's superior educational achievement and social status ("Whatever you think, doctor!"). The physical and emotional demands of illness reinforce this behavior.

Moreover, this perception of the sick role has been socially taught from childhood—and it is not easily altered even by the physician who ardently tries to engage the patient in decision making. Indeed, when patients are initially asked to participate in the decision-making process, some exhibit considerable confusion and anxiety. Thus, for many persons, the institutional role of patient requires the physician to assume the responsibilities of making decisions.

Ethicists typically condemn paternalistic practices in the therapeutic relationship, but fail to investigate the features that incline physicians to be paternalistic. Such behavior may be one way to assist persons whose autonomous behavior has been impaired by illness. Of course, it is an open moral question whether the constraints imposed by illness ought to be addressed in such a way. But only by coming to grips with the psychological and social dimensions of illness can we discuss how physicians can best respect persons who are patients.

RETURNING CONTROL TO PATIENTS

In the usual interpretation of respect for personal autonomy, noninterference is fundamental. In the medical setting, this means providing adequate information and competent care that accords with the patient's wishes. But if serious constraints upon autonomous behavior are intrinsic to the state of being ill, then noninterference is not the best course, since the patient's choices will be seriously limited. Under these conditions, real respect for autonomy entails a more inclusive understanding of the relationship between patients and physicians. Rather than restraining themselves so that patients can exercise whatever autonomy they retain in illness, physicians should actively seek to neutralize the impediments that interfere with patients' choices.

In *The Healer's Art*, Eric Cassell underscored the essential feature of illness that demands a revision in our understanding of respect for autonomy:

> If I had to pick the aspect of illness that is most destructive to the sick, I would choose the loss of control. Maintaining control over oneself is so vital to all of us that one might see all the other phenomena of illness as doing harm not only in their own right but doubly so as they reinforce the sick person's perception that he is no longer in control.[6]

Cassell maintains, "The doctor's job is to return control to his patient." But what is involved in "returning control" to patients? Pellegrino identifies two elements that are preeminent duties of the physician: to provide technically competent care and to fully inform the patient. The noninterference approach emphasizes these factors, and their importance is clear. Loss of control in illness is precipitated by a physical or mental defect. If technically competent therapy can fully restore previous health, then the patient will again be in control. Consider a patient who is treated with antibiotics for a routine throat infection of streptococcal origin. Similarly, loss of control is fueled by lack of knowledge—not knowing what is the matter, what it portends for life and limb, and how it might be dealt with. Providing information that will enable the patient to make decisions and adjust goals enhances personal control.

If physical and cognitive constraints were the only impediments to autonomous behavior, then Pellegrino's suggestions might be adequate. But providing information and technically competent care will not do much to alter psychological or social impediments. Pellegrino does not adequately portray the physician's role in ameliorating these.

How can the doctor offset the acute denial that prevented the adolescent patient from assessing the benefits and risks of intravenous feedings prior to his additional chemotherapy? How can he deal with the candidate for neurosurgery who clearly desired that attempts be made to restore his health, but feared cosmetic and functional impairments? Here strategies must go beyond the mere provision of information. Crucial information may have to be repeatedly shared with patients. Features of the situation that the patient has brushed over (as in denial) or falsely emphasized (as with acute anxiety) must be discussed in more detail or set in their proper perspective. And the physician may have to alter the tone of discussions with the patient, emphasizing a positive attitude with the overly depressed or anxious patient, or a more realistic, cautious attitude with the denying patient, in order to neutralize psychological constraints.

The physician may also need to influence the beliefs or attitudes of other people, such as family members, that limit their awareness of the patient's perspective. Such a strategy might have helped the parents of the dying child to conform with the patient's wishes. On the other hand, physicians may need to modify the patient's own understanding of the sick role. For example, they may need to convey that the choice of treatment depends not merely upon the physician's technical assessment, but on the quality of life and personal goals that the patient desires.

Once we admit that psychological and social constraints impair patient autonomy, it follows that physicians must carefully assess the psychological and social profiles and needs of patients. Thus, Pedro Lain-Entralgo insists that adequate therapeutic interaction consists in a combination of "objectivity" and "cooperation." Cooperation "is shown by psychologically reproducing in the mind of the doctor, insofar as that is possible, the meaning the patient's illness has for him."[7] Without such knowledge, the physician cannot assist patients in restoring control over their lives. Ironically, some critics have insisted that physicians are not justified in acting for the well-being of patients because they possess no "expertise" in securing the requisite knowledge about the patient.[8] But knowledge of the patient's psychological and social situation is also necessary to help the patient to act as a fully autonomous person.

BEYOND LEGALISM

Current notions of respect for autonomy are undergirded by a legal model of doctor-patient interaction. The relationship is viewed as a typical commodity exchange—the provision of technically competent medical care in return for financial compensation. Moreover, physicians and patients are presumed to have an equal ability to work out the details of therapy, *provided that* certain moral rights of patients are recognized. But the compromising effects of illness, the superior knowledge of physicians, and various institutional arrangements are also viewed as giving the physician an unfair power advantage. Since the values and interests of patients may conflict with those of the physician, the emphasis is placed upon noninterference.[9]

This legal framework is insufficient for medical ethics because it fails to recognize the impact of illness upon autonomous behavior. Even if the rights to receive adequate information and to provide consent are secured, affective and social constraints impair the ability of patients to engage in contractual therapeutic relationships. When people are sick, the focus upon equality is temporally misplaced. The goal of the therapeutic relationship is the "development" of the patient—helping to resolve the underlying physical (or mental) defect, and to deal with cognitive, psychological, and social constraints in order to restore autonomous functioning. In this sense, the doctor-patient interaction is not unlike the parent-child or teacher-student relationship.

The legal model also falls short because the therapeutic relationship is not a typical commodity exchange in which the parties use each other to accomplish mutually compatible goals, without taking a direct interest in each other. Rather, the status of patients as persons whose autonomy is compromised constitutes the very stuff of therapeutic art. The physician is attempting to alter the fundamental ability of patients to carry through their life plans. To accomplish this delicate task requires a personal knowledge about and interest in the patient. If we accept these points, then we must reject the narrow focus of medical ethics upon noninterference and emphasize patterns of interaction that free patients from constraints upon autonomy.

I hasten to add that I am criticizing the legal model only as a *complete* moral framework for therapeutic interaction. As case studies in medical ethics suggest, physicians and patients *are* potential adversaries. Moreover, the disability of the patient and various institutional controls provide physicians with a distinct "power advantage" that can be abused. Thus, a legitimate function of medical ethics is to formulate conditions that assure noninterference in patient decision making. But various positive interventions must also be emphasized, since the central task in the therapeutic process is assisting patients to reestablish control over their own lives.

In the last analysis, the crucial matter is how we view the patient who enters into the therapeutic relationship. Cassell points out that in the typical view "...the sick person is seen simply as a well person with a disease, rather than as qualitatively different, not only physically but also socially, emotionally, and even cognitively." In this view, "...the physician's role in the care of the sick is primarily the application of technology...and health can be seen as a commodity."[10] But if, as I believe, illness renders sick persons "qualitatively different," then respect for personal autonomy requires a therapeutic interaction considerably more complex than the noninterference strategy.

Thus the current "Principles of Medical Ethics" simply exhort physicians to be honest. But the crucial requirement is that physicians tell the truth in a way, at a time, and in whatever increments are necessary to allow patients to effectively use the information in adjusting their life plans.[11] Similarly, respecting a patient's refusal of treatment maximizes autonomy only if a balanced and thorough deliberation precedes the decision. Again, the "Principles" suggest that physicians observe strict confidentiality. But the more complex moral challenge is to use confidential information in a way that will help to give the patient more freedom. Thus, the doctor can keep a patient's report on family dynamics private, and still use it to modify attitudes or actions of family members that inhibit the patient's control.

At its root, illness is an evil primarily because it compromises our efforts to control our lives. Thus, we must preserve an understanding of the physician's art that transcends noninterference and addresses this fundamental reality.

REFERENCES

1 American Medical Association, *Current Opinions of the Judicial Council of the American Medical Association* (Chicago, Illinois: American Medical Association, 1981), p. ix. Also see Robert Veatch, "Professional Ethics: New Principles for Physicians?," *Hastings Center Report* 10 (June 1980), 16–19.

2 The National Commission for the Protection of Human Subjects of Biomedical and Behavioral Research, *The Belmont Report: Ethical Principles and Guidelines for the Protection of Human Subjects of Research* (Washington, D.C.: U.S. Government Printing Office, 1978), p. 58.

3 Tom Beauchamp and James Childress, *Principles of Biomedical Ethics* (New York: Oxford University Press, 1980), p. 59.

4 Edmund Pellegrino, "Toward a Reconstruction of Medical Morality: The Primacy of the Act of Profession and the Fact of Illness," *The Journal of Medicine and Philosophy* 4 (1979), 44–45.

5 Talcott Parsons, *The Social System* (Glencoe, Illinois: The Free Press, 1951), p. 437.

6 Eric Cassell, *The Healer's Art* (New York: Lippincott, 1976), p. 44. Although Cassell aptly describes the goal of the healer's art, it is unclear whether he considers it to be based upon the obligation to respect the patient's autonomy or the duty to enhance the well-being of the patient. Some parts of his discussion clearly suggest the latter.

7 Pedro Lain-Entralgo, *Doctor and Patient* (New York: McGraw-Hill, 1969), p. 155.

8 See Allen Buchanan, "Medical Paternalism," *Philosophy and Public Affairs* 7 (1978), 370–90.

9 My formulation of the components of the legal model differs from, but is highly indebted to, John Ladd's stimulating analysis in "Legalism and Medical Ethics," in John Davis et al., editors, *Contemporary Issues in Biomedical Ethics* (Clifton, N.J.: The Humana Press, 1979), pp. 1–35. However, I would not endorse Ladd's position that the moral principles that define our duties in the therapeutic setting are of a different logical type from those that define our duties to strangers.

10 Eric Cassell, "Therapeutic Relationship: Contemporary Medical Perspective," in Warren Reich, editor, *Encyclopedia of Bioethics* (New York: Macmillan, 1978), p. 1675.

11 Cf. Norman Cousins, "A Layman Looks at Truthtelling," *Journal of the American Medical Association* 244 (1980), 1929–30. Also see Howard Brody, "Hope," *Journal of the American Medical Association* 246 (1981), pp. 1411–12.

Truth-Telling

On Lying to Patients
Mack Lipkin

Mack Lipkin, M.D. (1907–1989), retired after 38 years in the private practice of internal medicine in New York City, where he also taught at the Medical College of Cornell University as well as at other medical schools. Following retirement, he joined the faculty of the University of Oregon School of Medicine and, in 1980, the faculty of the University of North Carolina School of Medicine at Chapel Hill where he was professor of medicine at the time of his death. He was the author of *The Care of Patients—Perspectives and Practices* and many papers in various medical publications.

   Lipkin argues that physicians should sometimes deceive their patients or withhold information from them. On his view, telling the "whole truth" is a practical impossibility. Furthermore, patients (1) do not have sufficient information about how their bodies function to interpret medical information accurately and (2) sometimes do not want to know the truth about their illness. For Lipkin, the crucial question is, "Is the deception intended to benefit the patient or the doctor?"

Should a doctor always tell his patients the truth? In recent years there has been an extraordinary increase in public discussion of the ethical problems involved in this question. But little has been heard from physicians themselves. I believe that gaps in understanding the complex interactions between doctors and patients have led many laymen astray in this debate.

It is easy to make an attractive case for always telling patients the truth. But as L. J. Henderson, the great Harvard physiologist-philosopher of decades ago, commented:

> To speak of telling the truth, the whole truth and nothing but the truth to a patient is absurd. Like absurdity in mathematics, it is absurd simply because it is impossible.... The notion that the truth, the whole truth, and nothing but the truth can be conveyed to the patient is a good specimen of that class of fallacies called by Whitehead "the fallacy of misplaced concreteness." It results from neglecting factors that cannot be excluded from the concrete situation and that are of an order of magnitude and relevancy that make it imperative to consider them. Of course, another fallacy is also often involved, the

Newsweek (June 4, 1979), p. 13. Reprinted with permission.

belief that diagnosis and prognosis are more certain than they are. But that is another question.

Words, especially medical terms, inevitably carry different implications for different people. When these words are said in the presence of anxiety-laden illness, there is a strong tendency to hear selectively and with emphases not intended by the doctor. Thus, what the doctor means to convey is obscured.

Indeed, thoughtful physicians know that transmittal of accurate information to patients is often impossible. Patients rarely know how the body functions in health and disease, but instead have inaccurate ideas of what is going on; this hampers the attempts to "tell the truth."

Take cancer, for example. Patients seldom know that while some cancers are rapidly fatal, others never amount to much; some have a cure rate of 99 percent, others less than 1 percent; a cancer may grow rapidly for months and then stop growing for years; may remain localized for years or spread all over the body almost from the beginning; some can be arrested for long periods of time, others not. Thus, one patient thinks of cancer as curable, the next thinks it means certain death.

How many patients understand that "heart trouble" may refer to literally hundreds of different abnormalities ranging in severity from the trivial to the instantly fatal? How many know that the term "arthritis" may refer to dozens of different types of joint involvement? "Arthritis" may raise a vision of the appalling disease that made Aunt Eulalee a helpless invalid until her death years later; the next patient remembers Grandpa grumbling about the damned arthritis as he got up from his chair. Unfortunately but understandably, most people's ideas about the implications of medical terms are based on what they have heard about a few cases.

The news of serious illness drives some patients to irrational and destructive behavior; others handle it sensibly. A distinguished philosopher forestalled my telling him about his cancer by saying, "I want to know the truth. The only thing I couldn't take and wouldn't want to know about is cancer." For two years he had watched his mother die slowly of a painful form of cancer. Several of my physician patients have indicated they would not want to know if they had a fatal illness.

Most patients should be told "the truth" to the extent that they can comprehend it. Indeed, most doctors, like most other people, are uncomfortable with lies. Good physicians, aware that some may be badly damaged by being told more than they want or need to know, can usually ascertain the patient's preferences and needs.

Discussions about lying often center about the use of placebos. In medical usage, a "placebo" is a treatment that has no specific physical or chemical action on the condition being treated, but is given to affect symptoms by a psychologic mechanism, rather than a purely physical one. Ethicists believe that placebos necessarily involve a partial or complete deception by the doctor, since the patient is allowed to believe that the treatment has a specific effect. They seem unaware that placebos, far from being inert (except in the rigid pharmacological sense), are among the most powerful agents known to medicine.

Placebos are a form of suggestion, which is a direct or indirect presentation of an idea, followed by an uncritical, i.e., not thought-out, acceptance. Those who have studied suggestion or looked at medical history know its almost unbelievable potency; it is involved to a greater or lesser extent in the treatment of every conscious patient. It can induce or remove almost any kind of feeling or thought. It can strengthen the weak or paralyze the strong; transform sleeping, feeding, or sexual patterns; remove or induce a vast array of symptoms; mimic or abolish the effect of very powerful drugs. It can alter the function of most organs. It can cause illness or a great sense of well-being. It can kill. In fact, doctors often add a measure of suggestion when they prescribe even potent medications for those who also need psychologic support. Like all potent agents, its proper use requires judgment based on experience and skill.

Communication between physician and the apprehensive and often confused patient is delicate and uncertain. Honesty should be evaluated not only in terms of a slavish devotion to language often misinterpreted by the patient, but also in terms of intent. *The crucial question is whether the deception was intended to benefit the patient or the doctor.*

Physicians, like most people, hope to see good results and are disappointed when patients do poorly. Their reputations and their livelihood depend on doing effective work; purely selfish reasons would dictate they do their best for their patients. Most important, all good physicians have a deep sense of responsibility toward those who have entrusted their welfare to them.

As I have explained, it is usually a practical impossibility to tell patients "the whole truth." Moreover, often enough, the ethics of the situation, the true moral responsibility, may demand that the naked facts not be revealed. The now popular complaint that doctors are too authoritarian is misguided more often than not. Some patients who insist on exercising their right to know may be doing themselves a disservice.

Judgment is often difficult and uncertain. Simplistic assertions about telling the truth may not be helpful to patients or physicians in times of trouble.

Lies to the Sick and Dying
Sissela Bok

Sissela Bok is associate professor of philosophy at Brandeis University, specializing in moral and political philosophy. Bok has served on human-experimentation committees in hospitals and on the Ethics Advisory Board to the Secretary of Health, Education, and Welfare (1979– 1980). She is the author of *Lying: Moral Choice in Public and Private Life* (1978), from which this article is excerpted, *Secrets: On the Ethics of Concealment and Revelation* (1983), and *A Strategy for Peace: Human Values and the Threat of War* (1989).

Bok challenges the following claims that physicians often make: (1) patients do not want bad news; and (2) truthful information harms patients. Against (1) Bok argues: (a) studies have shown that physicians and patients differ widely on the factual question of whether patients want to know the truth in the case of serious illness; and (b) physicians are only partly correct in their claim that patients who *say* they want to know the truth deny the truth even when given it repeatedly. Against (2) Bok argues: (a) the harm resulting from the disclosure of bad news or risks to patients is much less than physicians think; and (b) the benefits resulting from such disclosures are much more substantial than physicians believe. In responding to the two claims, Bok also brings out some of the other possible bad consequences of lying to patients with serious illnesses.

A forty-six-year-old man, coming to a clinic for a routine physical check-up needed for insurance purposes, is diagnosed as having a form of cancer likely to cause him to die within six months. No known cure exists for it. Chemotherapy may prolong life by a few extra months, but will have side effects the physician does not think warranted in this case. In addition, he believes that such therapy should be reserved for patients with a chance for recovery or remission. The patient has no symptoms giving him any reason to believe that he is not perfectly healthy. He expects to take a short vacation in a week.

For the physician, there are now several choices involving truthfulness. Ought he to tell the patient what he has learned, or conceal it? If asked, should he deny it? If he decides to reveal the diagnosis, should he delay doing so until after the patient returns from his vacation? Finally, even if he does reveal the serious nature of the diagnosis, should he mention the possibility of chemotherapy and his reasons for not recommending it in

From *Lying: Moral Choice in Public and Private Life*, by Sissela Bok. Copyright © 1978 by Sissela Bok. Reprinted by permission of Pantheon Books, a Division of Random House, Inc.

this case? Or should he encourage every last effort to postpone death?

In this particular case, the physician chose to inform the patient of his diagnosis right away. He did not, however, mention the possibility of chemotherapy. A medical student working under him disagreed; several nurses also thought that the patient should have been informed of this possibility. They tried, unsuccessfully, to persuade the physician that this was the patient's right. When persuasion had failed, the student elected to disobey the doctor by informing the patient of the alternative of chemotherapy. After consultation with family members, the patient chose to ask for the treatment.

Doctors confront such choices often and urgently. What they reveal, hold back, or distort will matter profoundly to their patients. Doctors stress with corresponding vehemence their reasons for the distortion or concealment: not to confuse a sick person needlessly, or cause what may well be unnecessary pain or discomfort, as in the case of the cancer patient; not to leave a patient without hope, as in those many cases where the dying are not told the truth about their condition; or to improve the chances of cure, as where unwarranted optimism is expressed about some form of therapy. Doctors use information as part of the therapeutic regimen; it is given out in amounts, in admixtures, and according to timing believed best for patients. Accuracy, by comparison, matters far less.

Lying to patients has, therefore, seemed an especially excusable act. Some would argue that doctors, and *only* doctors, should be granted the right to manipulate the truth in ways so undesirable for politicians, lawyers, and others.[1] Doctors are trained to help patients; their relationship to patients carries special obligations, and they know much more than laymen about what helps and hinders recovery and survival.

Even the most conscientious doctors, then, who hold themselves at a distance from the quacks and the purveyors of false remedies, hesitate to forswear all lying. Lying is usually wrong, they argue, but less so than allowing the truth to harm patients. B.C. Meyer echoes this very common view:

> [O]urs is a profession which traditionally has been guided by a precept that transcends the virtue of uttering truth for truth's sake, and that is, "so far as possible, do no harm."[2]

Truth, for Meyer, may be important, but not when it endangers the health and well-being of patients. This has seemed self-evident to many physicians in the past—so much so that we find very few mentions of veracity in the codes and oaths and writings by physicians through the centuries. This absence is all the more striking as other principles of ethics have been consistently and movingly expressed in the same documents.

The two fundamental principles of doing good and not doing harm—of beneficence and nonmaleficence—are the most immediately relevant to medical practitioners, and the most frequently stressed. To preserve life and good health, to ward off illness, pain, and death—these are the perennial tasks of medicine and nursing. These principles have found powerful expression at all times in the history of medicine. In the Hippocratic Oath physicians promise to:

> use treatment to help the sick...but never with a view to injury and wrong-doing.[3]

And a Hindu oath of initiation says:

> Day and night, however thou mayest be engaged, thou shalt endeavor for the relief of patients with all thy heart and soul. Thou shalt not desert or injure the patient even for the sake of thy living.[4]

But there is no similar stress on veracity. It is absent from virtually all oaths, codes, and prayers. The Hippocratic Oath makes no mention of truthfulness to patients about their condition, prognosis, or treatment. Other early codes and prayers are equally silent on the subject. To be sure, they often refer to the confidentiality with which doctors should treat all that patients tell them; but there is no corresponding reference to honesty toward the patient. One of the few who appealed to such a principle was Amatus Lusitanus, a Jewish physician widely known for his skill, who, persecuted, died of the plague in 1568. He published an oath which reads in part:

> If I lie, may I incur the eternal wrath of God and of His angel Raphael, and may nothing in the medical art succeed for me according to my desires.[5]

Later codes continue to avoid the subject. Not even the Declaration of Geneva, adopted in 1948 by the World Medical Association, makes any reference to it. And the Principles of Medical Ethics of the American Medical Association[6] still leave the matter of informing patients up to the physician.

Given such freedom, a physician can decide to tell as much or as little as he wants the patient to know, so long as he breaks no law. In the case of the man mentioned at the beginning of this [article], some physicians might feel justified in lying for the good of the patient, others might be truthful. Some may conceal alternatives to the treatment they recommend; others not. In each case, they could appeal to the A.M.A. Principles of Ethics. A great many would choose to be able to lie. They would claim that not only can a lie avoid harm for the patient, but that it is also hard to know whether they have been right in the first place in making their pessimistic diagnosis; a "truthful" statement could therefore turn out to hurt patients unnecessarily. The concern for curing and for supporting those who cannot be cured then runs counter to the desire to be completely open. This concern is especially strong where the prognosis is bleak; even more so when patients are so affected by their illness or their medication that they are more dependent than usual, perhaps more easily depressed or irrational.

Physicians know only too well how uncertain a diagnosis or prognosis can be. They know how hard it is to give meaningful and correct answers regarding health and illness. They also know that disclosing their own uncertainty or fears can reduce those benefits that depend upon faith in recovery. They fear, too, that revealing grave risks, no matter how unlikely it is that these will come about, may exercise the pull of the "self-fulfilling prophecy." They dislike being the bearers of uncertain or bad news as much as anyone else. And last, but not least, sitting down to discuss an illness truthfully and sensitively may take much-needed time away from other patients.

These reasons help explain why nurses and physicians and relatives of the sick and dying prefer not to be bound by rules that might limit their ability to suppress, delay, or distort information. This is not to say that they necessarily plan to lie much of the time. They merely want to have the freedom to do so when they believe it wise. And the reluctance to see lying prohibited explains, in turn, the failure of the codes and oaths to come to grips with the problems of truth-telling and lying.

But sharp conflicts are now arising. Doctors no longer work alone with patients. They have to consult with others much more than before; if they choose to lie, the choice may not be met with approval by all who take part in the care of the patient. A nurse expresses the difficulty which results as follows:

> From personal experience I would say that the patients who aren't told about their terminal illness have so many verbal and mental questions unanswered that many will begin to realize that their illness is more serious than they're being told.[. . .]
>
> Nurses care for these patients twenty-four hours a day compared to a doctor's daily brief visit, and it is the nurse many times that the patient will relate to, once his underlying fears become overwhelming. [. . .]This is difficult for us nurses because being in constant contact with patients we can see the events leading up to this. The patient continually asks you, "Why isn't my pain decreasing?" or "Why isn't the radiation treatment easing the pain?"[. . .]We cannot legally give these patients an honest answer as a nurse (and I'm sure I wouldn't want to) yet the problem is still not resolved and the circle grows larger and larger with the patient alone in the middle.[7]

The doctor's choice to lie increasingly involves co-workers in acting a part they find neither humane nor wise. The fact that these problems have not been carefully thought through within the medical profession, nor seriously addressed in medical education, merely serves to intensify the conflicts.[8] Different doctors then respond very differently to patients in exactly similar predicaments. The friction is increased by the fact that relatives often disagree even where those giving medical care to a patient are in accord on how to approach the patient. Here again, because physicians have not worked out to common satisfaction the question of whether relatives have the right to make such requests, the problems are allowed to be haphazardly resolved by each physician as he sees fit.

THE PATIENT'S PERSPECTIVE

The turmoil in the medical profession regarding truth-telling is further augmented by the pressures that patients themselves now bring to bear and by empirical data coming to light. Challenges are growing to [two] major arguments for lying to patients: . . . Patients do not want bad news; and truthful information harms them. . . .

The [first] argument for deceiving patients refers specifically to giving them news of a frightening or depressing kind. It holds that patients do not, in fact, generally want such information, that they prefer not to have to face up to serious illness and death. On the basis of such a belief, most doctors in a number of surveys stated that they do not, as a rule, inform patients that they have an illness such as cancer.

When studies are made of what patients desire to know, on the other hand, a large majority say that they *would* like to be told of such a diagnosis.[9] All these studies need updating and should be done with larger numbers of patients and non-patients. But they do show that there is generally a dramatic divergence between physicians and patients on the factual question of whether patients want to know what ails them in cases of serious illness such as cancer. In most of the studies, over 80 percent of the persons asked indicated that they would want to be told.

Sometimes this discrepancy is set aside by doctors who want to retain the view that patients do not want unhappy news. In reality, they claim, the fact that patients say they want it has to be discounted. The more someone asks to know, the more he suffers from fear which will lead to the denial of the information even if it is given. Informing patients is, therefore, useless; they resist and deny having been told what they cannot assimilate. According to this view, empirical studies of what patients say they want are worthless since they do not probe deeply enough to uncover this universal resistance to the contemplation of one's own death.

This view is only partially correct. For some patients, denial is indeed well established in medical experience. A number of patients (estimated at between 15 percent and 25 percent) will give evidence of denial of having been told about their illness, even when they repeatedly ask and are repeatedly informed. And nearly everyone experiences a period of denial at some point in the course of approaching death.[10] Elisabeth Kübler-Ross sees denial as resulting often from premature and abrupt information by a stranger who goes through the process quickly to "get it over with." She holds that denial functions as a buffer after unexpected shocking news, permitting individuals to collect themselves and to mobilize other defenses. She describes prolonged denial in one patient as follows:

> She was convinced that the X-rays were "mixed up"; she asked for reassurance that her pathology report could not possibly be back so soon and that another patient's report must have been marked with her name. When none of this could be confirmed, she quickly asked to leave the hospital, looking for another physician in the vain hope "to get a better explanation for my troubles." This patient went "shopping around" for many doctors, some of whom gave her reassuring answers, others of whom confirmed the previous suspicion. Whether confirmed or not, she reacted in the same manner; she asked for examination and reexamination....[11]

But to say that denial is universal flies in the face of all evidence. And to take any claim to the contrary as "symptomatic" of deeper denial leaves no room for reasoned discourse. There is no way that such universal denial can be proved true or false. To believe in it is a metaphysical belief about man's condition, not a statement about what patients do and do not want. It is true that we can never completely understand the possibility of our own death, any more than being alive in the first place. But people certainly differ in the degree to which they can approach such knowledge, take it into account in their plans, and make their peace with it.

Montaigne claimed that in order to learn both to live and to die, men have to think about death and be prepared to accept it.[12] To stick one's head in the sand, or to be prevented by lies from trying to discern what is to come, hampers freedom—freedom to consider one's life as a whole, with a beginning, a duration, an end.

Some may request to be deceived rather than to see their lives as thus finite; others reject the information which would require them to do so; but most say that they want to know. Their concern for knowing about their condition goes far beyond mere curiosity or the wish to make isolated personal choices in the short time left to them; their stance toward the entire life they have lived, and their ability to give it meaning and completion, are at stake.[13] In lying or withholding the facts which permit such discernment, doctors may reflect their own fears (which, according to one study,[14] are much stronger than those of laymen) of facing questions about the meaning of one's life and the inevitability of death.

Beyond the fundamental deprivation that can result from deception, we are also becoming increasingly aware of all that can befall patients in the course of their illness when information is denied or distorted. Lies place them in a position where they no longer participate in choices concerning their own health, including the choice of whether to be "patient" in the first place. A terminally ill person who is not informed that his illness is incurable and that he is near death cannot make decisions about the end of his life; about whether or not to enter a hospital, or to have surgery; where and with whom to spend his last days; how to put his affairs in order—these most personal choices cannot be made if he is kept in the dark, or given contradictory hints and clues.

It has always been especially easy to keep knowledge from terminally ill patients. They are most vulnerable, least able to take action to learn what they need to know, or to protect their autonomy. The very fact of being so ill greatly increases the likelihood of control by others. And the fear of being helpless in the face of such control is growing. At the same time, the period of dependency and slow deterioration of health and strength that people undergo has lengthened. There has been a dramatic shift toward institutionalization of the aged and those near death. (Over 80 percent of Americans now die in a hospital or other institution.)

Patients who are severely ill often suffer a further distancing and loss of control over their most basic functions. Electrical wiring, machines, intravenous administration of liquids, all create new dependency and at the same time new distance between the patient and all who come near. Curable patients are often willing to undergo such procedures; but when no cure is possible, these procedures merely intensify the sense of distance and uncertainty and can even become a substitute for comforting human acts. Yet those who suffer in this way often fear to seem troublesome by complaining. Lying to them, perhaps for the most charitable of purposes, can then cause them to slip unwittingly into subjection to new procedures, perhaps new surgery, where death is held at bay through transfusions, respirators, even resuscitation far beyond what most would wish.

Seeing relatives in such predicaments has caused a great upsurge of worrying about death and dying. At the root of this fear is not a growing terror of the *moment* of death, or even the instants before it. Nor is there greater fear of *being* dead. In contrast to the centuries of lives lived in dread of the punishments to be inflicted after death, many would now accept the view expressed by Epicurus, who died in 270 B.C.:[15]

> Death, therefore, the most awful of evils, is nothing to us, seeing that, when we are, death is not come, and, when death is come, we are not.

The growing fear, if it is not of the moment of dying nor of being dead, is of all that which now precedes dying for so many: the possibility of prolonged pain, the increasing weakness, the uncertainty, the loss of powers and chance of senility, the sense of being a burden. This fear is further nourished by the loss of trust in health professionals. In part, the loss of trust results from the abuses which have been exposed—the Medicaid scandals, the old-age home profiteering, the commercial exploitation of those who seek remedies for their ailments;[16] in part also because of the deceptive practices patients suspect, having seen how friends and relatives were kept in the dark; in part, finally, because of the sheer numbers of persons, often strangers, participating in the care of any one patient. Trust which might have gone to a doctor long known to the patient goes less easily to a team of strangers, no matter how expert or well-meaning.

It is with the working out of all that *informed consent*[17] implies and the information it presupposes that truth-telling is coming to be discussed in a serious way for the first time in the health professions. Informed consent is a farce if the information provided is distorted or withheld. And even complete information regarding surgical procedures or medication is obviously useless unless the patient also knows what the condition is that these are supposed to correct.

Bills of rights for patients, similarly stressing the right to be informed, are now gaining acceptance.[18] This right is not new, but the effort to implement it is. Nevertheless, even where patients are handed the most elegantly phrased Bill of Rights, their right to a truthful diagnosis and prognosis is by no means always respected.

The reason why even doctors who recognize a patient's right to have information might still not provide it brings us the [second] argument against telling all patients the truth. It holds that the information given might hurt the patient and that the concern for the right to such information is therefore a threat to proper health care. A patient, these doctors argue, may wish to commit suicide after being given discouraging news, or suffer a cardiac arrest, or simply cease to struggle, and thus not grasp the small remaining chance for recovery. And even where the outlook for a patient is very good, the disclosure of a minute risk can shock some patients or cause them to reject needed protection such as a vaccination or antibiotics.

The factual basis for this argument has been challenged from two points of view. The damages associated with the disclosure of sad news or risks are rarer than physicians believe; and the *benefits* which result from being informed are more substantial, even measurably so. Pain is tolerated more easily, recovery from surgery is quicker, and cooperation with therapy is greatly improved. The attitude that "what you don't know won't hurt you" is proving unrealistic; it is what patients do not know but vaguely suspect that causes them corrosive worry.

It is certain that no answers to this question of harm from information are the same for all patients. If we look, first, at the fear expressed by physicians that informing patients of even remote or unlikely risks connected with a drug prescription or operation might shock some and make others refuse the treatment that would have been best for them, it appears to be unfounded for the great majority of patients. Studies show that very few patients respond to being told of such risks by withdrawing their consent to the procedure and that those who do withdraw are the very ones who might well have been upset enough to sue the physician had they not been asked to consent beforehand.[19] It is possible that on even rarer occasions especially susceptible persons might manifest physical deteriorations from shock; some physicians have even asked whether patients who die after giving informed consent to an operation, but before it actually takes place, somehow expire because of the information given to them.[20] While such questions are unanswerable in any one case, they certainly argue in favor of caution, a real concern for the person to whom one is recounting the risks he or she will face, and sensitivity to all signs of distress.

The situation is quite different when persons who are already ill, perhaps already quite weak and discouraged, are told of a very serious prognosis. Physicians fear that such knowledge may cause the patients to commit suicide, or to be frightened or depressed to the point that their illness takes a downward turn. The fear that great numbers of patients will commit suicide appears to be unfounded.[21] And if some do, is that a response so unreasonable, so much against the patient's best interest that physicians ought to make it a reason for concealment or lies? Many societies have allowed suicide in the past; our own has decriminalized it; and some are coming to make distinctions among the many suicides which ought to be prevented if at all possible, and those which ought to be respected.[22]

Another possible response to very bleak news is the triggering of physiological mechanisms which allow death to come more quickly—a form of giving up or of preparing for the inevitable, depending on one's outlook. Lewis Thomas, studying responses in humans and animals, holds it not unlikely that:

> [...]there is a pivotal movement at some stage in the body's reaction to injury or disease, maybe in aging as well, when the organism concedes that it is finished and the time for dying is at hand, and at this moment the events that lead to death are launched, as a coordinated mechanism. Functions are then shut off, in sequence, irreversibly, and, while this is going on, a neural mechanism, held ready for this occasion, is switched on....[23]

Such a response may be appropriate, in which case it makes the moments of dying as peaceful as those who have died and been resuscitated so often testify. But it may also be brought on inappropriately, when the organism could have lived on, perhaps even induced malevolently, by external acts intended to kill. Thomas speculates that some of the deaths resulting from "hexing" are due to such responses. Lévi-Strauss describes deaths from exorcism and the casting of spells in ways which suggest that the same process may then be brought on by the community.[24]

It is not inconceivable that unhappy news abruptly conveyed, or a great shock given to someone unable to tolerate it, could also bring on such a "dying response," quite unintended by the speaker. There is every reason to be cautious and to try to know ahead of time how susceptible a patient might be to the accidental triggering—however rare—of such a response. One has to assume, however, that most of those who have survived long enough to be in a situation where their informed consent is asked have a very robust resistance to such accidental triggering of processes leading to death.

When, on the other hand, one considers those who are already near death, the "dying response" may be much less inappropriate, much less accidental, much less unreasonable. In most societies, long before the advent of modern medicine, human beings have made themselves ready for death once they felt its approach. Philippe Ariès describes how many in the Middle Ages prepared themselves for death when they "felt the end approach." They awaited death lying down, surrounded by friends and relatives. They recollected all they had lived through and done, pardoning all who stood near their deathbed, calling on God to bless them, and finally praying. "After the final prayer all that remained was to wait for death, and there was no reason for death to tarry."[25]

Modern medicine, in its valiant efforts to defer disease and to save lives, may be dislocating the conscious as well as the purely organic responses allowing death to come when it is inevitable, thus denying those who are dying the benefits of the traditional approach to death. In lying to them, and in pressing medical efforts to cure them long past the point of possible recovery, physicians may thus rob individuals of an autonomy few would choose to give up.

Sometimes, then, the "dying response" is a natural organic reaction at the time when the body has no further defense. Sometimes it is inappropriately brought on by news too shocking or given in too abrupt a manner. We need to learn a great deal more about this last category, no matter how small. But there is no evidence that patients in general will be debilitated by truthful information about their condition.

Apart from the possible harm from information, we are coming to learn much more about the benefits it can bring patients. People follow instructions more carefully if they know what their disease is and why they are asked to take medication; any benefits from those procedures are therefore much more likely to come about.[26] Similarly, people recover faster from surgery and tolerate pain with less medication if they understand what ails them and what can be done for them....[27]

NOTES

1 Plato, *The Republic*, 389 b.

2 B. C. Meyer, "Truth and the Physician," *Bulletin of the New York Academy of Medicine* 45 (1969): 59–71. See, too, the quotation from Dr. Henderson in Chapter 1 of this book [original source of this selection], p. 12.

3 W. H. S. Jones, trans., *Hippocrates*, Loeb Classical Library (Cambridge, Mass.: Harvard University Press, 1923), p. 164.

4 Reprinted in M. B. Etziony, *The Physician's Creed: An Anthology of Medical Prayers, Oaths and Codes of Ethics* (Springfield, Ill.: Charles C. Thomas, 1973), pp. 15–18.

5 See Harry Friedenwald, "The Ethics of the Practice of Medicine from the Jewish Point of View," *Johns Hopkins Hospital Bulletin*, no. 318 (August 1917), pp. 256–261.

6 "Ten Principles of Medical Ethics," *Journal of the American Medical Association* 164 (1957): 1119–20.

7 Mary Barrett, letter, *Boston Globe*, 16 November 1976, p. 1.

8 Though a minority of physicians have struggled to bring them to our attention. See Thomas Percival, *Medical Ethics*, 3d ed. (Oxford: John Henry Parker, 1849), pp. 132–41; Worthington Hooker, *Physician and Patient* (New York: Baker and Scribner, 1849), pp. 357–82; Richard C. Cabot, "Teamwork of Doctor and Patient Through the Annihilation of Lying," in *Social Service and the Art of Healing* (New York: Moffat, Yard & Co., 1909), pp. 116–70; Charles C. Lund, "The Doctor, the Patient, and the Truth," *Annals of Internal Medicine* 24 (1946): 955; Edmund Davies, "The Patient's Right to Know the Truth," *Proceedings of the Royal Society of Medicine* 66 (1973): 533–36.

9 For the views of physicians, see Donald Oken, "What to Tell Cancer Patients," *Journal of the American Medical Association* 175 (1961): 1120–28; and tabulations in Robert Veatch, *Death, Dying, and the Biological Revolution* (New Haven and London: Yale University Press, 1976), pp. 229–38. For the view of patients, see Veatch, *ibid.*; Jean Aitken-Swan and E.C. Easson, "Reactions of Cancer Patients on Being Told Their Diagnosis," *British Medical Journal*, 1959, pp. 779–83; Jim McIntosh, "Patients' Awareness and Desire for Information About Diagnosed but Undisclosed Malignant Disease," *The Lancet* 7 (1976): 300–303; William D. Kelly and Stanley R. Friesen, "Do Cancer Patients Want to Be Told?," *Surgery* 27 (1950): 822–26.

10 See Avery Weisman, *On Dying and Denying* (New York: Behavioral Publications, 1972); Elisabeth Kübler-Ross, *On Death and Dying* (New York: The Macmillan Co., 1969); Ernest Becker, *The Denial of Death* (New York: Free Press, 1973); Philippe Ariès, *Western Attitudes Toward Death*, trans. Patricia M. Ranum (Baltimore and London: Johns Hopkins University Press, 1974); and Sigmund Freud, "Negation," *Collected Papers*, ed. James Strachey (London: Hogarth Press, 1950), 5: 181–85.

11 Kübler-Ross, *On Death and Dying*, p. 34.

12 Michel de Montaigne, *Essays*, bk. 1, chap. 20.

13 It is in literature that these questions are most directly raised. Two recent works where they are taken up with striking beauty and simplicity are May Sarton, *As We Are Now* (New York: W.W. Norton & Co., 1973); and Freya Stark, *A Peak in Darien* (London: John Murray, 1976).

14 Herman Feifel et al., "Physicians Consider Death," *Proceedings of the American Psychoanalytical Association*, 1967, pp. 201–2.

15 See Diogenes Laertius, *Lives of Eminent Philosophers*, p. 651. Epicurus willed his garden to his friends and descendants, and wrote on the eve of dying:

   "On this blissful day, which is also the last of my life, I write to you. My continual sufferings from strangury and dysentery are so great that nothing could augment them; but over against them all I set gladness of mind at the remembrance of our past conversations." (Letter to Idomeneus, *Ibid.*, p. 549).

16 See Ivan Illich, *Medical Nemesis* (New York: Pantheon, 1976), for a critique of the iatrogenic tendencies of contemporary medical care in industrialized societies.

17 The law requires that inroads made upon a person's body take place only with the informed voluntary consent of that person. The term "informed consent" came into common use only after 1960, when it was used by the Kansas Supreme Court in *Nathanson vs. Kline*, 186 Kan. 393,350, p.2d,1093 (1960). The patient is now entitled to full disclosure of risks, benefits, and alternative treatments to any proposed procedure, both in therapy and in medical experimentation, except in emergencies or when the patient is incompetent, in which case proxy consent is required.

18 See, for example, "Statement on a Patient's Bill of Rights," reprinted in Stanley Joel Reiser, Arthur J. Dyck, and William J. Curran, *Ethics in Medicine* (Cambridge, Mass. and London: MIT Press, 1977), p. 148.

19 See Ralph Alfidi, "Informed Consent: A Study of Patient Reaction," *Journal of the American Medical Association* 216 (1971): 1325–29.

20 See Steven R. Kaplan, Richard A. Greenwald, and Arvey I. Rogers, Letter to the Editor, *New England Journal of Medicine* 296 (1977): 1127.

21 Oken, "What to Tell Cancer Patients"; Veatch, *Death, Dying, and the Biological Revolution*; Weisman, *On Dying and Denying*.

22 Norman L. Cantor, "A Patient's Decision to Decline Life-Saving Treatment: Bodily Integrity Versus the Preservation of Life," *Rutgers Law Review*, 26: 228–64; Danielle Gourevitch, "Suicide Among the Sick in Classical Antiquity," *Bulletin of the History of Medicine* 18 (1969): 501–18; for bibliography, see Bok, "Voluntary Euthanasia."

23 Lewis Thomas, "A Meliorist View of Disease and Dying," *The Journal of Medicine and Philosophy*, I (1976): 212–21.

24 Claude Lévi-Strauss, *Structural Anthropology* (New York: Basic Books, 1963), p. 167; See also Eric Cassell, "Permission to Die," in John Behnke and Sissela Bok, eds., *The Dilemmas of Euthanasia* (New York: Doubleday, Anchor Press, 1975), pp. 121–31.

25 Ariès, *Western Attitudes Toward Death*, p. 11.

26 Barbara S. Hulka, J. C. Cassel, et al., "Communication, Compliance, and Concordance between Physicians and Patients with Prescribed Medications," *American Journal of Public Health*, Sept. 1976, pp. 847–53. The study shows that of the nearly half of all patients who do not follow the prescriptions of the doctors (thus forgoing the intended effect of these prescriptions), many will follow them if adequately informed about the nature of their illness and what the proposed medication will do.

27 See Lawrence D. Egbert, George E. Batitt, et al., "Reduction of Postoperative Pain by Encouragement and Instruction of Patients," *New England Journal of Medicine* 270 (1964), pp. 825–827. See also: Howard Waitzskin and John D. Stoeckle, "The Communication of Information about Illness," *Advances in Psychosomatic Medicine*, vol. 8, 1972, pp. 185–215.

Lying and Deception: The Solution to a Dilemma in Medical Ethics
Joseph S. Ellin

Joseph S. Ellin is professor of philosophy at Western Michigan University. His specializations are philosophy of law and ethics. Ellin is the coeditor of *Profits and Professions* (1983) and author of "Special Professional Morality and the Duty of Veracity" and "Hume on the Morality of Princes."

Ellin poses the following apparent dilemma: "Either we say that veracity is an absolute duty, which is too strict; or we admit that it is prima facie only, which seems ad hoc, useless, and mushy." Ellin suggests that the resolution of the dilemma lies in the distinction drawn in morality between lying and deception. Conceiving the relationship between the patient and the physician as a "fiduciary" relationship, on the model of the lawyer-client relationship, Ellin proceeds to argue that physicians have an absolute duty not to lie to patients; however, they do not have even a prima facie duty not to deceive.

Should doctors deceive their patients? Should they ever lie to them? Situations arise in the practice of medicine in which it appears that a medically desirable course of treatment cannot be undertaken, or cannot succeed, unless the patient is deceived; or that a patient's health or

Reprinted with permission of the publisher from *Westminster Institute Review*, vol. 1 (May 1981), pp. 3–6.

state of mind would be damaged unless some information is concealed from him, at least temporarily. Sometimes medical personnel feel justified in practicing deceit for reasons which do not directly benefit patients; for example, Veatch's case of the medical students who are instructed to introduce themselves to hospital patients as "Doctor Smith" (instead of "Medical Student Smith") so as to overcome more quickly the anxiety they feel as they begin the transformation from layperson to physician.[1] Since in such cases most writers concede that patients ought not to be deceived unless something more important than truth is at stake, the problem is typically analyzed as determining the relative weight of the rights and interests involved: the patient's interest in the truth versus his or her interest in health and peace of mind, or perhaps the patient's right to the truth versus someone else's right to or interest in something else. When, however, the problem is posed in this way, the patient's right to the truth seems relatively unimportant, especially compared to an interest as obviously important as health, so that it seems evident that deception is justified, or even obligatory. The principle of not deceiving patients seems to have little weight when deception is thought necessary to achieve some desirable end.

The alternative, however, would seem to be to adopt the rigorist position that the duty of veracity is absolute, and this seems even less attractive. Most writers concede that the duty of veracity is prima facie only, at least as a principle of medical ethics where life and suffering are at stake; it does not appear plausible to adopt an ethic in which it is made obligatory to inflict avoidable anguish on someone already sick, especially where hope and good spirits, in addition to being desirable in themselves, may promote healing and help prolong life. One could hope to avoid this dilemma by holding that the duty of veracity, though not absolute, is to be given very great weight, and may be overridden only in the gravest cases; but this line conflicts with many of our intuitions about actual cases and will probably prove useless because ad hoc. There is a temptation to deceive, or at the very least to conceal information and blur the truth, not only to prevent anxiety and stimulate hope and good spirits, but to make possible the use of placebos, to persuade patients to abandon harmful habits, to generate confidence in the medical team and the like. The whole problem is to determine what counts as a sufficiently important end to justify an exception to the veracity principle. Hence the dilemma: either we say that veracity is an absolute duty, which is too strict; or we admit that it is prima facie only, which seems ad hoc, useless, and mushy.

I would like to suggest that the solution to this dilemma is to be found in the simple distinction between lying and deception. Writers on medical ethics do not seem to acknowledge this distinction, though it is commonly made in ordinary morality. But if we allow it, assuming also that we adopt a certain conception of the doctor-patient relationship, we can say that the duty not to lie is indeed absolute, but that there is no duty at all not to practice deception. Deception, on this view, is not even wrong prima facie, but is simply one tool the doctor may employ to achieve the ends of medicine. The conception of the doctor-patient relationship which allows us to reach this result is that of a fiduciary relationship, and the argument I wish to make is that two principles, the one prohibiting lying and the other allowing deception, may be defended through this conception.

A little reflection will make clear that in ordinary morality we do distinguish between lying and deception. Most of us would not lie, but we are much less scrupulous about deceiving. We might even make it a point of honor not to actually lie when we feel justified in planting false ideas in other people's minds. You ask me how my book is coming. I have done nothing on it in a month. I reply, "The work is very difficult." This is not a lie (the work *is* very difficult); but I have managed to convey a false impression. I prefer such evasion even to a white lie or harmless fiction ("Very well." "Slowly."). Countless examples suggest themselves. An amusing story is told of a certain St. Athanasius. His enemies coming to kill him, but mistaking him for another, asked, "Where is the traitor Athanasius?" The Saint replied, "Not far away."[2]

One reason we do not distinguish between lying and deception in the medical context is that deception is sometimes used for unacceptable ends. An example of such malignant deception is given by Marsha Millman. A doctor performs a liver biopsy (a procedure not without risk) under circumstances in which the procedure is probably not justified. He avoids telling the patient the results for some days. Finally he says, "Don't worry, the biopsy didn't show anything wrong with your liver." When the patient after much agitation is allowed to read her chart, she discovers that the report on the biopsy reads, "No analysis, specimen insufficient for diagnosis."[3]

When doctors deceive for self-interested motives, to cover up their bad judgment or their failures, we are apt to think the distinction between lying and deception is mere hair-splitting. Millman asserts that the doctor "had evasively lied." Though strictly speaking inaccurate, this characterization is correct from the moral point of view, since because of the doctor's bad motive, the evasion may be considered morally no different from a lie. But the situation is different when the motives are benevolent. James Childress gives the interesting case of a patient who, due to constant pain caused by chronic intestinal problems, injects himself six times daily with a strong (but allegedly non-addictive) pain-killer. When the patient is admitted to the hospital with another complaint, the staff decides to wean him from the drug by gradually diluting the dosage with saline solution. After a time, when the pain does not recur, the patient is told that he is no longer receiving the medication.[4]

Here we have a treatment plan that can work only through deception; if the patient knows he is not receiving the usual dosage, his pain will recur. Hence the staff does not have the option of simply telling him what they intend to do and then doing it over his objections. The staff's alternatives therefore are: comply with the patient's wishes and administer medication they believe to be unnecessary and harmful; promise to do what he wants and then follow their withdrawal plan anyway, i.e., lie; avoid telling him what they are doing without actually lying about it. If it were not possible to carry out the plan without lying, if for example the patient asked direct questions about his medication, the choice thus posed between abandoning the plan and lying to him would seem far more difficult than the choice between abandoning the plan and simply deceiving him. It seems preferable to carry out the plan without actually lying; so much so that we are tempted to say that if the staff could not avoid lying, it would be better to abandon the plan, whereas employing the plan using deception is quite justifiable, given the alternative.

The distinction between lying and deception may, however, seem unjustified from what Sissela Bok has called "the perspective of the deceived." As far as the deceived is concerned, deception can be just as bad as a lie. Both give rise to resentment, disappointment and suspicion. Those deceived, as Bok says, "feel wronged; ...They see that they were manipulated, that the deceit made them unable to make choices for themselves ...unable to act as they would have wanted to act."[5] The deceived has been led to have false beliefs, has been deprived of control of a situation, has been subjected to manipulation, and so suffers a sense of betrayal and wounded dignity. Like lying, deception harms many interests. We have an interest in acquiring true beliefs, in having the information needed to make wise decisions about our lives, in being treated as trustworthy and intelligent persons, in being able to trust those in whom we put our trust. The deceiver, either intentionally or inadvertently, harms these interests. To the person whose interests are harmed by deceit, it is small comfort that the deceit did not involve an actual lie.

Those who find the lying/deception distinction objectionable are probably thinking of the harm each does

to the deceived. Their argument is that if it is equally harmful to deceive and to lie, then no distinction between the two should be allowed. However, such a view oversimplifies the moral situation, as analysis of deception will reveal.

Intentional deception, short of lying, involves two elements: a statement or action from which it is expected that the person who is the target of the deception will draw a false conclusion, and failure to provide information which would prevent the conclusion from being drawn. The important thing is that the false information itself is not actually presented to the person deceived: everything said and done is in a sense innocent and within the rights of the deceiver. Because of this, it is possible to take the view that intentional deception is no moral wrong at all. No less a moralist than Kant writes: "I can make believe, make a demonstration from which others will draw the conclusion I want, though they have no right to expect that my action will express my real mind. In that case, I have not lied to them...I may, for instance, wish people to think that I am off on a journey, and so I pack my luggage."[6] Kant evidently sees nothing wrong with this; his view seems to be that he has every right to pack his luggage if he chooses and if others draw certain conclusions (however reasonable) which turn out to be false, they have only themselves to blame. This, however, is too lenient on deceivers. If a person says or does something, knowing or believing that others are likely to draw false conclusions from it, and if the person refrains from providing them information he knows would prevent the false conclusions from being drawn, then he is at least in part responsible for the deception. But though he is partly responsible, he is not as responsible as he would be were he to present the false conclusion himself. Even when there is a lie, of course, the victim must bear some of the blame for being deceived, since he has imprudently trusted the liar and failed to confirm the statements made. But when a victim is deceived without a lie, he is more to blame, since he has not only failed to investigate a situation, but has also drawn or jumped to a conclusion which goes beyond the statements made to him. Even where the conclusion is a very natural inference from the statements or actions, the fact that it is an inference shows that the deceived participates in his own deception.

However, this is not the only reason why deception is considered less bad than lying. When I lie, I tell you something which, since it is false, ought not to be believed; this harms your interest in having true beliefs. When I deceive, however, I merely give you grounds for an inference which does not actually follow; this harms your interest in having good grounds for inferences, but does not directly harm your interest in having true beliefs.

The third reason why deception is not as bad as lying is that lying violates the social contract in a way that deception does not. In a sense, the social contract is renewed by every act of speech (more properly by every assertion), since to speak is implicitly to give an assurance that what one says is true. Every statement implies a promise or certification of its truth. A lie, which with a single act both implies a promise and violates it, thus involves a self-contradiction. It could be said that the social contract prohibits deception generally, on the rule-utilitarian ground that social life would be unduly burdened if, as in a spy novel, every apparently innocent action were a potential source of misinformation. But though deception may be a violation of the rules (lying, too, is a violation of the rules in this sense), it is not at the same time a reaffirmation of the rules, and hence is not an implicit self-contradiction. We can understand this when we see that although the social contract may prohibit deception, it cannot prohibit deceptive statements, since deceptive statements which are not lies are true, and the social contract cannot prohibit true statements. The contract does prohibit making true statements with the intent to deceive, or in circumstances such that the speaker does or should realize that the statement is likely to deceive. But an intention is not a promise, not even an implicit promise, hence there is nothing self-contradictory about deception. To the extent that the deceiver affirms the contract by his statement, he also obeys the contract, since his statement is true.

This analysis has an important consequence for the theory of professional morality I am defending here, since it enables us to see the difference between lying and deception with regard to trust. In everyday life we have the feeling that the liar is less trustworthy than the deceiver. Why is this, since they both intend to mislead? The conceptual basis of this perception is that the liar reaffirms the promise of the social contract in the very act (the lie) by which he violates that promise. The deceiver may violate the social contract but does not promise to obey it in the very act of violation. Doubtless a deceiver should not be trusted, but it seems reasonable that we would be even more wary, more on guard against a person who not only deceives, but breaks a promise in the very act of reaffirming it. The significance of this distinction for professional morality I shall explain shortly.

So far I have argued that morality draws a distinction between lying and intentional deception. Now I must address the more controversial question of what the doctor's obligations are with respect to the duty of veracity. I will argue that if we conceive the doctor-patient relationship as a fiduciary relationship, then the doctor has an absolute duty not to lie, but not even a prima facie duty not to deceive. This is different from the view of ordinary morality which condemns both lying and deception, holds both wrong prima facie only, but holds lying morally worse. My defense of the above propositions as principles of medical ethics rests partly on conceptual points, and partly on contingent psychological facts having to do with the conditions of trust. It is because trust is more important in the doctor-patient relationship, conceived as fiduciary, than in ordinary life, that there is a difference between ordinary and professional morality.

As is well-known, there are many conceptions of the doctor-patient relationship. One can think of doctors as priests, friends, engineers, business partners, or partners in health. One can think of the relationship with patients as contractual, philanthropic, collegial, even exploitive. Doubtless there is merit in each of these points of view; each represents some significant truth about some doctor-patient relationships. Such conceptions or models are useful because they illuminate ethical principles; there are connections between the model of the relationship and the ethical principles which should govern it. A doctor who thinks of himself as a body mechanic will have different views about providing information to patients than one who thinks of himself as engaged with the patient in a partnership in healing. (It is unlikely that the doctors in the previous examples thought of themselves as engaged in a partnership with their patients.) Similarly, a doctor who imagines himself to be a patient's friend takes a different view of how much time he should spend with a patient than one who believes he is merely fulfilling a contract for services.

Undoubtedly many medical personnel think of themselves as having a fiduciary relationship, or something like it, with their patients or clients. The fiduciary conception is based on the legal notion of someone, the fiduciary, who has certain responsibilities for the welfare of another, the beneficiary. It is important to recognize that a fiduciary's responsibilities are limited to the specific goals of the relationship. A lawyer, for example, has responsibility for the client's legal affairs (or some of them), an accountant for his financial affairs, etc. Every beneficiary will have many interests which are external to the responsibilities of the fiduciary. This is not to say that these other interests might not impinge on the content of that relationship, but only that since the relationship was established for certain purposes relative to the specific competencies of the professional, the professional's responsibilities stop at the edges of these purposes.

If I seek legal assistance, it is because I want my legal interests to be protected; I do not expect my lawyer to take responsibility for my emotional stability, the strength of my marriage, how I use my leisure time, etc., though of course these other interests of mine might be affected by my legal condition. Where my legal interests conflict with some of my other interests, it is up to me, not my lawyer, to make the necessary choices. Those who expect their lawyer or doctor to look after a broad range of their interests, perhaps even their total welfare, obviously do not have a fiduciary conception of the professional relationship; they think of the professional as priest, friend, or some similarly broad model.

Since a fiduciary relationship is limited by specific defining goals, it is not a contractual relationship, although a legal contract may be the instrument that binds the relationship. A contractual relationship is more open, in that the parties may write anything they please into the contract. The responsibilities of the professional are exactly those stated in the contract, neither more nor less. In a contractual relationship, the professional's decisions will be guided by his interpretation of what the contract requires. Thus if a doctor believes he has agreed with the patient to do everything possible to restore the patient's health and preserve the patient's life, he will take one course of action. If, however, he believes he has also agreed to protect the patient's family from prolonged worry and exhaustion of resources, though these are not strictly speaking medical goals, he may well do or recommend something else.

Now in addition to one's interests in health, financial condition, etc., a person has moral interests. I have an interest not to be lied to, not to be manipulated, not to be treated with contempt. There is no theoretical reason why these moral interests could not conflict with other interests such as health. But since under the fiduciary conception a professional's responsibility is to foster only those interests which define the relationship, the professional is not obligated to foster the client's moral interests. Normally, of course, there will not be a conflict, and no doubt in certain professions, such as law, opportunity for conflict is small. But such conflicts do arise in the practice of medicine (the Childress example is a clear case). The fiduciary conception imposes no

professional obligation on the doctor to be concerned with these interests. This is not to say that a doctor ought not to be concerned with such interests. But if he should be, this is either because the doctor-patient relationship ought not to be construed as fiduciary, or because under certain circumstances, the commands of ordinary morality ought to override the commands of medical ethics.

Since a patient's interest in not being deceived is a moral interest and not a health interest, the doctor-patient relationship, construed as fiduciary, does not even prima facie exclude deception. To argue that it does, is to construe the relationship as priestly, friendly, contractual or something else. One could hold that if general moral obligations take precedence over professional obligations, the doctor has a general moral obligation not to deceive, even if he has no such professional obligation. That general moral obligations take precedence over professional obligations is a proposition many professionals would dispute, however; lawyers for example will argue that their general moral obligation not to harm or pain innocent people is overridden by their professional obligation to do everything possible to protect their client's legal interests.[7]

It may seem to follow from this that doctors also have no obligation to avoid actual lying when, in their best judgment, a patient's health might be injured were he to learn some truth. To see why this is not the case we have to distinguish between the obligations *of* the doctor-patient relationship, and the obligations which make the relationship possible. In a fiduciary relationship, the only obligation *of* the relationship is to do whatever is necessary to further the goals by which the relationship is defined. But it might be the case that the relationship could not be established unless other obligations were respected. If this is the case, it follows that obligations which make the relationship possible override, in cases of conflict, obligations *of* the relationship, since the latter could not exist without the former (if the relationship is not established, then neither are any of its obligations). Hence, if the obligation not to lie is an obligation which makes the relationship possible, it follows that this obligation overrides even the obligation to protect health, and is thus an absolute.

The argument that lying destroys the doctor-patient relationship, conceived as fiduciary, is partly a conceptual argument, partly an argument based on judgment and experience. It is often said that the doctor-patient relationship depends heavily on trust. The patient puts himself (often literally) in the hands of his doctor. Although this could be true to an extent of any interpretation of the relationship, it is less true of some interpretations than others. Contracts, for example, do not depend on trust so much as on an understanding of mutual self-interest; a contractual relationship succeeds when each party understands that it is not in either party's best interest to violate the contract. Even the priest or friend roles do not require trust as their foundation, though they do generate trust. A priest is someone who has a special calling or vocation; his entire life is dedicated to an ideal of service. We trust him because his life witnesses his trustworthiness.[8] A friendship relation is based on personal satisfactions and mutual compatibility; these generate trust but do not rest on it. It is the fiduciary relationship which depends heavily on trust. A fiduciary must be trusted to act with the true interests of the beneficiary in view; the law recognizes this by defining trust as "a fiduciary relationship."[9] If, however, we were to allow the fiduciary to lie, the trust basis of the relationship would be undermined and the relationship itself jeopardized. A lie, it will be recalled, violates a kind of implicit assurance we give when we speak, namely, that our words will be used to state the truth. Deception through evasive or misleading statements which are nonetheless true, does not violate such an assurance but accords with it. The deceiver can thus be trusted at least to speak the truth, while the liar violates the very assurance he is giving with his speech.

Although the argument that the liar undermines the basis of the fiduciary relationship by showing himself to be untrustworthy is empirical, it is not open to one kind of objection commonly brought against empirical arguments in ethics. The objection is that if the only reason to avoid a certain practice is that the practice leads to undesirable consequences, then the solution is to employ the practice anyway, but do so in such a way that the consequences are avoided. Thus Alan Goldman criticizes arguments which oppose lying or deceiving by "appeal to certain systematic disutilities that might be projected, e.g., effects upon the agent's trustworthiness and upon the trust that other people are willing to accord him if his lies are discovered." According to Goldman, "The only conclusion that I would draw from the empirical points...is that doctors should perhaps be better trained in psychology in order to be able to judge the effects..." of the decision to lie or not.[10]

Goldman's argument is good not against those who oppose lying on the ground that it destroys trust, but only against those who hold this and *also* hold (as Goldman himself holds) that lying would be wrong even if it didn't affect trust. If lying is wrong whether it affects trust or not, then the fact that it affects trust obviously cannot be the reason why it is wrong. But as I do not claim that lying is wrong (in the professional-client relationship) if it does not affect trust, I need not deny that the tendency of lying to destroy trust might from time to time be countered by certain clever psychological tactics on the part of liars. This does not in the least show that lying does not tend to destroy trust. However, I maintain that the tendency of lying to destroy trust is considerably greater than the tendency of deception to destroy trust, and this I argue partly on the basis of the conceptual difference between lying and deception, partly on the basis of experience. Lying is more destructive to trust than deception because lying is a greater violation of the social contract. The liar by his false speech violates the very promise that he makes in speaking, the promise to speak the truth. And it is for this reason, as I think experience reveals, that we find ourselves less trusting of someone who has lied to us, than of someone who has misled us or created a false impression.

Given this threat to trust, it seems plausible to hold that lying is too dangerous ever to be allowed in a relationship founded on trust. Suppose we adopted a rule which made lying only prima facie wrong, and thus permitted lying in certain very serious cases. The patient would know that the doctor could not be trusted to tell the truth, even in response to a direct question, when the doctor deemed it unwise to do so; and therefore the patient would know that the doctor could never be believed, since even an apparently trivial matter might in fact be serious enough for the doctor to feel justified in lying about. Of course the fact that the patient would know this does not necessarily mean that the patient would not trust the doctor anyway. But a patient who has been lied to has been given very strong grounds to conclude that the doctor is not to be trusted, so that even a single justified lie is likely to undermine the patient's trust.

Let us test the prohibition of lying against a case where our intuitions seem to lead us to the opposite conclusion. Gert and Culver give the following case: "Mrs. E is in extremely critical condition after an automobile accident which has taken the life of one of her four children and severely injured another. Dr. P believes that her very tenuous hold on life might be weakened by the shock of hearing of her children's conditions, so he decides to deceive her for a short period of time."[11] According to these authors, a rational person would choose to be deceived in such circumstances, so there is nothing wrong with the doctor's decision to deceive her. As is typical of the medical ethics literature, the authors do not distinguish between lying and deception. On our principles, there is nothing even prima facie wrong with the doctor's use of evasive or misleading statements to conceal the truth. But suppose Mrs. E demands a straight answer from which evasion offers no escape. Gert and Culver seem to propose that the question to be answered is whether a rational person would want to be lied to in these circumstances, but as there does not seem to be any way to arrive at an answer to this question, their proposal does not really advance beyond our intuitions. In this case, our intuitions strongly suggest that lying would be justified in order to protect the woman's health, but on the principles advanced in this essay, lying is not permitted, since if Dr. P lies in response to Mrs. E's direct question, she will eventually discover that he cannot be trusted, and that therefore they cannot enjoy a relationship based on trust. Of course this is not to say that the doctor must tell her the truth in the bluntest or most painful way, but only that he must not lie. Where a harmful truth cannot be concealed, it is up to the doctor to reveal it in a way least damaging to the patient. To take a different view is to hold that the doctor-patient relationship is not a fiduciary relationship based on trust, but something else, friendship perhaps, or maybe some form of paternalism, in which the doctor has the responsibility of balancing all of the patient's interests and making decisions in light of his conception of the patient's total welfare. If, however, these conceptions of the relationship seem unattractive to us (and I have not argued that they should seem unattractive) we will have to take the view, intuitions to the contrary notwithstanding, that even in the situation just described, the doctor's duty is to tell the truth.

NOTES

1 Robert Veatch, *Case Studies in Medical Ethics* (Cambridge: Harvard University Press, 1977), pp. 147f.
2 I found this example in an unpublished paper by James Rachels, "Honesty." Rachels evidently borrowed it from P. T. Geach, *The Virtues* (Cambridge: Cambridge University Press, 1977), p. 115.
3 Marcia Millman, *The Unkindest Cut* (New York: William Morrow and Co., 1977), pp. 138f.
4 James Childress, "Paternalism and Health Care," in *Medical Responsibility*, ed. Wade L. Robison and Michael S. Pritchard (New York: Humana Press, 1979), pp. 15–27.
5 Sissela Bok, *Lying* (New York: Pantheon Books, 1978), ch. 2.
6 Immanuel Kant, *Lectures on Ethics*, trans. Louis Infeld (New York: Harper and Row, 1963), pp. 147–154.
7 The contention that, as a general rule, professional obligations override ordinary moral obligations, is critically examined and disputed by Alan H. Goldman, *The Moral Foundations of Professional Ethics* (Totowa, N.J.: Littlefield, Adams and Co., 1980).
8 On the idea of medicine as a calling founded on "covenant" which transforms the doctor, see William F. May, "Code, Covenant, Contract or Philanthropy," *Hastings Center Report* 5, 6 (December, 1975): 29–38.
9 "Trust. Noun: a fiduciary relationship; a matter of confidence." *Ballantine's Law Dictionary*, 3rd ed.
10 Goldman, *Professional Ethics*, p. 176.
11 Bernard Gert and Charles Culver, "The Justification of Paternalism" in Robison and Pritchard, *Medical Responsibility*, p. 7.

Informed Consent

Opinion in *Canterbury v. Spence*
Judge Spotswood W. Robinson III

Spotswood W. Robinson III is a circuit court judge serving on the U.S. Court of Appeals, District of Columbia. Prior to his appointment to the bench, Judge Robinson served as an associate professor of law at Howard University (1939–1949) and as the dean of the Law School (1960–1963).

A 19-year-old man, John W. Canterbury, developed paraplegia after a laminectomy (a surgical procedure). Prior to the surgery, his physician, William Thornton Spence, did not inform Canterbury that the operation involved the risk of paralysis. Canterbury brought an action against the physician and the hospital. In defending his decision to withhold the information from the patient, Dr. Spence testified that communicating the 1 percent risk "is not good medical practice because it might deter patients from undergoing needed surgery and might produce adverse psychological reactions which could preclude the success of the operation." In this selection, Judge Robinson argues that an adult patient of sound mind has the right to determine what should be done to his or her body. Because of this right, a physician has the duty to inform the patient about those dangers that "are material" to the patient's decision. The Court allows two exceptions to this rule of disclosure. It holds, however, that a physician cannot remain silent simply because divulgence might prompt the patient to forgo therapy that the physician perceives as necessary.

Suits charging failure by a physician adequately to disclose the risks and alternatives of proposed treatment are not innovations in American law. They date back a good half-century, and in the last decade they have multiplied rapidly. There is, nonetheless, disagreement among the courts and the commentators on many major questions, and there is no precedent of our own directly in point. For the tools enabling resolution of the issues on this appeal, we are forced to begin at first principles.

The root premise is the concept, fundamental in American jurisprudence, that "[e]very human being of adult years and sound mind has a right to determine what shall be done with his own body...." True consent to what happens to one's self is the informed exercise of a choice, and that entails an opportunity to evaluate knowledgeably the options available and the risks attendant upon each. The average patient has little or no understanding of the medical arts, and ordinarily has only his physician to whom he can look for enlightenment

U.S. Court of Appeals, District of Columbia Circuit; May 19, 1972. 464 Federal Reporter, 2nd Series, 772. Reprinted with permission of West Publishing Company.

with which to reach an intelligent decision.[1] From these almost axiomatic considerations springs the need, and in turn the requirement, of a reasonable divulgence by physician to patient to make such a decision possible.[2]

A physician is under a duty to treat his patient skillfully, but proficiency in diagnosis and therapy is not the full measure of his responsibility. The cases demonstrate that the physician is under an obligation to communicate specific information to the patient when the exigencies of reasonable care call for it. Due care may require a physician perceiving symptoms of bodily abnormality to alert the patient to the condition. It may call upon the physician confronting an ailment which does not respond to his ministrations to inform the patient thereof. It may command the physician to instruct the patient as to any limitations to be presently observed for his own welfare, and as to any precautionary therapy he should seek in the future. It may oblige the physician to advise the patient of the need for or desirability of any alternative treatment promising greater benefit than that being pursued. Just as plainly, due care normally demands that the physician warn the patient of any risks to his well-being which contemplated therapy may involve.

The context in which the duty of risk-disclosure arises is invariably the occasion for decision as to whether a particular treatment procedure is to be undertaken. To the physician, whose training enables a self-satisfying evaluation, the answer may seem clear, but it is the prerogative of the patient, not the physician, to determine for himself the direction in which his interests seem to lie. To enable the patient to chart his course understandably, some familiarity with the therapeutic alternatives and their hazards becomes essential.

A reasonable revelation in these respects is not only a necessity but, as we see it, is as much a matter of the physician's duty. It is a duty to warn of the dangers lurking in the proposed treatment, and that is surely a facet of due care. It is, too, a duty to impart information which the patient has every right to expect.[3] The patient's reliance upon the physician is a trust of the kind which traditionally has exacted obligations beyond those associated with arms-length transactions. His dependence upon the physician for information affecting his well-being, in terms of contemplated treatment, is well-nigh abject. As earlier noted, long before the instant litigation arose, courts had recognized that the physician had the responsibility of satisfying the vital informational needs of the patient. More recently, we ourselves have found "in the fiducial qualities of [the physician-patient] relationship the physician's duty to reveal to the patient that which in his best interests it is important that he should know." We now find, as a part of the physician's overall obligation to the patient, a similar duty of reasonable disclosure of the choices with respect to proposed therapy and the dangers inherently and potentially involved....

Once the circumstances give rise to a duty on the physician's part to inform his patient, the next inquiry is the scope of the disclosure the physician is legally obliged to make. The courts have frequently confronted this problem but no uniform standard defining the adequacy of the divulgence emerges from the decisions. Some have said "full" disclosure, a norm we are unwilling to adopt literally. It seems obviously prohibitive and unrealistic to expect physicians to discuss with their patients every risk of proposed treatment—no matter how small or remote—and generally unnecessary from the patient's viewpoint as well. Indeed, the cases speaking in terms of "full" disclosure appear to envision something less than total disclosure, leaving unanswered the question of just how much.

The larger number of courts, as might be expected, have applied tests framed with reference to prevailing fashion within the medical profession. Some have measured the disclosure by "good medical practice," others by what a reasonable practitioner would have bared under the circumstances, and still others by what medical custom in the community would demand. We have explored this rather considerable body of law but are unprepared to follow it. The duty to disclose, we have reasoned, arises from phenomena apart from medical custom and practice. The latter, we think, should no more establish the scope of the duty than its existence. Any definition of scope in terms purely of a professional standard is at odds with the patient's prerogative to decide on projected therapy himself. That prerogative, we have said, is at the very foundation of the duty to disclose, and both the patient's right to know and the physician's correlative obligation to tell him are diluted to the extent that its compass is dictated by the medical profession.[4]

In our view, the patient's right of self-decision shapes the boundaries of the duty to reveal. That right can be effectively exercised only if the patient possesses enough information to enable an intelligent choice. The scope of the physician's communications to the patient, then, must be measured by the patient's need, and that need is the information material to the decision. Thus the test for determining whether a particular peril must be divulged is its materiality to the patient's decision: all risks potentially affecting the decision must be unmasked. And to safeguard the patient's interest in achieving his own determination on treatment, the law must itself set the standard for adequate disclosure.

Optimally for the patient, exposure of a risk would be mandatory whenever the patient would deem it significant to his decision, either singly or in combination with other risks. Such a requirement, however, would summon the physician to second-guess the patient, whose ideas on materiality could hardly be known to the physician. That would make an undue demand upon medical practitioners, whose conduct, like that of others, is to be measured in terms of reasonableness. Consonantly with orthodox negligence doctrine, the physician's liability for nondisclosure is to be determined on the basis of foresight, not hindsight; no less than any other aspect of negligence, the issue on nondisclosure must be approached from the viewpoint of the reasonableness of the physician's divulgence in terms of what he knows or should know to be the patient's informational needs. If, but only if, the fact-finder can say that the physician's communication was unreasonably inadequate is an imposition of liability legally or morally justified.

Of necessity, the content of the disclosure rests in the first instance with the physician. Ordinarily it is only he who is in position to identify particular dangers; always he must make a judgment, in terms of materiality, as to whether and to what extent revelation to the patient is called for. He cannot know with complete exactitude what the patient would consider important to his decision, but on the basis of his medical training and experience he can sense how the average, reasonable patient expectably would react. Indeed, with knowledge of, or ability to learn, his patient's background and current condition, he is in a position superior to that of most others—attorneys, for example—who are called upon to make judgments on pain of liability in damages for unreasonable miscalculation.

From these considerations we derive the breadth of the disclosure of risks legally to be required. The scope of the standard is not subjective as to either the physician or the patient; it remains objective with due regard for the patient's informational needs and with suitable leeway for the physician's situation. In broad outline, we agree that "[a] risk is thus material when a reasonable person, in what the physician knows or should know to be the patient's position, would be likely to attach significance to the risk or cluster of risks in deciding whether or not to forgo the proposed therapy."

The topics importantly demanding a communication of information are the inherent and potential hazards of the proposed treatment, the alternatives to that treatment, if any, and the results likely if the patient remains untreated. The factors contributing significance to the dangerousness of a medical technique are, of course, the incidence of injury and the degree of the harm threatened. A very small chance of death or serious disablement may well be significant; a potential disability which dramatically outweighs the potential benefit of the therapy or the detriments of the existing malady may summon discussion with the patient.

There is no bright line separating the significant from the insignificant; the answer in any case must abide a rule of reason. Some dangers—infection, for example—are inherent in any operation; there is no obligation to communicate those of which persons of average sophistication are aware. Even more clearly, the physician bears no responsibility for discussion of hazards the patient has already discovered, or those having no apparent materiality to patients' decision on therapy. The disclosure doctrine, like others marking lines between permissible and impermissible behavior in medical practice, is in essence a requirement of conduct prudent under the circumstances. Whenever nondisclosure of particular risk information is open to debate by reasonable-minded men, the issue is for the finder of the facts.

Two exceptions to the general rule of disclosure have been noted by the courts. Each is in the nature of a physician's privilege not to disclose, and the reasoning underlying them is appealing. Each, indeed, is but a recognition that, as important as is the patient's right to know, it is greatly outweighed by the magnitudinous circumstances giving rise to the privilege. The first comes into play when the patient is unconscious or otherwise incapable of consenting, and harm from a failure to treat is imminent and outweighs any harm threatened by the proposed treatment. When a genuine emergency of that sort arises, it is settled that the impracticality of conferring with the patient dispenses with need for it. Even in situations of that character the physician should, as current law requires, attempt to secure a relative's consent if possible. But if time is too short to accommodate discussion, obviously the physician should proceed with the treatment.

The second exception obtains when risk-disclosure poses such a threat of detriment to the patient as to become unfeasible or contraindicated from a medical point of view. It is recognized that patients occasionally become so ill or emotionally distraught on disclosure as to foreclose a rational decision, or complicate or hinder the treatment, or perhaps even pose psychological damage to the patient. Where that is so, the cases have generally held that the physician is armed with a privilege to keep the information from the patient, and we think it clear that portents of that type may justify the physician in action he deems medically warranted. The critical inquiry is whether the physician responded to a sound medical judgment that communication of the risk information would present a threat to the patient's well-being.

The physician's privilege to withhold information for therapeutic reasons must be carefully circumscribed, however, for otherwise it might devour the disclosure rule itself. The privilege does not accept the paternalistic notion that the physician may remain silent simply because divulgence might prompt the patient to forgo therapy the physician feels the patient really needs. That attitude presumes instability or perversity for even the normal patient, and runs counter to the foundation principle that the patient should and ordinarily can make the choice for himself. Nor does the privilege contemplate operation save where the patient's reaction to risk information, as reasonably foreseen by the physician, is menacing. And even in a situation of that kind, disclosure to a close relative with a view to securing consent to the proposed treatment may be the only alternative open to the physician. . . .

NOTES

1 Patients ordinarily are persons unlearned in the medical sciences. Some few, of course, are schooled in branches of the medical profession or in related fields. But even within the latter group variations in degree of medical knowledge specifically referable to particular therapy may be broad, as for example, between a specialist and a general practitioner, or between a physician and a nurse. It may well be, then, that it is only in the unusual case that a court could safely assume that the patient's insights were on a parity with those of the treating physician.

2 The doctrine that a consent effective as authority to form therapy can arise only from the patient's understanding of alternatives to and risks of the therapy is commonly denominated "informed consent." The same appellation is frequently assigned to the doctrine requiring physicians, as a matter of duty to patients, to communicate information as to such alternatives and risks. See, *e.g.*, Comment, Informed Consent in Medical Malpractice, 55 Calif. L. Rev. 1396 (1967). While we recognize the general utility of shorthand phrases in literary expositions, we caution that uncritical use of the "informed consent" label can be misleading. See, *e.g.*, Plante, An Analysis of "Informed Consent," 36 Ford. L. Rev. 639, 671–72 (1968).

In duty-to-disclose cases, the focus of attention is more properly upon the nature and content of the physician's divulgence than the patient's understanding or consent. Adequate disclosure and informed consent are, of course, two sides of the same coin—the former a *sine qua non* of the latter. But the vital inquiry on duty to disclose relates to the physician's performance of an obligation, while one of the difficulties with analysis in terms of "informed consent" is its tendency to imply that what is decisive is the degree of the patient's comprehension. As we later emphasize, the physician discharges the duty when he makes a reasonable effort to convey sufficient information although the patient, without fault of the physician, may not fully grasp it. Even though the factfinder may have occasion to draw an inference on the state of the patient's enlightenment, the fact-finding process on performance of the duty ultimately reaches back to what the physician actually said or failed to say. And while the factual conclusion on adequacy of the revelation will vary as between patients—as, for example, between a lay patient and a physician-patient—the fluctuations are attributable to the kind of divulgence which may be reasonable under the circumstances.

3 Some doubt has been expressed as to ability of physicians to suitably communicate their evaluations of risks and the advantages of optional treatment, and as to the lay patient's ability to understand what the physician tells him. Karchmer, Informed Consent: A Plaintiff's Medical Malpractice "Wonder Drug," 31 Mo. L. Rev. 29, 41 (1966). We do not share these apprehensions. The discussion need not be a disquisition, and surely the physician is not compelled to give his patient a short medical education; the disclosure rule summons the physician only to a reasonable explanation. That means generally informing the patient in non-technical terms as to what is at stake: the therapy alternatives open to him, the goals expectably to be achieved, and the risks that may ensue from particular treatment and no treatment. So informing the patient hardly taxes the physician, and it must be the exceptional patient who cannot comprehend such an explanation at least in a rough way.

4 For similar reasons, we reject the suggestion that disclosure should be discretionary with the physician.

The Values Underlying Informed Consent
President's Commission for the Study of Ethical Problems in Medicine and Biomedical and Behavioral Research

The President's Commission, created in 1978, began its deliberations early in 1980 and ended them in 1983. Its task was to consider several issues raised by the practice of medicine and the distribution of health care. The Commission issued reports on the informed consent requirement, the definition of death, genetic screening and counseling, the compensation of research subjects, and the distribution of health care. During its life, the Commission included twenty-one commissioners. It was chaired by Morris B. Abraham; its executive director was Alexander Morgan Capron, who is Norman Topping Professor of Law, Medicine, and Public Policy at the University of Southern California, Los Angeles.

The Commission identifies and discusses two values that should guide decision making in the health-care provider-patient relationship: the promotion of a patient's well-being and respect for a patient's self-determination. The Commission locates the ethical foundation of informed consent in the promotion of these two values and makes recommendations intended to ensure that these values are respected and enhanced. In making its recommendations, the Commission rejects the idea that obtaining informed consent is simply a matter of reciting the contents of a form and getting a signature. It sees ethically valid consent as a *process* of shared decision making based on mutual respect and participation. Although stressing the importance of self-determination, the Commission recognizes that some people may be permanently incapable of making their own decisions and that others may be temporarily unable to exercise their right of self-determination. It, therefore, provides some recommendations about making decisions for those unable to do so.

What are the values that ought to guide decisionmaking in the provider-patient relationship or by which the success of a particular interaction can be judged? The Commission finds two to be central: promotion of a patient's well-being and respect for a patient's self-determination.

SERVING THE PATIENT'S WELL-BEING

Therapeutic interventions are intended first and foremost to improve a patient's health. In most circumstances, people agree in a general way on what "improved health" means. Restoration of normal functioning (such as the repair of a fractured limb) and

Reprinted from President's Commission for the Study of Ethical Problems in Medicine and Biomedical and Behavioral Research, *Making Health Care Decisions*, Volume One: Report (1982), pp. 41–46, 2–6.

avoidance of untimely death (such as might occur without the use of antibiotics to control life-threatening infections in otherwise healthy persons) are obvious examples. Health care is, in turn, usually a means of promoting patients' well-being. The connection between a particular health care decision and an individual's well-being is not perfect, however. First, the definition of health can be quite controversial: does wrinkled skin or uncommonly short stature constitute impaired health, such that surgical repair or growth hormone is appropriate? Even more substantial variation can be found in ranking the importance of health with other goals in an individual's life. For some, health is a paramount value; for others—citizens who volunteer in time of war, nurses who care for patients with contagious diseases, hang-glider enthusiasts who risk life and limb—a different goal sometimes has primacy.

Absence of Objective Medical Criteria Even the most mundane case—in which there is little if any disagreement that some intervention will promote health—may well have no objective medical criteria that specify a single best way to achieve the goal. A fractured limb can be repaired in a number of ways; a life-threatening infection can be treated with a variety of antibiotics; mild diabetes is subject to control by diet, by injectable natural insulin, or by oral synthetic insulin substitutes. Health care professionals often reflect their own value preferences when they favor one alternative over another; many are matters of choice, dictated neither by biomedical principles or data nor by a single, agreed-upon professional standard.

In the Commission's survey it was clear that professionals recognize this fact: physicians maintained that decisional authority between them and their patients should depend on the nature of the decision at hand. Thus, for example, whether a pregnant woman over 35 should have amniocentesis was viewed as largely a patient's decision, whereas the decision of which antibiotic to use for strep throat was seen as primarily up to the doctor. Furthermore, on the question of whether to continue aggressive treatment for a cancer patient with metastases in whom such treatment had already failed, two-thirds of the physicians felt it was not a scientific, medical decision, but one that turned principally on personal values. And the same proportion felt the decision should be made jointly (which 64% of the doctors claimed it usually was).

Patients' Reasonable Subjective Preferences Determining what constitutes health and how it is best promoted also requires knowledge of patients' subjective preferences. In pursuit of the other goals and interests besides health that society deems legitimate, patients may prefer one type of medical intervention to another, may opt for no treatment at all, or may even request some treatment when a practitioner would prefer to follow a more conservative course that involved, at least for the moment, no medical intervention. For example, a slipped disc may be treated surgically or with medications and bed rest. Which treatment is better can be unclear, even to a physician. A patient may prefer surgery because, despite its greater risks, in the past that individual has spent considerable time in bed and become demoralized and depressed. A person with an injured knee, when told that surgery has about a 30% chance of reducing pain but almost no chance of eliminating it entirely, may prefer to leave the condition untreated. And a baseball pitcher with persistent inflammation of the el-

bow may prefer to take cortisone on a continuing basis even though the doctor suggests that a new position on the team would eliminate the inflammation permanently. In each case the goals and interests of particular patients incline them in different directions not only as to how, but even as to whether, treatment should proceed.

Given these two considerations—the frequent absence of objective medical criteria and the legitimate subjective preferences of patients—ascertaining whether a health care intervention will, if successful, promote a patient's well-being is a matter of individual judgment. Societies that respect personal freedom usually reach such decisions by leaving the judgment to the person involved.

The Boundaries of Health Care This does not mean, however, that well-being and self-determination are really just two terms for the same value. For example, when an individual (such as a newborn baby) is unable to express a choice, the value that guides health care decisionmaking is the promotion of well-being—not necessarily an easy task but also certainly not merely a disguised form of self-determination.

Moreover, the promotion of well-being is an important value even in decisions about patients who can speak for themselves because the boundaries of the interventions that health professionals present for consideration are set by the concept of well-being. Through societal expectations and the traditions of the professions, health care providers are committed to helping patients and to avoiding harm. Thus, the well-being principle circumscribes the range of alternatives offered to patients: informed consent does not mean that patients can insist upon anything they might want. Rather, it is a choice among medically accepted and available options, all of which are believed to have some possibility of promoting the patient's welfare, including always the option of no further medical interventions, even when that would not be viewed as preferable by the health care providers.

In sum, promotion of patient well-being provides the primary warrant for health care. But, as indicated, well-being is not a concrete concept that has a single definition or that is solely within the competency of health care providers to define. Shared decisionmaking requires that a practitioner seek not only to understand each patient's needs and develop reasonable alternatives to meet those needs but also to present the alternatives in a way that enables patients to choose one they prefer. To participate in this process, patients must engage in a dialogue with the practitioner and make their views on well-being clear. The majority of physicians (56%) and the public (64%) surveyed by the Commission felt that increasing the patient's role in medical decisionmaking would improve the quality of health care.[1]

Since well-being can be defined only within each individual's experience, it is in most circumstances congruent to self-determination, to which the Report now turns.

RESPECTING SELF-DETERMINATION

Self-determination (sometimes termed "autonomy") is an individual's exercise of the capacity to form, revise, and pursue personal plans for life. Although it clearly has a much broader application, the relevance of self-determination in health care decisions seems undeniable. A basic reason to honor an individual's choices about health care has already emerged in this Report: under most circumstances the outcome that will best promote the person's well-being rests on a subjective judgment about the individual. This can be termed the instrumental value of self-determination.

More is involved in respect for self-determination than just the belief that each person knows what's best for him- or herself, however. Even if it could be shown that an expert (or a computer) could do the job better, the worth of the individual, as acknowledged in Western ethical traditions and especially in Anglo-American law, provides an independent—and more important—ground for recognizing self-determination as a basic principle in human relations, particularly when matters as important as those raised by health care are at stake. This non-instrumental aspect can be termed the intrinsic value of self-determination.

Intrinsic Value of Self-Determination The value of self-determination readily emerges if one considers what is lost in its absence. If a physician selects a treatment alternative that satisfies a patient's individual values and goals rather than allowing the patient to choose, the absence of self-determination has not interfered with the promotion of the patient's well-being. But unless the patient has requested this course of conduct, the individual will not have been shown proper respect as a person nor provided with adequate protection against arbitrary, albeit often well-meaning, domination by others. Self-

determination can thus be seen as both a shield and a sword.

Freedom from Interference Self-determination as a shield is valued for the freedom from outside control it is intended to provide. It manifests the wish to be an instrument of one's own and "not of other men's acts of will."[2] In the context of health care, self-determination overrides practitioner-determination even if providers were able to demonstrate that they could (generally or in a specific instance) accurately assess the treatment an informed patient would choose. To permit action on the basis of a professional's assessment rather than on a patient's choice would deprive the patient of the freedom not to be forced to do something—whether or not that person would agree with the choice. Moreover, denying self-determination in this way risks generating the frustration people feel when their desires are ignored or countermanded....

SUMMARY OF CONCLUSIONS AND RECOMMENDATIONS

...The ethical foundation of informed consent can be traced to the promotion of two values: personal well-being and self-determination. To ensure that these values are respected and enhanced, the Commission finds that patients who have the capacity to make decisions about their care must be permitted to do so voluntarily and must have all relevant information regarding their condition and alternative treatments, including possible benefits, risks, costs, other consequences, and significant uncertainties surrounding any of this information. This conclusion has several specific implications:

1. Although the informed consent doctrine has substantial foundations in law, it is essentially an ethical imperative.

2. Ethically valid consent is a process of shared decisionmaking based upon mutual respect and participation, not a ritual to be equated with reciting the contents of a form that details the risks of particular treatments.

3. Much of the scholarly literature and legal commentary about informed consent portrays it as a highly rational means of decisionmaking about health care matters, thereby suggesting that it

may only be suitable for and applicable to well-educated, articulate, self-aware individuals. Whether this is what the legal doctrine was intended to be or what it has inadvertently become, it is a view the Commission unequivocally rejects. Although subcultures within American society differ in their views about autonomy and individual choice and about the etiology of illness and the roles of healers and patients,[3] a survey conducted for the Commission found a universal desire for information, choice, and respectful communication about decisions.[4] Informed consent must remain flexible, yet the process, as the Commission envisions it throughout this Report, is ethically required of health care practitioners in their relationships with all patients, not a luxury for a few.

4. Informed consent is rooted in the fundamental recognition—reflected in the legal presumption of competency—that adults are entitled to accept or reject health care interventions on the basis of their own personal values and in furtherance of their own personal goals. Nonetheless, patient choice is not absolute.

• Patients are not entitled to insist that health care practitioners furnish them services when to do so would violate either the bounds of acceptable practice or a professional's own deeply held moral beliefs or would draw on a limited resource on which the patient has no binding claim.

• The fundamental values that informed consent is intended to promote—self-determination and patient well-being—both demand that alternative arrangements for health care decisionmaking be made for individuals who lack substantial capacity to make their own decisions. Respect for self-determination requires, however, that in the first instance individuals be deemed to have decisional capacity, which should not be treated as a hurdle to be surmounted in the vast majority of cases, and that incapacity be treated as a disqualifying factor in the small minority of cases.

• Decisionmaking capacity is specific to each particular decision. Although some people lack this capacity for all decisions, many are incapaci-

tated in more limited ways and are capable of making some decisions but not others. The concept of capacity is best understood and applied in a functional manner. That is, the presence or absence of capacity does not depend on a person's status or on the decision reached, but on that individual's actual functioning in situations in which a decision about health care is to be made.

• Decisionmaking incapacity should be found to exist only when people lack the ability to make decisions that promote their well-being in conformity with their own previously. expressed values and preferences.

• To the extent feasible people with no decisionmaking capacity should still be consulted about their own preferences out of respect for them as individuals.

5. Health care providers should not ordinarily withhold unpleasant information simply because it is unpleasant. The ethical foundations of informed consent allow the withholding of information from patients only when they request that it be withheld or when its disclosure per se would cause substantial detriment to their well-being. Furthermore, the Commission found that most members of the public do not wish to have "bad news" withheld from them.

6. Achieving the Commission's vision of shared decisionmaking based on mutual respect is ultimately the responsibility of individual health care professionals. However, health care institutions such as hospitals and professional schools have important roles to play in assisting health care professionals in this obligation. The manner in which health care is provided in institutional settings often results in a fragmentation of responsibility that may neglect the human side of health care. To assist in guarding against this, institutional health care providers should ensure that ultimately there is one readily identifiable practitioner responsible for providing information to a particular patient. Although pieces of information may be provided by various people, there should be one individual officially charged with responsibility for ensuring that all the necessary information

is communicated and that the patient's wishes are known to the treatment team.

7. Patients should have access to the information they need to help them understand their conditions and make treatment decisions. To this end the Commission recommends that health care professionals and institutions not only provide information but also assist patients who request additional information to obtain it from relevant sources, including hospital and public libraries.

8. As cases arise and new legislation is contemplated, courts and legislatures should reflect this view of ethically valid consent. Nevertheless, the Commission does not look to legal reforms as the primary means of bringing about changes in the relationship between health care professionals and patients.

9. The Commission finds that a number of relatively simple changes in practice could facilitate patient participation in health care decisionmaking. Several specific techniques—such as having patients express, orally or in writing, their understanding of the treatment consented to—deserve further study. Furthermore, additional societal resources need to be committed to improving the human side of health care, which has apparently deteriorated at the same time there have been substantial gains in health care technology. The Department of Health and Human Services, and especially the National Institutes of Health, is an appropriate agency for the development of initiatives and the evaluation of their efficacy in this area.

10. Because health care professionals are responsible for ensuring that patients can participate effectively in decisionmaking regarding their care, educators have a responsibility to prepare physicians and nurses to carry out this obligation. The Commission therefore concludes that:

- Curricular innovations aimed at preparing health professionals for a process of mutual decisionmaking with patients should be continued and strengthened, with careful attention being paid to the development of methods for evaluating the effectiveness of such innovations.
- Examinations and evaluations at the professional school and national levels should reflect the importance of these issues.
- Serious attention should be paid to preparing health professionals for team practice in order to enhance patient participation and well-being.

11. Family members are often of great assistance to patients in helping to understand information about their condition and in making decisions about treatment. The Commission recommends that health care institutions and professionals recognize this and judiciously attempt to involve family members in decisionmaking for patients, with due regard for the privacy of patients and for the possibilities for coercion that such a practice may entail.

12. The Commission recognizes that its vision of health care decisionmaking may involve greater commitments of time on the part of health professionals. Because of the importance of shared decisionmaking based on mutual trust, not only for the promotion of patient well-being and self-determination but also for the therapeutic gains that can be realized, the Commission recommends that all medical and surgical interventions be thought of as including appropriate discussion with patients. Reimbursement to the professional should therefore take account of time spent in discussion rather than regarding it as a separate item for which additional payment is made.

13. To protect the interests of patients who lack decisionmaking capacity and to ensure their well-being and self-determination, the Commission concludes that:

- Decisions made by others on patients' behalf should, when possible, attempt to replicate the ones patients would make if they were capable of doing so. When this is not feasible, decisions by surrogates on behalf of patients must protect the patients' best interests. Because such decisions are not instances of personal self-choice, limits may be placed on the range of acceptable decisions that surrogates make beyond those that apply when a person makes his or her own decisions.

- Health care institutions should adopt clear and explicit policies regarding how and by whom decisions are to be made for patients who cannot decide.
- Families, health care institutions, and professionals should work together to make health care decisions for patients who lack decisionmaking capacity. Recourse to courts should be reserved for the occasions when concerned parties are unable to resolve their disagreements over matters of substantial import, or when adjudication is clearly required by state law. Courts and legislatures should be cautious about requiring judicial review of routine health care decisions for patients who lack capacity.
- Health care institutions should explore and evaluate various informal administrative arrangements, such as "ethics committees," for review and consultation in nonroutine matters involving health care decisionmaking for those who cannot decide.
- As a means of preserving some self-determination for patients who no longer possess decisionmaking capacity, state courts and legislatures should consider making provision for advance directives through which people designate others to make health care decisions on their behalf and/or give instructions about their care.

The Commission acknowledges that the conclusions contained in this Report will not be simple to achieve. Even when patients and practitioners alike are sensitive to the goal of shared decisionmaking based on mutual re-

spect, substantial barriers will still exist. Some of these obstacles, such as long-standing professional attitudes or difficulties in conveying medical information in ordinary language, are formidable but can be overcome if there is a will to do so. Others, such as the dependent condition of very sick patients or the ever-growing complexity and subspecialization of medicine, will have to be accommodated because they probably cannot be eliminated. Nonetheless, the Commission's vision of informed consent still has value as a measuring stick against which actual performance may be judged and as a goal toward which all participants in health care decisionmaking can strive....

NOTES

1 Many physicians and patients said they believed an increased patient role would give the patient a better understanding of the medical condition and treatment, would improve physician performance in terms of the honesty and scope of discussion, and would generally improve the doctor-patient relationship. However, a number of physicians claimed that greater patient involvement would improve the quality of care because it would improve compliance and would make patients more cooperative and willing to accept the doctor's judgment.

2 Isaiah Berlin, "Two Concepts of Liberty," in *Four Essays on Liberty*, Clarendon Press, Oxford (1969) at 118–38.

3 Robert A. Hahn, *Culture and Informed Consent: An Anthropological Perspective* (1982), Appendix F, in Volume Three of this Report.

4 The Commission's survey of the public broke down these responses on the basis of variables such as age, gender, race, education, and income.

The Many Faces of Competency
James F. Drane

James F. Drane is the Russell B. Roth Professor of clinical medical ethics at Edinboro University of Pennsylvania. He is the author of *Becoming a Good Doctor: The Place of Virtue and Character in Medical Ethics* (1988) and "Medical Paternalism and a New Style of Medical Ethics."

Drane focuses on the notion of competence and standards for competency assessment. He notes that although patient competence is recognized as a necessary condition for any valid consent, no agreement exists about acceptable standards of competence. Drane suggests a sliding-scale model for competency, such that different standards apply to different kinds of medical decisions. The first, least stringent standard has minimal competency requirements. Patients must be aware of their medical situation, and their assent may be either explicit or implied. This standard applies, for example, when medical decisions are made regarding treatments that pose no danger to a patient and are objectively in the patient's best interests. The second standard requires a higher level of comprehension and consent. The patient must (1) understand the medical situation and the risks and outcomes of different options and (2) be capable of making decisions based on this understanding. This standard applies, for example, where the diagnosis is doubtful or the diagnosis is certain but the treatment is dangerous. The third, strictest standard requires a critical reflective understanding of illness and treatment and the ability to make rational decisions based on relevant implications including articulated beliefs and values. This standard applies, for example, when the treatment in question is very dangerous and runs counter to both professional and public rationality.

The doctrine of informed consent, less than twenty-five years old, creates many dilemmas because it tries to balance very different values—specifically, on one side beneficence (health or well-being); on the other, autonomy (or self-determination). Most of the ethical commentary on informed consent and a majority of the court cases deciding consent questions have focused on the physician's responsibilities to disclose information and to keep the medical setting free of coercion. But more and more frequently clinical questions arise about the capacity or competence of a specific patient to give an informed consent.

If the patient is not competent, then his or her consent does not constitute an authorization to treat, no matter how thorough the disclosure or how free from coercion the medical setting. Incompetence also calls into

Reprinted with permission of the author and the publisher from *Hastings Center Report*, vol. 15 (April 1985), pp. 17–21.

question a patient's refusal of treatment. Patient competence in effect is a condition for the validity of consent. Incompetence both creates a new obligation to identify a surrogate and provides a basis for the physician to set aside the informed consent requirement in favor of what he or she thinks is best for the patient.

Only recently have scholars begun to pay attention to this element in the informed consent doctrine. Loren Roth, Paul Appelbaum, Alan Meisel, and Charles Lidz found that different clinicians use very different tests to judge competence.[1] They reduced these to five categories: (1) making a choice; (2) reasonable outcome of choice or ability to produce a reasonable choice; (3) choice based on rational reasons; (4) ability to understand the decision-making process; and (5) actual understanding of the process. Later, Appelbaum and Roth suggested four possible standards for judging competency: (1) evidencing a choice; (2) factual understanding of issues; (3) rational manipulation of information; and

(4) appreciation of the nature of the situation. They found any one of the four to be acceptable, as long as it was justified by a reasonable policy perspective.[2] Other authors have argued for a single standard: For Grace A. Olin and Harry S. Olin, competence means ability to retain information. For Howard Owens reality testing is the standard. Bernard Gert and Charles Culver in their book, *Philosophy in Medicine*, helped clarify the term by showing different ways competence is used in ordinary and professional language. Alan A. Stone has written extensively on informed consent and severely criticized court decisions that extended competency even of involuntary mental patients to refuse treatment. Mark Siegler made important conceptual points about the meaning of competency, and more than any other writer connected the issue to the medical setting in which it emerges.[3]

Finally, the President's Commission for the Study of Ethical Problems in Medicine and Biomedical and Behavioral Research in a recently published report discussed competency, which the Commission prefers to call decision-making capacity.[4] The Commission spelled out the components of competency or decisional capacity: the possession of a set of values and goals, the ability to communicate and understand information, and the ability to reason and deliberate. Although they did not adopt any one of the standards listed by Roth and Appelbaum, the Commissioners were very critical of the first two tests: "evidencing a preference" and "reasonable outcome" of the patient's decision.

Despite all the work done to date, the competency question remains unsettled. What should the standard for competence be in order to ensure valid consent or refusal of consent to medical procedures? To be acceptable, any standard of competence must meet several important objectives. It must incorporate the general guidelines set out in legal decisions; it must be psychiatrically and philosophically sound; it must guarantee the realization of ethical values on which the consent requirement is based; and it must be applicable in a clinical setting.

In practice some tests seem too lenient and expose patients to serious harm. Others seem too stringent and turn almost all seriously ill patients into incompetents, thereby depriving them of rights and dignity. The solution proposed here is based on no one standard, but works out a sliding scale for competency. Accordingly as the medical decision itself (the task) changes, the standards of competency to perform the task also change.

THE COMPETENCY ASSESSMENT

As long as a patient does or says nothing strange and acquiesces to treatment recommended by the medical professional, questions of competency do not arise. These questions arise usually when the patient refuses treatment or chooses a course of action which, in the opinion of the physician in charge, threatens his or her well-being. Either consenting to treatment or refusing consent may raise a suspicion of unreasonableness. More careful evaluation is then called for before a final determination of competency is made.

Competency assessment usually focuses on the patient's mental capacities: specifically the mental capacities to make a particular medical decision. Does this patient understand what is being disclosed? Can this patient come to a decision about treatment based on that information? How much understanding and rational decision-making capacity is sufficient for this patient to be considered competent? Or how deficient must this patient's decision-making capacity be before he or she is declared incompetent? A properly performed competency assessment should eliminate two types of error: preventing competent persons from deciding their own treatments; and failing to protect incompetent persons from the harmful effects of a bad decision.

The assessment process leads to a decision about a decision. A good clinical determination must balance the different and sometimes competing values of rationality, beneficence and autonomy. Rationality, or reasonableness, is an underlying assumption in competency determinations. In an emergency we presume that a rational person would want treatment and the informed consent requirement is set aside. But rationality cannot be set aside in nonemergency settings. A particular medical setting establishes certain expectations about what a reasonable person would do, and these expectations play an important role in competency determinations.

The patient's well-being (beneficence) also has to be considered in assessing competence. The same laws that establish the right to give or refuse informed consent express concern about protecting patients from the harm that could result from serious defects in decision-making capacity. Finally, a competency assessment must respect the value of autonomy. Patients must be permitted to determine their own fate, and a decision cannot be set aside simply because it differs from what other persons think is indicated.

A SLIDING-SCALE MODEL

How should the physician proceed when deciding on a patient's competence? The model proposed here posits three general categories of medical situations; in each category, as the consequences flowing from patient decisions become more serious, competency standards for valid consent or refusal of consent become more stringent. The psychiatric pathologies most likely to undermine the mental capacities required for each type of decision are listed in the tables on pp. 102–103.

A number of assumptions underlie the use of a sliding scale or variable standard rather than one ideal competency test. First, the objective content of the decision must be taken into consideration so that competency determinations remain linked to the decision at hand. Second, the value of reasonableness operates at every level. When people sit down to play chess, certain expectations are created even though no particular decisions are required. If, however, one player makes peculiar moves, the other will have to wonder whether his partner is competent or knows what he is doing. Something similar is assumed in the patient-physician partnership. Third, the reasonableness assumption justifies some paternalistic behavior. The physician or another surrogate is authorized by this model to decide what is best for the patient who is incompetent. In more cases than a patient-rights advocate would prefer, the patient's decision is set aside in favor of beneficence. The clinical values of health and patient well-being are balanced with the libertarian values of autonomy and self-determination.

EASY, EFFECTIVE TREATMENTS

Standard No. 1   The first and least stringent standard of competence to give a valid consent applies to medical decisions that are not dangerous and are objectively in the patient's best interest. Even though these patients are seriously ill, and therefore impaired in cognitive and volitional functioning, their consent to an effective, safe treatment is considered informed so long as the patient is aware of what is going on. *Awareness*, in the sense of being in contact with one's situation, satisfies the cognitive requirement of informed consent. *Assent* alone to the rational expectations of others satisfies the volitional component. When an adult goes along with what is considered appropriate and rational, then the presumption of competency holds. Higher standards for capacity to give

a valid consent to this first type of medical intervention would be superfluous.

Consider the following two examples. Betty Campbell, a twenty-five-year-old secretary who lives alone, has an accident. She arrives at the hospital showing signs of mild shock and suffering from the associated mental deficiencies; but her consent to blood transfusion, bone-setting, or even to some minor surgery need not be questioned. Even though there is no emergency, if she is aware of her situation and assents to receiving an effective, low-risk treatment for a certain diagnosis, there is no reason to question her competence to consent.

Phil Randall's situation is quite different. A twenty-three-year-old veteran who has been addicted to drugs and alcohol, he is on probation and struggling to survive in college. When Phil stops talking and eating for almost a week, his roommate summons a trusted professor. By this time Phil is catatonic, but the professor manages to get him on his feet and accompanies him in a police car to the state hospital. The professor gets through to Phil sufficiently to explain the advantages of signing in as a voluntary patient. Phil signs his name to the admission form, authorizing commitment and initial treatment. His consent to this first phase of therapy is valid because Phil is sufficiently aware of his situation to understand what is happening, and he assents to the treatment. Later on, when his condition improves, another consent may be required, especially if a more dangerous treatment or a long-term hospitalization is required. The next decision will require a higher degree of competence because it is a different type of task.

Having a lenient standard of competence for safe and effective treatments eliminates the ambiguity and confusion associated with phrases like "virtually competent," "marginally competent," and "competent for practical purposes." Such phrases are used to excuse the common sense practice of holding certain decisions to be valid even though the patients are considered incompetent by some abstract standard, which ignores the specific task or type of medical decision at hand.

The same modest standard of competence should apply to a dying patient who refuses to consent to treatments that are ineffective and useless. This is the paradigm case in the refusal-of-ineffective-treatment category.

Most of the patients who would be considered incompetent to make treatment decisions under this first category are legally incompetent. Those who use psychotic defenses that impede the awareness of their situation and any decision making ability are the only other patients who fall outside the wide first criterion. Even children who have reached the age of reason can be considered competent. According to law however, those below the ages of twenty-one or sometimes eighteen are presumed incompetent to make binding contracts, including health care decisions.

But exceptions are common. The Pennsylvania Mental Health Procedures Act (1976), for example, decided that fourteen-year-old adolescents were competent to give informed consent to psychiatric hospitalization. Adolescents are also considered competent in many jurisdictions to make decisions about birth control and abortion. I am suggesting that, for this first type of decision, children as young as ten or eleven are competent.

Authors like Alexander M. Capron, Willard Gaylin, and Ruth Macklin support a lowering of the age of competency to make some medical decisions.[5] The President's Commission also endorses a lower age of competence. The physician, however, cannot ignore the law and must obtain the consent of the child's legal guardian. But if a minor is competent or partially competent, there is good reason to involve him or her in the decision-making process.

LESS CERTAIN TREATMENTS

Standard No. 2 If the diagnosis is doubtful, or the condition chronic; if the diagnosis is certain but the treatment is more dangerous or not quite so effective; if there are alternative treatments, or no treatment at all is an alternative, then a different type of task is involved in making an informed treatment decision. Consequently, a different standard of competence is required. The patient now must be able to understand the risks and outcomes of the different options and then be able to make a decision based on this understanding. In this setting competence means ability to understand the treatment options, balance risks and benefits, and come to a deliberate decision. In other words, a higher standard of competence is required than the one discussed above. Let me give some examples of this type of decision, and the corresponding competency standards.

Antonio Marachal is a retired steel worker who has been hospitalized with a bad heart valve. Both the surgeon and his family doctor recommend an operation to replace the valve. Mr. Marachal understands what they tell him, but is afraid of undergoing the operation. He thinks he'll live just as long by taking good care of him-

self. His fear of surgery may not be entirely rational, but the option he prefers is real and there is no basis for considering his refusal to be invalid because of incompetence.

Or consider Geraldine Brown, a forty-year-old unmarried woman who is diagnosed as having leukemia. Chemotherapy offers a good chance for remission, but the side effects are repugnant and frightening to her. After hearing and understanding the diagnosis, alternatives, risks, and prognosis, she refuses, deciding instead to follow a program that centers on diet, exercise, meditation, and some natural stimulants to her immune system. Objectively, the standard medical treatment is preferable to what she decides, but informed consent joins objective medical data with subjective personal factors such as repugnance and burden. In this case the objective and subjective components balance out. A decision one way or the other is reasonable, and a person who can understand the options and decide in light of them is competent.

Although ability to understand is not the same as being capable of conceptual or verbal understanding, some commentators assume that the two are synonymous in every case. Many would require that patients remember the ideas and repeat what they have been told as a proof of competence. Real understanding, however, may be more a matter of emotions. Following an explanation, the patient may grasp what is best for her with strong feelings and convictions, and yet be hard pressed to articulate or conceptualize her understanding or conviction.

Competence as capacity for an understanding choice can also be reconciled with a decision to let a trusted physician decide what is the best treatment. Such a choice (a waiver) may be made for good reasons and represent a decision in favor of one set of values (safety or anxiety reduction) over another (independence and personal initiative). As such, it can be considered an informed consent and create no suspicion about competence.

Ignorance or inability to understand, however, does incapacitate a person for making this type of decision. This is especially so when the ignorance extends to the options and persists even after patient and careful explanation. Patience and care may sometimes require that more than one person be involved in the disclosure process before a person is judged incompetent to understand. An explanation by someone from the same ethnic, religious, or economic background may also be necessary.

..

A Sliding-Scale Model for Competency

STANDARD NO. 1

Objective Medical Decisions

effective treatment for acute illness
diagnostic certainty
high benefit/low risk
limited alternatives
severe disorder/major distress/immediately life-threatening

consent — *refusal*

ineffective treatment

A. Incompetent
unconscious
severe retardation
small children
total disorientation
severe senile dementia
autism
psychotic defenses
denial of self and situation
delusional projection

B. Competent
children (10 and above)
retarded (educable)
clouded sensorium
mild senile dementia
intoxicated
conditions listed under #2 and #3 (A & B)

Competency Standards

Minimal requirements:
1. *Awareness:* orientation to one's medical situation
2. *Assent:* explicit or implied

STANDARD NO. 2

Objective Medical Decisions

chronic condition/doubtful diagnosis
uncertain outcome of therapy for acute illness
balanced risks and benefits:
possibly effective, but burdensome
high risk, only hope

consent or refusal

A. Incompetent
severe mood disorders
phobia about treatment
mutis
short-term memory loss
thought disorders
ignorance
incoherence
delusion
hallucination
delirium
conditions listed under #1 (A & B)

B. Competent
adolescent (16 and over)
mildly retarded
personality disorders:
narcissistic, borderline and obsessive
conditions listed under #3 (A & B)

Competency Standards

Median requirements:
1. *Understanding:* of medical situation and proposed treatment
2. *Choice:* based on medical outcomes

STANDARD NO. 3

Objective Medical Decisions

A. Incompetent
indecisive or ambivalent
    over time
false beliefs about reality
hysteria
substance abuse
neurotic defenses:
intellectualization
repression
dissociation
acting out
mild depression
hypomania
conditions listed under
    #1 and #2 (A & B)

ineffective treatment

consent

refusal

effective treatment for acute
    illness
diagnostic certainty
high benefit/low risk
    limited alternatives
severe disorder/major
    distress/immediately
    life-threatening

B. Competent
above legal age
reflective and self-critical
mature coping devices:
    altruism
    anticipation
    sublimation

Competency Standards

Maximum Requirements:
1. *Appreciation:* critical and reflective understanding of illness and treatment
2. *Rational decision:* based on relevant implications including articulated beliefs and values

103

DANGEROUS TREATMENTS

Standard No. 3   The most stringent and demanding criterion for competence is reserved for those treatment decisions that are very dangerous, and run counter to both professional and public rationality. Here the decision involves not a balancing of what are widely recognized as reasonable alternatives or a reasonable response to a doubtful diagnosis, but a choice that seems to violate reasonableness. The patient's decision now appears irrational, indeed life-threatening. And yet, according to this model, such decisions are valid and respectable as long as the person making them satisfies the most demanding standards of competence. The patient's decision is a different type of task than the others we have considered. As such, different and more stringent criteria of capacity are appropriate.

Competence in this context requires an ability on the part of the decision maker to appreciate what he or she is doing. Appreciation requires the highest degree of understanding, one that grasps more than just the medical details of the illness, options, risks, and treatment. To be competent to make apparently irrational and very dangerous choices, the patient must appreciate the implications of the medical information for his or her life. Competence here requires an understanding that is both technical and personal, intellectual and emotional.

Because such decisions contravene public standards of rationality, they must be subjectively critical and reflective. The competent patient must be able to give reasons for the decision, which show that he has thought through the medical issues and related this information to his personal values. The patient's personal reasons need not be scientific or publicly accepted, but neither can they be purely private or idiosyncratic. Their intelligibility may derive from a minority religious view, but they must be coherent and follow the logic of that belief system. This toughest standard of competence demands a more rational understanding: one that includes verbalization, consistency, and the like. Some examples will illustrate.

Bob Cassidy, an eighteen-year-old high school senior and an outstanding athlete, is involved in an automobile accident which has crushed his left foot. Attempts to save the limb are unsuccessful, and infection threatens the boy's life. Surgeons talk to his parents who immediately give permission for amputation of the leg below the knee. Since Bob is legally no longer a minor, however, his consent is required for the surgery, but he refuses. "If I cannot play sports, my life is meaningless," he says. First the doctors try to talk to him, then his parents, finally some of his friends. But he refuses to discuss the matter. When anyone comes to his room he simply closes his eyes and lies motionless. "If they cannot make my foot as good as before, I want to die," he tells them. "What good is it to live with only one leg? Without sports I can't see anything worth living for." Bob is using unhealthy coping behavior to handle his situation. He refuses to consider the implications of what he is doing and shows signs of being seriously depressed. No arguments or justifications are offered to counter the indications of immaturity and mild emotional illness. For these reasons he is incompetent for the task he presumes to undertake.

Charles Kandell is a Jehovah's Witness and refuses a blood transfusion after a bad accident at his job. He is not yet in shock, but will shortly be in danger of death. His wife and family support his refusal and pledge to help care for his children. The doctor asks Charles if he fears judgment from God if blood were given against his will. He is adamant, explaining to the medical group that he has lived his life by these beliefs, knows the possible consequences, and holds eternal life to be more important than life here on earth. This decision meets the high standards required for such a decision, and should be respected as a competent refusal.

A patient need not have a serious psychiatric pathology in order to be considered incompetent to make such serious decisions. On the other hand, not every mental or emotional disturbance would constitute incompetence. A certain amount of anxiety, for example, accompanies any serious decision. A patient may suffer some pain, which would not necessarily impair such a decision. Even a degree of reactive depression may not incapacitate a patient for this type of decision. But any mental or emotional disorder that compromises appreciation and rational decision making would make a person incompetent. Persons, for example, who are incapable of controlling their destructive behavior cannot be considered competent to decide about treatments that have destructive features. Consequently, a patient who is hospitalized for a self-inflicted injury would not be considered competent to refuse a life-saving treatment. And dangerous decisions that are inconsistent with life-long values are strongly suspect as being products of incompetence.

The paradigm case of consent to ineffective treatment is a decision to engage in a high-risk drug trial unrelated to one's own illness.

OBJECTIONS TO THE SLIDING SCALE

Certain objections to this sliding scale notion are easy to anticipate. Libertarian thinkers will see it as justifying paternalistic behavior on the part of physicians and diminishing the patient's discretion to do whatever he or she prefers no matter what the consequence. True, by these standards some patient decisions would not be respected, but competency was originally required and continues to be needed in order to set aside certain dangerous and harmful decisions. This model provides guidelines for determining which patient decisions fall within the original purpose for a competency requirement. Besides, the sliding scale provides a justification even for decisions that are considered by some to be irrational. Instead of limiting freedom, it safeguards patient autonomy while balancing this value with well-being.

Admittedly, in the least stringent category the outcome, which is beneficial to the patient, plays a role in establishing the rationality of the decision and the competency of the decision maker. The President's Commission rejected a standard based on outcome for the following reason: if only the physician can determine outcome, and outcome constitutes the only test of a competent choice, then competence is a matter of doing what the doctor thinks best. But outcome is not *the* standard of competence in this model. Rather it is an important factor in only one class of medical decisions. In other decisions patients may competently go against medical assessments of outcome. In fact, a decision that leads to an outcome that professionals and nonprofessionals alike would consider the most unacceptable—unnecessary death—can be considered a valid and competent option according to this model.

Objections will also be raised against the most stringent standard for judging competence. If every patient must understand thoroughly and make a rational decision in order to be considered competent, then too many people will be considered incompetent. Consequently, the medical delivery system will be clogged with surrogate decision making, and many patients will be robbed of dignity and self-determination. The most stringent standard in this model requires just such capacities for competence, but only in cases where the patient has most to lose from his or her choice. If patients in category three suffer a decline in autonomy (and they do because some decisions will not be respected), this is balanced by a gain in beneficence.

BALANCING VALUES

A balancing of values is the cornerstone of a good competency assessment. Rationality is given its place throughout this model. Not only does the sliding scale reflect a rational ordering of things, but reasonableness is an underlying assumption for each standard of competence. Maximum autonomy, however, is also guaranteed because patients can choose to do even what is not at all beneficial (participate in an experiment which has little chance of improving their condition) or refuse to do what is most beneficial. Finally, beneficence is respected because patients are protected against harmful choices, when these are more the product of pathology than of self-determination.

REFERENCES

1 Loren H. Roth, Charles W. Lidz, and Alan Meisel, "Toward a Model of the Legal Doctrine of Informed Consent," *American Journal of Psychiatry* 134 (1977), 285–89; Loren H. Roth, Alan Meisel, and Charles W. Lidz, "Test of Competency to Consent to Treatment," *American Journal of Psychiatry* 134 (1977), 279–84; Paul S. Appelbaum and Loren H. Roth, "Clinical Issues in the Assessment of Competency," *American Journal of Psychiatry* 138 (1981), 1462–67; and Loren H. Roth and Paul S. Appelbaum, "The Dilemma of Denial in the Assessment of Competency to Refuse Treatment," *American Journal of Psychiatry* 139 (1982), 910–13.

2 Paul S. Appelbaum and Loren H. Roth, "Competency to Consent to Research," *Archives of General Psychiatry* 39 (1982), 951–58.

3 G.A. Olin and H.S. Olin, "Informed Consent in Voluntary Mental Hospital Admission," *American Journal of Psychiatry* 132 (1975), 938–41; H. Owens, "When Is a Voluntary Commitment Really Voluntary?" *American Journal of Orthopsychiatry* 47 (1977), 104–10; Charles Culver and Bernard Gert, *Philosophy in Medicine* (New York: Oxford University Press, 1982); Alan Stone, "The Right to Refuse Treatment," *Archives of General Psychiatry* 38 (1981), 358–62; Alan Stone, "Informed Consent: Special Problems for Psychiatry," *Hospital and Community Psychiatry* 30 (1979), 231–37; Mark Siegler, "Critical Illness: the Limits of Autonomy," *Hastings Center Report* 7 (Oc-

tober 1977), 12–15; and Mark Siegler and A.D. Goldblatt, "Clinical Intuition: A Procedure for Balancing the Rights of Patients and the Responsibilities of Physicians," in S.F. Spicker, J.M. Healey, and H.T. Engelhardt, eds., *The Law-Medicine Relation: A Philosophical Exploration* (Dordrecht, Holland: D. Reidel Publishing Co., 1981).

4 The President's Commission for the Study of Ethical Problems in Medicine and Biomedical and Behavioral Research, *Making Health Care Decisions*, Vol. 1 (Washington: U.S. Government Printing Office, 1982).

5 Willard Gaylin and Ruth Macklin, eds., *Who Speaks for the Child?* (New York: Plenum Press, 1982).

Two Models of Implementing Informed Consent
Charles W. Lidz, Paul S. Appelbaum, and Alan Meisel

Charles W. Lidz is professor of psychiatry and sociology at the University of Pittsburgh Center for Medical Ethics. Alan Meisel, J.D., is professor of psychiatry and professor of law at the same university. Lidz and Meisel are coauthors of *Informed Consent: A Study of Decisionmaking in Psychiatry* (1984). Paul S. Appelbaum is professor of psychiatry at the University of Massachusetts Medical Center. He is the coauthor, along with Lidz and Meisel, of *Informed Consent: Legal Theory and Clinical Practice* (1987).

Lidz, Appelbaum, and Meisel describe two ways in which the informed consent doctrine can be implemented. The *event model* of informed consent treats the giving and obtaining of informed consent and the provision of the requisite information as a discrete act that takes place at a single point in time. On the contrasting *process model*, giving patients information and obtaining their consent is an ongoing process integrated into the continuing physician-patient dialogue that is a routine part of ongoing diagnosis and treatment. The authors, arguing in favor of the process model, discuss some of its ethical and clinical benefits. Although they caution that the model is not universally applicable (e.g., in the case of emergency-care specialists), they maintain that even in such cases, patients should have full information about physicians' thinking and should be referred back to their attending physicians for additional information.

Since the concept of "informed consent" was first used in 1957,[1] it has become central to both legal and ethical regulation of American medicine, and much of the new subdiscipline of bioethics has been built around it.[2–6] The legal doctrine of informed consent specifies that physicians should disclose to patients all information "material" to making a decision whether to undergo or forgo a proposed treatment or diagnostic procedure. Thus, physicians must disclose the nature, purpose, risks, benefits, and alternatives of the proposed treat-

Reprinted with permission from *Archives of Internal Medicine*, vol. 148 (June 1988), pp. 1385–1389. Copyright © 1988, American Medical Association.

ment. The patient is then allowed to consent to or refuse this recommendation.[5,6] In contrast, the ethical "idea of informed consent," developed largely by theorists from the underlying values and goals that informed consent is intended to promote, contemplates that patients should collaborate with physicians in developing and evaluating treatment options, with patients having a veto over any proposed treatment.[7,8] Both legal and ethical commentators have argued that informed consent will produce many benefits, ranging from a reduction in medical mistakes to greater compliance with treatment.[9–11]

In spite of its enthusiastic reception in bioethics and law, the doctrine's reception in medical circles has been mixed. Many have noted that the legal requirements have led to few positive changes in the physician-patient relationship.[12,13] Indeed, both empirical research and clinical observations indicate that informed consent often becomes an empty ritual in which patients are presented with complex information that they cannot understand and that has little impact on their decision making.[14,15] Many see informed consent as directly interfering with the care of patients by wasting valuable time and leading patients to reject medically desirable care.[16,17]

While some elements of this critique are legitimate, we suggest that the problem lies not so much in the idea of informed consent, or even in its legal requirements, as in its *implementation* in the clinical setting. This article contrasts two models of implementing informed consent. Although both of these models may satisfy the legal requirements and thereby provide some protection against suit, their effects on physician-patient relationships are quite different. Clinicians employing the first model approach the task of obtaining informed consent as an event that occurs at a single point in time. We refer to this as the *event model* of obtaining informed consent. The second model treats informed consent as an integral and continuous part of the relationship between patients and physicians embedded in the treatment process. For this reason, we call it the *process model*.

CONSENT AS AN EVENT

The event model of informed consent treats medical decision making as a discrete act that takes place in a circumscribed period of time, usually shortly before the administration of treatment, and emphasizes the provision of information to patients at that time. Physicians are expected to provide patients with material information about treatment and then allow patients to decide whether to accept their recommendations.

The event model emphasizes the importance of complete, accurate information and thus satisfies most legal requirements. The law of informed consent has also focused on the validity and comprehensiveness of the disclosure and has shied away from evaluating such considerations as whether patients actually understand the disclosure.[5,6] The consent form, with its detailed recital of risks and benefits, can be seen as the central symbol of the event model.

Implementation of the event model contains little process. Consent begins when the "time to get consent" arrives and the physician introduces the consent form and lists the risks of treatment. Anything said prior to this point is usually considered irrelevant to consent. Anything that is said after the form is signed is also irrelevant. In the event model, informed consent is not directly concerned with improving the quality of the decision-making process or the patient's comprehension of treatment; rather, the emphasis is on the physician's provision of the information that a hypothetically rational person would want.

The event model has several advantages. First, it provides both physicians and patients with a clear idea of their responsibilities and privileges. Moreover, except for the form signing, informed consent does not interfere with the ordinary relationship between physician and patient. Also, the consent form is a clear-cut document for attorneys to use in the event of litigation; a well-crafted consent form may provide some protection for physicians against a lawsuit claiming that informed consent was not obtained.

Finally, the event model fits easily into the organization of hospital- and clinic-based medicine. Most modern health care organizations divide the care of patients into specialized tasks assigned to different care givers. House staff may be in charge of admission paperwork; attending physicians are responsible for overseeing patients' care; laboratory technicians perform the tests used in diagnosis. Likewise, informed consent is usually assigned to one member of the health care team, often a house-staff physician or nurse.[14]

There are, however, problems with the event model. Since patients often fail to understand the information they receive, and sense that their participation in decision making is not really desired, the event model fails to implement fully the idea of informed consent, although it may meet the minimal legal requirements. Physicians, too, sense the futility of the event model, which reinforces their disdain for informed consent as a waste of time. Furthermore, the event model often seems to make the interaction between physicians and patients more bureaucratic and less humane. For physicians who are committed to improved care for patients, this model of informed consent often seems detrimental to patient care.

If we ignore the ideals of patient participation espoused in the idea of informed consent and are simply concerned about protection from legal liability, the event model may be acceptable. However, there is an alternative approach that satisfies both sets of desiderata.

CONSENT AS A PROCESS

The process model of informed consent is built on a vision of active patient participation in decision making. While the event model inserts an extra step—informed consent—into otherwise unchanged decision making, the process model, by contrast, integrates informed consent into the physician-patient relationship as a facet of all stages of medical decision making.

If patients are to participate in the decision-making process, we must recognize that medical decisions are rarely made at one point in time. Rather, decisions about care frequently begin with the suspicion that something is wrong and that medical treatment may be necessary, and end only when the patient leaves follow-up care. Although some points in treatment involve more active decision making than others, treatment decisions are being made continually, even if the decision is merely to continue to observe patients' progress.

CONDITIONS OF THE PROCESS MODEL

There are three conditions that must be met before a process model can be implemented. First, the role expectations of both patients and physicians need to be modified. The classic physician-patient relationship involves a diffuse acceptance of the physician's authority to direct treatment and the patient's obligation to cooperate, predicated on psychological regression by the patient and re-creation of many features of the parent-child relationship.[18] This relationship works for patients with acute illnesses, but continuous dependency can injure patients' sense of autonomy and lead to a type of behavior vis-à-vis physicians that shares many features of adolescent rebellion. Moreover, the role of passive patient interferes with the type of decision making envisioned by the idea of informed consent.[19]

The goal of patient participation in medical decision making is aided by role expectations that view patients as members of treatment teams with specific expertises. Levy and Howard[20] identified four types of patient expertise, including (1) knowledge of important historical and contextual facts unavailable to other treatment team members; (2) the ability to evaluate symptoms within complex contexts only patients understand (eg, differentiating heartburn from angina pectoris depends, in part, on patient assessments, such as whether their pain feels like heartburn, on how anxiety-producing the day has

been, and on a subjective sense of the quantity of pain involved); (3) the responsibility for initiating health care in most situations; and (4) the responsibility for implementing self-care and life-style changes critical to the success of long-term treatment.

A second condition for successful participation by patients in decision making is a matching of illness models between patients and physicians. Physicians and patients often have very different ideas about medical problems and their ramifications. For example, physicians' expectations about the course of juvenile-onset diabetes differ substantially from those of new diabetics, whose concerns are likely to focus on the discomforts of insulin injections.

Patients enter their doctors' offices with a great deal of "folk wisdom" about medical problems. Some sectors of our society hold theories of disease that emphasize causation through spirits, nutritional deficiencies, energy imbalances, and spinal blockages.[21] Even when pieces of patients' knowledge are correct, they are often combined in ways that are not. Unless physicians recognize that their models of illness may differ from their patients' and adjust their discussions accordingly, they will lack much of the basis for collaboration on the selection of treatment.

The final condition for an informed consent process is a clarification of the values and expectations of both participants. For example, in treating chronic pancreatitis, a disease that is often a result of alcohol abuse, the acute pain can sometimes be alleviated by removing all or part of the pancreas. However, such a decision often leads to considerable morbidity of its own. Moreover, the effectiveness of a partial pancreatectomy is highly dependent on patients refraining from further alcohol abuse. Only with some clarification of the relative values each participant places on life span, pain relief, and alcohol use, will doctor and patient be able to reach agreement on treatment. Often, patients will not be able to identify their values about issues they have not previously considered; they must be given time to reflect and discuss the issues with friends and relatives, as well as with their physicians.[22]

THE ROLE OF MUTUAL MONITORING

A successful collaborative decision-making process requires that role expectations be modified, that illness models be matched, and that the values of both parties be made explicit. This can be accomplished only if both parties engage in a continual dialogue that we call *mutual monitoring*.[5] This involves using the routine, ongoing discussions of patients' problems as an opportunity to discuss both sides' expectations; understandings of the illness, values, and expectations for the treatment; and, of course, their views of the advantages and disadvantages of the various treatment options.

Current practice often involves only limited mutual monitoring. Physicians begin by asking for descriptions of the problems (or their current status) that brought patients in. Patients respond with simple accounts of their symptoms. Physicians then ask a long series of "close-ended" questions about patients' current physical condition and their history. An examination usually follows. Finally, physicians either announce what the problems are and prescribe treatment or state that further workup will be necessary. Sometimes physicians will ask if patients have any questions, or patients may ask on their own initiative, but these are typically brief and focus on details of compliance rather than on the choice of treatment. Evidence that patients do not understand the problem or have unrealistic goals for treatment is often ignored.[23]

While these interactions involve tacit discussion of the goals of treatment, and an observant physician may be able to pick up some information about the illness model that the patient uses, there is little place in this type of interaction for either patients or physicians to explain in any depth what they are thinking about.[24] Even when patients are given clear, reliable information on a single occasion and are allowed to ask questions, it is no substitute for mutual monitoring over the course of treatment, because both patients' and physicians' understandings of the problems are constantly changing.

The continued changes in both patients' and physicians' perceptions of medical problems occur, in part, because the medical problems evolve and, in part, because patients and physicians, like everyone else, continue to ruminate on what they know. While continual reordering of knowledge facilitates human creativity, it also makes for a great deal of misunderstanding between physicians and patients. Each new event, each new comment from a colleague or a friend, may become the occasion to rethink and reconsider what each party already knows about the disorder and the treatment. Even in the absence of new stimuli, both parties reorganize and rethink their knowledge about the treatment so as to build a relatively simple cognitive field consistent with the decisions that have already been made.[25] Moreover, the

course of the illness itself will change patients' perceptions of their problems. At the extreme, a patient facing death may find that what seemed important before is now trivial, and new issues and concerns arise. Thus a process model of informed consent requires continual dialogue between physicians and patients.

INFORMED CONSENT AND THE PHASES OF PATIENT CARE

The process model can be clarified by describing its effect on the different phases of treatment. Treatment of individual patients follows unique patterns, making generalization difficult, but for our purposes we will refer to five phases in the treatment process: establishing responsibility, defining the problem, setting goals, selecting an appropriate treatment, and extended treatment and follow-up.

Establishing Responsibility

An essential part of the beginning of any treatment relationship is the establishment of the physician's responsibilities for the patient's care. The extent of that process varies. When a profusely bleeding patient arrives in an emergency room, responsibility is usually established tacitly. More commonly, however, physicians will want to establish overtly three basic points: (1) the physician's role in treatment, (2) the substantive area of responsibility, and (3) the expected duration of the responsibility.

Sometimes these will be obvious. A patient who appears in an emergency room with a cut hand will probably assume that the physician who is providing care will focus on the cut and that the duration of the physician's responsibility will be short. Often, however, these issues will not be obvious. In all cases, patients need to know whether the particular physician will be in charge of care, will act as a consultant, or is only assisting others. Moreover, patients need to understand the areas of physicians' expertise and responsibility so that they can direct their questions appropriately. Finally, patients must know whether they will see a physician repeatedly or whether the present moment is the only chance to ask questions.

Defining the Problem

Diagnosing patients' problems may seem a purely technical matter in which patients play no roles. In fact, however, most nonemergency treatment involves a complex negotiation between physicians and patients about the definition of patients' problems.[23,24] Physicians who ignore patients' definitions of their problems often find that patients are dissatisfied and resistant to medical recommendations. Conversely, when physicians and patients share a definition of the problem and thus an orientation to particular treatment approaches, patients are more likely to follow through with treatment.[26]

Appropriate physician approaches to patients can facilitate an open negotiation about the problem to be treated. First, it is important for physicians to ask open-ended questions about the nature of a problem.[27] Although it is often useful to review the functioning of all organ systems with patients, this should only be done following open-ended questions directed at eliciting patients' complaints. Equally important, physicians must listen to the responses and not simply view the interaction as an opportunity to correct errors in patients' thinking. Patients are often more concerned with an illness' interference in their daily lives than with underlying pathologic processes. Although the response to the problem cannot ignore the underlying pathology, treatment is much more likely to gain patients' acceptance if it addresses the problems that trouble the patient most.

Setting Goals for Treatment

Even once physicians and patients agree about problems, there is still often substantial misunderstanding between them about the goals of treatment. Patients' expectations of treatment are often based on surgery or on the therapy of acute infectious diseases. They expect to be "cured" of their problems with little work on their part and often assume that treatment has failed if they are not.

Yet, assessing the risks and the benefits of particular treatments depends critically on what sort of goals can reasonably be expected. The potential benefits and risks of treatment are quite different if the patient has acute bronchitis and may have no lasting problems than if the problem is end-stage, metastatic cancer.

Selecting an Approach to Treatment

Once the goals of treatment have been defined, patients and physicians must reach a decision on how to achieve them. This aspect of treatment decision making has attracted the most attention in informed consent law, and

the legal requirements must play a part in determining physician behavior. Physicians must address the nature, purpose, risks, and benefits of the proposed treatment and any alternative treatments. Determining exactly which information to disclose is not a simple matter. The legal standards—information that a reasonable patient would find material to making a decision, or information that a reasonably prudent physician would disclose—are not particularly helpful in this regard.

Regardless of what standard applies, the emphasis should not be merely on the disclosure of "risks" but on a broader approach that describes both the advantages and disadvantages of treatment. Another critical part of choosing treatment is discussion of the therapeutic options. In most cases, treating physicians will have preferences for particular approaches to care. Indeed, in many cases there may be no medically acceptable alternatives. Provided physicians continue to understand that patients may see the matter differently, and that such views must be respected even if not agreed with, there is no reason why physicians should hesitate to state their point of view. One reason patients go to physicians is to gain access to their judgments about what should be done.

Extended Treatment and Follow-Up

The informed consent process during extended treatment and follow-up can be integrated into the ordinary process of monitoring patients' conditions. The standard question, "How is it going?" provides patients with an opportunity to express ideas about what continuing problems should be the focus of treatment. It needs to be remembered, however, that some patients hesitate to introduce their thoughts about treatment and that it is often necessary to ask repeatedly about patients' current views of their problems, goals, and preferred approaches. These may change for many reasons, including the effects of the disorder, pain and other side effects of treatment, and changes in patients' personal lives.

Patients' ruminations about the problem have the potential to provide insights that will help both patients and physicians better to understand the disorder, but initially they may leave patients confused about what is happening. A few strategic questions concerning what patients think about any new problem can help monitor patients' understanding of their disorders and treatment.

To maintain the informed consent process, a description of the next step in the treatment plan is essential. This may come to no more than explaining to a patient the need to stay in bed a few more days, or it may involve explaining what additional tests are needed and why. In either case, such an explanation provides an opportunity for patients to make sense of the seemingly chaotic series of procedures that they are expected to undergo.

Most interactions between physicians and patients should be terminated with a review of the overall treatment plan and how it contributes to the maintenance or improvement of patients' conditions. If physicians and patients meet frequently, it may become a test of a physician's ingenuity to keep the review from becoming monotonous. Nonetheless, such a review helps patients to keep a hopeful eye on the future and to justify the often painful present.

As episodes of treatment come to a close, the final task is to reestablish patients' responsibility for their own health care. Because illness, particularly illness that involves hospitalization, often induces profound emotional regression and dependence on the physician, follow-up care must concentrate on the reestablishment of patients' responsibility for themselves. This is the final phase of implementing an idea of the physician-patient relationship that seeks to maintain patients' sense of autonomy.

The reestablishment of personal autonomy is a normal part of the process of getting well again, and patients will generally undertake much of this emotional work on their own. Unfortunately, this is sometimes accomplished by projecting their anger at their dependence onto their physicians. The result is, occasionally, a lawsuit. Much more often it is an abiding sense of bitterness and selection of a new physician. It is important to understand that whether or not the anger is justified by the facts, its roots are often based in discomfort about the dependency that patients who are very ill typically feel.

THE LIMITS OF THE PROCESS MODEL

In spite of the ethical and clinical advantages of the process model, it is not universally applicable. Many physicians, eg, anesthesiologists or emergency care specialists, provide specialized services to their patients and have almost no relationship with their patients before or after the procedure is performed. In other cases, eg, house staff in an academic center, physicians may have quite brief relationships with their patients. In these instances, practices regarding disclosure and consent will, of necessity, closely approximate the event model. However, it is important that, even in these discussions, patients be fully informed of the physicians' thinking and that they be referred back to their attending physicians for further information. Especially when responsibility for care is diffused, the attending physician and the patient should be certain to review periodically the progress of treatment.

Another substantial limit on the process model concerns the economics of physicians' time. While there is reason to believe that such discussions are cost-effective, third-party payers have been reluctant to accept their importance. Although the process model need not consume great amounts of time, it is nonetheless important to begin modifying the reimbursement system to allow for such discussions. Current efforts to increase reimbursement from third-party payers for nonprocedural, "cognitive" services may be a step in the right direction.

CONCLUSIONS

Informed consent has been praised as "therapy" for the physician-patient relationship,[10] but it has also been criticized for not having had any substantial positive effect on that relationship. The idea of informed consent emphasizes the need for patient participation in treatment decision making. There is ample reason to believe that such participation is not to be valued merely for its own sake, but that it contributes to therapeutic outcomes. However, the typical implementation of informed consent, bolstered by a narrow vision of the legal doctrine, focuses on the presentation of information at one time, on what we have called the "event model" of informed consent. This information presentation is often too complex for the patient to understand without reflection and dialogue, and frequently constitutes a formalistic effort to comply with the law, at the expense of real collaboration.

We have emphasized that more effective implementation of the doctrine of informed consent requires its integration into the decision-making process, which takes place over time. The resulting process is neither an arbitrary legal imposition on clinical care nor a ritual disclosure that the patient cannot understand.

We recognize that no physician perfectly implements the standards for interacting with patients that we have described here and that sometimes there are practical impediments to their implementation. Nonetheless, we hope that we have provided a direction in which to move.

REFERENCES

1 *Salgo v Leland Stanford Jr University Board of Trustees*, 154 Cal App2d 560, 317 P2d 170 (1957).

2 Engelhart HT: *The Foundations of Bioethics*. New York, Oxford University Press, 1980, pp 250–335.

3 Beauchamp TL, Childress JF: *Principles of Biomedical Ethics*. New York, Oxford University Press, 1979, pp 56–96.

4 Faden RF, Beauchamp TL: *A History and Theory of Informed Consent*. New York, Oxford University Press, 1986.

5 Appelbaum PS, Lidz CW, Meisel AM: *Informed Consent: Legal Theory and Clinical Practice*. New York, Oxford University Press, 1987.

6 US Department of Health and Human Services: Final regulations amending basic HHS policy for protecting human research subjects. *Federal Register* 1981;46(Jan 26):8366–8386.

7 Katz J: *The Silent World of Doctor and Patient*. New York, Free Press, 1984.

8 President's Commission for the Study of Ethical Problems in Medicine and Biomedical and Behavioral Research: *Making Health Care Decisions*. Government Printing Office, 1982, vol 1: *Report*.

9 Katz J: Informed consent: A fairy tale? Law's vision. *Univ Pittsburgh Law Rev* 1977;39:137–174.

10 Restructuring informed consent: Legal therapy for the doctor-patient relationship. *Yale Law J* 1970;79:1533–1576.

11 Stone GC: Patient compliance and the role of the expert. *J Soc Iss* 1979;35:34–59.

12 Ingelfinger FJ: Informed (but uneducated) consent. *N Engl J Med* 1972;287;465–466.

13 Faden RR, Beauchamp TL: Decision making and informed consent: A study of the impact of disclosed information. *Soc Indicators Res* 1980;7:314–336.

14 Lidz CW, Meisel AM, Zerubavel E, et al: *Informed Consent: A Study of Decision Making in Psychiatry*. New York, Guilford Press, 1983.

15 Lidz CW, Meisel AM: Informed consent and the structure of medical care, in *President's Commission for the Study of Ethical Problems in Medicine and Biomedical and Behavioral Research: Making Health Care Decisions*. Government Printing Office, 1982, vol 2, pp 317–410.

16 Katz RL: Informed consent: Is it bad medicine? *West J Med* 1977;126:426–428.

17 Patten BM, Stump W: Death related to informed consent. *Tex Med* 1978;74:49–50.

18 Parson TD: *The Social System*. Glencoe, Ill, Free Press, 1951, chap 10.

19 Lidz CW, Meisel AM, Munetz M: Chronic disease and patient participation. *Cult Med Psychiatry* 1985;9:1–17.

20 Levy S, Howard J: Patient-centric technologies: A clinical-cultural perspective, in Millon T, Green C, Meagher R (eds): *Handbook of Clinical Health Psychology*. New York, Plenum Publishing Corp, 1982, pp 221–256.

21 Gillick MR: Common sense models of health and disease. *N Engl J Med* 1985;313:700–703.

22 Lidz CW: The weather report model of informed consent. *Bull Am Acad Psychiatry Law* 1980;8:152–170.

23 Lazare A, Eisenthal S, Frank A, et al: Studies on a negotiated approach to patient hospitalization, in Gallagher EB (ed): *The Doctor-Patient Relationship in the Changing Health Scene*, US Dept of Health, Education, and Welfare publication 28-183. Government Printing Office, 1978, pp 119–139.

24 Fisher S: Doctor talk/patient talk: How treatment decisions are negotiated in doctor-patient communication, in Fisher S, Todd AD (eds): *The Social Organization of Doctor-Patient Communication*. Washington, DC, Center for Applied Linguistics, 1983, pp 135–158.

25 Festinger L: *A Theory of Cognitive Dissonance*. Evanston, Ill, Row Peterson, 1957.

26 DiMatteo MR, DiNicola DD: *Achieving Patient Compliance*. Elmsford, NY, Pergamon Press Inc, 1982.

27 Mischler EG: *Discourse of Medicine: Dialectics of Medical Interviews*. Norwood, NJ, Ablex Publishing Corp, 1984.

Physicians' Duty to Treat

Altruism, Self-Interest, and Medical Ethics
Edmund D. Pellegrino

Edmund D. Pellegrino, a physician specializing in the philosophy of medicine, is the director of the Georgetown University Center for the Advanced Study of Ethics. Widely published, he is the coauthor of *A Philosophical Basis of Medical Practice* (1981) and *For the Patient's Good* (1988). He is also the coeditor of *Catholic Perspectives on Medical Morals* (1989).

Pellegrino argues that there are two conceptions of medicine today and each has different implications regarding physicians' duty to treat AIDS patients. The first conception sees medicine as an occupation like any other and the physician as having the same "rights," including the right to refuse services, as any other individual engaged in a business or a craft. The second, advanced by the author, distinguishes between medicine and other careers or forms of livelihood on three grounds: (1) the nature of illness itself; (2) the fact that the physician's knowledge is not individually owned and ought not to be used primarily for personal benefit; and (3) the physician's public acknowledgment, in taking an oath on graduation, of a collective covenant to use the acquired competence in the interests of the sick. In Pellegrino's account, these grounds give rise to an obligation on the part of physicians to make their knowledge available to all who need it, even if that involves effacing their own self-interests.

Nothing more exposes a physician's true ethics than the way he or she balances his or her own interests against those of the patient. Whether the physician is refusing to care for patients with the acquired immunodeficiency syndrome...or withdrawing from emergency department service for fear of malpractice suits, striking for better pay or fees, or earning a gatekeeper's bonus by blocking access to medical care, the question raised is the same. Does medicine entail effacement of the physician's self-interests—even to the point of personal and financial risk? Is some degree of altruism a moral obligation, or is nonmaleficence the limit of the physician's mandatory beneficence? How far does physician advocacy go?[1] What does the concept of physician as advocate mean?[2]

...Although the question is not new, the historic and ethical precedents are inconsistent. Even now, with respect to caring for AIDS patients, the guidelines are confusing. Item VI of the current American Medical Association Principles affirms the physician's right to choose whom to treat. The Ethical and Judicial Council

acknowledges the tradition to treat but permits "alternate arrangements" for physicians emotionally unable to comply. On the other hand, the American College of Physicians and the Infectious Disease Society of America are unequivocal about the physician's duty to treat.[3]

These inconsistencies cannot be resolved without a more explicit choice between two fundamentally opposed conceptions of medicine itself. One conception calls for self-effacement by the physician, while the other accommodates physician self-interest. Not to choose between these two is to reinforce the cynics, discourage the conscientious, and undermine the moral credibility of our whole enterprise. Some of us would argue that there is a right answer, but that a wrong answer is more honest than no answer at all.

The arguments of those who defend refusals to care for AIDS patients are several: AIDS was not in the social contract when they entered medicine, obligations to self and family override obligations to patients, physicians who contract AIDS are permanently lost to society and their patients, treating patients when one is fearful or hostile only compromises their care, some physicians are emotionally unable to cope, and house staff carry an unfair share of the risks.

Leaving aside the fact that the risks of contagion are disproportionate to the fear, these arguments are cogent

Reprinted with permission of the author and the publisher from *Journal of the American Medical Association*, vol. 258 (October 9, 1987), 1939–1940. Copyright © 1987, American Medical Association.

only if we accept the conception of medicine that undergirds them, ie, medicine is an occupation like any other, and the physician has the same "rights" as the businessman or the craftsman. Medical knowledge belongs to the physician to be dispensed in the marketplace on terms set by its owner. Being ill and in need of care is no different from needing any other service or commodity. Competence and avoidance of harm are all that can legitimately be demanded of physicians....

There are at least three things specific to medicine that impose an obligation of effacement of self-interest on the physician and that distinguish medicine from business and most other careers or forms of livelihood.[4]

First is the nature of illness itself. The sick person is in a uniquely dependent, anxious, vulnerable, and exploitable state. Patients must bare their weakness, compromise their dignity, and reveal intimacies of body and mind. The predicament forces them to trust the physician in a relationship of relative powerlessness. Moreover, physicians invite that trust when offering to put knowledge at the service of the sick. A medical need in itself constitutes a moral claim on those equipped to help.

Second, the knowledge the physician offers is not proprietary. It is acquired through the privilege of a medical education. Society sanctions certain invasions of privacy such as dissecting the human body, participating in the care of the sick, or experimenting with human subjects. The student is permitted access to the world's medical knowledge, much of it gained by observation and experiment on generations of sick persons. All of this, and even financial subsidization for medical education, is permitted for one purpose—that society have an uninterrupted supply of trained medical personnel.

The physician's knowledge, therefore, is not individually owned and ought not be used primarily for personal gain, prestige, or power. Rather, the profession holds this knowledge in trust for the good of the sick. Those who enter the profession are automatically parties to a collective covenant—one that cannot be interpreted unilaterally.

Finally, this covenant is publicly acknowledged when the physician takes an oath at graduation. This—not the degree—is the graduate's formal entry into the profession. The oath—whichever one is taken—is a public promise that the new physician understands the grav-

ity of this calling and promises to be competent and to use that competence in the interests of the sick. Some degree of effacement of self-interest is thus present in every medical oath. That is what makes medicine truly a profession.

These three things—the nature of illness, the nonproprietary character of medical knowledge, and the oath of fidelity to the patients' interests—generate strong moral obligations. To refuse to care for AIDS patients, even if the danger were much greater than it is, is to abnegate what is essential to being a physician. The physician is no more free to flee from danger in performance of his or her duties than the fireman, the policeman, or the soldier. To be sure, society and the profession have complementary obligations to reduce the risks and distribute the obligation fairly. However, physicians and other health professionals cannot avoid the obligation to make their knowledge available to all who need it.

Two divergent conceptions of medicine oppose each other in medical ethics today. One entails self-effacement, the other rejects it. What the AIDS epidemic and, in their own ways, the commercialization of medicine have done is to force an explicit choice. To make that choice, we need something we do not yet have—a moral philosophy of medicine, something that goes beyond professional codes, or the analysis of ethical puzzles. What is called for is a return to the normative quest of classic ethics—the quest for what it is to be a good physician and for what kind of person the physician should be....

NOTES

1 Sade R: Medical care as a right: A refutation. *N Engl J Med* 1971;285:1288–1292.

2 Hotchkiss WS: Doctor as patient advocate. *JAMA* 1987;258:947–948.

3 Health and Public Policy Committee, American College of Physicians and the Infectious Disease Society of America: Acquired immune deficiency syndrome. *Ann Intern Med* 1986;104:575–581.

4 Pellegrino ED, Thomasma DC: *The Good of the Patient: The Restitution of Beneficence in Medical Ethics.* New York, Oxford University Press Inc, in press.

AIDS and the Duty to Treat
John D. Arras

John D. Arras is associate professor of bioethics, Albert Einstein College of Medicine and Montefiore Medical Center. Arras is the coeditor of *Ethical Issues in Modern Medicine* (3d ed., 1989). His published articles include "Quality of Life in Neonatal Ethics: Beyond Denial and Evasion."

Arras, like Pellegrino, raises the question: Do physicians have an obligation to place themselves at risk in the service of patients? Arras criticizes those who have stressed the voluntary nature of the physician-patient "contract," finding voluntarism an unacceptable basis for medical practice in the age of AIDS. He discusses and criticizes some attempts to establish a duty to provide care, including the attempt to use the notion of a social contract between society and the medical profession as a basis for the duty. Dissatisfied with the social contract approach, Arras focuses on a virtue-based approach to the problem. He briefly discusses the moral tradition found in the history of the medical profession and maintains that recent history reveals a very strong commitment on the part of physicians to place patients' needs first even at the risk of their own health. Arras concludes by responding to the question, "Can or should the traditional duty to treat be extended to include HIV-infected patients?"

Do physicians, by virtue of their role as health care professionals, have a duty to treat HIV-infected patients? Must they subject themselves to the very small, but nonetheless terrifying, risk of becoming infected themselves in order to live up to the ethical demands of their calling? For most physicians toiling in the front lines against AIDS, this is a new and totally unanticipated moral question that has yet to receive a clear and satisfying answer.

The current generation of physicians has experienced very little exposure to serious occupational risk. Well protected by antiseptic techniques and antibiotics for a period of roughly thirty years, doctors in developed countries have come to believe (with some justification) that they are exempt from the riskier aspects of medicine that had claimed the lives of so many of their predecessors. Prior to this *pax antibiotica*, risk and fear accompanied physicians daily, especially during the all-too-frequent periods of plague and virulent infectious disease. For many, if not most, of these physicians, to be a doctor *meant* that one was willing to take personal risks for the benefit of patients. One entered the profession

with a keen appreciation of the hazards. By abruptly dispelling this perception of relative safety, AIDS has compelled today's physicians to reopen the traditional inquiry into the moral relationship between hazard and professional duty.

AIDS has likewise highlighted the limits of most contemporary bioethical inquiries into the physician-patient relationship. In their singleminded campaign against the excesses of medical paternalism, most bioethicists have been content merely to refute physicians' claims to moral expertise and special prerogatives based upon their Hippocratic duty to benefit the patient. In undermining this claim, bioethicists have completely ignored the question of whether physicians might still have special *responsibilities* as healers.

Moreover, the bioethicists' favorite metaphor for describing the physician-patient relationship, the contract between free and equal moral agents, has further obscured the issue of physicians' obligations to place themselves at risk in the service of their patients. By stressing the voluntary nature of the physician-patient "contract," bioethicists have inadvertently reinforced the notion that physicians, as free moral agents, have a perfect right to choose whomever they wish to serve. This claim to contractual freedom, enshrined in the 1957 AMA Code of Ethics,[1] likewise fails to address the ques-

Reprinted with permission of the author and the publisher from *Hastings Center Report*, vol. 18 (April/May 1988), Special Supplement, pp. 10–14, 16–18.

tion of whether physicians have a special duty to enter into contracts with hazardous patients.

Although there are many ways in which physicians can fail to discharge their putative duty to care for HIV-infected patients, ranging from outright refusal to foot-dragging, I shall focus on the central problem of categorical refusal to treat due to fear of infection. Do all physicians have an ethical duty to treat HIV-infected patients in spite of the risk, or can physicians fully discharge their moral duty to such persons by referring them to other physicians who are willing and capable of treating them? In short, is voluntarism an ethically acceptable basis for medical practice in the age of AIDS?

PROTECTING THE VULNERABLE: INDIVIDUAL RIGHTS AND PROFESSIONAL OBLIGATIONS

One promising starting point for our inquiry is to focus on the medical need of HIV-infected patients. These persons harbor a potentially lethal virus and may already be manifesting symptoms of ARC (AIDS Related Complex) or AIDS. They may require treatment of AIDS related conditions—such as Kaposi's sarcoma and pneumocystis pneumonia—or they may incidentally have other health problems requiring attention, such as kidney failure, heart defects, or dental problems. Although the diagnosis of HIV disease renders their plight particularly poignant, these patients resemble all patients with serious illnesses insofar as they are sick, vulnerable, and needy.

One compelling, though still contested, response to such health needs is to claim that they establish either an individual right to health care or at least a social duty to provide it.[2] This approach holds that because of the pivotal importance of health needs, including those needs created by AIDS, each person either infected with the virus or manifesting symptoms has a claim, grounded in justice, to the provision of needed health care.

The obvious drawback of this approach for our purposes is that it entirely avoids the question of physicians' individual or collective responsibility for HIV-infected patients. Whether we accept the language of individual rights or the language of societal obligation, the duty to provide care could be interpreted to fall squarely upon society through the vehicle of government, not on physicians as individuals or as a professional group. A voluntaristic system, with special incentives for those willing to treat, is compatible with this kind of societal duty.

A closely related argument makes use of the notion of a social contract between society and the medical profession. In exchange for the performance of a vital public service—that is, ministering to the needs of the sick and vulnerable—physicians as a group are granted monopolistic privileges over the practice of medicine. By seeking and receiving such a benefit, physicians incur a corresponding obligation founded on the notion of reciprocity.[3] If physicians are granted a monopoly over medical practice and then refuse to treat certain patients who are perhaps the most vulnerable members of society, who else will treat them? Just as the police have a duty to protect defenseless citizens based on their monopoly over the legitimate use of force, so physicians have a duty to treat those in medical need, even in the face of some personal risk.

By establishing some sort of duty to treat, the social contract approach thus improves upon the right-to-health-care argument, but we must concede immediately that it locates the duty not on the shoulders of each and every physician, but rather at the level of the medical profession. Since the parties to this contract are society and the profession, the social contract cannot generate, at least in the first instance, the kind of responsibility that goes through the profession to each individual member. So long as society's vital interest in caring for the vulnerable is secured, the social contract is upheld, no matter what the response of individual physicians.

This is where the analogy between physicians and the police breaks down. Whereas both groups have a professional monopoly on providing a vital public service, as well as the corresponding professional duty to provide it, individual police officers are also expected to take risks in the course of their ordinary duties. Whether they like it or not, they have to go down that dark alley where danger lurks. The reason for this disparity in the terms of these two social contracts is that police officers cannot usually delegate their risky business to others. Except for medical emergencies and personnel at public hospitals—the two obvious exceptions to the social contract's inattention to individual performance—physicians can usually refer undesirable or especially hazardous cases to others.

The sort of duty to treat generated by the social contract strategy is thus clearly compatible, at least in theory, with a voluntaristic system. Indeed, some might argue that such a voluntaristic system provides an optimal solution to the problem of AIDS: the patients get respectful care from physicians who really wish to provide it; unwilling doctors are freed from professional or legal coercion; and willing physicians are rewarded either by their own virtue or by incentives. In theory, everyone's needs and interests are thus secured by the social contract under conditions of maximal freedom of choice.

In practice, however, there is reason to believe that such a voluntaristic system might prove to be either unstable or inadequate. In the first place, such systems might place unfair demands upon those physicians who are willing to treat HIV-infected patients. If the majority of hospital-based physicians exempt themselves from the care of such patients, thereby dumping the burden upon a willing few, the resulting division of labor might easily be perceived as being grossly unfair. Those who undertook the nearly exclusive care of AIDS patients would thereby expose themselves to higher risk of both psychological burnout and eventual infection. In response to this perception, recalcitrant physicians might well agree to treat their fair share of AIDS patients so that the burden might be more or less equally distributed among the staff. Even so, it must be conceded that this shift from voluntarism to egalitarianism would be attributable, not to any putative individual duty to patients, but rather to a perceived duty to treat one's *colleagues* fairly.

An individualized duty to treat HIV-infected patients might nevertheless be empirically derived from the social contract if we could demonstrate that a voluntaristic system failed to perform according to the terms of the contract. Indeed, if it could be shown that voluntaristic systems tended to harm HIV-infected patients or failed to meet their needs, then the social contract could consistently call for the imposition of a duty to treat upon each and every doctor.

Demonstrating likely harms to HIV-infected patients under a purely voluntaristic system is not difficult. First, refusing to treat a person because he or she has AIDS or HIV infection ordinarily constitutes an insult of monumental proportions. The prospective patient is stigmatized and made to feel like an outcast. In itself this amounts to a significant injury.[4]

Secondly, the delays inherent in any system of widespread referrals might themselves cause significant harms. If patients suffering from severe or painful maladies are refused care by a physician or clinic and referred elsewhere, their conditions may well be exacerbated by the time they find someone willing and able to treat them.[5]

But perhaps the most obvious and serious problem with any voluntaristic system is that it would in all probability lead to lack of access and to substandard care. The dental profession provides an interesting case in point. A recent informal poll of the 4,100 member Chi-

cago Dental Society revealed only three dentists, all from the same clinic, who were willing to accept new AIDS referrals.[6]

Even if a voluntaristic system were able to produce enough willing physicians to solve the problem of access, the quality of the care received would remain an open question. Although it is possible (but not likely) that such a system could find the right incentives to achieve acceptable levels of quality, the history of our treatment of poor, stigmatized, and unpopular groups indicates that AIDS patients, like the insane and criminals, will most likely receive inadequate and substandard care. In either case, if the system were unable to secure either access or quality, the social contract through the conditions of licensure would justify the imposition of an individualized duty to treat.[7]

An individual duty to treat can thus be empirically derived from the collective duty ascribed to the profession, and this duty can justifiably be imposed by the state in conformity with the social contract. Perhaps this is enough to get the job done, and perhaps in the long run that is what matters most to AIDS patients; but it is certainly not the stuff on which legends of professional virtue are based. In order to ground the sort of individualized and unmediated duty to treat patients—despite substantial hazard—that we associate with the historical tradition of medicine, we have to shift our focus from the specific task of meeting social needs to understanding traditional conceptions of the virtuous physician.

CONCEPTIONS OF PROFESSIONAL VIRTUE

In general, virtue-based accounts of the physician-patient relationship depend upon both a specific conception of the goal or good of the medical art and an account of the virtues (for example, competence, courage, fidelity) necessary to attain that good.[8] In contrast to the more standard bioethical methodologies that attempt to marshall rules and principles toward the resolution of specific quandaries or dilemmas, virtue ethics is more concerned with articulating the character and role-specific duties of the good physician. There are two different approaches to virtue ethics that speak to the issue of physicians' duty to treat. One relies on a rather abstract end-means relationship; the other attempts to ground the notion of the virtuous physician in an analysis of the commitments endorsed by the profession historically....

Moral Tradition and Medical Virtue

[The latter] virtue-based approach relies, not on the nature or essence of medicine *sub specie aeternitatis*, but rather on the notion of a moral tradition embedded in the on-going history of the profession. Proponents of this view would agree with Alasdair MacIntyre's claim that we cannot answer the question "What am I to do?" without first answering the prior question "Of what story or stories do I find myself a part?"[9] They would then proceed to tell a story, to relate a history, of a profession that has incorporated a willingness to take risks for the benefit of patients as a constitutive element in physicians' self-understanding. Over time, this account would explain, the profession elevated the ideal of steadfast devotion to the well being of patients to the status of a fundamental duty, a definitive element inherent in the very role of physician. According to this story, physicians, if queried about their commitment to accept risk in the line of duty, would simply respond, "This is who we are; this is what we do. Those who fail to treat are cowards and not true physicians."

1. The Problem of Evidence   Incredibly, however, this is a history that has yet to be written. Apart from two pertinent articles that adopt contradictory positions, there are no focused, comprehensive, historical studies of physicians' duty to treat.[10] This is obviously a major problem for the virtue-based approach, since it attempts to ground the duty to treat in the historical practice and traditional self-understandings of physicians. In the absence of a reliable historical record, the status of the virtue-based duty is problematical.

To be sure, there is some historical evidence attesting to the existence of a self-perceived duty. Darrel M. Amundsen notes, for example, that as early as the 14th century, flight in the face of plague was regarded, both by physicians and the public at large, as a dereliction of duty and a shameful thing.[11] Although many physicians did, in fact, flee the plague, Amundsen contends that a standard of behavior had emerged according to which their retreat would be harshly judged. In support of this view, he quotes Guy de Chauliac, the Pope's physician at Avignon, who ruefully declared, "And I, to avoid infamy, dared not absent myself but with continual fear preserved myself as best I could."

Another important example of self-sacrificial behavior motivated by medical duty is provided by Benjamin Rush during the great yellow fever epidemic at Philadelphia in 1793.[12] Although Rush's extraordinary devotion to patients during the epidemic has become the stuff of

legend—as opposed, sadly, to the efficacy of his violent treatments—it is crucial to note that his courage was perceived by himself and others as required by duty. His acts were courageous, not because they went beyond the call of duty, but rather because he did his duty when others might be sorely tempted to flee from it.[13]

In spite of this "oral tradition" attesting to a duty to treat, we still lack rigorous historical studies that would establish an unbroken chain of professional duty stretching from the advent of the Black Death in Europe to modern times. Moreover, it is noteworthy that the only medical historian who has attempted to focus on this vast stretch of time has come to a very different conclusion. According to Daniel Fox, the history of medicine is marked, not so much by an unbroken tradition of risk taking for patients, as by a tradition of negotiation between civic leaders and the medical profession to provide for the needs of patients during epidemics. In short, Fox claims that voluntarism, rather than any individualized professional duty to treat, has been the historical norm.[14]

2. The Burden of Proof   Notwithstanding the absence of hard historical data on the duty to treat throughout the past six centuries, two salient facts suggest that the burden of proof should lie with those who would deny the existence of this duty. First, the persistence of an oral tradition or "folk wisdom" among physicians attesting to a duty to take risks for patients tells us a good deal about how physicians have traditionally understood their professional role. This sort of narrative tradition can still speak powerfully to us even if it does not meet the exacting standards of contemporary historiography.

Second, even if historians eventually demonstrate that voluntarism, rather than individual duty, best describes the behavior and beliefs of most physicians from the Middle Ages to the 20th century, they will most likely have to concede that, from the latter half of the 19th century onwards, tales of heroism eclipse accounts of flight as a sense of individual duty became indisputably rooted in the medical conscience. Even Zuger and Miles, who eventually conclude that the duty to treat cannot be firmly grounded in the vast canvass of medical history, admit that from the 1850s onwards "it becomes far more difficult to find recorded instances of physicians' reluctance to accept the risks that epidemics entailed for them. The stories of the cholera pandemics of the 19th century, the plague in the Orient, the influenza pandemic of 1918, polio in the 1950s, are largely ones of medical heroism."[15]

This firm understanding of the physician's duty was explicitly recognized as early as 1847 in the first code of ethics of the American Medical Association, which stated that "...when pestilence prevails, it is their duty to face the danger, and to continue their labors for the alleviation of the suffering, even at the jeopardy of their own lives."[16] Language to this effect remained in the Code until 1957, when it was dropped on account of medicine's (ultimately provisional) conquest of pestilential diseases.[17] Following a prolonged period of indecision on the physician's duty to treat HIV-infected patients, the A.M.A. in November 1987 unambiguously reaffirmed the duty to treat in the face of risk.[18] Although such codes are by no means infallible guides to the moral sensibilities of physicians, they at least provide good evidence of a profession's considered ethical judgments and of its own sense of identity.

Thus, although the historical record is woefully incomplete and physicians' track record is markedly inconsistent, our recent history reveals a very strong professional commitment to place the needs of the patient first, even at the risk of one's own health or life. This historical understanding, based perhaps more on *story* than on *historiography*, is aptly captured in Arnold Relman's claim that "the risk of contracting the patient's disease is one of the risks that is inherent in the profession of medicine. Physicians who are not willing to accept that risk....ought not to be in the practice of medicine."[19]...

AIDS AND THE DUTY TO TREAT

Can or should the traditional duty* to treat be extended to include HIV-infected patients? To answer this question, we must ask additional questions about the nature of the risks posed by AIDS to physicians. What exactly is the risk of transmission through occupational exposure? And, how should this risk be evaluated?

What is the Risk?   Since physicians do not usually have sex or share needles with their patients, the most likely routes of transmission are needle-stick accidents and blood splashing. In contrast to the risk of acquiring hepatitis B through an errant needle stick, the risk of HIV infection from similar accidents is very small— probably no more than one per every 200 incidents.[20] Even this low level of risk can be essentially eliminated for many physicians by scrupulous attention to established infection-control recommendations.

This is not to say that there is no risk at all. By February 1988, at least eight health care workers had acquired HIV infection through occupational exposure, and those who go on to develop full-blown AIDS will almost certainly die. Moreover, some physicians may be at higher risk for HIV infection. Surgeons, obstetricians and emergency room personnel, for example, appear to be disproportionately vulnerable to needle sticks and exposure to blood. Significantly, however, existing studies do not indicate a higher rate of occupational HIV transmission among these "high blood profile" specialties.[21]

Evaluating the Risk of AIDS   In addition to the task of scientifically estimating their actual exposure to risk, physicians must also evaluate this risk. Is it worth running? At first glance, this would appear to be an easy question for a historically based virtue ethics, since the objective risk of death from occupational exposure to HIV simply pales in comparison with the risks run by previous generations of physicians. But we must recall that the threshold separating duty from supererogation depends upon culturally relative definitions of reasonable or acceptable risks. What if risks that were acceptable thirty, sixty, or one hundred years ago are no longer deemed reasonable by physicians and the society at large?

*Editors' note: In a section not included in this excerpt from his article, Arras identifies six features of this duty to treat. (1) It is *a particularistic duty*—a duty based on a particular shared vision of the good animating a particular moral tradition. (2) It is a duty that may be grounded in several factors: (*a*) an empathetic response to patients' needs and medical vulnerability by those who, by virtue of their medical skills, possess an exclusive and awesome power; (*b*) physicians' indebtedness to society for the social contributions that enable physicians to acquire the necessary knowledge and skills; and (*c*) a shared ideal of medicine as a profession dedicated to the good of others. (3) It is *an individualized duty*—a duty that binds each and every physician to treat regardless of whether other physicians might be available. (4) In keeping with the previous feature, this duty to treat *rules out volunteerism*. Those who refuse to treat are bad physicians even if they succeed in referring all of their patients to others who satisfy all their medical needs. (5) It *has not been entirely self-imposed* but forged in an ongoing dialogue with society at large and thus has been subject to *social reinforcement*. (6) It is a duty that has a limit, one set by the level of risk involved. The problem is to determine the threshold of "acceptable risk," which is the dividing line between duty and supererogation.

Conditions certainly have changed, and these changes are responsible for much of our current perplexity regarding the limits of the duty to treat. Perhaps most importantly, the world (or at least the industrialized, affluent part of it) is now a much safer place. Prior to the development of antibiotics, antisepsis, and vaccines, the entire population of the world might be said to have constituted a gigantic "high risk group" for early death from pestilence and other killer diseases. Life for most people, including physicians, was on average much shorter than it is today.

Thus, to a 19th century physician, death from yellow fever would no doubt have seemed a tragic but not extraordinary possibility. By contrast, present day physicians fully expect to live a long life; they no longer believe that anyone, especially themselves, should die from an infectious disease.

Notwithstanding this displacement of the threshold of supererogation, today's medical profession appears to be extending its historical commitment to encompass those who suffer from HIV and AIDS. As the A.M.A. policy statement recently made clear, "that tradition must be maintained.... A physician may not ethically refuse to treat a patient whose condition is within the physician's current realm of competence solely because the patient is seropositive."[22] Although some physicians have privately or publicly engaged in categorical refusals to care for HIV-infected patients,[23] they appear to constitute, in the words of Surgeon General Koop, "a fearful and irrational minority."[24] To be sure, many physicians, especially the younger ones who bear most of the burden of caring for AIDS patients, tread a narrow path like Guy de Chauliac between fear of AIDS and fear of infamy; but very few are driven by fear to renounce the care of AIDS patients altogether.

Thus, while our altered perceptions of relative risk may help to account for resistance to treating AIDS patients, it appears that the medical profession has collectively decided, albeit with a significant amount of internal dissent, to view most occupational exposures to HIV disease as at least comparable to other risks inherent in the practice of medicine—that is, as "acceptable risks."

Notwithstanding this consensus on the basic issue, a significant number of physicians, especially those who are no longer subjected to the discipline of internship and residency programs, have come to the conclusion that for them the risk is not worth running, even if they concur with the CDC's low estimates. How can this be explained?

The answer lies, at least in part, in the way some of these physicians perceive those afflicted with HIV disease. In refusing to deal with such patients, many physicians seem not merely to be saying, "Why should I risk my life?" but rather, "Why should I risk my life for the likes of homosexuals and intravenous drug abusers?" In other words, these physicians want to know why they must incur even small risks of serious harm for the benefit of morally suspect groups. It is one thing, they say, to risk one's life for an "innocent" child afflicted with AIDS through no fault of his own, but it is quite another thing to expose oneself to risks for patients who have "brought it upon themselves" through behaviors that are either illegal, immoral, or both.[25]

This attempt to turn the HIV-infected person into a complete Other by means of distancing and devaluation is often supplemented by a simultaneous movement of imaginative identification. As he evaluates the risks, the physician places himself in the shoes of the AIDS patient, but instead of achieving sympathy, this act of identification often yields only horror. The physician must contemplate not only the risk of death, however small, but also the risk of dying as people often die of AIDS in our society—that is, as outcasts, as stigmatized objects of fascination and disgust.

The appropriate societal response to a reluctance to treat based on this kind of fear should be a renewed effort to extend compassion and humane services to *all* AIDS sufferers. The fear of stigmatization is real and a matter of legitimate concern. Although it does not justify categorical refusals to treat, such fear is not a shameful response to societal intolerance. If physicians are to be expected to put their lives on the line, the least society can do is to treat them and their families with gratitude and the utmost respect if they become infected.

But as for those physicians who refuse to treat because they do not deem the lives and health of homosexuals and drug addicts to be worth the slightest exposure to risk, it would seem that they violate an even more basic duty traditionally espoused by the medical profession: the duty to treat all patients with respect for their human dignity, irrespective of considerations of their personal attributes, their social or economic status, or the nature of their disease....

ACKNOWLEDGMENTS

This paper accumulated numerous debts. I am grateful to Michael Alderman, Ronald Bayer, Nancy Dubler, Liz Emrey, Robert Klein, Dorothy Levenson, Tom Murray, Kathleen Nolan, Nancy Rhoden, David Willis, Peter

Williams, and the members of The Hastings Center's project on "AIDS and Professional Responsibility," for many trenchant criticisms and helpful suggestions. I gratefully acknowledge the support of the New York Council for the Humanities.

REFERENCES

1 *Judicial Council of the American Medical Association: Current Opinions of the Judicial Council of the American Medical Association* (Chicago: American Medical Association, 1986), ix.

2 For a general discussion of the comparative merits of "rights-based" and "social duty" approaches to equity, see John Arras, "Retreat from the Right to Health Care," *Cardozo Law Review* 6:2 (Winter 1984), 321–45.

3 Compare John Rawls, *A Theory of Justice* (Cambridge, MA: Harvard University Press, 1971), 102–03.

4 Richard Goldstein, "AIDS and the Social Contract," *The Village Voice* 32:52 (December 29, 1987), 14ff.

5 See *Report on Discrimination Against People with AIDS* (January 1986–June 1987) and *AIDS and People of Color: The Discriminatory Impact* (August 1987).

6 "AIDS Clinic Being Weighed by Chicago Dental Society," *New York Times* (July 21, 1987), B4.

7 Since most state licensure laws do not address the issue of physicians' refusal to initiate treatment contracts, this imposition would most likely require fresh legislation.

8 Cf. Earl Shelp, ed., *Virtue and Medicine* (Boston: Reidel Publishing Company, 1985).

9 Alasdair MacIntyre, *After Virtue* (Notre Dame: Notre Dame University Press, 1981), 201.

10 Darrel M. Amundsen, "Medical Deontology and Pestilential Disease in the Late Middle Ages," *Journal of the History of Medicine and Allied Sciences 32* (1977), 403–21; and Daniel M. Fox, "The Politics of Physicians' Responsibility in Epidemics: A Note on History," *Hastings Center Report* 18:2 (April/May 1988).

11 Amundsen, "Medical Deontology," 408.

12 See generally, J.H. Powell, *Bring Out Your Dead: The Great Plague of Yellow Fever in Philadelphia in 1793* (Philadelphia: University of Pennsylvania Press, 1949).

13 On the relationships between courage, duty, and supererogation, see Douglas N. Walton, *Courage: A Philosophical Investigation* (Berkeley: University of California Press, 1986).

14 Fox, "The Politics of Physicians' Responsibility in Epidemics."

15 Abigail Zuger and Steven H. Miles, "Physicians, AIDS, and Occupational Risk," *Journal of the American Medical Association* 258, No. 14 (October 9, 1987), 1924–1928.

16 *Code of Ethics of the American Medical Association, 1847.* Reprinted in Chauncey D. Leake, ed., *Percival's Medical Ethics* (Huntington, NY: Krieger Publishing Company, 1975).

17 This interpretation of the A.M.A.'s decision to drop this provision was recently confirmed by Nancy Dickey, M.D., a member of the A.M.A. Council on Ethical and Judicial Affairs, at a meeting of the Hastings Center's project on "AIDS and Professional Responsibilities."

18 American Medical Association Council on Ethical and Judicial Affairs, *Report on Ethical Issues Involved in the Growing AIDS Crisis* (November 1987).

19 *Cardiovascular News* (August 1987), 7.

20 James R. Allen, "Health Care Workers and the Risk of HIV Transmission," *Hastings Center Report* 18:2 (April 1988).

21 See M.D. Hagen, et al., "Routine Preoperative Screening for HIV," *JAMA* 259:9 (March 4, 1988), 1357–59.

22 AMA Council on Ethical and Judicial Affairs, "Issues Involved in the Growing AIDS Crisis," December 1987.

23 "AIDS Fear Spawns Ethics Debate as Some Doctors Withhold Care," *New York Times* (July 11, 1987), A1, 12.

24 "Doctors Who Shun AIDS Patients are Assaulted by Surgeon General," *New York Times* (September 10, 1987), A1.

25 As a family practitioner from Illinois put it, "I would not knowingly treat a homosexual patient with AIDS, but I would treat patients who got the disease by blood transfusion, and I would treat children with AIDS." "What Doctors Think About AIDS," *MD* (January 1987), 95.

Conflicts of Obligations

The Physician as Gatekeeper
Edmund D. Pellegrino and David C. Thomasma

A biographical sketch of Edmund D. Pellegrino is found on page 113. David C. Thomasma is professor of medicine and philosophy and director of the medical humanities program at Loyola University Stritch School of Medicine. He is the author of *An Apology for the Value of Human Life* (1983) as well as the coauthor, with Pellegrino, of *A Philosophical Basis of Medical Practice* (1981) and *For the Patient's Good* (1988), from which this selection is excerpted.

Pellegrino and Thomasma examine the conflicts of interest that arise for physicians when they are given either negative or positive financial incentives to force them to act as gatekeepers—"rationers" of services such as tests, treatments, and operations. In their discussion, the authors distinguish among the following: (1) some de facto conflicts of interest that are impossible to eliminate; (2) de facto gatekeeping, the sort of rational use of resources whereby ineffective and nonbeneficial measures are not provided; (3) negative gatekeeping, where the physician is placed under constraints of self-interest to restrict the use of medical resources, especially expensive ones; and (4) positive gatekeeping, where the physician's interest lies in increasing rather than decreasing access to services. In the last two kinds of gatekeeping, the physician's self-interest, or the interest of institutions such as hospitals, rather than the patient's well-being becomes the standard for what services will be provided or withheld. Pellegrino and Thomasma condemn both negative and positive gatekeeping because they generate a conflict between the interests of physicians and patients, foster social injustice, and involve an erosion and a violation of the commitment to patient welfare that they identify as the primary moral imperative in medical care.

An ethically perilous line of reasoning is gaining wide currency in our country today. It starts with a legitimate concern for rising health care costs, finds them uncontrollable by any means except some form of rationing, and concludes that the physician must become the "gatekeeper," the designated guardian of society's resources. Through both negative and positive financial incentives, it is reasoned, the physician can be forced to conserve tests, treatments, operations, hospitalizations, and referrals for consultation. In this way, supposedly, costs will be cut by eliminating "unnecessary" medical care.

From an economic point of view, this argument is attractive to those who must shoulder a good part of our more-than-a-billion-dollars-a-day health care bill. Policy-

makers, corporation executives, insurance carriers, affluent patients, and some physicians have already accepted the economic inevitability of rationing. The ethical implications are brushed aside as secondary, given the size of the problem and the fact that it is, indeed, physicians who are responsible for 75 percent of all health care expenditures.

Before committing ourselves to a course of action that will drastically alter the already strained trust between patients and physicians, some of the ethical questions associated with gatekeeping need closer examination.

To what extent can, or should, the physician serve simultaneously his or her own needs, the needs of patients, and those of society? To what extent should the physician be a double, triple, or even quadruple agent? Under what conditions would such divided advocacy be necessary, desirable, or morally licit? What are the implications for our traditional understanding of medical ethics? How is the physician to resolve the conflicts of obligations built into divided advocacies?...

We start with an examination of the conflict of interest that is a de facto aspect of physician-patient relationships. We then define three kinds of gatekeeping roles [and] the moral issues inherent in each....

DE FACTO CONFLICT OF INTEREST

When the first physician requested a fee for his services, economics and conflict of interest entered medicine.[1] Ever since, the physician's fee and the degree to which he could point to the necessity for his services to justify maintaining his own income have been sources of suspicion and contention between physicians and patients. Socrates, in his dialogue with the cynical Thrasymachus, was forced to admit that the physician was engaged in two "arts"—the art of medicine, which had as its end the health of the patient, and the art of making money, which had the physician's self-interest as its end and did not, in itself, contribute to the patient's welfare at all.

> Then isn't it the case that the doctor insofar as he is the doctor considers or commands not the doctor's advantage but that of the sick man? For the doctor in the precise sense was agreed to be a ruler of bodies and not a money maker.[2]
>
> Do you call the medical art the wage earner's art even if a man practicing medicine should earn wages?[3]
>
> The medical art produces health, the wage earner's art wages.[4]

Plato admitted through the voice of Socrates that these two arts could be in conflict, indeed had to be, given their disparate ends. For a more modern version of the fee dilemma, no one has more tellingly exposed the inevitability of a certain amount of conflict of interest in the physician's work than Shaw.[5]

This de facto conflict of interest is difficult or impossible to eliminate, given that physicians must earn a living, support families, and have access to the same material goods as others. What mitigates the conflict is the ethical commitment of the physician to the patient's good, that is, to the principle of beneficence.

Beneficence has always implied some degree of effacement of the physician's self-interest in favor of the interest of the patient. For centuries, good physicians have treated patients who could not pay, have exposed themselves to contagion or physical harm in responding

to the call of the sick, and have sacrificed their leisure and time with their own families—sometimes too liberally—all out of commitment to serve the good of the sick.

Indeed, it is this effacement of self-interest that distinguishes a true profession from a business or craft.[6] And it is the expectation that physicians will, by and large, practice some degree of self-effacement that warrants the trust that society and individual patients place in them. It is the physician's public commitment to service beyond self-interest that constitutes the real entry of the medical graduate into the profession. The awarding of a medical degree signifies only successful completion of a course of study, but the oath is a public act of commitment to a special way of life demanded by the nature of medicine and the specific obligations that bind those who enter it.[7]

Ethical commitments can, and do, mitigate the conflicts of interest inherent in medical practice, but they do not eliminate them—except perhaps in the heroic examples of self-sacrifice we expect only of saints and martyrs. Surely, the salaried physician is not free of this impediment. If his financial incentives are reduced, other motives, including prestige, power, professional advancement, self-indulgence, unionization, and family obligations, can conflict with the care owed the patient. These can be just as detrimental to the patient's well-being as can the physician's monetary interests.

While there has always been some irreducible quantum of self-interest in medicine, rarely, if ever, has self-interest been socially sanctioned, morally legitimated, or encouraged as it is in the rationing approach to cost containment. Today the physician's self-interest is deliberately used by policymakers to contain the availability, accessibility, and quality of services to the patient. It is against this background of how they accentuate the de facto conflict of interest in medicine that the several forms of gatekeeping, licit and illicit, must be examined.

THREE FORMS OF GATEKEEPING

De Facto Gatekeeping: The Traditional Role

As with de facto conflict of interest, there is in the nature of the medical transaction an unavoidable gatekeeping function that the physician has always exercised and, indeed, is under compulsion to exercise in a morally defensible way. The unavoidable fact is that the physician recommends that tests, treatments, medications, operations, consultations, periods of stay in hospitals and nursing homes, and so forth meet the patient's needs.

This fact imposes a serious positive moral obligation on the physician to use both the individual's and society's resources optimally. In the case of the individual patient, the physician is obligated by his or her promise to act for the patient's welfare to use only those measures appropriate to cure the patient or alleviate his or her suffering. What the physician recommends must be *effective*, that is, it must materially modify the natural history of the disease, and it must also be *beneficial*, that is, it must be to the patient's benefit. Some measures—such as treatments for pneumonia—are highly effective, but may not be always beneficial if they unnecessarily prolong the act of dying and thus impose the burden of futility and expense without benefit for the patient. Other treatments benefit the patient but are not effective in altering the course of the disease—pain relief, nursing or home care, or intravenous fluids and nutrition.

The same distinction applies to diagnostic procedures. The physician has a moral obligation to use laboratory tests, X rays, and imaging procedures only if they contribute materially to the certitude of the diagnosis or the nature of the clinical decision. Marginally helpful tests, especially if they are expensive, or tests that are simply for teaching purposes (if the patient is in a teaching hospital) are not justifiable.

The physician, therefore, has a legitimate, indeed, a morally binding, responsibility to function as a gatekeeper. He must use his knowledge to practice competent, scientifically rational medicine. His guidelines should be diagnostic elegance (just the right degree of economy of means in diagnosis) and therapeutic parsimony (just those treatments that are demonstrably beneficial and effective). In this way the physician automatically fulfills several moral obligations: He avoids unnecessary risk to the patient from dubious treatment and he conserves the financial resources of both the patient and society.

The physician remains the patient's advocate. As the de facto gatekeeper, the physician is obliged to obtain tests and use treatments that are beneficial to his patient and not to restrict access for purely financial or economic reasons. The physician may withhold treatment if the patient decides that he does not wish to consume his family's resources. Thus, limiting access can be part of a legitimate gatekeeper role.

The role of de facto gatekeeper, when ethically performed, entails no conflict with the patient's good. Economics and ethics, individual and social good, and the doctor's and the patient's interests are all in congruence. In rational medicine, as we have defined it, the mode of the payment—whether by salary or fee—should make no difference. Properly conceived and practiced, rational medicine in a sense solves the dilemma posed in the first book of Plato's *Republic*. It subjects both the physician's art as physician and his art as wage earner to a higher standard—the standard of rational medicine that, in turn, derives its justification from the fact that it is in the patient's best interests. In the morally defensible gatekeeper role, the physician uses his de facto position to advance the good of his patient. In contrast, two new versions of gatekeeping have been introduced, each with attendant serious moral objection because their primary intent is economic, not ethical, obligation.

The Negative Gatekeeper Role

In the negative version of the gatekeeper role, the physician is placed under the constraints of self-interest to restrict the use of medical services of all kinds, but particularly those that are most expensive. A variety of measures is used, each of which interjects economic considerations into the physician's clinical decisions and limits his discretionary latitude in making decisions.

One way to do this is through the diagnostic-related group (DRG) program, which assigns in advance to more than four hundred disease categories a fixed sum or a fixed number of days of hospitalization. If the number of days (or tests, procedures, and so forth) is exceeded, the institution or the physician loses the difference; if the number of days of hospitalization is less than the standard allotment, then the institution or physician makes a profit.

In other plans the physician or institution contracts to provide care for some prescribed number of patients for a fixed annual sum. This can be an HMO or a preferred provider organization. Again, if the total costs for care exceed the contracted amount, the provider bears the loss; if the costs are less, the provider makes a profit. Variations on these themes are several, and they need not be detailed here. The essence of each is to motivate the provider to limit access to care by appealing to his or her self-interest.[8]

With all these plans the physician becomes the focus of incentives and disincentives in several ways: as a private practitioner when she hospitalizes a patient under the DRG system, and as the employee or partner in a prepayment insurance plan, such as an HMO, independent practice association, or primary care network. Increasingly, in each case, the physician's economic efficiency is monitored, and her deviations from the norm are rewarded or punished. The rewards may be in the form of profit sharing, bonuses, promotion in the organization, or other perquisites and preferments. The disincentives are loss of profit, limits on admitting privileges, or nonrenewal of a coemployment contract. In some instances productivity and efficiency schedules, and other quantitative measures, not only of cost containment but of profit making, are used to evaluate the physician's performance.

The major pressure in these plans at present is upon the primary care physician, the first contact within the health care system who makes the majority of decisions about entry into the system. The primary care physician may be the family primary practitioner, general internist, or pediatrician. The primary physician, as the "person in the trenches," has the greatest influence over access to expensive resources of hospitalization, testing, and consulting. For this reason, many prepayment plans insist that the patient stay with one primary care physician within the system, lest they shop around for one who might be more compliant. Gradually, as pressures for cost containment increase, the consultant and tertiary care specialists will very likely also be included as gatekeepers, with constraints and criteria suited to the nature of their specialties.

Positive Gatekeeping

The positive version of gatekeeping is less well defined and not usually explicitly formalized. In this version the physician is constrained to increase rather than decrease access to services. The purpose here is not containing costs but enhancing profits. For those who can pay, the latest and most expensive diagnostic or therapeutic services are offered; services are provided based on market "demand" rather than medical need. The aim is to "penetrate" or "dominate" the market to eliminate services that are not profitable. Increasing the demand for services is an implicit goal. Here the physician becomes virtually a salesperson. Already, we see this most blatantly in television and newspaper advertisements soliciting clients for elective surgery and all sorts of other services, some authentic and some quite useless.

With the positive gatekeeping role, the physician uses his or her de facto position as gatekeeper to his own financial advantage or to that of his employer. He shares in the profit directly if he is an owner of, or investor in,

the service provided; he is rewarded by pay increases, advancement, and so on if he is employed.

THE MORAL ISSUES IN MEDICAL GATEKEEPING

Moral Issues in Negative Gatekeeping

Both the positive and negative versions of gatekeeping exploit the de facto position of the physician as the filter through which patients gain access to services. The purposes to be served, however, are not primarily in the patient's interests. The moral issues arise from the degree to which these other interests dilute the trust the patient places in the physician as his or her primary agent advocate. The motives of self-interest upon which the newer gatekeeping roles depend complicate and accentuate the irreducible quanta of self-interest that have always existed in the physician-patient relationship.

Efforts at cost containment are not, in themselves, immoral and, as noted above, are morally mandatory when they are in the best interests of the patient. They violate those interests if, for whatever reason, they deny needed services or induce the patient to demand, or the physician to provide, unneeded services. The ethical dilemmas of gatekeeping therefore arise out of the way economic incentives and disincentives modify the physician's freedom to act in the patient's behalf. While in the past the physician was largely responsible for defining necessary and unnecessary care, those determinations are now formularized by policy. In applying the formulae the physician becomes the agent of the hospital or the system, rather than the patient. And her medical criteria of necessary treatment are subject to modification or veto by economic considerations.

Many of these ethical dilemmas are illustrated in the Medicare prospective payment system now in force in the majority of states. In this system the cost-based per diem reimbursement system of the past is replaced by a prospective payment system based on fixed prices for 471 DRGs. The initial motivation behind this transition was to improve quality of care by linking it directly to reimbursement. Thus, it was reasoned that the DRG system would cut costs by closer scrutiny of care, aimed especially at limiting "unnecessary" tests, drugs, procedures, and hospitalization. Besides being economically wasteful, unneeded care is sometimes dangerous to patients.

These cost-containment measures are not intrinsically immoral. Certainly, we cannot consider them unethical simply because they limit the physician's latitude in decision making. Rather, it is the effect of this limitation on the patient that is ethically crucial, as is the moral responsibility of the physician operating within such a system when she deems its impact to be harmful for her patient.

The difficulty in the application of present DRG policies arises in the determination of what is "necessary" for quality care for a particular patient. In a system based on average lengths of stay for each disease, individual patients may suffer, since no two diseases manifest themselves in the same way in every patient. As a result, disease entities, not individual patients, are treated, and the original aim of quality care is compromised. Sometimes this is dangerous to patients who may be transferred or "dumped" as their reimbursement runs out.[9]

Further, the needs for hospitalization, tests, and medical care for a previously healthy, middle-aged head of a household with a comfortable home and a good job who is diagnosed as having pneumonia are very different from the needs of a chronically ill, elderly widow, living alone and far from her family, who has the same disease. Given the variable nature of patient responses to illness, a certain number of individual cases must fall outside the statistical projections. These are termed *outliers*—those who need lengthier stays, more procedures, more medications, and so on than the DRG plan allows.

Two tendencies that are deleterious to patients are already manifested in the way the DRG system is being administered in many hospitals. One is the fact that patients are being discharged "quicker and sicker." The second is the failure to provide the extra funds needed by the outlier. In both instances it is often the frail, elderly patient who is sent "home" with no adequate provision for posthospital care in a nursing home, at home, or elsewhere. (The American Association of Retired Persons has a hot line to call in case the elderly think they have been discharged too early.[10]) In fact, the trend in public policy at the moment is to curtail payment for nonhospital and long-term care, further aggravating the harm caused by premature discharge. This system is also reported to endanger the poor.[11]

In prospective payment systems the physician is automatically a negative gatekeeper. To the extent that unnecessary care is avoided and the quality of care receives closer scrutiny, the good of the patient is served. But when the system harms the patient, the question of the physician's primary agency arises. If she is primarily the patient's advocate, agent, and minister, she must protect the patient's interest against the system, even at the cost of some risk and damage to her own self-interest.

In addition to the intrinsic difficulties of gatekeeping, the physician's judgments are beclouded by a variety of pressures and motives inimical to the patient's interests.[12] There is, first of all, the tendency to underutilization since this rewards the physician or hospital. The temptation, therefore, is great to cut corners, to declare as "frills" what might otherwise be necessities, or to be less sensitive to the more subtle, but equally important, needs of patients for psychosocial support. A study of British physicians showed that, because of social pressure, what were once considered medically indicated treatments are now deemed unnecessary and not in the patient's best interests. All that has changed is the determination to ration.[13] Further, the primary care physician is encouraged to temporize in her workup and to delay expensive tests, treatments, or consultations. This is especially the case in HMOs. The physician may even stretch her competence dangerously to do certain procedures herself in order to contain costs.

Another pressure in prospective payment plans is to disfavor or disenfranchise the sicker patients, those with chronic illnesses and those who need more expensive care. A study of Rush St. Luke's Hospital in Chicago demonstrated that the elderly in the intensive care unit will have to receive a much lower quality of care because the DRG system pays the hospital an average of twelve thousand dollars per patient less than it costs to treat them.[14] Less admirable still is the way cost containment can be used, consciously and unconsciously, to justify the exclusion or denial of services to difficult, troublesome, or obnoxious patients, or to other categories of patients one prefers not to see—the neurotic, the "complainers," the "hypochondriacs"—or, worst of all, the ethnic or social groups one dislikes personally.

Another deleterious effect of negative gatekeeping is to cultivate competition among providers on the wrong grounds. Instead of competition to provide the highest-quality care, as judged by the standards of rational medicine, there is competition for the best records of savings, productivity, and efficiency, the shortest hospital stays, or the least number of procedures done. Granted that excesses of care exist and are deleterious, it still does not follow that underutilization is beneficial, especially with certain very effective though costly high-technology procedures (for example, renal dialysis, organ transplant, coronary angioplasty, CAT scanning, and nuclear magnetic resonance examinations).

To be effective, many prospective payment plans insist that patients be locked into receiving care from one primary care physician. The choice of physicians and the freedom to switch is severely limited. The most sensitive part of the healing relationship, the confidence one must have in one's personal physician, is thus ignored or compromised. Especially in chronic or recurrent disease, this confidence is essential to effective care.

These factors converge to drive the physician's self-interest into conflict with the patient's. These conflicts are heightened by the rather drastic changes occurring in the economic status of the medical professional, which make the physician more vulnerable to economic pressure. Currently, there is an oversupply of physicians in urban areas and in many specialties.[15] Many physicians now graduate with debts for their education in the neighborhood of one hundred thousand dollars. The high cost of malpractice premiums must be laid out before anyone dares risk even a day of medical practice. Competition from corporately owned and operated clinics forces even conscientious physicians into "survival" tactics of questionable moral defensibility.

The result of all this is that many young, and even older, physicians are driven into salaried group practices and automatically become negative gatekeepers. The physician's independence, as Starr has shown, is rapidly eroding, and with it her ability to withstand the institutional and corporate strictures on her judgment about what is good for her patient.[16] It is becoming ever more costly, personally and financially, for even the most morally sensitive physician to practice the effacement of self-interest that beneficence-in-trust requires.

Moral Issues in Positive Gatekeeping

The moral conflicts in the positive version of gatekeeping are less subtle. Here the profit motive is primary. The transaction between physician and patient becomes a commodity transaction. The physician becomes an independent entrepreneur or the hired agent of entrepreneurs and investors who themselves have no connection with the traditions of medical ethics. The physician begins to practice the ethics of the marketplace, to think of his or her relationship with the patient not as a covenant or trust, but as a business and a contract relationship. Ethics becomes not a matter of obligations or virtue, but of legality. The metaphors of business and law

replace those of ethics. Medical knowledge becomes proprietary, the doctor's private property to be sold to whom he chooses at whatever price and condition he chooses.

When positive gatekeeping is employed, the dependence, anxiety, lack of knowledge, and vulnerability of the sick person (or even the healthy person) are exploited for personal profit. To encourage unnecessary cosmetic surgery, hysterectomies, CAT scans, or sonograms, even if the patient believes he or she ought to have "the latest and the best," is to defect from even the most primordial concept of stewardship of the patient's interest. Here the conflict of interest is more blatant than in the negative version of gatekeeping. The patient becomes primarily a source of income. The more crass financial motives that have motivated selfish physicians are legitimated and even given social sanction.

In the positive version of gatekeeping, there is not, as there may be in the negative version, any defensible moral argument. Some defend the profit motive as necessary to medical progress, to maintain quality of service or even to provide charitable care. It would be unrealistic to deny that for some physicians these are the only effective motives and that some good can come of them. But, ultimately, when a conflict occurs between profit and patient welfare, patient welfare is sure to suffer. The unrestrained monetary instinct corrupts medicine as surely as do unrestrained instincts for power or prestige....

On grounds of the conflict it generates between physician and patient interests and the social injustice it fosters, the role of gatekeeper entails an erosion and a violation of the commitment to patient welfare that must be the primary moral imperative in medical care. This commitment flows from the nature of illness and the promise to service made by individual physicians and the profession as a whole. That commitment has a basis in the empirical nature of the healing relationship, in which a sick person—dependent, vulnerable, exploitable—must seek out the help of another who has the necessary knowledge, skill, and facilities to effect a cure. It is inevitably a relationship of unequal freedom and power, in which the stronger party is obligated to protect the interest of the weaker.[17]...

For the dishonest or incompetent physician, the ethical dilemmas are inconsequential. It is the physician committed to the good of his patient, the one who practices rational medicine, for whom divided loyalties are a genuine ethical problem.

NOTES

1 Fees for service—in goods, preferments, or money—are as old as medicine. Fees, their level, problems in collection, and the like are found in many of the books of the Hippocratic corpus.

2 Plato *Republic*, I, 342d.

3 Ibid., I, 346b.

4 Ibid., I, 346d.

5 G. B. Shaw, *The Doctor's Dilemma* (Baltimore: Penguin, 1965). Note especially the acerbic but, sadly, too often accurate, "Preface on Doctors."

6 Cushing, *Consecratio Medici*, pp. 3–13. Also see E. D. Pellegrino, "What Is a Profession?" *Journal of Allied Health*, Vol. 12, No. 3 (1983), 168–176.

7 The Hippocratic oath is still the most common public declaration of voluntary assumption of ethical obligations inherent in medicine. Other oaths, such as the so-called oath of Maimonides, the oath of Geneva, and the World Health Organization, all carry the same message of commitment to the good of others....

8 Studies of experiences with physician gatekeeping are beginning to appear. Examples of such studies are these: J. M. Eisenberg, "The Internist as Gatekeeper," *Annals of Internal Medicine*, Vol. 102, No. 4 (1985), 537–543; A. R. Somers, "And Who Shall Be the Gatekeeper? The Role of the Primary Physician in the Health Care Delivery System," *Inquiry*, Vol. 20, No. 4 (1983), 301–313; J. K. Inglehart, "Medicaid Turns to Prepaid Managed Care," *New England Journal of Medicine*, Vol. 308, No. 16 (1983), 976–980; and S. H. Moore, "Cost Containment Through Risk Sharing by Primary Care Physicians," *New England Journal of Medicine*, Vol. 300, No. 24 (1979), 1359–1362.

9 U. Reinhardt, "Health and Hot Potatoes," editorial, Washington *Post*, March 16, 1985, sec. A, p. 20.

10 AARP hot line for insurance and information: 1-800-523-5800.

11 R. Kotulak, "Program to Cut Medicaid Cost May Hurt Poor," Chicago *Tribune*, Sunday, March 9, 1986, sec. 2, pp. 1–2.

12 Some of the tendencies, dangers, and conflicts potentially harmful to patients and ethically suspect are discussed in the following: R. A. Rosenblatt and I. S. Moscovice, "The Physician as Gatekeeper," *Medical Care*, Vol. 22, No. 2 (1984), 150–159; A. S. Relman, "The Allocation of Medical Resources by Physicians," *Journal of Medical Education*, Vol. 55 No. 2 (1980), 99–104; S. H. Moore, D. Martin, and W. C. Richardson, "Does the Primary Gatekeeper Control the Costs of Health Care?" *New England Journal of Medicine*, Vol. 309, No. 22 (1983), 1400–1404; and B. F. Overholt, "The Socioeconomic and Political Future of Gastroenterology. Part II: Primary Care Network—The Gatekeeper," *American Journal of Gastroenterology*, Vol. 78, No. 7 (1983), 456–460.

13 W. B. Schwartz and H. J. Aaron, "Rationing Hospital Care: Lessons from Britain," *New England Journal of Medicine*, Vol. 310, No. 4 (1984), 52–56.

14 P. W. Butler, R. C. Bone, and T. Field, "Technology Under Medicare Diagnosis-Related Groups Prospective Payment: Implications for Medical Intensive Care," *Chest*, Vol. 87, No. 2 (1985), 229–234.

15 Department of Health and Human Services, *Summary Report of the Graduate Medical Education National Advisory Committee to the Secretary* (Washington, DC: U.S. Government Printing Office, 1980).

16 P. Starr, *The Social Transformation of American Medicine* (New York: Basic Books, 1982).

17 Pellegrino, "Toward a Reconstruction of Medical Morality," 32–56.

ANNOTATED BIBLIOGRAPHY: CHAPTER 2

Ad Hoc Committee on Medical Ethics, American College of Physicians: "American College of Physicians Ethics Manual," *Annals of Internal Medicine* 101 (1984), pp. 129–137 (Part I), pp. 263–274 (Part II). This is a position paper published by the American College of Physicians. It is an extended presentation of the college's thinking on the physician-patient relationship, the physician-society relationship, and on other ethical issues including the ethics of research. The document can be seen as the fruition of much of the reflection that had taken place during the 10 to 15 years before its formulation.

Brody, Howard: "The Physician-Patient Relationship: Models and Criticisms," *Theoretical Medicine* 8 (1987), pp. 205–220. This article includes a very useful overview of some of the theoretical models for the physician-patient relationship. Brody suggests that an amalgamation of a contractarian model with elements from a virtue-based approach, combined with appropriate empirical investigation, may yield richer models.

Edelstein, Ludwig: *Ancient Medicine* (Baltimore: Johns Hopkins, 1967). In this book, Edelstein discusses "The Hippocratic Oath" and shows that it contains two distinct sets of obligations—those pertaining to the patient and those owed to the physician's teacher and the teacher's progeny.

Etziony, M. B., ed.: *The Physician's Creed* (Springfield, Ill.: Charles C Thomas, 1973). This is subtitled "An Anthology of Medical Prayers, Oaths and Codes of Ethics Written and Recited by Medical Practitioners through the Ages." The collection reveals the aims and ethical orientation of medicine during its history.

Faden, Ruth R., and Tom L. Beauchamp: *A History and Theory of Informed Consent* (New York: Oxford University Press, 1986). This ambitious work spans the history, theory, and practice of informed consent in medicine, human behavior research, philosophy, and law.

Fox, Daniel M.: "The Politics of Physicians' Responsibility in Epidemics: A Note on History," *Hastings Center Report* 18 (April/May 1988), pp. 5–10 of supplement. Fox addresses the following historical question: "How did the medical profession, collectively, behave toward patients with contagious diseases and how did public policy affect that behavior?"

Humber, James M., and Robert F. Almeder: *Biomedical Ethics Reviews, 1988: AIDS and Ethics* (Clifton, NJ: Humana Press, 1989). Among the articles in this issue, which is devoted to some of the most challenging questions raised by AIDS, is David T. Ozar's "AIDS, Risk, and the Obligations of Health Professionals." Ozar maintains that health-care professionals do have an obligation to run more than ordinary risks to their lives in the interest of those who need their care. However, he considers various scenarios to bring out the limits of this obligation.

Jennings, Bruce, Daniel Callahan, and Arthur L. Caplan: "Ethical Challenges of Chronic Illness," *Hastings Center Report* 18 (February/March 1988), pp. 3–10 of supplement. The authors explore the possibility that the special nature of chronic care and the experience of chronic illness may require a change in some of the assumptions made in biomedical ethics about the goals of medicine as well as a revision of central concepts such as patients' autonomy and best interests.

Ladd, John: "Legalism in Medical Ethics," *Journal of Medicine and Philosophy* 4 (March 1979), pp. 70–80. Ladd criticizes the recent trend in biomedical ethics that tends to reduce all moral relationships to rule-following and rights claims. He proposes an alternative "ethic of responsibility."

Masters, Roger D.: "Is Contract an Adequate Basis for Medical Ethics?" *Hastings Center Report* 5 (December 1975), pp. 24–28. Masters argues that contract theory is not an adequate basis for medical ethics. He examines the differences between the physician-patient relationship and the contractual relationship that usually holds between buyers and sellers of other types of services. Masters argues that we should not base medical ethics on some "presumed rights" of isolated individuals. We must focus instead on the entire social context and formulate theories about patients' rights and professional obligations within a broader ethical theory that will balance the interests and obligations of human beings as they relate to the whole community.

President's Commission for the Study of Ethical Problems in Medicine and Biomedical and Behavioral Research: *Making Health Care Decisions: The Ethical and Legal Implications of*

Informed Consent in the Patient-Practitioner Relationship, Vol. 1: Report (Washington, D.C.: U.S. Government Printing Office, 1982). This report presents the Commission's conclusions and recommendations regarding both the role of informed consent in the patient-practitioner relationship and the means which might be used to promote a fuller understanding by patients and professionals of their common enterprise.

————: *Making Health Care Decisions, Vol. 2: Appendices: Empirical Studies of Informed Consent.* This volume contains the empirical studies used by the President's Commission in formulating its conclusions.

————: *Making Health Care Decisions, Vol. 3: Studies in the Foundations of Informed Consent.* Viewpoints represented in this volume are those of a psychologist, a historian, an anthropologist, a sociologist, a pediatrician-oncologist, a philosopher, and a medical student.

Relman, Arnold S.: "Dealing with Conflicts of Interests," *The New England Journal of Medicine* 313 (1985), pp. 749–751. Relman condemns what he sees as a new entrepreneurialism on the part of physicians that serves to generate conflicts of interests between physicians' commercial interests and their loyalty to and treatment of patients.

Rosoff, Arnold J.: *Informed Consent: A Guide for Health Care Providers* (Rockville, Md.: Aspen, 1981). This is a reference book that contains a great deal of practical information. It (1) sets forth the law in the informed consent area; (2) provides a philosophical framework for understanding legal developments; and (3) lays a foundation for researching questions of patient-consent law in particular states.

Van Kirk, Carol A., and Edward D. Schreck: "Truth-Telling and Placebos: A Conflict of Duties," *Listening* 22 (1987), pp. 52–65. Van Kirk and Schreck first review W. D. Ross's ethical theory and then use the theory to resolve the conflict between physicians' duties of veracity and duties of beneficence. They conclude by applying this resolution to questions about the ethical use of placebos.

CHAPTER 3

PROFESSIONALS' OBLIGATIONS, INSTITUTIONS, AND PATIENTS' RIGHTS

INTRODUCTION

Many who receive medical care today do so in hospitals, nursing homes, clinics, and other large institutions. Providers of health care include nurses, interns, staff physicians, operating room technicians, and other health-care professionals and paraprofessionals. Many medical care providers are not private practitioners but employees of the kinds of institutions mentioned above. Under these circumstances, a discussion of patients' rights and health professionals' responsibilities must encompass much more than the moral considerations raised in Chapter 2, which center primarily on the physician-patient relationship. This chapter explores some of the rights of hospital patients, the correlative responsibilities of professionals, and some ethical issues raised regarding elderly patients, especially in extended-care facilities. It also examines some of the moral dilemmas faced by nurses and other health-care professionals because of possible conflicts of obligation (other than those discussed in Chapter 2) as well as questions about the appropriate role of institutional ethics committees.

Patients' Rights

What rights do hospital patients have? Recent statements of patients' rights, such as the American Hospital Association's "A Patient's Bill of Rights," included in this chapter, attempt to answer this question. These documents, however, usually say nothing about the nature of the rights in question. They do not specify whether the statements of "rights" function: (1) as analogues of professional codes of ethics intended to provide moral guidelines for professional behavior, (2) as explicit formulations of moral rights, carrying correlative obligations, which the framers of these statements believe to be among the moral rights of all autonomous individuals, or (3) simply as statements of legal rights granted by a particular legal system. Despite this ambiguity, statements of patients' rights do serve as reminders to both hospital patients and health professionals that patients are persons; they are neither "mere objects" to be manipulated by professionals nor subservient beings who have waived their right of self-determination and other rights simply by becoming hospital patients.

Statements of hospital patients' rights have been explicitly formulated only recently. Most of us would take the rights asserted for granted. They include, for example, patients' rights to confidentiality and to adequate information regarding their condition. The apparent need to make these rights explicit, however, may be due to an increased awareness of their importance and of their almost routine institutional abuses. Any recent hospital patient suspects that hospital routines are often organized around staff convenience rather than patient comfort and that patients are often treated as "cases" rather than as "persons." One critic of hospital practices, Willard Gaylin, describes the situation as follows:

> A stay in a hospital exposes an individual to a condition of passivity and impotence unparallelled in adult life, this side of prison. You are dressed in an uncomfortable garment, leaving you exposed and ludicrous; told when you must sleep and when you must rise; informed of what you may eat and when you have to eat it; notified as to when you can have visitors, who they shall be, and how long they can stay. You are discussed in the third person in your presence as though you were some idiot child or inanimate object. If you are unfortunate enough to have an interesting case, you will be presented to a group of strangers who may take the invasion of your privacy as their privilege. Your chart, at the foot of the bed, will contain all the vital information that you would seem to be entitled to have; yet, should you attempt to examine it, you will be treated like a pre-pubescent caught with a copy of *Portnoy's Complaint*.
>
> Some of this may be necessary for health and some for convenience, but most of it is simply the inevitable result of an authoritative person dealing with people who unquestionably accept his authority.[1]

Gaylin is not impressed by the American Hospital Association's statement of rights. He considers it a weak document that simply reminds patients of their rights but does not take hospitals to task for their failure to respect patients' rights. George Annas, in contrast, in a reading in this chapter, maintains that although the document can be criticized on grounds of incompleteness, lack of specificity, and unenforceability, it does have tremendous symbolic value, especially since the rights it espouses are currently under attack. Critics question both the advisability of asserting these rights and patients' interest in exercising them. For Annas, the grounds for the attack lie in the tension, discussed in Chapter 2, between health professionals' desires to promote patients' medical well-being, *as it is perceived by those professionals*, and patients' right of self-determination. Annas, arguing that patients do have rights and do want to exercise them, proposes and discusses five rights intended to humanize hospitals and to promote hospital patients' self-determination.

The Nurse: Professional Obligations and Patients' Rights

Nurses face both a special set of moral problems with regard to patients' rights and a set of moral problems similar to those faced by physicians. Nurses, like physicians, for example, are sometimes forced to choose between doing what they believe will promote patients' well-being and respecting patients' right of self-determination. In this chapter, Sheri Smith discusses three possible models of the nurse-patient relationship, analogous to three of the models of the physician-patient relationship presented by Robert Veatch in Chapter 2. Rejecting paternalism, she argues for a contracted-clinician model, which respects both a patient's right of self-determination and a nurse's right of conscientious refusal. She notes, however, that nurses often face moral dilemmas that are not faced by physicians. These dilemmas result from the nurse's position in the hospital health-care hierarchy. Nurses in hospitals care for patients and supervise others giving that care. Usually, they are directly responsible both for patient care and for the implementation of therapy. At the same time, nurses have very little influence in decision making regarding patients. Furthermore, they are subordinate to doctors who make diagnoses and issue orders that nurses are obligated to carry out. Under these circumstances, nurses are sometimes confronted with situations in which their obligations to patients seem to conflict with their obligations to physicians. The following questions exemplify the kinds of problems nurses face: (1) Should nurses follow physicians' orders when (a) they have good reason to believe that the orders are mistaken, (b) the physicians refuse to admit that they might be mistaken, and (c) following orders will jeopardize a patient's safety or well-being? (2) What should nurses do if they have good reason to believe that physicians are violating their patients' right of self-determination? For example, what should a nurse do when a physician lies or withholds information from a patient? E. Joy Kroeger Mappes focuses on these sorts of questions in this chapter. She stresses the difficulties faced by nurses in our society when protecting patients' interests requires them to "buck" the hierarchical system. Mappes attributes a major part of this difficulty to the classist and sexist forces in society. In a related reading in this chapter, Marsha D. M. Fowler discusses the relationship between nurses' obligations and nurses' rights. Beginning with the nursing profession's view of itself as a patient advocacy profession, Fowler presents four emerging models of nursing advocacy and identifies the nursing responsibilities associated with each. She then discusses the correlative rights that nurses must have if they are to fulfill their responsibilities to patients.

Confidentiality and Conflicting Obligations

Whatever the full complement of patients' rights may be, the right of privacy and the related principle of confidentiality deserve special discussion. The importance of the principle of confidentiality in the medical context has long been recognized. It is affirmed in the "Hippocratic Oath" as well as in more recent medical ethical codes such as those of the American Medical Association and the American Nurses' Association. It is also recognized by the ethical codes of medical record librarians and medical social workers. Even the law recognizes the importance of the patient's right to retain control of the information held by health professionals. It does so in two ways: (1) Physicians and psychotherapists are subject to legal sanctions if they reveal confidential information about patients; (2) Physicians and psychotherapists are exempt from giving testimony about their patients before a court of law. Most discussions of the moral significance of the principle of confidentiality in the health-care context stress either the importance of protecting the trust essential to the professional-patient relationship or respect for the patient's autonomy and privacy. Both LeRoy Walters and Morton E. Winston in this chapter discuss the justifications advanced for the rule of confidentiality in the medical context.

Most commentators, including Walters and Winston, believe that, despite the importance of medical confidentiality, the duty to respect confidentiality is a prima facie one, that is, one that may sometimes be justifiably overridden when it conflicts with other moral duties. In this chapter the articles by Walters and Winston, as well as the opinions in *Tarasoff v. Regents of the University of California*, focus on the moral dilemmas posed for health-care professionals when such conflicts arise. Winston's article deals with the moral problems posed for health-care professionals by patients who either have AIDS or are carriers of the AIDS virus. Under what conditions, if any, may physicians and nurses, for example, disclose confidential information about HIV carriers and other patients to prevent harm to others? In the *Tarasoff* case, the conflict at issue was between a psychologist's duty to respect the confidence of a patient, Prosenjit Poddar, and his possible obligation to warn a young woman, Tatiana Tarasoff, that Poddar might try to kill her. He did not warn the woman or her family, and Poddar did kill her. Should the psychologist have violated the principle of confidentiality in respect to his patient? Did he have an obligation to protect the life of a woman who was not his patient? If he did, should this obligation have taken precedence over his duty to respect Poddar's confidences? The contrast between the majority and the dissenting opinions in the case serves to heighten awareness of the moral dilemmas raised for the professional who must choose between violating a patient's rights and failing to perform an act that might save the life of another human being or otherwise prevent serious harm.

Additional problems are raised for the traditional right to confidentiality by current developments in medical care. Hospital medicine, the need to share information among the members of health-care teams, the existence of third-party insurance programs, and the expanding limits of medicine all result in a fairly wide dissemination of "confidential" information about patients. Mark Siegler, in this chapter, discusses some of these problems.

Hospital (Institutional) Ethics Committees

As the provision of medical care has become more complex and as technological advances have necessitated the reexamination of the values implicit in medical decision making, more and more health-care institutions, including hospitals, have established institutional ethics committees (IECs) to help them address the related ethical issues. IECs are usually composed of both medical and nonmedical members. A typical IEC consists of physicians, nurses, social workers, hospital administrators, attorneys, psychologists, and lay persons as well as members of the clergy and/or ethicists. The possible major functions of IECs include the following:

1. Education: educating the hospital staff about the ethical aspects of medical care

2. Policy and guideline formulation: developing mandatory or suggested institutional guidelines and policies regarding ethical issues

3. Consultation: reviewing cases, either prospectively or retrospectively, and making recommendations to those directly involved, as well as to hospital administrators and others should that be necessary; prospective reviews usually examine the options available in a single case, and retrospective reviews usually look at a group of cases as a class

Despite the proliferation of IECs, their proper role is still a matter of dispute. Mark Siegler in this chapter argues, for example, that their only proper role is education. He is especially concerned with denying IECs any role in medical decision making, either prospectively or retrospectively. In contrast, those who see the IEC's consultative role as valuable sometimes note the following benefits: In the case of retrospective reviews, the IEC can identify inappropriate decisions so that future similar cases can be better handled. In the case of prospective reviews, the IEC can facilitate communication by identifying ethical issues and spelling out the conflicting values and interests that may be at the heart of the disagreements. An IEC can provide a forum in which disagreements among staff, patients, and patients' families can be discussed and resolved; an IEC can also provide support when hard decisions have to be made. In addition, the committee may help to prevent unnecessary litigation by aiding in the resolution of disagreements that might otherwise require judicial handling. However, in another reading in this chapter, Bernard Lo, whose attitude toward the consultative role of IECs is much more favorable than Siegler's, raises some important questions about their efficacy and ethicality. He expresses concern about the actual process of committee decision making and sees a need to ensure that patient interests and wishes are adequately represented when IEC decisions are made.

Elderly Patients and Autonomy

Hospitals are not the only health-care institutions in which ethical dilemmas regarding patient care arise. Nursing homes, for example, which are becoming more prevalent in our society as the number of elderly and very old people increases, are also faced with the need to address important ethical concerns. Issues associated with patient autonomy are, perhaps, especially important in typical nursing home settings and other extended-care facilities. Although many geriatric patients are as capable of making fully autonomous decisions as other competent adults, the issue of patient competence may often arise with respect to those geriatric patients who suffer some degree of cognitive impairment ranging from the very slight to the severe. As Drane points out in Chapter 2, competence is not an all or nothing affair, yet there is often a tendency to treat elderly individuals in paternalistic ways even when their cognitive impairments are minor. In one of this chapter's readings, Ruth Macklin brings out some of the complexities involved in making judgments about the competence of the elderly and some of the assumptions underlying judgments about their diminished capacity. In another reading in this chapter, Marshall B. Kapp expresses concern that an overemphasis on the autonomy of the elderly may lead to forcing autonomous decision making on those competent elderly individuals who may prefer not to make their own decisions and who may even have a long history of letting others make them. Although Kapp focuses on the elderly, his reasoning can be more widely applied, since it raises questions for anyone who would maintain that individuals who are competent to make their own decisions cannot be acting morally if they decide to delegate their decision-making rights and responsibilities.

J.S.Z.

NOTE

1 Willard Gaylin, "The Patient's Bill of Rights," *Saturday Review of the Sciences* 1 (February 24, 1973), p. 22.

Hospitals and Patients' Rights

A Patient's Bill of Rights
American Hospital Association

This statement, issued by the American Hospital Association, was affirmed by the AHA House of Delegates on February 6, 1973. It makes explicit some "moral rights" that many would take for granted (such as the right to considerate and respectful care) and some legal rights that hospitals, as well as other institutions, must respect.

The American Hospital Association presents a Patient's Bill of Rights with the expectation that observance of these rights will contribute to more effective patient care and greater satisfaction for the patient, his physician,

Reprinted with the permission of the American Hospital Association.

and the hospital organization. Further, the Association presents these rights in the expectation that they will be supported by the hospital on behalf of its patients, as an integral part of the healing process. It is recognized that a personal relationship between the physician and the patient is essential for the provision of proper medical care. The traditional physician-patient relationship takes on a new dimension when care is rendered within an organizational structure. Legal precedent has established that the institution itself also has a responsibility to the patient. It is in recognition of these factors that these rights are affirmed.

(1) The patient has the right to considerate and respectful care.

(2) The patient has the right to obtain from his physician complete current information concerning his diagnosis, treatment, and prognosis in terms the patient can be reasonably expected to understand. When it is not medically advisable to give such information to the patient, the information should be made available to an appropriate person in his behalf. He has the right to know, by name, the physician responsible for coordinating his care.

(3) The patient has the right to receive from his physician information necessary to give informed consent prior to the start of any procedure and/or treatment. Except in emergencies, such information for informed consent should include but not necessarily be limited to the specific procedure and/or treatment, the medically significant risks involved, and the probable duration of incapacitation. Where medically significant alternatives for care or treatment exist, or when the patient requests information concerning medical alternatives, the patient has the right to such information. The patient also has the right to know the name of the person responsible for the procedures and/or treatment.

(4) The patient has the right to refuse treatment to the extent permitted by law and to be informed of the medical consequences of his action.

(5) The patient has the right to every consideration of his privacy concerning his own medical care program. Case discussion, consultation, examination, and treatment are confidential and should be conducted discreetly. Those not directly involved in his care must have the permission of the patient to be present.

(6) The patient has the right to expect that all communications and records pertaining to his care should be treated as confidential.

(7) The patient has the right to expect that within its capacity a hospital must make reasonable response to the request of a patient for services. The hospital must provide evaluation, service, and/or referral as indicated by the urgency of the case. When medically permissible, a patient may be transferred to another facility only after he has received complete information and explanation concerning the needs for and alternatives to such a transfer. The institution to which the patient is to be transferred must first have accepted the patient for transfer.

(8) The patient has the right to obtain information as to any relationship of his hospital to other health care and educational institutions insofar as his care is concerned. The patient has the right to obtain information as to the existence of any professional relationships among individuals, by name, who are treating him.

(9) The patient has the right to be advised if the hospital proposes to engage in or perform human experimentation affecting his care or treatment. The patient has the right to refuse to participate in such research projects.

(10) The patient has the right to expect reasonable continuity of care. He has the right to know in advance what appointment times and physicians are available and where. The patient has the right to expect that the hospital will provide a mechanism whereby he is informed by his physician or a delegate of the physician of the patient's continuing health care requirements following discharge.

(11) The patient has the right to examine and receive an explanation of his bill regardless of source of payment.

(12) The patient has the right to know what hospital rules and regulations apply to his conduct as a patient.

No catalog of rights can guarantee for the patient the kind of treatment he has a right to expect. A hospital has many functions to perform, including the prevention and treatment of disease, the education of both health professionals and patients, and the conduct of clinical research. All these activities must be conducted with an overriding concern for the patient, and, above all, the recognition of his dignity as a human being. Success in achieving this recognition assures success in the defense of the rights of the patient.

The Emerging Stowaway, Patients' Rights in the 1980s
George J. Annas

George J. Annas is Utley Professor of Health Law and Chief of the Health Law Section at Boston University School of Public Health. Annas is the author of *The Rights of Hospital Patients* (1975), coauthor of *Informed Consent to Human Experimentation* (1977), *The Rights of Doctors, Nurses, and Allied Health Professionals* (1981), and *Reproductive Genetics and the Law* (1987), and coeditor of *Genetics and the Law III* (1985). He also writes a regular column on "Law and the Life Sciences" for the *Hastings Center Report*.

Annas maintains that the majority of physicians favor medical paternalism because they value their patients' health and continued life more than patients' right to self-determination. This general view, he argues, affects their attitudes to "patients' rights" and tends to make them accept the conclusions of sloppy studies that downgrade the importance of some of the rights asserted and throw doubt on patients' interest in exercising them. Annas discusses some of these studies to bring out their inadequacies and then asserts five rights intended to humanize the hospital environment and give patients more of a voice regarding their treatment.

At one point in Edgar Allan Poe's *Narrative of Arthur Gordon Pym of Nantucket*, Pym, who has stowed away in the hold of a whaling vessel, believes he has been abandoned and that the hold will be his tomb. He expressed sensations of "extreme horror and dismay," and "the most gloomy imaginings, in which the dreadful deaths of thirst, famine, suffocation, and premature interment, crowded in as the prominent disasters to be encountered."

It is probably uncommon for hospitalized patients to feel as gloomy as Pym. Nevertheless, installed in a strange institution, separated from friends and family, forced to wear a degrading costume, confined to bed, and attended to by a variety of strangers who may or may not keep the patient informed of what they are doing, the average patient is intimidated and disoriented. Such an atmosphere encourages dependence and discourages the assertion of individual rights.

As the physician-director of Boston's Beth Israel Hospital has warned: "today's hospital stands increasingly to become a jungle, whose pathways to the uninitiated are poorly marked and fraught with danger...."[1]

In this jungle the notion that patients have rights that demand respect is often foreign.

The movement for enhanced patients' rights is based on two premises: (1) citizens possess certain rights that are not automatically forfeited by entering into a relationship with a physician or health care facility; and (2) most physicians and health care facilities fail to recognize these rights, fail to provide for their protection or assertion, and limit their exercise without recourse.[2]

The primary argument against patients' rights is that patients have "needs" and defining these needs in terms of rights leads to the creation of an unhealthy adversary relationship.[3] It is not, however, the creation of rights, but the disregard of them, that produces adversaries. When provider and patient work together in an atmosphere of mutual trust and understanding, the articulation of rights can only enhance their relationship....

THE AHA BILL OF RIGHTS

It must strike most people as ironic that the first major health care organization to put forward a patients' bill of rights was the American Hospital Association (AHA), an organization composed primarily of hospital administrators. One would not expect landlords to pen a bill of rights for tenants, police for suspects, or wardens for prisoners. Nor would one reasonably expect that the hospital administrator's view on rights for patients would be the same as either the patient's or society's. Nevertheless, physicians and nurses should be ashamed that the administrators were well out in front of them on this issue. Even though it leaves much to be desired in terms of completeness, specificity, and enforceability, the AHA Bill has tremendous symbolic value in legitimizing the notion of rights in the health care institution.[4] On the other hand, fewer than half of all AHA member hospitals have formally adopted even this bill, and the symbolic victory of the 1970s is currently under attack.

THE ATTACK ON PATIENTS' RIGHTS

Physicians, who perhaps value their own professional autonomy more than any other group, nevertheless devalue it for their own patients. Instead, paternalism is the norm with the majority of physicians believing that the health and continued life of their patients is much more important than their patients' right to self-determination. This belief system not only leads to conflicts with individual patients about their own care, but also to a general view that sees patients' rights as being a luxury item in medicine rather than a necessity.

A few examples illustrate the point. Two particular rights of patients have recently come under attack in the medical literature: access to medical records and informed consent. In an attack on "record reading," four psychiatrists at Boston's Peter Bent Brigham Hospital interviewed the 11 out of 2,500 patients at that hospital in a one year period who asked to see their medical records.[5] It is doubtful that anything of general importance about a patient's reactions to reading their charts can be learned from an uncontrolled, nonblind, clinically impressionistic study of those few individuals who, for whatever reason, buck a system that routinely fails to inform them of their right of access to their records. Nonetheless, the authors' conclusion that such patients have a variety of personality defects, usually manifesting themselves in mistrust of and hostility toward the hospital staff, should not be permitted to go uncontested. In a setting where trusting patients are not routinely told of their right to access, it seems reasonable to assume that only the least trusting or most angry will ask to see their

records. To locate the source of mistrust in the patient's personality style or in the stress of illness and hospitalization is to forget, as Dr. Lipsett perceptively suggests, that "the doctor-patient relationship cannot be understood simply in terms of the patient's side of the equation."[6] Altman et al. thus fall into what Professor Robert Burt of the Yale Law School has referred to as "the conceptual trap of attempting to transform two-party relationships, in which mutual self-delineations are inherently confused and intertwined, by conceptually obliterating one party...."[7] Thus, it would seem that the ten women who asked to read their charts "to confirm the belief that the staff harbored negative personal attitudes toward them..." were correct in the belief; the psychiatrists labelled them "of the hysterical type with demanding, histrionic behavior and emotional overinvolvement with the staff."

Altman et al. also seem unaware of the wide variety of settings in which patients have *benefited* from routine record access, and incorrectly assert that there were no strikingly beneficial effects in the two studies they do cite. In the first study, for example, two patients expressed their completely unfounded fear that they had cancer only after their record was reviewed with them, and one pregnant patient noted an incorrect Rh typing that permitted RhoGam to be administered at the time of delivery.[8] In the other study they cite, 50 percent of the patients made some factual correction in the record.[9]

In short, the study seems to have been done and published for the primary purpose of proving that the right to record access is unimportant since it is only exercised by "mentally disturbed" people who are not improved by reading their charts. It fails to prove this, and even if it succeeded, I would still be unwilling to deprive the other 2,489 patients of their right to access in the future. If we believe in individual freedom and the concept of self-determination, we must give all citizens the right to make their *own* decisions and to have access to information that is widely available to those making decisions about them. It is as irrelevant in this connection that 2,489 patients at the Peter Bent Brigham Hospital did not ask to see their records as it is that more than 200 million Americans never have had to exercise their right to remain silent when arrested. Rights serve us all, whether we exercise them or not.

The attack on informed consent, which many physicians have long considered a "legal fiction,"[10] most recently surfaced in a study often used to "prove" that informed consent was not an important patients' right in practice, because patients could not remember what they were informed of.[11] The methodology involved interviewing 200 consecutive cancer patients who had consented to chemotherapy, surgery, or radiation therapy for their cancers within 24 hours after they had signed consent forms. Upon questioning, most could not recall the procedure consented to, its major risks, or the alternatives to it. From this the authors conclude that the process is not working and that informed consent itself is suspect. Although this may seem to be a reasonable conclusion (an alternative one is simply that patients have poor recall), it turns out that the authors presumed their major premise. Approximately two-thirds of their sample group (66 percent) opted for radiation therapy. That group signed a consent form that said "the procedure, its risks and benefits and alternatives have been explained to me." Maybe they were, but maybe they were not. The authors did not know, so their entire study was based on a premise that was unsubstantiated. Such a poorly designed study, it seems to me, could only be published if the editors agreed so strongly with the conclusion that they did not even review the methodology.

A perhaps more interesting part of the study asked the patients some general questions about informed consent. The first was, "What are consent forms for?" Approximately 80 percent responded: "To protect the physicians' rights." The authors were upset at this response, but the patients of course were correct. That *is* the primary function of *forms*. If one wants these forms also to protect the patient, three simple steps are necessary: (1) the forms must be complete; (2) they must be in lay language; and (3) the patients must be given a copy of the form and time to think over the information it contains.[12] The reason none of these is usually done is clear: Informed consent is not taken seriously in the hospital setting. It is, like record access, a luxury that is secondary to caring for the medical "needs" of the patient, and besides, it really doesn't matter anyway because patients can't remember anything they've been told....

Other significant findings that indicate the extent to which patients understand and appreciate the consent process are: 80 percent thought the forms were necessary; 76 percent thought they contained just the right amount of information; 84 percent understood all or most of the information; 75 percent thought the explanations given were important; and 90 percent said they would try to remember the information contained on the forms. To me, this suggests that the patients surveyed, understood, and appreciated the informed consent pro-

cess much better than the researchers did. Their data are certainly not flawless, but one can conclude from the data just the opposite of what the researchers did: For almost all patients, informed consent is seen as very important.

Related to this general attack on rights is an attack on the patient population itself. The notion is that the major problems with the health care delivery system are not problems with providers, but with patients. We eat too much, smoke too much, do not exercise enough, take too many risks, and it serves us right if we get sick. The American health care enterprise must deal with a bad class of patients that (on top of everything) now not only wants access to care, but also wants some say in what kind of care is provided! As Lewis Thomas has put it in a related vein, this is "becoming folk doctrine about disease. You become ill because of not living' right. If you get cancer it is, somehow or other, your own fault. If you didn't cause it by smoking or drinking, or eating the wrong things, it came from allowing yourself to persist with the wrong kind of personality in the wrong environment."[13]

This attitude would be humorous if it was not so pervasive and did not affect patient care so profoundly. Martha Lear has given us some excellent and telling examples in her deeply moving book, *Heartsounds*, that chronicles the final four years of life of her physician-husband who goes through eight operations and eleven hospitalizations during that period. Together they identify the "it's your fault ploy," which means that no matter what goes wrong in the hospital setting, it is the fault of the patient, not the health care system.

> Why did the operation take so long?
> Because you lost so much blood.
> *Not*: Because the surgeon blew it.
> Why do you keep making these tests?
> Because you have a very stubborn infection.
> *Not*: Because I can't diagnose your case.
> Why did I get sick again?
> Because you were very weak.
> *Not*: Because I did not treat you competently the first time.[14]

Dr. Lear is constantly asking himself if he treated patients that way, and usually admits that he did. He suggests that every physician be required to spend at least a week a year in a hospital bed: "That would change some things in a hurry."[15]

AN AGENDA FOR THE 80s

Since patients *do* have rights and *do* want to exercise them, and since the major attacks on the notion of patients' rights have been based on sloppy studies and false premises, the patients' rights movement is likely to gain momentum. Indeed, the 1970s can be most properly viewed as a decade in which the notion of rights has become legitimized through basic education of health care providers to the existence of patients' rights. I suggest that the 1980s will be a decade in which the primary thrust will be working on ways to directly enhance the status of patients in the hospital as a means of humanizing the hospital environment so that patients can have a greater voice in how they are treated.

I suggest the following five point Patients' Rights Agenda for the 1980s:

1. No Routine Procedures

2. Open Access to Medical Records

3. Twenty-Four-Hour-a-Day Visitor Rights

4. Full Experience Disclosure

5. Effective Patient Advocate

1 *No Routine Procedures*   It is all too common for nurses and others to respond to the question, "Why is this being done?" with, "Don't worry, it's routine." This should not be an acceptable response. No procedure should *ever* be performed on a patient because it is routine; it should only be performed if it is *specifically* indicated for that patient. Thus, routine admission tests, routine use of johnnies, routine use of wheelchairs for in-hospital transportation, and routine use of sleeping pills, to name a few notable examples, would be abolished. Use of these procedures means patients are treated as fungible robots rather than individual human beings. These procedures are often demeaning and unnecessary.

2 *Open Access to Medical Records*   Although currently provided for by federal law and many state statutes and regulations, open access to medical records by patients remains difficult, and patients often assert their right to see their records at the peril of being labeled "distrustful" or "trouble-maker." The information in the hospital chart is about the patient and properly belongs to the

patient. The patient must have access to it, both to enhance his or her own decision-making ability and to make it clear that the hospital is an "open" institution that is not trying to hide things from the patient. Surely if hospital personnel are making decisions about the patient on the basis of information in the chart, the patient also deserves access to the information.

3 *Twenty-Four-Hour-a-Day Visitor Rights*   One of the most important ways to both humanize the hospital and enhance patient autonomy is to ensure that at least one person of the patient's choice has unlimited access to the patient at any time of the day or night. This person should also be permitted to stay with the patient during any procedure (e.g., childbirth, induction of anesthesia), as long as the person does not interfere with the care of other patients.

4 *Full Experience Disclosure*   The most important gain of the past decade has been the almost universal acknowledgment of the need for the patient's informed consent. Nevertheless, some information that is material to the patient's decision is still withheld: the experience of the person doing the procedure.[16] Patients have a right to know if the person asking permission to draw blood, take blood gases, do a bone marrow aspiration, or do a spinal tap has ever performed the procedure before, and if so, what the person's complication rate is. This applies not only to student nurses, but also to board certified surgeons—we all do things for the first time, and not every patient wants to take such an active role in our education.

5 *An Effective Patient Advocate*   Although a patients' bill of rights is necessary, it is not sufficient. Rights are not self-actualizing. Patients are sick and desire relief from pain and discomfort more than they demonstrate a desire to exercise their rights; they are also anxious, and may hold back complaints for fear of retaliation. It is critical that patients have access to a person whose job it is to work *for the patient* to help the patient exercise the rights outlined in the institution's bill of rights. This person should sit in on all major hospital committees that deal with patient care, have authority to obtain medical records for patients, call consultants, launch complaints directly with all members of the hospital, medical, nursing, and administrative staff, and be able to delay discharges. Although there appear to be some successful "patient representatives" that are hired by the

hospitals, it is not fair to give them this title since they must represent the hospital, and it is likely that ultimately effective representation can only be obtained by someone who is hired by a consumer group or governmental agency outside of the hospital in which the representative works.

CONCLUSION

We have made a beginning in the long journey toward humanizing the hospital and promoting patient self-determination in it. But more specific measures are needed before patients will be assured that they can effectively exercise their rights in institutional settings.

Like Poe's Arthur Gordon Pym, the notion that patients have rights has survived the days of darkness, isolation, and starvation. It is now generally accepted (although sporadically attacked), and it is up to patients and providers alike to see to it that these rights become a reality for every citizen.

NOTES

1 M. Rabkin, quoted in G. J. Annas, "The Hospital: A Patient Rights Wasteland," *Civil Liberties Review* (Fall 1974): 11.

2 See generally, G. J. Annas, *The Rights of Hospital Patients* (New York: Avon, 1975).

3 E. G. Margolis, "Conceptual Aspects of a Patient's Bill of Rights," *Connecticut Medicine Supplement* 43, no. 9 (October 1979): 9–11. Also see Ladd, "Legalism and Medical Ethics," in Davis, Hoffmaster, and Shorten, eds., *Contemporary Issues in Biomedical Ethics* (New Jersey, Humana Press, 1978), pp. 1–35.

4 Reprinted in Annas, pp. 25–27.

5 J. H. Altman, P. Reich, M. J. Kelly, and M. P. Rogers, "Patients Who See Their Medical Record," *New England Journal of Medicine* 302, no. 3 (1980): 169.

6 D. Lipsett, "The Patient and the Record," *New England Journal of Medicine* 302, no. 3 (1980): 167.

7 R. Burt, *Taking Care of Strangers: The Rule of Law in Doctor-Patient Relations* (New York: The Free Press, 1979), p. 43.

8 D. P. Stevens, R. Staff, and I. MacKay, "What Happens When Hospitalized Patients See Their Own Records," *Annals of Internal Medicine* 86 (1977): 474, 476.

9 A. Golodetz, J. Ruess, and R. Milhous, "The Right to Know: Giving the Patient His Medical Record," *Archives of Physical Medicine and Rehabilitation* 57 (1976): 78, 81. And experience under the new record access regulation enacted by the Board of Registration in Medicine indicates that patients want access to their records for a variety of reasons. In the period from October 13, 1978 (when the regulation went into effect) to January 31, 1980, the Medicine Board received more phone calls from consumers asking about the medical records regulation (approximately ten a month) than about any other single issue dealt with by the Board. There were also 33 formal complaints filed concerning record access during this period. Of this number, almost half (16) needed help from the Board to get their physician to forward a copy of their record directly to another physician. Of the remaining 17, 6 needed information for insurance purposes, 6 wanted to review the record for various reasons, one alleged negligence, one wanted the record sent to a school nurse, one was moving to another state, one wanted a second opinion, and one wanted her contact lens prescription. (Statistics compiled by Judy Miller, a student at Boston College Law School.)

10 See, for example, E. G. Laforet, "The Fiction of Informed Consent," *Journal of the American Medical Association* 235 (April 12, 1976): 1579.

11 B. R. Cassileth et al., "Informed Consent—Why Are Its Goals Imperfectly Realized?" *New England Journal of Medicine* 302, no. 16 (1980): 896.

12 See, generally, chapter on informed consent in G. J. Annas, L. H. Glantz, and B. F. Katz, *The Rights of Doctors, Nurses and Allied Health Professionals* (New York: Avon, 1981); and G. J. Annas, L. H. Glantz, and B. F. Katz, *Informed Consent to Human Experimentation: The Subject's Dilemma* (Cambridge, Mass.: Ballinger, 1977). And see D. Rennie, "Informed Consent by 'Well-Nigh Abject' Adults," *New England Journal of Medicine* 302, no. 16 (1980): 916. I suggest that the physician accept far more than simply the duty to improve consent forms. Physicians should accept education of the patient through the process of consent as a worthwhile therapeutic goal. To deny the possibility of informed consent is to ensure that it will never be achieved—an attitude that is immoral and illegal.

13 L. Thomas, "On Magic in Medicine," *New England Journal of Medicine* 299 (August 31, 1978): 461, 462.

14 M. L. Lear, *Heartsounds* (New York: Simon and Schuster, 1980), p. 47.

15 *Ibid.*, p. 44.

16 G. J. Annas, "The Care of Private Patients in Teaching Hospitals: Legal Implications," *Bulletin of the New York Academy of Medicine* 56, no. 4 (May 1980): 403–11.

Nurses' Obligations and Patients' Rights

American Nurses' Association Code for Nurses

This code of ethics, adopted by the American Nurses' Association, states some of the obligations nurses have to (1) their patients, (2) the nursing profession, and (3) the public. The word "patient," however, is never used. Throughout the document, the recipient of nurses' professional services is referred to as the "client." Unlike other codes of nursing ethics, this code does not explicitly assert any obligation "to carry out physicians' orders." Rather, it emphasizes nurses' obligations to clients and views both nurses and clients as the bearers of both basic rights and responsibilities.

PREAMBLE

A code of ethics makes explicit the primary goals and values of the profession. When individuals become nurses, they make a moral commitment to uphold the values and special moral obligations expressed in their code. The Code for Nurses is based on a belief about the nature of individuals, nursing, health, and society. Nursing encompasses the protection, promotion, and restoration of health; the prevention of illness; and the alleviation of suffering in the care of clients, including individuals, families, groups, and communities. In the context of these functions, nursing is defined as the diagnosis and treatment of human responses to actual or potential health problems.

Since clients themselves are the primary decision makers in matters concerning their own health, treatment, and well-being, the goal of nursing actions is to support and enhance the client's responsibility and self-determination to the greatest extent possible. In this context, health is not necessarily an end in itself, but rather a means to a life that is meaningful from the client's perspective.

When making clinical judgments, nurses base their decisions on consideration of consequences and of universal moral principles, both of which prescribe and justify nursing actions. The most fundamental of these principles is respect for persons. Other principles stemming from this basic principle are autonomy (self-determination), beneficence (doing good), nonmaleficence (avoiding harm), veracity (truth-telling), confidentiality (respecting privileged information), fidelity (keeping promises), and justice (treating people fairly).

In brief, then, the statements of the code and their interpretation provide guidance for conduct and relationships in carrying out nursing responsibilities consistent with the ethical obligations of the profession and with high quality in nursing care.

CODE FOR NURSES

1. The nurse provides services with respect for human dignity and the uniqueness of the client, unrestricted by considerations of social or eco-

nomic status, personal attributes, or the nature of health problems.

2. The nurse safeguards the client's right to privacy by judiciously protecting information of a confidential nature.

3. The nurse acts to safeguard the client and the public when health care and safety are affected by the incompetent, unethical, or illegal practice of any person.

4. The nurse assumes responsibility and accountability for individual nursing judgments and actions.

5. The nurse maintains competence in nursing.

6. The nurse exercises informed judgment and uses individual competence and qualifications as criteria in seeking consultation, accepting responsibilities, and delegating nursing activities to others.

7. The nurse participates in activities that contribute to the ongoing development of the profession's body of knowledge.

8. The nurse participates in the profession's efforts to implement and improve standards of nursing.

9. The nurse participates in the profession's efforts to establish and maintain conditions of employment conducive to high quality nursing care.

10. The nurse participates in the profession's effort to protect the public from misinformation and misrepresentation and to maintain the integrity of nursing.

11. The nurse collaborates with members of the health professions and other citizens in promoting community and national efforts to meet the health needs of the public.

Three Models of the Nurse-Patient Relationship
Sheri Smith

Sheri Smith is associate professor of philosophy at Rhode Island College. Her areas of specialization are ethics and professional ethics. Smith is a member of the scientific staff at the Roger Williams General Hospital in Providence, Rhode Island. She is also a member of the hospital's Institutional Review Board and serves on its Ethics Advisory Committee. Smith is a founding member of the Society for the Study of Professional Ethics and served as its first president (1978–1982).

Smith presents three possible models of the nurse-patient relationship. (1) *The Surrogate Mother Model*: On this model—analogous to Robert Veatch's priestly model of the physician—the nurse, like a mother, stands in a "paternalistic" relation to the patient. (2) *The Nurse-Technician Model*: On this model—analogous to Veatch's engineering model—the nurse is an ethically neutral provider of technical assistance paid for by patients, with patients retaining ultimate responsibility for identifying their needs and determining their best interests. (3) *The Contracted-Clinician Model*: On this model—analogous to Veatch's contractual model—both

---

From *Nursing: Images and Ideals*, edited by Stuart F. Spicker and Sally Gadow (New York: Springer Publishing Company, 1980), pp. 176–188. Copyright © 1980 by Stuart F. Spicker. Reprinted with permission.

the patient's right of self-determination and the nurse's right of conscientious objection are emphasized. Smith concludes by arguing in favor of the contracted-clinician model. She notes, however, that although both the physician-patient and nurse-patient relationships may be conceptualized in contractual terms, there may be a significant difference between the two sets of relationships because of nurses' obligations to obey physicians.

A critical philosophical issue about nursing is raised in several of the essays in this volume [*Nursing: Images and Ideals*], but it has been left unresolved. That issue is the question of the nature of the nurse-patient relationship. The failure to resolve the issue is critical, for the solution of ethical dilemmas in nursing practice often depends upon the definition of nursing and the responsibilities and rights thought to be inherent in the nurse-patient relationship.[1] My purpose in this [article] is to characterize three views of the nature of the nurse-patient relationship—the surrogate mother, nurse technician, and contracted clinician models—and to show the strengths and weaknesses of those models and their consequences for nursing practice. I will contend that assumptions about the nature of the nurse-patient relationship pervade the discussion of ethical dilemmas in nursing practice. In order to support that contention I will use examples from the essays by Dan Brock, who argues for the contracted clinician model; Mila Aroskar, who discusses the surrogate mother model in commenting on historical images of nurses; and Sally Gadow, whose conceptualizations of nursing can be shown to provide a philosophical basis for the models presented herein. My discussion of nursing models owes much to Robert Veatch's description of analogous models for the patient-physician relationship.[2] The question of how far the analogy between nurse-patient and physician-patient relationships can be drawn, and how the nature of the nurse-patient relationship might be altered by the relationship the patient has with his physician, is one on which I will comment briefly at the end of this discussion.

THE NURSE AS SURROGATE MOTHER

We can distinguish the three major models of the nurse-patient relationship by their conceptualizations of the extent and nature of the nurse's ethical responsibility and the assumptions made concerning patients and illness. In the surrogate mother model the nurse's primary responsibility and commitment is to the patient. (It should be noted here that, for the purposes of this discussion, "patient" will be understood to mean a competent adult.) The ethical responsibility of the nurse is defined by this commitment to the patient, as it is spelled out in nursing codes of ethics such as the American Nurses' Association Code. The nurse is even urged by the ANA code to serve as protector of the patient when his care and safety are in jeopardy through the actions of others. Other ethical responsibilities which nurses have, for example, in relation to physicians, are derived from this primary commitment to the patient.

It is the model of the nurse as a surrogate mother which has exerted greatest influence in the history of nursing and nursing education.[3] On this model, the nurse's ethical responsibility is understood as an unlimited commitment to the patient. It is the nurse's obligation to provide nursing care, to take care of the patient, and to act in his or her best interests at all times. The nurse has ultimate responsibility for the care which the patient receives. This means that the nurse also has an obligation to determine what constitutes the best care for the patient, and to act in his or her behalf if that care is not being provided. The nurse, then, has a kind of total commitment to patient care and ultimate responsibility for determining that the patient's best interests are served.

However, this commitment to the patient alone would not give rise to the surrogate mother model. It is only when joined with observations about the nature of sickness and patients that the model is derived. Patients, generally, are sick, suffering, fearful, dependent individuals. Because of illness and hospitalization, patients may be unable to exercise emotional control or to make important decisions, and, in at least some respects, may be irrational.[4] Consequently, the patient cannot be trusted to make the best decisions about his or her care, if able to make decisions at all. The patient needs someone to provide care and to make the decisions, i.e., decisions for his or her own good. The nurse's commitment to care for the patient, then, is a commitment to an individual who is sick, dependent, and perhaps unable to understand what his or her best interests are. The nurse's relationship to the patient should be that of a surrogate mother to her child.

It should be noted here that, on this model, the values of the nurse carry great weight, since nurses will make critical decisions in terms of their own values, i.e., their ideas about what constitutes the best interests of the patient. For example, a nurse might attempt to persuade a patient to accept a treatment for the patient's own good. She might withhold information if she believed that a patient would make the "wrong" choice if the information were provided. She might even make decisions concerning the appropriate goals for a patient's treatment. In short, acting on her responsibility for the care of the patient, the nurse may impose her own judgments and decisions about care.

On this model, then, the nurse's concern for the patient's welfare and intervention in his life are similar to a parent's concern for a child's welfare and intervention in the child's life. It is this conceptualization of nursing that is revealed by the stereotype of the nurse as mother described by Mila Aroskar in her essay "The Fractured Image: The Public Stereotype of Nursing and the Nurse." She suggests that traditionally nursing has implied a mother's relationship to her children, caring for her family and managing her home.[5] Moreover, Aroskar points out, in the first American nursing schools, the family was the model for the hospital, a model in which the nurse is seen as mother, the physician as father and patients as children.[6]

In her comments on the image of the nurse Aroskar supports the conclusions of JoAnn Ashley in *Hospitals, Paternalism, and the Role of the Nurse*. Ashley observes, "The role of women (nurses) was very early conceived as that of caring for the 'hospital family.' Their purpose was to provide efficient economical production in the form of patient care; they were to be loyal to the institution and devoted to preserving its reputation. Through service and self-sacrifice, they were to work continuously to keep the 'family' happy.... Like mothers in a household, nurses were responsible for meeting the needs of all members of the hospital 'family'—from patients to physicians."[7]

Thus, traditionally, the "mother" image has been the prevailing image of the nurse. The corresponding philosophical assumption is that the nature of the nurse-patient relationship is fundamentally like that of a mother to a child. This assumption has had profound impact on our beliefs about the character of nursing dilemmas, and our expectations concerning appropriate solutions of ethical issues in nursing practice, for it includes the belief that the nurse should always act in what is perceived to be the patient's interest.

This belief, that the nurse should always act in the patient's interest, as Sally Gadow points out, implies a conceptualization of nursing as paternalism. She notes that paternalism is often defended as the belief that, for an individual's own good, decisions should be made by those most capable of knowing what is in his best interest.[8] In actuality, however, paternalistic acts and attitudes limit the rights or freedom of individuals in their own interests.[9] Paternalism thus involves the intent to obtain what is believed to be a good for the other person, with the effect of violating his known wishes.[10] To accept the surrogate mother model of the nurse-patient relationship, therefore, with its assumptions about the extent of the nurse's ethical responsibility to the patient, and the helplessness and need of the patient, is to conceive of nursing as paternalism.

THE NURSE AS TECHNICIAN

If the two primary assumptions of the surrogate mother model concerning the extent of the nurse's ethical responsibility and the nature of patients are rejected, the resulting model of the nurse-patient relationship is a view which could be called the technical model. This model is derived from the contemporary view of nursing as a clinical science.[11] The nurse, it is suggested, should provide scientific care; that is, the nurse should apply scientific methods and scientific treatment to the care of patients. The nurse's commitment to the patient is a commitment to provide the best nursing care possible, meeting the patient's needs to the best of her ability. Further, the nurse is committed to the objective, nonjudgmental, noninterfering application of nursing knowledge and skills in treating patients. The nurse must respect the values and beliefs of patients, and be fair and unbiased in the treatment of patients. A nurse should not impose her own values or make value judgments in administering nursing care; on the contrary, she must remain ethically neutral. Thus the extent of the nurse's ethical responsibility is limited to the correct application of knowledge and skills to meet the needs of the patient.

The needs of the patient are biological phenomena with which a nurse must deal factually and objectively by providing care as requested by the patient. It is assumed that the patient's ability to make decisions and to judge his own best interests is not impaired by illness or hospitalization. Consequently, the patient retains ultimate responsibility for identifying his needs and determining his best interests. The nurse has no role in determining those interests and needs, either by attempting to influence the patient, or by refusing to help him attain his goals.

If the patient is regarded as completely capable of making his own decisions about what is good for him, and the nurse's obligation to the patient is to provide the scientific care he requests (or the physician requests for him), then the model of the nurse-patient relationship is as follows. It is a relationship between a technician, the nurse, and an individual who receives technical assistance, the patient. The nurse should merely apply knowledge and technical skills as requested by the patient. Her only concern as a professional should be to apply those skills correctly and objectively. That is to say, she should not be concerned with the decisions which the patient might make about his treatment or health, even if her involvement in his decisions would be for the patient's own good.[12] She should just provide the patient with any information and technical advice which he needs in order to make decisions concerning his health. It is a consequence of this model that the nurse would simply supply nursing care as requested, regardless of the foolishness or moral repugnance of the patient's requests and decisions. The nurse's moral values and judgments would be irrelevant to her function as a provider of nursing care.[13]

Belief in the nurse's ethical neutrality, her concern and obligation to provide the best, correct care, and the unimpaired rational abilities of the patient produce this model of the nurse-patient relationship. If the nurse's responsibility on this model is construed to include protecting the patient's interests as he has determined them, then the nurse's role is to serve as an advocate for the patient. This image of nursing as technical assistance to patients is the conceptualization which Gadow calls consumerism.[14]

THE NURSE AS CONTRACTED CLINICIAN

The third model of the nurse-patient relationship follows from the assumption that the patient is capable of determining his own best interests, a premise about patients which is also assumed by the technical model, and the belief that the ethical responsibility of the nurse is defined by the rights of the patient. The patient's right to

self-determination is essential to the rights-based moral view of the nurse-patient relationship which Dan Brock develops in his essay "The Nurse-Patient Relation: Some Rights and Duties." Brock argues that a nurse's unique relation to the patient can be explained only by viewing the nurse-patient relationship as arising from an agreement between nurse and patient, an agreement in which the patient contracts to have specified care provided by the nurse and the nurse incurs an obligation to the patient to provide that care.[15] On this model of the nurse-patient relationship, the patient has the right to control both what happens to his body and the role which the nurse takes with him in providing nursing care;[16] "...the right to determine what is done to and for the patient, and to control, within broad limits, the course of the patient's treatment and care, originates and generally remains with the patient."[17] Thus the nurse's commitment to the patient is a commitment to provide the nursing care which he chooses. Nurses are not justified in doing something because it is in the best interests of the patient, moreover, since the right to act in the patient's interest is "...*created* and *limited* by the permission or consent (from the patient-nurse/physician agreement) the patient has given."[18] Therefore, it is the patient's right to control the course of his treatment, his right to self-determination, which defines the ethical responsibility of the nurse.

An important consequence of the contracted clinician model is that the nurse is not required to be ethically neutral. Since the nurse-patient relationship arises from an agreement, the nurse can refuse to participate in the relationship, if her own ethical values would be compromised. For example, the nurse can refuse to care for abortion patients if she believes abortion is unethical. Therefore, the nurse's commitment to the patient is limited by her own permission or consent as well as by the rights of the patient.

The patient's right to self-determination, which is essential in this model, is also essential for Sally Gadow's conceptualization of nursing as existential advocacy. This conceptualization is based on the belief that "freedom of self-determination is the most fundamental and valuable human right, and therefore is a greater good than any which health care can provide."[19] Nurses must assist patients in authentically exercising that freedom of self-determination, that is, in making decisions which express the full complexity of their values.[20] The nurse is obligated to act in the patient's interest, but she cannot define what the patient's "best interest" is. She must assist patients to determine their best interests and to become clear about what they want to do.[21] "Existential advocacy, as the essence of nursing, is the nurse's participation with the patient in determining the unique meaning which the experience of health, illness, suffering, or dying is to have for that individual."[22]

Gadow argues for existential advocacy as the philosophical foundation of nursing. This conceptualization of nursing supports Brock's model of the nurse-patient relationship in its central features. Both Brock and Gadow agree that the fundamental value to be preserved in the nurse-patient relationship is the patient's right to self-determination. They are agreed that the patient determines what his best interests are and that the patient has the right to decide which role the nurse takes with him.[23] The conceptualization of nursing as advocacy, in Gadow's sense, could therefore serve as a basis for the contracted clinician model of the nurse-patient relationship. It is important to note here that it is not patients' rights advocacy which supports the contracted clinician model. For, as Gadow suggests, patients' rights advocacy is really what she calls consumerism, that is, the belief that the nurse should just obey the patient's wishes. Consumerism thus forces the patient to make a decision autonomously. It involves the paternalistic assumption that patients should make important decisions with only technical assistance and information.[24] However, Brock and Gadow both argue that the patient's right to self-determination is inviolate. That is, it is the patient's right to determine what he needs from the nurse; whether he makes a decision autonomously is his choice. The patient can, if he wishes, receive advice from the nurse; he can even choose a paternalistic relationship with the nurse. The patient's freedom to determine his relationship with the nurse is the key to the contracted clinician model.

AN ETHICAL DILEMMA

I have attempted to show that different beliefs about the ethical responsibilities of nurses and assumptions about patients yield three models of the nurse-patient relationship. These models have implications for nursing practice which are of critical importance. I will argue that, on the basis of these ethical implications, the contracted clinician model should be accepted. In order to establish that, it will be necessary to consider an example. The implications for nursing practice will be most clearly revealed if we consider a case which will show the essential differences concerning the responsibility of the nurse with regard to the patient's best interests, and the role of the nurse's personal values and beliefs.

> Mr. A. is a 56-year-old man who has had leukemia for one year. He has again voluntarily admitted himself for control of hemorrhaging and intractable pain. He also suffers from very high fevers and an oral infection with open sores. He is depressed and anxious about the future. During the past six months he has been hospitalized frequently to receive chemotherapy and blood transfusions. On recent hospitalizations, however, the chemotherapy has been discontinued because of Mr. A.'s lowered white blood count. Though he is aware of his deteriorating condition, he is optimistic about the possibility of another remission.
>
> When he is examined by the physician, the physician informs him that he is in the terminal phase of leukemia. The physician explains that he will receive painkillers and will be treated with intravenous fluids to combat the dehydration. Blood transfusions and a bone marrow aspiration will also be used to stabilize the progress of the disease. The physician, however, does not hold out any hope of prolonging Mr. A.'s life for a significant period of time. He indicates that there is only a remote hope of remission.
>
> Mr. A., extremely upset at this prognosis, exclaims that he cannot bear the pain any longer, and expresses a wish to die. Mr. A. explains his situation to his family and again expresses his wish to die without any prolonged suffering. Mrs. A. disagrees vehemently with him, and argues that any means available should be used to prolong Mr. A.'s life.
>
> Consequently, Mr. A. is admitted to the hospital, the intravenous treatment is begun, and he is left to rest. Several minutes later Nurse B., who has been present throughout Mr. A.'s examination and treatment, enters his room to discover that Mr. A. is unconscious; the flow of intravenous fluids has been mistakenly adjusted so that all of the intravenous fluids have been absorbed. As a result it is very unlikely that Mr. A. will regain consciousness. Moreover, the rapid infusion of the fluids will have immediate fatal consequences if action is not taken. What should Nurse B. do?[25]

As with all case descriptions, there is some ambiguity in this situation. It is unclear why Mr. A. voluntarily admitted himself under the circumstances or why he consented to the treatment. Since there are many aspects of this case that deserve more careful description and analysis, it cannot be adequately discussed within the scope of this [article]. It will serve, however, to illustrate the ethical implications of the three nurse-patient models.

It is necessary for the purposes of clarifying the implications of these models to make an assumption about the judgments and personal moral values of Nurse B. Let us assume that she disagrees with Mr. A.; she is convinced Mr. A. has valuable life remaining, and she believes that preserving life is a duty. In this situation there are essentially two options open to Nurse B. Nurse B. can respect Mr. A.'s wish to die and refrain from initiating any treatment, or Nurse B. can do everything possible to keep Mr. A. alive—for example, she can page the physician and immediately begin extraordinary emergency procedures. The critical element in Nurse B.'s decision in this case will be her own philosophical view of the nature of the nurse-patient relationship, that is, the role which she believes her values should play in that relationship, as well as her beliefs about her ethical responsibility for the patient.

If Nurse B. assumes the surrogate mother model of the nurse-patient relationship, there are important consequences for her practice of nursing. The strength of this model is that it clearly recognizes the vulnerability, suffering, and need of the patient. It recognizes that patients may not make the best decisions in situations such as Mr. A.'s situation. Nurse B., consequently, will be aware of Mr. A.'s vulnerability; she will be sympathetic, understanding, and willing to provide the mothering care and concern which Mr. A. may need.

Moreover, Nurse B. will regard her ethical commitment to the patient, Mr. A., as an all-encompassing responsibility to do what she believes is in Mr. A.'s best interests. Consequently, in this situation, she will act according to her perception of what is best for Mr. A. Even though Mr. A. has expressed a wish to die, she will page the physician and initiate emergency procedures in an attempt to save Mr. A.'s life.

If Nurse B. accepts the technical model, on the other hand, her action in this situation will be quite different. On the technical model, Nurse B.'s own beliefs about the sanctity of life are irrelevant, since she is required to be ethically neutral in her practice of nursing. Her skills are to be utilized to satisfy the patient's wishes and requests. If a patient requests an abortion, for example, the nurse's obligation is to supply good nursing care, regardless of her own judgments about the desirability or morality of abortion. In this case, since Mr. A. has expressed a wish to die, Nurse B. would ignore her own judgment about the best interests of Mr. A. and the immorality of letting him die. Nurse B. has no obligation to undertake any actions aimed at saving his life, for Mr. A. clearly does not wish to have his life saved. Therefore, Nurse B. will not initiate treatment.

Similarly, if Nurse B. accepts the contracted clinician model, she will not initiate treatment. On this model her ethical responsibility will be defined by Mr. A.'s right to control and determine what happens to him. Though Nurse B. disagrees with Mr. A.'s wish to die, she will not impose her own judgments and values in this situation. She will allow Mr. A. to die.

The differences between the technical model and the contracted clinician model are not obvious in this case, for though they involve quite different assumptions, they result in the same action. The key difference between these models is the role of the nurse's values in the nurse-patient relationship. On the technical model, the nurse's values are irrelevant, for she must remain ethically neutral. However, on the contracted clinician model, the nurse's values are important factors in the relationship with the patient. The nurse can refuse to participate in that relationship if her values are compromised. Thus this model allows the nurse's values to become an important aspect of the relationship with the patient.

Only the general features of the surrogate mother, technical, and contracted clinician models of the nurse-patient relationship have been outlined here. However, some significant conclusions can be drawn. First, the surrogate-mother model of the nurse-patient relationship is inadequate for the same reasons that a paternalistic model of the physician-patient relationship is unacceptable, i.e., it condones actions which violate a patient's right to self-determination. It is clearly ethically objectionable for the nurse to impose her beliefs about the patient's best interests and in effect to make an important decision for the patient. Secondly, it seems evident to me that the technical model is also inadequate. The nurse, in caring for patients and making decisions about nursing care, is not functioning solely as a technician. An acceptable model for the nurse-patient relationship must recognize the ethical aspects of nursing practice.

Because it recognizes the ethical aspects of nursing practice and the patient's right to self-determination, the contracted clinician model is the best of these three models. There is, however, one consequence of this which deserves comment. As Brock points out, the implication of his model is that the nurse-patient relationship is essentially the same as the physician-patient relationship.

It seems to me, though, that there is a significant difference. Though both nurse and physician are viewed as having a contractual relationship with the patient, there is an additional factor which complicates the nurse-patient relationship. The nurse is obligated to provide nursing care because of her agreement with the patient; furthermore, she is also obligated to obey the physician because of her agreement with the patient. That is, this obligation is imposed by the agreement with the patient because the nurse agrees to provide the nursing care necessary to the patient's needs as he or she identifies them. She is therefore obligated to assist the physician in providing care necessary to the patient's needs. The physician, however, does not have a similar obligation to the nurse. This suggests to me that these relationships may be significantly different in some respects. The question of how the nature of the nurse-patient relationship is altered by the relationship the patient has with his physician is an issue which deserves careful analysis, for these relationships are central to some of the most difficult ethical dilemmas in nursing practice.

NOTES

1 Sally Gadow argues that nursing can be defined in terms of the nurse-patient relationship in "Existential Advocacy: Philosophical Foundation of Nursing," in Stuart F. Spicker and Sally Gadow, eds., *Nursing: Images and Ideals*, New York: Springer, 1980, chapter 4.

2 Robert Veatch discusses his models of the patient-physician relationship in "Models for Ethical Medicine in a Revolutionary Age," *Hastings Center Report*, June 1972, pp. 5–7.

3 The influence of this image of nurses as surrogate mothers has been reported by several nurses and sociologists. For example, Hans O. Mauksch, "Nursing: Churning for Change," in Freeman, Howard E., *et al.* (eds.), *Handbook of Medical Sociology*, 2nd ed.,

Englewood Cliffs, N.J.: Prentice-Hall, Inc., 1972, and most recently Myra E. Levine in "Nursing Ethics and the Ethical Nurse," *American Journal of Nursing*, May 1977, p. 845.

4 Some interesting observations concerning patients are made by Henry J. Lederer, "How the Sick View Their World," in *The Journal of Social Issues*, 8(4), 1952, pp. 4–15.

5 Mila Aroskar, "The Fractured Image: The Public Stereotype of Nursing and the Nurse," in Spicker and Gadow, *Nursing*, chapter 2.

6 *Ibid.*

7 JoAnn Ashley, *Hospitals, Paternalism, and the Role of the Nurse* (New York: Teachers College Press, 1976), p. 17.

8 Gadow, "Existential Advocacy."

9 *Ibid.*

10 *Ibid.*

11 The view presented here about the nature of the nurse-patient relationship is that expressed by Gerene Major in her paper "The Abortion Patient and the Nurse." My thinking concerning the issues discussed herein was developed in response to her paper.

12 Gadow, "Existential Advocacy."

13 *Ibid.*

14 *Ibid.*

15 Dan Brock, "The Nurse-Patient Relation: Some Rights and Duties," in Spicker and Gadow, *Nursing*, chapter 5.

16 *Ibid.*

17 *Ibid.*

18 *Ibid.*

19 Gadow, "Existential Advocacy."

20 *Ibid.*

21 *Ibid.*

22 *Ibid.*

23 Gadow believes that the patient and nurse can freely decide what their relationship will be.

24 *Ibid.*

25 This case is based upon a case presented to me by Gertrude Mulvey, R.N.

Ethical Dilemmas for Nurses: Physicians' Orders versus Patients' Rights
E. Joy Kroeger Mappes

E. Joy Kroeger Mappes is assistant professor of philosophy at Frostburg State University (Maryland). Her areas of specialization are ethics and social philosophy. Mappes also serves as a member of a hospital ethics committee. In the past, she has worked as a registered nurse.

Mappes identifies two kinds of ethical dilemmas that arise for the hospital nurse. One kind of ethical dilemma arises in cases in which following a physician's orders (explicit or implicit) would violate the patient's right to adequate medical treatment. Although Mappes makes clear that the nurse can be faced with some difficult matters of judgment, she argues that the nurse is morally obligated to act on behalf of the patient in those cases in which there is good reason to think that the physician's orders are not in the best medical interest of the patient. A second kind of ethical dilemma arises in cases in which following a physician's orders would violate the patient's right of self-determination. In Mappes' view, this second class of cases is less problematic than the first, since the nurse is not faced with problematic judgments about the patient's best medical interest. She contends that the nurse is morally obliged to act to protect the patient's right of self-determination. However, emphasizing the classist and sexist forces that typically make it difficult for the nurse to act on behalf of the patient, she goes on to suggest that "changes must be made in the workplace."

The American Hospital Association in a widely promulgated statement entitled "A Patient's Bill of Rights," makes explicit a number of the generally recognized rights of hospitalized patients.[1] Among the rights expressly articulated in the AHA statement is a cluster of rights closely associated with a more general right, the right of self-determination. The "self-determination cluster" includes: (1) the right to information concerning diagnosis, treatment, and prognosis; (2) the right to information necessary to give informed consent; and (3) the right to refuse treatment. The AHA statement duly recognizes several other important patient rights but, importantly, fails to explicitly recognize the patient's right to adequate medical care.[2] Surely, if the purpose of a statement of patients' rights is to catalogue patients' rights, we ought not to overlook this one. After all, the patient has agreed to enter the hospital setting precisely for the purpose of obtaining medical treatment. To the extent that adequate medical care is not forthcoming, the patient has been done an injustice. That is, the patient's right to adequate medical care has been violated.

This paper explores two types of ethical dilemmas related to patients' rights that arise for the hospital nurse.[3] (1) The first set of dilemmas is related to the patient's basic right to adequate medical care. (2) The second set of dilemmas is related to the cluster of rights closely associated with the patient's right of self-determination. Dilemmas arise for a nurse if adequate medical care for a patient would be jeopardized by following the expressed or understood orders of a physician. Dilemmas also arise for a nurse if the patient's right to self-determination would be violated by following the expressed or understood orders of a physician. In each case, the logic of the dilemma is similar. The dilemma arises because the nurse's apparent obligation to follow the physician's order conflicts with his or her obligation to act in the interest of the patient. To carry out the physician's order would be to act against the interest of the patient. To act in the interest of the patient would be to disobey the physician's order.[4] I will argue that when this conflict arises the nurse's obligation to the patient is overriding and that nurses must act and be allowed and encouraged to act to protect the rights of the patient.

I NURSING DILEMMAS AND THE PATIENT'S RIGHT TO ADEQUATE MEDICAL CARE

In a hospital the primary responsibility for a patient's care rests with a physician. Physicians determine the medical diagnosis, treatment, and prognosis of patients' illnesses and write orders to arrive at and effect these determinations. In general, physicians' orders govern what a patient is to do and what is to be done for a patient, i.e., the degree of activity, diet, medication, diagnostic and treatment procedures to be performed. Nurses carry out physicians' orders themselves, delegate tasks to others, or make the orders known to those responsible for carrying them out. They are not generally allowed by law to diagnose or prescribe.[5] Although this is a greatly oversimplified picture of what goes on, as anyone familiar at all with the functioning of a hospital will realize, at least some of the complexities involved in the interaction among physicians, nurses, and patients in a hospital setting will emerge as we proceed.

The complexity of the ethical dilemmas arising for nurses regarding the patient's right to adequate medical care can best be understood by examining various examples. The following are suggested as being not atypical of situations arising in hospitals:

(1) A patient who has had emphysema for a number of years is admitted to a cardiac unit for observation with a tentative diagnosis of myocardial infarction. Oxygen is ordered in a concentration commonly given for patients with this diagnosis. The nurse, knowing that oxygen is contraindicated for patients with emphysema, must decide whether to carry out or question the order through appropriate channels.

(2) A patient admitted to the hospital for a diagnostic work-up has been on a special and fairly extensive drug therapy regimen. This regimen is common to patients of a particular private physician, seemingly regardless of their diagnosis. The private physician orders the drug therapy program continued after admission. However, accepted medical practice would ordinarily call for ceasing as many drugs as is safely possible, thus avoiding unnecessary variables in arriving at an accurate diagnosis. In general the private physician is viewed by other physicians as incompetent. The nurse is aware that the orders do not reflect good medical practice, but also realizes that she[6] will be dealing with this physician as long as she works at that hospital. The nurse must decide whether to follow the orders or refuse to carry out

the orders, attempting through channels to have the orders changed.

(3) A frail patient recovering from recent surgery has been receiving intra-muscular antibiotic injections four times a day. The injection sites are very tender, and though the patient now is able to eat without problems, the intern refuses to change the order to an oral route of administration of the antibiotic because the absorption of the medication would be slightly diminished. The nurse must decide whether to follow the order as it stands or continue through channels to try to have the order changed.

(4) A nurse on the midnight shift of a large medical center is closely monitoring a patient's vital signs (blood pressure, pulse rate, respiratory rate). The physicians have been unable to diagnose the patient's illness. In reviewing the patient's record, the nurse thinks of a possible diagnosis. The patient's condition begins to worsen and the nurse phones the intern-on-call to notify him of the patient's condition. The nurse mentions that the record indicates that diagnosis X is possible. The intern dismisses the nurse's suggested diagnosis and instructs the nurse to follow existing orders. Concerned that the patient's condition will continue to deteriorate, the nurse contacts her supervisor who concurs with the intern. The patient's blood pressure gradually but steadily falls and the pulse increases. The nurse has contacted the intern twice since the initial call but the orders remain unchanged. The nurse must decide whether to pursue the matter further, e.g., calling the resident-on-call and/or the patient's private physician.[7]

What are the obligations of nurses in such cases? Under what circumstances are nurses obligated to rely on their judgment and to question the physician's order? To what extent must nurses pursue the questioning when, in their view, the patient's right to adequate medical care is being violated? It is often taken for granted that when the medical assessments of physician and nurse differ, "the physician knows best." In order to see both why this is thought, perhaps correctly so, to be generally true and yet why it is surely not always true, it is necessary to consider some of the factors that account for the difference in physician and nurse assessments.

A nurse's assessment of what constitutes adequate medical treatment may differ from a physician's assessment for at least three reasons. (a) There is a difference in the amount and the content of their formal training. Physicians generally have a number of years more formal training than nurses, though that difference is not as great as it once was. More nurses now continue formal training in various ways, i.e., by pursuing graduate work and/or by becoming nurse practitioners, nurse clinicians, or nurse anesthetists. In addition, proportionately more nurses than ever before are college graduates. However, a physician's formal training is more extensive and detailed. Moreover, and perhaps most importantly, physicians are explicitly trained in the diagnosis and treatment of illness, with the emphasis of the training placed on the hard sciences. Nurses are trained to be knowledgeable about illness in general, the symptoms and treatment of illness, and the complications and side effects of various forms of therapy. While this formal training includes both the hard sciences and the social (primarily behavioral) sciences, there is an emphasis on the behavioral sciences. Nurses are trained to concentrate on the overall well-being of the patient. (*b*) There may be a difference in the length or concentration of their experience. For example, nurses who have worked in special care units (in medical and surgical cardiac units, burn units, renal units, intensive care units) for a number of years acquire a great deal of knowledge which may not be possessed by interns, and perhaps even residents and nonspecialty private physicians. Nurses who have worked for years in small community hospitals may well be more knowledgeable in some areas than some physicians. (*c*) There may be a difference in their knowledge of the patient. Nurses often have more detailed knowledge about patients than do physicians, who often see a patient only once a day. Nurses who are "at the bedside" are thus in a position to recognize small changes as they happen. Because of the possibility of more detailed knowledge, nurse assessments may be more accurate than physician assessments. Where physician and nurse assessments differ then, it is not necessarily the case that the physician's assessment is the correct one simply because of the amount and content of the physician's formal training. Physicians do make mistakes and, when they do, nurses must be in a position to protect the patient.[8]

Ethical dilemmas of the kind typified in the above four examples arise when to follow physician's orders would be to act against the medical interest of the patient. Given the fact that the *basic* obligation of both the physician and the nurse is to act in the medical interest of the patient, it is rather striking that anyone should suppose that the nurse's obligation to follow the physician's orders should ever take precedence. What, after all, is the foundation of the nurse's obligation to follow the physician's orders? Presumably, the nurse's obligation to follow the physician's orders is grounded on the

nurse's obligation to act in the medical interest of the patient. The point is that the nurse has an obligation to follow physicians' orders because, ordinarily, patient welfare (interest) thereby is ensured. Thus when a nurse's obligation to follow a physician's order comes into *direct* conflict with the nurse's obligation to act in the medical interest of the patient, it would seem to follow that the patient's interests should always take precedence.

For instance, Example 1 provides a clear case of a medically unsound order. In fact, it is such a clear case that a nurse not questioning the order would be judged incompetent. The medically unsound order may be the result of a medical mistake or of medical incompetence. If the order is the result of an oversight, the physician is likely to be grateful when (if) a nurse questions the order. If the order is a result of incompetence, the physician is not likely to be grateful. Whatever the reason for the medically unsound order, the nurse is obligated to question an order if it is clearly medically unsound. The nurse must refuse to carry out the order if it is not changed, and to press the matter through channels in order to protect the medical interest of the patient. Example 2 is similar to Example 1 in that it involves a medical practice that is clearly unsound. If the orders are questioned, the physician here again is not likely to be grateful. Indeed, since the physician's practice may ultimately be at stake, the pressures brought to bear on a nurse may be overwhelming, particularly if the physician's colleagues choose to defend him or her. It is undeniable, however, that medical incompetence is not in the best medical interest of patients, and thus that the nurse's obligation is to question the order. It is of course true that a nurse acting on behalf of the patient in this situation may pay a heavy price, perhaps his or her job, for protecting the medical interests of patients. However, the nurse's moral obligation is no less real on this account.

With Example 3 the murkiness begins, since it does not provide a clear case of unsound medical practice, though perhaps it presents us with a case in which the physician is operating with a too-narrow view of good medical practice. As I mentioned earlier, nurses often are more concerned with the overall well-being of the patient. Physicians often are concerned only with identifying the illness, treating it, and determining how responsive the illness is to the treatment. To the extent that Example 3 resembles Example 1, i.e., the lumps are very bad and the difference in the absorption of the medication in the two routes of administration is small, the nurse has an obligation to question the order. Example 4 is like Example 3 in that it does not provide a clear case of a medically unsound order. However, in Example 4, much more is at stake. Since life itself is involved, any decision must be considered very carefully. The problem here is not a problem of weighing or balancing but a problem of being either right or wrong. Both Examples 3 and 4 force a nurse to assess this question: "How strong are my grounds for thinking that the orders are not in tune with the patient's best medical interest?" The murkiness comes in knowing exactly when the physician's order is in direct conflict with the patient's medical interest. As the last two examples illustrate, it can be very difficult to know exactly what is in the best medical interest of the patient. To the extent that the nurse has carefully considered the situation and is sure that his or her view is in accord with good medical care, the order should be questioned. The less sure one is, the less clear it becomes whether the order should be questioned and the matter pressed through channels.

In arguing the above, I am not advocating uncritical questioning. Clearly, questioning at some point must cease. Otherwise, hospitals could not function efficiently and as a result the medical interest of all patients would suffer. But if there is little or no opportunity for nurses and other health professionals to contribute their knowledge to the care of the patient, or if they are directly or indirectly discouraged from contributing, it would seem that they will find it difficult, if not impossible, to fulfill their obligations with respect to the patient's right to adequate medical care.

II NURSING DILEMMAS AND THE PATIENT'S RIGHT OF SELF-DETERMINATION

The complexity of the ethical dilemmas arising for nurses regarding the patient's right of self-determination can best be understood by examining various cases. Again, the following are suggested as being not atypical of situations arising in hospitals:

(1) A patient is scheduled for prostate surgery (prostatectomy) early in the morning. Because he is generally unaware of what is happening to him due to senility, he is judged incompetent to give informed consent for surgery. The patient's sister visits him in the evenings, but the physicians have not been available during those times for her to give consent. The physicians have asked the nurses to obtain consent from the patient's sister. When she arrives the evening before surgery is

scheduled, the nurses explain to her that her brother is to have surgery and what it would entail. The sister had not been told that surgery was being considered and questions its necessity for her brother who has not experienced any real problems due to an enlarged prostate. She does not feel she can sign the consent form without talking with one of his physicians. Should the nurses encourage her to sign the consent form, as the physicians have requested, or call one of the physicians to speak with the patient's sister?

(2) A patient in the cardiac unit who was admitted with a massive myocardial infarction begins to show signs of increased cardiac failure. The patient and the family have clearly expressed their desire to the medical and nursing staff to refrain from "heroics" should complications arise. The patient stops breathing and the intern begins to intubate the patient, requests the nurse's assistance, and orders a respirator. Should the nurse follow orders or attempt to convince the intern to reconsider, calling the resident-on-call should the intern refuse?

(3) A patient is hospitalized for a series of diagnostic tests. The tests, history, and physical pretty clearly indicate a certain diagnosis. The physicians only tell the patient that they are not yet sure of the diagnosis, reassuring the patient that he is in good hands. Each day after the physicians leave, the patient asks the nurse, coming in to give medications, what the tests have shown and what his diagnosis is. When the nurse encourages the patient to ask the physicians these questions, he says he feels intimidated by them and that when he does ask questions they simply say that everything will be fine. Should the nurse reinforce what the physicians have said or attempt to convince the physicians that the patient has a right to information about his illness, pressing the matter through channels if they do not agree?

(4) A patient suffering from cancer is scheduled for surgery in the morning. While instructing the patient not to eat or drink after a certain hour, the nurse realizes that the patient is unaware of the risks involved in having the surgery and of those involved in not having the surgery. In talking further, the nurse sees clearly that the option of not having surgery was never presented and that the patient has only a vague idea of what the surgery will entail. She also appears to be unaware of her diagnosis. The patient has signed the consent form for surgery. Should the nurse proceed in preparing the patient for surgery, or, proceeding through channels, attempt to provide for a genuinely informed consent for the surgery?

What are the obligations of nurses in examples such as these? To what extent must nurses pursue questioning when, in their view, the patient's right of self-determination is being violated? Unless we are willing to say that a patient upon entering a hospital surrenders the right of self-determination, it seems clear that physicians' orders, explicit and implied, should be questioned in all of the above examples. After all, in each of the above examples, one of the rights expressly outlined by the American Hospital Association is in danger of being abridged. The rights involved are (or should be) known by all to be possessed by all. Here a difference in the formal training and knowledge based on experience is not relevant in any difference between a physician's and a nurse's assessment. No formal training in medicine is necessary to arrive at the conclusion that the patient's right of self-determination is endangered.

The tension that exists for nurses in situations typified in the above four examples is not really that of a moral dilemma, but rather, a tension between doing what is morally right and what is least difficult practically, a tension common in everyday life. The problem is not that the nurse's obligation is unclear, but that in actual situations fulfilling this moral obligation is extremely difficult. What we must consider now in some detail are the social forces that make it so difficult for a nurse to act on behalf of the patient.

III NURSING DILEMMAS AND THE IMPORTANCE OF A CLASSIST AND SEXIST CONTEXT

I have argued that when following a physician's order would violate the patient's right to adequate medical care or the patient's right of self-determination, the nurse's moral obligation is to question the order. If necessary, the matter should be pressed through channels. It is well and good to say what nurses should do. It is quite another thing, given the forces at work in the everyday world in which nurses must work, to expect nurses to do what they ought to do.

To begin with, we must recognize that there is an important class difference between physicians and nurses, the difference between the upper middle class or upper class of physicians and the lower middle class of nurses.[9] A large proportion of physicians both start out and end their lives in the upper class. Though the economic status of a physician is not as high as that of a high-level corporation executive, the social status of a physician is very high because of the prestige of the profession of medicine in the United States today.[10] Physicians have a high social status in American society and they understand and identify with people who have a similarly high status.[11] "Physicians talked with physicians; nurses talked with nurses," is an observation of one sociological study.[12] Generally physicians do not understand or identify with nurses (or with most patients), in part because of a difference in social status. Correspondingly there is an educational difference between physicians and nurses. As mentioned earlier, the formal educational training necessary for a physician is generally much longer than that necessary for a nurse, and their training differs in content.

The differences in the composition of each profession on the basis of sex is clear. Most physicians are male (93.1 percent) and most nurses are female (97.3 percent).[13] In accordance with traditional sex roles, physicians are encouraged to be decisive and to act with authority. Studies indicate that physicians view themselves as omnipotent.[14] Nurses are encouraged to be tactful, sensitive, and diplomatic. Tact and diplomacy are necessary to make a physician feel in control. Put another way, nurses' recommendations for patient treatment must take a particular form. These recommendations must appear to be initiated by the physician. Nurses are expected to take the initiative and are responsible for making recommendations, but at the same time must appear passive.[15] Nurses who see their roles, partially at least, as one of consultant must follow certain rules of the "game."[16] If they refuse to follow the rules, they will be made to suffer consequences such as snide remarks, ostracism, harassment, or job termination.

Again, in accordance with traditional sex roles, nurses in hospitals are viewed much the same as are wives and mothers in the family. This is the view of nursing held both by society and by physicians. Nurses as women are expected to be subservient to physicians as men, to provide "tender loving care" to whoever may be in need, and to be responsible and competent in the absence of physicians but to relinquish that responsibility upon request, i.e., when physicians are present.[17]

As in society, women in hospitals (here women nurses) are typically viewed as sex objects, a situation which encourages physicians to discount the input of nurses with regard to patient care. The observation that women are viewed by male physicians as sexual objects was prevalent in a project which studied the discriminatory practices and attitudes against women in forty-one United States medical schools as seen from questionnaires completed by 146 women medical students. As the author notes, "The open expression of the notion that any woman—even if she is a patient—is fair game for lecherous interests of all men (including physicians) is in some ways the most distressing fact of these student observations."[18] Responses showing the prevalent attitude of physicians toward women in general or toward women as patients included: "[I] often hear demeaning remarks, usually toward nurses offered by clinicians...." "[There is] superficial discussion of topics related to women....Basic assumption: women are not worth serious consideration." "[The] most frequent remarks concern female patients—women's illnesses are assumed psychosomatic until proven otherwise."[19] Perhaps the most frequent response of women medical students depicting the attitudes of male medical students, professors, and clinicians centered around the use of slides in class of parts of women's anatomy and slides of nude women from magazine centerfolds. Those slides were introduced by medical-student colleagues or instructors often to bait women medical students or belittle them. One student relates, "My own experience with [a professor who had included a "nudie" slide in his lecture] was an interesting and emotional comment ending on, 'Men need to look down on women, and that's why I show the slide.' "[20] The response of the male members of the class to the slides was generally one of unmitigated laughter and approval. With such a negative and restricted view of women as persons, nurses, not to mention all women, are at a disadvantage in dealing with most male physicians.

Another aspect of the sexism that permeates the physician-nurse relationship is reflected in divergent standards of mental health for men and women. A study of thirty-three female and forty-six male psychiatrists, psychologists, and social workers showed that they held a different standard of mental health for women and men. The standard agreed upon for mentally healthy men was basically the same as the standard for mentally healthy adults. The standard for mentally healthy women included being more easily influenced, less objective, etc., in general characteristics which are less socially desirable.[21] Women then who are mentally healthy women are mentally unhealthy adults and women who are mentally healthy adults are mentally unhealthy women. This is clearly a "no win" situation for all women. Women nurses are no exception.

It is the just described classist and sexist economic and social context of the physician-nurse relationship that often inhibits the nurse from effectively functioning

on behalf of the patient. Nurses have a moral responsibility to act on behalf of the patient, but in order to expect them to carry out that responsibility, changes must be made in the workplace. Nurses must be in a position to act to protect the rights of patients. They must be allowed and encouraged to do so. Therefore, those operating and managing hospitals and those responsible for hospital policies must establish policies which make it possible for nurses to protect patients' rights without risking their present and future employment. Those operating and managing hospitals cannot eradicate classism and sexism, but they must be aware of the impact it has on patient care, for again the ultimate goal of everyone connected with hospitals is adequate medical care within the framework of patients' rights. As potential patients it is important to all of us.[22]

NOTES

1 The statement can be found, for example, in *Hospitals*, vol. 4 (Feb. 16, 1973).

2 I am aware of the difficulties in determining what constitutes adequate medical care. For example, is adequate medical care determined solely by reference to past and present medical practices, by the established wisdom of knowledgeable health professionals, or by knowledgeable recipients of medical care? And how is the standard for knowledgeability determined? I am presuming that problems such as these, though difficult, are not insoluble. I am also aware of the related difficulty in distinguishing medical care from health care. And what distinguishes medical care and health care from nursing care? In this paper, "medical care" will refer to the diagnosis and treatment of illness. Health professionals then, who aid physicians in the process of diagnosing and treating illness, aid in providing medical care.

3 A large majority of all working nurses work in hospitals.

4 The International Code of Nursing Ethics is ambiguous in addressing such a dilemma. The relevant section (#7) of the code merely states: "The nurse is under an obligation to carry out the physician's orders intelligently and loyally and to refuse to participate in unethical procedures." What exactly is the nurse supposed to do when to carry out the physician's orders is in effect to participate in unethical procedures? The most recent (1976) version of the *Code for Nurses* (available from the American Nurses' Associ-

ation) adopted by the American Nurses' Association directly addresses this problem. Section 3 states, "The nurse acts to safeguard the client and the public when health care and safety are affected by the incompetent, unethical, or illegal practice of any person." The interpretive statement of section 3 begins, "The nurse's primary commitment is to the client's care and safety. Hence, in the role of client advocate, the nurse must be alert to and take appropriate action regarding any instances of incompetent, unethical, or illegal practice(s) by any member of the health-care team or the health-care system itself, or any action on the part of others that is prejudicial to the client's best interests."

5 The area of practice which is solely that of the nurse and the area of practice which is solely that of the physician is presently in a state of flux. The submissive role that nursing has held in relation to the physician's practice of medicine is being rejected by the nursing profession. Nurse practice acts, which regulate the practice of nursing, in many states reflect the change toward an expanded and more independent role for nurses. For example, a definition of a nursing diagnosis, as distinct from a medical diagnosis, is a part of some nurse practice acts. Daniel A. Rothman and Nancy Lloyd Rothman, *The Professional Nurse and the Law* (Boston: Little, Brown, 1977), pp. 65–81.

6 The overwhelming majority of nurses are women and the overwhelming majority of physicians are men. Because the examples are intended to reflect the hospital situation as it exists, I will use the feminine pronoun to refer to nurses and the masculine pronoun to refer to physicians.

7 In an actual case of this description, the intern dismissed the nurse's diagnosis by asking if her woman's intuition told her that diagnosis X was the correct one. The nurse's decision was to not pursue the matter, and early in the morning the patient sustained a cardiac arrest and was unresponsive to resuscitation efforts by the resuscitation team.

8 Obviously, nurses also make mistakes, but physicians are clearly in a position to protect the patient when they become aware of nurses' mistakes.

9 Vicente Navarro, "Women in Health Care," *New England Journal of Medicine*, vol. 292 (Feb. 20, 1975), p. 400.

10 Barbara Ehrenreich and John Ehrenreich, "Health Care and Social Control," *Social Policy*, vol. 5 (May/June 1974), p. 33.

11 Raymond S. Duff and August Hollingshead, *Sickness and Society* (New York: Harper & Row, 1968), p. 371.

12 *Ibid.*, p. 376.

13 Navarro, p. 400.

14 Robert L. Kane and Rosalie A. Kane, "Physicians' Attitudes of Omnipotence in a University Hospital," *Journal of Medical Education*, vol. 44 (August 1969), pp. 684–690; and Trucia Kushner, "Nursing Profession: Condition Critical," *Ms*, vol. 2 (August 1973), p. 99.

15 Kushner, p. 99.

16 Leonard I. Stein, "The Doctor-Nurse Game," in Edith R. Lewis, ed., *Changing Patterns of Nursing Practice: New Needs, New Roles* (New York: American Journal of Nursing Company, 1971), p. 227.

17 JoAnn Ashley, *Hospitals, Paternalism, and the Role of the Nurse* (New York: Teachers College, 1976), p. 17.

18 Margaret A. Campbell, *Why Would A Girl Go into Medicine?* (Old Westbury, N.Y.: Feminist Press, 1973), p. 73.

19 *Ibid.*, p. 74.

20 *Ibid.*, p. 26.

21 Inge K. Broverman, Donald M. Broverman, Frank E. Clarkson, Paul S. Rosenkrantz, and Susan R. Vogel, "Sex-Role Stereotypes and Clinical Judgments of Mental Health," *Journal of Consulting and Clinical Psychology*, vol. 34 (February 1970), pp. 1–7.

22 I wish to thank Jorn Bramann, Marilyn Edmunds, Jane Zembaty, and especially Tom Mappes for their helpful comments on earlier versions of this paper.

The Nurse's Role: Responsibilities and Rights
Marsha D. M. Fowler

Marsha D. M. Fowler is professor of theology and nursing, Azusa Pacific University, and staff affiliate for spirituality, pastoral care, and aging, Pasadena Presbyterian Church, Pasadena, California. She specializes in religious social ethics, bioethics, and pastoral care. Fowler is the coeditor of *Ethics at the Bedside: A Source Book for the Critical Care Nurse* (1987) and the author of numerous articles, including "Ethical Decision Making in Clinical Practice" and "Nursing's History."

Fowler first identifies the root concepts of nursing as nursing, health, person, and environment or society, defines nursing as "the diagnosis and treatment of human responses to actual or potential health problems," and links nursing autonomy and accountability with the nurse's patient-advocacy role. She then focuses on four emerging models of nursing advocacy and the nursing responsibilities related to each: (1) the legal rights model, (2) the values-based model, which is sometimes called the existential advocacy model, (3) the respect-for-persons model, and (4) the social advocacy model. The fourth model is a more political one than the first three. Its advocacy responsibilities include working to bring about social changes when these are necessary to correct systemwide inequities and injustices that result in care that does not respect the rights, values, or dignity of patients. Fowler concludes by discussing the rights that nurses must have if they are to fulfill their patient-advocate responsibilities.

There is general agreement among nursing theorists that the root concepts of nursing are: nursing, health, person, and environment or society.[1] These concepts, together, comprise the metaparadigm of nursing and identify its distinctive scientific focus. In contrast, the metaparadigm concepts of medicine are: physician, pathophysiology, person, and society or environment. Every theory or model of nursing or of medicine will incorporate and define the profession's metaparadigm concepts and their linkages. Thus, although theories of medicine will differ among themselves, and theories of nursing will likewise differ, they will remain theories of medicine or nursing, by virtue of their incorporation of all of the particular root concepts of the profession.

Conceptually, nursing is defined as "the diagnosis and treatment of human responses to actual or potential health problems."[2] The phenomena of concern to nurses are, then, responses to health problems, rather than the problems or diseases that cause them. Thus, the focus of nursing *qua* nursing is rather different from the focus of

Reprinted with permission of the publisher from *Biomedical Ethics Reviews 1987*, edited by James M. Humber and Robert F. Almeder (Clifton, N.J.: Humana Press, 1988), pp. 145–155.

medicine, though there are areas of overlapping concern. The definition, fundamental enterprise, concerns, ends, and goals of nursing differ from those of medicine. With difference comes a difference in the role, rights, responsibilities, and moral perspectives of nursing.

Contemporary nursing identifies itself as a "patient advocacy" profession that includes a primary commitment to the patient. (In general, nursing identifies the "patient" as the individual with an actual or potential health problem plus that person's relational web. In some instances, the patient may be a group or a community, depending upon the nature of the nursing specialty.) Patient advocacy and a primary commitment to the patient are not new with nursing; this focus can be found in the earliest moral literature of the profession in this country.

As early as 1893, when Lystra Gretter wrote the Florence Nightingale Pledge, the first moral code for American nursing, one can see strands of commitment to the patient. The Pledge states "with loyalty will I aid the physician in his work and will devote myself to the welfare of those committed to my care."[3] The pledge does not state, as it has often been interpreted, that the nurse is devoted to the physician and loyal to the patient, and by implication that nursing is based upon an historical ethics of obedience. The object of nursing's concern and devotion was and remains the patient; nursing's ethics is rooted in a relationship with the patient and the well-being of that patient, not in an ethics of obedience. Where nursing has differed historically has been in its determination of how one goes about assuring the well-being of the patient. In earlier days it was often held that nursing best served the patient by adherence to the physician's orders. Contemporary nursing observes that the patient is best served by the independent (autonomous) practice of nursing as nursing, and collaborative practice with medicine where medical issues are of concern.

Both the Code for Nurses of the International Council of Nurses (ICN) and the American Nurses' Association (ANA) Code for Nurses support this position. The ICN code states that "The nurse's primary responsibility is to the people who require nursing care."[4] The ANA code declares that:

> The nurse's primary commitment is to the health, welfare, and safety of the client. As an advocate of the client, the nurse must be alert to and take appropriate action regarding any instances of incompetent, unethical, or illegal practice by any member of the health care team or the health care system, or any action on the part of others that places the rights or best interests of the client in jeopardy.[5]

The ANA Code additionally states that "professional autonomy and self-regulation in the control of conditions of practice are necessary for implementing nursing standards."[6] In the ethics of the profession today, nursing inextricably links advocacy for the patient with nursing autonomy and accountability as well.

Despite the fact that nursing so strongly aligns itself with the patient, in the role of advocate, the actual definition and development of models of advocacy is as yet not well formulated. In general, there are four emerging models of nursing advocacy; the specification of the nurse's role and responsibilities within each model differs somewhat.

MODELS OF NURSING ADVOCACY FOR THE PATIENT: THE NURSE'S RESPONSIBILITIES

One model, as propounded by Annas, Winslow, and others, proposes an essentially legal understanding of

nursing advocacy as the appropriate metaphor for nursing practice.[7] It "is associated with virtues such as courage and norms such as the defense of the patient against the infringement of his or her rights."[8] Those rights include the patient's right to information about procedures, diagnosis, and treatment; the right to accept or refuse medical intervention, the right to leave the hospital, the right to be treated with respect, and so forth.[9] In this form of advocacy, the nurse is responsible to be well informed of the legal rights of the patient, and is willing to enter into disputes to fight for those rights when they have been or will be abridged.

This rights-based protection model of nursing advocacy is, in part, supported by the Code for Nurses, which calls for the nurse to act when "any action on the part of others...places the rights or best interests of the patient in jeopardy."[10] Even so, the "best interests" clause muddies the waters somewhat, since the patient's best interests are not the focus of the rights-based model.[4] Despite Winslow's support of this model, Fry and others decry the use of a legal-rights conception of advocacy as the ideal for the nurse-patient relationship.[11,12]

Historically nursing has tended to consider itself to be based in an interpersonal, or perhaps even a moral, relationship to the patient rather than a legal one. Thus, a rights-protection model of advocacy strains at the boundaries of nursing's self identity and is much less comfortable a metaphor than one rooted in a more existential and less legal understanding of nursing's relationship with the patient.

Kohnke favors a values-based model of advocacy with a decisional counseling type of process of enactment. In this view of advocacy, the responsibility of the nurse is to seek to assist the patient in identifying or clarifying his or her own values, and to make a decision that is most congruent with, and the best expression of, those values.[13] Steps in this process would include supporting the patient and assisting the patient to clarify values, appraise the situation, survey and evaluate alternatives, and act upon (and adhere to) that position even in the face of negative feedback.[14,15]

Gadow espouses a variant form of this view of advocacy. She sees advocacy as "existential advocacy," and proposes that:

> The philosophical foundation and ideal of nursing is that of advocacy—not the concept of advocacy implied in the patients' rights movement, in which any health professional potentially is a consumer advocate, but a fundamental, existential advocacy for which the nurse alone, among

all the health professionals, is uniquely suited, and which is as distinct from consumer advocacy as it is from paternalism.[16]

For Gadow, the role of the nurse in existential advocacy does not "consist in protecting the individuals' rights to do what they want," but rather:

> To help persons become clear about what they want to do, by helping them discern and clarify their values in the situation, and on the basis of that self-examination, to reach decisions which express their reaffirmed, perhaps recreated (by the illness), complex of values.[17]

Unfortunately, the values-based decisional model of nursing advocacy requires a patient who is self-determining (as an expression of values), or whose values could be known either through the family or through an instrument such as the durable power of attorney for health care. Thus, it is not sufficient as a model to encompass the patient who cannot participate in the decisional process or whose values can not be known.

Such a patient makes a third model of advocacy necessary. Fry has referred to this model as the "respect-for-persons" model and cites Murphy's perspective on this model.[18] Murphy has referred to the respect-for-persons model as the "patient-advocate model," a designation that is now insufficiently descriptive. This model demands that the nurse respect the dignity and personhood of the patient whether or not the patient is self-determining or autonomous. When the patient is self-determining (or has a surrogate decision maker), the nurse functions in a fashion similar to the values-based decisional model. However, when the patient is nonautonomous, and there is no one to speak for the patient, the nurse is called to act in the "best interests" of the patient, as defined by the nurse. Murphy maintains that the nurse is in the best position to make these judgments, largely owing to the amount of time the nurse spends with the individual patient, and the continuous, caring nature of the nurse-patient relationship.[19]

It is ultimately this model of advocacy that the Code for Nurses supports, despite its mention of protection of patient rights. This model demands that the nurse advocate be accountable directly to the patient for having served in his or her best interests, and accountable to society for the judgments made as an advocate for either the autonomous or nonautonomous patient.

Not all advocacy, however, takes place at the bedside. A "larger," more political perspective on nursing advocacy forms a fourth model. It is best typified by Freeman's notion of "practice as protest," which contains an element of bedside advocacy, but extends to social advocacy as a form of social criticism and social change. Freeman envisions three major ways in which nurses can practice/protest:

1. We can engage in public contest and confrontation, sharing the cause of the aggrieved.

2. We can act as advocates for those we serve, fighting the battles little and big—that they are ill prepared to fight for themselves.

3. We can, through the practice of nursing itself, build the capability of those we serve so they are able to fend for themselves, to earn their own place in the sun or fight for rights withheld.[20]

For Freeman, this form of advocacy does more than secure care for an individual. It is a means of calling to the attention of providers of care the inconsistencies and inadequacies of care.[21] It is rooted in a concept of social justice and is an attempt to get at and correct system-wide inequities and injustices that lead to care that fails to respect the rights, values, or dignity of the patient.

None of the four models above has been fully developed; they are emerging models of advocacy that have yet to be articulated in theory and tested in practice. Elements of each of these models can be seen throughout the nursing literature, and it remains to be seen which will emerge as the model with the greatest explanatory power in the light of the ethical norms and tradition of the profession.

THE NURSE'S RIGHTS AS PATIENT ADVOCATE

The Right to Protection from Reprisal

In a recent statement of the ANA Committee on Ethics, entitled "Ethics of Safeguarding Client Health and Safety," elements of each of the models of advocacy are evident, though there is a very strong emphasis on collective nursing action for social change. Collective action is not, however, merely for the purposes of bringing about social change through the power of a unified voice. Collective action also serves to protect individual nurses from possible retaliation for acting upon the moral norms of the profession.

The issue of the protection of the nurse who questions the moral or legal or medical appropriateness of another's actions has been a consistent concern within the profession. As the Code notes,

> There should be an established process for the reporting and handling of incompetent, unethical, or illegal practice within the employment setting so that such reporting can go through official channels without fear of reprisal.[22]

So too, the Committee notes that "collective action by the nursing profession is required in order to minimize the individual heroism and risk-taking often required in 'whistle-blowing' situations."[23] If the advocacy role of the nurse generates responsibilities toward or on behalf of the patient, and both the profession and the institution demand fulfillment of those responsibilities, the nurse has a right to act in accord with those duties without fear of reprisal.

The Nurse's Right to Institutional Processes and Procedures

Advocacy as a contemporary metaphor for nursing practice is sufficiently large to encompass other role obligations addressed by the Code for Nurses and the ethical literature of the profession. Such responsibilities include duties of acting nonprejudicially toward patients, maintaining confidentiality, respecting privacy, assuming accountability and responsibility for nursing judgments, maintaining competence, refusing an inappropriate assignment, developing the profession's body of knowledge, maintaining and improving the standards of the profession, assuring working conditions conducive to high-quality nursing care, maintaining the integrity of the profession, and collaborating with other health professionals to meet the health needs of the public.

In all this, however, the nurse cannot act upon the moral obligations the profession propounds without having adequate safeguards, as noted above, and viable processes or mechanisms in place. Herein lie, at least in part, the nurse's rights correlative to responsibilities. If a nurse is enjoined to act upon moral judgments, that nurse has a right to expect established processes for such action. The Code states that:

> To function effectively in this role [as patient advocate] nurses must be aware of the employing institution's policies and procedures, nursing standards of practice, the Code for Nurses, and laws governing nursing and health

care practice with regard to incompetent, unethical, or illegal practice.[24]

As an aside, it is clear that in order to judge the appropriateness of the actions of others (whether physician, nurse, or family member) relative to the patient's best interests, nurses must have extensive knowledge of professional codes and standards, laws that govern nursing and health care practice, and medical therapeutics. Note that although the law may declare a nurse not legally qualified to judge medical competence, the ethics of the profession nonetheless requires it.

The nurse's judgments are to be made over against these and other standards. Action based upon such judgments is dependent upon the existence of institutional processes. Generally, either or both of two major avenues of pursuit are available.

The Traditional Route of Patient Advocacy

The first route of patient advocacy is the traditional, upward, hierarchical reporting within the institution, with resort to noninstitutional authorities within the health care system when the various levels of the hierarchy are refractory to expressions of concern. This particular process involves immediate communication with the person judged not to be acting in the patient's best interests, factual documentation, memoranda of concern, and other written instruments as directed by the institution's policies. These rise to succeeding levels within the hierarchy, until such time as the situation is resolved.

A process of this nature is generally cumbersome, laborious, subject to interruption or delay, and often ineffectual. It is, however, accessible to all nurses. Every nurse has a right to expect that an institution will have formalized policies and procedures for reporting illegal, incompetent, or morally inappropriate behavior, and perhaps a different mechanism for each kind of problem. The nurse has both a right and responsibility to utilize the mechanisms in place, and to use them without penalty, before going outside established lines of communication.

Emerging Routes

A second and increasingly more efficient and effective avenue for patient advocacy is the institutional ethics committee (IEC), which is meant to address issues or problems of an ethical nature. (Questions of competence are often better addressed by peer review or quality assessment committees. Questions of lawfulness should be directed to other groups, depending upon the nature and context of the presumed illegal practice. In some instances, illegal practice should be reported to licensing boards; in others to the district attorney or other legal bodies.)

In 1984, the House of Delegates of the ANA adopted a resolution that encouraged state nurses' associations to:

> promote nurses' active participation in the development, implementation, and evaluation of formal mechanisms for multidisciplinary institutional ethical review such as institutional ethics committees.[25]

The ANA Committee on Ethics subsequently prepared guidelines to assist nurses in establishing and participating in the work of an IEC. The Committee noted that:

> The impetus for the development of such mechanisms arises out of ethical, legal, and social concerns that include an increasing dissatisfaction on the part of both health care professionals and consumers with existing institutional decision-making processes, and the difficult moral choices that directly and indirectly affect patient/client care and welfare.[26]

Nursing's concern for the development of IECs is specifically to protect the quality of patient care and the welfare, well-being, and interests of the patient.

Although in the stage of clinical trial, the IEC is proving a useful mechanism for the resolution or prevention of moral dilemmas that affect the quality of patient care. IECs are perhaps most effective in quasi-legislative, rather than quasi-judicial, functions. Some categories of moral dilemmas in nursing practice, which jeopardize either the rights or best interests of the patient, are recurrent. When nurses raise these issues to an IEC, that group can prepare general guidelines for efficiently and effectively handling a specific category of problem. When nurses remain silent, guidelines may never be developed.

Although the nurse has the right to expect that institutions will have procedures for reporting illegal, incompetent, or unethical behavior, and mechanisms (such as IECs) for their resolution, the nurse also has a duty to utilize the procedures that do exist and to assist in their development when they do not. That is, the nurse is expected to actively participate in establishing the work environment, moral milieu, or procedures

wherein the right of nurses to practice as patient advocates can be realized.

"Patient advocacy" is clearly the watchword of this era of nursing. It is not, of course, an end in itself, but rather a means to effect the nurturative, generative, and supportive practices of nursing, which focus the profession's attention on "health"; for health is "the center of nursing attention, not as an end in itself, but as a means to life that is meaningful and manageable."[27] The nurse is responsible to the patient and to society insofar as she or he has worked toward achieving that end.

NOTES AND REFERENCES

1 Jacqueline Fawcett (1984) *Analysis and Evaluation of Conceptual Models of Nursing* F. A. Davis, Philadelphia.
2 American Nurses' Association (1980) *Nursing: A Social Policy Statement* American Nurses' Association, Kansas City, MO.
3 Lystra Gretter (1893) *The Florence Nightingale Pledge* Lystra Gretter.
4 International Council of Nurses (1973) *Code For Nurses* Geneva, ICN.
5 American Nurses' Association (1985) *Code for Nurses with Interpretive Statements*, Kansas City, MO, ANA.
6 Ibid.
7 Winslow, G. (1984) From Loyalty to Advocacy: A New Metaphor for Nursing, *Hastings Center Report* 14(3), pp. 32–40.
8 Ibid., p. 32.
9 Ibid., p. 36.
10 Code p. 6.
11 Fry, S. T. (1984) Ethics in Community Health Nursing Practice, in *Community Health Nursing* (L. Lancaster and M. Stanhope, eds.) St. Louis, MO, Mosby, pp. 77–96.
12 Fowler, M. D. M. (1984) *Ethics in Nursing, 1893–1984: The Ideal of Service, The Reality of History* Los Angeles, University of Southern California.
13 Kohnke, M. E. (1980) The Nurse as Advocate. *American Journal of Nursing*, 80: 2038–2040.
14 Uustal, D. (1987) Values: Cornerstone of Nurses' Moral Art, in *Ethics at the Bedside* (M. Fowler and J. Levine-Ariff, eds.) Philadelphia, Lippincott, pp. 136–170.
15 Janis, I. (1983) *Short-Term Counseling*. New Haven, Yale University Press, p. 137.

16 Spicker, S. and Gadow, S. (1980) *Nursing Images and Ideals: Opening Dialogue with the Humanities* New York, Springer, p. 81.

17 Ibid., p. 85.

18 Fry, S. T. (1987) Autonomy, Advocacy, and Accountability: Ethics at the Bedside, *Ethics at the Bedside* (M. Fowler and J. Levine-Ariff, eds.) Philadelphia, Lippincott, pp. 39–50. I am indebted to Dr. Fry for her typology of models of advocacy.

19 Murphy, C. P. (1983) Models of the Nurse-Patient Relationship, in *Ethical Problems in the Nurse-Patient Relationship* (C. P. Murphy and H. Hunter, eds.) Boston, Allyn and Bacon, pp. 9–24.

20 Freeman, R. (1971) Practice as Protest. *American Journal of Nursing* 71: 5, 918–921.

21 Ibid., p. 920.

22 Code, p. 6.

23 Committee on Ethics, American Nurses' Association (December 1986) *Ethics of Safeguarding Client Health and Safety*, Kansas City, MO, ANA.

24 Code, p. 6.

25 American Nurses' Association (1986) *Guidelines for Nurses' Participation and Leadership in Institutional Ethical Review Processes*, Kansas City, MO, ANA.

26 Ibid.

27 ANA, Social Policy Statement, p. 6.

Confidentiality

The Principle of Medical Confidentiality
LeRoy Walters

LeRoy Walters is director of the Center for Bioethics, Kennedy Institute of Ethics, Georgetown University. He is also a member of Georgetown's department of philosophy. Walters is the editor of the annual *Bibliography of Bioethics* and coeditor of *Contemporary Issues in Bioethics* (3d ed., 1989). In addition, he has published articles on topics such as fetal research, the just-war tradition, and technology assessment and genetics. Among these articles are "Technology Assessment and Genetics" and "Ethical Issues in the Prevention and Treatment of AIDS."

Walters presents (1) the philosophical arguments for the preservation of the principle of medical confidentiality and (2) the kinds of reasons that could justify violations of the principle. Walters, while insisting upon the importance of the principle, holds that the health-care professional has only a prima facie and not an absolute obligation to preserve the principle. In Walters's view, the following sorts of considerations are relevant in determining whether this prima facie obligation may be overridden in a particular case: (1) The principle may come into conflict with the rights of the patient; (2) it may conflict with the interests of an innocent third party; and (3) there may be a serious conflict between the principle and the rights of society in general.

I

... There are two primary philosophical arguments in favor of preserving medical confidentiality. The first argument is utilitarian and refers to possible long-term consequences. The second argument is non-utilitarian and speaks of respect for the rights of persons.

The utilitarian argument for the preservation of medical confidentiality is that without such confidentiality the physician-patient relationship would be seriously impaired. More specifically, the promise of confidentiality encourages the patient to make a full disclosure of his symptoms and their causes, without fearing that an embarrassing condition will become public knowledge.[1] Among medical professionals, psychotherapists have been particularly concerned to protect the confidentiality of their relationship with patients. In the words of one psychiatrist:

> The patient in analysis must learn to free associate and to break down resistances to deal with unconscious threatening thoughts and feelings. To revoke secrecy after encouraging such risk-taking is to threaten all future interactions.[2]

A second argument for the principle of medical confidentiality is that the right to a sphere of privacy is a basic human right. In what is perhaps the classic essay concerning the right of privacy, Samuel Warren and Louis Brandeis wrote in 1890 that the common law secured "to each individual the right of determining, ordinarily, to what extent his thoughts, sentiments, and emotions shall be communicated to others."[3] Present-day advocates of the right of privacy frequently employ the imagery of concentric circles or spheres. In the center is the "core self," which shelters the individual's "ultimate secrets"—"those hopes, fears, and prayers that are beyond sharing with anyone unless the individual comes under such stress that he must pour out these ultimate secrets to secure emotional release."[4] According to this image, the next largest circle contains intimate secrets which can be shared with close relatives or confessors of various kinds. Successively larger circles are open to intimate friends, to casual acquaintances, and finally to all observers.

The principle of medical confidentiality can be based squarely on this general right of privacy. The patient, in distress, shares with the physician detailed information concerning problems of body or mind. To employ the imagery of concentric circles, the patient admits the physician to an inner circle. If the physician, in turn, were to make public the information imparted by the patient—that is, if he were to invite scores or thousands of other persons into the same inner circle—we would be justified in charging that he had violated the patient's right of privacy and that he had shown disrespect to the patient as a human being.

These two arguments for the principle of medical confidentiality—the argument based on probable consequences of violation and the argument based on the right of privacy—seem to constitute a rather strong case for the principle. However, we have not yet faced the question whether the principle of confidentiality is a moral

absolute, or whether it can be overridden by other considerations....

II

There are, in my view, three general reasons which might conceivably justify violating the principle of confidentiality.[5] The first is that the principle may come into conflict with the rights of the patient himself. To illustrate, one can envision a situation in which a patient, in a temporary fit of depression, threatens to kill himself or herself or to perform an irrational act which will almost certainly destroy the patient's reputation. In the case of threatened suicide, one finds oneself weighing a secret vs. a life. Perhaps the physician should feel free, in such a case, to violate the principle of confidentiality and to involve a third party for the protection of the patient himself or herself.

A second possible ground for violating the principle of confidentiality is that it may conflict with the right of an innocent third party. In older textbooks of moral theology, one can discover hypothetical cases constructed to illustrate this dilemma. Often the case involves a physician and a young couple about to be married. Because of his professional relationship with the husband-to-be, the physician knows that the man is concealing a condition of infective syphilis or permanent impotence from his future wife. The question then arises whether the physician should violate the principle of confidentiality in order to warn the unsuspecting innocent party.[6]

In our own time the physician's dilemma is more likely to concern the case of a "battered child." If the abused child is brought to the physician by the battering parents, the physician faces an immediate conflict of loyalties. Does he or she owe it to his adult patients to keep confidential the fact that they have abused the child? Or, is the physician under the obligation to protect the child from further harm by disclosing the child's injuries to the proper public authorities? It should perhaps be noted in passing that most states in the United States require that the physician report child-abuse cases to the appropriate governmental agency.[7]

A third possible ground for violating the principle of confidentiality is a serious conflict between the principle and the rights or interests of society in general. The possibility of such a conflict was formally recognized in 1912, when the American Medical Association revised its code of ethics. A new clause was introduced into the confidentiality section of the code, specifically authorizing the physician to report communicable diseases, even if such reports were based on confidential information. The justification for this type of disclosure was, of course, the protection of society at large from the spread of infectious disease.[8]

At present, various states require reports of particular types of contagious disease. Almost universally, the physician is legally obligated to report cases of venereal disease to the proper government authorities. The reporting of tuberculosis is also frequently required. State provisions for protecting the confidentiality of such public health reports vary widely, with about half of the states taking measures to prevent public disclosure of the data.[9] Whenever states require physicians to report such data concerning communicable diseases, the general justification for the violation of physician-patient confidentiality is that society at large must be protected.

There is a second type of situation in which the principle of confidentiality and the public good seem to come into sharp conflict. In these cases the physician discovers a serious medical problem in a patient whose occupation makes him responsible for the lives of many other persons. Two standard examples are a railroad signalman who is discovered to be subject to attacks of epilepsy, or an airline pilot with failing eyesight. A case reported in a recent essay on medical secrecy reads as follows:

> Last year, 30 people were killed when a bus driver had a heart attack and plunged his bus into the East River in New York City. The driver's physician had known about the bad heart, had cautioned him not to drive, but felt he could not report it to the company since the patient might lose his job.[10]

In cases involving such critical occupations, some would argue that the physician's duty to protect the lives of many persons overrides his obligation to observe the principle of medical confidentiality.

In the future we are likely to see vigorous battles waged over the question of medical confidentiality vs. the public good. Three examples can be briefly cited. Already one hears rhetoric which implies that genetic disorders are quasi-contagious diseases.[11] According to this viewpoint, members of future generations will be "infected" if decisive action is not taken now. Is it possible that such pressures will lead to the requirement that physicians routinely report genetic defects to public health authorities? To cite a second example, epidemiologists constantly pursue new correlations between chronic diseases and particular environmental factors or medical conditions. Their studies frequently require surveys of total populations or random samples of such populations.[12] Will the desire of patients to keep their medical records confidential and their refusal to take part in such epidemiological studies come to be seen as an anti-social act or as a failure to perform a civic duty? Third, it is at least conceivable that the concept of public health could be expanded to include "economic contamination." According to this view, any disease which prevents a person from being a fully-productive member of the labor force would be seen as a hazard to the society's overall economic health, particularly if public funds were being used to defray the expenses of the illness. Cost-benefit analysis would indicate that because of the illness, other persons in the society would need to work to subsidize the relatively-less-productive ill person. As one economist put it, well persons would become, at least partially, the "economic slaves" of the patient.[13] If the concept of public health is expanded in this economic direction, it seems likely that there will be tremendous pressure directed against maintaining the medical confidentiality of patients whose treatment is subsidized by public funds.

My own view is that the physician has a prima facie obligation to preserve the principle of medical confidentiality.[14] This obligation is based on the two considerations mentioned...above, a concern for protecting the physician-patient relationship and a desire to respect the patient's right of privacy. Thus, the burden of proof must be assumed by anyone who wishes to argue that the principle of medical confidentiality should be violated. However, there are some cases in which this prima facie obligation can be overridden because of other very weighty considerations, for example, the desire to protect the patient's own life or the lives of other persons. According to this view, then, the physician's duty to observe the principle of medical confidentiality is a very important moral obligation, but not an absolute obligation or one's only obligation....

NOTES

1 A similar line of argument was advanced in favor of testimonial privilege for physicians in *Randa v. Bear*, 50 Wash. 2d 415, 312 P. 2d 640 (1957); cited by William J. Curran and E. Donald Shapiro, *Law, Medicine, and Forensic Science* (2nd ed.; Boston: Little, Brown, 1970), p. 377.

2 Harvey L. Ruben and Diane D. Ruben, "Confidentiality and Privileged Communications: The Psychotherapeutic Relationship Revisited," *Medical Annals of the District of Columbia* 41 (6): 365, June 1972.

3 The Warren-Brandeis article appeared in the *Harvard Law Review*, vol. 4, 1890, at p. 193. This quotation is taken from Susan Beggs-Baker, *et al.*, "Individual Privacy Considerations for Computerized Health Information Systems," *Medical Care* 12 (1): 79, January 1974. For a perceptive recent treatment of the right to privacy see Charles Fried, *An Anatomy of Values: Problems of Personal and Social Choice* (Cambridge, Mass.: Harvard University Press, 1970), chap. 9. The constitutional right of privacy has recently been affirmed by the U.S. Supreme Court in the cases *Griswold v. Connecticut* [381 U.S. 479, 85 S. Ct. 1678 (1965)] and *Katz v. United States* [389 U.S. 347, 88 S. Ct. 507 (1967)].

4 Alan F. Westin, *Privacy and Freedom* (New York: Atheneum, 1967), p. 33.

5 The following analysis parallels, in part, Robert E. Regan's discussion of "various conflicts between the duty of medical secrecy and other rights and duties" in *Professional Secrecy in the Light of Moral Principles: with an Application to Several Important Professions* (Washington, D.C.: Augustinian Press, 1943), pp. 138–148.

6 This illustration is drawn from Regan, *Professional Secrecy*, pp. 143–147.

7 Dennis Helfman, *et al.*, "Access to Medical Records," in the *Appendix* to U.S. Department of Health, Education and Welfare, *Report of the Secretary's Commission on Medical Malpractice* (Washington, D.C.: U.S. Government Printing Office, 1973), pp. 180–181.

8 Regan, *Professional Secrecy*, p. 116. A similar, although more general, exception to the confidentiality obligation is included in the current AMA "Principles of Medical Ethics," (Judicial Council, *Opinions and Reports*, p. vii).

9 Helfman, *et al.*, "Access to Medical Records," p. 181. State laws requiring that cases of drug addiction be reported would be justified by means of analogous arguments (*ibid*).

10 Henry A. Davidson, "Professional Secrecy," in E. Fuller Torrey, ed., *Ethical Issues in Medicine: The Role of the Physician in Today's Society* (Boston: Little, Brown, 1968), p. 194.

11 See for example, Amitai Etzioni, *Genetic Fix* (New York: Macmillan, 1973), especially chap. 4.

12 Great Britain, Medical Research Council, "Responsibility in the Use of Medical Information for Research," *British Medical Journal* 1 (5847): 213–216, 27 January 1973.

13 See the comments of the economist Lester Thurow on a related issue in Betty Cochran, "Conference Report: Conception, Coercion, and Control," *Hospital and Community Psychiatry* 25 (5), 287, May 1974.

14 William Frankena, *Ethics* (2nd ed.; Englewood Cliffs, N.J.: Prentice-Hall, 1973), pp. 26–28.

Majority Opinion in *Tarasoff v. Regents of the University of California*
Justice Mathew O. Tobriner

Mathew O. Tobriner was an associate justice of the Supreme Court of California from 1962 until 1981. Prior to his appointment to the Supreme Court of California, Justice Tobriner served as a judge in the District Court of Appeals, 1st District of California (1959–1962) and as a professor at the Hastings Law School (1958–1959). Justice Tobriner contributes to legal journals.

Tatiana Tarasoff was murdered by Prosenjit Poddar, who was a patient of psychotherapists employed by the University of California Hospital. Her parents brought an action against the university regents, doctors, and campus police. The Tarasoffs complained that the doctors

California Supreme Court; July 1, 1976. 131 California Reporter 14. Reprinted with permission of West Publishing Co.

and police had failed to warn them that their daughter was in danger from Poddar. In finding for the Tarasoffs, Justice Tobriner argues that a doctor or psychotherapist treating a mentally ill patient has a duty to warn third parties of threatened dangers arising out of the patient's violent intentions. Responding to the defendants' appeal to the important role played by the principle of confidentiality in the psychotherapeutic situation, Tobriner argues that the public interest in safety from violent assault must be weighed against the patient's right to privacy.

On October 27, 1969, Prosenjit Poddar killed Tatiana Tarasoff. Plaintiffs, Tatiana's parents, allege that two months earlier Poddar confided his intention to kill Tatiana to Dr. Lawrence Moore, a psychologist employed by the Cowell Memorial Hospital at the University of California at Berkeley. They allege that on Moore's request, the campus police briefly detained Poddar, but released him when he appeared rational. They further claim that Dr. Harvey Powelson, Moore's superior, then directed that no further action be taken to detain Poddar. No one warned plaintiffs of Tatiana's peril....

We shall explain that defendant therapists cannot escape liability merely because Tatiana herself was not their patient. When a therapist determines, or pursuant to the standards of his profession should determine, that his patient presents a serious danger of violence to another, he incurs an obligation to use reasonable care to protect the intended victim against such danger. The discharge of this duty may require the therapist to take one or more of various steps, depending upon the nature of the case. Thus it may call for him to warn the intended victim or others likely to apprise the victim of the danger, to notify the police, or to take whatever other steps are reasonably necessary under the circumstances....

PLAINTIFFS' COMPLAINTS

...Plaintiffs' first cause of action, entitled "Failure to Detain a Dangerous Patient," alleges that on August 20, 1969, Poddar was a voluntary outpatient receiving therapy at Cowell Memorial Hospital. Poddar informed Moore, his therapist, that he was going to kill an unnamed girl, readily identifiable as Tatiana, when she returned home from spending the summer in Brazil. Moore, with the concurrence of Dr. Gold, who had initially examined Poddar, and Dr. Yandell, assistant to the director of the department of psychiatry, decided that

Poddar should be committed for observation in a mental hospital. Moore orally notified Officers Atkinson and Teel of the campus police that he would request commitment. He then sent a letter to Police Chief William Beall requesting the assistance of the police department in securing Poddar's confinement.

Officers Atkinson, Brownrigg, and Halleran took Poddar into custody, but, satisfied that Poddar was rational, released him on his promise to stay away from Tatiana. Powelson, director of the department of psychiatry at Cowell Memorial Hospital, then asked the police to return Moore's letter, directed that all copies of the letter and notes that Moore had taken as therapist be destroyed, and "ordered no action to place Prosenjit Poddar in 72-hour treatment and evaluation facility."

Plaintiffs' second cause of action, entitled "Failure to Warn on a Dangerous Patient," incorporates the allegations of the first cause of action, but adds the assertion that defendants negligently permitted Poddar to be released from police custody without "notifying the parents of Tatiana Tarasoff that their daughter was in grave danger from Prosenjit Poddar." Poddar persuaded Tatiana's brother to share an apartment with him near Tatiana's residence; shortly after her return from Brazil, Poddar went to her residence and killed her.

Plaintiffs' third cause of action, entitled "Abandonment of a Dangerous Patient," seeks $10,000 punitive damages against defendant Powelson. Incorporating the crucial allegations of the first cause of action, plaintiffs charge that Powelson "did the things herein alleged with intent to abandon a dangerous patient, and said acts were done maliciously and oppressively."

Plaintiffs' fourth cause of action, for "Breach of Primary Duty to Patient and the Public," states essentially the same allegations as the first cause of action, but seeks to characterize defendants' conduct as a breach of duty to safeguard their patient and the public. Since such conclusory labels add nothing to the factual allegations of the complaint, the first and fourth causes of action are legally indistinguishable....

...We direct our attention...to the issue of whether plaintiffs' second cause of action can be amended to state a basis for recovery.

PLAINTIFFS CAN STATE A CAUSE OF ACTION AGAINST DEFENDANT THERAPISTS FOR NEGLIGENT FAILURE TO PROTECT TATIANA

The second cause of action can be amended to allege that Tatiana's death proximately resulted from defendants' negligent failure to warn Tatiana or others likely to apprise her of her danger. Plaintiffs contend that as amended, such allegations of negligence and proximate causation, with resulting damages, establish a cause of action. Defendants, however, contend that in the circumstances of the present case they owed no duty of care to Tatiana or her parents and that, in the absence of such duty, they were free to act in careless disregard of Tatiana's life and safety.

In analyzing this issue, we bear in mind that legal duties are not discoverable facts of nature, but merely conclusory expressions that, in cases of a particular type, liability should be imposed for damage done. "The assertion that liability must...be denied because defendant bears no 'duty' to plaintiff 'begs the essential question—whether the plaintiff's interests are entitled to legal protection against the defendant's conduct.... [Duty] is not sacrosanct in itself, but only an expression of the sum total of those considerations of policy which lead the law to say that the particular plaintiff is entitled to protection.' "

In the landmark case of *Rowland v. Christian* (1968), Justice Peters recognized that liability should be imposed "for an injury occasioned to another by his want of ordinary care or skill" as expressed in section 1714 of the Civil Code. Thus, Justice Peters, quoting from *Heaven v. Pender* (1883) stated: " 'Whenever one person is by circumstances placed in such a position with regard to another...that if he did not use ordinary care and skill in his own conduct...he would cause danger of injury to the person or property of the other, a duty arises to use ordinary care and skill to avoid such danger.' "

We depart from "this fundamental principle" only upon the "balancing of a number of considerations"; major ones "are the foreseeability of harm to the plaintiff, the degree of certainty that the plaintiff suffered injury, the closeness of the connection between the defen-

dant's conduct and the injury suffered, the moral blame attached to the defendant's conduct, the policy of preventing future harm, the extent of the burden to the defendant and consequences to the community of imposing a duty to exercise care with resulting liability for breach, and the availability, cost and prevalence of insurance for the risk involved."

The most important of these considerations in establishing duty is foreseeability. As a general principle, a "defendant owes a duty of care to all persons who are foreseeably endangered by his conduct, with respect to all risks which make the conduct unreasonably dangerous." As we shall explain, however, when the avoidance of foreseeable harm requires a defendant to control the conduct of another person, or to warn of such conduct, the common law has traditionally imposed liability only if the defendant bears some special relationship to the dangerous person or to the potential victim. Since the relationship between a therapist and his patient satisfies this requirement, we need not here decide whether foreseeability alone is sufficient to create a duty to exercise reasonable care to protect a potential victim of another's conduct.

Although, as we have stated above, under the common law, as a general rule, one person owed no duty to control the conduct of another nor to warn those endangered by such conduct, the courts have carved out an exception to this rule in cases in which the defendant stands in some special relationship to either the person whose conduct needs to be controlled or in a relationship to the foreseeable victim of that conduct. Applying this exception to the present case, we note that a relationship of defendant therapists to either Tatiana or Poddar will suffice to establish a duty of care; as explained in section 315 of the Restatement Second of Torts, a duty of care may arise from either "(a) a special relation...between the actor and the third person which imposes a duty upon the actor to control the third person's conduct, or (b) a special relation...between the actor and the other which gives to the other a right of protection."

Although plaintiffs' pleadings assert no special relation between Tatiana and defendant therapists, they establish as between Poddar and defendant therapists the special relation that arises between a patient and his doctor or psychotherapist. Such a relationship may support affirmative duties for the benefit of third persons. Thus, for example, a hospital must exercise reasonable care to control the behavior of a patient which may endanger other persons. A doctor must also warn a patient if the patient's condition or medication renders certain conduct, such as driving a car, dangerous to others.

Although the California decisions that recognize this duty have involved cases in which the defendant stood in a special relationship *both* to the victim and to the person whose conduct created the danger, we do not think that the duty should logically be constricted to such situations. Decisions of other jurisdictions hold that the single relationship of a doctor to his patient is sufficient to support the duty to exercise reasonable care to protect others against dangers emanating from the patient's illness. The courts hold that a doctor is liable to persons infected by his patient if he negligently fails to diagnose a contagious disease, or having diagnosed the illness, fails to warn members of the patient's family.

Since it involved a dangerous mental patient, the decision in *Merchants Nat. Bank & Trust Co. of Fargo v. United States* (1967) comes closer to the issue. The Veterans Administration arranged for the patient to work on a local farm, but did not inform the farmer of the man's background. The farmer consequently permitted the patient to come and go freely during non-working hours; the patient borrowed a car, drove to his wife's residence and killed her. Notwithstanding the lack of any "special relationship" between the Veterans Administration and the wife, the court found the Veterans Administration liable for the wrongful death of the wife.

In their summary of the relevant rulings Fleming and Maximov conclude that the "case law should dispel any notion that to impose on the therapists a duty to take precautions for the safety of persons threatened by a patient, where due care so requires, is in any way opposed to contemporary ground rules on the duty relationship. On the contrary, there now seems to be sufficient authority to support the conclusion that by entering into a doctor-patient relationship the therapist becomes sufficiently involved to assume some responsibility for the safety, not only of the patient himself, but also of any third person whom the doctor knows to be threatened by the patient." [Fleming & Maximov, *The Patient or His Victim: The Therapist's Dilemma* (1974) 62 Cal. L. Rev. 1025, 1030.]

Defendants contend, however, that imposition of a duty to exercise reasonable care to protect third persons is unworkable because therapists cannot accurately predict whether or not a patient will resort to violence. In support of this argument amicus representing the American Psychiatric Association and other professional societies cites numerous articles which indicate that therapists, in the present state of the art, are unable reliably to predict violent acts; their forecasts, amicus claims, tend consistently to overpredict violence, and indeed are more often wrong than right. Since predictions of violence are often erroneous, amicus concludes, the courts should not render rulings that predicate the liability of therapists upon the validity of such predictions.

The role of the psychiatrist, who is indeed a practitioner of medicine, and that of the psychologist who performs an allied function, are like that of the physician who must conform to the standards of the profession and who must often make diagnoses and predictions based upon such evaluations. Thus the judgment of the therapist in diagnosing emotional disorders and in predicting whether a patient presents a serious danger of violence is comparable to the judgment which doctors and professionals must regularly render under accepted rules of responsibility.

We recognize the difficulty that a therapist encounters in attempting to forecast whether a patient presents a serious danger of violence. Obviously we do not require that the therapist, in making the determination, render a perfect performance; the therapist need only exercise "that reasonable degree of skill, knowledge, and care ordinarily possessed and exercised by members of [that professional specialty] under similar circumstances." Within the broad range of reasonable practice and treatment in which professional opinion and judgment may differ, the therapist is free to exercise his or her own best judgment without liability; proof, aided by hindsight, that he or she judged wrongly is insufficient to establish negligence.

In the instant case, however, the pleadings do not raise any question as to failure of defendant therapists to predict that Poddar presented a serious danger of violence. On the contrary, the present complaints allege that defendant therapists did in fact predict that Poddar would kill, but were negligent in failing to warn.

Amicus contends, however, that even when a therapist does in fact predict that a patient poses a serious danger of violence to others, the therapist should be absolved of any responsibility for failing to act to protect the potential victim. In our view, however, once a therapist does in fact determine, or under applicable professional standards reasonably should have determined, that a patient poses a serious danger of violence to others, he bears a duty to exercise reasonable care to protect the foreseeable victim of that danger. While the discharge of this duty of due care will necessarily vary with the facts of each case, in each instance the adequacy of the therapist's conduct must be measured against the traditional negligence standard of the rendition of reasonable care under the circumstances. As explained in Fleming and Maximov, *The Patient or His Victim: The Therapist's Dilemma* (1974), "...the ultimate question of resolving the tension between the conflicting interests of patient and potential victim is one of social policy, not professional expertise.... In sum, the therapist owes a legal duty not only to his patient, but also to his patient's would-be victim and is subject in both respects to scrutiny by judge and jury."...

The risk that unnecessary warnings may be given is a reasonable price to pay for the lives of possible victims that may be saved. We would hesitate to hold that the therapist who is aware that his patient expects to attempt to assassinate the President of the United States would not be obligated to warn the authorities because the therapist cannot predict with accuracy that his patient will commit the crime.

Defendants further argue that free and open communication is essential to psychotherapy; that "unless a patient...is assured that...information [revealed by him] can and will be held in utmost confidence, he will be reluctant to make the full disclosure upon which diagnosis and treatment...depends." The giving of a warning, defendants contend, constitutes a breach of trust which entails the revelation of confidential communications.

We recognize the public interest in supporting effective treatment of mental illness and in protecting the rights of patients to privacy and the consequent public importance of safeguarding the confidential character of psychotherapeutic communication. Against this interest, however, we must weigh the public interest in safety from violent assault. The Legislature has undertaken the difficult task of balancing the countervailing concerns. In Evidence Code section 1014, it established a broad rule of privilege to protect confidential communications between patient and psychotherapist. In Evidence Code section 1024, the Legislature created a specific and limited exception to the psychotherapist-patient privilege: "There is no privilege...if the psychotherapist has reasonable cause to believe that the patient is in such mental or emotional condition as to be dangerous to himself or to the person or property of another and that disclosure

of the communication is necessary to prevent the threatened danger."

We realize that the open and confidential character of psychotherapeutic dialogue encourages patients to express threats of violence, few of which are ever executed. Certainly a therapist should not be encouraged routinely to reveal such threats; such disclosures could seriously disrupt the patient's relationship with his therapist and with the persons threatened. To the contrary, the therapist's obligations to his patient require that he not disclose a confidence unless such disclosure is necessary to avert danger to others, and even then that he do so discreetly, and in a fashion that would preserve the privacy of his patient to the fullest extent compatible with the prevention of the threatened danger.

The revelation of a communication under the above circumstances is not a breach of trust or a violation of professional ethics; as stated in the Principles of Medical Ethics of the American Medical Association (1957), section 9: "A physician may not reveal the confidence entrusted to him in the course of medical attendance... *unless he is required to do so by law or unless it becomes necessary in order to protect the welfare of the individual or of the community.*" (Emphasis added.) We conclude that the public policy favoring protection of the confidential character of patient-psychotherapist communications must yield to the extent to which disclosure is essential to avert danger to others. The protective privilege ends where the public peril begins.

Our current crowded and computerized society compels the interdependence of its members. In this risk-infested society we can hardly tolerate the further exposure to danger that would result from a concealed knowledge of the therapist that his patient was lethal. If the exercise of reasonable care to protect the threatened victim requires the therapist to warn the endangered party or those who can reasonably be expected to notify him, we see no sufficient societal interest that would protect and justify concealment. The containment of such risks lies in the public interest. For the foregoing reasons, we find that plaintiffs' complaints can be amended to state a cause of action against defendants Moore, Powelson, Gold, and Yandell and against the Regents as their employer, for breach of a duty to exercise reasonable care to protect Tatiana....

Dissenting Opinion in *Tarasoff v. Regents of the University of California*
William P. Clark

William P. Clark, who began practicing law in 1958, served as associate justice of the Supreme Court of California from 1973 to 1981. Subsequently, he was assistant to the president of the United States for national security affairs (1982–1983) and secretary of the interior (1983–1985).

Justice Clark, dissenting from Justice Tobriner's majority opinion, argues that confidentiality in the psychiatrist-patient relationship must be assured for three reasons. (1) Without the promise of such confidentiality, people needing treatment will be deterred from seeking it. (2) Effective therapy requires the patient's full disclosure of his or her innermost thoughts. Without the assurance that the thoughts disclosed will not be revealed by the therapist, the patient could not overcome the psychological barriers standing in the way of such revelations. (3) Successful treatment itself requires a relationship of trust between psychiatrist and patient. In light of these three reasons, Clark argues that if a duty to warn is imposed on psychiatrists, the result will be an increase in violent acts by persons who either don't seek help or whose therapy is unsuccessful. Furthermore, Clark holds, imposing such a duty on psychiatrists will result in an increase in the involuntary civil commitment of patients.

Until today's majority opinion, both legal and medical authorities have agreed that confidentiality is essential to effectively treat the mentally ill, and that imposing a duty on doctors to disclose patient threats to potential victims would greatly impair treatment. Further, recognizing that effective treatment and society's safety are necessarily intertwined, the Legislature has already decided effective and confidential treatment is preferred over imposition of a duty to warn.

The issue whether effective treatment for the mentally ill should be sacrificed to a system of warnings is, in my opinion, properly one for the Legislature, and we are bound by its judgment. Moreover, even in the absence of clear legislative direction, we must reach the same conclusion because imposing the majority's new duty is certain to result in a net increase in violence....

COMMON LAW ANALYSIS

Entirely apart from the statutory provisions, the same result must be reached upon considering both general tort principles and the public policies favoring effective

California Supreme Court; July 1, 1976. 131 California Reporter 14. Reprinted with permission of West Publishing Co.

treatment, reduction of violence, and justified commitment.

Generally, a person owes no duty to control the conduct of another. Exceptions are recognized only in limited situations where (1) a special relationship exists between the defendant and injured party, or (2) a special relationship exists between defendant and the active wrongdoer, imposing a duty on defendant to control the wrongdoer's conduct. The majority does not contend the first exception is appropriate to this case.

Policy generally determines duty. Principal policy considerations include foreseeability of harm, certainty of the plaintiff's injury, proximity of the defendant's conduct to the plaintiff's injury, moral blame attributable to defendant's conduct, prevention of future harm, burden on the defendant, and consequences to the community.

Overwhelming policy considerations weigh against imposing a duty on psychotherapists to warn a potential victim against harm. While offering virtually no benefit to society, such a duty will frustrate psychiatric treatment, invade fundamental patient rights and increase violence.

The importance of psychiatric treatment and its need for confidentiality have been recognized by this court. "It is clearly recognized that the very practice of psychiatry vitally depends upon the reputation in the community that the psychiatrist will not tell." [Slovenko, *Psychiatry and a Second Look at the Medical Privilege* (1960) 6 Wayne L. Rev. 175, 188.]

Assurance of confidentiality is important for three reasons.

Deterrence from Treatment

First, without substantial assurance of confidentiality, those requiring treatment will be deterred from seeking assistance. It remains an unfortunate fact in our society that people seeking psychiatric guidance tend to become stigmatized. Apprehension of such stigma—apparently increased by the propensity of people considering treatment to see themselves in the worst possible light—creates a well-recognized reluctance to seek aid. This reluctance is alleviated by the psychiatrist's assurance of confidentiality.

Full Disclosure

Second, the guarantee of confidentiality is essential in eliciting the full disclosure necessary for effective treatment. The psychiatric patient approaches treatment with conscious and unconscious inhibitions against revealing his innermost thoughts. "Every person, however well-motivated, has to overcome resistances to therapeutic exploration. These resistances seek support from every possible source and the possibility of disclosure would easily be employed in the service of resistance." (Goldstein & Katz, *Psychiatrist-Patient Privilege: The GAP Proposal and the Connecticut Statute*, 36 Conn. Bar J., 175, 179; see also, 118 Am. J. Psych. 734, 735.) Until a patient can trust his psychiatrist not to violate their confidential relationship, "the unconscious psychological control mechanism of repression will prevent the recall of past experiences." [Butler, *Psychotherapy and Griswold: Is Confidentiality a Privilege or a Right?* (1971) 3 Conn. L. Rev. 599, 604.]

Successful Treatment

Third, even if the patient fully discloses his thoughts, assurance that the confidential relationship will not be breached is necessary to maintain his trust in his psychiatrist—the very means by which treatment is effected. "[T]he essence of much psychotherapy is the contribution of trust in the external world and ultimately in the

self, modelled upon the trusting relationship established during therapy" (Dawidoff, *The Malpractice of Psychiatrists*, 1966 Duke L. J. 696, 704). Patients will be helped only if they can form a trusting relationship with the psychiatrist. All authorities appear to agree that if the trust relationship cannot be developed because of collusive communication between the psychiatrist and others, treatment will be frustrated.

Given the importance of confidentiality to the practice of psychiatry, it becomes clear the duty to warn imposed by the majority will cripple the use and effectiveness of psychiatry. Many people, potentially violent—yet susceptible to treatment—will be deterred from seeking it; those seeking it will be inhibited from making revelations necessary to effective treatment; and, forcing the psychiatrist to violate the patient's trust will destroy the interpersonal relationship by which treatment is effected.

VIOLENCE AND CIVIL COMMITMENT

By imposing a duty to warn, the majority contributes to the danger to society of violence by the mentally ill and greatly increases the risk of civil commitment—the total deprivation of liberty—of those who should not be confined. The impairment of treatment and risk of improper commitment resulting from the new duty to warn will not be limited to a few patients but will extend to a large number of the mentally ill. Although under existing psychiatric procedures only a relatively few receiving treatment will ever present a risk of violence, the number making threats is huge, and it is the latter group—not just the former—whose treatment will be impaired and whose risk of commitment will be increased.

Both the legal and psychiatric communities recognize that the process of determining potential violence in a patient is far from exact, being fraught with complexity and uncertainty.[1]

In fact precision has not even been attained in predicting who of those having already committed violent acts will again become violent, a task recognized to be of much simpler proportions.

This predictive uncertainty means that the number of disclosures will necessarily be large. As noted above, psychiatric patients are encouraged to discuss all thoughts of violence, and they often express such thoughts. However, unlike this court, the psychiatrist does not enjoy the benefit of overwhelming hindsight in seeing which few, if any, of his patients will ultimately become violent. Now, confronted by the majority's new duty, the psychiatrist must instantaneously calculate potential violence from each patient on each visit. The difficulties researchers have encountered in accurately predicting violence will be heightened for the practicing psychiatrist dealing for brief periods in his office with heretofore nonviolent patients. And, given the decision not to warn or commit must always be made at the psychiatrist's civil peril, one can expect most doubts will be resolved in favor of the psychiatrist protecting himself.

Neither alternative open to the psychiatrist seeking to protect himself is in the public interest. The warning itself is an impairment of the psychiatrist's ability to treat, depriving many patients of adequate treatment. It is to be expected that after disclosing their threats, a significant number of patients, who would not become violent if treated according to existing practices, will engage in violent conduct as a result of unsuccessful treatment. In short, the majority's duty to warn will not only impair treatment of many who would never become violent but worse, will result in a net increase in violence.[2]

The second alternative open to the psychiatrist is to commit his patient rather than to warn. Even in the absence of threat of civil liability, the doubts of psychiatrists as to the seriousness of patient threats have led psychiatrists to overcommit to mental institutions. This overcommitment has been authoritatively documented in both legal and psychiatric studies. This practice is so prevalent that it has been estimated that "as many as twenty harmless persons are incarcerated for every one who will commit a violent act." [Steadman & Cocozza, *Stimulus/Response: We Can't Predict Who Is Dangerous* (Jan. 1975) 8 Psych. Today 32, 35.]

Given the incentive to commit created by the majority's duty, this already serious situation will be worsened....

NOTES

1 A shocking illustration of psychotherapists' inability to predict dangerousness...is cited and discussed in Ennis, *Prisoners of Psychiatry: Mental Patients, Psychiatrists, and the Law* (1972): "In a well-known study, psychiatrists predicted that 989 persons were so dangerous that they could not be kept even in civil mental hospitals, but would have to be kept in maximum security hospitals run by the Department of Correc-

tions. Then, because of a United States Supreme Court decision, those persons were transferred to civil hospitals. After a year, the Department of Mental Hygiene reported that one-fifth of them had been discharged to the community, and over half had agreed to remain as voluntary patients. During the year, only 7 of the 989 committed or threatened any act that was sufficiently dangerous to require retransfer to the maximum security hospital. Seven correct predictions out of almost a thousand is not a very impressive record.

"Other studies, and there are many, have reached the same conclusion: psychiatrists simply cannot predict dangerous behavior." (*Id.* at p. 227).

2 The majority concedes that psychotherapeutic dialogue often results in the patient expressing threats of violence that are rarely executed. The practical problem, of course, lies in ascertaining which threats from which patients will be carried out. As to this problem, the majority is silent. They do, however, caution that the therapist certainly "should not be encouraged routinely to reveal such threats; such disclosures could seriously disrupt the patient's relationships with his therapist and with the persons threatened."

Thus, in effect, the majority informs the therapists that they must accurately predict dangerousness—a task recognized as extremely difficult—or face crushing civil liability. The majority's reliance on the traditional standard of care for professionals that "therapist need only exercise 'that reasonable degree of skill, knowledge, and care ordinarily possessed and exercised by members of [that professional specialty] under similar circumstances' " is seriously misplaced. This standard of care assumes that, to a large extent, the subject matter of the specialty is ascertainable. One clearly ascertainable element in the psychiatric field is that the therapist cannot accurately predict dangerousness, which, in turn, means that the standard is inappropriate for lack of a relevant criterion by which to judge the therapist's decision. The inappropriateness of the standard the majority would have us use is made patent when consideration is given to studies, by several eminent authorities, indicating that "[t]he chances of a second psychiatrist agreeing with the diagnosis of a first psychiatrist 'are barely better than 50–50; or stated differently, there is about as much chance that a different expert would come to some different conclusion as there is that the other would agree.' " (Ennis & Litwack, *Psychiatry and the*

Presumption of Expertise: Flipping Coins in the Courtroom, 62 Cal. L. Rev. 693, 701, quoting Ziskin, Coping with Psychiatric and Psychological Testimony, 126.) The majority's attempt to apply a normative scheme to a profession which must be concerned with problems that balk at standardization is clearly erroneous.

In any event, an ascertainable standard would not serve to limit psychiatrist disclosure of threats with the resulting impairment of treatment. However compassionate, the psychiatrist hearing the threat remains faced with potential crushing civil liability for a mistaken evaluation of his patient and will be forced to resolve even the slightest doubt in favor of disclosure or commitment.

AIDS, Confidentiality, and the Right to Know
Morton E. Winston

Morton E. Winston is assistant professor and chair of the department of philosophy and religion at Trenton State College. He specializes in ethics, philosophy of science, and philosophy of mind. He is the coauthor of a related article, "AIDS and the Duty to Protect," and the coeditor of *The Philosophy of Human Rights* (forthcoming).

Winston addresses questions regarding the limits of medical confidentiality when third parties are at risk. He begins by discussing four arguments for the rule of medical confidentiality which are based respectively on (1) the individual's right to control personal information and to protect privacy; (2) and (3) the special moral relationship which exists between physicians and patients; and (4) utilitarian or broadly pragmatic considerations. Maintaining that the four arguments establish at least a prima facie obligation to maintain confidentiality, Winston proceeds to argue that two principles can be used to delimit those cases where the strict observance of confidentiality cannot be ethically justified. The first principle, which he calls the "harm principle," "requires moral agents to refrain from acts and omissions which would foreseeably result in preventable wrongful harm to innocent others." The second, which he calls the "vulnerability principle," is used to give a more precise analysis of those circumstances in which there is a strict duty to protect others. The vulnerability principle states that "the duty to protect against harm tends to arise most strongly in contexts in which someone is specially dependent on others or in some way specially vulnerable to their choices and actions." Using these principles, Winston distinguishes cases in which breaches of confidentiality in regard to AIDS carriers are justified from other cases in which they are not.

In June of 1987, a young woman who was nine months pregnant was shot with an arrow fired from a hunting bow on a Baltimore street by a man who was engaged in an argument with another person. Emergency workers from the city fire fighting unit were called to the scene, administered resuscitation to the profusely bleeding woman and took her to a local hospital where she died shortly afterwards. Her child, delivered by emergency Caesarean section, died the next day.

This tragedy would have been quickly forgotten as yet another incident of random urban violence if it had not been later learned that the woman was infected with the AIDS virus. A nurse at the hospital decided on her own initiative that the rescue workers who had brought the woman to the emergency room should be informed

Reprinted with permission from *Public Affairs Quarterly*, vol. 2 (April 1988), pp. 91–104.

that they had been exposed to HIV-infected blood and contacted them directly. Several days after this story hit the newspapers two state legislators introduced a bill adding AIDS to the list of diseases that hospitals would be required to inform workers about. A hospital spokeswoman was quoted in the newspaper as opposing the proposed legislation on the grounds that it would violate patient confidentiality, and that, "People taking care of patients should assume that everyone is a potential AIDS patient and take precautions. The burden is on you to take care of yourself."[1]

This case, and others like it, raises difficult and weighty ethical and public policy issues. What are the limits of medical confidentiality? Who, if anyone, has a right to know that they may have been exposed to AIDS or other dangerous infectious diseases? Whose responsibility is it to inform the sexual contacts of AIDS patients or others who may have been exposed to the infection? Can public health policies be framed which will effectively prevent the spread of the epidemic while also protecting the civil and human rights of its victims?

I   THE LIMITS OF CONFIDENTIALITY

The rule of medical confidentiality enjoins physicians, nurses, and health care workers from revealing to third parties information about a patient obtained in the course of medical treatment. The rule protecting a patient's secrets is firmly entrenched in medical practice, in medical education, and receives explicit mention in all major medical oaths and codes of medical ethics. Sissela Bok has argued that the ethical justification for confidentiality rests on four arguments.[2]

The first and most powerful justification for the rule of confidentiality derives from the individual's right, flowing from autonomy, to control personal information and to protect privacy. The right of individuals to control access to sensitive information about themselves is particularly important in cases where revelation of such information would subject the individual to invidious discrimination, deprivation of rights, or physical or emotional harm. Since persons who are HIV-infected or who have AIDS or ARC (AIDS-Related Complex), are often subjected to discrimination, loss of employment, refusal of housing and insurance, many physicians believe that the confidentiality of HIV antibody test results and diagnoses of AIDS should be safeguarded under all circumstances. Since many infected persons and AIDS pa-

tients are members of groups which have traditionally been subject to discrimination or social disapproval—homosexuals, drug users, or prostitutes—the protection of confidentiality of patients who belong to these groups is especially indicated.

The second and third arguments for confidentiality concern the special moral relationship which exists between physicians and their patients. Medical practice requires that patients reveal intimate personal secrets to their physicians, and that physicians live up to the trust that is required on the part of patients to reveal such information; to fail to do so would violate the physician's duty of fidelity. Additionally, since medical practice is normally conducted under a tacit promise of confidentiality, physicians would violate this expectation by revealing their patients' secrets.

The fourth argument for confidentiality is based on utilitarian or broadly pragmatic considerations. Without a guarantee of confidentiality, potential patients in need of medical care would be deterred from seeking medical assistance from fear that sensitive personal information will be revealed to third parties thereby exposing the individual to the risk of unjust discrimination or other harm. Many physicians who work with AIDS patients find such pragmatic arguments particularly compelling, believing, perhaps correctly, that breaches of medical confidentiality concerning antibody status or a diagnosis of AIDS, would have a "chilling effect" preventing people in high-risk groups from seeking voluntary antibody testing and counselling. Since programs of education designed to encourage voluntary testing and voluntary behavior change are widely believed to be the only effective and ethically acceptable means to curtail the spread of the AIDS epidemic, measures which mandate testing for members of certain groups, and which permit disclosure of test results to third parties, are viewed as inimical to the medical communities' effort to control and treat this disease.[3]

Together, these four arguments present a compelling rationale for treating confidentiality as sacrosanct, particularly in the context of AIDS, and according to Bok, help to "explain the ritualistic tone in which the duty of preserving secrets is repeatedly set forth in professional oaths and codes of ethics."[4] But, she continues,

Not only does this rationale point to links with the most fundamental grounds of autonomy and relationship and trust and help; it also serves as a rationalization that helps deflect ethical inquiry. The very self-evidence that it claims can then expand beyond its legitimate applications.

Confidentiality, like all secrecy, can then cover up for and in turn lead to a great deal of error, injury, pathology, and abuse.[5]

Bok believes that confidentiality is at best a prima facie obligation, one that while generally justified, can be overridden in certain situations by more compelling moral obligations. Among the situations which license breaches of confidentiality Bok cites are: cases involving a minor child or incompetent patient who would be harmed if sensitive information were not disclosed to a parent or guardian, cases involving threats of violence against identifiable third parties, cases involving contagious sexually transmitted diseases, and other cases where identifiable third parties would be harmed or placed at risk unknowingly by failure to disclose information known to a physician obtained through therapeutic communication.

In general, personal autonomy, and the derivative right of individuals to control personal information, is limited by the "Harm Principle" [HP], which requires moral agents to refrain from acts and omissions which would foreseeably result in preventable wrongful harm to innocent others. Bok argues that when HP (or a related ethical principle which I will discuss shortly) comes into play, "the prima facie premises supporting confidentiality are overridden,"...[6] If this argument is correct, then the strict observance of confidentiality cannot be ethically justified in all cases, and physicians and nurses who invoke the rule of confidentiality in order to justify their not disclosing information concerning threats or risks to innocent third parties may be guilty of negligence.

Before accepting this conclusion, however, it is necessary that we clarify the force of HP in the context of the ethics of AIDS, and refine the analysis of the conditions under which breaches of confidentiality pertaining to a patient's antibody status or a diagnosis of AIDS may be ethically justifiable.

II VULNERABILITY, DISEASE CONTROL, AND DISCRIMINATION

Defenders of HP typically hold that all moral agents have a general moral obligation with respect to all moral patients to (a) avoid harm, (b) prevent or protect against harm, and (c) remove harm. One problem with HP is that not all acts and omissions which result in harm to others appear to be wrong. For instance, if I buy the last pint of Haagen-Daz coffee ice cream in the store, then I have, in some sense, harmed the next customer who wants to buy this good. Similarly, if one baseball team defeats another, then they have harmed the other team. But neither of these cases represent *wrongful* harms. Why then are some harms wrongful and others not?

Robert Goodin has recently developed a theory which provides at least a partial answer to this question. According to Goodin, the duty to protect against harm tends to arise most strongly in contexts in which someone is specially dependent on others or in some way specially vulnerable to their choices and actions.[7] He dubs this the Vulnerability Principle [VP]. Vulnerability, implying risk or susceptibility to harm, should be understood in a relational sense: being vulnerable to another is a condition which involves both a relative inability of the vulnerable party to protect themselves from harm or risk, and a correlative ability of another individual to act (or refrain from actions) which would foreseeably place the vulnerable party in a position of harm or risk or remove them from such a position.

No one is completely invulnerable, and we are all to some extent dependent on the choices and actions of others. However, where there exists a rough parity of power among the parties to protect their own interests, VP does not apply. It only applies in cases where one party is *specially* vulnerable, the parties are unequal in their powers or abilities to protect their own interests, or where an inequality in knowledge or power gives one party an unfair advantage over the other.

The Vulnerability Principle is related to the Harm Principle in giving a more precise analysis of the circumstances in which a strict duty to protect others arises. For example, under HP it might be thought that individuals, qua moral agents, have a duty to insure that persons be inoculated against contagious, preventable diseases, such as polio. However, while we have no strong obligations under HP to ensure that other adults have been inoculated, we *do* have a strong general obligation under VP to see to it that all young children are inoculated, and I have a special duty as a parent to see that my own children are inoculated. Children, as a class, are especially vulnerable and lack the ability to protect themselves. Being a parent *intensifies* the duty to prevent harm to children, by focussing the duty to protect the vulnerable on individuals who are specially responsible for the care of children. For other adults, on the other hand, I have no strong duty to protect, since I may generally assume that mature moral agents have both the ability and the responsibility to protect themselves.[8]

Viewed in this light, the remarks quoted earlier by the hospital spokeswoman take on new meaning and relevance. She argued that it is the responsibility of health care workers to protect themselves by taking appropriate infection control measures in situations in which they may be exposed to blood infected with HIV. This argument might be a good one if people who occupy these professional roles are trained in such measures and are equipped to use them when appropriate. If they were so equipped, then in the Baltimore case, the nurse who later informed the rescue workers of the patient's antibody status was *not* specially responsible to prevent harm; the paramedics were responsible for their own safety.

The main problem with this argument is that it is not always possible to assume that emergency workers and others who provide direct care to AIDS patients or HIV-infected individuals are properly trained and equipped in infection control, nor, even if they are, that it is always feasible for them to employ these procedures in emergency situations. The scene of an emergency is not a controlled environment, and while emergency and public safety workers may take precautions such as wearing gloves and masks, these measures can be rendered ineffective, say, if a glove is torn and the worker cut while wrestling someone from a mass of twisted metal that was a car. While *post hoc* notification of the antibody status of people whom public safety workers have handled may not prevent them from contracting infection, it can alert them to the need to be tested, and thus can prevent them from spreading the infection (if they are in fact infected) to others, e.g., their spouses.

Health care workers, public safety workers, paramedics, and others who come into direct contact with blood which may be infected with the AIDS virus represent a class of persons for whom the Vulnerability Principle suggests a special "duty to protect" is appropriate. It is appropriate in these cases because such workers are routinely exposed to blood in the course of their professional activities, and exposure to infected blood is one way in which people can become infected with the AIDS virus. Such workers could protect themselves by simply refusing to handle anyone whom they suspected of harboring the infection. Doing this, however, would mean violating their professional responsibility to provide care. Hence, morally, they can only protect themselves by reducing their risk of exposure, in this case, by employing infection control measures and being careful. In this respect, health care workers, whether they work inside or outside of the hospital, are

in a relevantly different moral situation than ordinary people who are not routinely exposed to blood and who have no special duty to provide care, and this makes them specially vulnerable. It thus appears that the nurse who informed the emergency workers of their risk of exposure did the right thing in informing them, since in doing so she was discharging a duty to protect the vulnerable.[9]

But do similar conclusions follow with respect to "ordinary" persons who need not expose themselves to infection in the course of their professional activities? Consider the case in which a patient who is known to have a positive antibody status informs his physician that he does not intend to break off having sexual relations and that he will not tell his fiancée that he is infected with the AIDS virus.[10]

In this case, we have a known, unsuspecting party, the fiancée, who will be placed at risk by failure to discharge a duty to protect. The fiancée is vulnerable in this case to the infected patient, since it is primarily *his* actions or omissions which place her at risk. According to HP + VP, the patient has a strong special responsibility to protect those with whom he has or will have sexual relations against infection. There are a number of ways in which he can discharge this duty. For instance, he can break off the relationship, abstain from sexual intercourse, practice "safe sex," or he can inform his fiancée of his antibody status. This last option protects the fiancée by alerting her to the need to protect herself. But does the physician in this case also have a special responsibility to protect the fiancée?

She does, in this case, if she has good reason to believe that her patient will not discharge his responsibility to protect his fiancée or inform her of his positive antibody status. Since the physician possesses the information which would alert her patient's fiancée to a special need to protect herself, and the only other person who has this information will not reveal it, the fiancée is specially dependent upon the physician's choices and actions. Were she to fail to attempt to persuade her patient to reveal the information, or if he still refused to do so, to see to it that the patient's fiancée was informed, she would be acting in complicity with a patient who was violating his duty to prevent harm, and so would also be acting unethically under the Vulnerability Principle.

It thus appears that the rule of confidentiality protecting a patient's HIV antibody status cannot be regarded as absolute. There are several sorts of cases where HP + VP override the rule of confidentiality. However, finding there are justified exceptions to a generally justified rule of practice does not allow for unrestricted disclosure of antibody status to all and sundry. The basic question which must be answered in considering revealing confidential information concerning a patient's HIV antibody status is: *Is the individual to be notified someone who is specially vulnerable? That is, are they someone who faces a significant risk of exposure to the infection, and, will revealing confidential information to them assist them in reducing this risk to themselves or others?*

Answering this question is not always going to be easy, and applying HP + VP, and balancing its claims against those of confidentiality will require an extraordinary degree of moral sensitivity and discretion. Because the rule of confidentiality describes a valid prima facie moral responsibility of physicians, the burden of proof must always fall on those who would violate it in order to accommodate the claims of an opposing ethical principle. Perhaps this is why physicians tend to assume that if the rule of confidentiality is not absolute, it might as well be treated as such. Physicians, nurses, and others who are privy to information about patients' antibody status, by and large, are likely to lack the relevant degree of ethical sensitivity to discriminate the cases in which confidentiality can be justifiably violated from those where it cannot. So if we must err, the argument goes, it is better to err on the side of confidentiality.

Aside from underestimating the moral sensitivity of members of these professional groups, this argument fails to take into account that there are two ways of erring—one can err by wrongfully disclosing confidential information to those who have no right to know it, and one can err by failing to disclose confidential information to those who do have a right to know it. The harm that can result from errors of the first kind are often significant, and sometimes irreparable. But so are the harms that result from errors of the second kind. While the burden of proof should be placed on those who would breach the prima facie rule of confidentiality, it should sometimes be possible for persons to satisfy this burden and act in accordance with HP + VP without moral fault.

The strength of conviction with which many physicians in the forefront of AIDS research and treatment argue for the protection of confidentiality can be explained partly by recognizing that they view themselves as having a special responsibility to prevent harm to AIDS patients. The harm which they seek to prevent, however, is not only harm to their patients' health. It is also social harm caused by discrimination that these physicians are trying to prevent. This is yet a different application of

HP + VP in the context of AIDS which merits close attention.

As was noted earlier, the particular strength of the pragmatic argument for confidentiality in the context of AIDS, derives from the fact that, because of the public hysteria about AIDS, HIV infected persons or those with AIDS or ARC are likely to be subjected to invidious discrimination in housing, employment, access to insurance and other services, should the information that they are AIDS patients or are HIV-infected become widely known. These are clearly wrongful harms, but whose responsibility is it to prevent such harms? Generally speaking, preventing the harms which arise from injustice and disregard of civil and human rights is the proper responsibility of public officials. However, at present, only a few municipalities, San Francisco, New York City, and Washington, D.C. have enacted AIDS anti-discrimination legislation, and recently, the Reagan Administration has taken the position that it is not a Federal responsibility to do so.[11]

Because the efforts of public officials to pass and enforce effective AIDS anti-discrimination measures have been lackadaisical, many physicians feel that they have inherited the responsibility to protect their patients against the social harms caused by discrimination, and have acted on that conviction in the only way readily available to them, by insisting that the rule of confidentiality be strictly observed with respect to persons infected with HIV. Confidentiality of HIV antibody test results and diagnoses of AIDS is currently seen as the only effective barrier against unjust discrimination.

By relying exclusively on a guarantee of absolute confidentiality to protect people with AIDS from discrimination, we acknowledge the problem of harm caused by discrimination but do not effectively address it. The passage of anti-discrimination standards applying to HIV-infected persons, people with AIDS, ARC, and members of groups who are perceived as being infected, should be the first priority of all those who are concerned to prevent the spread of this disease. Such measures are justified not only on the grounds of human dignity, and human rights, but because in the context of the AIDS epidemic, they will also tend to function as effective public health measures by removing (or diminishing) one reason which deters persons at risk from seeking testing and counselling. Medical personnel and public health authorities who take the position that confidentiality is absolute in order to shield their patients from discrimination, will increasingly find themselves in the uncomfortable position of being accomplices to the irresponsible behavior of known noncompliant positives. What is needed, then, is a finely drawn public policy that includes strong and effective anti-discrimination standards, a public education program which encourages individual and professional responsibility, and a set of clear effective guidelines for public health authorities concerning when and to whom confidential information necessary for disease control and the protection of those at risk may be revealed.

III   WHO HAS A RIGHT TO KNOW?

The Vulnerability Principle suggests that breaches of confidentiality may be justified in cases where the following conditions obtain: (1) there is an identifiable person or an identifiable group of people who are "at risk" of contracting AIDS from a known carrier, (2) the carrier has not or will not disclose his/her antibody status to those persons whom he/she has placed or will place at risk, and (3) the identity of the carrier and his/her antibody status is known to a physician, nurse, health care worker, public health authority, or another person privileged to this information. It is justifiable, under these circumstances, to reveal information which might enable others to identify an AIDS patient or HIV-infected person. Revelation of confidential information is justified under this rule by the fact that others are vulnerable to infection, or may be unknowingly infecting others, and the information to be revealed may serve as an effective means of protecting those at risk.

The phrase "at risk" is most significant since not everyone who comes into contact with AIDS patients and HIV-infected persons will be placed at risk. Those persons who are most at risk are sexual partners of persons who are infected, persons who are exposed to an infected person's blood, and the fetuses of infected women.[12] Because these are the only documented means of transmitting the disease, it is relatively easy in the case of AIDS to identify those individuals who are specially vulnerable, and to distinguish them from others who are not. In particular, persons who will at most have "casual contact" with the patient are not specially vulnerable.[13] Discrimination in housing or employment is, therefore, not justifiable since AIDS cannot be transmitted by merely working in the same office or living in the same house as an HIV-infected person. On the other hand, it is known that AIDS can be transmitted by sexual contact or by blood or blood products. Fears of contagion

via these routes are not irrational, and public policies should address ways of preventing the further spread of the disease.

A policy option which has been suggested is mandatory HIV antibody testing for everyone, or for everyone in certain risk groups, or for people applying for marriage licenses, or as a preemployment screen. However, mandatory testing programs are fraught with ethical problems and, in general, are neither cost-effective nor just.[14] HIV testing should remain voluntary, but, if it is voluntary, and the onus of informing the sexual contacts of those who test positive is also voluntary, then some HIV-infected individuals will not be tested, and of those who are tested and are found to be positive, some will not inform their sexual partners.

A more justifiable policy would be to keep testing voluntary, but to urge those who test positive to disclose their antibody status to their known sexual contacts, or if they do not wish to or will not do this themselves, to ask them to supply the names of their partners so that notification of those at risk can proceed by other means. A number of states have instituted such programs of voluntary partner notification.[15] The ethical rationale supporting such measures derives a "right to know" another person's HIV antibody status from HP + VP, the fact that sexual transmission of HIV has been documented, and the assumption that notification will enable those who may have been exposed to the infection to protect themselves, and, if they are already infected, to protect others.

The main problem with reliance on voluntary personal disclosure is that there is no way to check to see whether or not the infected person has indeed complied and informed all of their contacts. Another way to carry out partner notification is to have the carrier voluntarily reveal the names of their sexual and drug contacts to physicians or nurses who will then personally notify partners. This method of contacting those at risk is preferable on two grounds: it may be emotionally easier for some people to have partner notification handled by third parties, and secondly, there is a way of checking to see that all identified sexual contacts have been notified.

The main problem with this proposal is that it places primary care providers in an uncomfortable "dual role." Instead of leaving this matter to the discretion of direct health care providers, procedures should be devised whereby physicians, nurses and other primary care personnel can avoid "dual roles" as caregivers and public health officers. One way to do this is to establish a special office in the state public health administration and to have public health authorities notify persons known to be at risk. Physicians and nurses can confidentially report cases of HIV infection to this office, and public health officials can make the determination as to whether notification of partners is warranted in accordance with the Vulnerability Principle. Patients should always be informed that this is being done, and should sign a form releasing the information needed to notify contacts. Notification taking this form would not have to indicate the source of the information, a private physician or clinic, and this might help allay fears about a "chilling effect" on a particular physician's AIDS practice. The notification of contacts should also attempt to protect the identity of the carrier. In making a partner notification, personnel in the public health office can simply state that they have reason to believe that a person may have been exposed to HIV and to urge that they report for testing and counselling.

This method will work with respect to known positives who voluntarily comply, but can anything be done about those who refuse to reveal the names of their contacts, or reveal only some of them?

Noncompliance in supplying names of sexual or IV drug partners should not be associated with sanctions such as fines or short prison terms; we cannot extort or coerce this kind of information, and such measures will tend to discourage some persons from seeking testing and counselling. The appropriate response to this kind of noncompliance should be a warning that more active means of contact tracing which involve greater risk of disclosure or invasion of privacy, such as surveillance and investigation, may be employed. In extreme cases, e.g., where known carriers continue to engage in practices likely to infect others, e.g. prostitution, stronger remedies and sanctions, e.g. civil commitment, quarantine, or arrest, may be justified.

Some may argue that such programs of partner notification and limited contract tracing are unwise on the grounds that they will tend to deter individuals from being tested in the first place. The reply is that such programs will not deter individuals who are socially responsible and are willing to take steps to protect themselves and others from HIV infection, and it will tend to increase compliance with voluntary disease control measures among identified HIV-infected members of risk groups who are reluctant to accept their social responsibilities. However, such programs have little chance of success unless they are coupled with strong federal antidiscrimination policies which are strictly enforced.[16] Such measures would function analogously to infection control measures in reducing or removing the risk of harm caused by discrimination, thereby enabling people to act more responsibly.

Even so, programs of voluntary partner notification and limited contact tracing for sexual and IV drug partners of known noncompliant positives will not prevent the infection from being transmitted. It is estimated that there are 1.5 million people in the United States currently infected with the virus and therefore capable of transmitting it. The overwhelming majority of those infected do not know that they are infected. Thus, the onus of responsibility for protecting people who are "at risk" rests primarily with those persons who engage in high risk behaviors, and only secondarily with other persons who have knowledge of infection or infectiousness such as health care providers and public health authorities. In some other cases, for instance, cases of pediatric AIDS, parents and classroom teachers will also have a "right to know" because they will be the ones responsible for the care and protection of minors. However, except in these cases, i.e., in cases where other individuals should have knowledge of HIV infection in order to protect themselves or specially vulnerable others from risk of infection, there is no generalized "right to know." Confidentiality should be protected in all other cases.[17]

NOTES

1 *The Baltimore Sun* June 11, 1987, p. D1.
2 Sissela Bok, *Secrets: On the Ethics of Concealment and Revelation* (New York: Vintage Books, 1983); Chapter IX.
3 Sheldon Landesman presents this argument compellingly: "Any legally or socially sanctioned act that breaches confidentiality or imposes additional burdens (such as job loss or cancellation of insurance) acts as a disincentive to voluntary testing. Thus if all physicians were legally required to report HIV-positive persons to a health department or to inform sexual partners at risk from the HIV-positive person, no one would come forward for testing. This is especially true if the physician is known to treat many patients with AIDS and HIV infection. The public knowledge that such a physician has violated confidentiality would result (indeed, has resulted in several cases) in a sharp decline of potentially infected persons seeking counselling and testing. Conse-

quently, a growing number of persons would remain ignorant of their infectiousness as would their sexual partners," *The Hastings Center Report*, Vol. 17 (1987), p. 25.

4 Bok, *Op. Cit.*, p. 123.

5 *Ibid.*

6 *Ibid.*, pp. 129–130. In a note at the end of this passage Bok concedes that the fourth premise involves important "line-drawing" problems which may vary among cases, a point that I will address shortly in the context of AIDS prevention and treatment.

7 Robert E. Goodin, *Protecting the Vulnerable: A Reanalysis of Our Social Responsibilities* (Chicago: The University of Chicago Press, 1985).

8 It follows on this view that I also have a responsibility to protect myself, or my future selves, from such preventable harms. Cf. M. E. Winston, "Responsibility to Oneself," unpublished paper presented at the American Philosophical Association, Pacific Division Meetings, March 27, 1987.

9 In fact, the fire fighters who provided emergency care to the wounded Baltimore woman were not wearing gloves. In this particular case a further reason for condoning the nurse's action might be found in the fact that the patient died. Is it possible to violate confidentiality when the person whose secret is revealed is dead? The pragmatic justifications for the rule of confidentiality would still apply in such cases, but it is a moot question as to whether the deceased individuals themselves can be harmed or wronged by revealing confidential information. See Joan Callahan, "Harming the Dead," *Ethics*, Vol. 97 (1987), pp. 341–352.

10 Cf. "AIDS and a Duty to Protect," *The Hastings Center Report*, Vol. 17 (1987), pp. 22–23.

11 *The New York Times*, September 21, 1987, p. A1.

12 The Center for Disease Control lists persons belonging to certain groups or who engage in certain types of behavior as having "high risk" of contracting HIV, and these include: homosexual/bisexual males, IV drug users, persons born in countries where heterosexual transmission is prevalent (e.g., Haiti and Central African countries), hemophiliacs, male and female prostitutes, sexual partners of members of high-risk groups, infants born to women in high-risk groups, and persons receiving blood transfusions before 1985 when screening for HIV began. [CDC. Additional Recommendations to Reduce Sexual and Drug Abuse-Related Transmission of Human T-

Lymphotropic Virus Type III/Lymphadenopathy-Associated Virus. MMWR 1986 March 14; 152–155.] It is important to note that not everyone belonging to these groups is "at risk." Certain behaviors in certain contexts place individuals at risk, and other behaviors can reduce or remove these risks.

13 In an epidemiological study by Friedland, et al. of the family members of 39 AIDS patients it was found that there were no instances of horizontal transmission of HIV to family members living in the same household. [Friedland, G. H., Saltzman, B. R., Rogers, M. S., Kahl, P. A., Lesser, M. L., Mayers, M. M., and Klein, R. S., "Lack of transmission of HTLV-III/LAV infection to household contacts of patients with AIDS or AIDS-related complex with oral candidiasis," *New England Journal of Medicine*. Vol. 314 (1986), pp. 344–349.] Additionally, there is no known risk of transmission of HIV in settings such as offices, schools, factories, or by personal services workers, such as beauticians and barbers or food service workers. [CDC. Recommendations for preventing transmission of infection with T-lymphotropic virus type III/lymphadenopathy-associated virus in the workplace. MMWR 1985, vol. 34, no. 45, pp. 682–695.]

14 See Kenneth R. Howe, "Why Mandatory Screening for AIDS Is a Very Bad Idea." In Christine Pierce and Donald VanDeVeer (Eds.), *AIDS: Ethics and Public Policy*, (Belmont: Wadsworth Publishing Co., 1988), pp. 140–149.

15 In Maryland, the Governor's Task Force on AIDS has recently recommended that, "Health care providers should strongly encourage HIV-infected patients to speak directly to and refer their own sexual and needle-sharing contacts for counselling and medical evaluation. There are instances, however, when these professionals may be *obligated* to notify persons *known* to have had significant exposures to HIV infection. In such cases, the duty to notify is a matter of good medical practice and supersedes the need to maintain confidentiality." *AIDS and Maryland: Policy Guidelines and Recommendations*, Report of the Governor's Task Force on Acquired Immune Deficiency Syndrome. December 1986.

16 Cf. Larry Gostin, "Time for Federal Laws on AIDS Discrimination," Letter to the Editor, *The New York Times*, October 1, 1987.

17 I am indebted to David Newell and to an anonymous reviewer for helpful comments on this paper.

Confidentiality in Medicine—A Decrepit Concept
Mark Siegler

Mark Siegler is professor of medicine and director of the Center For Clinical Medical Ethics at the University of Chicago. His numerous published articles in biomedical ethics include "A Physician's Perspective on a Right to Health Care" and "Therapeutic Research Protocol: Should Patients Pay?"

Siegler argues that hospital medicine, the rise of health-care teams, the existence of third-party insurance programs, and the expanding limits of medicine will necessarily have to modify our traditional understanding of medical confidentiality. He identifies two functions of confidentiality in medicine: (1) respect for the patient's sense of individuality and privacy and (2) the improvement of the patient's health care, which requires a bond of trust between the health professional and the patient. Siegler then proposes possible solutions to the problems raised by the developments in medical care cited above. He concludes by criticizing those violations of a patient's right of privacy that are due to careless indiscretion on the part of professionals.

Medical confidentiality, as it has traditionally been understood by patients and doctors, no longer exists. This ancient medical principle, which has been included in every physician's oath and code of ethics since Hippocratic times, has become old, worn-out, and useless; it is a decrepit concept. Efforts to preserve it appear doomed to failure and often give rise to more problems than solutions. Psychiatrists have tacitly acknowledged the impossibility of ensuring the confidentiality of medical records by choosing to establish a separate, more secret record. The following case illustrates how the confidentiality principle is compromised systematically in the course of routine medical care.

A patient of mine with mild chronic obstructive pulmonary disease was transferred from the surgical intensive-care unit to a surgical nursing floor two days after an elective cholecystectomy. On the day of transfer, the patient saw a respiratory therapist writing in his medical chart (the therapist was recording the results of an arterial blood gas analysis) and became concerned about the confidentiality of his hospital records. The patient threatened to leave the hospital prematurely unless I could guarantee that the confidentiality of his hospital record would be respected.

This patient's complaint prompted me to enumerate the number of persons who had both access to his hos-

pital record and a reason to examine it. I was amazed to learn that at least 25 and possibly as many as 100 health professionals and administrative personnel at our university hospital had access to the patient's record and that all of them had a legitimate need, indeed a professional responsibility, to open and use that chart. These persons included 6 attending physicians (the primary physician, the surgeon, the pulmonary consultant, and others); 12 house officers (medical, surgical, intensive-care unit, and "covering" house staff); 20 nursing personnel (on three shifts); 6 respiratory therapists; 3 nutritionists; 2 clinical pharmacists; 15 students (from medicine, nursing, respiratory therapy, and clinical pharmacy); 4 unit secretaries; 4 hospital financial officers; and 4 chart reviewers (utilization review, quality assurance review, tissue review, and insurance auditor). It is of interest that this patient's problem was straightforward, and he therefore did not require many other technical and support services that the modern hospital provides. For example, he did not need multiple consultants and fellows, such specialized procedures as dialysis, or social workers, chaplains, physical therapists, occupational therapists, and the like.

Upon completing my survey I reported to the patient that I estimated that at least 75 health professionals and hospital personnel had access to his medical record. I suggested to the patient that these people were all involved in providing or supporting his health-care services. They were, I assured him, working for him. De-

Reprinted by permission of the *New England Journal of Medicine*, vol. 307, pp. 1518–1521; 1982.

spite my reassurances the patient was obviously distressed and retorted, "I always believed that medical confidentiality was a part of a doctor's code of ethics. Perhaps you should tell me just what you people mean by 'confidentiality'!"

TWO ASPECTS OF MEDICAL CONFIDENTIALITY

Confidentiality and Third-Party Interests

Previous discussions of medical confidentiality usually have focused on the tension between a physician's responsibility to keep information divulged by patients secret and a physician's legal and moral duty, on occasion, to reveal such confidences to third parties, such as families, employers, public-health authorities, or police authorities. In all these instances, the central question relates to the stringency of the physician's obligation to maintain patient confidentiality when the health, well-being, and safety of identifiable others or of society in general would be threatened by a failure to reveal information about the patient. The tension in such cases is between the good of the patient and the good of others.

Confidentiality and the Patient's Interest

As the example above illustrates, further challenges to confidentiality arise because the patient's personal interest in maintaining confidentiality comes into conflict with his personal interest in receiving the best possible health care. Modern high-technology health care is available principally in hospitals (often, teaching hospitals), requires many trained and specialized workers (a "health-care team"), and is very costly. The existence of such teams means that information that previously had been held in confidence by an individual physician will now necessarily be disseminated to many members of the team. Furthermore, since health-care teams are expensive and few patients can afford to pay such costs directly, it becomes essential to grant access to the patient's medical record to persons who are responsible for obtaining third-party payment. These persons include chart reviewers, financial officers, insurance auditors, and quality-of-care assessors. Finally, as medicine expands from a narrow, disease-based model to a model that encompasses psychological, social, and economic problems, not only will the size of the health-care team and medical costs increase, but more sensitive informa-

tion (such as one's personal habits and financial condition) will now be included in the medical record and will no longer be confidential.

The point I wish to establish is that hospital medicine, the rise of health-care teams, the existence of third-party insurance programs, and the expanding limits of medicine all appear to be responses to the wishes of people for better and more comprehensive medical care. But each of these developments necessarily modifies our traditional understanding of medical confidentiality.

THE ROLE OF CONFIDENTIALITY IN MEDICINE

Confidentiality serves a dual purpose in medicine. In the first place, it acknowledges respect for the patient's sense of individuality and privacy. The patient's most personal physical and psychological secrets are kept confidential in order to decrease a sense of shame and vulnerability. Secondly, confidentiality is important in improving the patient's health care—a basic goal of medicine. The promise of confidentiality permits people to trust (i.e., have confidence) that information revealed to a physician in the course of a medical encounter will not be disseminated further. In this way patients are encouraged to communicate honestly and forthrightly with their doctors. This bond of trust between patient and doctor is vitally important both in the diagnostic process (which relies on an accurate history) and subsequently in the treatment phase, which often depends as much on the patient's trust in the physician as it does on medications and surgery. These two important functions of confidentiality are as important now as they were in the past. They will not be supplanted entirely either by improvements in medical technology or by recent changes in relations between some patients and doctors toward a rights-based, consumerist model.

POSSIBLE SOLUTIONS TO THE CONFIDENTIALITY PROBLEM

First of all, in all nonbureaucratic, noninstitutional medical encounters—that is, in the millions of doctor-patient encounters that take place in physicians' offices, where more privacy can be preserved—meticulous care should be taken to guarantee that patients' medical and personal information will be kept confidential.

Secondly, in such settings as hospitals or large-scale group practices, where many persons have opportunities to examine the medical record, we should aim to provide access only to those who have "a need to know." This could be accomplished through such administrative changes as dividing the entire record into several sections—for example, a medical and financial section—and permitting only health professionals access to the medical information.

The approach favored by many psychiatrists—that of keeping a psychiatric record separate from the general medical record—is an understandable strategy but one that is not entirely satisfactory and that should not be generalized. The keeping of separate psychiatric records implies that psychiatry and medicine are different undertakings and thus drives deeper the wedge between them and between physical and psychological illness. Furthermore, it is often vitally important for internists or surgeons to know that a patient is being seen by a psychiatrist or is taking a particular medication. When separate records are kept, this information may not be available. Finally, if generalized, the practice of keeping a separate psychiatric record could lead to the unacceptable consequence of having a separate record for each type of medical problem.

Patients should be informed about what is meant by "medical confidentiality." We should establish the distinction between information about the patient that generally will be kept confidential regardless of the interest of third parties and information that will be exchanged among members of the health-care team in order to provide care for the patient. Patients should be made aware of the large number of persons in the modern hospital who require access to the medical record in order to serve the patient's medical and financial interests.

Finally, at some point most patients should have an opportunity to review their medical record and to make informed choices about whether their entire record is to be available to everyone or whether certain portions of the record are privileged and should be accessible only to their principal physician or to others designated explicitly by the patient. This approach would rely on traditional informed-consent procedural standards and might permit the patient to balance the personal value of medical confidentiality against the personal value of high-technology, team health care. There is no reason that the same procedure should not be used with psychiatric records instead of the arbitrary system now employed, in which everything related to psychiatry is kept secret.

AFTERTHOUGHT: CONFIDENTIALITY AND INDISCRETION

There is one additional aspect of confidentiality that is rarely included in discussions of the subject. I am referring here to the wanton, often inadvertent, but avoidable exchanges of confidential information that occur frequently in hospital rooms, elevators, cafeterias, doctors' offices, and at cocktail parties. Of course, as more people have access to medical information about the patient the potential for this irresponsible abuse of confidentiality increases geometrically.

Such mundane breaches of confidentiality are probably of greater concern to most patients than the broader issue of whether their medical records may be entered into a computerized data bank or whether a respiratory therapist is reviewing the results of an arterial blood gas determination. Somehow, privacy is violated and a sense of shame is heightened when intimate secrets are revealed to people one knows or is close to—friends, neighbors, acquaintances, or hospital roommates—rather than when they are disclosed to an anonymous bureaucrat sitting at a computer terminal in a distant city or to a health professional who is acting in an official capacity.

I suspect that the principles of medical confidentiality, particularly those reflected in most medical codes of ethics, were designed principally to prevent just this sort of embarrassing personal indiscretion rather than to maintain (for social, political, or economic reasons) the absolute secrecy of doctor-patient communications. In this regard, it is worth noting that Percival's Code of Medical Ethics (1803) includes the following admonition: "Patients should be interrogated concerning their complaint in a tone of voice which cannot be overheard."[1] We in the medical profession frequently neglect these simple courtesies.

CONCLUSION

The principle of medical confidentiality described in medical codes of ethics and still believed in by patients no longer exists. In this respect, it is a decrepit concept. Rather than perpetuate the myth of confidentiality and invest energy vainly to preserve it, the public and the profession would be better served if they devoted their attention to determining which aspects of the original principle of confidentiality are worth retaining. Efforts could then be directed to salvaging those.[2]

NOTES

1 Leake, C. D., ed., *Percival's medical ethics*. Baltimore, Williams & Wilkins, 1927.

2 Supported by a grant (OSS-8018097) from the Na-

tional Science Foundation and by the National Endowment for the Humanities. The views expressed are those of the author and do not necessarily reflect those of the National Science Foundation or the National Endowment for the Humanities.

Hospital Ethics Committees

Ethics Committees: Decisions by Bureaucracy
Mark Siegler

A biographical sketch of Mark Siegler is found on page 181.

Siegler sees decision making by institutional ethics committees as a threat to the traditional doctor-patient relationship and as an unjustified interference with physicians' autonomous medical decision making. He argues that the main role of ethics committees should be educational, including the development of formal programs that will train physicians, nurses, and staff from all clinical disciplines in sound ethical decision making. Once institutional ethics committees have discharged their educational chores, he argues, they should be disbanded and replaced by a number of small advisory groups. Such advisory groups would be composed of individuals having the necessary specialized clinical expertise related to specific clinical units recognized as "high-risk ethical areas" and not the kinds of individuals who usually constitute the more general institutional committees (e.g., nonmedical and noninvolved professional and moral "experts" such as ethicists, lawyers, and clergy).

The rise of institutional ethics committees (IECs) is, unfortunately, a sign of the times. Their development symbolizes the dreary, depressed, and disorganized state to which American medicine has fallen. Not only have physicians lost political and economic power; they have even lost the autonomy to reach medical decisions. Good physicians have always incorporated technical judgments, ethical reflections, and patient wishes in reaching difficult decisions. However, the increased frequency of ethical problems has encouraged some physicians and ethicists to suggest that these decisions may be too complex for practitioners and are best made by committees.

CONCERNS ABOUT IECs

IECs threaten to undermine the traditional doctor-patient relationship and to impose new and untested ad-

Reprinted with permission of the author and the publisher from *Hastings Center Report*, vol. 16 (June 1986), pp. 22–24.

ministrative and regulatory burdens on patients, families, and physicians. Their existence may shift the focus of decision-making from the office or bedside to the conference room or executive suite.

Such committees may expand the number of participants in the decision from those directly involved in the case to an unmanageable collection of noninvolved professional and moral "experts," including other physicians, nurses, lawyers, hospital administrators, ethicists, clergy, community representatives, and patient advocates. These committees also may have serious conflicts of interest between their responsibility to the individual patient and their efforts to minimize hospital risk, to develop sound hospital policies, and perhaps even to allocate economic resources most efficiently.

Most troubling of all, they may remove or at least attenuate the decision-making authority of the physician who is responsible—medically, morally, and legally—for the patient's care. Some physicians may abdicate their medical responsibility by delegating difficult clinical-ethical decisions, an intrinsic part of medical practice, to such committees. In contrast to individual physicians, committees lack specific medical knowledge, have not been trained in the ethic of caring, have little responsibility or accountability for decisions, and have not been sanctioned by the patient to make such decisions. Thus, to delegate decision making to the IEC may be unethical for physicians and hospitals. Christine Cassel has put the point nicely:

> The coming together of many different perspectives and areas of expertise may provide the "crucible" in which the best (i.e., most humane and most just) decisions are made. But a committee can also provide the setting in which immoral decisions can be made for which no one has ultimate responsibility. This is most likely to occur in a setting where most persons on the committee are relatively removed from the clinical setting, where conflict of interest with administrative needs exists, and where the group dynamic is bureaucratized. Such a committee is no longer a crucible for the tempering of apparently conflicting values, but rather a bureau whose primary value is not the anguish of moral dilemma but the efficiency of decision making, abiding by rules and adhering to regulations and legal proscriptions.[1]

To justify the existence of IECs, their proponents have suggested many possible roles for them, including: (1) developing educational programs on bioethical matters; (2) providing an interdisciplinary forum for discussions about bioethical issues; (3) advising persons who seek counsel from the committee; and (4) assessing and evaluating hospital policies that relate to bioethical matters.[2] In addition, many supporters of IECs state categorically that such committees should not make patient care decisions.[3] Despite the rhetoric that forswears the use of IECs as decision-making bodies, I fear that these committees will, directly or indirectly, become increasingly involved in patient care decisions and will thus usurp the role and responsibility of those who should be making such decisions.

CAN DECISION MAKING BE AVOIDED?

My concerns may seem unjustified or at least excessive in view of these guidelines and other statements. In a recent article Norman Fost and Ronald E. Cranford note:

> The most controversial role of an ethics committee is as a consulting group for urgent decisions about withholding, withdrawing, or continuing life-sustaining medical care....

While some might advocate investing decision-making authority in such committees, there has been little experience with such a role. The majority of existing ethics committees surveyed by the President's Commission [in 1982] did not view themselves as primary decision makers. This has also been our experience as we have worked with at least 20 hospital ethics committees around the country. The majority have emphasized their consultative, advisory, informational, and consensus-development roles rather than primary decision making.[4]

Nevertheless, they conclude:

Hospital ethics committees are increasingly becoming a part of decision making involving life support in critically ill patients.

Fost and Cranford wish to draw a fine distinction between "...investing decision-making authority in such committees...." and having such committees "...increasingly [become] a part of decision making involving life support in critically ill patients." This is a distinction without a substantial difference. Further, Fost and Cranford may be technically correct when they note that "...the majority of existing ethics committees surveyed by the President's Commission did not view themselves as primary decision makers," although, in fact, 31 percent of committees surveyed said that one of their "actual" functions was to "make final decisions about life support." In addition, those hospital committees surveyed noted that other "actual" functions included: 1. "to provide counsel and support to physicians" (69 percent); 2. "to make ethical/social policy for care of critically ill" (38 percent); 3. "to review ethical issues in patient care decisions" (56 percent); and 4. "to determine medical prognosis" (25 percent).

Clearly, there are many ways in which ethics committees can become "involved" implicitly or explicitly in clinical decisions and can influence patient-physician decisions, even if *only* 31 percent of the committees surveyed reported that they actually made final decisions about life support. Thus, hospital ethics committees can constrain and modify physician-patient decisions in at least the following ways:

1. By developing rules, regulations, and institutional policies that limit the prudential clinical-ethical discretion that normally could be exercised by the responsible physician;

2. By reviewing physician decisions retrospectively (presumably for the purpose of approving or disapproving the decision);

3. By consulting on cases and by having the opinion of the committees carry the authority of the institution;

4. By serving occasionally as a quasi-judicial body that actually makes decisions and thus wrests the authority from the physician;

5. By influencing physicians to make the "right" decision through moral suasion and group power. Fost has cited one example of a disagreement between an attending pediatrician and a neonatologist that was brought to the attention of a hospital ethics committee. Although the committee did not vote or issue a formal recommendation, its discussion "...appeared to show a slim majority favoring continuing treatment." Fost writes: "The committee chairman said to the attending, 'Of course, the committee has no power to make decisions; the choice is still up to you.' To which the attending replied, 'Poppycock!' Understandably, he felt enormous social pressure to continue treatment and knew that he would be going upstream against colleagues if he chose otherwise...."[5]

AN ALTERNATIVE TO COMMITTEES

Ethics committees should divorce themselves absolutely from involvement in patient decision making and from ethics consultations and should not even review and criticize decisions that have been made previously. Other appropriately constituted hospital and medical committees (including the quality assurance committee, the morbidity and mortality committee, and the medical-legal affairs committee) should continue to monitor and correct deficiencies in patient care, including those associated with clinical-ethical decisions.

The principal role of ethics committees should be a broadly conceived program of education. Ethics committees should develop and coordinate institutional resources in clinical ethics and should also develop formal training programs for physicians, nurses, and staff from all clinical disciplines in order to train them in the knowledge and behavioral skills required to make sound decisions in their own area of expertise. The ultimate goal of institutional ethics committees should be to put themselves out of business after having completed this ambitious training program and provided for the training of new personnel.

I would be greatly reassured if I thought that institutional ethics committees were a short-term, stop-gap measure designed to train a sufficient number of clinicians to assume the task of making sound clinical-ethical decisions. This is not the way most bureaucracies function, and I suspect that we are more likely to see a progressive bureaucratization of institutional ethics committees with all that this entails, including newsletters, new journals, and national organizations.

In place of ethics committees, I encourage the formation of many small advisory groups possessing great clinical expertise in their own particular specialty and composed primarily of involved clinicians but with occasional representation of other experts. These advisory groups would be organized in those clinical units that were regarded as "high-risk ethical areas." Thus, a large hospital might have separate advisory groups in, for example, its burn unit, medical oncology service, neurosurgical ICU, respiratory ICU, neonatal ICU, AIDS clinic, emergency room, and in the transplantation surgery unit. For medical centers that perform several types of transplantation there might be a separate advisory group for each team.

Each of these clinical disciplines is extremely complex and presents very different types of clinical-ethical dilemmas. Only a very few trained clinicians (physicians or nurses) would be so presumptuous as to think that their particular clinical training had prepared them to take care of the entire range of medical problems from medical oncology to neonatal intensive care and liver transplantation. A superb operating room nurse would probably be uncomfortable and ill-prepared if he were assigned to a neurology unit. Furthermore, if the operating nurse specialized in open heart surgery procedures, he might not be entirely competent as the scrub on a neurosurgery case.

Clinicians realize that even though cellular biochemistry and organ physiology are similar in all patients, profound differences remain between the basic sciences of medicine and the clinical application of these sciences to the care of individual patients. Similarly, ethical principles such as beneficence, truth telling, and autonomy that are taken as basic by various philosophic and religious groups often must be applied with great subtlety and discretion, based on clinical experience, in particular clinical situations.

IECs, on the other hand, often think they are capable of analyzing, adjudicating, and resolving the most delicate and complex clinical matters. I think they are wrong. The goal of such committees should be to develop clinicians from each of the clinical disciplines who have both the cognitive knowledge in ethics and law and the clinical experience to assist their colleagues in reaching sound clinical-ethical decisions.

REFERENCES

1 Christine Cassel, "Deciding to Forego Life-Sustaining Treatment: Implications for Policy in 1984," *Cardozo Law Review*, May 1985, pp. 287–302.

2 See, for example, American Hospital Association, "Hospital Committees on Biomedical Ethics," Chicago, 1984. Also, President's Commission, *Deciding to Forego Life-Sustaining Treatment*, March 1983, Washington, D.C., pp. 439–57.

3 See, in addition to the AHS guidelines, the American Medical Association's "Guidelines for Ethics Committees in Health Care Institutions," *Journal of the American Medical Association* 253 (1985), 2698–99.

4 Norman Fost and Ronald E. Cranford, "Hospital Ethics Committees: Administrative Aspects," *Journal of the American Medical Association* 253 (1985), 2687–92.

5 Norman Fost, "What Can a Hospital Ethics Committee Do for You?" *Contemporary Pediatrics*, February 1986, p. 125.

Behind Closed Doors: Promises and Pitfalls of Ethics Committees
Bernard Lo

Bernard Lo, M.D., teaches in the division of general internal medicine at the University of California Medical Center, San Francisco. He is the author of "The Clinical Use of Advanced Directives" and the coauthor of "Do Not Resuscitate Decisions: A Prospective Study at Three Teaching Hospitals."

Unlike Siegler, Lo supports the continued existence of hospital ethics committees. However, he raises important questions about their ethicality, their effectiveness, and even the desirability of agreement by committee. Lo stresses the need for committees to define their goals more clearly and to establish procedures—especially regarding who will have access to committee proceedings—that will adequately protect the interests of patients. In discussing the questionable nature of agreement by committee, Lo stresses the dangers of "groupthink," especially the fact that it may result in an inadequate consideration of patients' preferences. Lo concludes by recommending that ethics committees, like all other medical innovations, be subject to evaluation before consulting ethics committees is accepted as a standard decision-making procedure. He also suggests several criteria that could be used to evaluate both the process by which committees review cases and the results of their deliberations.

Hospital ethics committees have been hailed as providing a promising way to resolve ethical dilemmas in patient care. Although ethics committees may have various tasks, such as confirming prognoses, educating care givers, or developing hospital policies, their most innovative role is making recommendations in individual cases.[1–5] This role has been supported by the President's Commission for the Study of Ethical Problems in Medicine and Biomedical and Behavioral Research, the American Medical Association, and the American Hospital Association. Strictly speaking, such recommendations are not binding, but they undoubtedly carry great weight, especially if they are cogently justified.[6] It is predicted that most ethics committees will make recommendations in particular cases[3] and that the courts will respect them.[3]

Ethics committees may offer an attractive alternative to the courts.[3–5] The judicial system may be too slow for clinical decisions.[7,8] Moreover, the adversarial judicial process may polarize physicians, patients, and

Reprinted with permission from the *New England Journal of Medicine*, vol. 317 (1987), pp. 46–50. Copyright © Massachusetts Medical Society.

families,[9] whereas ethics committees may reconcile divergent views. The 1986 New York State Task Force on Life and the Law encouraged resolving patient care dilemmas at the hospital level, rather than turning to the courts, and suggested that ethics committees might mediate such disagreements.[10]

Although I support ethics committees, several questions trouble me. First, are these committees ethical? The goals and procedures of some committees may conflict with established ethical principles. Second, is agreement by committees always desirable? Group dynamics may lead to flawed information, reasoning, or recommendations. Third, are these committees effective? Like other medical innovations, they need to be rigorously evaluated.

GOALS AND PROCEDURES OF ETHICS COMMITTEES

The very name suggests that ethics committees base their recommendations on ethical principles and rational deliberation, rather than on mere custom, political power, or self-interest. A consensus on medical decision making has emerged in the medical literature, court decisions, and reports of the President's Commission.[1,7,8,11,12] According to this consensus, competent patients should give informed consent or refusal to the recommendations of physicians. Care givers need not accede to patient requests for treatments, however, if there are no medical indications. In cases in which patients are incompetent, decisions should be based on their previously expressed preferences or, if such preferences are unclear or unknown, on their best interests. The goals of some ethics committees, however, may conflict with these ethical guidelines. Goals vary substantially among committees.[1–3,13–15] Some do not have explicit goals. One committee has said, "We have never formally stated in writing the exact purpose or purposes of our committee but have decided to proceed in an informal manner.... We felt that to formalize our objectives might be counterproductive to the work of our committee."[14] But as ethics committees mature, and especially as they wish to serve as alternatives to the courts, they need to define their goals more clearly. Some so-called ethics committees have as goals confirming prognoses, providing emotional support for care givers, or reducing legal liability for physicians or hospitals.[1–3,13–15] One hospital administrator has even suggested that the ethics committee be used as a public relations "tool" for justifying unpopular decisions to discontinue unprofitable services.[16] Although committees

on quality assurance, staff support, risk management, or public relations are important, there is little reason for patients, their surrogates, or the public to accept their recommendations about patient care.

After clarifying goals, committees can establish procedures. Ethics committees must decide who can refer cases or attend meetings. Many committees limit participation by patients and families. According to a 1982 survey, only 25 percent of ethics committees that reviewed cases allowed patients to bring cases to the committee. Only 19 percent of committees allowed patients to attend meetings, whereas 44 percent allowed family members to do so.[17] Limiting access to committee proceedings may seem desirable. It may be sound political strategy to overcome initial resistance to the ethics committee within the hospital. For example, attending physicians may fear that their authority will be undermined if patients, families, or nurses can ask the committee to review cases. Restricting access may also facilitate frank discussions by care givers and committee members about sensitive topics. In addition, discussions with other health professionals may help physicians to clarify their thinking before they talk to patients or families.

Restricted discussions, however, may not be accepted by patients, families, and society. Patients or surrogates who disagree with physicians are unlikely to regard the committee as impartial if they may not convene the committee or present their views directly, whereas physicians may do so. Disagreements that reach ethics committees usually involve important personal issues—even questions of life and death. In such vital decisions, patients and their proxies are not likely to accept recommendations by a committee whose members they have not met or that seems to meet behind closed doors.

The composition of ethics committees may not reassure patients that their wishes and interests are represented. Typically, most members of ethics committees are physicians, who may assess the importance of medical problems or the risks and benefits of treatment differently from patients.[18,19] Patients or surrogates who disagree with the committee's recommendations may say that the composition of the committee was biased against them.

Some committees meet with patients or family members who take the initiative and request meetings. But people who need the most help in expressing their preferences or interests may be the least likely to request a meeting. They may be cognitively impaired or unable to navigate the medical system, or there may be cultural, language, or educational barriers. Hence, it is desirable for the committee to take steps to inform patients, as well as care givers, of its work. Such information is particularly important if the committee can review a case without the consent of the parties. Mandatory review has been recommended, for example, when withholding life-sustaining treatment from neonates or from incompetent adults without surrogates is being considered.[20] A pamphlet about the committee might be distributed when patients are admitted. Patients or surrogates who are concerned that committee discussions or recommendations may invade their privacy can then express those concerns in advance. Before the committee discusses a case, it should inform patients or surrogates and invite them to participate in the deliberations.

Most ethics committees also restrict the access of nurses. The 1982 survey found that only 31 percent of committees allowed nurses to present cases, and only 50 percent allowed nurses to attend meetings.[17] But it may be advisable to increase the access of nurses. Nurses have close contact with patients and families and may take the role of patient advocates.[21] They may raise previously overlooked issues, contribute new information, or express the questions and viewpoints of patients and families. Disagreements by nurses with physicians' orders often indicate a need to reconsider decisions.[22]

Because ethics committees are touted as an alternative to the courts, it may be useful to compare their safeguards with those in legal procedures.[23] The legal system notifies parties of the proceedings, allows them to give evidence, and ensures representation for patients. If the patient is incompetent, the court may appoint a guardian ad litem to represent the interests of the patient or to argue for continuing treatment. Moreover, parties are notified of the decision and the reasons for it, so that the decision can be reviewed or appealed. Ethics committees that make recommendations may not need safeguards that are as elaborate as those in a legal system that makes binding decisions. But for ethics committees to be accepted as a quicker and less acrimonious alternative to the courts, they must be perceived to be as fair as the courts.

In order for ethics committees to assist in decision making, their recommendations and the reasons for them must be known by all parties. In addition to communicating with the patient or surrogate and the attending physician, a representative of the committee might write a note in the medical record, so that nurses, consultants, and physicians understand the committee's recommendation and reasoning. Ethics committees, however, may seem reluctant to allow their recommendations to be reviewed. Some committees do not note their recommendations and reasoning in the medical record. In addition, articles about ethics committees discuss how to reduce the liability of individual committee members by keeping records from being "discoverable"—that is, from being subpoenaed in civil suits.[20,24] Such apparent secrecy may evoke the suspicion that the committee is more concerned with protecting physicians, the hospital, or itself than with helping patients.

PITFALLS OF COMMITTEE DISCUSSIONS

Pressures on ethics committees to reach agreement may lead to recommendations that are ethically questionable. Agreement or even consensus does not confer infallibility. For example, in the 1960s, hospital committees selected patients with chronic renal failure for treatment with life-prolonging dialysis machines, which were limited in number. When it was disclosed that criteria of social worth were implicitly applied, these committee decisions were criticized as being unfair and discriminatory.[25]

In some circumstances, committees may impair rather than improve decision making. Political scientists and psychologists have shown that committees may inadvertently pressure members to reach consensus, avoid controversial issues, underestimate risks and objections, or fail to consider alternatives or to search for additional information.[26,27] In other words, committees may not serve their intended function of considering diverse viewpoints and arguments. Such undesirable qualities of committee discussions, which have been called "groupthink," may lead to grave errors in judgment.

Ethics committees may fall victim to groupthink. First, these committees may reach consensus too easily, by not adequately considering patients' preferences. Despite the ideal of informed consent, patients are often not involved in decisions about their care.[28–30] Second, committees may accept secondhand information uncritically. Physicians appreciate that medical consultants should take new histories, examine patients, and review x-ray films and scans.[31,32] Similarly, an ethics committee should scrutinize information about the medical situation and the patient's preferences. Conclusions and inferences, rather than primary data, may be presented. For instance, patients may be described as "terminal" or "hopelessly ill," or it may be reported that an incompetent patient would not want "heroic care." Since such phrases are ambiguous and potentially misleading, committees should require and, if necessary, seek out more specific information. Third, ethics committees may overlook imaginative means of resolving disagreements. Disputes over patient care are not always caused by conflicts of ethical principles or obligations. They may also result from misunderstandings, stress, or lack of attention to the details of care.[22] Despite stalemates over conflicting ethical principles or duties, agreements on particular recommendations for patient care may be possible.[33]

Ethics committees should appreciate that they work under conditions that predispose them to groupthink. A rapid recommendation may be needed despite uncertain information and conflicting values and interests. Such clinical urgency may press the committee to reach agreement. The committee may feel attacked by various groups: attending physicians who fear that their power is being usurped, nurses who think that they are given unreasonable orders, administrators who wish to control costs, or risk managers who want to avoid legal difficulties. If committee chairpeople are forceful leaders who control discussions, they may unintentionally discourage frank debate and disagreement. Tendencies toward groupthink may be reinforced if access to the committee is limited.

Ethics committees that recognize the dangers of groupthink can take steps to avoid them. First, committees can guard against premature agreement. The chairperson may explicitly ask that doubts and objections be expressed or may appoint members to make the case against the majority. Second, committees can scrutinize any secondhand information they receive. To understand the patient's preferences, the committee might talk with the patient or proxy directly, invite the patient or surrogate to participate in some discussions, or assign a committee member to act as a patient advocate. Third, the committee can look for innovative ways to settle disputes. Improved communication may resolve disagreements. Families, nurses, or house staff may accept the attending physician's decision after they hear the reasons for it and have an opportunity to ask questions. Alternatively, a compromise may be negotiated.[34] For example, a patient who threatens to sign out of a cardiac care unit may agree to further treatment if he or she is given more control over the timing of the administration of medications and nursing care and if one physician and one nurse take responsibility for answering his or her questions.

EVALUATING ETHICS COMMITTEES

Ultimately, the question of whether ethics committees are useful is an empirical one. Before consulting ethics committees can be considered to be a standard decision-making procedure rather than a promising innovation, they need to be evaluated. Because enthusiastic anecdotes about innovations may not be confirmed in controlled trials, pleas have been made to evaluate new tech-

nological procedures, such as angioplasty, before they are accepted and put into wide use.[35] Institutional innovations should also be evaluated, even if they seem to be obviously beneficial. For instance, hospices were expected to provide more humane and less expensive care for patients with terminal illnesses. Controlled studies, however, suggest that hospice care may not differ substantially from current conventional care and may be more expensive.[36-38]

As in any evaluation, deciding on clinically meaningful outcomes and designing unbiased studies require thought and planning. I suggest several criteria for evaluating both the process by which ethics committees review cases and the results of their deliberations. First, patients and their surrogates should have access to the ethics committees. Specifically, they should be able to ask the committees to review their cases and to meet with the committees if they desire. Second, recommendations by the committee and the reasons for them should be available to the parties in each case. Generally, a note in the medical record would be required. Third, recommendations by ethics committees and actual decisions by attending physicians should be consistent with ethical and legal guidelines. The gold standard should be the widespread ethical consensus that has emerged on many issues.[39] Evaluations might focus on whether ethics committees reduce discrepancies between this consensus and actual decisions by physicians. For instance, studies indicate that care givers often fail to discuss management options with patients or the surrogates of incompetent patients.[28-30] Ethics committees should recommend such discussions when appropriate. If their recommendations have an effect on care givers, fewer decisions will be made without such discussions with patients or their surrogates. Committees should also increase informed refusals of care by patients. Moreover, committees should decrease decisions based on ambiguous or uncorroborated second-hand information about the indications for treatment or about patient preferences. Fourth, parties in disagreements should be satisfied with the process of review and with the recommendations of the ethics committee. Although the degree of satisfaction of care givers with ethics consultations has been studied,[40] it is also important to determine the reactions of patients or their surrogates. Finally, ethics committees that make recommendations should have their own internal systems of review, to ensure that the suggested criteria are met.

In summary, the promise that ethics committees will resolve dilemmas about patient care and avoid legal disputes needs to be examined critically. If recommendations by ethics committees are to be accepted by patients, families, society, and the courts, the wishes and interests of patients must be represented and ethical guidelines must be followed. Committees can take active steps to reduce the risk of groupthink. Empirical studies may indicate what kinds of committees improve decisions relating to patient care and in which clinical circumstances.

REFERENCES

1 President's Commission for the Study of Ethical Problems in Medicine and Biomedical and Behavioral Research. Deciding to forego life-sustaining treatment: a report on the ethical, medical, and legal issues in treatment decisions. Washington, D.C.: Government Printing Office, 1983.

2 Cranford RE, Doudera AE, eds. Institutional ethics committees and health care decision making. Ann Arbor, Mich.: Health Administration Press, 1984.

3 Bayley SC, Cranford RE. Ethics committees: what we have learned. In: Friedman E, ed. Making choices: ethics issues for health care professionals. Chicago: American Hospital Publishing, 1986:193–9.

4 Lynn J. Roles and functions of institutional ethics committees: the President's Commission's view. In: Cranford RE, Doudera AE, eds. Institutional ethics committees and health care decision making. Ann Arbor, Mich.: Health Administration Press, 1984:22–30.

5 Committee on Ethics and Medical-Legal Affairs. Institutional ethics committee's [sic]: roles, responsibilities, and benefits for physicians. Minn Med 1985; 68:607–12.

6 Siegler M. Ethics committees: decisions by bureaucracy. Hastings Cent Rep 1986; 16(3):22–4.

7 Lo B, Dornbrand L. The case of Claire Conroy: Will administrative review safeguard incompetent patients? Ann Intern Med 1986; 104:869–73.

8 Lo B. The Bartling case: protecting patients from harm while respecting their wishes. J Am Geriatr Soc 1986; 34:44–8.

9 Burt RA. Taking care of strangers: the rule of law in doctor-patient relations. New York: Free Press, 1979.

10 New York State Task Force on Life and the Law. Do not resuscitate orders: the proposed legislation and report of the New York State Task Force on Life and the Law, April 1986.

11 Wanzer SH, Adelstein SJ, Cranford RE, et al. The physician's responsibility towards hopelessly ill patients. N Engl J Med 1984; 310:955–9.

12 Lo B, Jonsen AR. Clinical decisions to limit treatment. Ann Intern Med 1980; 93:764–8.

13 Levine C. Questions and (some very tentative) answers about hospital ethics committees. Hastings Cent Rep 1984; 14(3):9–12.

14 Kushner T, Gibson JM. Institutional ethics committees speak for themselves. In: Cranford RE, Doudera AE, eds. Institutional ethics committees and health care decision making. Ann Arbor, Mich.: Health Administration Press, 1984:96–105.

15 Fost N, Cranford RE. Hospital ethics committees: administrative aspects. JAMA 1985; 253:2687–92.

16 Summers JW. Closing unprofitable services: ethical issues and management responses. Hosp Health Serv Adm 1985; 30:8–28.

17 Youngner SJ, Jackson DL, Coulton C, Juknialis BW, Smith E. A national survey of hospital ethics committees. Crit Care Med 1983; 11:902–5.

18 Friedin RB, Goldman L, Cecil RR. Patient-physician concordance in problem identification in the primary care setting. Ann Intern Med 1980; 93:490–3.

19 McNeil BJ, Weichselbaum R, Pauker SG. Fallacy of the five-year survival in lung cancer. N Engl J Med 1978; 299:1397–401.

20 Winslow GR. From loyalty to advocacy: a new metaphor for nursing. Hastings Cent Rep 1984; 14(3):32–40.

21 Robertson JA. Ethics committees in hospitals: alternative structures and responsibilities. Conn Med 1984; 48:441–4.

22 Lo B. The death of Clarence Herbert: withdrawing care is not murder. Ann Intern Med 1984; 101:248–51.

23 Baron C. The case for the courts. J Am Geriatr Soc 1984; 32:734–8.

24 Cranford RE, Hester FA, Ashley BZ. Institutional ethics committees: issues of confidentiality and immunity. Law Med Health Care 1985; 13:52–60.

25 Fox RC, Swazey JP, eds. The courage to fail: a social view of organ transplants and dialysis. Chicago: University of Chicago Press, 1974:240–79.

26 Janis IL, Mann L. Decision-making: a psychological analysis of conflict, choice, and commitment. New York: Free Press, 1977.

Supported in part by a grant (1 P50 MH42459-01) from the National Institute of Mental Health and a grant from the Commonwealth Foundation.

I am indebted to L. Dornbrand, J. Ungaretti, S. Cummings, S. Schroeder, and W. Strull for helpful suggestions.

27 George A. Towards a more soundly based foreign policy. In: Commission on the Organization of the Government for the Conduct of Foreign Policy, appendix B. Washington, D.C.: Government Printing Office, 1975.

28 Lidz CW, Meisel A, Osterweis M, Holden JL, Marx JH, Munetz MR. Barriers to informed consent. Ann Intern Med 1983; 99:539–43.

29 Bedell SE, Pelle D, Maher PL, Cleary P. Do-not-resuscitate orders for critically ill patients in the hospital: How are they used and what is their impact? JAMA 1986; 256:233–7.

30 Goldman L, Lee T, Rudd P. Ten commandments for effective clinicians. Arch Intern Med 1983; 143:1753–5.

31 Lo B, Saika G, Strull W, Thomas E, Showstack J. 'Do not resuscitate' decisions: a prospective study at three teaching hospitals. Arch Intern Med 1985; 145:1115–7.

32 Tumulty PA. The effective clinician: his methods and approach to diagnosis and care. Philadelphia: W.B. Saunders, 1973:45–8.

33 Beauchamp TL, Childress J. Principles of biomedical ethics. 2nd ed. New York: Oxford University Press, 1983.

34 Steinbrook R, Lo B. The case of Elizabeth Bouvia: Starvation, suicide, or problem patient? Arch Intern Med 1986; 146:161–4.

35 Mock MB, Reeder GS, Schaff HV, et al. Percutaneous transluminal coronary angioplasty versus coronary artery bypass: Isn't it time for a randomized trial? N Engl J Med 1985; 312:916–9.

36 Kane RL, Wales J, Bernstein L, Leibowitz A, Kaplan S. A randomised controlled trial of hospice care. Lancet 1984; 1:890–4.

37 Kane RL, Bernstein L, Wales J, Rothenberg R. Hospice effectiveness in controlling pain. JAMA 1985; 253:2683–6.

38 Birnbaum HG, Kidder D. What does hospice cost? Am J Public Health 1984; 74:689–97.

39 Jonsen AR. A concord in medical ethics. Ann Intern Med 1983; 99:261–4.

40 Perkins HS, Saathoff BS. How do ethics consultations benefit clinicians? Clin Res 1986; 34:831A, abstract.

Autonomy and the Rights of Geriatric Patients

The Geriatric Patient: Ethical Issues in Care and Treatment
Ruth Macklin

Ruth Macklin is professor of bioethics at Albert Einstein College of Medicine, New York. She is the author of *Man, Mind and Morality: The Ethics of Behavior Control* (1981), *Moral Choices: Bioethics in Today's World* (1987), and *Mortal Choices: Ethical Dilemmas in Modern Medicine* (1988).

Macklin is concerned with two questions: Are there special ethical problems that arise in caring for elderly patients? Are there special ethical problems that arise in caring for them in an extended-care facility? In exploring these questions, she (1) discusses the complexity of making judgments about the competency of the elderly, (2) examines possible ways of testing competency, and (3) brings out some of the assumptions underlying judgments of diminished capacity in the elderly. Macklin concludes by raising questions about the paternalistic control exercised in extended-care facilities for the elderly and suggests the need for appropriate changes.

In any discussion about medical ethics, it is always fair to ask whether the ethical issues that arise in a particular setting or regarding a particular patient population are unique to that setting or population, or whether the same ethical concerns mark the care of patients in other facilities or from other special groups. It would be an easy, if not rather boring, exercise if we could simply transfer the moral problems and any proposed solutions to them from one setting, or one patient population, to another. Yet it would be surprising if there were no common ethical problems among different areas of medical practice. After all, medical treatment and research, nursing services, administration of health care facilities, and other activities in the sphere of medical and health care all focus on the patient: ill, ailing, or injured people. With regard to geriatric patients, these questions need reply: Are there special ethical problems that arise in caring for elderly patients, problems that never or rarely occur in general medicine or with other special populations? Are there special ethical problems that arise in caring for such patients in an extended care facility, problems that never or rarely exist in the context of ambulatory care or short-term medical facilities?

It should come as no surprise to learn that the answers to these questions are both "yes" and "no." Similarities and differences between the situations that give rise to ethical issues in the care and treatment of geriatric patients can be found elsewhere in medicine. It is only very recently, with the rise of the medical specialty of geriatrics, that medically related ethical problems of the elderly as a special patient population have begun to receive attention. Like the typical adult patient, many elderly persons are perfectly capable of granting (or refusing) consent for medical treatment, and of making life choices following their release from the hospital. Like other special populations, most notably mental patients, those elderly who suffer from senile dementia lack the capacity to grant informed consent or to participate in decisionmaking regarding their care and treatment.

Yet in spite of these evident similarities, the elderly differ in a number of relevant respects from other patient populations. Elderly patients, as they near the end of the life span, often have a different set of values in their assessments of the quality of life than do younger persons. Furthermore, elderly persons who have begun to decline in their mental capacity nevertheless have a lifetime of experiences and accomplishments that inform their wants and perceived needs relating to medical treatment and aftercare. Since there is no expectation that they will reenter the work force, or enjoy a return to

productivity, their plight differs significantly from that of other hospitalized adults who are better able to exercise their autonomy as patients. Finally, like all residents of extended care facilities, the elderly in such settings are at risk for increased dependency and other typical consequences of institutionalization.

Key concepts in bioethics include paternalism, autonomy, and informed consent. These assume special importance in the care and treatment of geriatric patients because of the prevalence of dementing illness. When elderly persons suffer slight cognitive impairment, to what extent should they be permitted (or encouraged) to make decisions regarding their own medical care and treatment, as well as other life choices? Under what conditions is it justifiable to remove from people their decisionmaking autonomy about matters affecting primarily themselves, when they have enjoyed a lifetime of such autonomy? Should a finding of incompetence in one area automatically be transferred to or assumed to exist in, any other area? (Compare competency to manage one's financial affairs, competency to make a will, and competency to grant or refuse consent for a medical procedure.) Are the considerations that might support some form of paternalism (coercing people for their own good) the same for all special populations whose competency may be in doubt, or do special considerations obtain in the case of the elderly? When elderly persons of questionable capacity disagree with what others think is best for them regarding a medical or life choice decision, how should such differences be handled? What role should other family members play in the settlement of such disagreements? This last question is of crucial importance for geriatric patients, since if they have not been declared *legally* incompetent, family members are not automatically empowered to override their relative's medical decision (for example, a refusal of amputation).

According to one recent account, "estimates are that approximately 10% of persons older than 65 years have clinically important intellectual impairment. In a survey of nursing homes published in 1978, respondents to a questionnaire reported that 50% to 75% of the residents in their facilities were intellectually impaired."[1] Another set of figures reports that "one out of every six persons over the age of 65—about 1½ million people—is at least moderately demented. Sixty to eighty percent of nursing home patients are demented."[2] These figures are roughly the same, and they suggest that the problem of senile dementia is one of considerable magnitude.

The magnitude of the problem is only one dimension that gives rise to ethical concerns. Another is the uncertainty and variability of judgments about the mental status of elderly patients. Several factors contribute to the uncertainty and variability of such judgments, and at the risk of repeating what is well known, it is worth citing a number of those factors to illustrate the complexity of the problem of making judgments of competence.

The first factor is the reversibility or irreversibility of impaired intellectual function. Obviously, it is important to assess the causes of mental impairment whenever possible, whether or not there exist clear or uncontroversial criteria for determining what a person should be permitted to do or to decide at a particular level of competence. The fact that we lack such criteria points to still another problem, to be addressed shortly. It seems clear that if impaired mental functioning can be reversed, not only should efforts be made to reverse it, but also that an ethical requirement in such situations is that any decisions about life choices affecting the elderly should be postponed if possible until mental function is restored. Although these points may seem obvious, it remains true that demands on the time and resources of personnel in a hospital or extended care facility often prevent prompt or accurate diagnoses, especially in an area of emerging medical knowledge, such as the causes of dementia. Since these causes are numerous, and include everything from depression to deficiencies in nutrients, prompt and thorough diagnostic workups are vital for the prospects of reversing mental impairment.

A fact that bears directly on the broader ethical issues in treating geriatric patients in an extended care facility is that the most common causes of *reversible* impaired intellectual function are therapeutic drug intoxication, depression, and metabolic or infectious disorders.[3] This fact suggests that adequate knowledge on the part of physicians and other health care workers, and the devotion of sufficient time and effort to make timely and accurate diagnoses, can go a long way toward reversing this unfortunate condition in many elderly patients. Especially troubling are the facts about the adverse effects of medication. "An enormous number of drugs have been implicated, including diuretics, digitalis, oral antidiabetic drugs, analgesics, anti-inflammatory agents, sedatives, and psychopharmacologic agents."[4] Add to the sheer number of drugs having this effect the further consideration that the elderly metabolize drugs differently from younger persons and that they are often being treated with multiple drugs, leading to toxicity from drug interactions, and it is not hard to conclude that a significant cause of mental impairment in elderly patients is iatrogenic.

More problematic from another standpoint are the disorders that cause *irreversible* dementia. According to a report of the National Institute on Aging Task Force, two of them—Alzheimer's disease and multiinfarct dementia—account for approximately 80 percent of the dementias of old age.[5] Unlike the reversible causes of mental impairment, which must be diagnosed and treated promptly, but in which actions or decisions on the part of the elderly can often await their improvement, cases of irreversible mental decline pose a different set of problems. A poignant moral dilemma in such cases is when, how much, and in what manner to disclose to a patient the prognosis of the disease and the facts about impending decline. We need to develop a sensitive and humane approach both to informing Alzheimer's patients of the details and prognosis of their disease, and to working with families in preparing for the patient's decline in mental capacity—a decline that has both short-term and long-term implications for decisions and actions concerning legal, financial, and other life circumstances. The ethical questions surrounding disclosure are linked with the more general issue of paternalism toward elderly persons who are in physical and mental decline, and whose growing dependence on others demands a morally sound approach.

Another factor lending complexity to the problem of making judgments of competency in the elderly is the existence of several different tests of competency—tests that may yield conflicting results when applied to elderly persons suffering from dementia. The above-noted report mentions several tests commonly used in the mental status examination: orientation for time, place, and persons; short-term memory; arithmetic calculation; ability to name objects; comprehension of spoken and written language; ability to write a spontaneous sentence; and ability to copy simple geometric figures. The report asserts that the impression of progressively deteriorating mental function can be confirmed and documented by such tests, but that assertion may be misleading. Even if these commonly used tests succeed in confirming a supposition that a patient is undergoing progressive mental decline, they yield no clear picture of the tasks or judgments that the patient is able or unable to perform beyond those specifically measured in the tests themselves. What does a test for a patient's ability to do arithmetic calculations have to do with that patient's understanding of a proposed medical procedure for which the patient's consent is sought? What does an inability to copy simple geometric figures tell us about a person's ability to make changes in his or her will? One problematic example is that of an elderly patient suffering from senile dementia who exhibits severe impairment of short-term memory, yet scores 110 on a standard psychometric instrument for measuring IQ. When two different tests of competency yield conflicting results, which one should be selected as a measure of the patient's competency? Or do they not conflict at all because they measure discrete capacities?

The existence of multiple measures for evaluating competency is one consideration contributing to the complexity of this issue. A related but quite different issue is the value question of how strong or how weak tests of competency should be—a factor that bears directly on the ethics of paternalistic treatment of elderly persons of questionable capacity. Since these conceptual and ethical issues surrounding judgments of competency are directly related to a patient's ability to grant or refuse consent for a wide variety of biomedical interventions, as well as to engage in a number of different life tasks, it is important to look carefully at current practices and knowledge in related fields. Recent research has concentrated largely on psychiatric patients in an attempt to gain a better understanding of competency as it relates to various tasks. The trend in both law and medicine in the last few years has been toward developing a notion of variable competence, and toward selecting situation-specific criteria for judging competence, rather than viewing it as a global attribute of people.

In a recent article discussing currently used tests of competency to consent to treatment, the authors describe five basic categories into which such tests fall.[6] These are: (1) evidencing a choice; (2) "reasonable" outcome of choice; (3) choice based on "rational" reasons; (4) ability to understand; and (5) actual understanding. Noting that these categories overlap, the authors point out that the tests range from the weakest test of competency to the strongest, with the tests at the lowest level being most respectful of the autonomy of patient decisionmaking. Just which of these tests ought to be used to determine the competence of elderly patients is a question not easy to answer, and one that probably would elicit some controversy among caregivers, family members, and elderly patients themselves. These same authors argue that

> the test that is actually applied combines elements of all of the tests described above. However, the circumstances in which competency becomes an issue determine which elements of which tests are stressed and which are underplayed. Although in theory competency is an independent variable that determines whether or not the patient's decision to accept or refuse treatment is to be honored, in practice it seems to be dependent on the interplay of two other variables, the risk/benefit ratio of treatment and the valence of the patient's decision, i.e., whether he or she consents to or refuses treatment.[7]

Since questions of individual preference and personal values are often bound up in treatment refusals, it is crucial to try to assess the reasons behind an elderly person's refusal to consent. The stricter the standard of competence, in the interest of protecting patients from their own unwise decisions, the more autonomy is traded for a gain in benevolent paternalism. It is generally assumed that when elderly patients suffer diminished capacity, and thus cannot speak on their own behalf, caregivers and family have their "best interests" at heart and will act in accordance with those interests; yet the validity of this and related assumptions has yet to be adequately explored. The question of where the presumption ought to lie regarding elderly persons of questionable competence is more a matter for decision than a matter of scientific discovery of the precise attributes that constitute competency. Should the presumption lie in their ability to judge and decide for themselves, suggesting the adoption of a weak test of competency? Or should the presumption lie on the side of impaired ability to judge, suggesting the adoption of a strong test of competency? We seek to avoid erring in either of two opposite directions: being too paternalistic with the elderly, taking their dependency and "childlike" attributes as grounds for coercing them for their own good; and on the other hand, being too permissive in respecting their autonomy, thereby opening the door to self-destructive or other irresponsible acts. The one evil consists of violating the cherished value of individual freedom; the other evil is to allow harm, destruction, or even death to befall a helpless, dependent person with declining mental and physical faculties.

These ethical dilemmas point to a research agenda for studying problems of competency and informed consent in the elderly. For elderly persons of doubtful or declining competence, the following problem areas deserve further study. Current practices surrounding disclosure by physicians, other health care workers, and family members to elderly patients with declining mental functioning need to be analyzed, focusing on the values to be attained by adhering to any particular policy or practice. What are the conditions under which full and frank disclosure about a patient's condition should take place? Are there special circumstances under which information should be withheld? How can such patients be helped to prepare themselves, psychologically and emotionally, for a deterioration in their cognitive capacities? What supports can be offered to the families of patients such as those suffering from Alzheimer's disease, especially in regard to assessing the appropriate time and method of disclosure?

Further work is also called for concerning the problem of paternalism toward the elderly who suffer from growing incompetence, and of the autonomy of aging individuals to make decisions and perform tasks both related and unrelated to biomedical procedures. Where ought the presumption lie: with the elderly themselves, to demonstrate their continued competence? Or with those who challenge their competence, to show that the principle of beneficence dictates treating those with senile dementia as incompetent, and therefore no longer autonomous, agents? There is a special poignancy to the problem of the growing incompetence of elderly persons, stemming from their own awareness of that decline, and the fact that having once been normally functioning adults, they are witness to their own mental and physical deterioration and to changes in the attitudes and behavior of others toward them. Even in cases where mental functioning is clearly impaired, a morally sound approach dictates enlisting the participation of elderly patients as much as possible in decisions regarding their own care and treatment.

At the outset I mentioned the prospect of special ethical problems that arise in caring for patients in an extended care facility. Although the characteristics of "total institutions"—to use Erving Goffman's term—are by now well-known, it is worth repeating here that, especially in the case of elderly persons, residents of such facilities often respond to their environment in ways that exacerbate their already declining capacities. One writer describes the situation as follows:

> Many nursing homes, geriatric wards, and mental hospitals have the characteristics of total institutions: simply by their institutional structures and expectations, they determine the behavior of their residents. . . . According to one description (Citrin and Dixon, 1977), a radical alteration in life-style following institutionalization, joined with increasing demands by the institution's staff and decreasing physical functioning frequently brings about socially withdrawn, confused, or disoriented behavior among the elderly. Thus (Butler 1975), substantial numbers of patients in mental hospitals develop a chronic state of psychological dependence and deterioration. Infantilization and loss of self-image are frequently the result of institutionalization and interaction with the institution's staff. . . .[8]

The term "infantilization" is a key one here, and serves as a reminder that the elderly in decline are not, of course, literally "infants," in spite of many behavioral similarities. The ethical problem is to determine to what extent care and treatment of the elderly who exhibit "infantile behavior" in the metaphorical sense should be treated as we deem it proper to treat infants and small children—that is, in accordance with a justifiable pattern of paternalistic control. Insofar as the institutional structure of an extended care facility deepens those problems by reinforcing the dependency and childlike behavior of its residents, it seems possible—at least in principle—to make changes in that structure, and thereby lessen the ethical problems to some extent. Let me illustrate.

I recently learned of the existence of several nursing homes in Great Britain,[9] facilities that differ markedly from those in the United States and are not typical in Britain, either. One way of describing this difference is by reference to the overworked "medical model" as compared with a "social model" for setting policies and organizing practices and social life in the institution. Whereas the typical pattern of nursing home organization is largely similar to that of a hospital, or more generally, a medical facility, these British nursing homes are organized more as a social facility. As in the typical nursing home, the residents are ill, ailing, infirm, mentally impaired, or incontinent, yet are able to perform a variety of tasks for themselves, including, for some, meal preparation. The residents are not only allowed but encouraged to make virtually every decision that affects their daily life and activity, except, of course, those requiring medical expertise. Thus they have liberty to choose the furniture in their rooms, to decide for themselves when to wake up in the morning and when to retire at night (even if they wish to stay up as late as 2 A.M.), and to make various other choices and decisions in their everyday lives. These British nursing homes thus strive to maximize the privacy, the autonomy, and the decisionmaking of their residents in an effort to create an atmosphere as similar as possible to that which the elderly persons enjoyed prior to entering. One especially striking feature is that residents are allowed to fight and squabble with one another, which enables them to vent their frustrations and emotions in ways they have experienced all their lives.

This social model has its value trade-offs, of course: what is a gain for the residents in their freedom, autonomy, and privacy amounts to a loss for staff in being able to run things as smoothly and efficiently as possible. The more choices and decisions that are left to the residents, the harder it is for staff to plan and organize the daily routine, since individual residents' wants and needs may vary substantially. It is apparently also true that the bias against paternalism is frequently difficult for the staff to accept, accustomed as they are to the norm in extended care facilities and hospitals, where the staff gives orders and constructs a regimen, and patients are expected to comply. One very positive benefit for residents of these facilities is improvement in depression, one of the most troubling and intractable characteristics of elderly persons.

If careful, empirical observation reveals that changes of this sort in the social structure of a facility for the elderly do indeed yield such benefits, then it is ethically desirable to make an effort to bring about such changes. Benefits to the residents clearly would seem to outweigh inconvenience and reduced efficiency of the staff, and although practical difficulties must always be heeded in any recommendations for change, this particular experience suggests another area for further research that might improve care and treatment of the elderly in extended care facilities.

NOTES

1 National Institute on Aging Task Force, "Senility Reconsidered: Treatment Possibilities for Mental Impairment in the Elderly," *Journal of the American Medical Association* 244 (1980): 259.

2 G. B. Kolata, "Clues to the Cause of Senile Dementia," *Science* 211 (1981): 1032.

3 National Institute on Aging Task Force, "Senility Reconsidered," pp. 259–263.

4 *Ibid.*, p. 260.

5 *Ibid.*

6 L. H. Roth, et al. "Tests of Competency to Consent to Treatment," *American Journal of Psychiatry* 134 (1977): 279–284.

7 *Ibid.*, pp. 283–284.

8 W. T. Reich, "Ethical Issues Related to Research Involving Elderly Subjects," *Gerontologist* 18 (1978): 333.

9 Presentation by Dr. Marvin Rosenberg delivered at The Hastings Center, Institute of Society, Ethics and the Life Sciences, Project on Health Policy and Geriatrics, May 13, 1981.

Medical Empowerment of the Elderly
Marshall B. Kapp

Marshall B. Kapp, who has a J.D. as well as a master's degree in public health, is professor in the department of medicine in society at Wright State University. Kapp is the author of *Legal Guide for Office Managers* (1985), coauthor of *Geriatrics and the Law: Patient Rights and Professional Responsibilities* (1985), and coeditor of *Legal and Ethical Aspects of Health Care for the Elderly* (1985).

Kapp strikes a cautionary note regarding recent attempts to empower the elderly by encouraging them to be active advocates of their own rights and interests and to participate maximally in their own significant decisions. Through such self-advocacy and exercise of decisionmaking power, the autonomy, independence, and dignity of the elderly are greatly enhanced. Kapp grants that empowering the elderly to make their own decisions, including those regarding health care, is a noble goal. He maintains, however, that there are a significant number of elderly people, as well as other adults, who would not voluntarily accept responsibility for making some or all of their own difficult decisions, including those regarding medical interventions. In Kapp's view we are faced with a fundamental policy issue: Should we permit capable, informed older adults voluntarily to waive empowerment or should we force empowerment on them? He discusses several arguments on both sides of this issue and concludes by offering a few guidelines whose intent is to foster empowerment while averting the possibility that we might "deny the elderly their autonomy by forcing it upon them."

Reprinted with permission of the author and the publisher from *Hastings Center Report*, vol. 19 (July/August 1989), pp. 5–7.

"Empowerment" of the elderly has become a popular gerontological buzz-phrase of the 1980s.[1] It refers to the movement among advocates for older individuals to encourage activism among the capable elderly regarding their own rights and interests whenever possible, within a society in which rights are respected and acted upon only if one claims those rights personally or through a proxy.[2] There is widespread philosophical agreement among professionals concerned with the well-being of the elderly that political, legal, social, economic, and health-related services that support the capacity of older persons to speak for themselves—that is, that empower older persons—greatly enhance the autonomy, independence, and dignity of the older self-advocate.

Additionally, recent research underscores the relationship between a sense of control over one's decisions and life goals and positive outcomes in aging.[3] Many interpret such data to show that the extent to which individuals are encouraged to take more control over their lives and health may be a major determinant of satisfaction and well-being (that is, quality of life) in their later years.

The chief legal mechanism of empowerment in the health area is the doctrine of informed consent, the requirement that medical interventions be administered to a patient only if preceded by the voluntary, adequately informed agreement of a capable patient or that patient's legally authorized substitute decisionmaker. The depth of commitment to the notion of empowerment of the elderly in health care is manifested in the growing use of legal planning devices, such as the living will and the durable power of attorney, on a prospective basis to effectuate informed consent later in life.[4] Through these legal mechanisms as well as other means, professional advocates, family members, friends, physicians, and other health care providers all play an important role in helping the elderly to make and exercise their own life choices.

LIMITS OF EMPOWERMENT

The enthusiasm for empowerment must be tempered with caution, however. There are important limits and nuances to this concept that must be thoroughly considered.

First, power over one's life entails more than mere control over particular choices. In a real sense, it is knowledge that creates power. Hence, the older individual's purported right to make choices about matters affecting him or her acquires meaning only if those choices are accompanied by adequate information, both about the personal rights involved and the factual ramifications of one's decision, as well as the range of reasonable alternatives among which to choose. As our early experience with "Medigap" insurance policies teaches, the older person's right to choose should not be confused with the "right to be ripped off." Thus, insistence on adequate information is essential to meaningful (as opposed to apparent) empowerment.

Second, decision-making power must be accepted voluntarily (if at all) by the older person. We rightly start with a legal and ethical presumption that most elderly people wish to make their own decisions regarding health care. However, this presumption is rebuttable, not conclusive. There are a significant number of adults, including but by no means limited to a substantial percentage of the elderly, who would not voluntarily accept responsibility for making some or all of their own difficult decisions.[5]

This paradox—older individuals who would rather not make their own decisions—compels us to confront a fundamental policy issue of whether we should permit capable, informed older adults voluntarily to waive empowerment if they so wish, or instead force empowerment on them. Put more starkly, should we recognize a right of the elderly to be dependent on others? This dilemma invokes basic philosophical premises about the nature of personal choice and responsibility, and their interaction and tension. In the context of elderly empowerment, is the relationship of rights and duties one of polarity or correlativity?

FORCED EMPOWERMENT

There are several plausible arguments for forcing capable, informed older individuals to be empowered, that is, to advocate for themselves and participate maximally in their own significant decisions. Some would argue that there is a fundamental duty incumbent on all of us to be autonomous, to accept personal responsibility as masters of our own ship. This view sees that decisions concerning one's own health are of such a deeply personal character that they cannot ethically be delegated to anyone else. The decision—and its consequences—belong to the patient alone. Jay Katz has claimed, for example, that as a matter of universal ethical and social policy, he would never permit any capable patient to abdicate or waive his or her right to make final medical decisions.[6]

Moreover, under this philosophical view, older persons who are *capable* of being empowered to fend for themselves in medical decisionmaking have a duty to *assume* responsibility for decisionmaking as a matter of justice. Otherwise they will unnecessarily consume increasingly scarce resources that should instead be directed toward the growing number of involuntarily dependent elders who have no choice but to rely on others for basic advocacy and proxy decision-making services. The establishment, administration, and monitoring of a proxy decision-making apparatus requires substantial financial costs.

Further, Katz and others have suggested that forcing consumers of medical services, including the able elderly, to accept decision-making power is the only effective way to safeguard against health care professionals acting paternalistically and condescendingly toward the consumer.[7] This position suggests a skeptical, even cynical, perspective toward the helping professions, particularly toward physicians, but one that is not convincingly disproved by historical analyses of communication within the professional-patient relationship and failures in implementing the spirit of the doctrine of informed consent.

FORGOING EMPOWERMENT

Nevertheless, persuasive arguments can be asserted in favor of allowing capable, informed older persons the choice to forgo, to a greater or lesser extent, personal empowerment and thereby waive or abdicate responsibility for some of the decisions they are ethically and legally entitled to make. On this position, choosing dependence on others rather than independence would be a respected alternative for the capable elder.

It can, first of all, be argued that honoring the older person's autonomy logically encompasses that person's right to delegate to others his or her decision-making duties, just as much as does honoring his or her right to consent to or refuse offered medical services. There is no logical mistake in permitting a capable person knowingly and voluntarily to transfer some decision-making power to another of his or her choosing. As Arthur Dyck reminds us, autonomy is not synonymous with self-determination; rather, autonomy is the capacity for self-determination, a capacity that the individual may or may not choose to exercise.[8] Both ethically and legally, society clearly permits informed individuals voluntarily to choose not to exercise their fundamental rights in other

areas of life. For instance, few of us would object to an older person turning over to an attorney substantial power relating to management of his or her financial affairs. Since the attorney stands in a fiduciary relationship with the client, he or she is ethically and legally obligated to act in the client's best interests. Similarly, the fiduciary nature of the physician-patient relationship mandates a commitment to the patient's best interests; hence, appointing a physician as an agent for choosing the appropriate course of medical care to follow is neither unwise nor an unwarranted burden upon the physician.[9]

PERILS OF INDEPENDENCE

Nevertheless, placing too much reliance on empowerment of the elderly can lead, if we are not careful, to the implicit condoning of neglect of the elderly if they do not exercise their power sufficiently. Individualism and independence, if too rugged, may turn into health care nihilism. When our expectations about responsibility are shifted too radically from institutions and agencies to the older individual, we run the risk of letting those institutions and agencies escape their proper duties too easily. We may provide them with too ready a defense, in the face of neglect, harm, and deterioration of older patients, that the power belonged to the older person (that is, the victim), and that the institution or agency was merely carrying out the elder's explicit or implied orders.[10] To blend autonomy with beneficence effectively, empowerment ideally should entail a negotiated sharing, as opposed to a sequential transfer of authority.[11]

For instance, an older hospital patient may insist on being discharged to a home environment where he or she lives alone and refuses assistance from home care staff. The hospital and its staff who facilitate the discharge without giving sufficient attention to alternatives may be compromising their commitment to beneficence under the guise of respecting autonomy. The institution and its staff should instead make every reasonable effort to negotiate terms of home care that are palatable to the patient but that provide at least minimally adequate assistance and assurance of protection. The proper degree of cajoling, persuasion and—if necessary—legal intervention will vary from case to case.

Lastly, it frequently is difficult to ascertain and interpret older individuals' actual preferences regarding specific questions about their medical care or other services. Many may wish to receive certain services, or conversely may desire to reject those services, but are too embarrassed or afraid to announce their preferences. Even after barriers to effective communication and informed consent have been vigorously addressed, some persons still simply would rather be led by others than assert themselves. This phenomenon should not surprise us, considering how many young and middle-aged persons in our society in effect elect to forfeit their own empowerment in important matters in favor of passively relying on the presumed expertise, experience, charisma, or caring of professionals, family members, or friends.

We cannot reasonably expect people who have a long-standing personal history of attempting to "escape from freedom"[12] suddenly to embrace an ethic of individual empowerment upon reaching a certain chronological age. If anything, the physical and social infirmities of age tend to compel movement in the opposite direction. Several recently completed empirical studies regarding the process of geriatric decisionmaking, as well as a body of published research concerning do-not-resuscitate decisionmaking, strongly suggest that many elders both want and expect others, such as their physicians, family members, and friends, to take primary responsibility for making medical decisions. Frequently these surrogate decisionmakers are provided with little or no direction by the older person to aid them in fulfilling this responsibility.[13]

Of course, the empirical fact that some elderly persons refuse their own empowerment does not definitively settle the normative question of whether such dependency is acceptable, let alone desirable. Still, such data are a meaningful part of health policy formulation and cannot be merely dismissed; instead, the relevance of moral principles for the question of empowerment of the elderly must be tested against this empirical basis. Ethical questions are not resolved by popular plebiscite, but actual opinions and actions are relevant factors in the health policy-making calculus.

RESOLVING THE TENSION

How, then, may we begin to resolve the tension created between the emphasis on empowerment of the elderly and the persisting desire by certain capable, informed older adults voluntarily to delegate their decision-making rights and responsibilities? No solutions are hazarded here, but a few guidelines may prove helpful.

The common law regarding the doctrine of patient waiver as an exception to the ordinary medical informed consent requirement is generally sensible and instructive. Such allowances recognize that society has a duty to strive for and facilitate empowerment of the elderly without forcing it on unwilling persons. Physicians and others in positions of authority ought to presume that most older persons would desire to make, or at least extensively participate in, medical and other decisions having an impact on their own lives, reserving reliance on a waiver of decision-making rights to a special, extraordinary occurrence.

By the same token, physicians should also recognize that exceptions to this presumption are displayed in the lives of a sizable number of older patients. Some capable elderly individuals will voluntarily and authentically choose, based on adequate information, to refrain from exercising their decision-making rights and responsibilities and to delegate those rights and responsibilities to the physician, family, or friends. Respect for persons necessarily entails respect for such conscious decisions not to decide personally.

The key ethical and legal concern lies in achieving the delicate balance of recognizing and respecting the older person's right to transfer empowerment, but not doing so too quickly or facilely. Physicians and other health care professionals should ensure that any purported delegation of decision-making authority by an older patient is indeed intentional and voluntary, made in the context of adequate information conveyed (or at least a bona fide attempt to convey) to the patient about the decision itself, its likely ramifications, and the patient's right to make that decision.[14] Before accepting and acting on the older patient's transfer of decision-making power, the physician or other professional should insist that the patient's wishes be indicated expressly and unambiguously. As an element of risk management, all professional-patient interactions concerning empowerment or its delegation should be thoroughly documented in the patient's medical record. In these circumstances, the physician or other health care professional ought to openly acknowledge reliance on the waiver exception, rather than hollowly pretend to follow the standard informed consent ritual.[15]

Empowerment of the elderly in medical decision-making is a noble social, political, and ethical cause. Like other noble causes, however, excesses and intolerances can occur unless we are on guard against them. It would be ironic indeed if we were to deny the elderly their autonomy by forcing it upon them. Yet another exquisite challenge for health professionals lies in recognizing and respecting the older patient's right to forgo and thereby delegate choice, as well as the right to choose his or her own medical destiny.

REFERENCES

1 Philip G. Clark, "Individual Autonomy, Cooperative Empowerment, and Planning for Long-Term Care Decision Making," *Journal of Aging Studies* 1 (1987), 65–76.

2 Elias S. Cohen, "Nursing Homes and the Least-Restrictive Environment Doctrine," in *Legal and Ethical Aspects of Health Care for the Elderly*, Marshall B. Kapp, H.E. Pies, and A.E. Doudera, eds. (Ann Arbor, MI: Health Administration Press, 1986), 173–184, at 173, 177–78.

3 Judith Rodin, "Aging and Health: Effects on the Sense of Control," *Science*, 19 September 1986, 1271–1276, at 1271.

4 Society for the Right to Die, *The Physician and the Hopelessly Ill Patient: Legal, Medical, and Ethical Guidelines* (New York: Society for the Right to Die, 1985); Mark Fowler, "Appointing an Agent to Make Medical Treatment Choices," *Columbia Law Review* 84 (1984), 985–1031, at 985.

5 Arthur L. Caplan, "Can We Talk? A Review of Jay Katz, *The Silent World of Doctor and Patient*," *Western New England Law Review* 9:43 (1987), 43–52, at 47–48; Marie Haug, "Doctor-Patient Relationships and the Older Patient," *Journal of Gerontology* 34:6 (1979), 852–60, at 852.

6 Jay Katz, *The Silent World of Doctor and Patient* (New York: Free Press, 1984).

7 See Barry Furrow, "Informed Consent: A Thorn in Medicine's Side? An Arrow in Law's Quiver?" *Law, Medicine and Health Care* 12:6 (1984), 268–73, at 278.

8 Arthur Dyck, "Self-Determination and Moral Responsibility," *Western New England Law Review* 9 (1987), 53–65, at 53–54.

9 See Benjamin Freedman, "A Moral Theory of Informed Consent," *Hastings Center Report* 5:4 (August 1975), 32–39, at 32.

10 Sandra H. Johnson, "Sequential Domination, Autonomy and Living Wills," *Western New England Law Review* 9 (1987), 113–37, at 113, 119.

11 Harry R. Moody, "From Informed Consent to Negotiated Consent," Special Supplement *Gerontologist* 28 (1988), 64–70, at 64.

12 Eric Fromm, *Escape from Freedom* (New York: Rinehart and Company, 1941).

13 Terrie Wetle, Susan Levkoff, and Julie Cwikel, "Research in Nursing Homes: Ethics and Methods"; Nancy R. Zweibel and Christine K. Cassel, "Preferences of Older Patients and Their Children for Life-Extending Medical Care: An Empirical Analysis of Values in Geriatric Medicine"; papers presented at the 40th Annual Meeting of the Gerontological Society of America, Washington, DC, November 21, 1987.

14 Alan Meisel, "Informed Consent: Who Decides for Whom?" in *Medical Ethics and the Law: Implications for Public Policy*, M. Hiller, ed. (Cambridge: Ballinger Press, 1981).

15 Jay Katz, "Physician-Patient Encounters 'On a Darkling Plain'," *Western New England Law Review* 9 (1987), 207–226, at 207, 217.

ANNOTATED BIBLIOGRAPHY: CHAPTER 3

Annas, George N.: *The Rights of Hospital Patients* (New York: Avon, 1975). This American Civil Liberties Union handbook on the rights of hospital patients is intended as a guide for those who are directly affected by the problems discussed. Using a question-and-answer approach, the book provides a statement of the rights patients had under the law at the time the guidebook was written.

Aroskar, Mila, Josephine M. Flaherty, and James M. Smith: "The Nurse and Orders Not to Resuscitate," *Hastings Center Report* 7 (August 1977), pp. 27–28. Aroskar presents a factual case study to illustrate the kinds of ethical problems faced by nurses. Flaherty and Smith discuss the moral principles involved and make recommendations concerning the nurses' actions in such cases.

Ashley, JoAnn: *Hospitals, Paternalism and the Role of the Nurse* (New York: Teachers College, 1976). This book is a study of the development of nursing in the United States. Ashley gives extensive historical documentation in showing that hospitals were established by male physicians and male hospital administrators to offer nursing care provided by women. Ashley amply documents the overt and covert efforts made to deny nurses any voice or control in establishing and changing hospital policies and nursing practices.

Benjamin, Martin, and Joy Curtis: *Ethics in Nursing* (New York: Oxford University, 1981). The intent of this book is to give nursing students and nurses an introduction to the identification and analysis of ethical issues in nursing. The book includes a large number of actual cases, many of which are discussed in detail.

Corcoran, Sheila: "Toward Operationalizing an Advocacy Role," *Journal of Professional Nursing* 4 (July–August 1988), pp. 242–248. Corcoran begins by contrasting two models of nursing advocacy—the legal rights model and the existential advocacy model. Accepting the second model, Corcoran describes an approach that nurses might take when they attempt to perform one of their advocacy duties: helping patients to make decisions.

Cranford, Ronald E., and A. Edward Doudera, eds.: *Institutional Ethics Committees and Health Care Decision Making* (Ann Arbor, Mich.: Health Administration Press, 1984). Published in cooperation with the American Society of Law and Medicine, this collection of articles includes material on the development, roles, and functions of ethics committees as well as on their legal aspects, problems, and implementation. Descriptive summaries of existing institutional ethics committees and sample guidelines and policies also are included.

Daley, Dennis W.: "*Tarasoff v. Regents of the University of California* (Cal. 528 P2nd 553) and the Psychotherapist's Duty to Warn," *San Diego Law Review* 12 (July 1975), pp. 932–951. Daley provides an analysis of the practical problems and potential consequences for psychiatry stemming from the *Tarasoff* decision. He discusses in more detail the same types of issues set forth in Justice Clark's dissenting opinion in the case, such as the difficulty of predicting violence and the importance of confidentiality in the patient-therapist relationship.

De George, Richard T.: "The Moral Responsibility of the Hospital," *The Journal of Medicine and Philosophy* 7 (1982), pp. 87–100. De George addresses the question: Can a hospital be held morally responsible? He argues that hospitals do satisfy criteria for moral responsibility and, therefore, can have moral responsibilities. De George explores how moral responsibility can be intelligibly attributed to a hospital as well as how the responsibilities of the hospital, which are assumed by those within it who act for it (e.g., physicians, administrators), can be separated from the professional moral responsibilities and the personal moral responsibilities of doctors, nurses, and others working in the hospital.

Gadow, Sally: "Medicine, Ethics, and the Elderly," *Gerontologist* 20 (December 1980), pp. 680–685. Gadow presents some of the ethical problems in the medical care of the elderly and discusses a spectrum of contemporary views on aging and some relevant ethical principles. She concludes by suggesting how the ethical problems might be addressed in view of the various social/medical views on aging and different ethical principles.

Lazarus, Tracey, Ana Mejia-Dietche, and Pamela B. Shein: "Don't Make Them Leave Their Rights at the Door: A Recommended Model State Statute to Protect the Rights of the Elderly in Nursing Homes," *Journal of Contemporary Health Law and Policy* 4 (1988), pp. 321–374. This article describes the way in which the Medicaid program impacts on nursing home care and suggests language for a Model Nursing Home Act, based on the language in existing state statutes.

Muyskens, James: *Moral Problems in Nursing: A Philosophical Investigation* (Totowa, N.J.: Rowman and Littlefield, 1982). This book is written primarily for nurses and nursing students. Muyskens presents and defends a specific moral stance and discusses the moral problems faced by nurses from that stance.

Swenson, Sara, et al., compilers: "Bibliography of Ethics Committees." Briarcliff Manor, N.Y.: The Hastings Center, Fall 1988. This is an excellent annotated bibliography.

Thornton, James E., and Earl R. Winkler, eds.: *Ethics and Aging* (Vancouver, Canada: The University of British Columbia Press, 1988). The articles in this book are written by professionals in various fields, including philosophy, sociology, anthropology, economics, nursing, psychology, and law. An extensive bibliography is also included.

Veatch, Robert M.: *Case Studies in Medical Ethics* (Cambridge, Mass.: Harvard University Press, 1977). Veatch offers excellent studies of cases that pose ethical dilemmas for medical professionals. He also provides a general introduction on ethical theory as well as analyses of some of the cases presented.

Winslow, Gerald R.: "From Loyalty to Advocacy: A New Metaphor for Nursing," *Hastings Center Report* 14 (June 1984), pp. 32–39. Winslow argues that in nursing literature two dominant metaphors have served as basic models of ideal nursing practice—a military metaphor, with its language of loyalty and obedience, and a legal metaphor, with its language of advocacy and rights.

CHAPTER 4

ETHICAL ISSUES IN HUMAN AND ANIMAL EXPERIMENTATION

INTRODUCTION

The major focus of this chapter is some of the ethical issues raised by biomedical experimentation (or research) using human subjects. Analyses of these issues employ some of the same ethical concepts and principles discussed in the previous two chapters. Here, too, appeal is made to the value of individual autonomy and to the requirement of informed consent. In addition, other questions are raised about the justifiability of experimentation that puts human subjects at risk and about the obligations that individuals might have to participate as experimental subjects. This chapter also includes a discussion of some ethical issues raised by animal experimentation.

Conceptual Issues

Before examining some of the ethical issues raised by human experimentation, we should clarify the meaning of "human experimentation" (or "research using human subjects") and the distinction often made between therapeutic and nontherapeutic experimentation (or research). In the biomedical context, "therapy" ordinarily refers to a set of activities whose primary purpose is to relieve suffering and to restore or maintain health. Therapy takes many forms. Medical treatment, diagnosis, and even some preventive measures (e.g., vaccine injections) are all considered forms of therapy. It is important to notice that the primary aim of therapy is to benefit the recipient. By way of contrast, "research" or "experimentation" refers to a set of scientific activities whose primary purpose is to develop or contribute to generalizable knowledge about the chemical, physiological, or psychological processes involved in human functioning. Such experimentation is called "human experimentation" not simply because it attempts to expand our knowledge of human functioning but because it uses human beings as subjects.

In keeping with these explications of therapy and experimentation or research a distinction is often drawn between therapeutic and nontherapeutic research. *Therapeutic research*, like all research, is said to be concerned with the acquisition of generalizable knowledge. However, in therapeutic experimentation, the patient-subjects are themselves expected to benefit medically from the new drug, vaccine, treatment, or diagnostic procedure being tried. For example, the first patients on kidney dialysis machines and the first recipients of coronary bypass surgery were participants in medical experiments. The techniques involved had never been tried on human subjects, so the use of these techniques on these patient-subjects was experimental. Furthermore, the information gained by the medical professionals furthered their research and thus contributed to generalizable knowledge. At the same time, however, the new techniques provided a form of therapy designed to alleviate the patient-subjects' own medical problems. Thus the procedures were used on the patients for their benefit, because they promised to be more effective than any other therapy available, and not simply to provide information required by the research project. By contrast, *nontherapeutic research* is said to be research whose *sole* aim is to provide information required by the researchers. Nontherapeutic research is not concerned with providing therapy for the research subjects. An example will illustrate the difference between therapeutic and nontherapeutic research projects.

In 1963 three doctors injected live cancer cells into twenty-two seriously ill and debilitated patients in the Jewish Chronic Disease Hospital in Brooklyn, New York. The purpose of the experiment was to measure the subject's ability to reject foreign cells. These subjects were selected for the experiment because of their debilitated condition. During an earlier phase of the research project, two things had been established: (1) healthy human subjects rejected the injected substance in four to six weeks; and (2) human subjects already ill with advanced cancer took six weeks to several months to reject it. The researchers thought it necessary to use the patients in the Jewish Chronic Disease Hospital to test the following hypothesis: The slower rejection rate of the cancer patients used in the earlier phase of the study was due to the debilitated condition that usually accompanies chronic illness and not to their cancer. Since the test used in the research project was completely unrelated to the therapeutic program of the twenty-two patients in the Jewish Chronic Disease Hospital, this research project provides a clear example of nontherapeutic research.

Nontherapeutic research, of course, is not limited to projects that involve the use of new techniques, drugs, or vaccines. Some nontherapeutic research projects are designed simply to understand normal or abnormal physiological or psychological functions. In such projects, the research subjects may be required to do little more than contribute urine or blood samples, fill out forms, or take written or oral tests.

In practice, it is difficult to draw a clear-cut line between therapeutic and nontherapeutic research projects. Therapeutic research is not conducted *solely* to benefit the patient-subjects since the purpose of all research is to contribute to generalizable knowledge. In addition, the therapeutic project may require patient-subjects to undergo additional procedures unrelated to their own therapy. They may have to give blood samples or be catheterized, for example. Such additional procedures are nontherapeutic for the patients and may even carry some risks unrelated to their own therapy. Nontherapeutic research, in turn, may *indirectly* provide medical benefits (e.g., better medical care) for experimental subjects. Because of these and other difficulties, some writers in biomedical ethics reject the terminology that contrasts therapeutic and nontherapeutic research. They replace it with a three-fold classification: (1) research, (2) practice, and (3) nonvalidated practices (i.e., innovative therapies). Research, as noted previously, is designed to develop generalizable knowledge and is not intended to directly benefit the patient. *Practice* is directly intended to benefit patients and uses validated procedures to do so, that is, procedures known to carry a "reasonable expectation of success." Nonvalidated practices are also directly intended to benefit patient-subjects, but the therapies are innovative and may not have been tested sufficiently to have a reasonable expectation of success.[1] The therapeutic-nontherapeutic research distinction continues to be widely used, however, and is utilized in codes of research ethics in setting up guidelines for the conduct of research using human subjects.

The Justifiability of Experimentation Using Human Subjects

Many biomedical research projects involve at least some risk to patient-subjects. Drugs being tested may turn out to be toxic, for example. In some experiments, subjects may have to be deliberately exposed to a disease such as malaria before they can be used to test the efficacy of a new treatment. What moral justification can be given for experimentation that puts human subjects at risk?

Little is said in response to this question in the literature of biomedical ethics. When it is discussed, the primary justification advanced for human experimentation is a utilitarian one. This justification features two central claims:

1. Human experimentation enhances the discovery of new diagnostic and therapeutic techniques. Past research, for example, has made possible cardiovascular surgery, renal transplantation, and the control of poliomyelitis.

2. Controlled experimentation is necessary for sound medical practice. Possible iatrogenic illnesses will be prevented only if clinical research provides necessary knowledge about human reactions to specific therapies. In the past, physicians employed many techniques that were of no benefit and sometimes even harmed patients. For example, neither the blood-letting common in the eighteenth century nor the practice of freezing the stomachs of patients with ulcers in the twentieth century had any therapeutic value. Yet both practices were erroneously believed to be therapeutic. To take another example, X-rays in the twentieth century were much too widely used before it was learned that there was a connection between overexposure to X-rays and certain types of cancer. Well-designed, controlled research projects, it is argued, will help to minimize the employment of useless or harmful procedures.

The utilitarian conclusion is that human experimentation is not just morally permissible; rather, it is morally required because its harmful consequences for some will be far outweighed by its anticipated provision of future benefits and prevention of future harm to others. Maurice B. Visscher, in this chapter, argues in this vein in defense of a "Research Imperative."

Sometimes a different sort of argument, based on considerations of justice, is advanced to justify human experimentation and to defend the view that individuals have a duty to participate as research subjects in projects designed to advance medical knowledge. The argument is simple. We are the beneficiaries of the advances made by past biomedical research. Without the use of human subjects these advances would have been impossible. Since we have benefited from the sacrifices made by past research subjects, we have an obligation, in the interest of fairness, to see that such research continues. Since it cannot continue without research subjects, we ought to reciprocate for past sacrifices by serving as subjects ourselves. Hans Jonas attacks this argument in this chapter, claiming that we have no obligation to participate as research subjects, even if medical progress requires it. In his view, medical progress is only an optional goal and not an essential one.

Informed Consent and Proxy Consent

Most of the literature on the ethics of human experimentation is concerned with specifying the *conditions* under which human experimentation is ethically acceptable. Since World War II, at least thirty-three different guidelines and codes of ethics identifying these conditions have been formalized. Foremost among these are the two codes included in this chapter—"The Nuremberg Code" and the "Declaration of Helsinki." Common to all these codes is the principle that experimentation cannot be conducted on human subjects without their informed consent. Intensive discussions of the informed consent requirement are commonplace in the literature on human experimentation. Some writers offer justifications of the requirement. Others discuss the difficulties of applying it in practice. Still others focus on questions dealing with the use of research subjects who cannot meet the conditions for informed consent.

The Justification and Application of the Informed Consent Requirement   The *justifications* offered for the requirement that no human beings be used as experimental subjects without their informed consent are similar to those advanced to justify the requirement in the ordinary (nonresearch) biomedical context. The primary argument, advanced from a deontological perspective, rests on the principle of respect for persons. Respect for human beings as persons requires that their autonomy be promoted and protected. Research that uses human subjects without their consent violates that autonomy and is, therefore, morally unacceptable. Paul Ramsey, one of the main proponents of this position, holds that informed consent is the "chief canon of loyalty" between two persons—the biomedical researcher and the patient-subject. It serves as a deontological check on any attempt to justify the use of human subjects solely on utilitarian grounds, insofar as it affirms that human beings are not objects to be used, without their consent, for others' benefit. In Ramsey's view only individuals who (1) are capable of knowingly involving themselves in a common cause with the researcher and (2) are willing to participate as research subjects may serve in that capacity.

The problems raised in *applying* the informed consent requirement in the research context are similar to those raised by the requirement in the ordinary (nonresearch) biomedical context and are discussed in Chapter 2. The problems stem from the requirement's three components: (1) the consentee must be informed; (2) the consentee must be competent to give consent; and (3) the consent must be voluntary. In a reading in this chapter, Franz J. Ingelfinger argues that research subjects do not typically satisfy all these conditions even when they are capable of signing the necessary forms or giving oral assent. Such empirical claims about problems associated with the application of the informed consent requirement are parts of a larger discussion that also includes conceptual and ethical dimensions. The meanings of concepts such as "voluntary" must be explicated, for example, before it can be determined what counts as "voluntary" consent. Then in a particular case, it must be empirically determined whether the individuals giving consent can meet the conditions required for "voluntary" consent. Ethical issues are also intertwined with the conceptual and empirical ones. Take the geriatric patient, mentioned by Ruth Macklin in Chapter 3, who suffers from Alzheimer's disease. Without research, the development of cures or preventive measures will not be possible. If it is necessary to use those suffering from Alzheimer's as research subjects, what rules should be adopted to gauge whether they are capable of giving consent? Someone in the earlier stages of the disease may fluctuate between periods of "competency" and "incompetency," complicated by the effects of the disease and the influence of medication. Should assent given during a "competent" period override dissent expressed during an "incompetent" one? Neither conceptual analysis alone nor empirical studies can answer this kind of question.

Proxy Consent for Research Subjects Incapable of Informed Consent   Since children, especially young children, cannot give informed consent because they lack the competence to assess information about research procedures, any research using them as subjects apparently violates the informed consent requirement. When the research project is primarily therapeutic and is reasonably expected to benefit the child, it is less troublesome. Here, as in the case of validated therapies, it is usually agreed that proxies, such as parents and guardians, can legitimately consent on the child's behalf. However, when the procedure is not intended to directly benefit the child but to acquire knowledge that will benefit future patients, the child's participation in the research is morally problematic. Is it ever morally correct for parents and guardians to consent in their children's behalf to the latter's participation in nontherapeutic research?

Proponents of research using children cite its benefits to children as a group. Children are not just "little adults" in sickness or in health. Results of studies on adults cannot be simply extrapolated to children. To cite just one example, it would be disastrous to administer intravenous fluids to infants and children on the basis of adult requirements. Children would be given too much or too little. The requirements for specific age groups can only be identified by studying the normal constituents of body fluids and metabolism in normal infants and children. There are also a number of diseases, like infantile autism, that are unique to children. For these, as well as many other reasons, the use of children as research subjects is required for medical progress that will eventually benefit children as a group. In view of these potential gains, some proponents of research using children advance arguments to justify the validity of proxy consent.

One such proponent, Richard A. McCormick, argues that parents can give a valid proxy consent to nontherapeutic pediatric research when (1) the risks of such research are minimal and (2) the potential benefits to *children as a group* may be very great. McCormick's claim is based on his "natural law" ethics. Human beings are, by their very nature, social beings. As social beings, they are mutually interdependent. As mutually interdependent beings, they owe it to each other to perform certain minimal moral duties. Included in these moral duties is the duty to participate in minimally risky nontherapeutic research whose benefit to society as a whole may be very great. Children as members of society also have these obligations, although they are too young to recognize them. Since children, like adults, should want to promote the greater social good, it is morally acceptable for their parents to consent to their participation in minimally risky experiments.[2]

Perhaps no one is more opposed to using children as subjects in nontherapeutic research than Ramsey, whose argument is included in a reading in this chapter. In Ramsey's view, it is always wrong to subject children to procedures that are neither intended nor reasonably expected to directly benefit them. An experimental procedure holds the promise of directly benefiting a child if the procedure (1) is seen as the best means of effecting the child's recovery or (2) is intended to protect the child against some greater risk. Using young children in experimental trials of polio vaccines, for example, at a time when children were at risk of contracting the crippling disease summer after summer, was morally acceptable in Ramsey's view, because the risks of the experimental procedure had to be weighed against the dangers posed for the experimental subjects themselves by polio epidemics. Ramsey rejects the claim that using children as subjects in a nontherapeutic research project is morally acceptable when the intended beneficiaries are children as a group. His position is grounded in the claim (discussed earlier in this introduction) that all human experimentation must be a joint venture, freely undertaken by two autonomous persons. In keeping with this position, he refuses to recognize the validity of proxy consent to any nontherapeutic procedures. Although Ramsey's article focuses primarily on children, he extends the same line of reasoning to research involving incompetent adults, and he rejects the legitimacy of their use as research subjects in projects that hold no promise of benefiting them directly.

Barry F. Brown's argumentation in this chapter stands in sharp contrast to Ramsey's. Brown focuses on incompetent adults, specifically Alzheimer's patients, and defends their use in at least some nontherapeutic research projects. He develops a McCormick-type argument and maintains that proxy consent to participation in nontherapeutic research may be morally legitimate in the case of those who are in the advanced stages of Alzheimer's, so long as the intended beneficiaries of the research are potential Alzheimer's patients. In his view, what directly benefits the latter *indirectly* benefits the research subjects insofar as they are all members of a community or class with the same *common good*—the prevention of the harm resulting from the disease.

Experimental Design and Random Clinical Trials

Questions about informed consent are also raised in discussions of an especially important type of clinical trial—the randomized clinical trial (RCT). The RCT is a controlled comparison of two or more treatments in which the subjects are assigned at random or by chance to a particular treatment. In one of this chapter's readings, Bruce Miller explains what RCTs involve as well as the differences between them and other types of clinical trials. Miller also brings out some of the major ethical issues raised by RCTs, including those raised by the informed consent requirement when the patients, and often the professionals directly involved in their care, do not know just which treatment the patients are receiving. In a related article in this chapter, Paul S. Appelbaum et al. focus on the consent transaction involved in RCTs. They maintain that patients who supposedly give informed consent to participate in RCTs often still mistakenly believe that they are being given the therapy that is best for them as individuals, even though the experimental design may in fact preclude that.

Animal Experimentation

The use of animals in scientific experimentation intended to benefit human beings raises its own set of troubling questions. Is there any need to use animals in experiments intended to benefit human beings? Do animals have any moral status at all? If yes, do they have the same moral status as human beings so that whatever is morally illegitimate in the case of humans is also illegitimate in the case of animals? To answer the latter two questions, it is necessary to answer a prior question: What characteristic(s) must an entity possess if it is to be correctly described as having moral status? In this chapter's final reading, Arthur L. Caplan addresses these and other questions. He discusses the views of both proponents and opponents of animal experimentation before presenting his own reasoning regarding the moral status of animals and the implications of this reasoning for the morality of animal experimentation.

J.S.Z.

NOTES

1 On these distinctions, see Robert J. Levine, "Clarifying the Concepts of Research Ethics," *Hastings Center Report* 9 (June 1979), pp. 21–26.
2 Richard A. McCormick, "Proxy Consent in the Experimentation Situation," *Perspectives in Biology and Medicine* 18 (Autumn 1974), pp. 2–20.

Ethical Codes

The Nuremberg Code

"The Nuremberg Code of Ethics in Medical Research" was developed by the Allies after the Second World War. During the War Crimes Trials in Germany, this code provided the standards against which the practices of Nazis involved in human experimentation were judged. The Nuremberg Code emphasizes the essentiality of voluntary consent. Its first and longest article discusses consent in great detail. The code also sets forth other criteria that must be met before any experiment using human beings as subjects can be judged morally acceptable.

(1) The voluntary consent of the human subject is absolutely essential. This means that the person involved should have legal capacity to give consent; should be so situated as to be able to exercise free power of choice, without the intervention of any element of force, fraud, deceit, duress, overreaching, or other ulterior form of constraint or coercion; and should have sufficient knowledge and comprehension of the elements of the subject matter involved as to enable him to make an understanding and enlightened decision. This latter element requires that before the acceptance of an affirmative decision by the experimental subject there should be made known to him the nature, duration, and purpose of the experiment; the method and means by which it is to be conducted; all inconveniences and hazards reasonably to be expected; and the effects upon his health or person which may possibly come from his participation in the experiments.

The duty and responsibility for ascertaining the quality of the consent rests upon each individual who initiates, directs or engages in the experiment. It is a personal duty and responsibility which may not be delegated to another with impunity.

(2) The experiment should be such as to yield fruitful results for the good of society, unprocurable by other methods or means of study, and not random and unnecessary in nature.

(3) The experiment should be so designed and based on the results of animal experimentation and a knowledge of the natural history of the disease or other

Reprinted from *Trials of War Criminals before the Nuremberg Military Tribunals* (Washington, D.C.: U.S. Government Printing Office, 1948).

problem under study that the anticipated results [will] justify the performance of the experiment.

(4) The experiment should be so conducted as to avoid all unnecessary physical and mental suffering and injury.

(5) No experiment should be conducted where there is an a priori reason to believe that death or disabling injury will occur; except, perhaps, in those experiments where the experimental physicians also serve as subjects.

(6) The degree of risk to be taken should never exceed that determined by the humanitarian importance of the problem to be solved by the experiment.

(7) Proper preparations should be made and adequate facilities provided to protect the experimental subject against even remote possibilities of injury, disability, or death.

(8) The experiment should be conducted only by scientifically qualified persons. The highest degree of skill and care should be required through all stages of the experiment of those who conduct or engage in the experiment.

(9) During the course of the experiment the human subject should be at liberty to bring the experiment to an end if he has reached the physical or mental state where continuation of the experiment seems to him to be impossible.

(10) During the course of the experiment the scientist in charge must be prepared to terminate the experiment at any stage, if he has probable cause to believe, in the exercise of good faith, superior skill and careful judgment required of him that a continuation of the experiment is likely to result in injury, disability, or death to the experimental subject.

Declaration of Helsinki
World Medical Association

In 1964 the Eighteenth World Medical Assembly meeting in Helsinki, Finland, adopted an ethical code to be used as a guide by medical doctors involved in biomedical research involving human subjects. This code was revised at the Twenty-Ninth World Medical Assembly held in Tokyo, Japan, in 1975. The code reprinted here is the revised version. It has much in common with the Nuremberg Code (e.g., the informed consent requirement and the requirement that animal experimentation must precede human experimentation). The Helsinki Code, however, goes beyond the Nuremberg Code in certain important respects. Two differences are especially noteworthy: (1) The Helsinki Code distinguishes between clinical (therapeutic) and nonclinical (nontherapeutic) biomedical research and sets forth specific criteria of ethical acceptability for each, as well as other basic principles common to both. (2) The Nuremberg Code is silent regarding the informed consent requirement in the case of the legally incompetent. The Helsinki Code addresses itself to such cases, asserting the ethical acceptability of what is sometimes called "proxy consent."

INTRODUCTION

It is the mission of the medical doctor to safeguard the health of the people. His or her knowledge and conscience are dedicated to the fulfillment of this mission.

The Declaration of Geneva of The World Medical Association binds the doctor with the words, "The health of my patient will be my first consideration," and the International Code of Medical Ethics declares that, "Any act or advice which could weaken physical or mental resistance of a human being may be used only in his interest."

The purpose of biomedical research involving human subjects must be to improve diagnostic, therapeutic and prophylactic procedures and the understanding of the aetiology and pathogenesis of disease.

In current medical practice most diagnostic, therapeutic or prophylactic procedures involve hazards. This applies *a fortiori* to biomedical research.

Medical progress is based on research which ultimately must rest in part on experimentation involving human subjects.

In the field of biomedical research a fundamental distinction must be recognized between medical research in which the aim is essentially diagnostic or therapeutic for a patient, and medical research, the essential object of which is purely scientific and without direct diagnos-

tic or therapeutic value to the person subjected to the research.

Special caution must be exercised in the conduct of research which may affect the environment, and the welfare of animals used for research must be respected.

Because it is essential that the results of laboratory experiments be applied to human beings to further scientific knowledge and to help suffering humanity, The World Medical Association has prepared the following recommendations as a guide to every doctor in biomedical research involving human subjects. They should be kept under review in the future. It must be stressed that the standards as drafted are only a guide to physicians all over the world. Doctors are not relieved from criminal, civil and ethical responsibilities under the laws of their own countries.

I BASIC PRINCIPLES

(1) Biomedical research involving human subjects must conform to generally accepted scientific principles and should be based on adequately performed laboratory and animal experimentation and on a thorough knowledge of the scientific literature.

(2) The design and performance of each experimental procedure involving human subjects should be clearly formulated in an experimental protocol which should be transmitted to a specially appointed independent committee for consideration, comment and guidance.

(3) Biomedical research involving human subjects should be conducted only by scientifically qualified persons and under the supervision of a clinically competent medical person. The responsibility for the human subject must always rest with a medically qualified person and never rest on the subject of research, even though the subject has given his or her consent.

(4) Biomedical research involving human subjects cannot legitimately be carried out unless the importance of the objective is in proportion to the inherent risk to the subject.

(5) Every biomedical research project involving human subjects should be preceded by careful assessment of predictable risks in comparison with foreseeable benefits to the subject or to others. Concern for the interests of the subject must always prevail over the interests of science and society.

(6) The right of the research subject to safeguard his or her integrity must always be respected. Every precaution should be taken to respect the privacy of the subject and to minimize the impact of the study on the subject's physical and mental integrity and on the personality of the subject.

(7) Doctors should abstain from engaging in research projects involving human subjects unless they are satisfied that the hazards involved are believed to be predictable. Doctors should cease any investigation if the hazards are found to outweigh the potential benefits.

(8) In publication of the results of his or her research, the doctor is obliged to preserve the accuracy of the results. Reports of experimentation not in accordance with the principles laid down in this Declaration should not be accepted for publication.

(9) In any research on human beings, each potential subject must be adequately informed of the aims, methods, anticipated benefits and potential hazards of the study and the discomfort it may entail. He or she should be informed that he or she is at liberty to abstain from participation in the study and that he or she is free to withdraw his or her consent to participation at any time. The doctor should then obtain the subject's freely-given informed consent, preferably in writing.

(10) When obtaining informed consent for the research project the doctor should be particularly cautious if the subject is in a dependent relationship to him or her or may consent under duress. In that case the informed consent should be obtained by a doctor who is not engaged in the investigation and who is completely independent of this official relationship.

(11) In case of legal incompetence, informed consent should be obtained from the legal guardian in ac-

cordance with national legislation. Where physical or mental incapacity makes it impossible to obtain informed consent, or when the subject is a minor, permission from the responsible relative replaces that of the subject in accordance with national legislation.

(12) The research protocol should always contain a statement of the ethical considerations involved and should indicate that the principles enunciated in the present Declaration are complied with.

II MEDICAL RESEARCH COMBINED WITH PROFESSIONAL CARE (CLINICAL RESEARCH)

(1) In the treatment of the sick person, the doctor must be free to use a new diagnostic and therapeutic measure, if in his or her judgment it offers hope of saving life, reestablishing health or alleviating suffering.

(2) The potential benefits, hazards and discomfort of a new method should be weighed against the advantages of the best current diagnostic and therapeutic methods.

(3) In any medical study, every patient—including those of a control group, if any—should be assured of the best proven diagnostic and therapeutic method.

(4) The refusal of the patient to participate in a study must never interfere with the doctor-patient relationship.

(5) If the doctor considers it essential not to obtain informed consent, the specific reasons for this proposal should be stated in the experimental protocol for transmission to the independent committee (I, 2).

(6) The doctor can combine medical research with professional care, the objective being the acquisition of new medical knowledge, only to the extent that medical research is justified by its potential diagnostic or therapeutic value for the patient.

III NON-THERAPEUTIC BIOMEDICAL RESEARCH INVOLVING HUMAN SUBJECTS (NON-CLINICAL BIOMEDICAL RESEARCH)

(1) In the purely scientific application of medical research carried out on a human being, it is the duty of the doctor to remain the protector of the life and health of that person on whom biomedical research is being carried out.

Know (2) The subjects should be volunteers—either healthy persons or patients for whom the experimental design is not related to the patient's illness.

(3) The investigator or the investigating team should discontinue the research if in his/her or their judgment it may, if continued, be harmful to the individual.

(4) In research on man, the interest of science and society should never take precedence over considerations related to the well-being of the subject.

The Justifiability of Experimentation Using Human Subjects

Medical Research on Human Subjects as a Moral Imperative
Maurice B. Visscher

Maurice B. Visscher, M.D., is professor emeritus of physiology at the University of Minnesota Medical School. He is past president of the National Society for Medical Research. Visscher is the author of *Ethical Constraints and Imperatives in Medical Research* (1975), from which this selection is excerpted. He is also the editor of *Chemistry and Medicine* (1940) and *Humanistic Perspectives in Medical Ethics* (1972).

Visscher offers a justification for the use of human subjects in biomedical research. He maintains that such experimentation is necessary if physicians are to comply with the chief principle of traditional medical ethics, "First do no harm." If physicians are to avoid "unintentional" harm to their patients, Visscher argues, new therapies must be developed and tested. Since human beings differ physiologically from animals in other species, human subjects must ultimately be used as research subjects, even in those cases where animals can be used in the initial stages of research.

PRIMUM NON NOCERE

The use of human subjects in biomedical research is considered by scientists to be indispensable to progress in medical science and to consequent improvement in the art of medical practice, but the protection of the rights and welfare of every human being is equally a first priority of a civilized society. So long as these two basic precepts are not in conflict there are no major ethical problems in connection with scientific study on human subjects. However, there are situations in which the two objectives can clash, and then ethical problems arise.

In the practice of medicine the classic principle *primum non nocere* could be, if one knew what might be harmful, a simple rule to follow. Unfortunately even in ordinary medical practice such certainty is impossible. Intentional harm can be avoided, but unintentional

From Maurice B. Visscher, *Ethical Constraints and Imperatives in Medical Research*, 1975. Courtesy of Charles C. Thomas, Publisher, Springfield, Illinois.

harm cannot yet be avoided because of lack of adequate knowledge of human biology, broadly defined. Thus one comes, in attempting to fulfill the primary obligation of the medical profession, "first do no harm," to an ethical imperative to the profession as a whole and to the investigative physician specifically to make studies to learn how to avoid doing harm to patients. In other words, physicians frequently cannot properly perform their first function fully unless more research is done. This may be, to some, a different twist to the problem of ethics of medical practice, including the investigative use of human subjects, from the more simplistic views of the past. If it is, as seems obvious, obligatory upon physicians to learn how to do no harm, then scientific investigation, including that on human subjects, becomes a necessity for an ethical medical profession. Equally it becomes an activity [in] which society at large must, if it wishes to provide a milieu in which medicine can be practiced ethically, promote the conditions under which medical and related research can be carried out in harmony with humanistic ethics.

The learned pharmacologist, Nobel Laureate Professor B. N. Halpern,[1] who discovered and developed numerous widely used and important new therapeutic agents, has stated the case very convincingly. In a recent essay he wrote in connection with studies of drug toxicity and effectiveness:

I should like to stress yet again most forcefully that, in the interests of science and even of the protection of society against the absolutely unpredictable collective damage that the introduction of a new drug may cause, it is indispensable that trials in man should be included in pharmacological research.

The term "human experimentation" raises a sinister echo in each of us, for reasons known to us all. But fear solves no scientific problems. For my part, the recommendations...that safety tests of new drugs should be carried out on fully informed volunteers in conditions of almost absolute security—is more in conformity with the requirements of ethics than the thousands of such trials hypocritically carried out daily in hospitals in all countries on individuals who are totally ignorant of what is being done to them.

Writing on the topic, "Justification for the Human Trial," [Henry K.] Beecher[2] has said:

The importance of the project undertaken must be commensurate with the risk involved. The insurance of this is a cardinal responsibility of all who undertake experimentation in man. But having stated that important principle, there is still a vast area where judgment—one hopes sound judgment—must operate. Only the fanatic denies that animal experimentation must precede the human. As Sir Geoffrey Jefferson put it, "Man is too rare, too expensive, altogether too valuable an animal" to be first used in study of technical procedures or trial of even therapeutic agents. There are (nevertheless) species differences. Ultimately, the definitive test must be done in man.

This is obviously true because, although certain similarities are found in fundamental processes from the simplest organisms to man, as in the general mechanisms of information storage in the genetic apparatus, and in the basic building blocs of certain enzymes, there are also very important differences between species, becoming greater the farther they are apart in the phylogenetic tree. Even within a single genus the possibilities for variations in gene combinations are so great that aside from single ovum twins or the products of many generations of inbreeding important differences between individuals are evident in many characteristics. Histoincompatibility as a cause of the usual homograft rejection is evidence that even at the molecular level individuality is the rule. Fortunately for the applicability of blood transfusion in therapy is the existence, as first discovered by Landsteiner, of major blood types, within which differences in properties of agglutinins for red blood cells are ordinarily so small as to permit survival of the cells. An extension of Landsteiner's discovery, and others based upon it, into the field of tissue and organ transplantation is also yielding promising results.

It is, of course, not only in the area of immunology that individuality is important. Reactions to drugs of all sorts differ, not only in different species but among individuals of a single species or even a single genus. For example, the doses of digitalis glycosides required to produce a given effect in a rat are orders of magnitude higher than those needed per unit body weight in a cat or a man. Some drug effects seen in one species, or even in an entire family within a particular class, are not seen at all in another class. It is partly for these reasons that drug studies must be carried out in many species of lower animals before even planning to use them in man. And because of the intraspecies and intragenus variability of individuals, one must eventually study the effects of new agents on large numbers of humans in order to know what the limiting parameters for both efficacy and safety are. Furthermore the physician must know how to assess the idiosyncracies of individual patients in their responsiveness to pharmaceutical agents, and must understand as much as is known about the principles of action of such agents if he is to be a reliable physician.

There is also a need to study human subjects in connection with disease entities which are unique to man, or almost so. Likewise with respect to nervous and mental processes, although much can be learned by studies on lower animals, particularly with respect to basic neural mechanisms, there remain those features of function that are uniquely human which would forever remain shrouded in mystery if the scientific method were not to be employed to throw light upon them.

In other words, it is a fanciful dream concocted in the minds of scientific illiterates that medical science, or any other biological science, could progress without the study of actual living systems, and ultimately in the case of medicine, study of living human subjects.

There is a corollary to these lines of reasoning. It is that there is an ethical imperative for physicians as a group to promote medical research, including studies on human subjects. Obviously for various reasons not every physician can be an investigator, but at least every physician should give moral support to the enterprise of advancement of medical knowledge. The vast majority of physicians accept this view in principle, but in practice many fail to act to promote the medical research enterprise.

The conclusions of Claude Bernard[3] in his *Introduction to the Study of Experimental Medicine*, written a little more than a century ago, are undoubtedly pertinent today. He said, "For we must not deceive ourselves, morals do not forbid making experiments on one's neighbor or on one's self; in everyday life men do nothing but experiment on one another. Christian morals forbid only one thing, doing ill to one's neighbor. So, among the experiments that may be tried on man, those that can only harm are forbidden, those that are innocent are permissible, and those that may do good are obligatory."

REFERENCES

1 Halpern, B. N.: CIOMS round tables: 1. *Biomedical Science and the Dilemma of Human Experimentation.* Paris, UNESCO House, 1967, pp. 30, 31.
2 Beecher, Henry K.: *Experimentation in Man.* Springfield, Thomas, 1958, p. 32.
3 Bernard, Claude as translated by Henry Copley Greene: *An Introduction to the Study of Experimental Medicine.* U.S.A., Henry Schuman, 1927, p. 102.

Philosophical Reflections on Experimenting with Human Subjects
Hans Jonas

Hans Jonas is professor emeritus of philosophy at the New School for Social Research. His areas of specialization are ancient philosophy, metaphysics, and ethics. Jonas is the author of several works including *Phenomenon of Life* (1968), *The Phenomenon of Life: Toward a Philosophical Biology* (1983), and *The Imperative of Responsibility: In Search of an Ethics for the Technological Age* (1985). He has also published a collection of his essays, *Philosophical Essays: From Ancient Creed to Technological Man* (1974). This collection includes such articles as "Biological Engineering—A Preview" and "Against the Stream: Comments on the Definition and Redefinition of Death."

Jonas criticizes two arguments often given to justify using human beings as research subjects. (1) Medical experimentation is justified either because it will result in great benefits to society or because it will prevent great future harm. (2) Justice requires that we, who are the beneficiaries of past research, in turn accept the obligation to participate in such research. Jonas maintains against (1) that most of the biomedical research using human subjects is not essential to the well-being or survival of the species. Furthermore, he holds, we do not have a strict obligation to advance medical progress. Jonas maintains against (2) that past participants in medical research performed altruistic acts. If we owe *them* anything, we owe them a debt of gratitude. We do not owe any obligation to *society in general* to participate in medical research simply because we are the beneficiaries of past research. Jonas does not claim that all experimentation on human subjects is unjustified. He does hold, however, that the first volunteers for such experimentation should be the researchers themselves or other members of the scientific community. These are the individuals who are most capable of giving truly educated informed consent and who are best able to identify with the purposes of the research projects.

Experimenting with human subjects is going on in many fields of scientific and technological progress. It is designed to replace the over-all instruction by natural, occasional experience with the selective information from artificial, systematic experiment which physical science has found so effective in dealing with inanimate nature. Of the new experimentation with man, medical is surely the most legitimate; psychological, the most dubious; biological (still to come), the most dangerous. I have chosen here to deal with the first only, where the case *for* it is strongest and the task of adjudicating conflicting claims hardest....

THE PECULIARITY OF HUMAN EXPERIMENTATION

Experimentation was originally sanctioned by natural science. There it is performed on inanimate objects, and this raises no moral problems. But as soon as animate, feeling beings become the subjects of experiment, as they do in the life sciences and especially in medical research, this innocence of the search for knowledge is lost and questions of conscience arise. The depth to which moral and religious sensibilities can become aroused over these questions is shown by the vivisection issue. Human experimentation must sharpen the issue as it involves ultimate questions of personal dignity and sacrosanctity. One profound difference between the human experiment and the physical (besides that between animate and inanimate, feeling and unfeeling nature) is this: The physical experiment employs small-scale, artificially devised substitutes for that about which knowledge is to be obtained, and the experimenter extrapolates from these models and simulated conditions to nature at large. Something deputizes for the "real thing"—balls rolling down an inclined plane for sun and planets, electric discharges from a condenser for real lightning, and so on. For the most part, no such substitution is possible in the biological sphere. We must operate on the original itself, the real thing in the fullest sense, and perhaps affect it irreversibly. No simulacrum can take its place. Especially in the human sphere, experimentation loses entirely the advantage of the clear division between vicarious model and true object. Up to a point, animals may fulfill the proxy role of the classical physical experiment. But in the end man himself must furnish knowledge about himself, and the comfortable separation of non-committal experiment and definitive action vanishes. An experiment in education affects the lives of its

subjects, perhaps a whole generation of schoolchildren. Human experimentation for whatever purpose is always *also* a responsible, non-experimental, definitive dealing with the subject himself. And not even the noblest purpose abrogates the obligations this involves.

This is the root of the problem with which we are faced: Can both that purpose and this obligation be satisfied? If not, what would be a just compromise? Which side should give way to the other? The question is inherently philosophical as it concerns not merely pragmatic difficulties and their arbitration, but a genuine conflict of values involving principles of a high order. May I put the conflict in these terms? On principle, it is felt, human beings *ought* not to be dealt with in that way (the "guinea pig" protest); on the other hand, such dealings are increasingly urged on us by considerations, in turn appealing to principle, that claim to override those objections. Such a claim must be carefully assessed, especially when it is swept along by a mighty tide. Putting the matter thus, we have already made one important assumption rooted in our "Western" cultural tradition: The prohibitive rule is, to that way of thinking, the primary and axiomatic one; the permissive counter-rule, as qualifying the first, is secondary and stands in need of justification. We must justify the infringement of a primary inviolability, which needs no justification itself; and the justification of its infringement must be by values and needs of a dignity commensurate with those to be sacrificed....

HEALTH AS A PUBLIC GOOD

The cause invoked [for medical experimentation] is health and, in its more critical aspect, life itself—clearly superlative goods that the physician serves directly by curing and the researcher indirectly by the knowledge gained through his experiments. There is no question about the good served nor about the evil fought—disease and premature death. But a good to whom and an evil to whom? Here the issue tends to become somewhat clouded. In the attempt to give experimentation the proper dignity (on the problematic view that a value becomes greater by being "social" instead of merely individual), the health in question or the disease in question is somehow predicated on the social whole, as if it were society that, in the persons of its members, enjoyed the one and suffered the other. For the purposes of our problem, public interest can then be pitted against private interest, the common good against the individual good. Indeed, I have found health called a national resource, which of course it is, but surely not in the first place.

In trying to resolve some of the complexities and ambiguities lurking in these conceptualizations, I have pondered a particular statement, made in the form of a question, which I found in the *Proceedings* of the earlier *Daedalus* conference: "Can society afford to discard the tissues and organs of the hopelessly unconscious patient when they could be used to restore the otherwise hopelessly ill, but still salvageable individual?" And somewhat later: "A strong case can be made that society can ill afford to discard the tissues and organs of the hopelessly unconscious patient; they are greatly needed for study and experimental trial to help those who can be salvaged."[1] I hasten to add that any suspicion of callousness that the "commodity" language of these statements may suggest is immediately dispelled by the name of the speaker, Dr. Henry K. Beecher, for whose humanity and moral sensibility there can be nothing but admiration. But the use, in all innocence, of this language gives food for thought. Let me, for a moment, take the question literally. "Discarding" implies proprietary rights—nobody can discard what does not belong to him in the first place. Does society then own my body? "Salvaging" implies the same and, moreover, a use-value to the owner. Is the life-extension of certain individuals then a public interest? "Affording" implies a critically vital level of such an interest—that is, of the loss or gain involved. And "society" itself—what is it? When does a need, an aim, an obligation become social? Let us reflect on some of these terms.

WHAT SOCIETY CAN AFFORD

"Can society afford...?" Afford what? To let people die intact, thereby withholding something from other people who desperately need it, who in consequence will have to die too? These other, unfortunate people indeed cannot afford not to have a kidney, heart, or other organ of the dying patient, on which they depend for an extension of their lease on life; but does that give them a right to it? And does it oblige society to procure it for them? What is it that *society* can or cannot afford—leaving aside for the moment the question of what it has a *right* to? It surely can afford to lose members through death; more than that, it is built on the balance of death and birth decreed by the order of life. This is too general, of course, for our question, but perhaps it is well to re-

member. The specific question seems to be whether society can afford to let some people die whose death might be deferred by particular means if these were authorized by society. Again, if it is merely a question of what society can or cannot afford, rather than of what it ought or ought not to do, the answer must be: Of course, it can. If cancer, heart disease, and other organic, noncontagious ills, especially those tending to strike the old more than the young, continue to exact their toll at the normal rate of incidence (including the toll of private anguish and misery), society can go on flourishing in every way.

Here, by contrast, are some examples of what, in sober truth, society cannot afford. It cannot afford to let an epidemic rage unchecked; a persistent excess of deaths over births, but neither—we must add—too great an excess of births over deaths; too low an average life expectancy even if demographically balanced by fertility, but neither too great a longevity with the necessitated correlative dearth of youth in the social body; a debilitating state of general health; and things of this kind. These are plain cases where the whole condition of society is critically affected, and the public interest can make its imperative claims. The Black Death of the Middle Ages was a *public* calamity of the acute kind; the life-sapping ravages of endemic malaria or sleeping sickness in certain areas are a public calamity of the chronic kind. Such situations a society as a whole can truly not "afford," and they may call for extraordinary remedies, including, perhaps, the invasion of private sacrosanctities.

This is not entirely a matter of numbers and numerical ratios. Society, in a subtler sense, cannot "afford" a single miscarriage of justice, a single inequity in the dispensation of its laws, the violation of the rights of even the tiniest minority, because these undermine the moral basis on which society's existence rests. Nor can it, for a similar reason, afford the absence or atrophy in its midst of compassion and of the effort to alleviate suffering—be it widespread or rare—one form of which is the effort to conquer disease of any kind, whether "socially" significant (by reason of number) or not. And in short, society cannot afford the absence among its members of *virtue* with its readiness for sacrifice beyond defined duty. Since its presence—that is to say, that of personal idealism—is a matter of grace and not of decree, we have the paradox that society depends for its existence on intangibles of nothing less than a religious order, for which it can hope, but which it cannot enforce. All the more must it protect this most precious capital from abuse.

For what objectives connected with the medico-biological sphere should this reserve be drawn upon—for example, in the form of accepting, soliciting, perhaps even imposing the submission of human subjects to experimentation? We postulate that this must be not just a worthy cause, as any promotion of the health of anybody doubtlessly is, but a cause qualifying for transcendent social sanction. Here one thinks first of those cases critically affecting the whole condition, present and future, of the community we have illustrated. Something equivalent to what in the political sphere is called "clear and present danger" may be invoked and a state of emergency proclaimed, thereby suspending certain otherwise inviolable prohibitions and taboos. We may observe that averting a disaster always carries greater weight than promoting a good. Extraordinary danger excuses extraordinary means. This covers human experimentation, which we would like to count, as far as possible, among the extraordinary rather than the ordinary means of serving the common good under public auspices. Naturally, since foresight and responsibility for the future are of the essence of institutional society, averting disaster extends into long-term prevention, although the lesser urgency will warrant less sweeping licenses.

SOCIETY AND THE CAUSE OF PROGRESS

Much weaker is the case where it is a matter not of saving but of improving society. Much of medical research falls into this category. As stated before, a permanent death rate from heart failure or cancer does not threaten society. So long as certain statistical ratios are maintained, the incidence of disease and of disease-induced mortality is not (in the strict sense) a "social" misfortune. I hasten to add that it is not therefore less of a human misfortune, and the call for relief issuing with silent eloquence from each victim and all potential victims is of no lesser dignity. But it is misleading to equate the fundamentally human response to it with what is owed to society: it is owed by man to man—and it is thereby owed by society to the individuals as soon as the adequate ministering to these concerns outgrows (as it progressively does) the scope of private spontaneity and is made a public mandate. It is thus that society assumes responsibility for medical care, research, old age, and innumerable other things not originally of the public realm (in the original "social contract"), and they become duties toward "society" (rather than directly to-ward one's fellow man) by the fact that they are socially operated.

Indeed, we expect from organized society no longer mere protection against harm and the securing of the conditions of our preservation, but active and constant improvement in all the domains of life: the waging of the battle against nature, the enhancement of the human estate—in short, the promotion of progress. This is an expansive goal, one far surpassing the disaster norm of our previous reflections. It lacks the urgency of the latter, but has the nobility of the free, forward thrust. It surely is worth sacrifices. It is not at all a question of what society can afford, but of what it is committed to, beyond all necessity, by our mandate. Its trusteeship has become an established, ongoing, institutionalized business of the body politic. As eager beneficiaries of its gains, we now owe to "society," as its chief agent, our individual contributions toward its *continued pursuit*. I emphasize "continued pursuit." Maintaining the existing level requires no more than the orthodox means of taxation and enforcement of professional standards that raise no problems. The more optional goal of pushing forward is also more exacting. We have this syndrome: Progress is by our choosing an acknowledged interest of society, in which we have a stake in various degrees; science is a necessary instrument of progress; research is a necessary instrument of science; and in medical science experimentation on human subjects is a necessary instrument of research. Therefore, human experimentation has come to be a societal interest.

The destination of research is essentially melioristic. It does not serve the preservation of the existing good from which I profit myself and to which I am obligated. Unless the present state is intolerable, the melioristic goal is in a sense gratuitous, and this not only from the vantage point of the present. Our descendants have a right to be left an unplundered planet; they do not have a right to new miracle cures. We have sinned against them, if by our doing we have destroyed their inheritance—which we are doing at full blast; we have not sinned against them, if by the time they come around arthritis has not yet been conquered (unless by sheer neglect). And generally, in the matter of progress, as humanity had no claim on a Newton, a Michelangelo, or a St. Francis to appear, and no right to the blessings of their unscheduled deeds, so progress, with all our methodical labor for it, cannot be budgeted in advance and its fruits received as a due. Its coming-about at all and its turning out for good (of which we can never be sure) must rather be regarded as something akin to grace.

THE MELIORISTIC GOAL, MEDICAL RESEARCH, AND INDIVIDUAL DUTY

Nowhere is the melioristic goal more inherent than in medicine. To the physician, it is not gratuitous. He is committed to curing and thus to improving the power to cure. Gratuitous we called it (outside disaster conditions) as a *social* goal, but noble at the same time. Both the nobility and the gratuitousness must influence the manner in which self-sacrifice for it is elicited, and even its free offer accepted. Freedom is certainly the first condition to be observed here. The surrender of one's body to medical experimentation is entirely outside the enforceable "social contract."

Or can it be construed to fall within its terms—namely, as repayment for benefits from past experimentation that I have enjoyed myself? But I am indebted for these benefits not to society, but to the past "martyrs," to whom society is indebted itself, and society has no right to call in my personal debt by way of adding new to its own. Moreover, gratitude is not an enforceable social obligation; it anyway does not mean that I must emulate the deed. Most of all, if it was wrong to exact such sacrifice in the first place, it does not become right to exact it again with the plea of the profit it has brought me. If, however, it was not exacted, but entirely free, as it ought to have been, then it should remain so, and its precedence must not be used as a social pressure on others for doing the same under the sign of duty....

THE "CONSCRIPTION" OF CONSENT

...The mere issuing of the appeal, the calling for volunteers, with the moral and social pressures it inevitably generates, amounts even under the most meticulous rules of consent to a sort of *conscripting*. And some soliciting is necessarily involved....And this is why "consent," surely a non-negotiable minimum requirement, is not the full answer to the problem. Granting then that soliciting and therefore some degree of conscripting are part of the situation, who may conscript and who may be conscripted? Or less harshly expressed: Who should issue appeals and to whom?

The naturally qualified issuer of the appeal is the research scientist himself, collectively the main carrier of the impulse and the only one with the technical competence to judge. But his being very much an interested party (with vested interests, indeed, not purely in the public good, but in the scientific enterprise as such, in "his" project, and even in his career) makes him also suspect. The ineradicable dialectic of this situation—a delicate incompatibility problem—calls for particular controls by the research community and by public authority that we need not discuss. They can mitigate, but not eliminate the problem. We have to live with the ambiguity, the treacherous impurity of everything human.

SELF-RECRUITMENT OF THE COMMUNITY

To whom should the appeal be addressed? The natural issuer of the call is also the first natural addressee: the physician-researcher himself and the scientific confraternity at large. With such a coincidence—indeed, the noble tradition with which the whole business of human experimentation started—almost all of the associated legal, ethical, and metaphysical problems vanish. If it is full, autonomous identification of the subject with the purpose that is required for the dignifying of his serving as a subject—here it is; if strongest motivation—here it is; if fullest understanding—here it is; if freest decision—here it is; if greatest integration with the person's total, chosen pursuit—here it is. With the fact of self-solicitation the issue of consent in all its insoluble equivocality is bypassed *per se*. Not even the condition that the particular purpose be truly important and the project reasonably promising, which must hold in any solicitation of others, need be satisfied here. By himself, the scientist is free to obey his obsession, to play his hunch, to wager on chance, to follow the lure of ambition. It is all part of the "divine madness" that somehow animates the ceaseless pressing against frontiers. For the rest of society, which has a deep-seated disposition to look with reverence and awe upon the guardians of the mysteries of life, the profession assumes with this proof of its devotion the role of a self-chosen, consecrated fraternity, not unlike the monastic orders of the past, and this would come nearest to the actual, religious origins of the art of healing....

NOTE

1 *Proceedings of the Conference on the Ethical Aspects of Experimentation on Human Subjects*, November 3–4, 1967 (Boston, Massachusetts), pp. 50–51.

Informed Consent and Proxy Consent

Informed (but Uneducated) Consent
Franz J. Ingelfinger

Franz J. Ingelfinger (1910–1980) was a physician who taught in the department of medicine, Boston University. He was also the editor of the *New England Journal of Medicine*, the journal of the Massachusetts Medical Society, from 1967 to 1977. In his capacity as editor, Ingelfinger frequently wrote editorials dealing with issues in biomedical ethics. He was the coeditor of *Controversy in Internal Medicine* (1974). His articles include "Medicine: Meritorious or Meretricious?" and "Arrogance."

Ingelfinger discusses some of the problems raised in *applying* the informed consent requirement. He questions the capacity of most patient-subjects to adequately comprehend the information given by the physician-investigator. Ingelfinger also holds that any investigator-subject relation involves some coercion on the part of the investigator. If free choice requires the absence of all such coercion as well as adequate comprehension of the pertinent information, he contends, then in most cases the "process of obtaining informed consent is no more than elaborate ritual conferring no more than the semblance of propriety on human experimentation."

The trouble with informed consent is that it is not educated consent. Let us assume that the experimental subject, whether a patient, a volunteer, or otherwise enlisted, is exposed to a completely honest array of factual detail. He is told of the medical uncertainty that exists and that must be resolved by research endeavors, of the time and discomfort involved, and of the tiny percentage risk of some serious consequences of the test procedure. He is also reassured of his rights and given a formal, quasilegal statement to read. No exculpatory language is used. With his written signature, the subject then caps the transaction, and whether he sees himself as a heroic martyr for the sake of mankind, or as a reluctant guinea pig dragooned for the benefit of science, or whether, perhaps, he is merely bewildered, he obviously has given his "informed consent." Because established routines have been scrupulously observed, the doctor, the lawyer, and the ethicist are content.

But the chances are remote that the subject really understands what he has consented to—in the sense that the responsible medical investigator understands the goals, nature, and hazards of his study. How can the layman comprehend the importance of his perhaps not re-

ceiving, as determined by the luck of the draw, the highly touted new treatment that his roommate will get? How can he appreciate the sensation of living for days with a multi-lumen intestinal tube passing through his mouth and pharynx? How can he interpret the information that an intravascular catheter and radiopaque dye injection have an 0.01 per cent probability of leading to a dangerous thrombosis or cardiac arrhythmia? It is moreover quite unlikely that any patient-subject can see himself accurately within the broad context of the situation, to weigh the inconveniences and hazards that he will have to undergo against the improvements that the research project may bring to the management of his disease in general and to his own case in particular. The difficulty that the public has in understanding information that is both medical and stressful is exemplified by [a] report [in the *New England Journal of Medicine*, August 31, 1972, page 433]—only half the families given genetic counseling grasped its impact.

Nor can the information given to the experimental subject be in any sense totally complete. It would be impractical and probably unethical for the investigator to present the nearly endless list of all possible contingencies; in fact, he may not himself be aware of every untoward thing that might happen. Extensive detail, moreover, usually enhances the subject's confusion. Epstein

Reprinted by permission from the *New England Journal of Medicine*, vol. 287, no. 9 (August 31, 1972), pp. 465–466.

and Lasagna showed that comprehension of medical information given to untutored subjects is inversely correlated with the elaborateness of the material presented.[1] The inconsiderate investigator, indeed, conceivably could exploit his authority and knowledge and extract "informed consent" by overwhelming the candidate-subject with information.

Ideally, the subject should give his consent freely, under no duress whatsoever. The facts are that some element of coercion is instrumental in any investigator-subject transaction. Volunteers for experiments will usually be influenced by hopes of obtaining better grades, earlier parole, more substantial egos, or just mundane cash. These pressures, however, are but fractional shadows of those enclosing the patient-subject. Incapacitated and hospitalized because of illness, frightened by strange and impersonal routines, and fearful for his health and perhaps life, he is far from exercising a free power of choice when the person to whom he anchors all his hopes asks, "Say, you wouldn't mind, would you, if you joined some of the other patients on this floor and helped us to carry out some very important research we are doing?" When "informed consent" is obtained, it is not the student, the destitute bum, or the prisoner to whom, by virtue of his condition, the thumb screws of coercion are most relentlessly applied; it is the most used and useful of all experimental subjects, the patient with disease.

When a man or woman agrees to act as an experimental subject, therefore, his or her consent is marked by neither adequate understanding nor total freedom of choice. The conditions of the agreement are a far cry from those visualized as ideal. Jonas would have the subject identify with the investigative endeavor so that he and the researcher would be seeking a common cause: "Ultimately, the appeal for volunteers should seek... free and generous endorsement, the appropriation of the research purpose into the person's [i.e., the subject's] own scheme of ends."[2] For Ramsey, "informed consent" should represent a "covenantal bond between consenting man and consenting man [that] makes them ...joint adventurers in medical care and progress."[3] Clearly, to achieve motivations and attitudes of this lofty type, an educated and understanding, rather than merely informed, consent is necessary.

Although it is unlikely that the goals of Jonas and of Ramsey will ever be achieved, and that human research subjects will spontaneously volunteer rather than be "conscripted,"[2] efforts to promote educated consent are

in order. In view of the current emphasis on involving "the community" in such activities as regional planning, operation of clinics, and assignment of priorities, the general public and its political leaders are showing an increased awareness and understanding of medical affairs. But the orientation of this public interest in medicine is chiefly socioeconomic. Little has been done to give the public a basic understanding of medical research and its requirements not only for the people's money but also for their participation. The public, to be sure, is being subjected to a bombardment of sensation-mongering news stories and books that feature "break-throughs," or that reveal real or alleged exploitations—horror stories of Nazi-type experimentation on abused human minds and bodies. Muckraking is essential to expose malpractices, but unless accompanied by efforts to promote a broader appreciation of medical research and its methods, it merely compounds the difficulties for both the investigator and the subject when "informed consent" is solicited.

The procedure currently approved in the United States for enlisting human experimental subjects has one great virtue: patient-subjects are put on notice that their management is in part at least an experiment. The deceptions of the past are no longer tolerated. Beyond this accomplishment, however, the process of obtaining "informed consent," with all its regulations and conditions, is no more than elaborate ritual, a device that, when the subject is uneducated and uncomprehending, confers no more than the semblance of propriety on human experimentation. The subject's only real protection, the public as well as the medical profession must recognize, depends on the conscience and compassion of the investigator and his peers.

REFERENCES

1 Epstein, L. C., Lasagna, L.: "Obtaining informed consent: form or substance." *Arch Intern Med* 123:682–688, 1969.
2 Jonas, H.: "Philosophical reflections on experimenting with human subjects." *Daedalus* 98:219–247, Spring, 1969.
3 Ramsey, P.: "The ethics of a cottage industry in an age of community and research medicine." *N Engl J Med* 284:700–706, 1971.

Consent as a Canon of Loyalty with Special Reference to Children in Medical Investigations
Paul Ramsey

Paul Ramsey is Harrington Spear Paine Professor of Religion at Princeton University. His books include *The Patient as Person: Explorations in Medical Ethics* (1970), *Fabricated Man: The Ethics of Genetic Control* (1970), *Ethics at the Edges of Life* (1978), and *Deeds and Rules in Christian Ethics* (1980). He is also the editor of *Jonathan Edwards: Ethical Writings* (1989).

According to Ramsey, the principle of informed consent is the "cardinal canon of loyalty," which joins people together in medical practice and investigation. In his view, experimentation on a human subject, which is not for that subject's benefit, can never be justified if it is performed without the subject's free and informed consent. Since young children are incapable of giving such consent, research involving children should never be allowed unless participation in such research benefits the child. The use of an experimental procedure on children is morally justified only if the procedure is either (1) seen as the best means to effect the child's own recovery from an illness or disease or (2) intended to protect the child against some greater risk.

From consent as a canon of loyalty in medical practice it follows that children, who cannot give a mature and informed consent, or adult incompetents, should not be made the subjects of medical experimentation unless, other remedies having failed to relieve their grave illness, it is reasonable to believe that the administration of a drug as yet untested or insufficiently tested on human beings, or the performance of an untried operation, may further *the patient's own recovery*.

Now that is not a very elaborate moral rule governing medical practice in the matter of experiments involving children or incompetents as human subjects. It is a good example of the general claims of childhood specified for application in medical care and research. It is also a qualification immediately entailed by the meaning of consent in medical investigations as a joint undertaking between men. Again, one has to be prudent (which does not mean overcautious or scrupulous) in order to know how to care for child-patients in this way. One must know the possible relation of a proposed procedure to the child's own recovery, and also its likely effectiveness compared with other methods that have been or could be tried. These considerations may provide the doctor with necessary and sufficient reason for investiga-

tions upon children, perhaps even very hazardous ones. One has to proportion the peril to the diagnostic or therapeutic needs of the child.

Practical medical judgment has undeniable and ominous room for its determinations, since a "benefit" is whatever is *believed* to be of help to the child. Still the limits this rule imposes on practice are essentially clear; where there is no possible relation to the child's recovery, a child is not to be made a mere object in medical experimentation for the sake of good to come. The likelihood of benefits that could flow from the experiment for many other children is an equally insufficient warrant for child experimentation. The individual child is to be tended in illness or in dying, since he himself is not able to donate his illness or his dying to be studied and worked upon solely for the advancement of medicine. Again, future experience may tell us more about the meaning of this particular rule expressive of loyalty to a human child, and we may learn a great deal more about how to apply it in new situations with greater sensitivity and refinement—or we may learn more and more how to practice violations of it. But we are committed to refraining from morally significant exceptions to this rule defining impermissible medical experimentation upon children.

To experiment on children in ways that are not related to them as patients is already a sanitized form of barbarism; it already removes them from view and pays

Reprinted with permission of the publisher from Paul Ramsey, *The Patient as a Person* (New Haven, Conn.: Yale University Press, 1970).

no attention to the faithfulness-claims which a child, simply by being a normal or a sick or dying child, places upon us and upon medical care. We should expect no morally significant exceptions to this canon of faithfulness to the child. To expect future justifiable exceptions is, in some sense, already to have forgotten the child. . . .

To attempt to consent for a child to be made an experimental subject is to treat a child as not a child. It is to treat him as if he were an adult person who has consented to become a joint adventurer in the common cause of medical research. If the grounds for this are alleged to be the presumptive or implied consent of the child, that must simply be characterized as a violent and a false presumption. Nontherapeutic, nondiagnostic experimentation involving human subjects must be based on true consent if it is to proceed as a human enterprise. No child or adult incompetent can choose to become a participating member of medical undertakings, and no one else on earth should decide to subject these people to investigations having no relation to their own treatment. That is a canon of loyalty to them. This they claim of us simply by being a human child or incompetent. When he is grown, the child may put away childish things and become a true volunteer. This is the meaning of being a volunteer: that a man enter and establish a consensual relation in some joint venture for medical progress—where before he could not, nor could anyone else, "volunteer" him for submission to unknown possible hazards for the sake of good to come.

If the requirement of parents, investigators, and state authorities in regard to their wards is "Never subject children to the unknown possible hazards of medical investigations having no relation to their own treatment," we must understand that the maladies for which the individual needs treatment and protection need not already be resident within the compass of the child's own skin. He can properly be regarded as one of a population, and we can add to the foregoing words: "except in epidemic conditions." Dr. Salk tried his polio vaccine on himself and his own children first. Then it was tested on selected children within a normal population. This involved some risk for the children vaccinated, and for other children as well, that the disease *might* be contracted from the vaccine itself, or that there might be unexpected injurious results. But the normal population of children was already subjected to waves of crippling epidemic summer after summer. A parent consenting for his child to be used in this trial was balancing the risks from the trial against the hazards from polio itself for that same child.

Physician-investigators are often in a quandary in which they are torn between the warrants for giving an experimental drug, and the warrants for withholding it from anyone in order to test it. Neither act seems justified, or both acts are equally warranted, when there is no available remedy and the indications are that a new drug may succeed. This situation also justifies a parent or guardian in consenting for a child, since we are supposing the hazard of the proposed treatment to be less or no greater than the hazard of the disease itself when treated by the established procedures. That would be a medical trial having clear relation to the treatment or protection of the child himself. He is not made, without his consent, the subject of medical investigations of possible benefit only to other children, other patients, or for the future advancement of medical science.

These may have been the circumstances surrounding the field trial of the vaccine for rubella (German measles) made in Taiwan, if this was in epidemic conditions, or in expectation of epidemic conditions, early in 1968 by a medical team from the University of Washington, headed by Dr. Thomas Grayston.[1] The vaccine was given to 3,269 young grade-school boys in the cities of Taipei and Taichung, while roughly an equal number were left unvaccinated for comparison purposes. The latter group were given Salk polio vaccine so that they would derive some benefit from the experience to which they were subjected. This generous "payment" does not alter the moral dilemma of withholding the rubella vaccine from a selected group. Yet there may have been an equipoise between the hazards of contracting rubella or other damage from the vaccine and the hazards of contracting it if not vaccinated. There could have been a likelihood favoring the vaccinated of the two comparison groups.

These considerations, we may suppose, produced the quandary in the conscience of the investigators that was partially relieved by giving the unrelated Salk vaccine to the control group. Such equipoise alone would warrant—and it would sufficiently warrant—a parent or guardian in consenting that his child or ward be used for these research purposes. In the face of actual or predictable epidemic conditions, this would be medical investigation having some measurable or immeasurable relation to a child's own treatment or protection, as surely as the catheterization of the heart of a child with congenital heart trouble may be needed in his own diagnosis and treatment; and to this type of treatment a parent may venture to consent in his child's behalf. If no gulf is to be fixed between maladies beneath the skin and diseases afflicting children as members of a population, then the consent-requirement means: "Never submit children to medical investigation not related to their own treatment, except in face of epidemic conditions, endangering also each individual child." This is simply the meaning of the consent-requirement in application, not a "quantity-of-benefit-to-come" exception clause or a violation of this canon of loyalty to child-patients.

Indeed, a stricter construction of the necessary connection between proxy consent and the foreseeable needs of the child would permit the use of only girl children in field trials of rubella vaccine. Rubella is not the most contagious type of measles. The benefit to the subjects used in these trials (which plus the consent of parents legitimated subjecting them to experiment) was mainly to prevent their giving birth to children with congenital malformations should they later contract rubella during pregnancy. Therefore, there was stronger argument for considering only girl children as part of a population in establishing the necessary connection between experiment and "treatment."

More questionable were the earlier trials of the rubella vaccine performed upon the inmates of a retarded children's home in Conway, Arkansas. These subjects were not specially endangered by an epidemic of rubella. Few of the girls among them will ever be able to become part of the population of child-bearing women, or be in danger of pregnancy while in institutions. Using them simply had the advantage that they were segregated from the rest of the population, and any degree of risk to them would not spread to other people, including women of child-bearing age.

If children are incapable of truly consenting to experiments having unknown hazards for the sake of good to come, and if no one else should consent for them in cases unrelated to their own treatment, then medical research and society in general must choose a perhaps more difficult course of action to gain the benefits we seek from medical investigations. Surely it was possible to secure normal adult volunteers to consent to segregate themselves from the rest of the population for the duration of a rubella trial.[2] That method was simply more costly and inconvenient. At the same time, this illustrates the general fact that if we as a society are to proceed to the conquest of diseases, indeed, if we are to teach medical skills with fairness and justice to the poor and the ward patients, and with no violation of the basic claims of childhood, then there must be far greater encouragement generally in our society of a willingness to engage as joint adventurers for medical progress than has been achieved, or believed morally required by the principle of consent, in the past....

NOTES

1 *New York Times*, October 17, 1968.
2 *New York Times*, April 5, 1969, reported that a hundred monks and nuns, from both Anglican and Roman Catholic orders, living in enclosed communities, were the voluntary subjects in testing American, British, and Belgian vaccines against German measles. This project was organized and directed by Dr. J. A. Dudgeon of London's Great Ormond Street Hospital for Sick Children.

Proxy Consent for Research on the Incompetent Elderly
Barry F. Brown

Barry F. Brown is associate professor of philosophy at St. Michael's College, University of Toronto. His areas of specialization are metaphysics and ethics, including biomedical ethics. Brown is the author of *Accidental Beings: A Study in the Metaphysics of St. Thomas Aquinas* (1985).

Brown argues (1) that some research using borderline or definitely incompetent elderly patients is justified and (2) that relatives can legitimately give proxy consent for patients' use as research subjects even though the patients cannot directly benefit from their participation. The moral legitimacy of proxy consent to participation in research that benefits the participant is taken for granted in Brown's argument. However, he widens the scope of relevant benefits so that it includes certain indirect benefits. Brown's argument is based on a conception of the relationship between the individual good and the societal or common good. He argues that research ethics require a conception of the *common good* that (1) is narrower than that of society as a whole and yet transcends immediate benefit to an individual and (2) includes the individual's good rather than being in opposition to it. On Brown's analysis, if the "community" with which the research subject is identified consists of those who have a stake in the amelioration or prevention of the disease from which the individual suffers, then the subject who participates in research intended to benefit members of that community is indirectly benefited as a member of that group, since the good of the class is "his" good. Brown ends on a cautionary note, indicating the need for stringent protective procedures.

In the past decade, the ethical issues of research with the elderly have become of increasing interest in gerontology, medicine, law, and biomedical ethics. In particular, the issue has been raised whether the elderly deserve special protection as a dependent group (Ratzan 1980). One of the most profound difficulties in this area of reflection is that of the justification of proxy consent for research on borderline or definitely incompetent patients.

Some diseases of the elderly, such as Alzheimer's disease, cause senile dementia: devastating for the patient and family and, in future, a considerable burden for society. This condition, in turn, renders a patient incapable of giving informed, voluntary consent to research procedures designed to learn about the natural history of the disease, to control it, and to find a cure. The research must be done on human subjects, since there is not as yet a suitable animal model; indeed some feel that there never can be such a model. A protection of the patient, rooted in concern for his best interests, from procedures to which he cannot give consent gives rise to a paradox: "If we can only perform senile dementia research using demented patients, but should not allow them to participate because they are incompetent, then we are left in a quandary. We cannot ethically conduct senile dementia research using demented patients because they are incompetent; but we cannot technically perform it using competent subjects because they are not demented" (Ratzan 1980: 36). Such a position seems to protect demented patients at the expense of their exposure, as a class, to prolonged misery or death.

If the patient cannot give consent, is the proxy consent of relatives ethically valid? That is, do the relatives have the moral right or capacity to give consent for procedures that may not offer much hope for the patient in that they may not offer a direct benefit to him?

Such procedures have by recent convention been called non-therapeutic. They might offer a possible benefit for other sufferers in the future, but little hope of benefit for *this* patient, here and now.

At present, an impasse has developed regarding such research. It appears that such procedures might be illegal under criminal laws on assault. If the research is strictly non-therapeutic, then no benefit is to be found for the patient-subject. If the requirement of therapeutic experimentation is that a direct, or fairly immediate, improvement in the patient's condition is the sole benefit that could count, then it is difficult to see how this could be discovered. For unlike the case of a curable disease or research on preventive measures for childhood diseases, such as polio, the Alzheimer's patients suffer from a presently terminal illness. Studies of the causation of this condition may hold little or no hope of alleviating the condition in them. There appears to be no present or future benefit directly accruing to them. Others may benefit, but they likely will not. Thus, it seems, there is no benefit in view.

If, in fact, such procedures, even relatively innocuous ones, are illegal, then such research cannot go ahead. If so, such persons will remain "therapeutic orphans" just as surely as infants and children unless proxy consent is valid. If proxy consent is also legally invalid, then the legal challenge to this impasse may be either legislative or judicial. In either case, ethical arguments must be offered as justification for the case that proxy consent is or ought to be legally valid. The following explorations are a contribution to that debate.

Can some kind of benefit for the demented be found in research that offers no immediate hope of improvement? I believe that it can, but the nature of that benefit will be unfamiliar or unacceptable to those who are sure that there are only two mutually exclusive alternatives: a utilitarian conception of the social good pitted against a deontological notion of the individual's rights.

Contemporary biomedical ethics routinely employs three principles in its effort to resolve such dilemmas (Reich 1978; Beauchamp & Childress 1983). These are the principle of beneficence, which demands that we do good and prevent harm; the principle of respect for persons (or the principle of autonomy), from which flows the requirement of informed consent; and the principle of justice, which demands the equitable distribution of the benefits and burdens of research. But the first two obviously conflict with each other in human experimentation: the principle of beneficence, which mandates research to save life and restore health, especially if this is seen as directed to the good of society, is in tension with the principle of respect for persons, which requires us to protect the autonomy of subjects. Moreover, the principle of beneficence requires us not only to benefit persons as patients through research, but also to avoid harming them as research subjects in the process. So there is an internal tension between moral demands created by the same principle. Finally, demented patients are no longer fully or sufficiently autonomous. Standard objections to paternalism do not apply. Consequently paternalism of the parental sort is not inappropriate, but rather necessary in order to protect the interest of the patient.

Simple application of these principles, therefore, will not provide a solution. Underlying the manner in which they are applied are radically different conceptions of the relationship of the individual good to the societal or common good.

In the present framework of philosophical opinion, there appear to be two major positions. On the one hand, some consequentialist arguments for non-therapeutic research justify non-consensual research procedures on the grounds that individual needs are subordinate to the general good conceived as an aggregate of individual goods. This good, that of the society as a whole, can easily be seen to take precedence over that of individuals. This is especially so if the disease being researched is conceptualized as an "enemy" of society. On the other hand, a deontological position argues that the rights of the individual take precedence over any such abstract general good as the advancement of science, the progress of medicine, or the societal good. In this view, to submit an individual incapable of giving or withholding consent to research procedures not for his own direct benefit is to treat him solely as a means, not as an end in himself. In this debate, one side characterizes the general good proposed by the other as much too

broad and inimical to human liberty; the other sees the emphasis on individual rights as excessively individualistic or atomistic.

There are strengths and weaknesses in both approaches. The consequentialist rightly insists on a communal good, but justifies too much; the deontologist rightly protects individual interests, but justifies too little. I contend that if we are to resolve the dilemma concerning the incompetent "therapeutic orphan," it is necessary to go between these poles. In order to do so, I wish to draw upon and develop some recent explorations concerning non-therapeutic research with young children. In at least one important respect, that of incompetence, children and the demented are similar. We ought to treat similar cases similarly. I wish also to argue that research ethics requires: (1) a conception of the *common good* that is at once narrower than that of society as a whole and yet transcends immediate benefit to a single individual; and (2) a conception of the common good that sees it not in opposition to the individual good but including it, so that the good is seen as distributed to individuals.

THE LESSON OF RESEARCH WITH CHILDREN

As to the first, we may learn much from the discussions concerning research with children, particularly as they bear upon the distinction between therapeutic and non-therapeutic experimentation. In the 1970s a spirited debate took place between the noted ethicists Paul Ramsey and Richard McCormick on the morality of experimentation with children (Ramsey 1970, 1976, 1977; McCormick 1974, 1976). Ramsey presented a powerful deontological argument against non-therapeutic experimentation with children. Since infants and young children cannot give consent, an essential requirement of the canon of loyalty between researcher and subject, they cannot be subjected ethically to procedures not intended for their own benefit. To do so, he contended, is to treat children solely as means to an end (medical progress), not as ends in themselves (Ramsey 1970).

McCormick, arguing from a natural law position similar to that developed in the next section, argued that since life and health are fundamental natural goods, even children have an obligation to seek to preserve them. Medical research is a necessary condition of ensuring health, and this is a desirable social goal. Consequently children, as members of society, have a duty in social justice to wish to accept their share of the burdens of participating in research that promises benefit to society and is of minimal or no risk. Thus the parents' proxy consent is a reasonable presumption of the child's wishes if he were able to consent (McCormick 1974).

There are two major puzzles generated by this debate over non-therapeutic research in children. First, Ramsey stressed that the condition to which a child may be at risk need not reside within his skin, but could be an epidemic dread disease. Thus, testing of preventive measures such as polio vaccine on children is justified; indeed it counts for Ramsey as therapeutic. This is interesting for several reasons. First, the therapeutic benefit may be indirect or remote, not necessarily immediate. Second, it embodies the concept of a group or population at risk smaller than society as a whole. Third, it apparently allows for considerable risk. There was a risk of contracting polio from the vaccine. Although the risk might have been slight statistically, the potential damage was grave. By Ramsey's own account, a slight risk of grave damage is a grave risk. Thus, he was prepared to go beyond the limit of minimal or no risk on the grounds that the polio vaccine was *therapeutic*, while McCormick attempted to justify *non-therapeutic* research on children, but confined the risk to minimal or none. It is odd that in the subsequent protracted debate, this difference was not contested.

The second major puzzle arises from McCormick's view that fetuses, infants, and children ought to participate in low- or no-risk non-therapeutic research in order to share in the burden of social and medical progress in order that all may prosper. Note that only *burdens* are to be shared, not benefits. This is because the topic by definition was non-therapeutic experimentation. By putting it this way he seemed to many to be subordinating the interests of such subjects to a very broadly construed societal good. But let us remember that the argument for such research in the first place was that without it, infants and children would be "therapeutic orphans." That is, without pediatric research, there could be fewer and slower advances in pediatric therapy.

Although not of direct benefit, such research is intended for the long-term benefit of children, and is thus indirectly or remotely therapeutic. It is not conducted for "the benefit of society" or for "the advancement of medical science"; it is for children in the future. Otherwise, it could be carried out on adults. Thus, such research should be construed as done not in view of broad social benefit but for the benefit of children as a group or a sub-set of society. Of course, if advances are made in

medicine for the sake of children, society benefits as well, but this is incidental and unnecessary. The sole justification is provided by the benefits now and to come for *children*. At the same time, such benefits set one of the limits for such research: it should be confined to children's conditions, and should not be directed at conditions for which the research may be done on competent persons.

THE COMMON GOOD OF A DISEASE COMMUNITY

Some of the hints arising from the foregoing debate can now be developed. It is indeed wrong to experiment on an incompetent person for "the benefit of society" if the research is unrelated to that person's disease and he is made a subject simply because he is accessible and unresistant. But is it necessarily unethical to conduct experiments on an incompetent person which attempt to discover the cause of the condition which causes the incompetence, and which may cure it or prevent it in others, even if he will not himself be cured?

In a "third way" of conceptualizing the relation between the individual and the group, the good in view is neither that of society as a whole nor that of a single individual. It involves the group of persons with a condition, such as Alzheimer's disease. Here I turn to a conception of the common good articulated by John Finnis of Oxford. Finnis defines the common good not as the "greatest good for the greatest number" but as "a set of conditions which enables the members of a community to attain for themselves reasonable objectives, or to realize reasonably for themselves the value(s) for the sake of which they have reason to collaborate with each other (positively and/or negatively) in a community" (Finnis 1980: 155).

The community may be either the complete community or the political one, or it may be specialized, such as the medical community, the research community, or the community of children with leukemia, and so on. The common good is thus not the sum total of individual interests, but an ensemble of conditions which enable individuals to pursue their objectives or purposes, which enable them to flourish. The purposes are fundamental human goods: life, health, play, esthetic experience, knowledge, and others. Relevant to this discussion are life, health, especially mental integrity, and the consequent capacity for knowledge, all of which are threatened by diseases which cause dementia.

For my purposes, the community should be considered to be, at a minimum, those suffering from Alzheimer's disease. They have, even if they have never explicitly associated with each other, common values and disvalues: their lost health and the remaining health and vitality they possess. It could be said with McCormick that if they could do so, they would reasonably wish the good of preventing the condition in their relatives and friends.

But the community may be rightly construed more broadly than this. It naturally includes families with whom the patients most closely interact and which interact in voluntary agencies devoted to the condition, the physicians who treat them, the nurses, social workers, and occupational therapists who care for them, and the clinical and basic researchers who are working to understand, arrest, cure, and prevent the disease.

The participation of the patient, especially the demented patient, may be somewhat passive. He is a member of the specialized community by accident, not by choice, unless he has indicated his wish to become a research subject while still competent. Efforts to determine what a demented or retarded person would have wished for himself had he been competent have been made in American court decisions involving an incompetent patient's medical care. These "substituted judgment" approaches may have some worth, especially if the patient had expressed and recorded his wishes while still competent.

An individual might execute a document analogous to a human tissue gift—a sort of pre-dementia gift, in which he would officially and legally offer his person to medical research if and when he became demented. This might alleviate the problem of access to some extent, but it has its own difficulties. A pre-dementia volunteer cannot know in advance what types of research procedures will be developed in future, and so cannot give a truly informed consent except to either very specific procedures now known or to virtually anything. Such a precommitment may give some support to the decision to allow him to be a subject. But that decision, I contend, is justified by the claim, if valid, that it is for the common good of the dementia-care-research community, of which he is a member and to which, it is presumed, he would commit himself if he were capable of doing so at the time.

It is true, of course, that one might not ever have wished to participate in research procedures. In this case, the individual should be advised to register his or her objection in advance, along the lines that have been suggested for objection to organ donation in those countries that have a system of presumed consent for such donation. This can be achieved by carrying a card on which such an opt-out is recorded, or by placing one's name on a registry which might be maintained by support organizations. I suggest that unless one opt out in this manner, in the early stages of the disease, he or she be considered to have opted-in. That is, there should be a policy of presumed consent. In any event, as experience with organ retrieval has shown, in the final analysis it is the permission of relatives that is decisive in both those cases in which an individual has consented and those in which he or she has not made his or her wishes known.

The other members of the community may not all know each other. They do, however, have common values and, to a considerable degree, common objectives. There can be a high level of deliberate and active interaction, especially if there is close communication between the researchers, family, and volunteers in the voluntary health agencies.

What, then, is the ensemble of conditions which constitute the common good of the Alzheimer's community? Insofar as the purposes of collaboration include the effort to cure or to alleviate the disease, the common good would embrace, in addition to caring health professionals, a policy of promoting research, its ethical review, a sufficient number of committed clinical and scientific researchers, the requisite physical facilities and funding (some or all of which may be within other communities such as hospitals and medical schools), availability of volunteers for research, an atmosphere of mutual trust between researcher and subject, and finally ongoing research itself. This list is not exhaustive.

If access to the already demented is not allowed, and if this is essential for research on the disease to continue, it may well be impossible to find the answers to key questions about the disease. The common good of the Alzheimer's community would be damaged or insufficiently promoted. Since the goods of life and mental health are fundamental goods, this insufficiency would be profound.

One essential aspect of this common good is distributive justice. Each patient-subject shares not only in the burdens of research in order that all may prosper, but also the benefits. The benefits are not necessarily improved care or cure for the subject, but generally improved conditions for all such patient-subjects: a more aggressive approach to research, improved knowledge of the disease, increased probabilities for a cure, and others. Since the individual participates wholly in that good, he will be deprived of it in its entirety if it is not pursued. The common good is not so much a quantity of benefits as a quality of existence. It can therefore be distributed in its fullness to each member of the community. So, too, each can suffer its diminution.

Richard McCormick (1974) left his description of the common good unnecessarily broad and sweeping. According to some natural law theorists (Maritain 1947) the common good is always a distributed good, not simply the sum of parts. It is construed as flowing back upon the individual members of the community, who are not simply parts of a whole but persons, to whom the common good is distributed in its entirety. Thus, not only can the common good of which McCormick speaks be narrowed to that of children as a group (equivalent to Ramsey's population at risk) but the benefits of such research can be seen as redistributed to the individuals of the group. The benefits are not to be taken in the sense of an immediately available therapy, but in the sense of improved general conditions under which a cure, amelioration, or prevention for all is more likely.

CONCLUSION

Some of these observations can now be applied to the case of the elderly demented. First, the debate showed the inadequacy of the simple distinction between therapeutic and non-therapeutic experimentation, which has been challenged on several grounds in past years. For example, May (1976: 83) includes diagnostic and preventive types of research under therapeutic experimentation, whereas Reich (1978: 327) observes that the terms "therapeutic" and "non-therapeutic" are inadequate because they do not seem to include research on diagnostic and preventive techniques. In the area of the development of experimental preventive measures such as vaccines for epidemic diseases, and in the area of diseases in which research is carried out on terminal patients with little or no expectation of immediate benefit for these patients, the distinction is somewhat blurred. In each case, there is a defined population at risk: one without the disease but at great risk of contracting it, the other with a disease but with little hope of benefiting from the research.

Such types of research seem to constitute an intermediate category: the "indirectly therapeutic," involving the hope of either prevention or alleviation or cure. This category as applied to dementia shows some char-

acteristics of therapeutic experimentation in the accepted sense, since it is carried out on persons who are ill and it is directed to their own illness. But it also shares some properties of non-therapeutic research, since it is not for their immediate treatment and, therefore, benefit. The good to be achieved is more remote, both in time and in application, since it is less sharply located in the individual than is therapy as such.

It must be admitted that there is a difference between the testing of a vaccine for prevention of disease in young, healthy children and research on elderly, seriously ill patients. In the former, the child-subjects will benefit if the vaccine is successful, or at least be protected from harm. In the latter, the subjects will not benefit by way of prevention or cure of their disease, but rather simply by being part of a community in which those goals are being actively pursued. The identification of the demented patient's good with that common good is doubtless less concrete than the identification of the child's good with that of his peers. But it seems to me that underlying both these cases is a notion of the common good required to justify all cases of research that do not promise a hope of direct benefit to a person who is, here and now, ill.

Years ago, Hans Jonas (1969) noted that a physician-researcher might put the following question to a dying patient: "There is nothing more I can do for you. But there is something you can do for me. Speaking no longer as your physician but on behalf of medical science, we could learn a great deal about future cases of this kind if you would permit me to perform certain experiments on you. It is understood that you yourself would not benefit from any knowledge we might gain; but future patients would." Although greatly vulnerable and deserving of maximum protection, such a patient might be ethically approached to be a research subject, because the benefits to future patients are in a way a value to him: "At least that residue of identification is left him that it is his own affliction by which he can contribute to the conquest of that affliction, his own kind of suffering which he helps alleviate in others; and so *in a sense it is his own cause*" (Jonas 1969: 532, emphasis mine).

In this case, the individual apprehends a good greater than his personal good, less than that of society: that of his disease class, which is *his* good. Of course, the identification of which Jonas speaks is psychological; he would likely not agree with the approach herein outlined and might require that such participation be through a conscious, free choice of the patient. Nevertheless, it is a real, objective good which justifies his choice and prevents us from asking him to participate in research unrelated to his disease. Can a relative, a son or daughter perhaps, ethically make that decision for an incompetent, demented Alzheimer's patient? If so, it is because, in a sense, it is the patient's cause, the patient's good as a member of a community which justifies that choice. It is not a matter of enforcing a social duty or minimal social obligation here, but seeking a good that lies in the relationship one has to others with the same disease. That same good, as noted above, limits the participation of the subject to research related precisely to his disease, not to anything else.

What is the implication of this for risk and the limits of risk? As has been seen, some wish to allow for exposure of subjects to greater than minimal risk provided only that it is classified as "therapeutic" (though the subjects are not ill). Others, in spite of the fact that the research is intended for the benefit of a group at risk, classify it as non-therapeutic and limit the acceptable risk to minimal levels. Are these the only alternatives? One advisory group has allowed, in the case of the mentally incompetent, for a "minor increase over minimal risk" in such circumstances (National Commission for the Protection of Human Subjects 1978: 16). This is presumably permitted because the research is "of vital importance for the understanding or amelioration of the type of disorder or condition of the subjects" or "may reasonably be expected to benefit the subjects in future" (17). But what counts as minor increase in risk? Proposed research into Alzheimer's might involve invasive procedures such as brain biopsies, implantation of electrodes, spinal taps, and injections of experimental drugs. Are these of greater risk than that specified by the National Commission simply because they are invasive of the human brain? Or is there clear statistical risk of serious added damage to the brain? These are matters for empirical study. The invasiveness per se should not rule out a procedure. The major limitations should be whether the procedure is painful, causes anxiety, or adds to the already serious damage to the brain. If research involving procedures of greater risk than "minor increase over minimal" is ever to be justified, it must be so by the intent to avert the proportional evils of death or mental incapacity. If these are insufficient, then I fail to see what grounds might be available upon which to base a case for legislative change.

It is clear, then, that should such research be acceptable, it also demands that stringent protective procedures be established in order to ensure that the demented are not drafted into research unrelated to their disease class. This is because the standard, being broader than that of "direct or fairly immediate benefit," is open to an accordionlike expansion, and therefore to abuse. Such safeguards could include: rigorous assurance that the proxy's consent (in reality, simply a permission) is informed and voluntary, the provision of a consent auditor, and various layers of administrative review and monitoring, from a local institutional review board up to a judicial review with a guardian appointed to represent the patient-subject's rights. These procedures may prove to be onerous. But we are on dangerous ground, and as we try to avoid overprotection, which may come at the expense of improved therapy for all, we must also avoid opening up a huge door to exploitation.

REFERENCES

Beauchamp, T.L., & Childress, J.F. (1983). *Principles of biomedical ethics.* 2nd ed. New York: Oxford University Press

Finnis, J. (1980). *Natural law and natural rights.* Oxford: Clarendon Press

Jonas, H. (1969). Philosophical reflections on experimenting with human subjects. In T. Beauchamp and L. Walters (Eds.), *Contemporary issues in bioethics.* 2nd ed. Belmont, CA: Wadsworth

Maritain, J. (1947). *The person and the common good.* New York: Charles Scribner's Sons

May, W. (1976). Proxy consent to human experimentation. *Linacre Quarterly, 43,* 73–84

McCormick, R. (1974). Proxy consent in the experimentation situation. *Perspectives in Biology and Medicine, 18,* 2–20

McCormick, R. (1976). Experimentation in children: sharing in sociality. *Hastings Center Report, 6,* 41–46

National Commission for the Protection of Human Subjects (1978). *Report and recommendations: Research involving those institutionalized as mentally infirm.* Washington, DC

Ramsey, P. (1970). *The patient as person.* New Haven: Yale University Press

Ramsey, P. (1976). The enforcement of morals: Non-therapeutic research on children. *Hastings Center Report, 4,* 21–30

Ramsey, P. (1977). Children as research subjects: a reply. *Hastings Center Report, 2,* 40–41

Ratzan, R. (1980). "Being old makes you different": The ethics of research with elderly subjects. *Hastings Center Report, 5*, 32–42

Reich, W. (1978). Ethical issues related to research involving elderly subjects. *Gerontologist, 18*, 326–37

The Ethics of Random Clinical Trials
Bruce Miller

Bruce Miller is professor and chair of the department of philosophy at Michigan State University. He specializes in philosophy of law and medical ethics. He is also assistant coordinator of the medical humanities program in the College of Human Medicine at the university. Miller's published articles include "Autonomy and the Refusal of Life Saving Treatment."

Miller explains the structure of a random clinical trial (RCT) and the differences between noncontrolled and controlled trials, providing examples of each. He identifies and discusses three categories of ethical issues raised by clinical trials: (1) issues dealing with the initiation of a trial, (2) issues regarding the termination of a trial, and (3) issues regarding informed consent. Miller concludes that the use of RCTs is not justifiable unless the patient-subjects are competent and knowingly and voluntarily risk their own interests.

INTRODUCTION

Before a medical treatment is approved today as effective and safe, a controlled trial of the treatment must be done. This is frequently done in a random clinical trial (RCT), the gold standard of medical research methods. The RCT is a controlled comparison of two treatments whose design uses the techniques of modern statistics. The aim of this [article] is to explore the ethical issues in the use of RCTs.

THE STRUCTURE OF A RANDOM CLINICAL TRIAL

The purpose of an RCT is to determine which of two or more treatments is safer or more effective for a given illness. The subjects are selected for admission to a trial on

From *Health Care Ethics: An Introduction*, edited by Donald VanDeVeer and Tom Regan, pp. 128–138, 152–157. Copyright © 1987 by Temple University. Reprinted by permission of Temple University Press.

the basis of diagnostic criteria formulated as precisely as possible in order to ensure that they all have the same illness. Next, the subjects are randomly assigned to the treatment alternatives. If an RCT is double-blind, neither the patients nor physicians know which treatment a patient is receiving. Results of the treatments are collected and these data then are analyzed using appropriate statistical techniques. Finally, conclusions are drawn regarding the relative effectiveness of the treatments. The effectiveness of a treatment is measured by relief of symptoms as reported by the subjects or observed by a physician, or by more objective features such as a reduction in the incidence of death, nonrecurrence of the disease, or an alteration in laboratory tests such as blood counts, X-rays, and biopsies. The risks in a treatment are the side effects, which can be anything from death to minor matters like nausea and dizziness. Other items may include whether the two groups of subjects were comparable with respect to influencing factors such as age, sex, prior illness, and severity of illness, whether the results of the research show that one treatment is always to be preferred over the other, or whether one treatment seems best only for a certain class of patients.

Aspects of a Random Clinical Trial

Five aspects of the RCT need further explanation: (1) the use of a control group; (2) the placebo effect; (3) double-blinding; (4) random assignment; and (5) statistical significance. One of the reasons for a control group is that the knowledge sought is whether the new treatment is better than existing treatments. A trial without a control may show that the new treatment has some effect and that it has certain side effects, but that may not indicate whether it is more effective or safer than an existing treatment. Sometimes there is no existing treatment, or none that has any significant effect; the control group then may be given a placebo. A placebo is something that is believed to have no biological effect on a patient's illness. In drug therapy, a placebo will be a substance like a sugar pill or an injection of sterile water or saline solution.

The reason for using a placebo control group is that there is a placebo effect to every medical treatment. A person who is ill and who believes that a physician can do something that will relieve the illness typically will have some improvement from the belief alone. The physician's belief that he or she is doing something beneficial to the patient may contribute to the patient's improvement. Part of the effect of every treatment is a result of these symbolic aspects of the patient-physician relationship. To determine the effectiveness of a medical treatment in a research trial, the trial must be structured to distinguish the placebo effect of the treatment from the biological effect of the treatment.

Another reason for the use of a control group is to distinguish the effects of the treatment from the effects of other factors. Suppose that a group of patients is diagnosed as having a certain disease to a certain degree; let's call that condition A. Suppose all these patients are given a drug and six weeks later none of them has condition A. One might conclude that the drug caused this, but condition A may have disappeared independent of the drug rather than because of it. Condition A may simply have run its natural course. If the patients were hospitalized, the environmental change may have been the cause. A methodological postulate of science is that if all we know is that one set of events or conditions preceded another event or condition, we cannot conclude that one particular preceding event or condition was the cause of the subsequent event or condition. The RCT attempts to construct two groups that are identical in all respects except that one group receives one treatment and the other group another. If one group shows significantly more improvement than the other, this improvement can be attributed to the treatment, because that is the only relevant difference between the two groups.

Random assignment to alternative treatments randomly distributes the many possible influencing factors so that it can be assumed that the groups of subjects are alike in all respects, and differences in outcome can be attributed to the difference in treatments. Another reason for using random assignments of subjects is to eliminate bias in the selection of treatment. If a decision must be made whether each patient will receive treatment A or treatment B, physicians may assign a greater portion of the less ill patients to one of the treatments without being conscious of doing so.

The reason for using a double-blind is to avoid any bias of subjects or physicians in reporting or recording patients' symptoms. If a patient knows that he or she is receiving a placebo, he or she may not expect to get well and therefore may not. However, if a patient knows that he or she is receiving a newly discovered treatment that is thought by physicians to hold out great promise of a cure, this may influence the patient's beliefs and reports about how the treatment is working. If the physician who examines the patient knows which of the treatments the patient is receiving, this can influence the physician's reports on the patient. A physician need not have a conscious belief that one treatment is better than another to be biased; a mere hunch, or a personal interest in the results of the trial, may be sufficient to cause lack of uniformity in the observation and care of patients in the trial.

The concept of *statistical significance* is of importance in discussions of the ethical issues of RCTs. There are many different methods of determining statistical significance. They will be described briefly and intuitively here. Consider a simple coin-tossing example. Suppose I toss a coin twice and both times it comes up heads. Prior to any toss of this particular coin, the chances of tossing a head and of tossing a tail are equal. This is expressed by saying that the probability of a head is .5 and the probability of a tail is .5. After two successive heads are tossed, suppose someone claims that the coin is rigged so that it always comes up heads. We probably would reply that the conclusion is not warranted because there have only been two tosses; a nonrigged coin might produce two heads in a row. Suppose eight more heads are tossed. Now it is more plausible to say that the coin is rigged, because it is very unlikely that one would toss ten heads in a row. The statistical significance of the claim that the coin is rigged is greater after ten heads in a row than after two heads in a row.

The concept of statistical significance is fairly easy to understand in the coin-tossing example; in other contexts, the notion of statistical significance is more complicated. We now will consider a simple medical example to explain the notion in a more relevant context. Suppose there are two drugs, A and B. Suppose we wish to know whether A or B is more effective in reducing mortality from a given disease. A and B are randomly assigned to patients with the disease, and we determine whether the patients are dead or alive at some particular period of time after receiving the drug. Suppose four patients enter into the trial, and two of them receive drug A and die, while two receive drug B and survive. Prior to the trial, the hypotheses that we might form about drug A and drug B are that there is no difference in their effect on mortality, that there is a 100 percent difference in their effect on mortality, or anything in between. Based on the results in four patients, the no-difference hypothesis seems unsupported, while the alternatives have received some support. We would not have much warrant to conclude that B is 100 percent more effective than A, for there is not much support from the four instances of administering the drugs. Suppose the drugs are administered sixteen more times, with ten patients receiving drug A and ten patients receiving drug B, and, as before, all the patients on A die and all the patients on B survive. Now we could be much more confident of the claim that B is 100 percent more effective than A in preventing death.

This hypothetical example is more clear-cut than the usual result of medical research; rarely is there a 100 percent difference in mortality for two treatments. This is because of the biological variability of individuals. We are not exactly alike biologically, and thus diseases and treatments affect us differently. A more common result in a trial of the sort we are imagining is that the survival rate for B was 60 percent, and the survival rate for drug A was 40 percent. However, the same point applies regarding the number of subjects in the trial (the sample size). If the 60–40 percent difference were obtained after five patients were put on each drug, that would be less significant statistically than if the same difference were obtained after twenty patients were put on each drug. Statisticians are able to determine the number of patients required in a trial in order to reach a given level of significance. There is a consensus that a certain level of significance is desired. In one version of the test of statistical significance, that level is expressed as $P \leq .05$. This

means that there is less than a one in twenty chance (probability of .05) that there is no difference in the medical effects of the two treatments, and that the difference is the result of the chance allocation of more good-prognosis patients to one treatment than another (this assumes that the patients are being randomly assigned to the two treatments). If the significance level is less than .05, then more confidence can be placed in the view that the difference is the result of the treatment, if it is greater than .05, then less confidence is justifiable. Statisticians admit that a significance level of .05 is somewhat arbitrary. Since significance is a matter of degree, no strong arguments can be given that a medical researcher ought to strive for a level of .05 rather than .06 or .07. The importance of this point will be discussed later.

There are many alternatives to the RCT. Some of them are elaborate adaptations of modern techniques of statistical analysis and will not be discussed in this paper. The procedures which will be considered are the RCT and consecutive trials. In a trial of the latter sort, as the name suggests, each subject enrolled, in succession, is given the experimental treatment. Consecutive trials do not have the same kind of controls as the RCTs mentioned above. The next section discusses research on the treatment of a disease, first by a consecutive trial and then by an RCT.

Examples of a Noncontrolled and a Controlled Trial

A group of researchers were working on the possible beneficial effects of cryogenic therapy (i.e., treating disease by lowering the temperature of all or part of the body). Among the diseases studied was peptic ulcer, a lesion or wound in the stomach wall caused by excess gastric secretion of acid. It is a common disease that can cause death. The technique developed was "gastric freezing." A tube was inserted into the stomach; at the end of the tube was a balloon. The tube was constructed so that a cold liquid could be circulated through the balloon and thereby lower the temperature of the stomach. The procedure initially was tried with dogs, and it was discovered that the freezing reduced the secretion of acids and caused structural changes in the tissue of the stomach wall. The procedure was then tried on patients who had been admitted to the hospital for surgical treatment of peptic ulcer. Thirty-one patients received the gastric freeze. The treatment lasted for about one hour with temperature maintained at -12 to -20 degrees centigrade. The investigators stated that all patients reported a marked or complete relief of subjective symptoms (e.g., stomach pain), and thirty of the thirty-one patients showed a significant decrease in the secretion of acid, an objective measure. The researchers concluded that the treatment appeared simple, effective and safe. In an addendum to the article, they reported that 120 patients had now received the treatment without complication.[1]

In the years immediately following this report, the procedure was introduced in many hospitals. Reports began to arise regarding complications, and many physicians raised questions about the long-term effectiveness of the treatment. A prominent medical journal surveyed physicians using the procedure and reported that although there was an initial decrease in acid secretion, there was a return to the previous level of secretion within six weeks to six months. Nonetheless, patients continued to report a significant improvement in symptoms.

At this point, the evidence on the effectiveness of gastric freezing for peptic ulcer was ambiguous. Although the treatment did provide relief of symptoms, the fact that the reduction of acid secretion does not persist raises doubts about the effectiveness. The symptoms of peptic ulcer, abdominal pain and nausea, are the result of excess secretion of acid, but since the treatment did not maintain reduced levels of acid secretion, there were doubts that the symptomatic improvement was a result of the freezing of the stomach. It may be that there was some other physiological mechanism bringing about the improvement in symptoms, or it may have been a placebo effect. To resolve these issues, a controlled trial was needed.

In a controlled trial of gastric freezing, one group of patients would have to receive the treatment and another group would have to receive a treatment that resembles the gastric freezing so closely that neither they nor the physicians examining them could know which they received. It would be easy to keep the examining physicians in ignorance: just don't tell them. The problem was to make the patients in the control group believe that they were receiving a real gastric freeze. The researchers designed a tube and balloon that resembled the equipment for the gastric freeze except that cold liquid did not circulate in the balloon. In the sham procedure, the temperature in the balloon was at 37 degrees Centigrade. Cold liquid did circulate in the tube, so the patients felt the cold in their mouth and throat, and believed their stomachs were being cooled.

One hundred and sixty patients were randomly assigned. Eighty-two received the freeze treatment; seventy-eight received the sham treatment. All patients were followed for thirteen months. Six weeks after the treatment, 47 percent of the freeze patients reported that they were improved or symptom free compared with 39 percent of the sham patients. However, as time passed, most patients in both groups relapsed or became worse: at 12 months, 28 percent in the freeze group and 30 percent in the sham group relapsed. At no time was there a significant difference in the two groups. Measurement of acid secretion was done before and immediately after treatment and at every follow-up visit. There was no significant difference in the levels of gastric secretion before and after treatment. The researchers concluded that "this study demonstrates conclusively that the 'freezing' procedure was no better than the sham in the treatment of duodenal ulcer.... It is reasonable to assume that the relief of pain and subjective improvement reported by early investigators was probably due to the psychologic effect of the procedure."[2]

ETHICAL ISSUES ABOUT CLINICAL TRIALS

The ethical issues in the two trials of gastric freezing can be divided into three categories: first, issues about the initiation of a trial; second, issues regarding the termination of a trial; and third, issues regarding informing patients and obtaining their consent to be subjects in the trial of a medical procedure.

Issues of Initiation

When the uncontrolled trial of gastric freezing was started, was it ethical to treat the patients with a procedure whose effectiveness and safety were not determined? There are standard surgical treatments for patients with ulcers, and the effectiveness and safety of those treatments are known; they are not fully satisfactory, since they do not prevent recurrence and there is a significant risk to any patient who undergoes surgery with general anesthesia. Still, a patient and his or her physician have evidence on which to judge whether or not it is in the interest of the patient to undergo the standard surgical treatments. Though there is some evidence that the gastric freeze will be effective and safe, a patient with an ulcer cannot be assured that the gastric freeze is the best treatment.

Whether the interests of patients were being sacrificed was also a question in the controlled trial of the gastric freeze treatment. After the noncontrolled trial was published, many physicians who adopted the procedure reported that although there was symptomatic relief, there was no evidence that the level of acid secretion was reduced for a significant time. There may have been enough evidence from these reports to determine that gastric freezing was not an effective treatment. The fact that several controlled trials were done shows that medical researchers believed that either (1) there was insufficient evidence to show that the treatment was not effective, or (2) though the evidence was sufficient, a controlled trial had to be done to persuade others. The freeze treatment is more convenient and safer than the usual surgical treatment, and some distinguished medical researchers believed it to be effective; thus, there was some ground for a physician to use the treatment. In order to stop these physicians from using the treatment, a controlled study was done to show conclusively that the treatment is not effective. If it is not, then the patients who were entered into the controlled trial of gastric freezing had their interests sacrificed in the interest of future patients.

A crucial ethical issue in clinical research emerges: *Is it justifiable to sacrifice the interest of current patients by making them subjects in an RCT to determine what is most beneficial for future patients?* If the answer to this question is no, then a significant restraint is placed on progress in medicine. Research on new treatments would not be totally forbidden, but it would be permissible only in those cases in which it could be shown that everything that was done to a patient was in the best interest of *that patient*. Just how much current research would be unjustified is difficult to say. Research on fatal diseases for which there is no effective life-saving treatment would be permissible, as would research on patients whose condition is terminal because they have not responded to conventional treatments. Experimentation with treatments for nonfatal diseases for which there is no effective treatment would be justifiable provided the side effects of the new treatment were known, and known not to be more severe than allowing the disease to run its course.

Another ethical question emerges from consideration of the idea that the justification for medical research is the benefit of future patients. The researchers who did the initial trials of gastric freezing chose to do a noncontrolled trial. Animal trials were done, but all researchers know that such results are not directly transferable to human beings. The researchers also knew, or should have known, that all treatments have a placebo effect; this is especially true for the symptoms of ulcers.

Any effectiveness shown in a noncontrolled trial may be the result largely, or entirely, of the placebo effect. To benefit future patients, researchers must show that a treatment has more than a placebo effect and more effect than treatments currently in use. The noncontrolled trial of gastric freezing is not only questionable regarding the interests of patients in the trial, but also questionable regarding the interests of future patients.

Two more ethical issues about the initiation of clinical trials should be mentioned in connection with the gastric freezing research: whether it was justifiable to use a sham treatment for a control, and whether it was justifiable to randomly assign the patients to the sham or real gastric freeze. With regard to the sham control, the physicians had no reason to believe that the procedure could have more than a placebo effect. Since there are treatments that have a real biologic effect on ulcers, it seems clear that the interests of the patients assigned to the sham treatment were being sacrificed. With regard to random assignment, patients usually expect that a physician's decision is based on a judgment of what is best for the patient; when the treatment decision is made by a random method, this expectation of the patient, and obligation of the physician, is not being met.

Issues Regarding Termination

One hundred and sixty patients were studied in the controlled trial of the gastric freeze procedure; at the end of the trial, the researchers concluded that the gastric freeze was an ineffective treatment for peptic ulcer. During the course of the study, data were available on the two treatments. Suppose that after eighty patients there was evidence that the real freeze was no more effective than the sham freeze. In that case, the next 120 patients were receiving a treatment that the researchers had evidence to believe was ineffective. At what point in a controlled trial is there sufficient evidence to reach a conclusion and stop the trial?

When a controlled trial is designed, a determination is made on how many patients will be included in the study. Many factors are used in this determination. An important one is the level of statistical significance. Statisticians can calculate how many patients will be needed in the trial in order to reach an .05 level of significance. Generally, and setting other aspects aside, the larger the number of patients in a trial, the more likely it is that a result significant at the .05 level will be reached.

The researchers in the controlled trial of gastric freezing only reported the results for the total 160 patients. Suppose that after eighty patients were treated, the null hypothesis (that there is no difference in the treatments) is confirmed at the .07 level. This is not the level that statisticians recommend as good enough. The question is, "Good enough for what?" A level of .07 may be enough for a judgment that it is not in the interest of the eighty-first patient to have a gastric freeze rather than one of the standard surgical treatments. The argument for continuing the trial to 160 patients is that the researcher wants to show that the treatment has no more than placebo effect—with as much certainty as is widely accepted in medical research—so that future physicians will have no grounds at all to use the gastric freeze. Again, the conflict is between the interests of patients in the trial and those of future patients....

Issues of Informed Consent

There are several distinct issues regarding informed consent to participation in an RCT. First, must the subjects be informed that they will be assigned to a treatment at random? Second, if a placebo is being used in the trial, must subjects be told of that fact? Third, should the subjects be informed of the preliminary results of a clinical trial and have the option of withdrawing?

The Food and Drug Administration and the Department of Health and Human Services have extensive regulations concerning informed consent to participation in research. Their purpose is recognition of the right of potential subjects to self-determination. The elements of informed consent specified in the regulations include a statement that the study involves research; an explanation of the purposes of the research and the expected duration of the subject's participation; a description of the procedures to be followed; identification of any procedures that are experimental; a description of any reasonably foreseeable risks or discomforts; a description of any benefits to the subject or others; a disclosure of appropriate alternative procedures or courses of treatment; a statement that participation is voluntary, refusal to participate will involve no penalty or loss, and the subject may discontinue participation at any time. None of these clearly requires that subjects be informed of randomization, placebo control, or preliminary results.

The ethical issue that must be answered here is whether the general right of self-determination requires that the doctrine of informed consent be interpreted to mandate that a subject in an RCT be informed of randomization, placebos, and preliminary results. The right of self-determination, like any other right, has a scope that must be determined—that is, it must be determined how far the right goes before other considerations have

more weight. A familiar example will help here. The right to speak one's own mind does not have an unlimited scope; a person does not have the right to speak in a manner that is libelous or slanderous, or to speak with the intent to cause a public disturbance. There comes a point at which speaking one's mind can cause harm to others, and the right to free speech does not extend that far.

The following ethical issues about RCTs have been identified in the preceding discussion of the two trials of gastric freezing. Because they are common to many different kinds of clinical research, it will be useful to state them here in a summary manner.

1. Is it justifiable to treat patients with a new and unproven therapy?

2. Is it justifiable to randomize patients to treatments?

3. Should clinical trials be done with an RCT or a consecutive trial?

4. Is uncontrolled research justifiable?

5. Are placebos or sham treatments justifiable in an RCT?

6. Is the random assignment of subjects justifiable?

7. Should a trial be continued when one treatment appears favorable?

8. Should subjects be informed of random assignment, placebo, and preliminary results?

We have also seen that the central issue that underlies all of this is the justifiability of sacrificing the interests of the patients who will be subjects in an RCT for the benefit of future patients....

Informed Consent

The problem of sacrificing the interests of subjects to the interests of future patients might be resolved by obtaining the informed consent of all subjects. Suppose the patients in the gastric freeze RCT were fully informed (i.e., they were told that the treatment might have only a placebo effect and that the purpose of the RCT was to discover if this were so, that subjects would be randomly assigned to a real freeze and a sham freeze, that they could choose not to participate in the RCT and then they would be offered standard treatments, that if they participated the trial would be continued to obtain a given level of statistical significance, that they would not be told of preliminary results because that might effect their results). If this were done, the patients who chose to be in the RCT would be voluntarily making a choice that might sacrifice their interests; this action would be a commendable, altruistic concern for the interests of future patients.

Defenders of RCTs might resist fully informing subjects. They might argue that if the subjects were told all of the above, very few patients would agree to participate, and that those who did may not be a representative sample of patients who are now receiving the treatment. The defenders might argue that the information should be limited so that a sufficiently large and representative sample of patients could be obtained.

The argument is plainly faulty. It simply assumes that it is justifiable to sacrifice the interests of current patients for the interests of future patients and thereby imposes on the current patients the researcher's view of the relationship between the interests of current and future patients. Even if certain information about the RCT is likely to result in refusals, it is relevant and should be given to the subjects.

Suppose the information is given; an important issue is whether it must also be understood and used by the potential subject. Most patients develop trust in physicians and accept their recommendations. When the recommendation is for a treatment that the physician believes is in the best interest of the patient, then the patient's trust may be justified and the patient is not being taken advantage of. But when the physician is also a researcher, or the cooperating agent of a researcher, the ground of the patient's trust has been tainted.

These points demonstrate that the process of obtaining consent for RCTs is very important. How, when, and by whom the consent is obtained will influence the patient's decision. A physician can present the opportunity to participate in such a way that the patient feels the physician wants the patient to do so and would be disappointed if the patient refused; the physician might indicate directly or indirectly to the patient, "Until now I have been doing everything for you and now it's your turn to do something for me." Alternatively, the physician might present the opportunity to participate as entirely up to the patient and indicate that she or he will be fully supportive of the patient whatever decision the latter makes. Clearly, this is the proper course.

Another matter of importance is whether patients can and do understand the information relevant to a decision to participate in an RCT. This is a factual matter that can be researched, but very little research has been done, and what there is provides no clear answers.[3] A primary issue is whether the relevant information is so technical that the average person could not understand it well. For example, can average persons understand the concept of statistical significance well enough to know what they are agreeing to when they agree to continue in an RCT and not be informed of the preliminary results because they may not be statistically significant to the .05 level? Further, a patient's illness may affect his or her ability to make an independent decision to become a subject in an RCT. If a patient is terminally ill, he or she may agree to an RCT because of a belief that it is a chance for a new miracle cure. A sick patient may be so vulnerable and dependent on physicians that he or she may agree to anything recommended by a physician for fear of losing the approval and support of a person who is of great importance to him or her at the time.

Although there are no researched answers to these questions, our common understanding indicates that these matters are serious....

Review of Risks and Benefits

A defender of RCTs may argue that the shortcomings of informed consent as a protection against unjustified sacrifice are overcome by the multiple reviews of risks and benefits. Under current government regulations, every RCT is reviewed at least four times. First, the researcher, with advice from colleagues and supervisors, must decide whether a particular research project is justifiable. The researcher's own beliefs about the risks of the procedure for subjects and the possible benefits to subjects and future patients will be part of this judgment. After the research is designed, it must be submitted to an institutional review board (IRB). In this submission, the researcher must describe the research, its expected risks and benefits, the process by which informed consent will be obtained, and what the subjects will be told. The IRB may approve, disapprove, or require modification of the research. The IRB's principal concern is to protect the rights and welfare of subjects. An IRB must apply the following criteria:

1. Risks to subjects are minimized.

2. Risks to subjects are reasonable in relation to anticipated benefits, if any, to subjects, and the importance of the knowledge that may reasonably be expected to result.

3. The selection of subjects is equitable.

4. Informed consent will be sought from each prospective subject or the subject's legally authorized representative.[4]

The regulations provide great detail about obtaining informed consent, but there is nothing on the matter of sacrifice of the interest of subjects to future patients other than the statement that the risks to subjects should be reasonable in relation to the possible benefits to future patients (concerning the knowledge that may be gained). The next level is a panel of scientists who review the project for its scientific merit. If a proposed project were so lacking in scientific merit that it could not lead to useful knowledge, presumably it would not be approved and subjects would not undergo risks. The final level of review is from prospective subjects; they must decide, perhaps with the advice of others, including their physician, whether they believe the risk-benefit relationship is a sacrifice they are willing to assume.

The fourth level, review by potential subjects, cannot itself resolve the concern about the justification of sacrifice. We must assume that there will be some patients who are recruited whose consent will be based on a less than adequate understanding of the research protocol or on a vulnerability and dependence resulting from illness or misplaced trust. With this in mind, how should an IRB determine that the risk-benefit relationship is justifiable?

One approach might be for IRB members to consider whether they would be willing to enter the RCT if they were in the patients' position. There are two problems with this approach. First, what a person sees as a justifiable sacrifice depends greatly on his or her general set of values and preferences. People vary on such things as risk taking, interest in medical research, avoidance of pain, inconvenience of hospital stays or outpatient clinic appointments, and numerous other relevant particulars. A decision by one person that he or she would find a sacrifice not unreasonable does *not* support the claim that it is justifiable to approve it for others. Second, the IRB members are not in the position of the patients asked to be subjects. Judgments about what one would do if...are frequently hedged by statements like, "But of course if I ever really faced the decision, I'm not sure what I would do." Thus, what an IRB member now believes he or she would consent to does not justify a sacrifice for others who will be subjects.

Another defense of the adequacy of an IRB review is that an IRB contains many members; some of them are not researchers and some of them must be persons not associated with the institution at which the research will be done. With a large and diverse membership, an IRB's decision carries the authority of a collective judgment. If the research placed an unjustified risk on some subjects, some members would notice that and the research would be disapproved or returned for modification. The problem with this argument is that it places undue confidence in a committee process, and it ignores the fact that committees of this sort tend to identify with the institution they work for or that appoints them, and that most of the members of an IRB are researchers. They may not be medical researchers, but they will tend to share the values and aspirations of the researchers who designed the RCT.

If neither informed consent or IRB review provides sufficient assurance that the sacrifice of the interests of subjects in RCTs is justifiable, is there any other alternative? Jonas[5] has argued that subjects in medical research should be recruited and selected in a descending order or priority. At the top of the list would be medical researchers themselves, and those who are in related sciences and other fields who can understand the research protocols and who share the researcher's commitment to new knowledge and the interests of future patients. At the bottom of the list would be those who are vulnerable because of illness, ignorance, or economic disadvantage. The priority is not attached to availability, so that if a sufficient number of subjects could not be recruited from the top of the list, it would be legitimate to drop down the list. Rather, the list is tied to the relative urgency of the research. If research is required to find a treatment for an epidemic disease that threatens nearly everyone, then those at the bottom can be recruited. The analogy Jonas gives is with conscription to defend a nation against an unjust aggressor. However, there are no research guidelines that have tried to incorporate ideas like these.

CONCLUSION

The object of this [article] has been to explore ethical questions about RCTs. The particular emphasis has been on the problems generated by decisions to initiate research with an RCT, to control the research with a placebo or other treatment, and to terminate an RCT. Most discussions of the ethics of medical research pay little attention to these problems and concentrate instead on questions about informed consent and IRB review.

The conclusions of the preceding section come down on the side of critics of RCTs. This should not be taken to imply that it is my view that RCTs are never justified or that medical research in general is unjustified....[However,] we must conclude that the use of RCTs in which competent subjects do not knowingly and voluntarily risk their own interests are not justifiable. Aggregate benefits to future patients fail to warrant the imposition of serious risks on less than fully informed "consenting" persons.

NOTES

1 O. H. Wangensteen, et al., "Achieving 'Physiological Gastrectomy' by Gastric Freezing: Preliminary Report of Experimental and Clinical Study," *Journal of the American Medical Association* 180 (1962): 439–444.

2 J. M. Ruffin, et al., "A Co-operative Double-Blind Evaluation of Gastric 'Freezing' in the Treatment of Duodenal Ulcer," *New England Journal of Medicine* 281 (1969): 16–19.

3 Alan Meisel and Loren Roth, "What We Do and Do Not Know About Informed Consent," *Journal of the American Medical Association* (1981): 2473–2477.

4 Department of Health and Human Services, *Policy for Protection of Human Subjects*, 45 Federal Register 46, 46.111.

5 Hans Jonas, "Philosophical Reflections on Experimentation with Human Subjects," in *Experimentation with Human Subjects*, ed. P. A. Freund (New York: George Braziller, 1970).

False Hopes and Best Data: Consent to Research and the Therapeutic Misconception

Paul S. Appelbaum, Loren H. Roth, Charles W. Lidz, Paul Benson, and William Winsdale

Biographical sketches of Paul S. Appelbaum and Charles W. Lidz are found on page 106. Loren H. Roth is professor of psychiatry, University of Pittsburgh. He is coauthor, with Appelbaum, of "The Structure of Informed Consent in Psychiatric Research" and, with Appelbaum and Lidz, of "The Therapeutic Misconception: Informed Consent in Psychiatric Research." Paul Benson is associate professor of sociology, University of Massachusetts, Boston, specializing in social interaction and deviance. William J. Winslade is professor of medical jurisprudence at the University of Texas Medical Branch at Galveston. He is the coauthor of *Choosing Life or Death: A Guide for Patients, Families, and Professionals* (1986). Benson, Roth, and Winslade are coauthors of "Informed Consent in Psychiatric Research: Preliminary Findings from an Ongoing Investigation."

The authors focus on one aspect of a central concern regarding RCTs: the potential conflict between the scientific methodology intended to provide generalizable knowledge and physicians' commitment to providing the personal care intended to serve patients' best interests. They argue that the "therapeutic misconception" is common among patient-subjects. To labor under a therapeutic misconception is to deny the possibility that participation in an RCT may be seriously disadvantageous to oneself because of the very nature of the research process. The authors maintain, however, that insofar as many potential subjects can be taught that research and ordinary treatment differ in significant ways, the therapeutic misconception can be avoided. When potential participants understand the differences, they can make informed decisions, avoiding the therapeutic misconception. The authors conclude by discussing the question, "Who should explain the therapeutic misconception to potential subjects?" They support the view that the explanatory task should be given to individuals who are not members of the research team. They suggest using trained educators such as nurses.

Reprinted with permission of the authors and the publisher from *Hastings Center Report*, vol. 17 (April 1987), pp. 20–24.

Following a suicide attempt, a young man with a long history of tumultuous relationships and difficulty controlling his impulses is admitted to a psychiatric hospital. After a number of days, a psychiatrist approaches the patient, explaining that he is conducting a research project to determine if medications may help in the treatment of the patient's condition. Is the patient interested, the psychiatrist asks? The answer: "Yes, I'm willing to do anything that might help me."

The psychiatrist returns over the next several days to explain the project further. He tells the patient that two medications are being used, along with a placebo; medications and placebo are assigned randomly. The trial is double-blinded; that is, neither physician nor patient will know what the patient is receiving until after the trial has been completed. The patient listens to the explanation and reads and signs the consent form. Since the process of providing information and obtaining consent seems, on the surface, exemplary, there appears to be little reason to question the validity of the consent.

Yet when the patient is asked why he agreed to be in the study, he offers some disquieting information. The medication that he will receive, he believes, will be the one most likely to help him. He ruled out the possibility that he might receive a placebo, because that would not be likely to do him much good. In short, this man, now both a patient and a subject, has interpreted, even distorted, the information he received to maintain the view—obviously based on his wishes—that every aspect of the research project to which he had consented was designed to benefit him directly. This belief, which is far from uncommon, we call the "therapeutic misconception." To maintain a therapeutic misconception is to deny the possibility that there may be major disadvantages to participating in clinical research that stem from the nature of the research process itself.

RESEARCH RISKS AND THE SCIENTIFIC METHOD

The unique aspects of clinical research include the goal of creating generalizable knowledge; the techniques of randomization; and the use of a study protocol, control groups, and double-blind procedures. Do these elements create a body of risks or disadvantages for research subjects? The answer lies in understanding how the scientific method is often incompatible with one of the first principles of clinical treatment—the value that the legal philosopher Charles Fried calls "personal care."[1]

According to the principle of personal care, a physician's first obligation is solely to the patient's well-being. A corollary is that the physician will take whatever measures are available to maximize the chances of a successful outcome. A failure to adhere to this principle creates at least a potential disadvantage for the clinical research subject: there is always a chance that the subject's interests may become secondary to other demands on the physician-researcher's loyalties.[2] And the methods of science inhibit the application of personal care.

Randomization, an important element of many clinical trials, demonstrates the problem. The argument is often made that comparisons of multiple treatment methods are legitimately undertaken only when the superiority of one over the other is unknown; thus the physician treating a patient in one of these trials does not abandon the patient's personal care, but merely allows chance to determine the assignment of treatments, each of which is likely to meet the patient's needs.[3]

But as Fried and others have noted, it is very unlikely that two treatments in a clinical trial will be identically desirable *for a particular patient*. The physician may have reason to suspect, for example, that a given treatment is more likely to be efficacious for a particular patient, even if overall evidence of greater efficacy is lacking. This suspicion may be based on the physician's previous experience with a subgroup of patients, the patient's own past treatment experience, the family history of responsiveness to treatment, or idiosyncratic elements in the patient's case. Subjects may have had previous unsatisfactory responses to one of the medications in a clinical trial, or may display clinical characteristics that suggest that one class of medications is more likely to benefit them than another.

Ordinarily, these factors would guide the therapeutic approach. But in a randomized study physicians cannot allow these factors to influence the treatment decision, and efforts to control for such factors in the selection of subjects, while theoretically possible, are cumbersome, expensive, and may bias the sample. Thus reliance on randomization represents an inevitable compromise of personal care in the service of attaining valid research results. There are at least two reports in the literature of physicians' reluctance to refer patients to randomized trials because of the possible decrement in the level of personal care.[4]

The use of a study protocol to regulate the course of treatment—essential to careful clinical research—also impedes the delivery of personal care. Protocols often indicate the pattern and dosages of medication to be administered or the blood levels to be attained. Even if they allow some individualization of medication, changes in time or magnitude may be limited. Thus patients who do not respond initially to a low dose of medication may not receive a higher dose, as they would if they were being treated without a protocol; on the other hand, patients experiencing side effects, which could be controlled by lowering their dosage, yet which are not so severe as to require withdrawal from the study, cannot receive the relief they would get in a therapeutic setting.

Analogously, adjunctive medications or forms of therapy, which may interfere with measurement of the primary treatment effect, are often prohibited. The exclusion of adjunctive medications, such as sleeping medications or decongestants, may increase a patient's discomfort. The requirement for a "wash-out" period, during which subjects are kept drug-free, may place previously stable patients at risk of relapse even before the experimental part of the project begins. And alternating placebo and active treatment periods may mean that a patient who responds well to a medication must be taken off that drug for the purposes of the study; conversely, patients who improve on placebo must be subject to the risks of active medication. In sum, the necessary rigidities of an experimental protocol often lead investigators to forgo individualized treatment decisions.

The need for control groups or placebos and double-blind procedures can produce similar effects. In the therapeutic setting patients will rarely receive medications that are deliberately designed to be pharmacologically ineffective; the ethics of those occasional situations when placebos are employed clinically are hotly disputed.[5] Yet, placebos are routinely employed in clinical investigations, without the intent of benefiting the individual subject.

Similarly, clinicians in a nonresearch setting will never allow themselves to remain ignorant of the treatment patients are receiving. Double-blind procedures, however, are necessary to ensure the integrity of a research study, even if they delay recognition of side effects or drug interactions, or have other adverse consequences.

Are these disadvantages so important that they should routinely be called to the attention of research subjects? That issue raises an empirical question: how prevalent is the therapeutic misconception?

STUDIES ON CONSENT

Our findings suggest that research subjects systematically misinterpret the risk/benefit ratio of participating in research because they fail to understand the underlying scientific methodology.[6]

This conclusion is based on our observations of consent transactions in four research studies on the treatment of psychiatric illness, and our interviews with the subjects immediately after consent was obtained. The studies varied in the extent of the information they provided to subjects. Two of the studies compared the effects of two medications on a psychiatric disorder (one used, in addition, a placebo control group). A third study examined the relative efficacy of two dosage ranges of the same medication. And a fourth examined two different social interventions in chronic psychiatric illness, compared with a control group.

The populations in these studies ranged from actively psychotic schizophrenic patients to nonpsychotic, and in some cases, minimally symptomatic, borderline, and depressed patients. Our questions were based on information included on the consent form with regard to the understanding of randomized or chance assignment; and the use of control groups, formal protocols, and double-blind techniques. Eighty-eight patients comprised the final data pool, but since all of the issues addressed here were not relevant to each project the sample size varied for each question.

We found that fifty-five of eighty subjects (69 percent) had no comprehension of the actual basis for their random assignment to treatment groups, while only twenty-two of eighty (28 percent) had a complete understanding of the randomization process. Thirty-two subjects stated their explicit belief that assignment would be made on the basis of their therapeutic needs. Interestingly, many of these subjects constructed elaborate but entirely fictional means by which an assignment would be made that was in their best interests. This was particularly evident when information about group assignment was limited to the written consent forms and not covered in the oral disclosure; subjects filled vacuums of knowledge with assumptions that decisions would be made in their best interests.

Similar findings were evident concerning other aspects of scientific design. With regard to nontreatment control groups and placebos, fourteen of thirty-three (44 percent) subjects failed to recognize that some patients who desired treatment would not receive it. Concerning use of a double-blind, twenty-six of sixty-seven subjects (39 percent) did not understand that their physician would not know which medication they would receive; an additional sixteen of sixty-seven subjects (24 percent) had only partially understood this. Most striking of all, only six of sixty-eight subjects (9 percent) were able to recognize a single way in which joining a protocol would restrict the treatment they could receive. In the two drug studies in which adjustment of medication dosage was tightly restricted, twenty-two of forty-four subjects (50 percent) said explicitly that they thought their dosage would be adjusted according to their individual needs.

Two cases illustrate how these flaws in understanding affect the patient's ability to assess the benefits of the research. The first demonstrates the effect of a complete failure to recognize that scientific methodology has other than a therapeutic purpose. The second demonstrates a more subtle influence of a therapeutic orientation on a subject who understands the overall methodology but has certain blindspots.

In the first case, a twenty-five-year-old married woman with a high-school education was a subject in a randomized, double-blind study that compared the use of two medications and a placebo in the treatment of a nonpsychotic psychiatric disorder. When interviewed, she was unsure how it would be decided which medication she would receive, but thought that the placebo would be given only to those subjects who "might not need medication." The subject understood that a double-blind procedure would be used, but did not see that the protocol placed any constraints on her treatment. She said that she considered this project not an "experiment," a term that implied using drugs whose effects were unknown. Rather, she considered this to be "research," a process whereby doctors "were trying to find out more about you in depth." She decided to participate because, "I needed help and the doctor said that other people who had been in it had been helped." Her strong conviction that the project would benefit her carried through to the end of the study. Although the investigators rated her a nonresponder, she was convinced that she had improved on the medication. She attributed her improvement in large part to the double-blind procedures, which kept her in the dark as to which medication she was receiving, thereby preventing her from persuading herself that the medication was doing no good. She was quite pleased about having participated in the study.

In the same study, another subject was a twenty-five-year-old woman with three years of college. At the time of the interview, she had minimal psychiatric symptoms and her understanding of the research was generally excellent. She recognized that the purpose of the project was to find out which treatment worked best for her group of patients. She spontaneously described the three groups, including the placebo group, and indicated that assignment would be at random. She understood that dosages would be adjusted according to blood levels and that a double-blind would be used. When asked directly, however, how *her* medication would be selected, she said she had no idea. She then added, "I hope it isn't by chance," and suggested that each subject would probably receive the medication she needed. Given the discrepancy between her earlier use of the word "random" and her current explanation, she was then asked what her understanding was of "random." Her definition was entirely appropriate: "by lottery, by chance, one patient who comes in gets one thing and the next patient gets the next thing." She then began to wonder out loud if this procedure was being used in the current study. Ultimately, she concluded that it was not.

In this case, despite a cognitive understanding of randomization, and a momentary recognition that random assignment would be used, the subject's conviction that the investigators would be acting in her best interests led to a distortion of an important element of the experimental procedure and therefore of the risk/benefit analysis.

The comments of colleagues and reports by other researchers have persuaded us that this phenomenon extends to all clinical research. Bradford Gray, for example, found that a number of subjects in a project comparing two drugs for the induction of labor believed, incorrectly, that their needs would determine which drug they would receive.[7] A survey of patients in research projects at four Veterans Administration hospitals showed that 75 percent decided to participate because they expected the research to benefit their health.[8] Another survey of attitudes toward research in a combined sample of patients and the general public revealed the thinking behind this hope: when asked why people in general should participate in research, 69 percent cited benefit to society at large and only 5 percent cited benefit to the subjects; however, when asked why *they* might participate in a research project, 52 percent said they would do it to get the best medical care, while only 23 percent responded that they would want to contribute to scientific knowledge.[9] Back in the psychiatric setting, Lee Park and Lino Covi found that a substantial percentage of patients who were told they were being given a placebo would not believe that they received inactive medication,[10] and Vincenta Leigh reported that the most common fantasy on a psychiatric research ward was that the research was actually designed to benefit the subjects.[11]

RESPONDING TO THE PROBLEM

Should we do anything about the therapeutic misconception? It could be argued that as long as the research project has been peer-reviewed for scientific merit and approved for ethical acceptability by an institutional review board (IRB), the problem of the therapeutic misconception is not significant enough to warrant intervention. In this view, some minor distortion of the risk/benefit ratio has to be weighed against the costs of attempting to alter subjects' appreciation of the scientific methods. Such costs include time expended and the delay in completing research that will result when some subjects decide that they would rather not participate.

Whether we accept this view depends on the value that we place on the principle of autonomy that underlies the practice of informed consent. Autonomy can be overvalued when it limits necessary treatment, as it may, for example, in the controversy over the right to refuse psychotropic medications. There, we believe, patients' interests would best be served by giving claims to autonomy lesser weight.[12] But when we enter the research setting, limiting subjects' autonomy becomes a tool not for promoting their own interests, but for promoting the interests of others, including the researcher and society as a whole. We are not willing to accept such limitations for the benefit of others, particularly when, as described below, there may exist an effective mechanism for mitigating the problem.

Assuming that one agrees that distortions of the type we have described in subjects' reasoning are troublesome and worthy of correction, is such an effort likely to be effective? One might point to the data just presented to argue that little can be done to ameliorate the problem. The investigator in one of the projects we studied offered his subjects detailed and extensive information in a process that often extended over several days and included one session in which the entire project was reviewed. Despite this, half the subjects failed to grasp that treatment would be assigned on a random basis, four of twenty misunderstood how placebos would be used, five of twenty were not aware of the use of a double-blind, and eight of twenty believed that medications would be adjusted according to their individual needs. Is it not futile, then, to attempt to disabuse subjects of the belief that they will receive personal care?

Various theoretical explanations of our findings could support this view. Most people have been socialized to believe that physicians (at least ethical ones) always provide personal care.[13] It may therefore be very difficult, perhaps nearly impossible, to persuade subjects that *this* encounter is different, particularly if the researcher is also the treating physician, who has previously satisfied the subject's expectations of personal care. Further, insofar as much clinical research involves persons who are acutely ill and in some distress, the well-known tendency of patients to regress and entrust their well-being to an authority figure would undercut any effort to dispel the therapeutic misconception.

In response, more of our data must be explored. In each of the studies we observed, one cell of subjects was the target of an augmented informational process, which supplemented the investigator's disclosures to subjects with a "preconsent discussion." This discussion was led by a member of our research team who was trained to teach potential subjects about such things as the key methodologic aspects of the research project, especially methods that might conflict with the principle of personal care.

By introducing a neutral discloser, distinct from the patient's treatment team, we shifted the emphasis of the disclosure to focus on the ways in which research differs from treatment. Of the subjects who received this special education, eight of sixteen (50 percent) recognized that randomization would be used, as opposed to thirteen of the fifty-one (25 percent) remaining subjects; five of five (100 percent) understood how placebos would be employed in the single study that used them, compared with eleven of the fifteen (73 percent) remaining subjects; nine of sixteen (56 percent) comprehended the use of a double blind while only fifteen of fifty-one (31 percent) remaining subjects did so; and five of seventeen (29 percent) initially recognized other limits on their treatment as a result of constraints in the protocol, compared with one of the fifty-one (2 percent) other subjects.

Our data suggest that many subjects can be taught that research *is* markedly different from ordinary treatment. Other efforts to educate subjects about the use of scientific methodology offer comparably encouraging results.[14] There is no reason to believe that subjects will refuse to hear clear-cut efforts to dispel the therapeutic misconception.

Novel approaches such as we employed may be one thing, of course, while routine procedures are something else. Perhaps our data derive from an unusually gifted group of patient-subjects. Will the complexity of explaining the principle of the scientific method defy understanding by most research subjects?

Undercutting the therapeutic misconception, thereby laying out some of the major disadvantages of any clinical research project, is probably much simpler than it seems. About the goals of research, subjects could be told: "Because this is a research project, we will be doing some things differently than we would if we were simply treating you for your condition. Not all the things we do are designed to tell us the best way to treat *you*, but they should help us to understand how people with your condition *in general* can best be treated." About randomization: "The treatment you receive of the three possibilities will be selected by chance, not because we believe that one or the other will be better for you." About placebos: "Some subjects will be selected at random to receive sugar pills that are not known to help the condition you have; this is so we can tell whether the medications that the other patients get are really effective, or if everyone with your condition would have gotten better anyway."

One can quibble about the wording of specific sections, and complexities can arise with particular projects, but the concepts underlying scientific methodology are in reality quite simple. And as long as subjects understand the key principles of how the study is being conducted, investigators can probably omit some of the detail that currently clogs consent forms and confuses subjects about the minor risks that accompany the experimental procedures, such as blood drawing. Overall, then, we may end up with a much simpler consent process when we focus on the issue of personal care.

Who should have the task of explaining the therapeutic misconception to subjects? Clearly, investigators should be encouraged to discuss such issues with subjects and to include them on consent forms, but several problems arise here. First, it is decidedly *not* in investigators' self-interest for them to disabuse potential subjects of the therapeutic misconception. Experienced investigators, as we have reported elsewhere,[15] view the recruitment of research subjects as an intricate and extended effort to win the potential subject's trust. One of our subjects in this study described the process in these words: "It was almost as if they were courting me.... everything was presented in the best possible light." One could argue that it is unrealistic to expect investigators to raise additional doubts about the benefits that subjects can expect; any effort in that regard will result in resistance by investigators, particularly those who have yet to internalize the justifications for informed consent in general.

Second, even investigators who recognize the desirability of subjects making informed decisions may have great trouble conveying this particular information. When a researcher tells subjects that he or she is not selecting the treatment that will be given or that the medications being used may be no more effective than a placebo, the researcher is confessing uncertainty over the best approach to treatment, as well as the likely outcome. Harold Bursztajn and colleagues have argued that the essential uncertainty of all medical practice is precisely what physicians need to convey in *both* research and treatment settings.[16] Yet, as Jay Katz points out, physicians have been systematically socialized to underplay or ignore uncertainty in their discussions with patients.[17] In a recent report of physicians' reluctance to enter patients in a multicenter breast cancer study, 22 percent of the principal investigators cited as a major obstacle to enrolling subjects difficulty in telling patients that they did not know which treatment was best.[18]

Third, few researchers who are also clinicians feel comfortable acknowledging, even to themselves, that the course of treatment may not be optimally therapeutic for the patient. Thus, there appear such statements as the following, which recently was published in *The Lancet*: "A doctor who contributes to randomized treatment trials should not be thought of as a research worker, but simply as a clinician with an ethical duty to his patients not to go on giving them treatments without doing everything possible to assess their true worth."[19] The author concludes that since randomized trials are not really research, there is no need to obtain *any* informed consent from research subjects. Although this conclusion may be extreme, the example emphasizes the difficulties of getting investigators to admit to themselves, much less to their patient-subjects, the limits they have accepted on the delivery of personal care.

If there is concern with particular protocols, IRBs might consider supplementing the investigators' disclosure and the "courtship" process with a session in which the potential subject reviews risks and benefits with someone who is not a member of the research team. (John Robertson has proposed a similar approach, albeit out of other concerns.[20]) The neutral explainer would be responsible to the IRB and would be trained to emphasize those aspects of the research situation about which the IRB has the greatest concern. This approach might be especially appropriate when the investigator is also the subject's treating physician and the methodology used is likely to be interpreted as therapeutic in intent. The model we employed of using a trained educator (nurses are natural candidates for the job) worked well. It is certainly more manageable and less disruptive than the oft-heard suggestions that patient advocates or consent monitors sit in on every interaction between subject and investigator.

There may be advantages to using a trained, neutral educator, apart from aiding subjects' decision-making. Subjects' perceptions of the research team as willing to "level with them," even to the point of explaining why it might not be in subjects' interests to participate in the study, may increase their trust and cooperation. On the other hand, failure to deal with the therapeutic misconception during the consent process could increase distrust of researchers and the health care system in general, if subjects later come to feel they were "deceived," as a few did in the studies we observed. Enough experiences of this sort could further heighten public antipathy to medical research, particularly if they are publicized as some have been.[21] The scientific method is a powerful tool for advancing knowledge, but like most potent clinical procedures it has side effects that must be attended to, lest the benefits sought be overwhelmed by the disadvantages that accrue. With careful planning, the therapeutic misconception can be dispelled, leaving the subjects with a much clearer picture of the relative risks and benefits of participation in research.

ACKNOWLEDGMENTS

The authors acknowledge the invaluable assistance of Paul Soloff, M.D., in the collection of the data described in this paper.

REFERENCES

1 Charles Fried, *Medical Experimentation: Personal Integrity and Social Policy* (New York: American Elsevier Publishing Co., 1974).

2 Arthur Schafer, "The Ethics of the Randomized Clinical Trial," *New England Journal of Medicine* 307 (Sept. 16, 1982), 719–24.

3 "Consent: How Informed?" *The Lancet* I (June 30, 1984), 1445–47.

4 Kathryn M. Taylor, Richard G. Margolese, and Colin L. Soskolne, "Physicians' Reasons for Not Entering Eligible Patients in a Randomized Clinical Trial of Surgery for Breast Cancer," *New England Journal of Medicine* 310 (May 24, 1984), 1363–67; Mortimer J. Lacher, "Physicians and Patients as Obstacles to Randomized Trial," *Clinical Research* 26 (December 1978), 375–79.

5 Sissela Bok, "The Ethics of Giving Placebos," *Scientific American* 231:5 (May 1974), 17–23.

6 Paul S. Appelbaum, Loren H. Roth, and Charles W. Lidz, "The Therapeutic Misconception: Informed Consent in Psychiatric Research," *International Journal of Law and Psychiatry* 5 (1982), 319–29; Paul Benson, Loren H. Roth, and William J. Winslade, "Informed Consent in Psychiatric Research: Preliminary Findings from an Ongoing Investigation," *Social Science and Medicine* 20 (1985), 1331–41.

7 Bradford H. Gray, *Human Subjects in Medical Experimentation: A Sociological Study of the Conduct and Regulation of Clinical Research.* (New York: John Wiley & Sons, 1975).

8 Henry W. Riecken and Ruth Ravich, "Informed Consent to Biomedical Research in Veterans Administration Hospitals," *Journal of the American Medical Association* 248 (July 16, 1982), 344–48.

9 Barrie R. Cassileth, Edward J. Lusk, David S. Miller, and Shelley Hurwitz, "Attitudes toward Clinical Trials among Patients and Public," *Journal of the American Medical Association* 248 (August 27, 1982), 968–70.

10 Lee C. Park and Lino Covi, "Nonblind Placebo Trial: An Exploration of Neurotic Patients' Responses to Placebo When Its Inert Content Is Disclosed," *Archives of General Psychiatry* 12 (April 1965), 336–45.

11 Vincenta Leigh, "Attitudes and Fantasy Themes of Patients on a Psychiatric Research Unit," *Archives of General Psychiatry* 32 (May 1975), 598–601.

12 Paul S. Appelbaum and Thomas G. Gutheil, "The Right to Refuse Treatment: The Real Issue is Quality of Care," *Bulletin of the American Academy of Psychiatry and the Law* 9 (1982), 199–202.

13 Cassileth et al., *op cit.*

14 Jan M. Howard, David DeMets, and the BHAT Research Group, "How Informed Is Informed Consent? The BHAT Experience," *Controlled Clinical Trials* 2 (1981), 287–303.

15 Paul S. Appelbaum and Loren H. Roth, "The Structure of Informed Consent in Psychiatric Research," *Behavioral Sciences and the Law* 1:3 (Autumn 1983), 9–19.

16 Harold Bursztajn, Richard I. Feinbloom, Robert M. Hamm, and Archie Brodsky, *Medical Choices, Medical Chances: How Patients, Families, and Physicians Can Cope with Uncertainty.* (New York: Free Press, 1984).

17 Jay Katz, *The Silent World of Doctor and Patient,* (New York: Free Press, 1984).

18 Taylor et al., *op cit.*

19 Thurston B. Brewin, "Consent to Randomized Treatment," *The Lancet* II (Oct. 23, 1982), 919–21.

20 John A. Robertson, "Taking Consent Seriously: IRB Intervention in the Consent Process," *IRB: A Review of Human Subjects Research* 4:5 (September-October 1982), 1–5.

21 Dava Sobel, "Sleep Study Leaves Subject Feeling Angry and Confused," *New York Times* (July 15, 1980), p. C-1.

Animal Experimentation

Beastly Conduct: Ethical Issues in Animal Experimentation
Arthur L. Caplan

Arthur L. Caplan is director, Center for Biomedical Ethics, and professor in the departments of philosophy and surgery at the University of Minnesota. He is the editor of *The Sociobiology Debate* (1978) and the coeditor of *Darwin, Marx, and Freud: Their Influence on Moral Theory* (1984) and *Scientific Controversies: Resolution and Closure of Disputes in Science and Technology* (1987). His articles include "Organ Procurement: It's Not in the Cards."

Caplan identifies three major areas of dispute in discussions of the moral legitimacy of animal research: (1) the need to conduct any research upon animals, (2) the moral value to be assigned to animals, and (3) the moral priority that ought to be accorded the issue when we face other problems such as human starvation, malnutrition, war, and crime. He compares and contrasts positions taken on these three issues by the "pro" and "anti" animal research camps. After bringing out their respective positions, Caplan discusses at length the appropriate criteria for the attribution of moral worth. He concludes that (1) purposiveness is the property that suffices for conferring moral worth upon entities; (2) animals, like humans, are so organized as to be purposive creatures having desires, drives, intentions, and aspirations; (3) it is prima facie wrong to frustrate these purposes. Nonetheless, Caplan concludes, it does not follow that animal experimentation is never justifiable but only that any such experimentation must be justified by compelling reasons that outweigh the wrongness of interfering with the efforts of purposive creatures to fulfill their desires.

THE LEGITIMACY OF MEANS AND THE LEGITIMACY OF ENDS IN ANIMAL EXPERIMENTATION

There has been a great deal of argument in recent years over the subject of animal experimentation. Few topics are able to elicit the degree of moral vehemence and passion that this topic does. Accusations of moral blindness fly back and forth between vivisectionists and antivivisectionists. Bills are submitted almost willy-nilly at

Reprinted with permission of the author and the publisher from *Annals of the New York Academy of Sciences*, vol. 406 (1983), pp. 159–169.

both the federal and state level, lobbying efforts on both sides of the issue are best described as fierce, and the disputants seem to delight in holding meetings and conferences at which their opponents are persona non grata—on both sides opponents are rarely invited, and, if they somehow manage to appear, they are made the object of calumny usually reserved only for criminals or even politicians.[12]

Despite the political and sociological vortex surrounding the issue of animal experimentation, it would be wrong for those on either side to underestimate the sincerity and thoughtfulness that can underlie much of the noise and rhetoric characteristic of current public debates over the issue. In recent years a rather rich philosophical literature[10,11] has developed on the subject of the moral responsibilities of human beings toward animals, and this literature surely must be reckoned with by all parties to the debate. Just as it is wrong to suppose that all vivisectionists are callous brutes, unconcerned about the effects of their work on their animal subjects, it is also wrong to assume that all antivivisectionists are misanthropic kooks who are too emotionally unstable to recognize the benefits that derive from research involving animals.

Before considering some of the moral questions that arise in the context of the practice of experimentation involving animals, it is important to make a distinction between two issues that are often conflated by parties on both sides of the issue. Oftentimes scientists go to great lengths to demonstrate to each other and the general public that they take every possible precaution to assure the humane treatment of any animals that may be used for experimental purposes. Scientists often note with pride that they have, through their own voluntary efforts, established clear codes of conduct about the care and handling of laboratory animals. Moreover, most reputable scientists in America and other nations go to great lengths to minimize, through the use of anesthetics, anesthesia, and other means, the pain or suffering that animals endure as a result of the process of experimentation.

The many efforts now made to reduce animal suffering and to ensure the proper care and handling of animals used for research purposes are often brought forward in response to criticisms leveled by antivivisectionists concerning the enterprise of animal research. Unfortunately, persons who question the moral legitimacy of animal experimentation are not likely to be dissuaded from their view by demonstrations of the care and concern shown by those engaged in the practice.

There are really two issues involved in thinking about research involving animals and questions of humane care are pertinent only to one of them—(1) is it morally legitimate to conduct research upon animals?; (2) if it is morally permissible to utilize animals for research purposes, what moral responsibilities must be discharged by those engaged in such research? Questions on what conduct constitutes humane care, guidelines on the handling and transport of animal subjects, and efforts to teach students and professionals techniques that will minimize animal suffering and pain consequent to research interventions are all only relevant to the question of professional duty within the research context. However, before these issues can be usefully discussed, it is necessary to examine the prior question of whether it is morally justifiable to conduct any research on animals. For if the answer to this question is no, then no amount of guidelines, restraint, educational effort, or codified standards will suffice in response to criticisms of the activity.

THE MAJOR AREAS OF CONTENTION CONCERNING THE MORAL LEGITIMACY OF ANIMAL RESEARCH

If one reviews the various public pronouncements[1,3,6,7,10,12] made about the issue of animal experimentation by parties on both sides of the issue, it quickly becomes evident that there exist three major areas of dispute. First, there is a good deal of disagreement about the need to conduct any research upon animals. Second, there is much disagreement about the moral value to be assigned to animals. Much of the attention to issues of animal sentience and consciousness in debates about the ethics of animal research are spin-offs from this issue since the more animals are felt to possess mental powers equivalent to or closely resembling those possessed by humans, the more various people feel disposed to assign moral worth to such creatures. Third, there is a good deal of tacit or between-the-lines argument about the moral priority that ought be accorded the whole issue of the ethics of animal experimentation. Many persons admit that the question of the legitimacy of animal experimentation is a vexing one, but there is no agreement over whether the topic is one that ought to command wide public attention and legislative concern. Other issues, such as human starvation, malnutrition, war, crime, poverty and the like are felt, oftentimes, to deserve precedence over the fates of animals in research laboratories.[12]

It is interesting to compare and contrast the positions taken by the 'pro' and 'anti' vivisection camps on these three major issues. To some degree some of the stereotyping and caterwauling so characteristic of disputes over this issue can be defused by a little reflection over the stances adopted by the parties to the debate on the major question surrounding the legitimacy of the research enterprise.

The Provivisection Point of View

Need   Provivisectionists argue that it is ludicrous to talk at the present time about the complete replacement or elimination of animals from the context of experimentation. If human health and well-being are to be improved, if human safety is to be assured in both medical and non-medical contexts, and if human knowledge is to advance, then some amount of animal experimentation must be conducted. It is simply not possible, given our present knowledge, to utilize alternatives to animals and simultaneously maintain publicly acceptable levels of human health and well-being. In part, this is due to the fact that testing chemicals or pharmaceutical substances on cells or other limited organic systems fails to capture the complexities involved in the processing of such substances by whole organisms. The pursuit of such universally recognized human goods, as health, safety, and knowledge, requires that some animals be utilized in research contexts.

Moral Equality   Most provivisectionists do not accept the equation of animals and humans as entities deserving of equal moral consideration and concern. Some believe that animals do not suffer or feel pain in ways analogous to that experienced by human beings, and, thus, do not deserve the same sort of protections and considerations as human beings do in experimental settings. Others favoring vivisection simply see human beings and their goals and purposes as more worthy of moral respect than the goals and purposes of members of the animal kingdom. Thus, the general health of human beings or the welfare of any specific individual human being counts for far more, in their view, than the well-being or health of any single animal or groups of animals. This view is reflected in the fact that scientists will often comment to each other in private that they have actually heard some antivivisectionists say that they would rather one baby be used for experimental purposes than one thousand rats. Such statements are held up as exemplifying the moral blindness of those who would equate animal welfare with human welfare.

Priority   Many persons involved with or supportive of the use of animals in experimental studies find it hard to believe that so much energy, money, and time is devoted to this issue by opponents of such practices. They note that there is plenty of misery about in both the human and animal kingdoms and that antivivisectionists might better devote their frenetic energies to obviating the many other clear injustices that exist in the world. Why, it is sometimes asked, don't antivivisectionists attempt to stop such practices as pet abuse, hunting, or meat-eating rather than focus as they do on animal research?

The numbers of animals who suffer at the hands of humans are surely greater in these other contexts, and these would therefore seem to be more appropriate places for political and legislative intervention by those concerned with animal welfare.

The Antivivisectionist Point of View

Need   Antivivisectionists believe that while it may be true that not all animal experimentation can be abolished (some believe that all could), it is nevertheless true that far more could be eliminated than is presently the case. They argue that there exist many techniques for replacing animals in experiments, including cellular studies, computer simulations, and careful field studies upon animals in natural settings. Moreover, they argue, even more could be done in the way of replacement and reduction in the number of animals used in scientific research but for the pernicious influence of the animal breeding industry, which has no obvious interest in seeing animal experimentation curbed or in developing suitable substitutes for whole live animals. Antivivisectionists see the continued and ongoing reliance of scientists upon animal studies as the natural outcome of an economic and political situation in which various parties have powerful vested interests in assuring the continuance of the status quo with regard to animal research.

It should also be noted that while most opponents of animal research do not challenge the legitimacy of such goals as the assurance of human health and safety or the advancement of human knowledge, they find defenses of animal research couched in terms of these broad social goals inadequate. First, they argue, it is not clear that human knowledge is likely to be advanced by the kinds of studies and experiments to which animals are currently put by scientists. There is simply too much waste, replication, and redundancy in scientific experimentation to justify the toll imposed on animals in the name of advancing scientific knowledge. Second, it is not clear that human health is always advanced by animal research since ultimately all drugs and procedures must be tried on humans anyway.

More importantly, they note, a good deal of animal experimentation is conducted in order to assure the American consumer a suitable range of cosmetics, toiletries, and other aesthetic paraphernalia. These are hardly indispensable aspects of human existence, and the antivivisectionists have been quick to note that safety with regard to perfumes and underarm deodorants is hardly an awe-inspiring moral imperative when assessing the legitimacy of the animal sacrifices involved in order to attain safety with regard to these frivolous ends.

Moral Equality Sophisticated critics of the entire enterprise of animal research argue that science itself is in many ways responsible for skepticism about the acceptability of animal research. While there have existed strong traditions within both science and religion committed to the view that animals are nothing more than dumb brutes or automata, the fact is that scientific research has, over the years, revealed essential similarities between humans and animals with respect to many physical and mental properties. Surely, such critics note, we know enough about the physiology, neurology and behavioral capacities of higher vertebrates to make us realize that these creatures can feel pain, can suffer, and that they ought not be treated any differently than we would treat any human being endowed with such capacities and traits. There is an implicit demand for consistency behind much of the antivivisectionist opposition to research on animals—what we would not dream of doing to a child, a fetus, a newborn, a demented person, a retarded person, a senile person, a comatose person, or a dead person, we ought not dream of doing to a sentient animal.

The argument from consistency does not commit the antivivisectionist to the equation of animals and humans in terms of their moral worth. Rather, the view held by most antivivisectionists is that animals have the minimal properties capable of conferring moral standing upon an entity—sentience, consciousness, or the capacity to feel pain. These properties, or some one of them, seem sufficient for according moral status to animals. Animals and humans both possess, on this view, minimally sufficient attributes for becoming the objects of moral concern. Both kinds of organisms satisfy minimal requirements for being valued, and in this sense they ought to be viewed as of equal moral worth.

Priority While antivivisectionists argue that animals and humans are equal in terms of their both possessing capacities that qualify them for moral concern and respect, antivivisectionists give a higher priority to the need to attend to animal suffering than do many proponents of research. The primary reason that seems to motivate the view that animal suffering deserves our legislative and regulatory attention is that animals are not in a position to avoid the types of suffering they encounter in the laboratory. While it is true that animals cause each

other harm in nature, the fact remains that the sorts of suffering they often encounter in research settings is entirely due to the activities of human beings. Human beings, thus, are responsible for inflicting an additional measure of pain and suffering upon creatures who are unable to protect themselves against these evils. While human beings can, assumedly, avoid at least some of the pain and misery they inflict on their fellows in various situations, animals in laboratories cannot and thus possess a special claim to human moral attention because they are so utterly dependent on humans for alleviating the suffering they encounter.

THE ISSUE OF MORAL EQUALITY

Having presented the basic outlines of the dispute about animal experimentation, the rest of this essay will focus on the thorny question of the moral worth of animals and humans. For, if it is true that at least some partisans on both sides of the issue are in basic agreement that human health, well-being, and safety are desirable goods, and, that the production of human knowledge that promotes these ends is also good, then it would seem that the real issue dividing 'pro' and 'anti' vivisectionists is the degree to which sacrifices and concessions have to be made with regard to these goods in order to promote animal well-being and decrease animal suffering. Both the level of priority accorded the enterprise of animal experimentation as a moral question and the zeal with which alternatives to animal use are pursued pivot around the degree to which animals are seen as worthy of moral concern. The moral equality of animals and humans is thus the crucial issue dividing the two sides in current disputes, and it is this question which merits close, critical scrutiny if any progress is to be made toward settling the issue.

Much of the basis for the belief that animals and humans have an equal claim to moral consideration arises from an awareness of recent history in the discipline of ethics.[11] During the past two hundred years or so, many human beings have come to realize that differences in sex, race, ethnic group, or sexual preference are not relevant properties for excluding individuals from the moral realm. The recent popularity of the story of the Elephant Man in the movies and on Broadway derives in part from the message conveyed by the leading character of the play, John Merrick, that despite his deformed and even ghastly appearance, he is still a person worthy of moral concern and respect. Physical form and appearance are not in themselves reasons for excluding someone or even something from the sphere of our moral concern. Thus, while animals are certainly different in their shape, form, and physical appearance from human beings, these differences are not in themselves sufficient for establishing a relevant moral difference between animals and humans any more than are the various shapes, colors, and sizes of human beings.

Some persons have turned to other criteria besides physical differences for distinguishing between the moral worth of animals and humans. Reason, language, intentionality, self-awareness, and a sense of personal identity have all been suggested as properties possessed by humans which distinguish them from animals with respect to their moral worth.[2] But there are problems in using these properties as a basis for distinguishing animals from humans concerning moral worth. Many human beings lack some or all of the aforementioned properties. Certainly fetuses, comatose persons, and dead persons can be said to lack all of them. Yet, we do not feel free to do as we please with individuals who are in one of these categories of humanhood. It is also the case that the mental powers of many humans are, at various times, often severely impaired or entirely absent, i.e., when they are asleep, under the influence of drugs, etc., and yet we do not believe that the moral worth of such persons evaporates with the temporary disappearance of their mental powers.

Nor is it evident that animals lack the capacities and abilities to manifest some or all of the mental properties often held to distinguish man and beast. There is a voluminous literature in ethology and comparative psychology that indicates that at least some animals are capable of primitive forms of reasoning, intentionality, language, and self-awareness.[1,3,5] Certainly enough evidence has accumulated in the behavioral and biological sciences to cast suspicions on claims for the complete absence of higher mental states and abilities in the animal world. Given the uncertainty surrounding the question of animal awareness, it seems reasonable, in light of what we know about other similarities and commonalities between humans and animals, to err in the direction of commonality when in doubt until definitive evidence can be produced—that what has proven true with regard to genetic, morphological, physiological, biochemical, and anatomical properties is not true with respect to mental properties.

Given the fact that not all humans always possess fully developed mental powers and the likely circumstance that at least some animals do, there would appear to be no basis for drawing a hard and fast line between animals and humans in terms of physical or mental properties. What is important about this claim is that the moral worth of entities does seem linked in important ways to abilities and capacities to suffer, feel pain, or have their goals and purposes frustrated. While it is evident that bodily form or physical appearance are unimportant in deciding whether one ought to be concerned about the welfare of another creature, it is true that certain properties must be presumed if talk about welfare is to make any sense. The ability to feel pain, to suffer anxiety or stress, and the capacity to have one's desires, purposes, or intentions frustrated, all seem to be grounds for speaking meaningfully about the welfare of something. If a creature can experience pain, then, other things being equal, it certainly seems wrong to inflict pain on that creature. Similarly, if an organism, be it human or animal, seeks to fulfill some purpose or end—to drink some water, return home, to rest—it seems wrong (again, other things being equal) to frustrate such desires or purposes.

Sentience and purposiveness seem to be the kinds of properties that confer moral worth on creatures. Any entity, human or non-human, terrestrial or non-terrestrial, that could reasonably be said to possess sentience or purpose seems to be the sort of thing to which it is reasonable to attribute moral worth.[4,6] Unless some reason can be given for interfering with or hindering a creature so endowed, it seems inherently wrong to inflict pain on a sentient entity or to frustrate the purposes and goals of such a creature.

It is with respect to the properties of sentience or purposiveness that humans and animals can be said to be of equal moral worth. Most humans and many animals seem to possess some degree of sentience. They are alert to stimuli and will seek those they find pleasant and attempt to avoid those they find noxious. Many animals and most humans seem to harbor any number of desires, aspirations, intentions, and purposes as can be inferred from the efforts they will make to attain certain goals or to overcome certain obstacles that may stand between them and the objects of their desires. While the issue of sentience and purposiveness is in part a scientific question, at least with regard to the distribution and degree of such properties in the biological world, there would seem to be good reasons for thinking that these properties represent excellent candidates for conferring moral worth upon entities.[4]

It should be noted that in arguing that sentience and purposiveness are sufficient properties for attributing moral worth to an entity, this does not mean that both or either property is necessary for having moral worth. Creatures may someday be found on this or other planets that lack these traits, but possess still others that might make them objects of our moral respect. Moreover, the fact that an entity possesses sentience or purposiveness only satisfies the minimal conditions requisite for having moral worth. It may be possible to distinguish further among various creatures as to which ones have more or higher degrees of these salient features. It would surely be a logical error to infer from the fact that animals meet minimal conditions for having moral worth that there are no relevant differences with respect to these properties that distinguish humans and animals— for example, few animals will modify their behavior toward other animals as a result of reading this paper, while it is possible that some human beings may do so.

If it is true that the existence of sentience and/or purposiveness are sufficient traits for imputing moral worth to someone/something, then it would seem there exist what philosophers term *prima facie* duties[2,9] that ought be exercised toward such creatures. Unless one can justify the behavior by an appeal to some higher moral reason or purpose, it would be wrong to harm or frustrate any creature, including an animal, for no reason. Perhaps the cruelest or meanest activity that humans can engage in is the harming or frustrating of others, human and animal, for no reason other than simple meanness of spirit. In some ways human beings are actually in a better position than minimally endowed animals to cope with the frustration and pain of being deceived, fooled, hindered, tricked, or duped since humans are at least bright enough to occasionally figure out what is going on and take steps to avoid or end their suffering. Animals, confronted with malevolent owners or mischievous children, are competent enough to serve as the objects of malevolent intentions (as the pet owners or children know all too well), but are not competent enough to avoid or evade their plight.

It is important to distinguish between an entity's having moral worth, a status I have argued derives from the properties of sentience and purposiveness, and an entity's being a moral agent. Or, in other words, to distinguish between being a moral object and a moral agent. It is true that many animals and some humans lack all of the properties of mentation we commonly associate with *Homo sapiens*. It would be ludicrous to think that we could hold all animals and humans morally responsible for their actions or that we should expect moral reciprocity from any creature capable of sentience

and purpose. What is sufficient in terms of properties that concern moral worth or standing is hardly sufficient in terms of properties that confer moral agency and moral responsibility. We need not determine the nature of the properties that would be sufficient for establishing moral competence among creatures (although it is interesting to note that historically not a few animals have been punished by their owners and even by courts as liable for the untoward outcomes of their behavior!) in this paper. All that need be noted is that the class of moral agents is far smaller than the class of moral objects, and that arguments about the moral equality of animals and humans concern the latter status and not the former.

SENTIENCE AND PURPOSIVENESS AS CRITERIA OF MORAL WORTH

I have argued thus far that both sentience and purposiveness seem to me to be properties sufficient for conferring moral worth on entities who possess them. However, I have not faced the question of whether these properties must both be present, or whether either one of them is sufficient by itself for establishing moral worth. Since moral considerableness entails a number of responsibilities on human agents in terms of their not harming or interfering with creatures that have moral worth, it is important to look carefully at these two properties to see whether they are independent and individually adequate for conferring moral worth.

In recent arguments about the ethics of animal experimentation, some philosophers,[10,11] notably and most vocally Peter Singer in his book *Animal Liberation*, have argued for the sufficiency of sentience as a property for conferring moral worth upon entities. Singer presents a four-part argument in this book that runs as follows: (1) Any creature that is sentient has an interest in not suffering and not feeling pain; (2) all interests must be taken into account in deciding how we ought to behave; (3) equal interests in not suffering or experiencing pain must be counted equally; (4) we should act to bring about the greatest amount of good and to minimize suffering and pain. Thus, if animals can suffer and feel pain as a result of being sentient, Singer argues we must treat them impartially in assessing the practice of animal experimentation. What counts is not only the degree to which human safety is assured and human health promoted, but the degree to which animal suffering is exacerbated by experimental procedures. We should not engage in any particular experiment where the degree of suffering or pain produced in sentient creatures is not outweighed by the amount of benefit to be produced for other sentient creatures, animal and human.

Singer's position is one of classical utilitarianism—the costs and benefits of every action must be computed as best as can be done and decisions about the acceptability or non-acceptability of any action or practice turn on the beliefs we have about the overall effects of the action or practice in terms of goods versus suffering produced. In most cases, Singer argues,[11] animal experiments fail to be justifiable since, given animal sentience, the degree of suffering involved cannot, with certainty, be predicted to be outweighed by the goods to be obtained by engaging in any given case of animal experimentation. Since we should be impartial as to the source of suffering when it occurs, animals and humans being equally deserving of moral consideration when they are capable of suffering or feeling pain, we ought to modify our current experimental practices accordingly and drastically decrease the use of animals in research.

The difficulties confronting Singer's criterion of sentience and his four-part argument are many.[9,10] For example, it is not clear that most scientists would disagree with the claim that human benefit ought outweigh animal suffering if animal experimentation is to be morally legitimated.[12] Indeed, as critics of Singer's view point out, the issue of how much suffering is caused by animal experiments is an empirical question and it is not clear that the benefits do not outweigh the harms in assessing most cases of animal research.

More seriously, Singer's argument against animal experiment founders on two other issues. First, his position would seem to permit experimentation on any creatures which cannot, for whatever reason, suffer or feel pain. Thus, if we can make animal experimentation, or human experimentation for that matter, pain-free, we would appear to be justified in conducting research that would produce benefits in terms of health, well-being, safety, or knowledge. Also, if we could produce vast benefits to animals or humans by utilizing only a few animals or humans in painful experiments, this practice would also escape moral condemnation since, on Singer's construction of the argument, it is only the net outcome of experimentation that legitimates the activity.

I suspect that sentience and the corresponding ability it confers upon animals to suffer or feel pain is a bit too lofty a standard to invoke in thinking about the question of moral worth. It seems wrong to treat humans or animals who are incapable of suffering or feeling pain as undeserving of moral respect and consideration. For example, even if a human being were rendered unable to feel pain or to suffer by surgical intervention or through the use of drugs, I doubt whether members of our society would want to say that such persons could then be used in any way scientists deemed useful in the process of research.

It is interesting to note that Singer's view, while popular in antivivisectionist circles these days, does not lead to the view that all animal experimentation is wrong. Nor does it lead to the view that animals have rights—a concept that is antithetical to a utilitarian analysis of moral worth. However, if we look to purposiveness and intentionality rather than sentience and the ability to suffer as the standard of moral worth, I think we come closer to locating the kind of criterion that motivates much of the moral concern about animal experimentation.

If animals and humans are so organized as to be purposive creatures with various desires, drives, intentions, and aspirations, it seems wrong to cavalierly frustrate these purposes. It might be argued that if animals and humans are biologically constituted so as to pursue their own existence, which is a fact quite consistent with current thinking in evolutionary theory, then it is morally wrong to interfere with or deprive animals of the opportunity to fulfill this basic drive. In other words, animals and humans, endowed by nature with a will to survive, have a right to survive—rights being consequent upon the purposiveness and teleological orientation of living things.[9] If all creatures who possess purposiveness have a right to be left alone to pursue their ends, then the basic moral repugnance felt by many people about animal experimentation can be easily understood—most experimentation deprives animals of the right to exist, or, at minimum, frustrates certain basic drives and intentions they manifest. While human beings are under no moral obligation to aid their fellows or animals in the pursuit of their basic purposes, they do appear to be under some constraint not to uncaringly interfere with other organisms.

I believe that purposiveness rather than sentience is a property that suffices for conferring moral worth upon entities. When organisms have sufficient organization to have basic drives, desires, and intentions, be they amoebas, bees, birds, or retarded humans, it is wrong to interfere with their efforts to fulfill these desires. It needs to be quickly added that such interference is wrong unless there exists some other reason or justification for doing so. The fact is that, as is the case with the abortion debate, most persons erroneously believe that once animal rights are established, the issue of animal experimentation is settled.[2] If it is wrong to interfere with purposive creatures, then no animal research could ever be morally legitimate. But such a view confuses the question of how moral worth and moral rights arise with the question of what to do when rights conflict—a common, ordinary, and unavoidable consequence of the nature of the world we live in.

No animals or humans capable of purposiveness should be interfered with by others, other things being equal. But other things are rarely equal. If humans are to survive, they must eat, and animals may have to suffer the consequences. If human beings are to fulfill their desires to have medicines, then some creatures will have to suffer in the course of discovering whether different substances have therapeutic value. While it is true that we ought not interfere with or hinder the bringing to fruition of the desires and purposes of others, animals and humans, in a world of limited resources and conflicting purposes, some creatures will, of necessity, have their basic rights overridden.

THE LEGITIMACY OF ANIMAL EXPERIMENTATION RECONSIDERED

It should be evident from the preceding discussion that science has no one to blame but itself for the existence of worries about the ethics of animal experimentation. Science has shown the degree to which sentience and purposiveness permeate the animal kingdom, and thus has raised doubts about the validity of causing harm to or interfering with creatures who may not differ all that much from human beings in the properties that count from a moral point of view. If sentience or, minimally, purposiveness are sufficient for conferring moral worth on things, and if we are to be consistent in our moral practices and beliefs, then we may have to rethink our ordinary attitudes about the legitimacy of animal experimentation.

Perhaps the strongest caveat to emerge from an analysis of the morality of animal research is that the burden of proof always rests upon the experimenter to justify the use of animals in experimental contexts. The antivivisectionist has nothing to prove; many animals used in experiments are sentient and purposive, and thus have *prima facie* rights to live and be left alone. Those who would override or abrogate these rights must provide compelling reasons for doing so. Humility and sen-

sitivity, not arrogance and hubris, must be the hallmarks of animal research since it is only out of ignorance and expediency that we put members of the animal kingdom to our purposes rather than theirs.

The other conclusion that follows from the analysis of the moral legitimacy of animal experimentation is that such activity is always morally tragic. No matter what goods are promoted by the process, some creatures who are unable to alter their circumstances will have their basic rights of life and fulfillment infringed. Since this is so, it would seem imperative that steps be taken to reduce waste and duplication in the use of animals for research purposes, put more funds toward the development of alternatives to animal testing, and make the public aware of the moral trade-offs that must be faced in deciding how best to achieve human well-being, health, safety, and knowledge at the expense of animal suffering. Ultimately, the public will have to decide what sorts of trade-offs are morally acceptable when animal and human interests conflict.

ACKNOWLEDGMENTS

I would like to thank De Anti-Vivisectie-Stichting of The Netherlands for providing me with the opportunity to present some of the material in this paper in a series of lectures at the Universities of Leiden, Groningen, Wachningen, Nijmegen and the Free University of Amsterdam. I am particularly grateful to Corrie Smid, Eleanor Seiling, Janet Caplan, and Peter Singer for helpful conversations regarding many of the ideas presented in this paper. I would also like to acknowledge the support of the Marilyn M. Simpson Charitable Income Trust in preparing this paper.

REFERENCES

1 Bowd, A. D. 1980. Ethical reservations about psychological research with animals. Psychol. Rec. 30(Spring): 201–210.
2 Caplan, A. L. 1978. Rights language and the ethical treatment of animals. *In* Implications of History and Ethics to Medicine—Veterinary and Human. L. McCullough & J. P. Morris, Eds.: 126–135. Texas A&M University Press. College Station, Tex.

3 Fox, M. S. 1981. Experimental psychology, animal rights, welfare and ethics. Psychopharm. Bull. 17(2): 80–84.

4 Goodpaster, K. E. 1978. On being morally considerable. J. Phil. 76(6): 308–324.

5 Griffin, D. R. 1976. The Question of Animal Awareness. Rockefeller University Press. New York.

6 Hoff, C. 1980. Immoral and moral uses of animals. N. Eng. J. Med. 302(2): 115–118.

7 Morris, R. K. & M. W. Fox, Eds. 1978. On the Fifth Day: Animal Rights and Human Ethics. Acropolis Books. Washington, D.C.

8 Passmore, J. 1976. Man's Responsibility for Nature. Scribner's. New York.

9 Regan, T. 1980. Animal rights, human wrongs. Environ. Ethics 2(2): 99–120.

10 Regan, T. & P. Singer, Eds. 1976. Animal Rights and Human Obligations. Prentice-Hall. Englewood Cliffs, N.J.

11 Singer, P. 1975. Animal Liberation. Avon Books. New York.

12 Visscher, M. B. 1979. Animal rights and alternative methods. The Pharos (Fall): 11–19.

ANNOTATED BIBLIOGRAPHY: CHAPTER 4

Annas, George J., Leonard H. Glantz, and Barbara F. Katz: *Informed Consent to Human Experimentation: The Subject's Dilemma* (Cambridge, Mass.: Ballinger, 1977). Annas, Glantz, and Katz trace and analyze the legal system's attempt to articulate the law of informed consent to human experimentation with different types of subjects and different types of research. The authors show that the research subject is not the only one faced with moral dilemmas. Lawyers and judges, as well as investigators, face numerous and complicated problems in attempting to determine how to implement the ethical and legal requirement of "competent, voluntary, informed, and understanding consent."

Beecher, Henry K.: *Research and the Individual* (Boston: Little, Brown, 1970). This is one of the earlier works dealing with the ethical problems raised by research involving human subjects. It includes a collection of codes of ethics for those involved in such research.

Capron, Alexander M.: "Medical Research in Prisons: Should a Moratorium Be Called?" *Hastings Center Report* 3 (June 1973), pp. 4–6. Capron argues that a moratorium should be called on prison research until the problems raised by the current conduct of such research are resolved.

Daedalus (Spring 1969). This entire issue focuses on the ethical aspects of experimentation with human subjects. Especially useful is David D. Rutstein's article, "The Ethical Design of Human Experiments."

Greenwald, Robert A., Mary Kay Ryan, and James E. Mulvihill: *Human Subjects Research: A Handbook for Institutional Review Boards* (New York: Plenum, 1982). This is a useful, practical handbook for members of institutional review boards (IRBs) as well as for those engaged in research using human subjects who plan to submit a project proposal to an IRB.

IRB: A Review of Human Subjects Research (Briarcliff Manor, N.Y.: The Hastings Center). This periodical, published ten times a year, is devoted to articles dealing with the ethical aspects of research using human subjects.

Journal of Medicine and Philosophy 11 (November 1986). This issue, "Ethical Issues in the Use of Clinical Controls," is edited by Kenneth F. Schaffner. Schaffner himself provides a historical and methodological context for the essays in this volume, and the essays deal with some of the problems posed by clinical trials in general as well as by RCTs and prerandomized clinical trials in particular.

Katz, Jay, with Alexander M. Capron and Eleanor Swift Glass, eds.: *Experimentation with Human Beings: The Authority of the Investigator, Subject, Professions, and State in the Human*

Experimentation Process (New York: Russell Sage, 1972). This is an excellent, well-organized collection of edited materials dealing with human experimentation. It includes discussions of the function and limitations of informed consent; discussions of experimentation on specific subject groups, such as dying and uncomprehending subjects; and a wealth of other material on the topic of experimentation.

Macklin, Ruth, and Susan Sherwin: "Experimenting on Human Subjects: Philosophical Perspectives," *Case Western Law Review* 25 (Spring 1975), pp. 434–471. Macklin and Sherwin examine the ethical problems raised by research on human subjects from various philosophical points of view. They are particularly concerned to show the shortcomings of the views of Immanuel Kant and John Stuart Mill. Macklin and Sherwin reject these two views and recommend using John Rawls's theory of social justice as a model for making ethical judgments.

Marquis, Don: "Leaving Therapy to Chance," *Hastings Center Report* 13 (August 1983), pp. 40–47. Marquis argues that RCTs as presently conducted are unethical although they clearly provide important benefits.

Melnick, Vijaya, and Nancy N. Dubler, eds.: *Alzheimer's Dementia: Dilemmas in Clinical Research* (Clifton, N.J.: Humana Press, 1985). This collection of articles by ethicists, lawyers, historians, and neurologists deals with many of the complex medical, ethical, and legal issues associated with a disease that affects more elderly people each year.

National Commission for the Protection of Human Subjects of Biomedical and Behavioral Research: *The Belmont Report: Ethical Principles and Guidelines for the Protection of Human Subjects of Research.* DHEW (OS) 78-0012. *The Belmont Report. Appendix*, vols. 1, 2. DHEW (OS) 78-0013, 78-0014. (Bethesda, Md., 1978). This report was put out by a commission established under the National Research Act (P.L. 93-348). The commission's purpose was to develop ethical guidelines for the conduct of research involving human subjects and to make recommendations for the application of these guidelines to research conducted or supported by the Department of Health, Education, and Welfare. *The Belmont Report* is the commission's final and most general report. Other reports, listed below, deal with narrower topics. The appendixes to this report and to the ones listed below contain many useful papers, reports, and other materials that were reviewed by the commission prior to formulating its recommendations.

————: *Report and Recommendations: Research Involving Children.* DHEW (OS) 77-0004. *Appendix: Research Involving Children.* DHEW (OS) 77-0005. (Bethesda, Md., 1977).

————: *Report and Recommendations: Research Involving Prisoners.* DHEW (OS) 76-131. *Appendix: Research Involving Prisoners.* DHEW (OS) 76-132. (Bethesda, Md., 1976).

————: *Report and Recommendations: Research Involving Those Institutionalized as Mentally Infirm.* DHEW (OS) 78-0006. *Appendix: Research Involving Those Institutionalized as Mentally Infirm.* DHEW (OS) 78-0007. (Bethesda, Md., 1978).

Sechzer, Jeri A.: *The Role of Animals in Biomedical Research* (New York: The New York Academy of Sciences, 1983). This issue of the *Annals of the New York Academy of Sciences* (vol. 406) contains papers, discussions, and summaries on a wide range of topics dealing with animal experimentation. Topics include the methodologies employed as well as some of the relevant ethical and public policy issues.

Tannenbaum, Jerrold, and Andrew N. Rowan: "Rethinking the Morality of Animal Research," *Hastings Center Report* 15 (October 1985), pp. 32–43. The authors argue that we need a clearer understanding of the ethical issues involved in animal research to provide the groundwork for public policy. Their article discusses some of these issues.

Taylor, Kathryn M., Richard G. Margolese, and Colin L. Soskolne: "Physicians' Reasons for Not Entering Eligible Patients in a Randomized Clinical Trial of Surgery for Breast Cancer," *The New England Journal of Medicine* 310 (May 24, 1984), pp. 1363–1367. This report illustrates some of the ethical problems raised by RCTs. The reasons identified for physician reluctance include (1) concern about the effect that the RCT would have on the doctor-patient relationship; (2) difficulties with informed consent; and (3) perceived conflicts between the roles of clinician and scientist.

Warren, John W., et al.: "Informed Consent by Proxy: An Issue in Research with Elderly Patients," *The New England Journal of Medicine* 315 (October 30, 1986), pp. 1124–1128. The authors studied the proxy decisions made in behalf of 168 nursing home patients whose participation was requested in a research study involving minimal risk. They bring out and discuss the reasons that led almost one-half of the proxies to refuse consent.

CHAPTER 5

ETHICAL ISSUES REGARDING THE MENTALLY ILL AND THE MENTALLY RETARDED

INTRODUCTION

What social policies should we adopt in regard to persons whose autonomy is diminished due to internal factors such as mental illness or mental retardation? The policies we adopt largely determine the roles played by professionals in the lives of mentally ill and mentally retarded individuals. This chapter focuses first on moral issues raised regarding some social policies dealing with the mentally ill, and then on moral issues raised regarding some social policies dealing with the mentally retarded.

Mental Illness and Involuntary Civil Commitment

Mental illness poses both personal and social problems. On the personal level, mental illness often disrupts family relationships, severely incapacitates individuals, and makes everyday living a hazardous, torturous affair. Mentally ill individuals who are severely disoriented or deluded may be unable to care for their routine needs and may thus pose a serious risk to their own well-being. Those who are sufficiently depressed may run the risk of committing suicide. Those who are extremely agitated or confused may pose a threat of serious harm not just to themselves but to their families as well. On a wider social level, the mentally ill may be nuisances, may disrupt social activities, and may engage in serious antisocial behavior. In light of all this, questions arise concerning the state's legitimate role regarding those classified as mentally ill. Does morality permit or, perhaps, even require laws that give representatives of the state, such as judges and psychiatrists, the power to control the lives of those diagnosed as mentally ill? This power is exercised when patients are committed to mental institutions against their "will" or when they are subjected to some form of therapy either without their consent or with "consent" that is given only because acceptance of therapy is a necessary condition for release.

The Concept of Mental Illness   Explorations of the moral correctness of state interference in the lives of the mentally ill are complicated by the difficulty of defining "mental illness." In modern physiological medicine, a patient might be diagnosed as suffering from leukemia. The patient is said to have a certain pathological condition, a physical disease. He or she is physically ill. In modern psychiatry, a patient might be diagnosed as suffering from some type of schizophrenia. The patient is said to have a certain psychopathological condition, a mental disease. He or she is mentally ill.

In our culture, when labels such as "insane" and "sick" are so readily predicated of human behavior, it is difficult not to feel a certain sense of puzzlement in the face of the concepts of mental health and mental illness. Our difficulty, however, is not limited to the confusion that is produced by the offhand misuse of such labels. If we had access to a firmly entrenched theory of mental health, we would probably feel ourselves to be on firmer ground. But that is just the problem. Mental health professionals subscribe to widely varying theories of mental health. As if that is not confusing enough, we are also confronted with the fact that psychiatrists in the same school of thought often find it difficult to agree whether or not a certain diagnostic label is applicable to an individual case.

It is sometimes alleged, most prominently in the work of the psychiatrist Thomas S. Szasz, that mental illness is a myth. According to Szasz, as reflected in his selection in this chapter, the concept of mental illness has no scientific or descriptive content whatsoever and thus ought to be abandoned. Although it masquerades as a scientific concept, it functions in an exclusively normative way. When someone is labeled "mentally ill," Szasz holds, it is solely because that individual has deviated from certain ethical, political, or social norms. Rem B. Edwards offers in this chapter a contrasting view. He advances a tentative definition of mental illness and argues that there are some cases that can be correctly described as involving insanity.

Involuntary Civil Commitment   Views on the justifiability of involuntary civil commitment often reflect underlying conceptions of mental illness. For example, in his book *Ideology and Insanity*, Szasz argues that involuntary civil commitment is a crime against humanity and should be abolished.[1] Szasz's stance is clearly related to his "social deviance model" of mental illness. However, those who believe that mental illness is a definable reality rather than a myth are typically inclined to consider involuntary civil commitment justifiable in at least some circumstances. Paul Chodoff, in a reading in this chapter, discusses both the abolitionist position on involuntary civil commitment and the contrasting views of those who adopt a medical model of mental illness.

Clearly, those involved in disputes about the morality of involuntary civil commitment often disagree about the concept of mental illness. They also often disagree on empirical issues, such as the "dangerousness" of the mentally ill or the extent of their competency. The bearing of these empirical disagreements on the moral positions taken regarding involuntary civil commitment emerges in the discussion below concerning the kinds of moral justifications that are advanced for the practice.

Explorations of the morality of involuntary civil commitment procedures usually involve implicit or explicit discussion of the liberty-limiting principles presented in Chapter 1. Should those classified as mentally ill be committed on any of the following grounds?

1. To keep them from seriously harming others (the harm principle);

2. To prevent them from offending others (the offense principle);

3. To keep them from harming themselves (the principle of paternalism);

4. To benefit them (the principle of extreme paternalism).

In assessing attempted justifications of involuntary civil commitment practices, we must keep two other questions in mind: (*a*) Which of the above principles are morally acceptable liberty-limiting principles? (*b*) Which principle is actually being used (explicitly or implicitly) to justify commitment? In regard to (*a*), for example, if the principles of paternalism a_e *not* acceptable liberty-limiting principles, involuntary civil commitment cannot be justified on paternalistic grounds. In regard to (*b*), critics of involuntary civil commitment often argue as follows: It is not uncommon to commit individuals to institutions simply because their behavior is offensive; but the attempt to justify their commitment is made on other inapplicable grounds, such as their supposed dangerousness. Much of the behavior that earns the mentally ill the label of "dangerous" is at most offensive to others. Shouting harangues on street corners and other bizarre behaviors, although offensive to some, pose no threat of serious harm. If offensive behavior is the real basis for committing someone to a mental institution, then the justifying ground would have to be provided by the offense principle and not the harm principle. But few of us would hold that offensive behavior alone is a sufficient ground for the deprivation of liberty. Therefore, exposing the actual reasons for commitment in certain cases may lead to the conclusion that interference in these cases is not justified.

Dangerousness and the Harm Principle   Since the harm principle is a widely accepted liberty-limiting principle, that principle alone would provide a strong ground for the involuntary civil commitment of mentally ill individuals *if* the mentally ill pose a serious threat of harm to others. It is not surprising, therefore, that the harm principle is often invoked, implicitly or explicitly, to justify involuntary civil commitment procedures. But are the mentally ill so dangerous that their commitment is necessary to protect others from harm? To answer this question it is necessary to distinguish between different kinds of cases.

In some cases there is very little doubt that those labeled "mentally ill" are dangerous and pose a *serious threat of physical harm to others*. One example is an individual, classified as schizophrenic perhaps, who attempts to carry out the commands of a disembodied voice ordering the execution of parents or siblings. Persons of this sort certainly pose a serious, imminent threat to others. Or another example is the individual, labeled paranoid perhaps, who has a history of violent and apparently irrational acts and who gives every indication of repeating such acts. Persons of this sort might also be correctly perceived as dangerous. Thus, in cases involving either imminent potential physical violence or actual physical violence, involuntary civil commitment would certainly seem to be justified by the harm principle. Still, not everyone would agree with this conclusion. Abolitionists like Szasz, for example, want no special treatment for those considered mentally ill. If they perform acts forbidden by law, they should be subject to the same legal sanctions as anyone else. But if they break no laws, the state has no moral right to interfere with their freedom.

Even if Szasz is wrong, however, and the harm principle is correctly invoked in justifying *some* involuntary civil commitments, it does not follow that it justifies the commitment of everyone who is labeled both "mentally ill and dangerous." Mental health workers often diagnose individuals as mentally ill when their behavior seems inexplicable, bizarre, or threatening. They then make predictions about their dangerousness. The purported dangerousness of *most of those* diagnosed as mentally ill, however, is unsupported by actual evidence. Studies have shown either that mental patients as a group are no more dangerous than others[2] or that, if they are, the differences are so small that they allow very little success in prediction.[3] If a psychiatrist's prediction of dangerousness is accepted as sufficient justification for involuntary commitment, the uncertainty of those predictions would result in the commitment of a very large number of nondangerous people.

Paternalism and Autonomy   As we saw in Chapter 1, taking decisions out of people's hands for their own good is paternalistic. When individuals are incapable temporarily or permanently of making decisions about their own well-being, there is no usurpation of autonomy, since the conditions for acting autonomously are absent. In these sorts of cases it would be incorrect to hold that the individual's autonomy has been infringed, interfered with, or limited. The problematic cases arise, however, when an individual's abilities to effectively deliberate and make decisions are diminished by delusions, compulsions, and other internal factors associated with mental illness; and yet the person is an adult capable of understanding enough about his or her situation to refuse to assent to commitment. When the organ responsible for the cognitive functions required for informed consent is itself considered to be malfunctioning, how much weight should be given to a person's refusal? Proponents of paternalistic interventions in such cases sometimes argue as follows. Suppose individuals reject commitment or psychiatric help because their present condition renders them incapable of realizing that these are in their own long-term interest. If they were thinking more clearly, if they were not confused or severely depressed by their illnesses, would they not want the benefits involved? Would they not want others to keep them from running the risks to their physical and mental well-being that they will continue to run if they are not committed? Would they not want the treatment that would restore their competency for rational decision making—a competency that is presently limited by internal factors? Those who argue in this way believe that the autonomy of those diagnosed as mentally ill is sometimes sufficiently diminished to justify their involuntary commitment not only to keep them from harming themselves but to help them in regaining lost autonomy.

The Mentally Ill and Deinstitutionalization

In the 1960s and 1970s, in the movement to deinstitutionalization, many of those who had been committed to mental hospitals were released and returned to the community. In contrast to involuntary civil commitment, the ideal of deinstitutionalization, which incorporates an emphasis on community health-care centers, held out a promise that the chronically mentally ill would receive care without infringement on their civil rights. Deinstitutionalization was officially defined by the director of the National Institute of Mental Health as follows:

> (1) The prevention of inappropriate mental hospital admissions through the provision of community alternatives for treatment, (2) the release to the community of all institutionalized patients who have been given adequate preparation for such a change, and (3) the establishment and maintenance of community support systems for noninstitutionalized people receiving mental health services in the community.[4]

Whatever the original ideal, deinstitutionalization has in fact resulted in a massive dumping of the chronically ill into communities with few facilities and little aftercare. Between 1955 and 1984, 433,407 mental hospital beds were taken out of use.[5] In addition, many state mental institutions were closed, in effect leaving many of the long-term mentally ill with nowhere to go.

In a recent book, *Nowhere to Go*, E. Fuller Torrey maintains that the effects of the policy of deinstitutionalization include the following:

(1) There are at least twice as many seriously mentally ill individuals living on streets and in shelters as there are in public mental hospitals. (2) There are increasing numbers of seriously mentally ill individuals in the nation's jails and prisons. (3) Seriously mentally ill individuals are regularly released from hospitals with little or no provision for aftercare or followup treatment. . . . [4] Laws designed to protect the rights of the seriously mentally ill primarily protect their right to remain mentally ill. . . . [5] The majority of mentally ill individuals discharged from hospitals have been officially lost. Nobody knows where they are.[6]

In one of this chapter's readings, H. Richard Lamb discusses deinstitutionalization. Although he believes that many things have gone right with deinstitutionalization, he points out some of its unfortunate results and discusses changes that need to be made. His article is addressed primarily to mental health professionals whose task he sees as maximizing the benefits of deinstitutionalization for those who suffer from long-term mental illness and yet are capable of living as part of the community. Like Chodoff, however, Lamb holds that there are some long-term mentally ill individuals who, for either long or short times, need highly structured care. Such care, Lamb notes, can only be provided in a hospital or in some alternative setting such as California's locked, skilled-nursing facilities, which have special programs for psychiatric patients.

The Mentally Retarded—Sterilization and Rights

The mentally ill are not the only group whose members have often been almost routinely institutionalized in the past or whose freedoms have been limited because of their presumed incompetency in decision making. Many mentally retarded persons have spent their lives in institutions. Many have been denied educational and other opportunities. Some have been sterilized without their consent. In many states today, even the mildly retarded, if considered legally incompetent, cannot decide to marry, have children, live alone, or enter into any contractual relations without the consent of a guardian. As in the case of the mentally ill, the usual reason given for denying even those who are mildly retarded the freedom of decision possessed by other adults is the purported danger posed by those with cognitive deficiencies to themselves and others. As some of the readings in previous chapters bring out, however, competency is not "all or nothing." Individuals may lack the cognitive skills to solve a geometric problem and yet have sufficient cognitive ability to make everyday decisions about housing, meals, and other practical affairs. Over three-quarters of those considered retarded in our society are classified as "mildly retarded." Those who fit this classification have an I.Q. range of 52 to 68 as measured on the Stanford-Binet Scale, and their ability to function on a day-to-day level differs widely, depending on their education, training, and experience.[7]

The routine paternalistic treatment of the mentally retarded, especially of the mildly retarded, has been increasingly challenged. One practice around which challenges have centered is involuntary sterilization. However, Robert Neville offers arguments in this chapter for sterilizing the mentally retarded without their consent. Neville sees involuntary sterilization as morally justified when it is in the best interests of mildly retarded persons who lack the capacity to give or withhold informed consent because they do not understand the issues involved. He grants, however, that many empirical questions about the competency of mentally retarded individuals remain to be answered. In another reading in this chapter, Elizabeth S. Scott brings out the changes that have taken place in U.S. sterilization laws. In the past, involuntary sterilization was used as a state weapon in a war against mental deficiency, but current laws have established very strong barriers against the sterilization of the mentally retarded. Scott criticizes the one-sidedness of many of these laws, which place retarded persons' interests in procreation above all their other interests, including an interest in avoiding pregnancy.

Recent developments in implantable drug-delivery systems may offer an alternative to surgical sterilization as a means of preventing pregnancies in the case of those who are mentally retarded. At face value, the implantable contraceptive device seems much less ethically problematic than surgical sterilization, since such a device neither requires a major medical intervention nor results in permanent sterilization. However, as Eric T. Juengst and Ronald A. Siegel bring out in a reading in this chapter, despite its advantages, the implantation of the device without the consent of the mentally retarded individual raises some of the same ethical problems as involuntary surgical sterilization.

The retarded have problems that require special attention if they are to develop and exercise their autonomy to the fullest extent possible. Yet advocates for the retarded sometimes argue that those who are intellectually disadvantaged should be treated just like everyone else, with the same basic rights as all other citizens. This point of view is expressed in a code of rights proclaimed at a 1981 conference on mental retardation. The code demands "the closing of all institutions for intellectually disadvantaged persons."[8] While this statement was not the first articulated demand for a shift from custodialism to community care for the mentally retarded, it was the first code incorporating such demands written by "intellectually handicapped" representatives. In asserting their right to make their own choices about employment, housing, and so forth, the delegates argued, "We are humans first and disadvantaged second."[9] Another code, proclaimed by the International League of Societies for the Mentally Handicapped and reprinted in this chapter, asserts both the same basic rights for the mentally retarded as those held by other citizens of the same country and age and a set of special rights.

T.A.M. and J.S.Z.

NOTES

1 Thomas S. Szasz, *Ideology and Insanity* (New York: Doubleday, 1970). See especially pp. 113–139.
2 Jonas R. Rappeport, ed., *The Clinical Evaluation of the Dangerousness of the Mentally Ill* (Springfield, Ill.: Charles C Thomas, 1967), pp. 72–80.
3 Alan A. Stone, *Mental Health and Law: A System in Transition* (Rockville, Md.: Center for Studies of Crime and Delinquency, National Institute of Mental Health, DHEW Publication No. [ADM] 75–176, 1975).
4 E. Fuller Torrey, *Nowhere to Go: The Tragic Odyssey of the Homeless Mentally Ill* (New York: Harper and Row, 1988), p. 4.
5 Ibid., p. 139.
6 Ibid., pp. 5–6.
7 The figures used in classifying the mentally retarded vary. One classification made on the basis of I.Q. and social adaptation tests classifies retardation as mild, moderate, severe, or profound as follows: *Mild*—I.Q. 50–70. The mildly retarded are often indistinguishable from other children until they show difficulty learning conceptual subjects. (About 80 percent of those classified as mentally retarded in the United States fall into this category.) *Moderate*—I.Q. 35–50. The moderately retarded do have the capacity to develop self-supportive and self-protective skills if they are given the proper training. *Severe*—I.Q. 20–35. The severely mentally retarded are often, but not always, physically handicapped. They show motor, speech, and language retardation and require custodial care. *Profound*—I.Q. less than 20. The profoundly retarded are often physically handicapped and need constant care or supervision if they are to survive. From David F. Allen and Victoria S. Allen, *Eth-*

ical Issues in Mental Retardation: Tragic Choices—Living Hope (Nashville, Tenn.: Abingdon Press, 1979), pp. 19–20.

8 The Australian Voice of Intellectually Disadvantaged Citizens, "Code of Rights" (Resolutions of the Second South Pacific Conference on Mental Retardation, Melbourne, Australia, presented by members of the Fifth Strand to Senator Fred Chaney, Federal Social Security Minister, August 28, 1981).

9 Stanley S. Herr, *Rights and Advocacy for Retarded People* (Lexington, Mass.: Lexington Books, 1983), p. 37.

The Concept of Mental Illness

The Myth of Mental Illness
Thomas S. Szasz

Thomas S. Szasz, M.D., is professor of psychiatry at the State University of New York Health Sciences Center in Syracuse. A cofounder of the American Association for the Abolition of Involuntary Mental Hospitalization, he has long been an outspoken critic of contemporary psychiatric practice. Among his numerous published works are *The Ethics of Psychoanalysis* (1965), *The Manufacture of Madness* (1970), *Heresies* (1976), and *Insanity: The Idea and Its Consequences* (1987).

Szasz contends that there is no such thing as mental illness. In his view, the concept of mental illness has no cognitive (descriptive) content, functioning instead as a myth. Although he maintains that the term "mental illness" is unnecessary and misleading when used to refer to brain diseases, he especially objects to employing the term "mental illness" to refer to alleged deformities of personality. Szasz maintains that, whereas physical illness may be ascribed on the basis of deviation from the norm of structural and functional integrity of the body, mental illness is ascribed solely on the basis that there is deviation (of personal behavior) from certain ethical, political, or social norms. According to Szasz, psychiatrists are mistaken in thinking that they are engaged in diagnosing and treating medical illness. Their patients do not have mental diseases but rather are experiencing "problems in living."

I

At the core of virtually all contemporary psychiatric theories and practices lies the concept of mental illness. A critical examination of this concept is therefore indispensable for understanding the ideas, institutions, and interventions of psychiatrists.

My aim in this essay is to ask if there is such a thing as mental illness and to argue that there is not. Of

Originally appeared in *The American Psychologist*, copyright © 1960 by the American Psychological Association. *Ideology and Insanity* by Thomas S. Szasz. Copyright © 1970 by Thomas S. Szasz. Reprinted by permission of Doubleday, a division of Bantam, Doubleday, Dell Publishing Group, Inc.

course, mental illness is not a thing or physical object; hence it can exist only in the same sort of way as do other theoretical concepts. Yet, to those who believe in them, familiar theories are likely to appear, sooner or later, as "objective truths" or "facts." During certain historical periods, explanatory concepts such as deities, witches, and instincts appeared not only as theories but as *self-evident causes* of a vast number of events. Today mental illness is widely regarded in a similar fashion, that is, as the cause of innumerable diverse happenings.

As an antidote to the complacent use of the notion of mental illness—as a self-evident phenomenon, theory, or cause—let us ask: What is meant when it is asserted that someone is mentally ill? In this essay I shall describe the main uses of the concept of mental illness, and I shall argue that this notion has outlived whatever cognitive usefulness it might have had and that it now functions as a myth.

II

The notion of mental illness derives its main support from such phenomena as syphilis of the brain or delirious conditions—intoxications, for instance—in which persons may manifest certain disorders of thinking and behavior. Correctly speaking, however, these are diseases of the brain, not of the mind. According to one school of thought, *all* so-called mental illness is of this type. The assumption is made that some neurological defect, perhaps a very subtle one, will ultimately be found to explain all the disorders of thinking and behavior. Many contemporary physicians, psychiatrists, and other scientists hold this view, which implies that people's troubles cannot be caused by conflicting personal needs, opinions, social aspirations, values, and so forth. These difficulties—which I think we may simply call *problems in living*—are thus attributed to physico-chemical processes that in due time will be discovered (and no doubt corrected) by medical research.

Mental illnesses are thus regarded as basically similar to other diseases. The only difference, in this view, between mental and bodily disease is that the former, affecting the brain, manifests itself by means of mental symptoms; whereas the latter, affecting other organ systems—for example, the skin, liver, and so on—manifests itself by means of symptoms referable to those parts of the body.

In my opinion, this view is based on two fundamental errors. In the first place, a disease of the brain, analogous to a disease of the skin or bone, is a neurological defect, not a problem in living. For example, a *defect* in a person's visual field may be explained by correlating it with certain lesions in the nervous system. On the other hand, a person's *belief*—whether it be in Christianity, in Communism, or in the idea that his internal organs are rotting and that his body is already dead—cannot be explained by a defect or disease of the nervous system. Explanations of this sort of occurrence—assuming that one is interested in the belief itself and does not regard it simply as a symptom or expression of something else that is more interesting—must be sought along different lines.

The second error is epistemological. It consists of interpreting communications about ourselves and the world around us as symptoms of neurological functioning. This is an error not in observation or reasoning, but rather in the organization and expression of knowledge. In the present case, the error lies in making a dualism between mental and physical symptoms, a dualism that is a habit of speech and not the result of known observations. Let us see if this is so.

In medical practice, when we speak of physical disturbances we mean either signs (for example, fever) or symptoms (for example, pain). We speak of mental symptoms, on the other hand, when we refer to a patient's communications about himself, others, and the world about him. The patient might assert that he is Napoleon or that he is being persecuted by the Communists. These would be considered mental symptoms only if the observer believed that the patient was *not* Napoleon or that he was *not* being persecuted by the Communists. This makes it apparent that the statement "X is a mental symptom" involves rendering a judgment that entails a covert comparison between the patient's ideas, concepts, or beliefs and those of the observer and the society in which they live. The notion of mental symptom is therefore inextricably tied to the social, and particularly the ethical, context in which it is made, just as the notion of bodily symptom is tied to an anatomical and genetic context.[1]

To sum up: For those who regard mental symptoms as signs of brain disease, the concept of mental illness is unnecessary and misleading. If they mean that people so labeled suffer from diseases of the brain, it would seem better, for the sake of clarity, to say that and not something else.

III

The term "mental illness" is also widely used to describe something quite different from a disease of the brain. Many people today take it for granted that living is an arduous affair. Its hardship for modern man derives, moreover, not so much from a struggle for biological survival as from the stresses and strains inherent in the social intercourse of complex human personalities. In this context, the notion of mental illness is used to identify or describe some features of an individual's so-called personality. Mental illness—as a deformity of the personality, so to speak—is then regarded as the cause of human disharmony. It is implicit in this view that social intercourse between people is regarded as something inherently harmonious, its disturbance being due solely to the presence of "mental illness" in many people. Clearly, this is faulty reasoning, for it makes the abstraction "mental illness" into a cause of, even though this abstraction was originally created to serve only as a shorthand expression for, certain types of human behavior. It now becomes necessary to ask: What kinds of behavior are regarded as indicative of mental illness, and by whom?

The concept of illness, whether bodily or mental, implies deviation from some clearly defined norm. In the case of physical illness, the norm is the structural and functional integrity of the human body. Thus, although the desirability of physical health, as such, is an ethical value, what health is can be stated in anatomical and physiological terms. What is the norm, deviation from which is regarded as mental illness? This question cannot be easily answered. But whatever this norm may be, we can be certain of only one thing: namely, that it must be stated in terms of psychosocial, ethical, and legal concepts. For example, notions such as "excessive repression" and "acting out an unconscious impulse" illustrate the use of psychological concepts for judging so-called mental health and illness. The idea that chronic hostility, vengefulness, or divorce are indicative of mental illness is an illustration of the use of ethical norms (that is, the desirability of love, kindness, and a stable marriage relationship). Finally, the widespread psychiatric opinion that only a mentally ill person would commit homicide illustrates the use of a legal concept as a norm of mental health. In short, when one speaks of mental illness, the norm from which deviation is measured is a *psychosocial and ethical* standard. Yet, the remedy is sought in terms of *medical* measures that—it is hoped and assumed—are free from wide differences of ethical value. The definition of the disorder and the terms in which its remedy are sought are therefore at serious odds with one another. The practical significance of this covert conflict between the alleged nature of the defect and the actual remedy can hardly be exaggerated.

Having identified the norms used for measuring deviations in cases of mental illness, we shall now turn to the question, Who defines the norms and hence the deviation? Two basic answers may be offered: First, it may be the person himself—that is, the patient—who decides that he deviates from a norm; for example, an artist may believe that he suffers from a work inhibition; and he may implement this conclusion by seeking help *for himself* from a psychotherapist. Second, it may be someone other than the "patient" who decides that the latter is deviant—for example, relatives, physicians, legal authorities, society generally; a psychiatrist may then be hired by persons other than the "patient" to do something *to him* in order to correct the deviation.

These considerations underscore the importance of asking the question, Whose agent is the psychiatrist? and of giving a candid answer to it. The psychiatrist (or non-medical mental health worker) may be the agent of the patient, the relatives, the school, the military services, a business organization, a court of law, and so forth. In speaking of the psychiatrist as the agent of these persons or organizations, it is not implied that his moral values, or his ideas and aims concerning the proper nature of remedial action, must coincide exactly with those of his employer. For example, a patient in individual psychotherapy may believe that his salvation lies in a new marriage; his psychotherapist need not share this hypothesis. As the patient's agent, however, he must not resort to social or legal force to prevent the patient from putting his beliefs into action. If his *contract* is with the patient, the psychiatrist (psychotherapist) may disagree with him or stop his treatment, but he cannot engage others to obstruct the patient's aspirations.[2] Similarly, if a psychiatrist is retained by a court to determine the sanity of an offender, he need not fully share the legal authorities' values and intentions in regard to the criminal, nor the means deemed appropriate for dealing with him; such a psychiatrist cannot testify, however, that the accused is not insane, but that the legislators are—for passing the law that decrees the offender's actions illegal.[3] This sort of opinion could be voiced, of course—but not in a courtroom, and not by a psychiatrist who is there to assist the court in performing its daily work.

To recapitulate: In contemporary social usage, the finding of mental illness is made by establishing a deviance in behavior from certain psychosocial, ethical, or legal norms. The judgment may be made, as in medicine, by the patient, the physician (psychiatrist), or others. Remedial action, finally, tends to be sought in a therapeutic—or covertly medical—framework. This creates a situation in which it is claimed that psychosocial, ethical, and legal deviations can be corrected by medical action. Since medical interventions are designed to remedy only medical problems, it is logically absurd to expect that they will help solve problems whose very existence have been defined and established on non-medical grounds.

IV

Anything that people *do*—in contrast to things that *happen* to them[4]—takes place in a context of value. Hence, no human activity is devoid of moral implications. When the values underlying certain activities are widely shared, those who participate in their pursuit often lose sight of them altogether. The discipline of medicine—both as a pure science (for example, research) and as an applied science or technology (for example, therapy)—contains many ethical considerations and judgments. Unfortunately, these are often denied, minimized, or obscured, for the ideal of the medical profession as well as of the people whom it serves is to have an ostensibly value-free system of medical care. This sentimental notion is expressed by such things as the doctor's willingness to treat patients regardless of their religious or political beliefs. But such claims only serve to obscure the fact that ethical considerations encompass a vast range of human affairs. Making medical practice neutral with respect to some specific issues of moral value (such as race or sex) need not mean, and indeed does not mean, that it can be kept free from others (such as control over pregnancy or regulation of sex relations). Thus, birth control, abortion, homosexuality, suicide, and euthanasia continue to pose major problems in medical ethics.

Psychiatry is much more intimately related to problems of ethics than is medicine in general. I use the word "psychiatry" here to refer to the contemporary discipline concerned with problems in living, and not with diseases of the brain, which belong to neurology. Difficulties in human relations can be analyzed, interpreted, and given meaning only within specific social and ethical contexts. Accordingly, the psychiatrist's socioethical orientations will influence his ideas on what is wrong with the patient, on what deserves comment or interpretation, in what directions change might be desirable, and so forth. Even in medicine proper, these factors play a role, as illustrated by the divergent orientations that physicians, depending on their religious affiliations, have toward such things as birth control and therapeutic abortion. Can anyone really believe that a psychotherapist's ideas on religion, politics, and related issues play no role in his practical work? If, on the other hand, they do matter, what are we to infer from it? Does it not seem reasonable that perhaps we ought to have different psychiatric therapies—each recognized for the ethical positions that it embodies—for, say, Catholics and Jews, religious persons and atheists, democrats and Communists, white supremacists and Negroes, and so on? Indeed, if we look at the way psychiatry is actually practiced today, especially in the United States, we find that the psychiatric interventions people seek and receive depend more on their socioeconomic status and moral beliefs than on the "mental illnesses" from which they ostensibly suffer.[5] This fact should occasion no greater surprise than that practicing Catholics rarely frequent birth-control clinics, or that Christian Scientists rarely consult psychoanalysts.

V

The position outlined above, according to which contemporary psychotherapists deal with problems in living, not with mental illnesses and their cures, stands in sharp opposition to the currently prevalent position, according to which psychiatrists treat mental diseases, which are just as "real" and "objective" as bodily diseases. I submit that the holders of the latter view have no evidence whatever to justify their claim, which is actually a kind of psychiatric propaganda: their aim is to create in the popular mind a confident belief that mental illness is some sort of disease entity, like an infection or a malignancy. If this were true, one could *catch* or *get* a mental illness, one might *have* or *harbor* it, one might *transmit* it to others, and finally one could *get rid* of it. Not only is there not a shred of evidence to support this idea, but, on the contrary, all the evidence is the other way and supports the view that what people now call mental illnesses are, for the most part, *communications* expressing unacceptable ideas, often framed in an unusual idiom.

This is not the place to consider in detail the similarities and differences between bodily and mental illnesses. It should suffice to emphasize that whereas the term "bodily illness" refers to physicochemical occurrences that are not affected by being made public, the term "mental illness" refers to sociopsychological events that are crucially affected by being made public. The psychiatrist thus cannot, and does not, stand apart from the person he observes, as the pathologist can and often does. The psychiatrist is committed to some picture of what he considers reality, and to what he thinks society considers reality, and he observes and judges the patient's behavior in the light of these beliefs. The very notion of "mental symptom" or "mental illness" thus implies a covert comparison, and often conflict, between observer and observed, psychiatrist and patient. Though obvious, this fact needs to be re-emphasized, if one wishes, as I do here, to counter the prevailing tendency to deny the moral aspects of psychiatry and to substitute for them allegedly value-free medical concepts and interventions.

Psychotherapy is thus widely practiced as though it entailed nothing other than restoring the patient from a state of mental sickness to one of mental health. While it is generally accepted that mental illness has something to do with man's social or interpersonal relations, it is paradoxically maintained that problems of values—that is, of ethics—do not arise in this process. Freud himself went so far as to assert: "I consider ethics to be taken for granted. Actually I have never done a mean thing."[6] This is an astounding thing to say, especially for someone who had studied man as a social being as deeply as Freud had. I mention it here to show how the notion of "illness"—in the case of psychoanalysis, "psychopathology," or "mental illness"—was used by Freud, and by most of his followers, as a means of classifying certain types of human behavior as falling within the scope of medicine, and hence, by fiat, outside that of ethics. Nevertheless, the stubborn fact remains that, in a sense, much of psychotherapy revolves around nothing other than the elucidation and weighing of goals and values— many of which may be mutually contradictory—and the means whereby they might best be harmonized, realized, or relinquished.

Because the range of human values and of the methods by which they may be attained is so vast, and because many such ends and means are persistently unacknowledged, conflicts among values are the main source of conflicts in human relations. Indeed, to say that human relations at all levels—from mother to child, through husband and wife, to nation and nation—are fraught with stress, strain, and disharmony is, once again, to make the obvious explicit. Yet, what may be obvious may be also poorly understood. This, I think, is the case here. For it seems to me that in our scientific theories of behavior we have failed to accept the simple fact that human relations are inherently fraught with difficulties, and to make them even relatively harmonious requires much patience and hard work. I submit that the idea of mental illness is now being put to work to obscure certain difficulties that at present may be inherent—not that they need to be unmodifiable—in the social intercourse of persons. If this is true, the concept functions as a disguise: Instead of calling attention to conflicting human needs, aspirations, and values, the concept of mental illness provides an amoral and impersonal "thing"—an "illness"—as an explanation for problems in living. We may recall in this connection that not so long ago it was devils and witches that were held responsible for man's problems of living. The belief in mental illness, as something other than man's trouble in

getting along with his fellow man, is the proper heir to the belief in demonology and witchcraft. Mental illness thus exists or is "real" in exactly the same sense in which witches existed or were "real."

VI

While I maintain that mental illnesses do not exist, I obviously do not imply or mean that the social and psychological occurrences to which this label is attached also do not exist. Like the personal and social troubles that people had in the Middle Ages, contemporary human problems are real enough. It is the labels we give them that concern me, and, having labeled them, what we do about them. The demonologic concept of problems in living gave rise to therapy along theological lines. Today, a belief in mental illness implies—nay, requires—therapy along medical or psychotherapeutic lines.

I do not here propose to offer a new conception of "psychiatric illness" or a new form of "therapy." My aim is more modest and yet also more ambitious. It is to suggest that the phenomena now called mental illnesses be looked at afresh and more simply, that they be removed from the category of illnesses, and that they be regarded as the expressions of man's struggle with *the problem of how he should live*. This problem is obviously a vast one, its enormity reflecting not only man's inability to cope with his environment, but even more his increasing self-reflectiveness.

By problems in living, then, I refer to that explosive chain reaction that began with man's fall from divine grace by partaking of the fruit of the tree of knowledge. Man's awareness of himself and of the world about him seems to be a steadily expanding one, bringing in its wake an even larger *burden of understanding*.[7] This burden is to be expected and must not be misinterpreted. Our only rational means for easing it is more understanding, and appropriate action based on such understanding. The main alternative lies in acting as though the burden were not what in fact we perceive it to be, and taking refuge in an outmoded theological view of man. In such a view, man does not fashion his life and much of his world about him, but merely lives out his fate in a world created by superior beings. This may logically lead to pleading non-responsibility in the face of seemingly unfathomable problems and insurmountable difficulties. Yet, if man fails to take increasing responsibility for his actions, individually as well as collectively, it seems unlikely that some higher power or being would assume this task and carry this burden for him. Moreover, this seems hardly a propitious time in human history for obscuring the issue of man's responsibility for his actions by hiding it behind the skirt of an all-explaining conception of mental illness.

VII

I have tried to show that the notion of mental illness has outlived whatever usefulness it may have had and that it now functions as a myth. As such, it is a true heir to religious myths in general, and to the belief in witchcraft in particular. It was the function of these belief-systems to act as social tranquilizers, fostering hope that mastery of certain problems may be achieved by means of substitutive, symbolic-magical, operations. The concept of mental illness thus serves mainly to obscure the everyday fact that life for most people is a continuous struggle, not for biological survival, but for a "place in the sun," "peace of mind," or some other meaning or value. Once the needs of preserving the body, and perhaps of the race, are satisfied, man faces the problem of personal significance: What should he do with himself? For what should he live? Sustained adherence to the myth of mental illness allows people to avoid facing this problem, believing that mental health, conceived as the absence of mental illness, automatically insures the making of right and safe choices in the conduct of life. But the facts are all the other way. It is the making of wise choices in life that people regard, retrospectively, as evidence of good mental health!

When I assert that mental illness is a myth, I am not saying that personal unhappiness and socially deviant behavior do not exist; what I am saying is that we categorize them as diseases at our own peril.

The expression "mental illness" is a metaphor that we have come to mistake for a fact. We call people physically ill when their body-functioning violates certain anatomical and physiological norms; similarly, we call people mentally ill when their personal conduct violates certain ethical, political, and social norms. This explains why many historical figures, from Jesus to Castro, and from Job to Hitler, have been diagnosed as suffering from this or that psychiatric malady.

Finally, the myth of mental illness encourages us to believe in its logical corollary: that social intercourse would be harmonious, satisfying, and the secure basis of a good life were it not for the disrupting influences of mental illness, or psychopathology. However, universal human happiness, in this form at least, is but another example of a wishful fantasy. I believe that human happiness, or well-being, is possible—not just for a select few, but on a scale hitherto unimaginable. But this can be achieved only if many men, not just a few, are willing and able to confront frankly, and tackle courageously, their ethical, personal, and social conflicts. This means having the courage and integrity to forego waging battles on false fronts, finding solutions for substitute problems—for instance, fighting the battle of stomach acid and chronic fatigue instead of facing up to a marital conflict.

Our adversaries are not demons, witches, fate, or mental illness. We have no enemy that we can fight, exorcise, or dispel by "cure." What we do have are problems in living—whether these be biologic, economic, political, or socio-psychological. In this essay I was concerned only with problems belonging in the last-mentioned category, and within this group mainly with those pertaining to moral values. The field to which modern psychiatry addresses itself is vast, and I made no effort to encompass it all. My argument was limited to the proposition that mental illness is a myth, whose function it is to disguise and thus render more palatable the bitter pill of moral conflicts in human relations.

NOTES

1 See Szasz, T. S.: *Pain and Pleasure: A Study of Bodily Feelings* (New York: Basic Books, 1957), especially pp. 70–81; "The problem of psychiatric nosology." *Amer. J. Psychiatry*, 114:405–13 (Nov.), 1957.

2 See Szasz, T. S.: *The Ethics of Psychoanalysis: The Theory and Method of Autonomous Psychotherapy* (New York: Basic Books, 1965).

3 See Szasz, T. S.: *Law, Liberty, and Psychiatry: An Inquiry into the Social Uses of Mental Health Practices* (New York: Macmillan, 1963).

4 Peters, R. S.: *The Concept of Motivation* (London: Routledge & Kegan Paul, 1958), especially pp. 12–15.

5 Hollingshead, A. B., and Redlich, F. C.: *Social Class and Mental Illness* (New York: Wiley, 1958).

6 Quoted in Jones, E.: *The Life and Work of Sigmund Freud* (New York: Basic Books, 1957), Vol. III, p. 247.

7 In this connection, see Langer, S. K.: *Philosophy in a New Key* [1942] (New York: Mentor Books, 1953), especially Chaps. 5 and 10.

Mental Health as Rational Autonomy
Rem B. Edwards

Rem B. Edwards is professor of philosophy and a senior member of the medical ethics faculty at the University of Tennessee. He is the author of *Pleasures and Pains: A Theory of Qualitative Hedonism* (1979), editor of *Psychiatry and Ethics: Insanity, Rational Autonomy, and Mental Health Care* (1982), and coeditor of *Bioethics* (1988).

Edwards proposes and explicates the following tentative definition: "'Mental illness' means only those undesirable mental/behavioral deviations which involve primarily an extreme and prolonged inability to know and deal in a rational and autonomous way with oneself and one's social and physical environment." On Edwards's analysis, Szasz is correct in condemning "mental illness" as a myth *in some cases*—those where values other than rationality and autonomy are at stake. However, he argues, Szasz is wrong in not seeing that there are some cases that can be correctly described as involving insanity. Edwards believes that his proposed definition can provide effective guidance, even though any definition of "mental illness" necessarily involves a value component as well as a descriptive component.

It has often been noted that psychiatric labeling has grave moral consequences, i.e. consequences which seriously affect the moral standing, rights, and quality of life of other people. In the name of supposedly scientific and objective medicine, it legitimizes the enormous power which psychiatrists and mental institutions have over other people, especially the weaker and more vulnerable members of society. Psychiatric labeling is a form of moral as well as medical behavior which has clear disadvantages as well as clear advantages. On the debit side, it serves to isolate socially those persons to whom labels of lunacy are applied; and it often generates enormous mistrust and alienation between them and their family and friends. It permanently stigmatizes those so characterized and negatively affects for years to come their opportunities for such basic amenities as self respect, employment, promotion, housing, education, marriage and general social trust and acceptance. It dehumanizes and degrades those to whom it is applied, allowing us to regard and treat the mentally ill as slightly less than human. Nevertheless, it may still be a rationally acceptable and justifiable mode of inter-personal interaction, despite its obvious moral liabilities. Recognizing that psychiatric labeling of individual persons may have grave

The Journal of Medicine and Philosophy 6 (1981), pp. 309–322. Copyright © 1981 by D. Reidel Publishing Co., Dordrecht, Holland and Boston, U.S.A. Reprinted by permission of Kluwer Academic Publishers.

consequences, we should also acknowledge that the very act of defining and providing a range of application for such concepts as 'mental health' and 'mental illness' is itself a moral act which greatly affects the lives of others.

There is both an evaluative and a descriptive dimension to our concepts of 'mental health' and 'mental illness.' The latter term applies to describable mental and/or behavioral deviations of which we strongly disapprove. In addition to statistical abnormality, the disapproval element is a necessary condition for applying the term; for there are many 'healthy' minority deviations of which we strongly approve, such as the rare but precious intellectual genius, creativity and sensitivity of our most outstanding artists, writers, scientists, philosophers, and moral and religious leaders. It is a great but often made mistake, however, to allow statistical deviation and the disapproval element to be sufficient conditions for applying the notion of 'mental illness,' for then we must allow every peculiar mental/behavioral process of which we disapprove to count as a mental illness. To avoid the excesses into which so much of psychiatry has lapsed in recent years, we must allow the notion to be applied only to a small sub-class of disapproved psychic processes, distresses and behaviors. The issue is: do we wish to medicalize the whole of life, or do we wish instead to recognize and preserve other evaluative realms of discourse such as that of intrinsic value and disvalue, as well as distinctive moral, political, and religious norms?

Our present problem is not merely of academic interest, for there is a powerful tendency at work in modern secular, scientific society to allow older religious and moral values simply to fade away and to medicalize the whole sphere of moral, political, and religious deviation. When confronted by conditions and behaviors of which we disapprove, so many of us no longer use such ethico-religious terms as 'ungodly,' 'sinful,' and 'immoral,' or even such political terms as 'unjust' or 'undemocratic.' Instead we apply such highly evaluative pseudo-scientific terms as 'sick,' 'unhealthy,' 'immature,' 'a sad case,' etc. We often do not realize that this whole way of talking tends to put ministers, political activists, and even serious minded moralists as such out of business. Physicians and psychiatrists become the secular priests and final arbiters of what we should value and disvalue—in the name of 'empirical' medicine. Many recent authors such as Réne Dubos, Ivan Illich, Nicholas Kittrie and Thomas Szasz have condemned such creeping medical imperialism and totalitarianism for a variety of reasons. Some protestors do so simply because they wish to make a place for moral, political and religious norms and deviations which should not be confused with or collapsed into an all embracing domain of 'mental health' and 'mental illness.' This may involve recognizing and respecting other intrinsic, moral, social, political and religious values and disvalues in their own right. E. Fuller Torrey was doing this when he criticized as follows the 1977 report of President Carter's Commission on Mental Health, which equated mental illness with the unhappiness which results from social injustice, discrimination and poverty:

> Certainly poverty and discrimination are terrible injustices that cause widespread anguish and unhappiness. But anguish and unhappiness are not mental illness, and herein lies the confusion. Poverty and discrimination are no more 'mental health' problems than famine and war. They are human problems and should be attacked as such, with all the governmental and private resources at our disposal: jobs must be created; opportunities equalized; housing built; food supplies fairly distributed. Labeling them mental-health problems not only obscures their true importance but also creates the illusion that they can be 'cured' if we will only put enough mental-health professionals into positions of power (Torrey, 1977, p. 10).

Resisting medical imperialism in psychiatric labeling may also involve an awareness of the grave moral consequences of psychiatric name calling, or an appreciation of the horrendous physical and psychic conse-

quences of much that passes for 'therapy,' or a sense of the desirability of protecting the integrity of language itself. Economic considerations also are very much involved in any decision to expand or restrict our notion of 'illness,' even of 'mental illness.' If a condition gets classified as an illness, insurance companies and government agencies such as Medicare and Medicaid will be expected to pay the bills in many cases; and if the condition is not so classified, these agencies will not pay. There are many good reasons for wanting to limit the scope of application for the notion of 'mental illness,' rather than allow it to swallow up *all* those states of mind, distresses and deviant behaviors of which we disapprove. Surely things have gotten way out of hand when a psychoanalyst such as Fine (1967, p. 95) tells us, "neurosis is defined in the analytic sense as distance from the ideal; then it can be said to affect 99 percent of the population. Thus, the essential thesis of this paper emerges: The ultimate goal of psychoanalysis is the reform of society."

I shall now make a conservative proposal for the proper limitation of the very notion of 'mental illness' which until recently has been a presupposition of our entire legal system, which is very close to what I have found many mental health professionals actually using in their work in mental hospitals, and which is also very close to what the term traditionally meant before the advent of the sort of medical imperialism which Kittrie (1971, pp. 340–410) has called "the therapeutic state," or which Illich (1976, pp. 31–60) has called "the medicalization of life." There is nothing final about this proposal. It is merely an attempt to generate a discussion of the proper limits of 'mental illness,' *recognizing that the lives of many people will be greatly affected by where we draw the line.*

Definition: 'Mental illness' means only those undesirable mental/behavioral deviations which involve primarily an extreme and prolonged inability to know and deal in a rational and autonomous way with oneself and one's social and physical environment. In other words, madness is extreme and prolonged practical irrationality and irresponsibility. Correspondingly, 'mental health' includes only those desirable mental/behavioral normalities and occasional abnormalities which enable us to know and deal in a rational and autonomous way with ourselves and our social and physical environment. In other words, mental health is practical rationality and responsibility. A number of other theorists such as Breggin (1974, 1975), Engelhardt, Jr. (1973), Fingarette (1972) and Moore (1975), have arrived at similar views.

There is much here that needs explaining. By 'mental/behavioral' I mean thinking, willing and feeling which may manifest itself in publicly observable bodily alterations and activities. By 'autonomy' I mean having and freely actualizing a capacity for making one's own choices, managing one's own practical affairs and assuming responsibility for one's own life, its station and its duties. Before defining 'rationality,' and specifying its relevant realm of application, let us first recognize that there is a large domain of human belief which falls quite legitimately into the category of contested beliefs and unanswered questions, and which should be regarded as only peripherally relevant to the identification of madness. Most of our political, philosophical and religious beliefs, many scientific and factual beliefs, and many questions of value and practice belong to the class of contested beliefs and unanswered questions. There is no clear answer to what it is and what it is not rational to believe in these areas. I keep telling my colleagues in philosophy that in such matters, there is very little difference between being around a mental hospital and being around a department of philosophy! Political, philosophical and religious beliefs especially should never provide us with *primary* grounds for diagnosing mental illness. If that restriction had been observed, attempts would not have been made to have Mary Baker Eddy declared insane and institutionalized involuntarily for being a Christian Scientist. Nor would Ezra Pound have been institutionalized for political dissent. Irrationality and irresponsibility with respect to knowing and dealing with oneself and one's social and physical environment should be the primary focus for defining and diagnosing mental illness. We cannot declare a Christian Scientist mentally ill for believing that a broken bone has been miraculously healed if indeed no fractures show up any longer on X-rays. However, if anyone for any reason insists that healing has occurred when the fractures are still showing up, or if a woman insists that she has a million children and spends all her time looking for them, or if someone insists that they no longer need to eat since they died yesterday and are now in Heaven, then questions of sanity may be very legitimately raised and would be so raised even by Christian Scientists. True, there will be some tough marginal cases such as that of the sociopath; but some cases will be clear enough. Situations will also arise in which philosophical and religious beliefs impinge upon personal, empirical and social realities, but mental illness should not be diagnosed unless it manifests itself in these practical areas.

Are we all just a little bit crazy, as some psychotherapists and much of our popular wisdom and humor insinuate? This depends in part on whether we are willing to call *any* momentary lapse into irrationality and irre-

sponsibility a form of 'mental illness,' or whether we wish to reserve the term only for extreme and persistent forms of such. Because of the grave consequences of psychiatric labeling, it seems morally desirable to limit it to the latter, and I am offering a moral argument for a very limited and conservative conception of 'mental illness.' As for the factors of duration and degree, there is no *precise* answer to the question of 'how long?' or 'how extreme?'. But it seems both socially undesirable and linguistically unconventional (at least prior to our recent medicalization of the whole of life) to count momentary and relatively superficial confusions, lapses of memory, emotional traumas and perceptual errors, etc. as indications of mental illness. A moment of confusion does not count as a mental illness any more than a single sneeze counts as a respiratory disease. The concept of duration belongs in our definitions of all diseases. On my analysis, mental illness will be a matter of degree of both time and severity of impairment and as such will be on a continuum with the whole of life; and there will be a grey area of controversial borderline cases. But some instances of it will be unmistakable in their duration and degree. If we take the duration factor seriously, there will be no such thing as temporary insanity, but this has never been anything more than a legal fiction invented for excusing certain persons when no other legal rationale for doing so could be found. It is important that we understand that only relatively extreme forms of such mental/behavioral malfunctions count as mental disorders. Though the question is worth exploring, we should be wary of altering this to mean that any such malfunction which is *capable* of taking an extreme form is a mental illness, for then we would be right back to the medicalization of the whole of life. It should also be noted that the factual claim that extreme mental/behavioral malfunctions are grounded in some 'underlying pathology,' located in the brain, the unconscious, the enduring structure of the mind itself, or what have you, has not been built into our definition of mental illness. This is a hotly contested issue, especially between behaviorally oriented psychologists and their adversaries; and such a consideration can be introduced only when it has been confronted head-on and found to be justified. All the data are not in on this one yet.

Now, what is meant by 'rational?' Whatever it is, mental disorders are shortcomings or departures from it, and only those disorders which involve the absence of it are to count as mental disorders. Other undesirable mental/behavioral deviations should be classified in other ways, such as intrinsically bad, immoral, criminal, irreligious, etc. There are a number of defining elements in our common notion of 'rationality.' This is an important word in our living languages, not a technical word invented by philosophers. But philosophers may contribute to its clarification, and there is widespread agreement among both philosophers and non-philosophers that rationality involves (1) being able to distinguish means from ends and being able to identify processes and manifest behaviors which likely will result in the realization of consciously envisioned goals; (2) thinking logically and avoiding logically contradictory beliefs; (3) having factual beliefs which are adequately supported by empirical evidence, or at least avoiding factual beliefs which are plainly falsified by experience; (4) having and being able to give reasons for one's behavior and beliefs; (5) thinking clearly and intelligibly, and avoiding confusion and nonsense; (6) having and exhibiting a capacity for impartiality or fair mindedness in judging and adopting beliefs; (7) having values which have been (or would be) adopted under conditions of freedom, enlightenment, and impartiality. Rationality is a function of how we know, not of what we know. Ignorance is not insanity, but irrationality is. Stupidity, the deliberate choice of self-defeating ends, is also not insanity.

I am fully aware that many books could be and have in fact been written explicating all the complications of and full conceptual significance of these seven defining features of 'rationality,' but I do not have space here to rewrite such books. I do think that the last element is so difficult to apply that it should never be used in diagnosing insanity, though it has very legitimate philosophical uses. For purposes of defining 'mental illness,' I hope that enough has been said to indicate the sort of direction in which the notions of 'rationality' and 'irrationality' as deviations from such, have been traditionally understood. Of course, there are all sorts of degrees in the development of our human capacity for rationality, and it is only fairly extreme and persistent departures from some of our seven defining features of rationality which count as mental illness. Only a few of these factors need be involved in any particular case. Most people are not *very* rational, but most people are nevertheless sane. *Extreme* departures from sanity are not as difficult to identify in practice as some skeptical critics, especially lawyers and philosophers who have never spent any time around mentally disturbed persons, would have us to believe. Cases on the borderline of such extremities are the ones which understandably give headaches to mental health professionals, but such professionals can also cite many clear cut cases involving extreme and prolonged incompetence and self-defeating performances in selecting effective means to avowed ends, of radically inconsistent practical belief systems, items of which are plainly controverted by empirical facts, of inability to cite reasons for belief and behavior, of persisting and pervasive conceptual confusions, and of intrenched inabilities to adopt fair minded perspectives on either factual or valuational beliefs.

Since being rational involves having and acting upon factual beliefs supported by common experience and avoiding beliefs clearly at odds with common experience, it is easy to understand how persisting hallucinations and perceptual distortions contribute to irrationality. They involve loss of contact with our common world and generate beliefs about and behaviors directed toward things that are just not there. To the extent that unconscious conflicts, powers and processes interfere with the functioning of conscious rational autonomy, they too are relevant for diagnosing mental illness.

No account of underlying pathology in the brain or in a Freudian psyche has been built into the definition here proposed of mental illness as loss of practical rational autonomy. Neither has the attempt to correlate mental illness with such pathology been excluded by such an analysis. Indeed, I wish to encourage an exploration of possible connections between mental illness so conceived and current concepts of and research on organic brain pathology, the standard functional psychoses and neuroses, and mental retardation. My suspicion is that standard (and desirable) brain structure, function and chemistry can be correlated with all manifestations of rational autonomy, even if the precise relation between them always remains shrouded in metaphysical mystery. Though we do not know precisely how conscious thought and decision processes are related to brain function, we might still find that predictable correlations can be made between consciousness and brain. We might discover, and to some extent have actually found, that physical therapies such as psychotropic drugs, electroshock and even carefully controlled psychosurgery have predictable connections with restoration to rational autonomy and mental health. True, drugs *may* be used as 'chemical straight jackets.' They may also be used to correct an imbalance in the dopamine circuit of the brain of the schizophrenic. A renewal of rational autonomy may thus be correlated experimentally with a return to more normal brain chemistry. The medical model is not included in our concept of mental illness/health, but its relevance is not excluded either. In this area much work remains to be done.

The problem of placing proper limits on the notion of mental disorder becomes especially acute when it is allowed to range over the whole spectrum of disapproved mental/behavioral phenomena, including those which have little or nothing to do with breakdowns of rational autonomy, but which still might be disapproved on moral, legal, or religious grounds. It is not very difficult to see that schizophrenics, paranoids, and manic depressives, etc. are irrational and have lost control; but many people certainly have great difficulty seeing that irrationality has much to do with many other conditions which are often classified as mental disturbances. An example of such a highly controversial classification would be homosexuality uncomplicated by distress, which was listed in 1968 as a mental disorder in the A.P.A.'s *Diagnostic and Statistical Manual of Mental Disorders, II*, but which is not listed in the new *DSM-III* in 1980. Has Anita Bryant persuaded us that this is really an ethico-religious problem after all, or have we been convinced that it is really no problem at all? In the 19th century, masturbation was regarded as a manifestation of madness and treated with the harshest of imaginable 'therapies,' but few persons even disapprove of it these days, much less classify it as madness. *DSM-III* includes caffeinism and excessive smoking as mental disorders. Will these have the same ultimate fate as masturbation? Anyone who has read Szasz (1972) knows that alcoholism and drug addictions are very debatable categories of mental illness. As he puts it, "Bad habits are not disease: a refutation of the claim that alcoholism is a disease." Is alcoholism a mental or a moral problem? My own view is that alcohol abuse begins as a moral problem and ends as a mental disease as it gradually becomes physically addictive, deprives the individual of much rational autonomy, and in some cases (Korsakov's psychosis) turns the brain to mush. I shall not attempt to work through *DSM-II* or *DSM-III* in detail to see which diagnostic categories might involve a confusion of irrationality with immorality or irreligion. Let the A.P.A. do that! I wish only to assert that not every disapproved mental/behavioral phenomenon should count as mental illness, that we should make a concerted effort to disentangle legitimate psychiatric valuations from moral and religious ones, and that we should attempt to put a screeching halt to the rampant proliferation of psychiatric diagnostic categories because of the grossly detrimental effects of the very act of psychiatric labeling if for no other reason. I am convinced that psychiatric labeling does have legitimate uses, but it also has illegitimate ones, and it will be the mark of the wise psychiatrist, psychologist and philosopher to be able to distinguish the two.

No doubt, many psychologists and psychiatrists will want to reject the definitions of 'mental illness' and 'mental health' here proposed. This is not a great embarrassment, however, for there is *no* definition of these terms anywhere in the literature that many psychologists and psychiatrists would not want to reject. One of the truly embarrassing aspects of this field of medicine is that there is so little agreement on theoretical fundamentals. This always adds fuel to the fire of those who insist that the 'medical model' has no legitimate application to mental/behavioral disorders. Why should anyone want to reject the conservative definition of 'mental illness' in terms of impairment of rational autonomy here being proposed? I am confident that most objections will be based upon the tendency inherent in all medical imperialism to engulf all disapproved mental/behavioral conditions and processes under the label of 'sick,' and to recognize no separate domains of intrinsic, social, moral, political, legal and religious values and disvalues.

The same imperialistic tendency is at work when we come to positive conceptions of 'mental health.' The tendency in so many cases is to equate this with *everything* desirable, not simply with the desirability of rational autonomy. *Every* desirable mode of experience, activity, self-realization, happiness and social organization are packed into imperialistic conceptions of 'mental health.' Consider and analyze for yourself the intrinsic, social, moral, religious, legal, etc. values which are packed into the following definitions.

1. "Health is a state of complete physical, mental and social well-being and not merely the absence of disease or infirmity" (The World Health Organization, 1978, p. 89).

2. "The crucial consideration in determining human normality is whether the individual is an asset or a burden to society and whether he is or is not contributing to the progressive development of man" (Alfred Adler as summarized by O. H. Mower in Boorse, 1976, p. 69).

3. "Let us define mental health as the adjustment of human beings to the world and to each other with a maximum of effectiveness and happiness. Not just efficiency, or just contentment—or the grace of obeying the rules of the game cheerfully. It is all of these together. It is the ability to maintain an even temper, an alert intelligence, socially considerate behavior, and a happy disposition. This, I think, is a healthy mind" (Karl Menninger in Boorse, 1976, p. 69–70).

4. "Mental health, in the humanistic sense, is characterized by the ability to love and to create, by the emergence from the incestuous ties to family and nature, by a sense of identity based on one's experience of self as the subject and agent of one's powers, by the grasp of reality inside and outside of ourselves, that is by the development of objectivity and reason.... The mentally

healthy person is the person who lives by love, reason and faith, who respects life, his own and that of his fellow man" (Fromm, 1955).

5. "...here we have to deal with those persons who fall ill as soon as they pass beyond the irresponsible age of childhood, and thus never attain a phase of health—that of unrestricted capacity in general for production and enjoyment" (Freud equating mental health with his 'genital phase' of personality development, in Rickman, 1957, p. 66).

6. "True Sanity entails in one way or another the dissolution of the normal ego, that false self competently adjusted to our alienated social reality; the emergence of the 'inner' archetypal mediators of divine power, and through this death a new kind of ego-functioning, the ego now being the servant of the divine, no longer its betrayer" (Laing, 1967).

Many wonderful things other than rational autonomy are mentioned in the foregoing imperialistic definitions of mental health, and we should realize that the judgment that they do not belong in such a definition is not by any means the same as the judgment that they are not wonderful! Nor is it the same as the judgment that we never need help and counseling in achieving these wonderful things. It simply recognizes that those who do such counseling should more honestly be termed applied axiologists, moral eductors, spiritual mentors, political activists, etc. Szasz (1974, p. 262) has a point in condemning 'mental illness' as a myth *where values other than those of rationality and autonomy are involved* in the therapist-patient relationship. *Beyond that point*, psychotherapists *are* dealing with what he terms "personal, social, and ethical problems in living." *Up to that point*, however, they are dealing with real insanity, which Szasz fails to see. The rationally autonomous person may *choose for himself* just how much value he will attach to social conformity and adjustment, productivity, pleasure, heterosexuality, socially considerate behavior, love, faith, creativity, introspection, mysticism and all such good things. The rationally autonomous person may still need value education in such matters, and it may be a perfectly legitimate function of psychotherapists and mental hospitals to provide such, though not in the name of treating mental illness or under the guise of *medical* expertise.

We should acknowledge that two great and interrelated goods have been built into our very conception of sanity—rationality and autonomy. It is quite possible, however, to agree that these are great goods without agreeing upon precisely what kind of goods they are, and

for most practical purposes it is not even necessary to agree upon the latter. Philosophers distinguish intrinsic goods, things worth having, experiencing, doing, preserving for their own sake from instrumental goods, things required for the actualization of other values beyond themselves. Are rationality and autonomy intrinsic ends in themselves? Are they merely indispensable means to other intrinsic goods such as enjoyment or long range happiness defined in terms of enjoyment? Is their actualization inherently enjoyable in itself, so that they become an integral part of our happiness, as John Stuart Mill suggested? We need not agree upon such abstruse philosophical questions in order to agree that rationality and autonomy are great and indispensable human goods, and that life is so greatly impoverished that it merits the labels 'insanity' or 'mental illness' where these functions are significantly diminished.

Rationality and autonomy are controversial goods, not universally prized, however. Blind faith and obedience to external authority are greatly preferred by many (but not all) religious thinkers and by totalitarian political regimes everywhere. A well functioning democracy must be heavily populated by citizens exemplifying a significant degree of rational autonomy, and in that sense there is a political dimension to our definitions of mental health and mental illness. And though *we* may conceive of rational autonomy as the very essence of moral agency, we should not forget that many religious and non-democratic political perspectives regard rational autonomy with dismay and insist that *their* ideal moral agents renounce it, or better yet never develop it, for blind, unthinking, inherited or emotionally induced devotion to unquestioned authority. In Russia, it is the rationally autonomous person who is involuntarily institutionalized in mental hospitals! Thus, it may not be possible to separate *completely* the values of mental health as rational autonomy from *all* political, moral and religious values. We can separate them from *most* such values, i.e. all the others, however; and it is necessary in a democratic society so to do.

Finally, we should realize that the value dimensions of how we conceive of 'mental illness' and 'mental health' are relevant to the practice of medicine in a mental hospital. If a mental hospital declares (as one with which I am acquainted has done) that "The goal of the institute is to restore its patients to an optimum level of social, intellectual, emotional, and vocational functioning in the community," we need to ask whether this is a realistic goal and just what it implies practically for patients. My own view is that 'optimum' is much too strong a word to use here, just as 'complete' was much too strong in the World Health Organization definition of 'health.' As a general affirmation of charity toward all and malice toward none, such formulations have a legitimate place. But as an avowal of realistic goals, such a statement is surely too strong. *All* the institutional and social arrangements and efforts of society and all the energies of the individual are required for the *summum bonum*, whatever that might be conceived to be; and no medical institution should claim or aspire to have the power and the resources required for its achievement. Reaching the *summum bonum* should certainly not be a prerequisite for discharge from such a hospital, for no one would ever be discharged! In that sense such a goal is not a realistic one, especially for involuntarily committed patients. It would be much more sensible for mental hospitals to aim at a restoration to minimal sanity in the present conservative sense of the term, i.e. a degree of rational autonomy which is minimally sufficient for 'making it' in society, recognizing that even this is relative to what any given society or functional segment thereof expects of its members and provides by way of support.

Although care for and cure of mental illness should be the primary functions of a mental hospital, they certainly need not be its sole legitimate functions, any more than the physical care for and cure of disease need be the sole legitimate function of general hospitals and other medical practitioners. Medical professionals both within and without mental hospitals may also willingly and legitimately accept the additional tasks of relieving and preventing pain even where there is no hope of a cure, of assisting in social adaptation, giving moral counsel, and even being religious mentors (chaplains have a place) if they find that their patients are willing to ask and pay voluntarily for such services, or that society is willing to provide such services for those who want them but cannot pay. My only concern is that they recognize and admit what they are doing and not confuse treating mental illness with every form of aiding in the pursuit of justice and happiness.

NOTE

Writing of this paper was supported by a N.E.H. Development Grant in Medical Ethics, ED-32672-78-652.

REFERENCES

Breggin, P. R.: 1974, 'Psychotherapy as applied ethics', *Psychiatry* 34, 59–74.

Breggin, P. R.: 1975, 'Psychiatry and psychotherapy as political processes', *American Journal of Psychotherapy* 29, 369–382.

Boorse, C.: 1976, 'What a theory of mental health should be', *Journal for the Theory of Social Behavior* 6, 61–84.

Engelhardt, Jr. H. T.: 1973, 'Psychotherapy as meta-ethics', *Psychiatry* 36, 440–445.

Fine, R.: 1967, 'The goals of psychoanalysis', in Alvin R. Mahrer (ed.), *The Goals of Psychotherapy*, Appleton-Century-Crofts, New York, pp. 73–98.

Fingarette, H.: 1972, 'Insanity and responsibility', *Inquiry* 15, 6–29.

Fromm, E.: 1955, *The Sane Society*, Fawcett Publications, Greenwich, Conn., pp. 180–181.

Illich, I.: 1976, *Medical Nemesis, The Expropriation of Health*, Bantam Books, New York, pp. 31–60.

Kittrie, N.: 1971, *The Right to be Different: Deviance and Enforced Therapy*, The Johns Hopkins Press, Baltimore, pp. 340–410.

Laing, R. D.: 1967, *The Politics of Experience*, Ballantine Books, New York.

Moore, M. S.: 1975, 'Some myths about "Mental illness" ', *Archives of General Psychiatry* 32, pp. 1483–1497.

Rickman, J. (ed.): 1957, *A General Selection from the Works of Sigmund Freud*, Doubleday & Co., Garden City, New York, p. 66.

Szasz, T. S.: 1972, 'Bad habits are not diseases: A refutation of the claim that alcoholism is a disease', *The Lancet* 2, 83–84.

Szasz, T. S.: 1974, *The Myth of Mental Illness*, Harper & Row, New York.

Torrey, Fuller E.: 1977, 'Carter's little pills', *Psychology Today* 11, 10–11.

World Health Organization: 1978, 'A definition of health', in T. Beauchamp, and Le Roy Walters (eds.), *Contemporary Issues in Bioethics*, Dickenson Publishing Co., Encino California, p. 89.

Involuntary Civil Commitment and Deinstitutionalization

Majority Opinion in *O'Connor v. Donaldson*
Justice Potter Stewart

Justice Potter Stewart served as an associate justice of the Supreme Court of the United States from 1958 until 1981. Prior to that appointment, he practiced law (1941–1954) and served as a judge on the United States Circuit Court of Appeals for the 6th District (1954–1958).

In 1943, Kenneth Donaldson's parents asked a judge to commit their 34-year-old son to a mental institution for treatment. They did this after Donaldson's fellow workers apparently knocked him unconscious after he made a political comment. Once Donaldson was institutionalized and his reactions to what he perceived as injustices were diagnosed as pathological, he was given electroconvulsive therapy. After eleven weeks of ECT, he was released. In 1956, Donaldson visited his parents in Florida. During his visit, he made some complaints, which led his father to request a sanity hearing for his son. The senior Donaldson argued that his son was suffering from a "persecution complex." As a result of this complaint, Donaldson was arrested, jailed, and diagnosed as "paranoid schizophrenic" by a sheriff and two physicians. The physicians, each of whom spoke to Donaldson for less than two minutes, were not psychiatrists. Later a judge visited him and informed him that he would be sent to Florida State Hospital. This decision was based on the physicians' conclusions. Donaldson's requests for a judicial hearing and a lawyer were granted; but the hearing was held in jail, the physicians did not attend, and Donaldson's lawyer left while Donaldson was still testifying. Donaldson was sent to the hospital for a "few weeks' rest." He remained there for fifteen years, never seeing a judge and seeing a psychiatrist only a few times a year. During those fifteen years, Donaldson petitioned various courts eighteen times, asking for a hearing. All but one of these requests were dismissed on the basis of physicians' reports and his previous institutionalization. When his case was finally going to be heard in 1971, Donaldson was released and certified as "no longer incompetent." However, he continued his suit, asking $100,000 in damages for the fifteen years he had been committed without treatment. He won his case against J. B. O'Connor, the superintendent of the institution, and a codefendant physician, although only $38,500 was granted in damages.

The case was ultimately appealed to the United States Supreme Court. In handing down its 1975 landmark decision, the court ruled that a finding of mental illness alone is insufficient grounds for confining a nondangerous individual who has the capacity to survive safely in freedom, either by himself or with the help of responsible and willing relatives or friends. Justice Potter Stewart wrote the majority opinion, which is partially reprinted here.

I

Donaldson's commitment was initiated by his father, who thought that his son was suffering from "delusions." After hearings before a county judge of Pinellas County, Fla., Donaldson was found to be suffering from "paranoid schizophrenia" and was committed for "care, maintenance, and treatment" pursuant to Florida statutory provisions that have since been repealed. The state

United States Supreme Court; June 26, 1975, 422 U.S. 563. 95 S.Ct. 2486.

law was less than clear in specifying the grounds necessary for commitment, and the record is scanty as to Donaldson's condition at the time of the judicial hearing. These matters are, however, irrelevant, for this case involves no challenge to the initial commitment, but is focused, instead, upon the nearly 15 years of confinement that followed.

The evidence at the trial showed that the hospital staff had the power to release a patient, not dangerous to himself or others, even if he remained mentally ill and had been lawfully committed. Despite many requests, O'Connor refused to allow that power to be exercised in

Donaldson's case. At the trial, O'Connor indicated that he had believed that Donaldson would have been unable to make a "successful adjustment outside the institution," but could not recall the basis for that conclusion. O'Connor retired as superintendent shortly before the suit was filed. A few months thereafter, and before the trial, Donaldson secured his release and a judicial restoration of competency, with the support of the hospital staff.

The testimony at the trial demonstrated, without contradiction, that Donaldson had posed no danger to others during his long confinement, or indeed at any point in his life. O'Connor himself conceded that he had no personal or secondhand knowledge that Donaldson had ever committed a dangerous act. There was no evidence that Donaldson had ever been suicidal or been thought likely to inflict injury upon himself. One of O'Connor's codefendants acknowledged that Donaldson could have earned his own living outside the hospital. He had done so for some 14 years before his commitment, and immediately upon his release he secured a responsible job in hotel administration.

Furthermore, Donaldson's frequent requests for release had been supported by responsible persons willing to provide him any care he might need on release. In 1963, for example, a representative of Helping Hands, Inc., a halfway house for mental patients, wrote O'Connor asking him to release Donaldson to its care. The request was accompanied by a supporting letter from the Minneapolis Clinic of Psychiatry and Neurology, which a codefendant conceded was a "good clinic." O'Connor rejected the offer, replying that Donaldson could be released only to his parents. That rule was apparently of O'Connor's own making. At the time, Donaldson was 55 years old, and, as O'Connor knew, Donaldson's parents were too elderly and infirm to take responsibility for him. Moreover, in his continuing correspondence with Donaldson's parents, O'Connor never informed them of the Helping Hands offer. In addition, on four separate occasions between 1964 and 1968, John Lembcke, a college classmate of Donaldson's and a longtime family friend, asked O'Connor to release Donaldson to his care. On each occasion O'Connor refused. The record shows that Lembcke was a serious and responsible person, who was willing and able to assume responsibility for Donaldson's welfare.

The evidence showed that Donaldson's confinement was a simple regime of enforced custodial care, not a program designed to alleviate or cure his supposed illness. Numerous witnesses, including one of O'Connor's codefendants, testified that Donaldson had received nothing but custodial care while at the hospital.

O'Connor described Donaldson's treatment as "milieu therapy." But witnesses from the hospital staff conceded that, in the context of this case, "milieu therapy" was a euphemism for confinement in the "milieu" of a mental hospital. For substantial periods, Donaldson was simply kept in a large room that housed 60 patients, many of whom were under criminal commitment. Donaldson's requests for ground privileges, occupational training, and an opportunity to discuss his case with O'Connor or other staff members were repeatedly denied.

At the trial, O'Connor's principal defense was that he had acted in good faith and was therefore immune from any liability for monetary damages. His position, in short, was that state law, which he had believed valid, had authorized indefinite custodial confinement of the "sick," even if they were not given treatment and their release could harm no one.

The trial judge instructed the members of the jury that they should find that O'Connor had violated Donaldson's constitutional right to liberty if they found that he had

> confined [Donaldson] against his will, knowing that he was not mentally ill or dangerous or knowing that if mentally ill he was not receiving treatment for his alleged mental illness....
>
> Now, the purpose of involuntary hospitalization is treatment and not mere custodial care or punishment if a patient is not a danger to himself or others. Without such treatment there is no justification from a constitutional stand-point for continued confinement unless you should also find that [Donaldson] was dangerous to either himself or others.

The trial judge further instructed the jury that O'Connor was immune from damages if he

> reasonably believed in good faith that detention of [Donaldson] was proper for the length of time he was so confined....
>
> However, mere good intentions which do not give rise to a reasonable belief that detention is lawfully required cannot justify [Donaldson's] confinement in the Florida State Hospital.

The jury returned a verdict for Donaldson against O'Connor and a codefendant, and awarded damages of $38,500, including $10,000 in punitive damages.

The Court of Appeals affirmed the judgment of the District Court in a broad opinion dealing with "the far-reaching question whether the Fourteenth Amendment guarantees a right to treatment to persons involuntarily civilly committed to state mental hospitals." The appellate court held that when, as in Donaldson's case, the rationale for confinement is that the patient is in need of treatment, the Constitution requires that minimally adequate treatment in fact be provided. The court further expressed the view that, regardless of the grounds for involuntary civil commitment, a person confined against his will at a state mental institution has "a constitutional right to receive such individual treatment as will give him a reasonable opportunity to be cured or to improve his mental condition." Conversely, the court's opinion implied that it is constitutionally permissible for a State to confine a mentally ill person against his will in order to treat his illness, regardless of whether his illness renders him dangerous to himself or others.

II

We have concluded that the difficult issues of constitutional law dealt with by the Court of Appeals are not presented by this case in its present posture. Specifically, there is no reason now to decide whether mentally ill persons dangerous to themselves or to others have a right to treatment upon compulsory confinement by the State, or whether the State may compulsorily confine a nondangerous, mentally ill individual for the purpose of treatment. As we view it, this case raises a single, relatively simple, but nonetheless important question concerning every man's constitutional right to liberty.

The jury found that Donaldson was neither dangerous to himself nor dangerous to others, and also found that, if mentally ill, Donaldson had not received treatment. That verdict, based on abundant evidence, makes the issue before the Court a narrow one. We need not decide whether, when, or by what procedures, a mentally ill person may be confined by the State on any of the grounds which, under contemporary statutes, are generally advanced to justify involuntary confinement of such a person—to prevent injury to the public, to ensure his own survival or safety,[1] or to alleviate or cure his illness. For the jury found that none of the above grounds for continued confinement was present in Donaldson's case.

Given the jury's findings, what was left as justification for keeping Donaldson in continued confinement? The fact that state law may have authorized confinement of the harmless mentally ill does not itself establish a constitutionally adequate purpose for the confinement. Nor is it enough that Donaldson's original confinement

was founded upon a constitutionally adequate basis, if in fact it was, because even if his involuntary confinement was initially permissible, it could not constitutionally continue after that basis no longer existed.

A finding of "mental illness" alone cannot justify a State's locking a person up against his will and keeping him indefinitely in simple custodial confinement. Assuming that that term can be given a reasonably precise content and that the "mentally ill" can be identified with reasonable accuracy, there is still no constitutional basis for confining such persons involuntarily if they are dangerous to no one and can live safely in freedom.

May the State confine the mentally ill merely to ensure them a living standard superior to that which they enjoy in the private community? That the State has a proper interest in providing care and assistance to the unfortunate goes without saying. But the mere presence of mental illness does not disqualify a person from preferring his home to the comforts of an institution. Moreover, while the State may arguably confine a person to save him from harm, incarceration is rarely if ever a necessary condition for raising the living standards of those capable of surviving safely in freedom, on their own or with the help of family or friends.

May the State fence in the harmless mentally ill solely to save its citizens from exposure to those whose ways are different? One might as well ask if the State, to avoid public unease, could incarcerate all who are physically unattractive or socially eccentric. Mere public intolerance or animosity cannot constitutionally justify the deprivation of a person's physical liberty.

In short, a State cannot constitutionally confine without more a nondangerous individual who is capable of surviving safely in freedom by himself or with the help of willing and responsible family members or friends. Since the jury found, upon ample evidence, that O'Connor, as an agent of the State, knowingly did so confine Donaldson, it properly concluded that O'Connor violated Donaldson's constitutional right to freedom.

III

O'Connor contends that in any event he should not be held personally liable for monetary damages because his decisions were made in "good faith." Specifically, O'Connor argues that he was acting pursuant to state law which, he believed, authorized confinement of the mentally ill even when their release would not compromise their safety or constitute a danger to others, and that he could not reasonably have been expected to know that the state law as he understood it was constitutionally invalid. A proposed instruction to this effect was rejected by the District Court.

The District Court did instruct the jury, without objection, that monetary damages could not be assessed against O'Connor if he had believed reasonably and in good faith that Donaldson's continued confinement was "proper," and that punitive damages could be awarded only if O'Connor had acted "maliciously or wantonly or oppressively." The Court of Appeals approved those instructions. But that court did not consider whether it was error for the trial judge to refuse the additional instruction concerning O'Connor's claimed reliance on state law as authorization for Donaldson's continued confinement. Further, neither the District Court nor the Court of Appeals acted with the benefit of this Court's most recent decision on the scope of the qualified immunity possessed by state officials.... [*Wood v. Strickland* (1975)]

Under that decision, the relevant question for the jury is whether O'Connor "knew or reasonably should have known that the action he took within his sphere of official responsibility would violate the constitutional rights of [Donaldson], or if he took the action with the malicious intention to cause a deprivation of constitutional rights or other injury to [Donaldson]." For the purposes of this question, an official has, of course, no duty to anticipate unforeseeable constitutional developments.

Accordingly, we vacate the judgment of the Court of Appeals and remand the case to enable that court to consider, in light of *Wood v. Strickland*, whether the District Judge's failure to instruct with regard to the effect of O'Connor's claimed reliance on state law rendered inadequate the instructions as to O'Connor's liability for compensatory and punitive damages.[2]

It is so ordered.

Vacated and remanded.

NOTES

1 The judge's instructions used the phrase "dangerous to himself." Of course, even if there is no foreseeable risk of self-injury or suicide, a person is literally "dangerous to himself" if for physical or other reasons he is helpless to avoid the hazards of freedom either through his own efforts or with the aid of willing family members or friends. While it might be argued that the judge's instructions could have been more detailed on this point, O'Connor raised no objection to them, presumably because the evidence clearly showed that Donaldson was not "dangerous to himself" however broadly that phrase might be defined.

2 Upon remand, the Court of Appeals is to consider only the question whether O'Connor is to be held liable for monetary damages for violating Donaldson's constitutional right to liberty. The jury found, on substantial evidence and under adequate instructions, that O'Connor deprived Donaldson, who was dangerous neither to himself nor to others and was provided no treatment, of the constitutional right to liberty. That finding needs no further consideration. If the Court of Appeals holds that a remand to the District Court is necessary, the only issue to be determined in that court will be whether O'Connor is immune from liability for monetary damages.

Of necessity our decision vacating the judgment of the Court of Appeals deprives that court's opinion of precedential effect, leaving this Court's opinion and judgment as the sole law of the case.

The Case for Involuntary Hospitalization of the Mentally Ill
Paul Chodoff

Paul Chodoff is clinical professor of psychiatry and behavioral sciences at George Washington University School of Medicine. Chodoff, who also maintains a private practice, is coeditor of *Psychiatric Ethics* (1981) and the author of numerous articles, including "The Diagnosis of

The American Journal of Psychiatry, vol. 133, no. 5 (May 1976), pp. 496–501. Copyright © 1976, The American Psychiatric Association. Reprinted by permission.

Hysteria: An Overview," "The Effect of Third-Party Payment on the Practice of Psychotherapy," and "Psychiatry and Fiscal Third Party."

Chodoff is concerned with the question of the justifiability of involuntary civil commitment. He presents a number of cases as examples of behavior which most of us would agree differ significantly from the norm. He uses these cases as a background for his analysis and evaluation of three stances that are often taken toward involuntary civil commitment. The three stances are those of (1) abolitionists, (2) medical-model psychiatrists, and (3) civil liberties lawyers.

I will begin this paper with a series of vignettes designed to illustrate graphically the question that is my focus: under what conditions, if any, does society have the right to apply coercion to an individual to hospitalize him against his will, by reason of mental illness?

Case 1 A woman in her mid 50s, with no previous overt behavioral difficulties, comes to believe that she is worthless and insignificant. She is completely preoccupied with her guilt and is increasingly unavailable for the ordinary demands of life. She eats very little because of her conviction that the food should go to others whose need is greater than hers, and her physical condition progressively deteriorates. Although she will talk to others about herself, she insists that she is not sick, only bad. She refuses medication, and when hospitalization is suggested she also refuses that on the grounds that she would be taking up space that otherwise could be occupied by those who merit treatment more than she.

Case 2 For the past 6 years the behavior of a 42-year-old woman has been disturbed for periods of 3 months or longer. After recovery from her most recent episode she has been at home, functioning at a borderline level. A month ago she again started to withdraw from her environment. She pays increasingly less attention to her bodily needs, talks very little, and does not respond to questions or attention from those about her. She lapses into a mute state and lies in her bed in a totally passive fashion. She does not respond to other people, does not eat, and does not void. When her arm is raised from the bed it remains for several minutes in the position in which it is left. Her medical history and a physical examination reveal no evidence of primary physical illness.

Case 3 A man with a history of alcoholism has been on a binge for several weeks. He remains at home doing little else than drinking. He eats very little. He becomes

tremulous and misinterprets spots on the wall as animals about to attack him, and he complains of "creeping" sensations in his body, which he attributes to infestation by insects. He does not seek help voluntarily, insists there is nothing wrong with him, and despite his wife's entreaties he continues to drink.

Case 4 Passersby and station personnel observe that a young woman has been spending several days at Union Station in Washington, D.C. Her behavior appears strange to others. She is finally befriended by a newspaper reporter who becomes aware that her perception of her situation is profoundly unrealistic and that she is, in fact, delusional. He persuades her to accompany him to St. Elizabeth's Hospital, where she is examined by a psychiatrist who recommends admission. She refuses hospitalization and the psychiatrist allows her to leave. She returns to Union Station. A few days later she is found dead, murdered, on one of the surrounding streets.

Case 5 A government attorney in his late 30s begins to display pressured speech and hyperactivity. He is too busy to sleep and eats very little. He talks rapidly, becomes irritable when interrupted, and makes phone calls all over the country in furtherance of his political ambitions, which are to begin a campaign for the Presidency of the United States. He makes many purchases, some very expensive, thus running through a great deal of money. He is rude and tactless to his friends, who are offended by his behavior, and his job is in jeopardy. In spite of his wife's pleas he insists that he does not have the time to seek or accept treatment, and he refuses hospitalization. This is not the first such disturbance for this individual; in fact, very similar episodes have been occurring at roughly 2-year intervals since he was 18 years old.

Case 6 Passersby in a campus area observe two young women standing together, staring at each other, for over an hour. Their behavior attracts attention, and eventually the police take the pair to a nearby precinct station for questioning. They refuse to answer questions and sit mutely, staring into space. The police request some type of psychiatric examination but are informed by the city attorney's office that state law (Michigan) allows persons to be held for observation only if they appear obviously dangerous to themselves or others. In this case, since the women do not seem homicidal or suicidal, they do not qualify for observation and are released.

Less than 30 hours later the two women are found on the floor of their campus apartment, screaming and writhing in pain with their clothes ablaze from a self-made pyre. One woman recovers; the other dies. There is no conclusive evidence that drugs were involved (1).

Most, if not all, people would agree that the behavior described in these vignettes deviates significantly from even elastic definitions of normality. However, it is clear that there would not be a similar consensus on how to react to this kind of behavior and that there is a considerable and increasing ferment about what attitude the organized elements of our society should take toward such individuals. Everyone has a stake in this important issue, but the debate about it takes place principally among psychiatrists, lawyers, the courts, and law enforcement agencies.

Points of view about the question of involuntary hospitalization fall into the following three principal groups: the "abolitionists," medical model psychiatrists, and civil liberties lawyers.

THE ABOLITIONISTS

Those holding this position would assert that in none of the cases I have described should involuntary hospitalization be a viable option because, quite simply, it should never be resorted to under any circumstances. As Szasz (2) has put it, "we should value liberty more highly than mental health no matter how defined" and "no one should be deprived of his freedom for the sake of his mental health." Ennis (3) has said that the goal "is nothing less than the abolition of involuntary hospitalization."

Prominent among the abolitionists are the "anti-psychiatrists," who, somewhat surprisingly, count in their ranks a number of well-known psychiatrists. For them mental illness simply does not exist in the field of psychiatry (4). They reject entirely the medical model of mental illness and insist that acceptance of it relies on a

fiction accepted jointly by the state and by psychiatrists as a device for exerting social control over annoying or unconventional people. The anti-psychiatrists hold that these people ought to be afforded the dignity of being held responsible for their behavior and required to accept its consequences. In addition, some members of this group believe that the phenomena of "mental illness" often represent essentially a tortured protest against the insanities of an irrational society (5). They maintain that society should not be encouraged in its oppressive course by affixing a pejorative label to its victims.

Among the abolitionists are some civil liberties lawyers who both assert their passionate support of the magisterial importance of individual liberty and react with repugnance and impatience to what they see as the abuses of psychiatric practice in this field—the commitment of some individuals for flimsy and possibly self-serving reasons and their inhuman warehousing in penal institutions wrongly called "hospitals."

The abolitionists do not oppose psychiatric treatment when it is conducted with the agreement of those being treated. I have no doubt that they would try to gain the consent of the individuals described earlier to undergo treatment, including hospitalization. The psychiatrists in this group would be very likely to confine their treatment methods to psychotherapeutic efforts to influence the aberrant behavior. They would be unlikely to use drugs and would certainly eschew such somatic therapies as ECT.* If efforts to enlist voluntary compliance with treatment failed, the abolitionists would not employ any means of coercion. Instead, they would step aside and allow social, legal, and community sanctions to take their course. If a human being should be jailed or a human life lost as a result of this attitude, they would accept it as a necessary evil to be tolerated in order to avoid the greater evil of unjustified loss of liberty for others (6).

THE MEDICAL MODEL PSYCHIATRISTS

I use this admittedly awkward and not entirely accurate label to designate the position of a substantial number of psychiatrists. They believe that mental illness is a mean-

---

Editors' note: Electroconvulsive therapy (ECT) involves direct intervention into the brain. In ECT, electric currents applied to the front of the patient's head induce convulsions and unconsciousness.

ingful concept and that under certain conditions its existence justifies the state's exercise, under the doctrine of parens patriae, of its right and obligation to arrange for the hospitalization of the sick individual even though coercion is involved and he is deprived of his liberty. I believe that these psychiatrists would recommend involuntary hospitalization for all six of the patients described earlier.

The Medical Model

There was a time, before they were considered to be ill, when individuals who displayed the kind of behavior I described earlier were put in "ships of fools" to wander the seas or were left to the mercies, sometimes tender but often savage, of uncomprehending communities that regarded them as either possessed or bad. During the Enlightenment and the early nineteenth century, however, these individuals gradually came to be regarded as sick people to be included under the humane and caring umbrella of the Judeo-Christian attitude toward illness. This attitude, which may have reached its height during the era of moral treatment in the early nineteenth century, has had unexpected and ambiguous consequences. It became overextended and partially perverted, and these excesses led to the reaction that is so strong a current in today's attitude toward mental illness.

However, reaction itself can go too far, and I believe that this is already happening. Witness the disastrous consequences of the precipitate dehospitalization that is occurring all over the country. To remove the protective mantle of illness from these disturbed people is to expose them, their families, and their communities to consequences that are certainly maladaptive and possibly irreparable. Are we really acting in accordance with their best interests when we allow them to "die with their rights on" (1) or when we condemn them to a "preservation of liberty which is actually so destructive as to constitute another form of imprisonment" (7)? Will they not suffer "if [a] liberty they cannot enjoy is made superior to a health that must sometimes be forced on them" (8)?

Many of those who reject the medical model out of hand as inapplicable to so-called "mental illness" have tended to oversimplify its meaning and have, in fact, equated it almost entirely with organic disease. It is necessary to recognize that it is a complex concept and that there is a lack of agreement about its meaning. Sophisticated definitions of the medical model do not require only the demonstration of unequivocal organic pathology. A broader formulation, put forward by sociologists

and deriving largely from Talcott Parsons' description of the sick role (9), extends the domain of illness to encompass certain forms of social deviance as well as biological disorders. According to this definition, the medical model is characterized not only by organicity but also by being negatively valued by society, by "nonvoluntariness," thus exempting its exemplars from blame, and by the understanding that physicians are the technically competent experts to deal with its effects (10).

Except for the question of organic disease, the patients I described earlier conform well to this broader conception of the medical model. They are all suffering both emotionally and physically, they are incapable by an effort of will of stopping or changing their destructive behavior, and those around them consider them to be in an undesirable sick state and to require medical attention.

Categorizing the behavior of these patients as involuntary may be criticized as evidence of an intolerably paternalistic and antitherapeutic attitude that fosters the very failure to take responsibility for their lives and behavior that the therapist should uncover rather than encourage. However, it must also be acknowledged that these severely ill people are not capable at a conscious level of deciding what is best for themselves and that in order to help them examine their behavior and motivation, it is necessary that they be alive and available for treatment. Their verbal message that they will not accept treatment may at the same time be conveying other more covert messages—that they are desperate and want help even though they cannot ask for it (11).

Although organic pathology may not be the only determinant of the medical model, it is of course an important one and it should not be avoided in any discussion of mental illness. There would be no question that the previously described patient with delirium tremens is suffering from a toxic form of brain disease. There are a significant number of other patients who require involuntary hospitalization because of organic brain syndrome due to various causes. Among those who are not overtly organically ill, most of the candidates for involuntary hospitalization suffer from schizophrenia or one of the major affective disorders. A growing and increasingly impressive body of evidence points to the presence of an important genetic-biological factor in these conditions; thus, many of them qualify on these grounds as illnesses.

Despite the revisionist efforts of the antipsychiatrists, mental illness *does* exist. It does not by any means include all of the people being treated by psychiatrists (or by non-psychiatrist physicians), but it does encompass those few desperately sick people for whom involuntary commitment must be considered. In the words of a recent article, "The problem is that mental illness is not a myth. It is not some palpable falsehood propagated among the populace by power-mad psychiatrists, but a cruel and bitter reality that has been with the human race since antiquity" (12, p. 1483).

Criteria for Involuntary Hospitalization

Procedures for involuntary hospitalization should be instituted for individuals who require care and treatment because of diagnosable mental illness that produces symptoms, including marked impairment in judgment, that disrupt their intrapsychic and interpersonal functioning. All three of these criteria must be met before involuntary hospitalization can be instituted.

1. Mental Illness This concept has already been discussed, but it should be repeated that only a belief in the existence of illness justifies involuntary commitment. It is a fundamental assumption that makes aberrant behavior a medical matter and its care the concern of physicians.

2. Disruption of Functioning This involves combinations of serious and often obvious disturbances that are both intrapsychic (for example, the suffering of severe depression) and interpersonal (for example, withdrawal from others because of depression). It does not include minor peccadilloes or eccentricities. Furthermore, the behavior in question must represent symptoms of the mental illness from which the patient is suffering. Among these symptoms are actions that are imminently or potentially dangerous in a physical sense to self or others, as well as other manifestations of mental illness such as those in the cases I have described. This is not to ignore dangerousness as a criterion for commitment but rather to put it in its proper place as one of a number of symptoms of the illness. A further manifestation of the illness, and indeed, the one that makes involuntary rather than voluntary hospitalization necessary, is impairment of the patient's judgment to such a degree that he is unable to consider his condition and make decisions about it in his own interests.

3. Need for Care and Treatment The goal of physicians is to treat and cure their patients; however, sometimes they can only ameliorate the suffering of their patients and sometimes all they can offer is care. It is not possible to predict whether someone will respond to treatment; nevertheless, the need for treatment and the availability of facilities to carry it out constitute essential preconditions that must be met to justify requiring anyone to give up his freedom. If mental hospital patients have a right to treatment, then psychiatrists have a right to ask for treatability as a front-door as well as a back-door criterion for commitment (7). All of the six individuals I described earlier could have been treated with a reasonable expectation of returning to a more normal state of functioning.

I believe that the objections to this formulation can be summarized as follows.

1. The whole structure founders for those who maintain that mental illness is a fiction.

2. These criteria are also untenable to those who hold liberty to be such a supreme value that the presence of mental illness per se does not constitute justification for depriving an individual of his freedom; only when such illness is manifested by clearly dangerous behavior may commitment be considered. For reasons to be discussed later, I agree with those psychiatrists (13, 14) who do not believe that dangerousness should be elevated to primacy above other manifestations of mental illness as a sine qua non for involuntary hospitalization.

3. The medical model criteria are "soft" and subjective and depend on the fallible judgment of psychiatrists. This is a valid objection. There is no reliable blood test for schizophrenia and no method for injecting grey cells into psychiatrists. A relatively small number of cases will always fall within a grey area that will be difficult to judge. In those extreme cases in which the question of commitment arises, competent and ethical psychiatrists should be able to use these criteria without doing violence to individual liberties and with the expectation of good results. Furthermore, the possible "fuzziness" of some aspects of the medical model approach is certainly no greater than that of the supposedly "objective" criteria for dangerousness, and there is little reason to believe that lawyers and judges are any less fallible than psychiatrists.

4. Commitment procedures in the hands of psychiatrists are subject to intolerable abuses. Here, as Peszke said, "It is imperative that we differenti-

ate between the principle of the process of civil commitment and the practice itself" (13, p. 825). Abuses can contaminate both the medical and the dangerousness approaches, and I believe that the abuses stemming from the abolitionist view of no commitment at all are even greater. Measures to abate abuses of the medical approach include judicial review and the abandonment of indeterminate commitment. In the course of commitment proceedings and thereafter, patients should have access to competent and compassionate legal counsel. However, this latter safeguard may itself be subject to abuse if the legal counsel acts solely in the adversary tradition and undertakes to carry out the patient's wishes even when they may be destructive.

Comment

The criteria and procedures outlined will apply most appropriately to initial episodes and recurrent attacks of mental illness. To put it simply, it is necessary to find a way to satisfy legal and humanitarian considerations and yet allow psychiatrists access to initially or acutely ill patients in order to do the best they can for them. However, there are some involuntary patients who have received adequate and active treatment but have not responded satisfactorily. An irreducible minimum of such cases, principally among those with brain disorders and process schizophrenia, will not improve sufficiently to be able to adapt to even a tolerant society.

The decision of what to do at this point is not an easy one, and it should certainly not be in the hands of psychiatrists alone. With some justification they can state that they have been given the thankless job of caring, often with inadequate facilities, for badly damaged people and that they are now being subjected to criticism for keeping these patients locked up. No one really knows what to do with these patients. It may be that when treatment has failed they exchange their sick role for what has been called the impaired role (15), which implies a permanent negative evaluation of them coupled with a somewhat less benign societal attitude. At this point, perhaps a case can be made for giving greater importance to the criteria for dangerousness and releasing such patients if they do not pose a threat to others. However, I do not believe that the release into the community of these severely malfunctioning individuals will serve their interests even though it may satisfy formal notions of right and wrong.

It should be emphasized that the number of individuals for whom involuntary commitment must be considered is small (although, under the influence of current pressures, it may be smaller than it should be). Even severe mental illness can often be handled by securing the cooperation of the patient, and certainly one of the favorable efforts. However, the distinction between voluntary and involuntary hospitalization is sometimes more formal than meaningful. How "voluntary" are the actions of an individual who is being buffeted by the threats, entreaties, and tears of his family?

I believe, however, that we are at a point (at least in some jurisdictions) where, having rebounded from an era in which involuntary commitment was too easy and employed too often, we are now entering one in which it is becoming very difficult to commit anyone, even in urgent cases. Faced with the moral obloquy that has come to pervade the atmosphere in which the decision to involuntarily hospitalize is considered, some psychiatrists, especially younger ones, have become, as Stone (16) put it, "soft as grapes" when faced with the prospect of committing anyone under any circumstances.

THE CIVIL LIBERTIES LAWYERS

I use this admittedly inexact label to designate those members of the legal profession who do not in principle reject the necessity for involuntary hospitalization but who do reject or wish to diminish the importance of medical model criteria in the hands of psychiatrists. Accordingly, the civil liberties lawyers, in dealing with the problem of involuntary hospitalization, have enlisted themselves under the standard of dangerousness, which they hold to be more objective and capable of being dealt with in a sounder evidentiary manner than the medical model criteria. For them the question is not whether mental illness, even of disabling degree, is present, but only whether it has resulted in the probability of behavior dangerous to others or to self. Thus they would scrutinize the cases previously described for evidence of such dangerousness and would make the decision about involuntary hospitalization accordingly. They would probably feel that commitment is not indicated in most of these cases, since they were selected as illustrative of severe mental illness in which outstanding evidence of physical dangerousness was not present.

The dangerousness standard is being used increasingly not only to supplement criteria for mental illness but, in fact, to replace them entirely. The recent Supreme Court decision in *O'Connor v. Donaldson* (17) is certainly a long step in this direction. In addition, "dangerousness" is increasingly being understood to refer to the probability that the individual will inflict harm on himself or others in a specific physical manner rather than in other ways. This tendency has perhaps been carried to its ultimate in the *Lessard v. Schmidt* case (18) in Wisconsin, which restricted suitability for commitment to the "extreme likelihood that if the person is not confined, he will do immediate harm to himself or others." (This decision was set aside by the U.S. Supreme Court in 1974.) In a recent Washington, D.C., Superior Court case (19) the instructions to the jury stated that the government must prove that the defendant was likely to cause "substantial physical harm to himself or others in the reasonably foreseeable future."

For the following reasons, the dangerousness standard is an inappropriate and dangerous indicator to use in judging the conditions under which someone should be involuntarily hospitalized. Dangerousness is being taken out of its proper context as one among other symptoms of the presence of severe mental illness that should be the determining factor.

1. To concentrate on dangerousness (especially to others) as the sole criterion for involuntary hospitalization deprives many mentally ill persons of the protection and treatment that they urgently require. A psychiatrist under the constraints of the dangerousness rule, faced with an out-of-control manic individual whose frantic behavior the psychiatrist truly believes to be a disguised call for help, would have to say, "Sorry, I would like to help you but I can't because you haven't threatened anybody and you are not suicidal." Since psychiatrists are admittedly not very good at accurately predicting dangerousness to others, the evidentiary standards for commitment will be very stringent. This will result in mental hospitals becoming prisons for a small population of volatile, highly assaultive, and untreatable patients (14).

2. The attempt to differentiate rigidly (especially in regard to danger to self) between physical and other kinds of self-destructive behavior is artificial, unrealistic, and unworkable. It will tend to confront psychiatrists who want to help their patients with the same kind of dilemma they were faced with when justification for therapeutic abortion on psychiatric grounds depended on evidence of suicidal intent. The advocates of the dangerousness standard seem to be more comfortable with and pay more attention to the factor of dangerousness to others even though it is a much less frequent and much less significant consequence of mental illness than is danger to self.

3. The emphasis on dangerousness (again, especially to others) is a real obstacle to the right-to-treatment movement since it prevents the hospitalization and therefore the treatment of the population most amenable to various kinds of therapy.

4. Emphasis on the criterion of dangerousness to others moves involuntary commitment from a civil to a criminal procedure, thus, as Stone (14) put it, imposing the procedures of one terrible system on another. Involuntary commitment on these grounds becomes a form of preventive detention and makes the psychiatrist a kind of glorified policeman.

5. Emphasis on dangerousness rather than mental disability and helplessness will hasten the process of deinstitutionalization. Recent reports (20, 21) have shown that these patients are not being rehabilitated and reintegrated into the community, but rather, that the burden of custodialism has been shifted from the hospital to the community.

6. As previously mentioned, emphasis on the dangerousness criterion may be a tactic of some of the abolitionists among the civil liberties lawyers (22) to end involuntary hospitalization by reducing it to an unworkable absurdity.

DISCUSSION

It is obvious that it is good to be at liberty and that it is good to be free from the consequences of disabling and dehumanizing illness. Sometimes these two values are incompatible, and in the heat of the passions that are often aroused by opposing views of right and wrong, the partisans of each view may tend to minimize the importance of the other. Both sides can present their horror stories—the psychiatrists, their dead victims of the failure of the involuntary hospitalization process, and the lawyers, their Donaldsons. There is a real danger that instead of acknowledging the difficulty of the problem, the two camps will become polarized, with a consequent rush toward extreme and untenable solutions rather than working toward reasonable ones.

The path taken by those whom I have labeled the abolitionists is an example of the barren results that ensue when an absolute solution is imposed on a complex problem. There are human beings who will suffer greatly if the abolitionists succeed in elevating an abstract principle into an unbreakable law with no exceptions. I find myself oppressed and repelled by their position, which seems to stem from an ideological rigidity which ignores that element of the contingent immanent in the structure of human existence. It is devoid of compassion.

The positions of those who espouse the medical model and the dangerousness approaches to commitment are, one hopes, not completely irreconcilable. To some extent these differences are a result of the vantage points from which lawyers and psychiatrists view mental illness and commitment. The lawyers see and are concerned with the failures and abuses of the process. Furthermore, as a result of their training, they tend to apply principles to classes of people rather than to take each instance as unique. The psychiatrists, on the other hand, are required to deal practically with the singular needs of individuals. They approach the problem from a clinical rather than a deductive stance. As physicians, they want to be in a position to take care of and to help suffering people whom they regard as sick patients. They sometimes become impatient with the rules that prevent them from doing this.

I believe we are now witnessing a pendular swing in which the rights of the mentally ill to be treated and protected are being set aside in the rush to give them their freedom at whatever cost. But is freedom defined only by the absence of external constraints? Internal physiological or psychological processes can contribute to a throttling of the spirit that is as painful as any applied from the outside. The "wild" manic individual without his lithium, the panicky hallucinator without his injection of fluphenazine hydrochloride and the understanding support of a concerned staff, the sodden alcoholic—are they free? Sometimes, as Woody Guthrie said, "Freedom means no place to go."

Today the civil liberties lawyers are in the ascendancy and the psychiatrists on the defensive to a degree that is harmful to individual needs and the public welfare. Redress and a more balanced position will not come from further extension of the dangerousness doctrine. I favor a return to the use of medical criteria by psychia-trists—psychiatrists, however, who have been chastened by the buffeting they have received and are quite willing to go along with even strict legal safeguards as long as they are constructive and not tyrannical.

REFERENCES

1 Treffert, D. A.: "The practical limits of patients' rights." *Psychiatric Annals* 5(4):91–96, 1971.
2 Szasz, T.: *Law, Liberty and Psychiatry*, New York, Macmillan Co., 1963.
3 Ennis, B.: *Prisoners of Psychiatry*, New York, Harcourt Brace Jovanovich, 1972.
4 Szasz, T.: *The Myth of Mental Illness*, New York, Harper & Row, 1961.
5 Laing, R.: *The Politics of Experience*, New York, Ballantine Books, 1967.
6 Ennis, B.: "Ennis on 'Donaldson'." *Psychiatric News*, Dec. 3, 1975, pp. 4, 19, 37.
7 Peele, R., Chodoff, P., Taub, N.: "Involuntary hospitalization and treatability. Observations from the DC experience." *Catholic University Law Review* 23:744–753, 1974.
8 Michels, R.: "The right to refuse psychotropic drugs." *Hastings Center Report*, Hastings-on-Hudson, NY, 1973.
9 Parsons, T.: *The Social System*. New York, Free Press, 1951.
10 Veatch, R. M.: "The medical model; its nature and problems." *Hastings Center Studies* 1(3):59–76, 1973.
11 Katz, J.: "The right to treatment—an enchanting legal fiction?" *University of Chicago Law Review* 36:755–783, 1969.
12 Moore, M. S.: "Some myths about mental illness." *Arch Gen Psychiatry* 32:1483–1497, 1975.
13 Peszke, M. A.: "Is dangerousness an issue for physicians in emergency commitment?" *Am J Psychiatry* 132:825–828, 1975.
14 Stone, A. A.: "Comment on Peszke, M. A.: Is dangerousness an issue for physicians in emergency commitment?" Ibid. 829–831.
15 Siegler, M., Osmond, H.: *Models of Madness, Models of Medicine*. New York, Macmillan Co., 1974.
16 Stone, A.: Lecture for course on The Law, Litigation, and Mental Health Services. Adelphi, Md., Mental Health Study Center, September 1974.
17 O'Connor v Donaldson, 43 USLW 4929 (1975).

18 Lessard v Schmidt, 349 F Supp 1078, 1092 (ED Wis 1972).

19 In re Johnnie Hargrove, Washington, DC, Superior Court Mental Health number 506–75, 1975.

20 Rachlin, S., Pam, A., Milton, J.: "Civil liberties versus involuntary hospitalization." *Am J Psychiatry* 132:189–191, 1975.

21 Kirk, S. A., Therrien, M. E.: "Community mental health myths and the fate of former hospitalized patients." *Psychiatry* 38:209–217, 1975.

22 Dershowitz, A. A.: "Dangerousness as a criterion for confinement." *Bulletin of the American Academy of Psychiatry and the Law* 2:172–179, 1974.

Deinstitutionalization at the Crossroads
H. Richard Lamb

H. Richard Lamb, M.D., is professor in the department of psychiatry at the University of Southern California School of Medicine. He is the editor of *The Homeless Mentally Ill: A Task Force Report of the American Psychiatric Association* (1984). His published articles include "Some Reflections on Treating Schizophrenics" and "Structure: The Neglected Ingredient of Community Treatment."

Lamb, while acknowledging that many things have gone right with deinstitutionalization, points out some of its unfortunate results—the problem of the homeless mentally ill, for example. His special concern is with the long-term mentally ill, a nonhomogeneous group whose various members have very different needs. A minority of the long-term mentally ill need a highly structured, locked, 24-hour environment for the adequate intermediate or long-term management of their illness. Deinstitutionalization for them may be a disservice. However, the majority of the long-term mentally ill are able to live in the community, although the needs of members of this group are also very diverse. Lamb argues that a comprehensive system of care for those able to live in the community must be established, but such a system must recognize their heterogeneity. He concludes with a number of recommendations for mental health professionals. The recommendations are calculated to maximize the benefits of deinstitutionalization for individuals with very different needs.

Probably nothing more graphically illustrates the problems of deinstitutionalization than the shameful and incredible phenomenon of the homeless mentally ill. The conditions under which they live are symptomatic of the lack of a comprehensive system of care for the long-term mentally ill in general. Though the homeless mentally ill have become an everyday part of today's society, they are nameless; the great majority are not on the caseload of any mental health professional or mental health agency. Hardly anyone is out looking for them, for they are not officially missing. By and large the system does not know who they are or where they came from.

We can see first hand society's reluctance to do anything definitive for them: for instance, stopgap measures such as shelters may be provided, but the underlying problem of a lack of a comprehensive system of care is not addressed (1). We can see our own ambivalence about taking the difficult stands that need to be taken—as, for instance, advocating changes in the laws for involuntary treatment and the ways these laws are administered.

When we get to know homeless mentally ill persons as individuals, we often find that they are not able to meet the criteria for the programs that most appeal to us

Hospital and Community Psychiatry, vol. 39 (September 1988), pp. 941–945. Copyright © 1988, The American Psychiatric Association. Reprinted by permission.

as professionals. For the citizenry generally, the homeless mentally ill represent everything that has gone wrong with deinstitutionalization, and their circumstances have persuaded many that deinstitutionalization was a mistake.

Many things have gone right with deinstitutionalization. For instance, the chronically mentally ill have much more liberty, in the majority of cases appropriately so, than when they were institutionalized; we have learned what is necessary to meet their needs in the community; and we have begun to understand the plight of families and how to enlist their help in the treatment process. But the purpose of this paper is twofold: to examine the problems of deinstitutionalization—not just with regard to the homeless mentally ill but for the long-term mentally ill generally—and to draw upon our experience, especially our clinical experience, in working with them in order to make recommendations about what we should do.

HOSPITAL AND COMMUNITY

Has deinstitutionalization gone too far in attempting to treat long-term mentally ill persons in the community? We now have more than three decades of experience to guide us. Some long-term mentally ill persons require a highly structured, locked, 24-hour setting for adequate intermediate or long-term management (2). For those who need such care, do we not have a professional obligation to provide it (3), either in a hospital or in an alternative setting such as California's locked skilled nursing facilities with special programs for psychiatric patients (4)?

Where to treat should not be an ideological issue; it is a decision best based on the clinical needs of each person. Unfortunately deinstitutionalization efforts have, in practice, too often confused locus of care and quality of care (5). Where mentally ill persons are treated has been seen as more important than how they are treated. Care in the community has often been assumed almost by definition to be better than hospital care. In actuality, poor care can be found in both hospital and community settings. But the other issue that requires attention is appropriateness. The long-term mentally ill are not a homogeneous population; what is appropriate for some is not appropriate for others.

For instance, what of those persons who are characterized by such problems as assaultive behavior; severe, overt major psychopathology; lack of internal controls; reluctance to take psychotropic medications; inability to

adjust to open settings; problems with drugs and alcohol; and self-destructive behavior? When attempts have been made to treat some of these persons in open community settings, they have required an inordinate amount of time and effort from mental health professionals, various social agencies, and the criminal justice system. Many have been lost to the mental health system and are on the streets or in jail.

Moreover, both mentally ill persons and mental health professionals have often considered these results as evidence of failures by both groups. As a consequence, many long-term mentally ill persons have become alienated from a system that has not met their needs, and some mental health professionals have become disenchanted with their treatment. Unfortunately the heat of the debate over whether to provide intermediate and long-term hospitalization for such patients has tended to obscure the benefits of community treatment for the great majority of the long-term mentally ill who do not require such highly structured 24-hour care.

SOME BASIC QUESTIONS

What about the majority of long-term mentally ill persons who are able to live in the community? First and foremost, we need to ask ourselves if we have truly established this group as the highest-priority population in public mental health.

If so, does this priority include commitments of our resources and our funding, as well as our concern? We have learned a great deal about the needs of the long-term mentally ill in the community. Thus we know that this population needs a comprehensive and integrated system of care (6); such a system would include an adequate number and range of supervised, supportive housing settings; adequate, comprehensive, and accessible crisis intervention, both in the community and in hospitals; and ongoing treatment and rehabilitative services, all provided assertively through outreach when necessary.

We know the importance of a system of case management in which every long-term mentally ill person is on the caseload of a mental health agency that will take full responsibility for individualized treatment planning, linking patients to needed resources and monitoring them so that they not only receive the services they need but are not lost to the system. Have we done enough to put our knowledge into practice? For most parts of this nation, the answer is clearly no (7).

THERAPEUTIC BUT REALISTIC OPTIMISM

Nothing is more important than therapeutic optimism if we are to work successfully with the long-term mentally ill. But equally important is a need for a realistic appraisal of these persons' capacities. With such an appraisal we can mount vigorous treatment and rehabilitation efforts for those with the potential for high levels of functioning and strive for other goals, such as improving quality of life, when patients have less potential.

An important issue related to goal setting is that the kinds of criteria that theorists, researchers, policy-makers, and clinicians use to assess social integration have a distinct bias in favor of the values held by these professionals and by middle-class society generally (8). Thus holding a job, increasing one's socialization and relationships with other people, and living independently may be goals that are not shared by a large proportion of the long-term mentally ill.

Likewise, what makes the patient happy may be unrelated to these goals. Patients may want (or need) to avoid the stress of competitive employment, or even sheltered employment, and of living independently. They may experience more anxiety than gratification from the threat of intimacy that accompanies increased involvement with other people. Furthermore, many relatives may be primarily interested in the simple provision of decent custodial care (9).

Moreover, if we use expectations applicable to the higher-functioning patients as our only model, we will neglect the large population who are lower functioning and cannot respond to these expectations. And, in fact, in many jurisdictions this population has been neglected. We can only speculate about why.

One possible reason is the failure by some mental health professionals to recognize that there are many different kinds of long-term patients who vary greatly in their capacity for rehabilitation and for change (10). Long-term mentally ill persons differ in their ability to cope with stress without decompensating and developing psychotic symptoms. They differ too in the kinds of stress and pressure they can handle; for instance, some who are amenable to social rehabilitation cannot handle the stresses of vocational rehabilitation, and vice versa. What may appear, at first glance, to be a homogeneous group turns out to be a group that ranges from persons who can tolerate almost no stress at all to those who can, with some assistance, cope with most of life's demands.

Such a view is supported by the very marked variations of course and outcome in both the shorter-term

follow-up studies of schizophrenia (11,12) and the longer-term studies discussed later. For some long-term patients, competitive employment, independent living, and a high level of social functioning are realistic goals; for others, just maintaining their present level of functioning should be considered a success (13).

Dependency, and the reactions of professionals to it, may well be another important factor. To gratify dependency needs and to nurture are crucial activities in the helping professions. And we learn to do this in such a way that patients do not experience a loss of self-esteem from knowing that they need our help and support (14). Not only may this process be draining to professionals, but in addition when we nurture, we expect growth, and we are sorely disappointed when we do not get it, even though the potential for the growth we seek may not be there. As a result, lower-functioning patients may receive less of our attention, our resources, and our efforts.

Moreover, most of us, as products of our culture and our society, tend to morally disapprove of persons who have "given in" to their dependency needs, who have adopted a passive, inactive life-style, and who have accepted public support instead of working (10). Perhaps this moral disapproval helps to explain why programs whose goals are rehabilitating patients to high levels of functioning, or "mainstreaming" them, attract the most attention and the most funding. Such programs are very much needed. If, however, professionals attempt to raise patients' low-functioning adaptations to the pressures of life, without making a realistic appraisal of the capabilities of each individual, an acute exacerbation of psychosis may result. Probably no problems are more difficult to overcome in the treatment of the long-term mentally ill than those of professionals having to come to terms with the fact that some persons are unable, or unwilling, or both to give up a life of dependency.

The matter of independence presents similar problems. Society generally, including professionals, highly values independence. And yet nothing is more difficult for many long-term mentally ill persons to attain and sustain (15). The issue of supervised versus unsupervised housing provides an example. Professionals want to see their patients living in their own apartments, managing on their own, perhaps with some outpatient support. But the experience of deinstitutionalization has been that most long-term mentally ill persons living in unsupervised settings in the community find the ordinary stresses of managing on their own more than they can handle. After a while they tend to not take their medications, to neglect their nutrition, and to let their lives unravel and become disorganized. Eventually they find their way back to the hospital or the streets (1).

Mentally ill persons highly value independence, but they very often underestimate their dependency needs. Professionals need to be realistic about their patients' potential for independence, even if the patients are not.

Still another factor that may contribute to the focus on higher-functioning patients is some professionals' lack of appreciation of the rewards of treating patients who function less well and of forming a relationship over many years with both patient and family. Even when the potential for higher functioning is limited, we can derive an immense amount of satisfaction from helping to transform chaotic, dysphoric life-styles into stable ones, with at least some opportunity for pleasure and contentment for both the mentally ill person and the family.

LONG-TERM OUTCOME AND EXPECTATIONS

Some mental health professionals believe that long-term follow-up studies of schizophrenia indicate that we should raise our expectations of how schizophrenics will function in the community. Such a conclusion requires closer scrutiny. These studies, with mean lengths of follow-up ranging from 22.4 to 36.9 years, have demonstrated considerable degrees of improvement and even "recovery" over time (16–20).

These findings are not surprising, for they are consistent with everyday clinical experience that schizophrenia in the patient's middle and later years tends to be more benign and far less stormy than in the earlier years. In contrast, younger schizophrenics are faced with the same concerns and life-cycle stresses as others in their age group. They strive for independence, satisfying relationships, a sense of identity, and vocational success. Many, lacking the ability to withstand stress and intimacy, struggle and often repeatedly fail. The result is anxiety, depression, psychotic episodes, and hospitalization. Denial of illness and the rebelliousness of youth often compound the problems.

As the years go by, schizophrenics and those around them tend to come to terms with the illness. Goals are lowered, and expectations are lessened. Under these circumstances many persons with limited abilities to cope and deal with stress gradually become able to function in both vocational and domestic roles, meeting lowered expectations of others and themselves. With time the fires of youth burn lower. Increasing maturity is still another

factor. Thus older patients with schizophrenia may present a far different picture than when they were younger, less mature, and striving to meet higher aspirations.

There is a danger, however, in using the word recovery rather than remission when referring to improved or even normal functioning. Recovery implies eradication of the illness. The evidence is compelling that schizophrenia, with its predisposition to decompensation under stress, is a genetically determined illness (21). There is no evidence that patients' genetic predisposition to decompensate under stress disappears. Moreover, as important as these long-term findings are, they should not mislead clinicians working with schizophrenics in their twenties or thirties to expect short- or intermediate-term results that are beyond individual patients' capabilities within shorter time frames.

PROBLEMS OF THE CITIES

What are the practical limits of what our nation, and in particular our largest cities, can and will do to serve the long-term mentally ill? The greatest number of these persons are in our largest cities, but it is here that the politics are most complex, the bureaucracies largest and most cumbersome, the battles for power and turf fiercest (22,23). Here too the administrative costs of providing care tend to be high, often more than 50 percent of the budget, leaving an insufficient amount for actual services to patients. It is in the largest cities, too, that resistance to change tends to be strongest and most stubborn. These factors, if not corrected, inevitably lead to inadequate care of the long-term mentally ill.

INVOLUNTARY TREATMENT

Involuntary treatment presents us with an extremely difficult dilemma. Our beliefs in civil liberties come into conflict with our concern for the welfare of our patients. This dilemma can be resolved if we believe that the mentally ill have a right to involuntary treatment (24,25) when, because of severe mental illness, they present a serious threat to their own welfare or that of others and at the same time are not mentally competent to make a rational decision about accepting treatment.

Reaching out to patients and working to encourage them to accept help on a voluntary basis is certainly an important first step. But if it fails and the patient is at serious risk, helping professionals need to see that ethically we cannot simply stop there. Is it not our obligation to advocate for changes in the laws that will facilitate involuntary treatment for such persons, or changes in the way the laws for involuntary treatment are administered? These changes would result in patients' prompt return to acute inpatient treatment when it is clinically indicated, and ongoing measures, such as conservatorship, court-mandated outpatient treatment, and appointment of a payee for the patient's Supplemental Security Income check, when they are indicated.

What is needed is a treatment philosophy recognizing that such external controls are a positive, even crucial, therapeutic approach for those in the long-term mentally ill population who lack the internal controls to deal with their impulses and to organize themselves to cope with life's demands. Such external controls may interrupt the self-destructive, chaotic life of a patient who is on the streets and in and out of jails and hospitals.

For instance, in some parts of California, conservatorship has become an important therapeutic modality for such persons. It is particularly useful when conservators are psychiatric social workers or persons with similar backgrounds and skills who use their court-granted authority to become a crucial source of stability and support for chronically mentally ill persons. Conservatorship thus can enable persons who might otherwise be long-term residents of hospitals to live in the community and achieve a considerable measure of autonomy and satisfaction in their lives.

If we do not take a firm stand on these issues, we risk being seen by society, not to mention by the long-term mentally ill themselves, as uncaring and even inhumane. The homeless mentally ill dramatically illustrate this issue.

THE TASKS AHEAD OF US

What do we need to do to get deinstitutionalization back on course? The following strategies should be considered.

- We should acknowledge that while deinstitutionalization was a positive step and the correct thing to do, it has gone too far.
- Of the long-term mentally ill now in the community, only some need intermediate or long-

term highly structured 24-hour residential care. For those who need such care, however, we should provide it. When we do not, the resulting problems and debate obscure the benefits of community treatment for the great majority who do not require highly structured 24-hour care.

- We should truly make the long-term mentally ill our highest priority in public mental health in terms of both resources and funding. In making this commitment, we should join witn our natural allies, the families.
- We should establish a comprehensive and coordinated system of care for the long-term mentally ill.
- We should not settle for stop-gap solutions, as, for instance, relying on a system of shelters for the homeless mentally ill instead of dealing with the underlying problem of the lack of a comprehensive system of care for the long-term mentally ill generally.
- We should have the needed therapeutic optimism to treat the long-term mentally ill, but temper this optimism with realistic, individualized goals.
- We should emphasize that the long-term mentally ill are a highly heterogeneous population.
- We should be aware that the values and goals of psychiatrically disabled persons may be different from those projected onto them by well-meaning professionals.
- We should continue to mount a vigorous rehabilitation effort aimed at achieving higher levels of functioning, both social and vocational, for those long-term mentally ill persons who can benefit from it.
- We should also give high priority to those among the long-term mentally ill who function at lower levels and not focus only on persons with higher functioning.
- We should realize the gratification we can derive from helping to change the chaotic and painful life of a patient who is on the streets and in and out of jails and hospitals into a stable life that offers the possibility of at least some contentment, even if we cannot rehabilitate that patient to a high level of functioning.
- We should not confuse the more favorable long-term outcome of schizophrenia over 20 or more years with the lesser improvements that can be

accomplished over the short or intermediate term.

- We should come to grips with the bureaucracy, politics, and inefficiency of our largest cities, where so many long-term mentally ill persons live. It may be that these problems cannot be solved and that in some instances the responsibility for the long-term mentally ill should be taken away from the cities and another administrative solution found—as, for instance, turning this responsibility over to the states.
- We as mental health professionals should actively advocate involuntary treatment, both emergency and ongoing, for persons for whom it is clinically indicated.

We have now had more than three decades of experience with deinstitutionalization. Most of what we know about community treatment of the long-term mentally ill we have learned the hard way—through experience. We need to be guided by that hard-won knowledge, look at each long-term mentally ill person as an individual with unique strengths, weaknesses, and needs, and do what our experience and clinical judgment tell us needs to be done to maximize the benefits of deinstitutionalization for each individual.

REFERENCES

1 Lamb HR (ed): The Homeless Mentally Ill: A Task Force Report of the American Psychiatric Association. Washington, DC, American Psychiatric Association, 1984

2 Dorwart RA: A ten-year follow-up study of the effects of deinstitutionalization. Hospital and Community Psychiatry 39:287–291, 1988

3 Group for the Advancement of Psychiatry: The Positive Aspects of Long Term Hospitalization in the Public Sector for Chronic Psychiatric Patients. New York, Mental Health Materials Center, 1982

4 Lamb HR: Structure: the neglected ingredient of community treatment. Archives of General Psychiatry 37:1224–1228, 1980

5 Bachrach LL: A conceptual approach to deinstitutionalization. Hospital and Community Psychiatry 29:573–578, 1978

6 Bachrach LL: The challenge of service planning for chronic mental patients. Community Mental Health Journal 22:170–174, 1986

7 Talbott JA: The fate of the public psychiatric system. Hospital and Community Psychiatry 36:46–50, 1985

8 Shadish WR Jr, Bootzin RR: Nursing homes and chronic mental patients. Schizophrenia Bulletin 7:488–498, 1981

9 Thomas S: A survey of the relative importance of community care facility characteristics to different consumer groups. Presented at the Midwestern Psychological Association, St Louis, 1980

10 Lamb HR: Treating the Long-Term Mentally Ill. San Francisco, Jossey-Bass, 1982

11 World Health Organization: Schizophrenia: An International Follow-Up Study. New York, Wiley, 1979

12 Hawk AB, Carpenter WT, Strauss JS: Diagnostic criteria and five-year outcome in schizophrenia: a report from the International Pilot Study of Schizophrenia. Archives of General Psychiatry 32:343–347, 1975

13 Solomon EB, Baird B, Everstine L, et al: Assessing the community care of chronic psychotic patients. Hospital and Community Psychiatry 31:113–116, 1980

14 Lamb HR: Some reflections on treating schizophrenics. Archives of General Psychiatry 43:1007–1011, 1986

15 Harris M, Bergman HC: Differential treatment planning for young adult chronic patients. Hospital and Community Psychiatry 38:638–643, 1987

16 Bleuler M: A 23-year longitudinal study of 208 schizophrenics and impressions in regard to the nature of schizophrenia, in The Transmission of Schizophrenia. Edited by Rosenthal D, Kety SS. Oxford, England, Pergamon, 1968

17 Huber G, Gross G, Schuttler R, et al: Longitudinal studies of schizophrenic patients. Schizophrenia Bulletin 6:592–605, 1980

18 Ciompi L: Catamnestic long-term study on the course of life and aging of schizophrenics. Schizophrenia Bulletin 6:606–618, 1980

19 Tsuang M, Woolson R., Fleming J: Long-term outcome of major psychoses, I: schizophrenia and affective disorders compared with psychiatrically symptom-free surgical conditions. Archives of General Psychiatry 36:1295–1301, 1979

20 Harding CM, Brooks GW, Ashikaga T, et al: The Vermont longitudinal study of persons with severe mental illness, II: long-term outcome of subjects who retrospectively met DSM-III criteria for schizophre-

nia. American Journal of Psychiatry 144:727–735, 1987

21 Kety SS, Rosenthal D, Wender PH, et al: Studies based on a total sample of adopted individuals and their relatives: why they were necessary, what they demonstrated and failed to demonstrate. Schizophrenia Bulletin 2:413–428, 1976

22 Keill SL: Politics and public psychiatric programs. Hospital and Community Psychiatry 36:1143, 1985

23 Elpers JR: Dividing the mental health dollar: the ethics of managing scarce resources. Hospital and Community Psychiatry 37:671–672, 1986

24 Rachlin S: One right too many. Bulletin of the American Academy of Psychiatry and the Law 3:99–102, 1975

25 Lamb HR, Mills MJ: Needed changes in law and procedure for the chronically mentally ill. Hospital and Community Psychiatry 37:475–480, 1986

Sterilization and the Rights of the Mentally Retarded

Sterilizing the Mildly Mentally Retarded Without Their Consent
Robert Neville

Robert Neville is professor of philosophy and religious studies at the State University of New York at Stonybrook. He is the editor of *New Essays in Metaphysics* (1987). His published articles include "Behavior Control: Ethical Analysis," "Philosophical Perspectives on Freedom of Inquiry," and "Pots and Black Kettles: A Philosopher's Perspective on Psychosurgery."

Neville maintains that it is sometimes morally permissible to sterilize mildly retarded individuals without their consent. He advances, and argues for, two claims: (1) involuntary sterilization is in the best interests of some mildly mentally retarded persons because it will maximize their freedom to enjoy heterosexual activity; (2) involuntary sterilization enhances the dignity of the mildly mentally retarded's position in the moral community insofar as it fosters and encourages their capacity for moral behavior.

Under certain specific circumstances it is morally permissible to sterilize some mildly mentally retarded people without their consent. At the outset of my argument I want to acknowledge that there is a grave difficulty, conceptually and empirically, in identifying which individuals belong to the relevant class of the mentally retarded. If that class is either conceptually so vague or empirically so confused that individuals who do not belong in it are inadvertently placed there, then it would be ethically impermissible to subject the class to involun-

tary sterilization. But let me put that difficulty aside until the end, and proceed with the argument as if we knew with acceptable exactness who the mildly mentally retarded are and which of them meet the specified requirements for sterilization.

THE HUMBLE ARGUMENT

My argument is really two arguments, one nested in the other. The first can be called the "humble argument" for involuntary sterilization, and it attempts to make the case that involuntary sterilization is in the best interest of certain mildly mentally retarded people. The second can be called the "philosophical argument," and it interprets the "humble argument" as a problem of rights and responsibilities, and attempts to show that involuntary sterilization in the right cases fosters rather than denies the membership of the mildly mentally retarded in the moral community.

The humble argument begins with certain observations. First, at least some mildly mentally retarded people are capable of engaging in and taking pleasure in heterosexual intercourse. My following remarks concern only this group; presumably those incapable of such intercourse would not need sterilization; those who, because of inexperience, do not know their capacities for pleasure should be viewed as capable of engaging in and taking pleasure from sexual activity until proved otherwise.

Second, for some mildly retarded people sexual activity is capable of being integrated into emotional aspects of affection, which can in turn contribute to positive, rewarding fulfillments of personal and social life. Freed from pregnancy, childbearing, and child rearing, an active heterosexual life can enrich the existence of some mildly mentally retarded people in much the way it can that of so-called "normals." Other things being equal, mildly mentally retarded people can benefit from and have a right to sexual activity and the social forms sexual relationships can involve, such as marriage. Capacities for marriage and long-lasting affection do not have to be clearly present, however, for the retarded to have a claim on sexual activity for purposes of pleasure alone.

Third, what begins to make the situation for the retarded "not equal" to that for "normals"? For mildly mentally retarded women the physiological and emotional changes that take place during pregnancy, and the violence of childbirth, are often experienced as disorienting and terrifying traumata. To the extent that a retarded man participates in the process, he too can be disoriented and lose his personal equilibrium.

Fourth, child rearing is sometimes beyond the capacities of mildly mentally retarded people precisely because of the characteristics of their retardation. The fact that child rearing is in practice also beyond the emotional capacities of many normal people should not obscure the overwhelming difficulty that it often poses for the retarded. Now it seems a prima facie argument that children ought not be conceived if there is not some reasonable expectation that they will receive minimal care. (Note that this is not an argument that conceived children should be aborted, which is more difficult to sustain.)

Fifth, mildly mentally retarded people have very great difficulty in managing impermanent forms of contraception. I am assuming that sterilization is the only permanent contraceptive; at least it cannot be reversed without medical help. Therefore, if these mildly mentally retarded people are to engage in sexual intercourse, which is otherwise desirable, without fear of the woman becoming pregnant, sterilization seems the only responsible contraceptive choice.

The humble argument, then, puts together these observations and says that the mildly mentally retarded people to whom these conditions apply should be sterilized so that they may enjoy heterosexual activity if they are so inclined. If they were not sterilized they would have to be prevented from engaging in sexual activity, or conditioned to homosexual or autoerotic sexual activity exclusively, which would be hard to guarantee. If their sex lives were not so controlled, they would run the risk of pregnancy with likely trauma for themselves and improper care for their child. If the retarded people do not or cannot give consent, then someone should have the standing to insist that the retarded be sterilized involuntarily.

An added consideration may be raised at the level of the humble argument. Who is to be sterilized, men, women, or both? The answer to that question clearly depends on the circumstances—whether the candidates are living in an institution, whether that institution is highly regulated or more informal in its management of personal associations; or, if the candidates are living outside institutions, in what kinds of settings. But generally the point of sterilization is to maximize the freedom of the mildly mentally retarded in sexual matters, and it is relevant to administer the procedure to any candidate meeting the conditions who stands to suffer harm or loss of freedom without it.

THE PHILOSOPHICAL ARGUMENT

The humble argument is a fairly straightforward, prudential argument operating within the limits and categories generally taken for granted when dealing with the mildly mentally retarded. The philosophical argument differs by calling into question the limits and categories otherwise taken for granted.

My philosophical argument consists of two main parts. The first considers the objection that sterilization of the mildly mentally retarded is wrong if done involuntarily because it would thereby deny the subjects their proper place in the moral community, treating them as means only and not ends in themselves. I shall argue on the contrary that the procedure enhances the dignity of their position in the moral community. The second part raises the very large problem of who decides about sterilization in the context of the mildly mentally retarded. Whereas some people might argue that no third party has sufficient standing in the matter to warrant doing violence to the candidate, I shall argue that it is the responsibility (a) of the moral community to establish policy creating such standing, and (b) of its properly delegated representatives to carry out the policy subject to a variety of checks.

Membership in the Moral Community

In that tradition of Western theory which takes most seriously the dignity of the human individual, the Kantian, one of the central concepts is that of the moral community. The dignity that should be accorded to each person as a human being consists in being regarded as a member of the moral community. Membership in that community means that a person is held to be morally responsible for his or her actions and life, and is to be held responsible by the rest of the community for assuming that responsibility.

With respect to human dignity, the grave danger is that a person will be treated as a thing rather than a responsible agent. This may happen when someone or some group treats a person merely as a means toward their own ends; this was Immanuel Kant's particular worry. It may also happen when the community simply fails to recognize the person as a moral agent, which happens most often when people's behavior is explained in such a way as to shift responsibility onto causes other than themselves. This objectification or alienation has been a primary worry of existentialists and many other social critics. In a strict philosophical sense (deriving from Aristotle), violence is done to people when they are prevented by external forces from fulfilling their basic or natural goals; one form of violence is to prevent someone from exercising membership in the moral community.

The mildly retarded suffer enough from their incapacities that special care should be taken to ensure them as full a membership in the moral community as possible. To sterilize them involuntarily, some people argue, is to do them unnecessary and dehumanizing violence. It is to regard them first of all as incapable of making a responsible decision about sterilization, thus ruling them

out of membership in this respect; no defender of involuntary sterilization could deny this fact. It is, second, to regard their sex lives and childbearing and child rearing lives as so controlled by irresponsible impulses that the people may just as well be managed like objects in those areas of life. Third, it is quite possible and indeed likely, according to this position, that sterilization is sought for the mildly mentally retarded in order to make their custody easier, in which cases the people are treated in that respect as means only, not as ends in themselves.

In answer to these arguments let me point out three characteristics of the moral community. First, membership in the moral community is relative to the capacity for taking moral responsibility; there is no membership in the moral community under ordinary circumstances in the respects in which there is no capacity for taking responsibility. Second, most capacities for taking moral responsibility need to be developed; ordinary socialization develops most of them. The state of moral adulthood can be defined as being in possession of the capacity to take responsibility for developing the other capacities for responsible action that might be called upon. Third, a general moral imperative for any community is that its structures and practices foster the development of the capacities for responsible behavior wherever possible, and avoid hindering that development.

The idea of a moral community is an ideal that exists in pure form only in the imagination. When the ideal is applied to actual communities, it must be tailored to the fact that some people can have only partial memberships because of limited capacity for morally responsible behavior. Children, for example, only slowly take on the capacities for full membership in the moral community, and come to be treated as full members by degrees. Ordinarily we think of young children as full human beings because of their potential to develop into adults with full capacity for responsible action; when the coherence of their lives is extended over a reasonable life span, they can be expected to have moral capacities in due season.

Other people have other sorts of limited capacities for responsible behavior, such as those resulting from mental illness or senility, in which certain areas of life may involve severe incapacities for responsible behavior whereas others do not. In these cases, we usually regard people as fully human members of the moral community by according them the rights of responsibility where they do in fact have the capacity and by assigning to other people the responsibilities of proxy in areas of incapacity. The concept of a proxy, in the restrictive use of my distinction, is that of an agent who fits into the patient's overall moral responsibility as a substitute in a certain area or under certain circumstances; the concept of proxy is used to maintain and support the notion that a person is a member of the moral community in circumstances where the direct capacity for that is lacking.

The case of the mildly mentally retarded is somewhat different from that of children and from the limited capacity of the mentally ill or senile. Like children, their capacities for development may be far greater than would have been imagined a few years ago. But unlike children, the pacing and sequencing of their development does not lead to emotional maturity at the same time they reach bodily maturity. For instance, the emotional and intellectual capacities to manage conventional birth control methods, to adjust to pregnancy, or to raise children do not develop by the time their physical development and their social peers among nonretarded people are ready for sexual activity.

Neither, sometimes, does the capacity to make informed decisions about sterilization. Indeed, if one were to say that heterosexual activity should be prevented among certain mildly mentally retarded people until such time as they develop the capacities for responsible behavior regarding pregnancy, or for consenting to surgical sterilization, the result is very likely to be the prevention of heterosexual activity altogether. As the humble argument says, this approach would amount to preventing the development of an important capacity for responsible behavior in areas that would be possible if an active sex life were possible, and would therefore be contrary to the imperative that the moral community foster such capacities.

Mildly mentally retarded people are like certain kinds of mentally ill people in that, from the adult perspective, there are certain areas of life in which they may lack capacities for responsible behavior and other areas where they may have them. But they are unlike mentally ill people in an important respect. A mentally ill person is conceived to be a member of the moral community because even though a proxy might exercise some of his or her responsibilities, he or she is believed to have the structure of a person who possesses the capacities for those responsibilities.

This belief is based on the fact, for instance, that the person once exercised those responsibilities before becoming ill. With the help of a proxy, almost as a prosthetic device, a mentally ill person can be presented to the moral community as a fully responsible moral agent. A mildly mentally retarded person, however, lacks the full personality structure that would come from having

had the capacities for morally responsible behavior in the past. Although another person might make decisions in areas in which the retarded person is incapacitated, that would not strictly speaking be a case of proxy because the retarded person does not have a personality structured around the capacity for which a proxy might have to substitute.

Paternalism and proxy are models for enabling persons—children and the mentally ill, respectively—to enjoy membership in the moral community when they themselves have capacities for only partial membership. Another model is needed for the limited capacity of mildly mentally retarded people, one which I propose to call the model of "involuntary restrictive conditions." The model depicts mildly mentally retarded people as members of the moral community on the condition that they meet certain restrictions. Just as people with bad eyesight may be licensed to drive with the restriction that they wear glasses, so mildly mentally retarded people may be required to meet certain restrictions in order to be members of the moral community.

The analogy with driver's licenses is imperfect, however, because a person with bad eyesight can always choose not to drive and thereby not to need to wear glasses. But a person cannot choose to be in or out of the moral community; one is either in the position to be held responsible or one is not. Mildly mentally retarded people, and perhaps other groups, must meet the restrictions as conditions for being in the community. Therefore, from the standpoint of mildly mentally retarded people, the restrictive conditions are involuntary.

In a moment I shall urge that sterilization may be a proper involuntary restrictive condition for membership in the moral community for mildly mentally retarded people, subject to the limitations mentioned in connection with the humble argument. Before that, however, I want to address the question of who decides about involuntary restrictive conditions.

Who Should Decide?

Whether a certain restrictive condition does indeed foster the capacity for responsible moral behavior is an empirical question. The suggestion has been made that, with sterilization, mildly mentally retarded people will be able to engage in the kind of sex life that can develop their capacities for responsible behavior in various human relationships. Without sterilization they either would be prevented from having sex, and therefore would not develop those capacities for sexual affection and comradeship, or they would have sex and find themselves in such trouble that sexual affection and companionship would again be beyond them.

Furthermore, this empirical argument suggests that behavior having to do with sexual affection and companionship is more important than what mildly mentally retarded people might gain from opportunities for pregnancy, childbirth, and child rearing. The first "who decides" question is: Who decides whether that empirical argument is right? I suggest that this decision is a broad social one, which should be as informed as possible by experts in all the relevant fields, including both mental retardation and ethics. Clearly that argument will always be under redefinition and refinement.

But the next "who decides" question is: Who sets the policies regarding the treatment of the mildly mentally retarded? The answer is that the decision must come from the political process (again informed by relevant experts, and formulated by broad intellectual dialogue). The reason for locating the decision in the political process is that that is the only legitimate way by which individuals can be dealt with against their wills by due process. But there are two normative factors within the political process. One is that the process should conform to whatever political norm structures it—for instance, that of a representative democracy. According to this factor, what the political process decides about mildly mentally retarded people is legitimate if due political procedures have been followed. The other normative factor, however, is the demands of being a moral community, since the political process is the vehicle for actualizing those demands. A political decision is moral if it accords with what is required as a minimum for a moral community.

If the sterilization of mildly mentally retarded people, subject to appropriate limitations, does indeed foster important capacities for morally responsible behavior, and if a moral community ought to foster such capacities where possible, the warrant for politically deciding to sterilize certain mildly mentally retarded people is a moral one, not merely one of political legitimacy. There is a prima facie obligation to foster people's capacity for responsibility, since this capacity is the basis of their membership in the moral community. Paradoxically, to refrain from sterilization is to do them the violence of preventing them from participating in the moral community in one of the important respects of which they are capable.

Assuming that the political process results in a sterilization policy, by what procedures and what officers

should decisions be made about particular candidates? That is a prudential political question that I shall not attempt to address. It is necessary at this point, however, to refer to what Hastings Center lore calls the "klutz factor," namely, that translating a theoretical moral argument into a public policy with significant effects is likely to lead to blunders and abuse. Because of the "klutz factor," prudence may very well dictate that policies should be far more conservative than morality otherwise would dictate.

For instance, as I stated in the "humble argument," the candidates for involuntary sterilization should include those who are capable of engaging in and taking pleasure in heterosexual activity, and yet who are incapable of taking responsibility for this activity in regards to pregnancy and the rest. This is a positive argument for sterilizing a class of people. In light of the "klutz factor," according to which the wrong people might be sent to the surgeon, perhaps it would be a prudent extra restriction to insist that candidates have demonstrated their need for sterilization by having already gotten into trouble by their sexual activity. I am not sure how to prevent such a restriction from being turned into a punitive measure against the retarded, however.

In general, with regard to all the "who decides" questions, it is important to make sure that the process of decision is self-critical and that opposition to any point of view is always funded as a corrective support.

UNIFYING THE ARGUMENTS

The philosophical side of the argument has intended to show that, contrary to the beliefs of some, involuntary sterilization does not involve treating the mildly mentally retarded as if they were not members of the moral community; rather, it acknowledges real incapacities and neutralizes their effects, thereby enabling other capacities to be realized. Furthermore, if sterilization does in some important ways lead to the development of greater capacities for responsibility, then it is part of the obligation a society owes to its potential members to provide it, subject to appropriate protections against abuse. If a mildly mentally retarded person lacks the capacity to give or withhold informed consent because he or she does not understand the subtle issues involved, then having the decision made by the society's agents is one of the involuntary restrictive conditions that might help place the person in the community. The society has the prima facie obligation to make that decision and should do so unless other considerations prevail.

The basic philosophical principle involved in this argument is that a moral community has the social responsibility to foster capacities for morally responsible behavior. It should do so paternalistically in the case of children; it should do so with appropriate proxies in the case of impaired capacities; and it should do so through the institution of involuntary restrictive conditions in the case of basic human capacities that are undevelopable only in a future that is too late for other valuable capacities to be developed that otherwise would have been possible.

This reasoning brings us back to the "humble argument." From a philosophical point of view, the humble argument might well be valid. At least it is not wrong by virtue of violating the canons of membership in the moral community; it does not deny human dignity. Indeed, the structure of the humble argument is to provide for the dignity of humane heterosexual relations by removing the unbearable complications of potential pregnancy. Whether its premises are valid is an empirical matter.

Let me close by dealing with the question of adequate diagnosis of the appropriate conditions for involuntary sterilization. Some structure must be worked out to determine appropriate subjects. We have seen that to do so requires two sorts of determinations. The first is whether informed and emotionally balanced decisions regarding sterilization are within the capacities of the candidates; if they are, then the candidates' word should be decisive, and if they prefer nonsterilization then society should respect that choice, whatever other compensatory restrictions it requires (such as no sexual activity). The second is whether the candidates are capable of heterosexual intercourse but not capable of coping adequately with pregnancy, childbirth, and child rearing. Not all mentally retarded people would fall into this category, and specific empirical criteria would have to be developed before a program of involuntary sterilization could be instituted.

If no mildly mentally retarded people can be found who fall into this category, then none of them should be involuntarily sterilized. The consequence of this requirement is that the validity of involuntary-sterilization programs depends upon the development of criteria and diagnostic skills sufficient to discriminate the proper category of people. There have been disagreements concerning whether the definitions of relevant characteristics, and diagnostic skills for discerning them, are sufficiently developed to provide a capacity for responsible programs. In the face of excessive modesty and caution it should be pointed out that people are now classified as mildly mentally retarded and subjected to programs intended to help them.

There is one final point. It is sometimes believed that there is a totalitarian impetus lurking in any social policy that might require people to be good—in this case, to submit to involuntary restrictive conditions in order to develop the amiable responsibilities of a decent sex life. I admit that there is a danger, but urge that it be guarded against by specific safeguards and internal critical mechanisms rather than by a blanket rejection. If people could be whole and fully responsible by themselves, society would have no positive responsibilities, only negative, peace-keeping ones. But because people become responsible through the grace of social life, and because some people need special help in exercising responsibility, society does have positive duties in developing the capacity for responsible moral behavior.

Current Sterilization Law: A Paternalism Model
Elizabeth S. Scott

Elizabeth S. Scott, J.D., is associate professor and director, Center for the Study of Children and the Law, University of Virginia School of Law. Her published articles include "Children's Preference in Adjudicated Custody Decisions" and "Sterilization of Mentally Retarded Persons: Reproductive Rights and Family Privacy," from which this selection is excerpted.

Reprinted with permission of the author and the publisher from *Duke Law Journal*, vol. 806 (1986), pp. 806–808, 817–825. Copyright © 1986, Duke University School of Law.

In Scott's review of current sterilization law, she explains how the law has been radically transformed in reaction to a time in the recent past when involuntary sterilization was used by the state as a weapon in a war against mental deficiency, but she criticizes current law as a one-sided response to earlier abuses. On her view, the well-intentioned paternalism reflected in current sterilization law, although correct in maintaining a strong presumption against sterilization, may hurt some retarded persons because it places their interest in procreation above all their other interests, including an interest in avoiding pregnancy.

Sterilization is one of the most frequently chosen forms of contraception in the world; many persons who do not want to have children select this simple, safe, and effective means of avoiding unwanted pregnancy. For individuals who are mentally disabled, however, sterilization has more ominous associations. Until recently, involuntary sterilization was used as a weapon of the state in the war against mental deficiency. Under eugenic sterilization laws in effect in many states, retarded persons were routinely sterilized without their consent or knowledge.

Sterilization law has undergone a radical transformation in recent years. Influenced by a distaste for eugenic sterilization and a desire to redress past injustices, the emerging law seeks to protect the interests of mentally disabled persons by erecting formidable barriers to sterilization. The policy goals of this reform movement are commendable. However, in its singleminded effort to prevent erroneous sterilizations, the law departs from what would be its underlying objectives: to protect where possible the individual's right to make her[1] own reproductive decisions and to ensure that any decision made by others will best protect her interests.

Current law purports to protect the individual's reproductive rights, but the focus is one-sided. Although the law protects the "right to procreate," it does so by unnecessarily burdening the reciprocal right not to procreate. The option of sterilization—seen as a legitimate exercise of the right of reproductive privacy when chosen by the normal person—may be unavailable to the retarded person. Despite rhetorical emphasis on the importance of reproductive autonomy, the paternalistic stance of the law improperly limits the freedom of some persons who may be capable of making their own reproductive choices. In many states, only a court acting as decisionmaker is deemed capable of protecting disabled persons from those who would violate their rights.

The assumption that the law's overriding purpose is to protect the right to procreate arises from the historical and political context of the reform movement. It is not based on a careful analysis of the retarded person's interest in reproductive autonomy and how this interest may be affected by her disability. There is an understandable reluctance to undertake such analysis; even asking the question implies differences in the interests of retarded and nonretarded people. However, the failure to discern the actual interests at stake can lead to erroneous decisions contrary to the normative objective of the law....

CURRENT STERILIZATION LAW

The preceding factors have stimulated the reform of sterilization law in recent years. A few jurisdictions have banned sterilization of incompetent persons altogether. Under most reform laws, however, the state may authorize sterilization under its parens patriae authority if certain conditions are met. Many of these laws follow a model derived from a Washington Supreme Court case, *In re Guardianship of Hayes.*[2] *Hayes* requires a two-part inquiry. First, the court must determine whether the individual is competent to make an informed medical decision about sterilization.[3] This inquiry seeks to protect the autonomy interest of the competent person who has no need for a surrogate decisionmaker. If the court determines that the person is incompetent, it must then consider specific factors and decide whether sterilization is in the person's best interest.

Most laws following the *Hayes* decision embody strict procedural and substantive requirements that create a strong presumption against sterilization. These laws presume that there is a conflict of interest between the child and the parent in this context and consequently exclude parents from any role in the decision. A court makes the sterilization decision in a formal "semiadversarial" proceeding. The retarded individual is represented by an attorney, usually a guardian ad litem, who may be directed to oppose the parents' petition for sterilization. Most of the reform laws allow a court to order sterilization only upon findings based on clear and convincing evidence.

In addition to procedural restrictions, these laws employ rigorous substantive criteria to guide the court's deliberations. Some require inquiries into whether the individual is able to reproduce and whether she is "imminently" likely to engage in sexual activity. The petitioner will be asked to demonstrate that less drastic forms of contraception have been tried and are not feasible. The court must also assess the individual's capacity to care for a child. Some states require a determination that sterilization is medically essential to preserve the life or the physical or mental health of the individual. In some states, the court must also inquire into the disabled person's understanding of reproductive functions and the relationship between sexual intercourse, pregnancy, and childbirth. Some laws direct the court to consider the psychological trauma associated with sterilization and alternatively with pregnancy and childbirth. Additionally, an inquiry into the individual's preferences about sterilization may be required, although her objection is not determinative. The *Hayes* decision and some later laws require findings that medical science is not on the verge of breakthroughs that will correct the individual's disability or make reversible sterilization available. These various criteria create formidable substantive barriers to the sterilization of mentally retarded persons.

Current law explicitly or implicitly excludes some variables from the court's consideration, such as the state's interest in protecting society from the genetic and financial burden of children produced by retarded persons. The parents' interest in protecting their child from unwanted pregnancy or in avoiding the inconvenience associated with menstrual hygiene is also excluded from consideration. Finally, the disabled individual's interest in promoting family stability by reducing the stress associated with her care may not be considered.

The substantive criteria that guide the decisionmaker are formulated into four kinds of legal rules. The *Hayes* opinion adopts the most common approach, which could be termed a "mandatory criteria" rule; under this type of rule a court can authorize sterilization only if several specific findings are clearly made.[4] This rule places a significant burden on the petitioner, limits judicial discretion, and makes it difficult to establish the desirability of sterilization. The "discretionary best interest" standard is a more flexible rule; instead of requiring specific findings, it directs judges to consider and weigh designated criteria in determining whether sterilization is in the incompetent person's best interest. A few states have adopted the "substituted judgment" ap-

proach first proposed by the New Jersey Supreme Court in *In re Grady*.[5] *Grady* directs the court to consider the *Hayes* criteria and any other relevant factors in order to make the decision that the disabled person would make for herself if she were competent. Finally, a few jurisdictions simply prohibit the sterilization of anyone found by the court to be incompetent to give informed consent to the medical procedure.

On a functional level, the various legal rules seem to promote different objectives. A rule prohibiting sterilization without the subject's informed consent apparently aims to protect only the right to procreate. Sterilization is by definition a violation of this right, regardless of the person's preferences. At the other extreme, the substituted judgment standard attempts, at least in theory, to approximate the choice that the individual would make if she were competent. Between these two extremes are laws that attempt to protect the individual's interest in procreation from parental or state interference. Despite variation, however, the reform laws are all based on a paternalism model. The model protects the mentally disabled person by establishing a heavy presumption against sterilization and by requiring a judicial decisionmaker.

THE LIMITS OF GOOD INTENTIONS: SOME PROBLEMS WITH THE PATERNALISM MODEL

The rigorously protective approach of the paternalism model may seem to offer a desirable level of protection when parents propose sterilization. The irreversibility of the medical procedure in itself justifies caution. Given the abuses of the past and lingering biases toward mentally retarded persons, a rule that constrains the surrogate decisionmaker by a strong presumption against sterilization would seem to be justified.

Some retarded persons, however, may be hurt by laws based on the paternalism model because that model places the interest in procreation above all other interests, including the interest in avoiding pregnancy. Like other people, a retarded person may have an interest in engaging in a sexual relationship without fear of pregnancy. This objective could often be most satisfactorily implemented through sterilization, but that option usually will be unavailable under current law. Current law also unnecessarily restricts the individual's interest in reproductive autonomy. Although accorded rhetorical deference, this interest is protected only if the individual is found to be intellectually capable of making the medical decision. If the person is found to be incompetent, a court decides whether sterilization is in her best interest. Yet it seems possible that some persons who may be incapable of informed *medical* decisions may be capable of meaningful *reproductive* choices (to produce a child or avoid pregnancy). The basis of the restricted conception of individual autonomy under the paternalism model is unclear. It may derive from a desire to protect vulnerable individuals from those who threaten their right to procreate. Alternatively, it may be based on a simplistic analysis of the mentally disabled person's interest in reproductive autonomy.

Another problematic aspect of this model is the presumed conflict of interest in all cases between parent and child. Because every disabled person is assumed to have an interest in procreation that conflicts with her parents' effort to obtain sterilization, parental or family interests are excluded from the decision calculus. This approach may protect the mildly disabled person who may have an interest in making her own choices about reproduction. But it could be harmful for the more severely retarded person. Parents who care for a severely disabled child assume a substantial burden. It is not clear that the law serves the interest of such a person by augmenting that burden, especially if the presumed interest in procreation in fact does not exist. It is also not clear that a surrogate will be a better decisionmaker than the parents, who presumably know and love the child.

It is unlikely that sterilization, the contraceptive choice of many normal persons, is only infrequently desirable for retarded persons. Yet sterilization will rarely be ordered in many states because most parents will be unable to meet the rigid criteria set out in the sterilization laws. These laws erect obstacles to sterilization in order to protect a possible interest in procreation, yet they do not grapple directly with the basic question: How can it be determined whether a given individual has this interest? In the absence of such an inquiry, it is unclear whether the purported safeguards serve an actual protective function or whether they simply burden the petitioning parent and ultimately the affected individual....

NOTES

1 This article uses the feminine pronoun to refer to the mentally retarded person for whom sterilization is proposed because it appears that the issue arises much more frequently with females than with males....
2 93 Wash. 2d 228, 608 P.2d 635 (1980).
3 The *Hayes* court explained that: "The judge must first find by clear, cogent and convincing evidence that the individual is (1) incapable of making his or her own decision about sterilization, and (2) unlikely to develop sufficiently to make an informed judgment about sterilization in the foreseeable future." Id. at 238, 608 P.2d at 641.
4 *See Hayes*, 93 Wash. 2d at 238–39, 608 P.2d at 641.
5 85 N.J. 235, 426 A.2d 467 (1981).

Subtracting Injury from Insult: Ethical Issues in the Use of Pharmaceutical Implants
Eric T. Juengst and Ronald A. Siegel

Eric T. Juengst is assistant professor of humanities (philosophy) at the Pennsylvania State University College of Medicine. His areas of specialization are medical ethics and philosophy of medicine. He is the author of "Prenatal Diagnosis and the Ethics of Uncertainty" and the co-editor of *The Meaning of AIDS* (1989). Ronald A. Siegel is assistant professor of pharmacy and pharmaceutical chemistry at the University of California at San Francisco. His research interests lie in the physical chemistry of polymers, the applications of these polymers in drug delivery, and the general design of drug delivery systems.

Juengst and Siegel discuss some ethical issues raised by implantable drug-delivery systems when those receiving the implants are the mentally ill and the mentally retarded. The first drug implant they consider works as a relatively long-term contraceptive and might be seen as an alternative to sterilization for mentally retarded adolescents. The second drug implant they

Reprinted with permission of the authors and the publisher from *Hastings Center Report*, vol. 18 (December 1988), pp. 41–46.

consider delivers a behavior control drug and might be seen as an alternative to psychosurgery for severely mentally ill patients whose behavior is consistently violent and yet who refuse to comply with a regimen of antipsychotic drugs. Juengst and Siegel strike a cautionary note. They maintain that the noninvasiveness and reversibility of pharmaceutical implants, although genuine virtues, are insufficient to eliminate all the ethical problems raised by involuntary sterilization and involuntary psychosurgery.

Ten years ago, psychosurgery...and surgical sterilization received considerable attention in bioethics. These interventions provided riveting examples of the kinds of questions that the young field took as its domain: questions about the ethical boundaries of biomedicine's power to modify bodies and minds. The focus of the field has since shifted. Soon, however, the concerns of the last decade may be raised again, from a quite different corner of biomedicine. Advances in biomedical engineering and pharmaceutical chemistry are converging to produce devices that can be implanted in the body to deliver controlled doses of drugs automatically for months at a time.[1] These implants could be used to produce the *effects* of psychosurgery [and] surgical sterilizations ...without their irrevocable invasions of bodily integrity. For contemporary pharmaceutical engineers, and for clinicians of the 1990s, the question is how well the earlier exploration of biomedicine's moral boundaries provides guidance in this new pharmacologic terrain.

In one respect, the discussion of the ethical issues raised by the surgeries does provide important precedents for the ethics of drug implantation: its analyses do map the relevant moral ground. However, the language of those analyses, while nicely crafted for their contexts, could seriously mislead efforts to evaluate the use of drug implants. Its dominant metaphors—trespass, unjust punishment, and irretractable offense—can be misread to imply that the clinical virtues of implantation—noninvasiveness, efficiency, and reversibility—allow this practice to escape the moral pitfalls encountered by the surgeries. To follow the lead of the earlier discussion successfully requires a critical rereading of its metaphors that can distinguish between their clinical and moral meanings.

IMPLANTABLE DRUG DELIVERY SYSTEMS

In the next two decades we may expect a revolution in drug therapy. In addition to the new hormones, en-

zymes, and vaccines that the biotechnology industry is producing, new techniques for drug delivery are being introduced. One idea that has received considerable attention from academic and industrial researchers is the development of implantable devices designed to release a drug into the body in a controlled manner. A well known example is the mechanical insulin pump carried by some diabetics.[2] Subcutaneous reservoirs, which deliver drugs passively into the blood stream, have been under development since the late 1960s.[3] "NORPLANT" (R), the implantable contraceptive device developed by The Population Council, is a more recent example. This small plastic rod infused with a contraceptive steroid is inserted subcutaneously under local anesthetic. The device is physically unobtrusive and can automatically release preset contraceptive doses for five years after implantation.[4] Current research is also aimed at developing self-regulated implants capable of interacting with their environment to meet the body's fluctuating pharmacologic needs.[5]

The reversibility and longevity of an implant depends on its design. In principle, implants can be designed to release drugs over virtually any duration, although most current devices have life spans measured in months rather than years. Some systems, like NORPLANT, are designed to remain intact throughout the release process and must be removed surgically when exhausted. Others are designed to degrade into nontoxic by-products as the drug is released. Because they often lose their mechanical integrity during erosion, degradable devices may not be removable once implanted. Thus, while they may be more convenient than nondegradable devices, they may preclude other treatment choices for considerable periods of time.

In part, implantation is attractive because the traditional routes for drug delivery—ingestion or injection—are not well suited to the administration of new, genetically engineered biologicals. Such drugs are usually proteins and would be digested if taken orally. They also usually require regular administration, burdening patients with the inconvenience and discomfort of living with a prolonged course of injections. Implantable devices, by providing for the measured, subcutaneous release of a drug, are designed to obviate these problems.

Implantation holds advantages for other classes of drugs as well. Because they can be implanted near their target organs, less drug is required to achieve the same effect as oral or intravenous administration. "Organ targeting" has also been shown to avoid many of the side effects of oral administration by reducing the drug's dispersal and absorption in other parts of the body.[6]

Finally, developing improved pharmaceutical implants is attractive for more prosaic reasons. The process of developing, screening, clinically testing, and obtaining regulatory approval for a new drug often requires decades. Yet patent protection is relatively short (seventeen years), and must often overlap with several stages of the process. Drug companies are finding it less lucrative to develop new drugs than to seek new delivery methods for existing ones.

All these considerations may drastically change our view of what it means to be "taking drugs" for a medical problem. The combination of implantation's efficiency (in terms of enhanced drug efficacy, reduced side effects, greater convenience, and better compliance), with its relative noninvasiveness and reversibility give the technology distinct clinical advantages. There is a danger, though, that these virtues could distract us from other problems that could arise in prescribing this technology.

THE DOUBLE-EDGED VIRTUES OF IMPLANTATION TECHNOLOGY

As a novel therapeutic tool, any new implantable drug delivery device will present the same ethical questions that attend other clinical innovations: Its introduction will be marked by uncertainty about safety and efficacy, and its use will entail predictable risks as well as benefits. Drug implantation, in other words, is a double-edged technology in the usual sense of having both virtues and vices as a clinical tool. But these are not the issues that we address here. Drug implantation may also face ethical questions precisely when its virtues recommend its use. To the extent that they cause us to neglect those questions, implantation's virtues themselves may be double-edged. Ironically, their distracting potential is probably greatest where these questions are most pressing, because of the way our moral metaphors exacerbate it. Under their influence, implantation's clinical virtues appear to condone its use in cases where any intervention would be morally problematic.

NONINVASIVENESS

One of the primary reasons contraceptive implants are attractive is that they provide the long-term prophylaxis of surgical sterilization without requiring a major medical intervention. But consider the following scenario:

> The parents of an eighteen-year-old girl with Down syndrome come to their physician for help. Their daughter is sexually mature, and has an IQ of sixty-five. She is able to get about on her own and attends a special school each day. Her parents had hoped to place her in an adult group home when she completed school, but fear that she may well become pregnant and that this will be a very upsetting experience for her. They have tried oral contraceptives, which the girl refuses to take without a daily struggle, and they do not wish to subject her to the risks of an IUD. They feel that sterilization through tubal ligation is the only answer. However, they are relieved to learn about the existence of a biologically implantable device like NORPLANT that will have the same effect, and request it from their physician.[7]

Ethical debate on surgical sterilization for retarded adolescents usually contrasts the psychological burden of pregnancy and the potential psychosocial benefits of sexual activity with the surgery's harm to the patient's reproductive capacity, the lack of her consent to the procedure, and the foreclosure of her future reproductive options.[8] The issue turns on which course seems better to promote the patient's autonomy: to exercise, on her behalf, her right to sterilization, or to defend, since she cannot, the privacy of her reproductive choices.[9]

All of these considerations would also be present in a decision to fit the patient with a long-term contraceptive implant. The patient would be rendered infertile without her consent, and in a way that she would be powerless to change for an extended period. The problem of determining her competency to make reproductive choices and raise children remains, as well as the prospect of infringing unjustifiably on a very important sphere of personal decisionmaking.

However, the implant will not sterilize the patient permanently, as tubal ligation would. Moreover, implantation entails neither the dramatic invasion of bodily integrity of surgery nor the recurrent struggle of administering oral contraceptives. It is a minor procedure, performed in the doctor's office and then forgotten. Do these clinical advantages help ameliorate the physician's ethical problem?

Those concerned about surgical sterilization of the retarded often cite the bodily injury of the procedure in the same breath with its insult to the patient's autonomy. For example, one cautious critic of sterilization argues that:

> A just cause is required because sterilization in the absence of consent constitutes a significant invasion of the body and a rather massive intrusion into the sphere of reproductive privacy.[10]

Here, the "trespass" metaphors of "invasion" and "intrusion" provide useful but complementary descriptions of both the physical harms and moral wrongs involved in involuntary sterilization.

Nevertheless, "trespass" metaphors do tend to focus on the consequences of surgery for (structural) bodily integrity rather than for (functional) reproductive capacity. The prospect of minimally invasive implantable contraceptive devices forces us to ask which of these harms is really of central concern. If the decisive ethical issue is how best to promote the subject's reproductive autonomy, how relevant is the fact that involuntary implantation can compromise reproductive function without a "significant invasion of the body"?

The "bodily invasion" of surgery provides a graphic symbol of trespass, but it is the intervention's *functional* effects that intrude furthest into the subject's reproductive privacy. Of course, invasive surgery is riskier than subcutaneous implantation: the noninvasiveness of the implant gives it a genuine clinical advantage, which counts ethically in its favor. However, to the extent that the noninvasiveness of the implantable contraceptive is viewed as the *decisive* ethical consideration in cases like this, the language of the surgical sterilization debate will have misled our moral reflection. In this debate, appeals to bodily integrity play a primarily rhetorical role; they are designed to invoke the metaphors of trespass that underscore the importance of the reproductive function at stake...

REVERSIBILITY

It is easy to see how invasiveness...play[s] [an] important symbolic [role] in ethical debates over involuntary sterilization....But is the clinical irreversibility of [the] intervention merely a rhetorically useful side issue as well? The reversibility of implantation seems to speak most directly to the ethical issues in [this case] because it

provides a way to proceed in the face of moral uncertainty. For example, consider the case for using implants as an alternative to psychosurgery....

> A long-term inpatient at a mental institution with a history of paranoia and violent behavior consistently refuses to comply with a regimen of anti-psychotic drugs. Electroencephalographic examination of the patient shows brain activity compatible with temporal lobe epilepsy. Because of this finding, the institution's medical staff discusses psychosurgery as an alternative to the patient's forced medication. However, since the patient's medications, once administered, do seem effective in controlling his behavior, they are hesitant to proceed. As a third option, a consulting pharmacologist suggests that an implantable drug delivery system be used to supply the patient's regimen of anti-psychotic medication automatically for months at a time.

The ethics of psychosurgical intervention oscillates around two related issues: distinguishing the cure of behavioral pathology from unjustified behavior control, and determining a psychiatric patient's authority to refuse (or consent to) this kind of treatment.[11] Neither of these issues is peculiar to psychosurgery and a decision to use a pharmaceutical implant raises exactly the same questions about how best to promote and protect this patient's interests. However, commentators usually argue that psychosurgery is a paradigm for ethical conflicts in behavior control techniques because of its invasiveness, destructiveness, and irreversibility:

> Psychosurgery is perhaps the most dramatic of all medically based individual therapies for mental and behavioral deviance. It goes directly to the physical seat of experience, and makes irreversible destructive lesions. Because of its dramatic quality, psychosurgery focuses with great intensity the fundamental problem of all behavior control: by what values should behavior be controlled?[12]

What is special about psychosurgery, then, is the way it metaphorically underscores its own moral dangers: Not only does it offend the patient's integrity, but its insult is one that can never be retracted. Psychosurgery's irreversibility, like its invasiveness, neatly dramatizes the seriousness of the moral hazards it shares with...surgical sterilization: the misuse of medical expertise and the violation of the patient's personal autonomy. The question raised by the prospect of a pharmaceutical implant is whether the permanence of psychosurgery has any other moral significance, against which the implant's reversibility measures favorably.

Clearly, there are clinical situations in which the implant's reversibility would make it the intervention of choice. For example, lucid patients might be given the opportunity to commit themselves to a "Ulysses contract," with the option of renegotiating at the end of each cycle.[13] However, in our case, the staff must still face the central issues of whether the goal of the intervention is therapeutic or coercive, and how to respond when the patient refuses it. If the staff's intent is coercive or the patient's refusal valid, the fact that the implant's behavioral effects are reversible will not undo the wrong that forced implantation would represent. Could we justify denying individuals the right to vote by pointing out that they will get another chance in the next election?

Of course, the implant could be proposed simply to test the validity of the patient's refusal. If it were used to enhance our confidence in the patient's capacity for self-determination and to allow him to make an authoritative decision about further treatment, the moral importance of its reversibility would increase. In fact, if the goal of such a test is to return control to the patient, the preference should be for the most readily reversible intervention that would work: for example, a course of traditionally administered medication. Here, the convenience of the implant may recommend its use..., but its relative longevity and irreversibility actually militate against it.

More important, just why does the moral significance of reversibility increase when implantation is used to resolve our uncertainty about the patient's capacity? In this situation, the implant's reversibility opens the possibility of making amends for the moral insult of its imposition on the patient. But the significance of this is only that it allows us to apologize for imposing the test, not that it renders apologies unnecessary. The implant's reversibility does not allow us to avoid inflicting the insult in the first place, any more than it speaks to the question of whether behavior control is the appropriate prescription for this patient's problems. Once again, it would be a mistake to let the prominence of the "irreversibility" rhetoric in the psychosurgery debate suggest that the reversibility of pharmaceutical implants allows us to avoid all the serious ethical concerns of psychosurgery.

MORAL AND CLINICAL MEANINGS

The noninvasiveness, increased efficiency, and reversibility of pharmaceutical implants will make implantation

technology the preferred approach to drug delivery in an increasing number of situations, and rightly so: they are genuine virtues. Implantable devices can accomplish the goals of surgical sterilization...and psychosurgery without the invasiveness...or irreversibility that serve as graphic reminders of the moral issues these latter interventions raise. But having subtracted the injuries of those interventions from their insults, drug implantation can still leave clinicians facing the most serious moral problems of the surgeries: the conflicts between visions of personal autonomy and difficulties in distinguishing the appropriate therapeutic uses of medical knowledge from its abuses on behalf of social prejudices and priorities.

To remain sensitive to these problems, it is important to be able to distinguish the moral and the clinical meanings of the metaphors that give implantation's virtues their appearance of moral force. It is natural that biomedicine should focus on the clinical interpretations of "trespass," "unjust punishment," and "irrevocable insult," and seek therapeutic strategies, like drug implantation, that can address them. But this search risks distracting us from the moral dangers the metaphors warn against. To the extent that drug implantation will be contemplated in cases like those examined above, these hazards still exist in the moral terrain this technology must cross. The charts of this terrain provided by its pioneers will be invaluable in that crossing, but only if we translate their signs and symbols correctly.

REFERENCES

1 See A.C. Tanquary and R.E. Lacey, eds., *Controlled Release of Biologically Active Agents* (New York: Plenum Press, 1974); Perry J. Blackshear, "Implantable Drug Delivery Systems," *Scientific American* 241:6 (December 1979), 66–73; Joseph Kost and Robert Langer, "Controlled Release of Bioactive Agents," *Trends in Biotechnology* 2 (1984), 47–51.

2 Michael Sefton, "Implantable Pumps," CRC *Critical Reviews in Biomedical Engineering* 14 (1987), 201–40.

3 Robert A. Ratcheson and Ayub K. Ommaya, "Experience with the Subcutaneous Cerebrospinal-Fluid Reservoir: Preliminary Report of 60 Cases," *New England Journal of Medicine* 279:19 (November 7, 1968), 1025–31.

4 Irving Civin, "Clinical Effects of NORPLANT Subdermal Implants for Contraception," *Advances in Human Fertility and Reproductive Endocrinology* 2 (1982), 89–116.

5 Seo Y. Jeong *et al.*, "Self-Regulating Insulin Delivery Systems," *Journal of Controlled Release* 2 (1985), 143–52.

6 B.B. Pharris *et al.*, "Progestasert: A Uterine Therapeutic System for Long Term Contraception," *Fertility and Sterility* 25:11 (November 1974), 915–21.

7 We are indebted to Adele Hoffman and James Morrissey for this case, which we have adapted for our purposes.

8 Ruth Macklin and Willard Gaylin, eds., *Mental Retardation and Sterilization: A Problem of Competency and Paternalism* (New York: Plenum Press, 1981).

9 Daniel Wikler, "Paternalism and the Mildly Retarded," *Philosophy and Public Affairs* 8 (1979), 915–21.

10 LeRoy Walters, "Sterilizing the Retarded Child," *Hastings Center Report* 6:2 (April 1976), 13–15.

11 Ruth Macklin, *Man, Mind and Morality: The Ethics of Behavior Control* (Englewood Cliffs, NJ: Prentice-Hall, 1982), 15–18.

12 Robert Neville, "Psychosurgery," in *The Encyclopedia of Bioethics*, ed. Warren Reich (New York: Macmillan, 1978), 1387.

13 See also Rebecca Dresser, "Bound to Treatment: The Ulysses Contract," *Hastings Center Report* 14:3 (June 1984), 13–17.

Declaration of General and Special Rights of the Mentally Retarded
International League of Societies for the Mentally Handicapped

The International League of Societies for the Mentally Handicapped, now known as the International League of Societies for Persons with Mental Handicap, was founded in 1960. Its founders included representatives of parent organizations and professional groups as well as individuals concerned with the interests of the mentally handicapped. Since proclaiming the rights below, the League has published *Step by Step: Implementation of the Rights of Mentally Retarded Persons*.

This declaration of rights was officially proclaimed in 1968 at a meeting of the League. In 1971 it was adopted almost word for word by the United Nations General Assembly. Among the positive rights it asserts are the rights to economic security, a decent standard of living, and the education, training, habilitation, and guidance requisite to develop abilities and potentials to the fullest possible extent.

Whereas the universal declaration of human rights, adopted by the United Nations, proclaims that all of the human family, without distinction of any kind, have equal and inalienable rights of human dignity and freedom;

Whereas the declaration of the rights of the child, adopted by the United Nations, proclaims the rights of the physically, mentally or socially handicapped child to special treatment, education and care required by his particular condition.

Now therefore, The International League of Societies for the Mentally Handicapped expresses the

general and special rights of the mentally retarded as follows:

ARTICLE I.

The mentally retarded person has the same basic rights as other citizens of the same country and same age.

ARTICLE II.

The mentally retarded person has a right to proper medical care and physical restoration and to such education, training, habilitation and guidance as will enable him to develop his ability and potential to the fullest possible extent, no matter how severe his degree of disability. No mentally handicapped person should be deprived of such services by reason of the costs involved.

ARTICLE III.

The mentally retarded person has a right to economic security and to a decent standard of living. He has a right to productive work or to other meaningful occupation.

ARTICLE IV.

The mentally retarded person has a right to live with his own family or with fosterparents; to participate in all aspects of community life, and to be provided with appropriate leisure time activities. If care in an institution becomes necessary it should be in surroundings and under circumstances as close to normal living as possible.

ARTICLE V.

The mentally retarded person has a right to a qualified guardian when this is required to protect his personal wellbeing and interest. No person rendering direct services to the mentally retarded should also serve as his guardian.

ARTICLE VI.

The mentally retarded person has a right to protection from exploitation, abuse and degrading treatment. If accused, he has a right to a fair trial with full recognition being given to his degree of responsibility.

ARTICLE VII.

Some mentally retarded persons may be unable, due to the severity of their handicap, to exercise for themselves all their rights in a meaningful way. For others, modification of some or all of these rights is appropriate. The procedure used for modification or denial of rights must contain proper legal safeguards against every form of abuse, must be based on an evaluation of the social capability of the mentally retarded person by qualified experts and must be subject to periodic reviews and to the right of appeal to higher authorities.

Above all—The mentally retarded person has the right to respect.

ANNOTATED BIBLIOGRAPHY: CHAPTER 5

Callahan, Joan C.: "Liberty, Beneficence, and Involuntary Confinement," *Journal of Medicine and Philosophy* 9 (August 1984), pp. 261–293. Callahan specifies a set of conditions that must be satisfied to justify paternalistic treatment of a mentally ill adult. She also provides a critique of contemporary commitment criteria.

"Changing Social and Psychological Concepts of Mental Illness," *Journal of Contemporary Issues* 1 (August 1973), pp. 31–56. This excellent review article examines a number of efforts to reevaluate both the nature of mental illness and the practice of psychiatry. A long and useful bibliography is also provided.

Edwards, Rem B., ed.: *Psychiatry and Ethics: Insanity, Autonomy, and Mental Health Care* (Buffalo, N.Y.: Prometheus Books, 1982). This well-organized collection of articles includes chapters on the concept of mental illness, the therapist-patient relationship and rights, the informed consent requirement, coercion in commitment and therapy, controversial behavioral control therapies, the insanity defense, and deinstitutionalization. The authors include psychologists, psychiatrists, sociologists, lawyers, surgeons, medical directors, and political scientists.

Forst, Martin L.: *Civil Commitment and Social Control* (Lexington, Mass.: Lexington Books, 1978). Forst offers an empirical investigation of the operation and functioning of one civil commitment statute (California's "Mentally Disordered Sex Offender [MDSO] Statute") and its relation to the criminal justice system. He does a comparative study of the relationship between the civil and criminal commitment systems.

Goffman, Erving: *Asylums* (New York: Doubleday Anchor, 1961). Goffman provides an analysis of life in total institutions in general and in mental institutions in particular.

Hasker, William: "The Critique of 'Mental Illness': Conceptual and/or Ethical Crisis?" *Journal of Psychology and Theology* 5 (Spring 1977), pp. 110–124. After analyzing Szasz's attack on the concept of mental illness, Hasker argues that Szasz's critique has not as yet received a satisfactory response. Hasker contends that the most promising strategy of response is to try to define "a limited concept of mental illness."

Herr, Stanley S.: *Rights and Advocacy for Retarded People* (Lexington, Mass.: Lexington Books, 1983). This is a comprehensive, coherent review of the legal and judicial processes that have shaped the field of mental retardation. Herr provides an historical background, brings out the assumptions that underlie our treatment of the mentally retarded, and suggests a future agenda for those who serve as advocates for the mentally retarded.

Livermore, Joseph M., Carl P. Malmquist, and Paul E. Meehl: "On the Justifications for Civil Commitment," *University of Pennsylvania Law Review* 117 (November 1968), pp. 75–96. The authors critique various philosophical justifications for the involuntary civil commitment of the mentally ill. They also present a range of cases to bring out the kinds of situations where involuntary civil commitment might be justified.

Macklin, Ruth: "Mental Health and Mental Illness: Some Problems of Definition and Concept Formation," *Philosophy of Science* 39 (September 1972), pp. 341–365. Macklin examines a number of difficulties associated with attempts to define mental health and mental illness. In part 5 of this article, she directly addresses the views of Szasz, concluding that there is no compelling reason to adopt his view that mental illness is a myth.

Macklin, Ruth, and Willard Gaylin, eds.: *Mental Retardation and Sterilization: A Problem of Competency and Paternalism* (New York: Plenum Press, 1981). In 1976–1977, the Hastings Center conducted a project titled "Ethical Issues in the Care and Treatment of the Mildly Mentally Retarded." This book is the result of the interdisciplinary meetings held as part of that project. Participants included philosophers, psychiatrists, psychologists, social scientists, and lawyers. The book has two parts and an appendix. Part I is a report of the outcome of the deliberations. Part II contains several articles written by seminar participants. The appendix contains excerpts from five court cases involving the sterilization of mentally retarded persons.

Moore, Michael S.: "Some Myths about 'Mental Illness,' " *Inquiry* 18 (Autumn 1975), pp. 233–265. Moore rejects the notion that mental illness is a myth. Committed to the view that mental illness is a "cruel and bitter reality," he identifies and rejects various versions of the myth argument.

Rosenhan, D.L.: "On Being Sane in Insane Places," *Science* 179 (January 19, 1973), pp. 250–258. This much discussed article describes the results of an experiment in which sane people gained admittance to mental hospitals. Once inside the hospital, they were perceived as insane, leading Rosenhan to conclude that in psychiatric hospitals we cannot distinguish sane from insane.

Schafer, Arthur: "Civil Liberties and the Elderly Patient." In James E. Thornton and Earl R. Winkler, eds., *Ethics and Aging: The Right to Live, the Right to Die* (Vancouver: The University of British Columbia Press, 1988), pp. 208–214. Schafer examines and criticizes some of the justifications used for limiting the freedom of elderly patients. His analysis shows the similarities between these justifications and those used for depriving the mentally ill of civil liberties.

Scott, Elizabeth S.: "Sterilization of Mentally Retarded Persons: Reproductive Rights and Family Privacy," *Duke Law Journal* 806 (1986), pp. 806–865. In this long article, from which an excerpt is reprinted in this chapter, Scott develops an alternative to the paternalistic approach in regard to the sterilization of retarded persons. Her approach is based on the primacy of individual and family autonomy.

Szasz, Thomas S.: "Involuntary Mental Hospitalization: A Crime against Humanity." In Thomas S. Szasz, *Ideology and Insanity* (New York: Doubleday, 1970), pp. 113–139. Szasz argues that the practice of involuntary mental hospitalization should be abolished. In his view, there is a strong analogy between the practice of involuntary mental hospitalization and the institution of slavery.

Torrey, E. Fuller: *Nowhere to Go: The Tragic Odyssey of the Homeless Mentally Ill* (New York: Harper and Row, 1988). Concerned with the effects of deinstitutionalization, Torrey discusses nineteenth- and twentieth-century U.S. social policies in regard to the mentally ill and the changes in our society's thinking regarding mental illness and mental health in this century. He condemns both the warehousing of patients in mental institutions when institutionalization was in vogue and the dumping of patients without adequate supporting mechanisms since the rush to deinstitutionalization. Torrey closes by describing the sorts of changes that should be made to improve the services available to the mentally ill.

CHAPTER 6

SUICIDE AND THE REFUSAL OF LIFE-SUSTAINING TREATMENT

INTRODUCTION

This chapter addresses the most prominent ethical questions about suicide and a closely related topic, the refusal of life-sustaining treatment. The occurrence of a suicide is, in typical cases, a rather grim reminder of the possibility of human despair. The suicide of a friend or relative usually occasions shock and almost always occasions sadness. However, many people say not only that suicide is tragic but also that it is immoral. Accordingly, one focal point of discussion in this chapter is the morality of suicide. Also under discussion is the justifiability of state intervention for the purpose of coercively preventing a person from committing suicide. In considering the refusal of life-sustaining treatment—the second pocket of ethical concern in this chapter—emphasis is placed on adult patients. The refusal of treatment by competent adults receives significant attention, but treatment decisions for adults who have lost decision-making capacity also receive extensive consideration.

What Is Suicide?

It is unwise to attempt to discuss the moral dimensions of suicide without paying some attention to the concept of suicide itself. Consider two people, one saying that suicide is always immoral and the other saying that suicide is sometimes morally acceptable. It is possible that these two people are in substantive moral agreement and differ only with regard to an operating definition of suicide. One of them may hold that suicide is immoral but say that a certain action is not suicide and is therefore morally acceptable, whereas the other may call the same action suicide but consider it a morally acceptable form of suicide. The following cases and the

310

accompanying analysis are presented in order to shed some measure of light on the concept of suicide.

(1) A woman, having despaired of achieving a satisfying life, leaps to her death from the top of a city skyscraper. (2) An elderly man dies from a massive overdose of sleeping pills, leaving behind a note explaining that he is not bitter but that life seems to have passed him by. He has outlived his friends, he has no employment, he finds no enjoyment in his pastimes, etc. (1) and (2) provide us with clear cases of suicide. In accordance with what might be called the standard definition of suicide, each of these cases is a suicide precisely because it features the *intentional termination of one's own life*. Consider a third case. (3) In time of war, a soldier is captured and subjected to torture. Feeling unable to resist any longer, but determined not to yield any information that would endanger the lives of his comrades, he hangs himself. This third case is noteworthy, in contrast to (1) and (2), in that it features an other-directed rather than a self-directed motivation. Still, it seems to be a clear case of the intentional termination of one's own life. It is sometimes said that the self-killing in such cases is sacrificial rather than suicidal, but to deny that (3) is a case of suicide is surely to abandon the standard definition of suicide.

(4) A truckdriver, foreseeing his own death, nevertheless steers his runaway truck into a concrete abutment in order to avoid hitting a schoolbus that has stopped on the roadway to discharge children. (5) In a somewhat similar and much discussed actual case, a certain Captain Oates fell ill and found himself physically unable to continue on with a party of explorers in the Antarctic. The explorers were struggling to find their way out of a blizzard. Captain Oates, determined not to further endanger his colleagues by hindering their progress, but unable to convince them to leave him to die, simply walked off to meet his death in the blizzard. One may feel some puzzlement as to whether (4) and (5) are to be identified as cases of suicide. As in (3), the notion of sacrificial death may come to mind. Presumably neither the truckdriver nor Captain Oates wanted to die; each sacrificed his own life so that the lives of others might be protected. In contrast to (3), however, it is plausible to say, in accordance with the standard definition, that (4) and (5) are not cases of suicide. On this view, it would be said that neither the truckdriver nor Captain Oates *intentionally terminated* his life. While each initiated a chain of events that was foreseen as leading to his own death, neither initiated the chain of events because he desired to die, but quite the contrary, because he desired to attain some other objective, that is, the protection of others. Thus the primary intention of the basic action (redirecting the truck, walking away from camp) was to protect others; one's own death, it is said, is foreseen but not intended. Still, many would insist, contrary to the line of thought just developed, that both the truckdriver and Captain Oates did *intentionally terminate* their lives, since it was in their power to avoid their deaths but they chose (seemingly in noble fashion) not to do so.

One final case must be introduced. (6) A Jehovah's Witness, as a matter of religious principle, refuses to consent to a blood transfusion and dies. Is (6) a case of suicide? This judgment turns, as does our judgment regarding (4) and (5), on the interpretation of the phrase "intentional termination." The Jehovah's Witness, in many ways similar to the traditional Christian martyr, refuses to sacrifice religious principle and thereby brings about his or her own death. Those who say that (6) is not a case of suicide point out that the Jehovah's Witness typically does not want to die. The Jehovah's Witness foresees but does not intend his or her own death. Those who say that (6) is a case of suicide point out that, in effect, the avoidance of death is within the power of the Jehovah's Witness. Thus choosing to refuse the blood transfusion constitutes an intentional termination of life.

Notice, under certain circumstances, that refusal of life-sustaining treatment is undeniably suicide. Suppose a person in good health is accidentally injured and needs a routine blood transfusion in order to recover. Suppose further that this person refuses life-sustaining treatment simply because he or she wants to die. In such a case, refusing life-sustaining treatment is simply a convenient way of committing suicide. The phrase "intentional termination," however it is to be finally analyzed, clearly incorporates passive as well as active means. A person can commit suicide just as effectively by (passively) refusing to eat as by (actively) taking an overdose of drugs.

The Morality of Suicide

The preceding discussion of the concept of suicide has been presented as a necessary prelude to a consideration of ethical questions about suicide. As previously indicated, the first focal point of discussion in this chapter is the question: Under what circumstances, if at all, is suicide morally acceptable? Classical literature on the morality of suicide provides a number of sources who issue a strong moral condemnation of suicide. St. Augustine, St. Thomas Aquinas, and Immanuel Kant are prominent examples. Augustine's arguments are dominantly theological in character, but Aquinas and Kant advance philosophical as well as religiously based arguments against suicide. According to Aquinas, suicide is to be condemned not only because it violates our duty to God but also because it violates the natural law, and, moreover, because it injures the community. Kant, in the first selection of this chapter, argues that suicide degrades human worth and is therefore always immoral. R. B. Brandt, in this chapter's second selection, critically analyzes the most influential of the classical arguments against suicide. Brandt also forcefully defends the view that suicide is not necessarily immoral. This more liberal viewpoint, it is important to note, is not unprecedented in the classical literature on suicide. The Roman Stoic Seneca and the eighteenth-century Scottish philosopher David Hume are quite notable in their explication and defense of such a view.

The more liberal view on the morality of suicide might be explicated in general terms as follows. Suicide, to the extent that it does no substantial damage to the interests of other individuals, is morally acceptable. Moreover, even in cases where suicide has some impact on others, no person is morally obliged to undergo extreme distress to save others some smaller measure of sadness, and so forth. In accordance with this line of thought, it can be argued that suicide is morally acceptable even in some cases where a person has some rather significant social obligations, such as the duty to care for minor children. Suppose that a person has fallen unaccountably into a profound and inescapable depression. Suppose further that psychiatric counseling provides no relief. If the person becomes so undermined as to be incapable of caring for the minor children anyway, the argument goes, then suicide is morally acceptable.

Suicide Intervention

A second focal point of discussion in this chapter is the question: Is it justifiable for some agent of the state, acting in the name of society, to intervene and coercively prevent a person from committing suicide? Consider first the case of a competent adult with a reasoned and settled intention to commit suicide. In such a case, state intervention for the purpose of coercively preventing suicide would seem to present a significant ethical difficulty. The libertarian,[1] committed to the rejection of paternalistic interferences with individual liberty, argues that a competent adult's self-determination must be respected, even if his or her decision to commit suicide is considered unwise by others. In contrast, those who are more sympathetic to the legitimacy of paternalism are likely to argue that it is justifiable for society to interfere paternalistically with an individual's liberty (even a competent adult's) in order to protect that person from *serious and irrevocable* kinds of harm. One other line of argument deserves mention in the context of paternalism. In order to undermine the force of the libertarian contention that a competent adult's decision to commit suicide must be respected, it is sometimes asserted that a suicidal intention is necessarily irrational, thus a symptom of mental illness and incompetence. In other words, it is impossible for a competent adult to have a suicidal intention. Although this point seems to be built into some psychiatric theories, it is considered by many philosophers to be an implausible contention. Brandt, in his discussion of the rationality of suicide, argues that suicide is surely a rational choice under certain kinds of circumstances.

Two other arguments may be presented in defense of societal intervention to prevent competent adults from committing suicide. First, it might be said that intervention is necessary in order to protect society's general interest in the sanctity of human life. The libertarian usually responds that such a vague interest cannot override individual self-determination. Second, it might be said that suicide is rightly prevented because it is immoral. Clearly, this second argument is asserted only by those who believe the law may rightly function to enforce morality. Needless to say, libertarians argue forcefully against this general principle.

In discussing the justifiability of state intervention for the purpose of coercively preventing a person from committing suicide, we should keep in mind that suicide attempts are very frequently not the result of a reasoned and settled intention. A humane social policy would certainly allow state intervention in cases where *temporary* disordering factors such as drugs, alcohol, or extreme (but fleeting) depression are operative. Indeed, libertarian principles are no more incompatible with intervention in the case of a temporarily disordered person than they are with intervention in the case of children or incompetent adults. In the case of a temporarily disordered person threatening suicide, intervention constitutes no substantive deprivation of liberty. The person involved, by hypothesis, is not acting in character; he or she does not really want to commit suicide. In typical cases, after the temporary crisis period, the individual is grateful for the (paternalistic) intervention. In one of this chapter's readings, David F. Greenberg argues in support of a suicide prevention policy that would allow temporary but not permanent intervention.

The Refusal of Life-Sustaining Treatment

In considering the refusal of life-sustaining treatment,[2] there seem to be noteworthy differences among the following: (1) cases in which a patient, by accepting life-sustaining treatment, would return to a state of health; (2) cases in which a patient, by accepting life-sustaining treatment, would simply continue a severely compromised existence; and (3) cases in which a terminally ill patient, by accepting life-sustaining treatment, would merely *prolong the dying process*. Surely "suicide" is a label that seems inappropriate for the refusal of treatment in (3), even if it is not inappropriate for the refusal of treatment in (1) and (2).

Refusal of treatment in cases of the first type is relatively uncommon but typically dramatic. The most discussed example involves a Jehovah's Witness who refuses to accept a blood transfusion for religious reasons. In one of this chapter's readings, Ruth Macklin argues—principally on the basis of individual autonomy—that the right of a competent adult Jehovah's Witness to refuse a life-sustaining blood transfusion should be respected.

In conjunction with continuing developments in the courts, refusal of treatment in cases of the second type is probably becoming increasingly common. By and large, the law now recognizes the right of a competent adult—and not just one who is terminally ill or in the process of dying—to refuse any life-sustaining treatment. Consider in this regard the example of a patient whose life is severely compromised by the presence of painful and debilitating arthritis. This patient is being treated for pneumonia and is temporarily respirator-dependent until the antibiotics have a chance to take effect. The pneumonia is entirely curable and the patient, however much compromised from a quality-of-life standpoint, is not in the process of dying. If the patient now decides to forgo the respirator, we cannot simply say that the patient has chosen not to prolong the dying process. Accordingly, although considerations of individual autonomy provide a strong moral warrant for the right to refuse life-sustaining treatment in general, a few commentators would take issue with the right to refuse treatment in this kind of case because they are concerned about the implications of accepting quality-of-life considerations.

Refusal of treatment in the third type of case has a strong foundation in both morality and law and is certainly very common. In many cases of terminal illness, "aggressive" treatment is capable of warding off death—for a time. However, it is often questionable whether such treatment is in a patient's best interest, and a competent adult is generally considered to have both a moral and legal right to refuse treatment that would merely prolong the dying process.

Some of the difficulties associated with life-sustaining treatment decisions can be illustrated through a consideration of cardiopulmonary resuscitation. When a terminally ill patient undergoes cardiac arrest, resuscitation techniques can sometimes restore heartbeat and thus prolong life. Yet, in many cases, the patient does not desire and cannot benefit from resuscitation. Of course, in other cases, the patient does desire and can benefit from resuscitation. In still other cases, the appropriateness of resuscitation is more in doubt. Perhaps the patient has been ambivalent in expressing a preference about resuscitation. Perhaps the physician is uncertain whether or not resuscitation would be of genuine benefit to the patient. Perhaps the physician believes that resuscitation is in the patient's best interest, but the patient has expressed a preference not to be resuscitated. Or perhaps the physician believes that resuscitation is not in the patient's best interest, but the patient has expressed a preference to be resuscitated. In one of this chapter's readings, the President's Commission for the Study of Ethical Problems in Medicine and Biomedical and Behavioral Research provides an extensive analysis of the ethical considerations relevant to resuscitation decisions—decisions that are ordinarily made within the framework of the physician-patient relationship. According to the Commission, patient self-determination is the single most important ethical consideration in resuscitation decisions, although the physician's assessment of benefit to the patient, which is sometimes in conflict with patient preference, is also relevant. In proposing an overall scheme to guide decision making, the Commission attempts to come to grips not only with the conflicts that may arise between patient preference and physician's assessment of benefit but also with the uncertainties that may arise from either perspective.

Some terminally ill patients willingly submit to any medical intervention thought to be capable of extending their lives. Many others, in the light of the seriously compromised character of their present existence, are more concerned to achieve what M. Pabst Battin in this chapter calls "the least worst death." Battin's principal point is that a patient, with the advice of a physician, has the best chance of achieving "the least worst death" by the *selective* refusal of treatment.

Treatment Decisions for Incompetent Patients

The rigors of incurable illness and the dying process frequently deprive previously competent patients of their decision-making capacity. How can a person best ensure that his or her personal wishes with regard to life-sustaining treatment will be honored even if decision-making capacity is lost? Although communication of one's attitudes about various forms of life-sustaining treatment to one's physician, family, and friends surely provides some measure of protection, it is frequently asserted that the most effective protection comes through the formation of *advance directives*.

There are two basic types of advance directives, and each has legal status in most but not all states. In executing an *instructional* directive, a person specifies instructions about her or his care in the event that decision-making capacity is lost. Such a directive dealing specifically with the dying process and refusal of various forms of life-sustaining treatment is usually called "a living will." In executing a *proxy* directive, a person specifies a surrogate decision maker to make health-care decisions for him or her in the event that decision-making capacity is lost. The legal mechanism for executing a proxy directive is called a "durable power of attorney." Since purging ambiguities from even the most explicit written directives is difficult, as is foreseeing all the contingencies that might give rise to a need for treatment decisions, many commentators recommend the execution of a durable power of attorney even if a person has already executed a living will.

If a patient lacks decision-making capacity, a surrogate decision maker must be identified, and this will ordinarily be a member of the family or a close personal friend. If the patient has provided instructional directives, the surrogate is of course expected to follow them, but often enough a surrogate decision maker must function in the absence of instructional directives. In applying the *substituted judgment* standard, the surrogate decision maker is expected to consider the patient's preferences and values and make the decision that the patient would make if she or he were able to choose. If no reliable basis exists to infer what the patient would have chosen, then the surrogate decision maker is expected to retreat to the *best-interests* standard. In applying the best-interests standard, the surrogate decision maker is expected to choose what a rational person in the patient's circumstances would choose.

In one of this chapter's selections, the Hastings Center Project Group on the Termination of Treatment suggests procedures for the identification of surrogate decision makers and focuses attention on life-sustaining treatment decisions for patients who lack decision-making capacity. In this chapter's final selection, John D. Arras explicitly considers the dilemmas of surrogate decision making that arise when decisions have to be made for elderly, severely demented patients who have left behind no significant instructional directives. In his view, since neither the substituted judgment standard nor the best-interest standard produces an acceptable result, "a procedural solution" is needed. In the course of his discussion, Arras also considers the problem of surrogate decision making for patients in a persistent vegetative state. A more extensive discussion of persistent vegetative state can be found in Chapter 7 in conjunction with a discussion of the definition of death.

T.A.M.

NOTES

1 The label "libertarian," in this context, refers to a person who asserts the primacy of individual liberty. In particular, a libertarian is reluctant to accept the principles of paternalism and the principle of legal moralism as legitimate liberty-limiting principles. (These principles are discussed in Chapter 1.)

2 In part, discussion of the refusal of life-sustaining treatment in this chapter effectively paves the way for the introduction of a complex set of issues under the heading of "Euthanasia" in Chapter 7.

The Morality of Suicide

Suicide
Immanuel Kant

Immanuel Kant (1724–1804), widely acknowledged to be one of the most influential figures in the history of Western philosophy, was a native of East Prussia. Kant largely dedicated his life to academic philosophy and was eventually appointed to the chair of logic and metaphysics at the University of Königsberg. His works are voluminous and address a very wide range of philosophical issues. Kant's ethical theory, discussed in Chapter 1, is a landmark of deontological thought. The *Groundwork of the Metaphysic of Morals* (1785) and *The Critique of Practical Reason* (1788) are two of his most notable works in ethics.

Kant issues a blanket moral condemnation of suicide: "Suicide is in no circumstances permissible." In his view, suicide is characterized by the intention to destroy oneself. Thus neither the "victim of fate" nor the person whose intemperance leads to a shortened life is guilty of suicide. Kant insists that suicide is self-contradictory, in the sense that the power of free will is used for its own destruction. In a related consideration, suicide is said to be a moral abomination because it degrades human worth. Kant also claims that suicide is rightly condemned on religious grounds.

DUTIES TOWARDS THE BODY IN REGARD TO LIFE

What are our powers of disposal over our life? Have we any authority of disposal over it in any shape or form? How far is it incumbent upon us to take care of it? These are questions which fall to be considered in connexion with our duties towards the body in regard to life. We must, however, by way of introduction, make the following observations. If the body were related to life not as a condition but as an accident or circumstance so that we could at will divest ourselves of it; if we could slip out of it and slip into another just as we leave one country for another, then the body would be subject to our free will and we could rightly have the disposal of it. This, however, would not imply that we could similarly dispose of our life, but only of our circumstances, of the movable goods, the furniture of life. In fact, however, our life is entirely conditioned by our body, so that we cannot conceive of a life not mediated by the body and we cannot make use of our freedom except through the body. It is, therefore, obvious that the body constitutes a

From Immanuel Kant, *Lectures on Ethics*, translated by Louis Infield (New York: Harper & Row, 1963), pp. 147–154. Reprinted by permission of Methuen & Co. Ltd.

part of ourselves. If a man destroys his body, and so his life, he does it by the use of his will, which is itself destroyed in the process. But to use the power of a free will for its own destruction is self-contradictory. If freedom is the condition of life it cannot be employed to abolish life and so to destroy and abolish itself. To use life for its own destruction, to use life for producing lifelessness, is self-contradictory. These preliminary remarks are sufficient to show that man cannot rightly have any power of disposal in regard to himself and his life, but only in regard to his circumstances. His body gives man power over his life; were he a spirit he could not destroy his life; life in the absolute has been invested by nature with indestructibility and is an end in itself; hence it follows that man cannot have the power to dispose of his life.

SUICIDE

Suicide can be regarded in various lights; it might be held to be reprehensible, or permissible, or even heroic. In the first place we have the specious view that suicide can be allowed and tolerated. Its advocates argue thus. So long as he does not violate the proprietary rights of others, man is a free agent. With regard to his body there are various things he can properly do; he can have a boil lanced or a limb amputated, and disregard a scar; he is, in fact, free to do whatever he may consider useful and advisable. If then he comes to the conclusion that the most useful and advisable thing that he can do is to put an end to his life, why should he not be entitled to do so? Why not, if he sees that he can no longer go on living and that he will be ridding himself of misfortune, torment and disgrace? To be sure he robs himself of a full life, but he escapes once and for all from calamity and misfortune. The argument sounds most plausible. But let us, leaving aside religious considerations, examine the act itself. We may treat our body as we please, provided our motives are those of self-preservation. If, for instance, his foot is a hindrance to life, a man might have it amputated. To preserve his person he has the right of disposal over his body. But in taking his life he does not preserve his person; he disposes of his person and not of its attendant circumstances; he robs himself of his person. This is contrary to the highest duty we have towards ourselves, for it annuls the condition of all other duties; it goes beyond the limits of the use of free will, for this use is possible only through the existence of the Subject.

There is another set of considerations which make suicide seem plausible. A man might find himself so placed that he can continue living only under circumstances which deprive life of all value; in which he can no longer live conformably to virtue and prudence, so that he must from noble motives put an end to his life. The advocates of this view quote in support of it the example of Cato. Cato knew that the entire Roman nation relied upon him in their resistance to Caesar, but he found that he could not prevent himself from falling into Caesar's hands. What was he to do? If he, the champion of freedom, submitted, every one would say, "If Cato himself submits, what else can we do?" If, on the other hand, he killed himself, his death might spur on the Romans to fight to the bitter end in defence of their freedom. So he killed himself. He thought that it was necessary for him to die. He thought that if he could not go on living as Cato, he could not go on living at all. It must certainly be admitted that in a case such as this, where suicide is a virtue, appearances are in its favour. But this is the only example which has given the world the opportunity of defending suicide. It is the only example of its kind and there has been no similar case since. Lucretia also killed herself, but on grounds of modesty and in a fury of vengeance. It is obviously our duty to preserve our honour, particularly in relation to the opposite sex, for whom it is a merit; but we must endeavour to save our honour only to this extent, that we ought not to surrender it for selfish and lustful purposes. To do what Lucretia did is to adopt a remedy which is not at our disposal; it would have been better had she defended her honour unto death; that would not have been suicide and would have been right; for it is no suicide to risk one's life against one's enemies, and even to sacrifice it, in order to observe one's duties towards oneself.

No one under the sun can bind me to commit suicide; no sovereign can do so. The sovereign can call upon his subjects to fight to the death for their country, and those who fall on the field of battle are not suicides, but the victims of fate. Not only is this not suicide, but the opposite; a faint heart and fear of the death which threatens by the necessity of fate, is no true self-preservation; for he who runs away to save his own life, and leaves his comrades in the lurch, is a coward; but he who defends himself and his fellows even unto death is no suicide, but noble and high-minded; for life is not to be highly regarded for its own sake. I should endeavor to preserve my own life only so far as I am worthy to live. We must draw a distinction between the suicide and the victim of fate. A man who shortens his life by intemperance is guilty of imprudence and indirectly of his own death; but his guilt is not direct; he did not intend to kill himself; his death was not premeditated. For all our offences are either *culpa* or *dolus*. There is certainly no *dolus* here, but there is *culpa*; and we can say of such a man that he was guilty of his own death, but we cannot say of him that he is a suicide. What constitutes suicide is the intention to destroy oneself. Intemperance and excess which shorten life ought not, therefore, to be called suicide; for if we raise intemperance to the level of suicide, we lower suicide to the level of intemperance. Imprudence, which does not imply a desire to cease to live, must, therefore, be distinguished from the intention to murder oneself. Serious violations of our duty towards ourselves produce an aversion accompanied either by horror or by disgust; suicide is of the horrible kind, *crimina carnis* of the disgusting. We shrink in horror from suicide because all nature seeks its own preservation; an injured tree, a living body, an animal does so; how then could man make of his freedom, which is the acme of life and constitutes its worth, a principle for his own destruction? Nothing more terrible can be imagined; for if man were on every occasion master of his own life, he would be master of the lives of others; and being ready to sacrifice his life at any and every time rather than be captured, he could perpetrate every conceivable crime and vice. We are, therefore, horrified at the very thought of suicide; by it man sinks lower than the beasts; we look upon a suicide as carrion, whilst our sympathy goes forth to the victim of fate.

Those who advocate suicide seek to give the widest interpretation to freedom. There is something flattering in the thought that we can take our own life if we are so minded; and so we find even right-thinking persons defining suicide in this respect. There are many circumstances under which life ought to be sacrificed. If I cannot preserve my life except by violating my duties towards myself, I am bound to sacrifice my life rather than violate these duties. But suicide is in no circumstances permissible. Humanity in one's own person is something inviolable; it is a holy trust; man is master of all else, but he must not lay hands upon himself. A being who existed of his own necessity could not possibly destroy himself; a being whose existence is not necessary must regard life as the condition of everything else, and in the consciousness that life is a trust reposed in him, such a being recoils at the thought of committing a breach of his holy trust by turning his life against himself. Man can only dispose over things; beasts are things in this sense; but man is not a thing, not a beast. If he disposes over himself, he treats his value as that of a beast. He who so behaves, who has no respect for human nature and makes a thing of himself, becomes for everyone an Object of freewill. We are free to treat him as a beast, as a thing, and to use him for our sport as we do a horse or a dog, for he is no longer a human being; he has made a thing of himself, and, having himself discarded his humanity, he cannot expect that others should respect humanity in him. Yet humanity is worthy of esteem. Even when a man is a bad man, humanity in his person is worthy of esteem. Suicide is not abominable and inadmissible because life should be highly prized; were it so, we could each have our own opinion of how highly we should prize it, and the rule of prudence would often indicate suicide as the best means. But the rule of morality does not admit of it under any condition because it degrades human nature below the level of animal nature and so destroys it. Yet there is much in the world far more important than life. To observe morality is far more important. It is better to sacrifice one's life than one's morality. To live is not a necessity; but to live honourably while life lasts is a necessity. We can at all times go on living and doing our duty towards ourselves without having to do violence to ourselves. But he who is prepared to take his own life is no longer worthy to live at all. The pragmatic ground of impulse to live is happiness. Can I then take my own life because I cannot live

happily? No! It is not necessary that whilst I live I should live happily; but it is necessary that so long as I live I should live honourably. Misery gives no right to any man to take his own life, for then we should all be entitled to take our lives for lack of pleasure. All our duties towards ourselves would then be directed towards pleasure; but the fulfillment of those duties may demand that we should even sacrifice our life.

Is suicide heroic or cowardly? Sophistication, even though well meant, is not a good thing. It is not good to defend either virtue or vice by splitting hairs. Even right-thinking people declaim against suicide on wrong lines. They say that it is arrant cowardice. But instances of suicide of great heroism exist. We cannot, for example, regard the suicides of Cato and Atticus as cowardly. Rage, passion and insanity are the most frequent causes of suicide, and that is why persons who attempt suicide and are saved from it are so terrified at their own act that they do not dare to repeat the attempt. There was a time in Roman and in Greek history when suicide was regarded as honourable, so much so that the Romans forbade their slaves to commit suicide because they did not belong to themselves but to their masters and so were regarded as things, like all other animals. The Stoics said that suicide is the sage's peaceful death; he leaves the world as he might leave a smoky room for another, because it no longer pleases him; he leaves the world, not because he is no longer happy in it, but because he disdains it. It has already been mentioned that man is greatly flattered by the idea that he is free to remove himself from this world, if he so wishes. He may not make use of this freedom, but the thought of possessing it pleases him. It seems even to have a moral aspect, for if man is capable of removing himself from the world at his own will, he need not submit to any one; he can retain his independence and tell the rudest truths to the cruellest of tyrants. Torture cannot bring him to heel, because he can leave the world at a moment's notice as a free man can leave the country, if and when he wills it. But this semblance of morality vanishes as soon as we see that man's freedom cannot subsist except on a condition which is immutable. This condition is that man may not use his freedom against himself to his own destruction, but that, on the contrary, he should allow nothing external to limit it. Freedom thus conditioned is noble. No chance or misfortune ought to make us afraid to live; we ought to go on living as long as we can do so as human beings and honourably. To bewail one's fate and misfortune is in itself dishonourable. Had Cato faced any torments which Caesar might have inflicted upon him with a resolute mind and remained steadfast, it would have been noble of him; to violate himself was not so. Those who advocate suicide and teach that there is authority for it necessarily do much harm in a republic of free men. Let us imagine a state in which men held as a general opinion that they were entitled to commit suicide, and that there was even merit and honour in so doing. How dreadful everyone would find them. For he who does not respect his life even in principle cannot be restrained from the most dreadful vices; he recks neither king nor torments.

But as soon as we examine suicide from the standpoint of religion we immediately see it in its true light. We have been placed in this world under certain conditions and for specific purposes. But a suicide opposes the purpose of his Creator; he arrives in the other world as one who has deserted his post; he must be looked upon as a rebel against God. So long as we remember the truth that it is God's intention to preserve life, we are bound to regulate our activities in conformity with it. We have no right to offer violence to our nature's powers of self-preservation and to upset the wisdom of her arrangements. This duty is upon us until the time comes when God expressly commands us to leave this life. Human beings are sentinels on earth and may not leave their posts until relieved by another beneficent hand. God is our owner; we are His property; His providence works for our good. A bondman in the care of a beneficent master deserves punishment if he opposes his master's wishes.

But suicide is not inadmissible and abominable because God has forbidden it; God has forbidden it because it is abominable in that it degrades man's inner worth below that of the animal creation. Moral philosophers must, therefore, first and foremost show that suicide is abominable. We find, as a rule, that those who labour for their happiness are more liable to suicide; having tasted the refinements of pleasure, and being deprived of them, they give way to grief, sorrow, and melancholy.

The Morality and Rationality of Suicide
R. B. Brandt

R. B. Brandt is professor emeritus of philosophy at the University of Michigan. He is the author of *Ethical Theory* (1959) and *A Theory of the Good and the Right* (1979), and he is the coeditor of *Meaning and Knowledge* (1965) and *The Problems of Philosophy* (3d ed., 1978). Brandt's article "Toward a Credible Form of Utilitarianism" is one prominent example of his many contributions to contemporary discussions of utilitarian theory.

Operating on the assumption that suicide is to be understood as the intentional termination of one's own life, Brandt sets himself firmly against the view that suicide is always immoral. He critically analyzes, and finds wanting, various classes of arguments that have been advanced to support the alleged immorality of suicide: (1) theological arguments, (2) arguments from natural law, and (3) arguments to the effect that suicide necessarily does harm to other persons or to society in general. Brandt does acknowledge that there is some obligaion to refrain from committing suicide when that act would be injurious to others, but he insists that this obligation may often be overridden by other morally relevant considerations. Clearly, for Brandt, suicide is sometimes morally acceptable. He also insists that a person's decision to commit suicide may be quite rational, although he is careful to warn of potential errors in judgment. He concludes by analyzing the various factors that are relevant in establishing the moral obligation of other persons toward those who are contemplating suicide.

THE MORAL REASONS FOR AND AGAINST SUICIDE

[Assuming that there is suicide if and only if there is intentional termination of one's own life,] persons who say suicide is morally wrong must be asked which of two positions they are affirming: Are they saying that *every* act of suicide is wrong, *everything considered*; or are they merely saying that there is always *some* moral obligation—doubtless of serious weight—not to commit suicide, so that very often suicide is wrong, although it is possible that there are *countervailing considerations* which in particular situations make it right or even a moral duty? It is quite evident that the first position is absurd; only the second has a chance of being defensible.

In order to make clear what is wrong with the first view, we may begin with an example. Suppose an army pilot's single-seater plane goes out of control over a heavily populated area; he has the choice of staying in the plane and bringing it down where it will do little damage but at the cost of certain death for himself, and of bailing out and letting the plane fall where it will, very possibly killing a good many civilians. Suppose he chooses to do the former, and so, by our definition, commits suicide. Does anyone want to say that his action is morally wrong? Even Immanuel Kant, who opposed suicide in all circumstances, apparently would not wish to say that it is; he would, in fact, judge that this act is not one of suicide, for he says, "It is no suicide to risk one's life against one's enemies, and even to sacrifice it, in order to preserve one's duties toward oneself."[1] St. Thomas Aquinas, in his discussion of suicide, may seem to take the position that such an act would be wrong, for he says, "It is altogether unlawful to kill oneself," admitting as an exception only the case of being under special command of God. But I believe St. Thomas would, in fact, have concluded that the act is right because the basic intention of the pilot was to save the lives of civilians, and whether an act is right or wrong is a matter of basic intention.[2]

In general, we have to admit that there are things with some moral obligation to avoid which, on account of other morally relevant considerations, it is sometimes right or even morally obligatory to do. There may be some obligation to tell the truth on every occasion, but surely in many cases the consequences of telling the truth would be so dire that one is obligated to lie. The same goes for promises. There is some moral obligation to do what one has promised (with a few exceptions); but, if one can keep a trivial promise only at serious cost to another person (i.e., keep an appointment only by failing to give aid to someone injured in an accident), it is surely obligatory to break the promise.

The most that the moral critic of suicide could hold, then, is that there is *some* moral obligation not to do what one knows will cause one's death; but he surely cannot deny that circumstances exist in which there are obligations to do things which, in fact, will result in one's death. If so, then in principle it would be possible to argue, for instance, that in order to meet my obligation to my family, it might be right for me to take my own life as the only way to avoid catastrophic hospital expenses in a terminal illness. Possibly the main point that critics of suicide on moral grounds would wish to make is that it is never right to take one's own life *for reasons of one's own personal welfare*, of any kind whatsoever. Some of the arguments used to support the immorality of suicide, however, are so framed that if they were supportable at all, they would prove that suicide is *never* moral.

One well-known type of argument against suicide may be classified as *theological*. St. Augustine and others urged that the Sixth Commandment ("Thou shalt not kill") prohibits suicide, and that we are bound to obey a divine commandment. To this reasoning one might first reply that it is arbitrary exegesis of the Sixth Commandment to assert that it was intended to prohibit suicide. The second reply is that if there is not some consideration which shows on the merits of the case that suicide is morally wrong, God had no business prohibiting it. It is true that some will object to this point, and I must refer them elsewhere for my detailed comments on the divine-will theory of morality.[3]

Another theological argument with wide support was accepted by John Locke, who wrote: "...Men being all the workmanship of one omnipotent and infinitely wise Maker; all the servants of one sovereign Master, sent into the world by His order and about His business; they are His property, whose workmanship they are made to last during His, not one another's pleasure ...Every one...is bound to preserve himself, and not to quit his station wilfully...."[4] And Kant: "We have been placed in this world under certain conditions and for specific purposes. But a suicide opposes the purpose of his Creator; he arrives in the other world as one who has deserted his post; he must be looked upon as a rebel against God. So long as we remember the truth that it is God's intention to preserve life, we are bound to regulate our activities in conformity with it. This duty is upon us until the time comes when God expressly commands us to leave this life. Human beings are sentinels on earth and may not leave their posts until relieved by another beneficent hand."[5] Unfortunately, however, even if we grant that it is the duty of human beings to do what God commands or intends them to do, more argument is required to show that God does *not* permit human beings to quit this life when their own personal welfare would be maximized by so doing. How does one draw the requisite inference about the intentions of God? The difficulties and contradictions in arguments to reach such a conclusion are discussed at length and perspicaciously by David Hume in his essay "On Suicide," and in view of the unlikelihood that readers will need to be persuaded about these, I shall merely refer those interested to that essay.[6]

A second group of arguments may be classed as arguments *from natural law*. St. Thomas says: "It is altogether unlawful to kill oneself, for three reasons. First, because everything naturally loves itself, the result being that everything naturally keeps itself in being, and resists corruptions so far as it can. Wherefore suicide is contrary to the inclination of nature, and to charity whereby every man should love himself. Hence suicide is always a mortal sin, as being contrary to the natural law and to charity."[7] Here St. Thomas ignores two obvious points. First, it is not obvious why a human being is morally bound to do what he or she has some inclination to do. (St. Thomas did not criticize chastity.) Second, while it is true that most human beings do feel a strong urge to live, the human being who commits suicide obviously feels a stronger inclination to do something else. It is as natural for a human being to dislike, and to take steps to avoid, say, great pain, as it is to cling to life.

A somewhat similar argument by Immanuel Kant may seem better. In a famous passage Kant writes that the maxim of a person who commits suicide is "From self-love I make it my principle to shorten my life if its continuance threatens more evil than it promises pleasure. The only further question to ask is whether this principle of self-love can become a universal law of nature. It is then seen at once that a system of nature by whose law the very same feeling whose function is to stimulate the furtherance of life should actually destroy life would contradict itself and consequently could not subsist as a system of nature. Hence this maxim cannot possibly hold as a universal law of nature and is therefore entirely opposed to the supreme principle of all duty."[8] What Kant finds contradictory is that the motive of self-love (interest in one's own long-range welfare) should

sometimes lead one to struggle to preserve one's life, but at other times to end it. But where is the contradiction? One's circumstances change, and, if the argument of the following section in this [paper] is correct, one sometimes maximizes one's own long-range welfare by trying to stay alive, but at other times by bringing about one's demise.

A third group of arguments, a form of which goes back at least to Aristotle, has a more modern and convincing ring. These are arguments to show that, in one way or another, a suicide necessarily does harm to other persons, or to society at large. Aristotle says that the suicide treats the *state* unjustly.[9] Partly following Aristotle, St. Thomas says: "Every man is part of the community, and so, as such, he belongs to the community. Hence by killing himself he injures the community."[10] Blackstone held that a suicide is an offense against the king "who hath an interest in the preservation of all his subjects," perhaps following Judge Brown in 1563, who argued that suicide cost the king a subject—"he being the head has lost one of his mystical members."[11] The premise of such arguments is, as Hume pointed out, obviously mistaken in many instances. It is true that Freud would perhaps have injured society had he, instead of finishing his last book, committed suicide to escape the pain of throat cancer. But surely there have been many suicides whose demise was not a noticeable loss to society; an honest man could only say that in some instances society was better off without them.

It need not be denied that suicide is often injurious to other persons, especially the family of a suicide. Clearly it sometimes is. But, we should notice what this fact establishes. Suppose we admit, as generally would be done, that there is some obligation not to perform any action which will probably or certainly be injurious to other people, the strength of the obligation being dependent on various factors, notably the seriousness of the expected injury. Then there is *some* obligation not to commit suicide, when that act would probably or certainly be injurious to other people. But, as we have already seen, many cases of *some* obligation to do something nevertheless are *not* cases of a duty to do that thing, *everything considered*. So it could sometimes be morally justified to commit suicide, even if the act will harm someone. Must a man with a terminal illness undergo excruciating pain because his death will cause his wife sorrow—when she will be caused sorrow a month later anyway, when he is dead of natural causes? Moreover, to repeat, the fact that an individual has some obligation not to commit suicide when that act will probably injure other persons does not imply that, everything considered, it is wrong for him to do it, namely, that in all circumstances suicide *as such* is something there is some obligation to avoid.

Is there any sound argument, convincing to the modern mind, to establish that there is (or is not) *some moral obligation* to avoid suicide *as such*, an obligation, of course, which might be overridden by other obligations in some or many cases? (Captain Oates may have had a moral obligation not to commit suicide as such, but his obligation not to stand in the way of his comrades getting to safety might have been so strong that, everything considered, he was justified in leaving the polar camp and allowing himself to freeze to death.)

To present all the arguments necessary to answer this question convincingly would take a great deal of space. I shall, therefore, simply state one answer to it which seems plausible to some contemporary philosophers. Suppose it could be shown that it would maximize the long-run welfare of everybody affected if people were taught that there is a moral obligation to avoid suicide—so that people would be motivated to avoid suicide just because they thought it wrong (would have anticipatory guilt feelings at the very idea), and so that other people would be inclined to disapprove of persons who commit suicide unless there were some excuse.... One might ask: how could it maximize utility to mold the conceptual and motivational structure of persons in this way? To which the answer might be: feeling in this way might make persons who are impulsively inclined to commit suicide in a bad mood, or a fit of anger or jealousy, take more time to deliberate; hence, some suicides that have bad effects generally might be prevented. In other words, it might be a good thing in its effects for people to feel about suicide in the way they feel about breach of promise or injuring others, just as it might be a good thing for people to feel a moral obligation not to smoke, or to wear seat belts. However, it might be that negative moral feelings about suicide as such would stand in the way of action by those persons whose welfare really is best served by suicide and whose suicide is the best thing for everybody concerned.

WHEN A DECISION TO COMMIT SUICIDE IS RATIONAL FROM THE PERSON'S POINT OF VIEW

The person who is contemplating suicide is obviously making a choice between future world-courses; the world-course that includes his demise, say, an hour from now, and several possible ones that contain his demise at a later point. One cannot have precise knowledge about many features of the latter group of world-courses, but it is certain that they will all end with death some (possibly short) finite time from now.

Why do I say the choice is between *world*-courses and not just a choice between future life-courses of the prospective suicide, the one shorter than the other? The reason is that one's suicide has some impact on the world (and one's continued life has some impact on the world), and that conditions in the rest of the world will often make a difference in one's evaluation of the possibilities. One *is* interested in things in the world other than just oneself and one's own happiness.

The basic question a person must answer, in order to determine which world-course is best or rational for him to choose, is which he *would* choose under conditions of optimal use of information, when *all* of his desires are taken into account. It is not just a question of what we prefer *now*, with some clarification of all the possibilities being considered. Our preferences change, and the preferences of tomorrow (assuming we can know something about them) are just as legitimately taken into account in deciding what to do now as the preferences of today. Since any reason that can be given today for weighting heavily today's preference can be given tomorrow for weighting heavily tomorrow's preference, the preferences of any time-stretch have a rational claim to an equal vote. Now the importance of that fact is this: we often know quite well that our desires, aversions, and preferences may change after a short while. When a person is in a state of despair—perhaps brought about by a rejection in love or discharge from a long-held position—nothing but the thing he cannot have seems desirable; everything else is turned to ashes. Yet we know quite well that the passage of time is likely to reverse all this; replacements may be found or other types of things that are available to us may begin to look attractive. So, if we were to act on the preferences of today alone, when the emotion of despair seems more than we can stand, we might find death preferable to life; but, if we allow for the preferences of the weeks and years ahead, when many goals will be enjoyable and attractive, we might find life much preferable to death. So, if a choice of what is best is to be determined by what we want not only now but later (and later desires on an equal basis with the present ones)—as it should be—then what is the best or preferable world-course will often be quite different from what it would be if the choice, or what is best for one, were fixed by one's desires and preferences now.

Of course, if one commits suicide there are no future desires or aversions that may be compared with present ones and that should be allowed an equal vote in deciding what is best. In that respect the course of action that results in death is different from any other course of action we may undertake. I do not wish to suggest the rosy possibility that it is often or always reasonable to believe that next week "I shall be more interested in living than I am today, if today I take a dim view of continued existence." On the contrary, when a person is seriously ill, for instance, he may have no reason to think that the preference-order will be reversed—it may be that tomorrow he will prefer death to life more strongly.

The argument is often used that one can never be *certain* what is going to happen, and hence one is never rationally justified in doing anything as drastic as committing suicide. But we always have to live by probabilities and make our estimates as best we can. As soon as it is clear beyond reasonable doubt not only that death is now preferable to life, but also that it will be every day from now until the end, the rational thing is to act promptly.

Let us not pursue the question of whether it is rational for a person with a painful terminal illness to commit suicide; it is. However, the issue seldom arises, and few terminally ill patients do commit suicide. With such patients matters usually get worse slowly so that no particular time seems to call for action. They are often so heavily sedated that it is impossible for the mental processes of decision leading to action to occur; or else they are incapacitated in a hospital and the very physical possibility of ending their lives is not available. Let us leave this grim topic and turn to a practically more important problem: whether it is rational for persons to commit suicide for some reason other than painful terminal physical illness. Most persons who commit suicide do so, apparently, because they face a nonphysical problem that depresses them beyond their ability to bear.

Among the problems that have been regarded as good and sufficient reasons for ending life, we find (in addition to serious illness) the following: some event that has made a person feel ashamed or lose his prestige and status; reduction from affluence to poverty; the loss of a limb or of physical beauty; the loss of sexual capacity; some event that makes it seem impossible to achieve things by which one sets store; loss of a loved one; disappointment in love; the infirmities of increasing age. It is not to be denied that such things can be serious blows to a person's prospects of happiness.

Whatever the nature of an individual's problem, there are various plain errors to be avoided—errors to which a person is especially prone when he is depressed—in deciding whether, everything considered, he prefers a world-course containing his early demise to one in which his life continues to its natural terminus. Let us forget for a moment the relevance to the decision of preferences that he may have tomorrow, and concentrate on some errors that may infect his preference as of today, and for which correction or allowance must be made.

In the first place, depression, like any severe emotional experience, tends to primitivize one's intellectual processes. It restricts the range of one's survey of the possibilities. One thing that a rational person would do is compare the world-course containing his suicide with his *best* alternative. But his best alternative is precisely a possibility he may overlook if, in a depressed mood, he thinks only of how badly off he is and cannot imagine any way of improving his situation. If a person is disappointed in love, it is possible to adopt a vigorous plan of action that carries a good chance of acquainting him with someone he likes at least as well; and if old age prevents a person from continuing the tennis game with his favorite partner, it is possible to learn some other game that provides the joys of competition without the physical demands.

Depression has another insidious influence on one's planning; it seriously affects one's judgment about probabilities. A person disappointed in love is very likely to take a dim view of himself, his prospects, and his attractiveness; he thinks that because he has been rejected by one person he will probably be rejected by anyone who looks desirable to him. In a less gloomy frame of mind he would make different estimates. Part of the reason for such gloomy probability estimates is that depression tends to repress one's memory of evidence that supports a nongloomy prediction. Thus, a rejected lover tends to forget any cases in which he has elicited enthusiastic response from ladies in relation to whom he has been the one who has done the rejecting. Thus his pessimistic self-image is based upon a highly selected, and pessimistically selected, set of data. Even when he is reminded of the data, moreover, he is apt to resist an optimistic inference.

Another kind of distortion of the look of future prospects is not a result of depression, but is quite normal. Events distant in the future feel small, just as objects distant in space look small. Their prospect does not have the effect on motivational processes that it would have if it were of an event in the immediate future. Psychologists call this the "goal-gradient" phenomenon; a rat, for instance, will run faster toward a perceived food box than a distant unseen one. In the case of a person who has suffered some misfortune, and whose situation now is an unpleasant one, this reduction of the motivational influence of events distant in time has the effect that present unpleasant states weigh far more heavily than probable future pleasant ones in any choice of world-courses.

If we are trying to determine whether we now prefer, or shall later prefer, the outcome of one world-course to that of another (and this is leaving aside the questions of the weight of the votes of preferences at a later date), we must take into account these and other infirmities of our "sensing" machinery. Since knowing that the machinery is out of order will not tell us what results it would give if it were working, the best recourse might be to refrain from making any decision in a stressful frame of mind. If decisions have to be made, one must recall past reactions, in a normal frame of mind, to outcomes like those under assessment. But many suicides seem to occur in moments of despair. What should be clear from the above is that a moment of despair, if one is seriously contemplating suicide, ought to be a moment of reassessment of one's goals and values, a reassessment which the individual must realize is very difficult to make objectively, because of the very quality of his depressed frame of mind.

A decision to commit suicide may in certain circumstances be a rational one. But a person who wants to act rationally must take into account the various possible "errors" and make appropriate rectification of his initial evaluations.

THE ROLE OF OTHER PERSONS

What is the moral obligation of other persons toward those who are contemplating suicide? The question of their moral blameworthiness may be ignored and what is rational for them to do from the point of view of personal welfare may be considered as being of secondary concern. Laws make it dangerous to aid or encourage a suicide. The risk of running afoul of the law may partly determine moral obligation, since moral obligation to do something may be reduced by the fact that it is personally dangerous.

The moral obligation of other persons toward one who is contemplating suicide is an instance of a general obligation to render aid to those in serious distress, at least when this can be done at no great cost to one's self.

I do not think this general principle is seriously questioned by anyone, whatever his moral theory; so I feel free to assume it as a premise. Obviously the person contemplating suicide is in great distress of some sort; if he were not, he would not be seriously considering terminating his life.

How great a person's obligation is to one in distress depends on a number of factors. Obviously family and friends have special obligations to devote time to helping the prospective suicide—which others do not have. But anyone in this kind of distress has a moral claim on the time of any person who knows the situation (unless there are others more responsible who are already doing what should be done).

What is the obligation? It depends, of course, on the situation, and how much the second person knows about the situation. If the individual has decided to terminate his life if he can, and it is clear that he is right in this decision, then, if he needs help in executing the decision, there is a moral obligation to give him help. On this matter a patient's physician has a special obligation, from which any talk about the Hippocratic oath does not absolve him. It is true that there are some damages one cannot be expected to absorb, and some risks which one cannot be expected to take, on account of the obligation to render aid.

On the other hand, if it is clear that the individual should not commit suicide, from the point of view of his own welfare, or if there is a presumption that he should not (when the only evidence is that a person is discovered unconscious, with the gas turned on), it would seem to be the individual's obligation to intervene, prevent the successful execution of the decision, and see to the availability of competent psychiatric advice and temporary hospitalization, if necessary. Whether one has a right to take such steps when a clearly sane person, after careful reflection over a period of time, comes to the conclusion that an end to his life is what is best for him and what he wants, is very doubtful, even when one thinks his conclusion a mistaken one; it would seem that a man's own considered decision about whether he wants to live must command respect, although one must concede that this could be debated.

The more interesting role in which a person may be cast, however, is that of adviser. It is often important to one who is contemplating suicide to go over his thinking with another, and to feel that a conclusion, one way or the other, has the support of a respected mind. One thing one can obviously do, in rendering the service of advice, is to discuss with the person the various types of issues discussed above, made more specific by the concrete circumstances of his case, and help him find whether, in view, say, of the damage his suicide would do to others, he has a moral obligation to refrain, and whether it is rational or best for him, from the point of view of his own welfare, to take this step or adopt some other plan instead.

To get a person to see what is the rational thing to do is no small job. Even to get a person, in a frame of mind when he is seriously contemplating (or perhaps has already unsuccessfully attempted) suicide, to recognize a plain truth of fact may be a major operation. If a man insists, "I am a complete failure," when it is obvious that by any reasonable standard he is far from that, it may be tremendously difficult to get him to see the fact. But there is another job beyond that of getting a person to see what is the rational thing to do; that is to help him *act* rationally, or *be* rational, when he has conceded what would be the rational thing.

How either of these tasks may be accomplished effectively may be discussed more competently by an experienced psychiatrist than by a philosopher. Loneliness and the absence of human affection are states which exacerbate any other problems; disappointment, reduction to poverty, and so forth, seem less impossible to bear in the presence of the affection of another. Hence simply to be a friend, or to find someone a friend, may be the largest contribution one can make either to helping a person be rational or see clearly what is rational for him to do; this service may make one who was contemplating suicide feel that there is a future for him which it is possible to face.

NOTES

1 Immanuel Kant, *Lectures on Ethics*, New York: Harper Torchbook (1963), p. 150.

2 See St. Thomas Aquinas, *Summa Theologica*, Second Part of the Second Part, Q. 64, Art. 5. In Article 7, he says: "Nothing hinders one act from having two effects, only one of which is intended, while the other is beside the intention. Now moral acts take their species according to what is intended, and not according to what is beside the intention, since this is accidental as explained above" (Q. 43, Art. 3: I–II,

Q. 1, Art. 3, as 3). Mr. Norman St. John-Stevas, the most articulate contemporary defender of the Catholic view, writes as follows: "Christian thought allows certain exceptions to its general condemnation of suicide. That covered by a particular divine inspiration has already been noted. Another exception arises where suicide is the method imposed by the state for the execution of a just death penalty. A third exception is *altruistic* suicide, of which the best known example is Captain Oates. Such suicides are justified by invoking the principles of double effect. The act from which death results must be good or at least morally indifferent; some other good effect must result: The death must not be directly intended or the real means to the good effect, and a grave reason must exist for adopting the course of action" [*Life, Death and the Law*, Bloomington, Ind.: Indiana University Press (1961), pp. 250–51]. Presumably the Catholic doctrine is intended to allow suicide when this is required for meeting strong moral obligations; whether it can do so consistently depends partly on the interpretation given to "real means to the good effect." Readers interested in pursuing further the Catholic doctrine of double effect and its implications for our problem should read Philippa Foot, "The Problem of Abortion and the Doctrine of Double Effect," *The Oxford Review*, 5:5–15 (Trinity 1967).

3 R. B. Brandt, *Ethical Theory*, Englewood Cliffs, N.J.: Prentice Hall (1959), pp. 61–82.

4 John Locke, *Two Treatises of Government*, Ch. 2.

5 Kant, *Lectures on Ethics*, p. 154.

6 This essay appears in collections of Hume's works.

7 For an argument similar to Kant's, see also St. Thomas Aquinas, *Summa Theologica*, II, II, Q. 64, Art. 5.

8 Immanuel Kant, *The Fundamental Principles of the Metaphysic of Morals*, trans H. J. Paton, London: The Hutchinson Group (1948), Ch. 2.

9 Aristotle, *Nicomachaean Ethics*, Bk. 5, Ch. 10., p. 1138a.

10 St. Thomas Aquinas, *Summa Theologica*, II, II, Q. 64, Art. 5.

11 Sir William Blackstone, *Commentaries*, 4:189; Brown in Hales v. Petit, I Plow. 253, 75 E.R. 387 (C. B. 1563). Both cited by Norman St. John-Stevas, *Life, Death and the Law*, p. 235.

Suicide Intervention

Interference with a Suicide Attempt
David F. Greenberg

David F. Greenberg, after receiving a Ph.D. in physics and serving as senior fellow, Committee for the Study of Incarceration (Washington, D.C.), is presently professor of sociology at New York University. He is the author, coauthor, or editor of *University of Chicago Graduate Problems in Physics* (1965), *Struggle for Justice* (1971), *Mathematical Criminology* (1979), *Crime and Capitalism: Essays in Marxist Criminology* (1981), and *The Construction of Homosexuality* (1988).

Greenberg sets out to design an appropriate suicide prevention policy. He suggests, as an aid to impartial thinking, that we consider this matter from behind a "veil of ignorance," in accordance with the theory of John Rawls. We would be willing, he argues, to authorize some measure of interference, yet would also insist that such interference not be unlimited. After identifying the main objectives of an ideal suicide prevention policy, he argues in support of a policy that would allow temporary intervention.

REFORMULATING THE SUICIDE DEBATE

...The advocate of intervention typically assumes that the individual under consideration *is* suicidal, not someone mistakenly thought to be suicidal or maliciously and wrongfully accused of being suicidal. Consequently, he may pay insufficient attention to the problem of screening. In addition, he is likely to assume that intervention motivated by the goal of preventing suicides will, at least some of the time, attain its goal. Yet this need not be the case. The effectiveness of any given measure in preventing suicides is an empirical question the answer to which may not simply be assumed. The libertarian, on the other hand, assumes, perhaps with no greater justification, that suicide attempters want to die, so that abstaining from interference conforms to their wishes. This assumption, too, may be wide of the mark. These hidden assumptions require careful examination before an objective look at the suicide prevention debate may be had.

A   Do Suicide Attempters Want to Die?

Unlike early research on suicide, recent studies have considered the conscious, self-perceived motivations of

Reprinted with permission of the author and the publisher from *New York University Law Review*, 49 (May–June 1974), pp. 227–269.

suicide attempters to be worthy of study, and have attempted to situate these motivations in the life experiences and circumstances of the attempters. Researchers are in agreement that most attempters do not unequivocally want to die. For example, sociologist Jack Douglas concludes:

> In the vast majority of cases,...individuals committing dangerous acts against themselves do have what they themselves see as some degree of intention to die....But there is also every indication that in the great majority of cases where there is such an intention to die, there is also an intention to use suicide, through the construction of certain meanings for others involved, so that they can live better either in this world or the next. Suicide, then, is generally a highly ambivalent action. Even those individuals with very serious intentions of dying by suicide rarely give up hope of living. After taking pills, they call for help or move toward others; when cutting their throats they make "hesitation" cuts; and most individuals who attempt or commit suicide have given their friends and relations serious warnings of their intentions to kill themselves.[1]

In accord with the foregoing observations is the report of a team of psychiatrists: "[W]e have come to regard attempted suicide not as an effort to die but rather as a communication to others in an effort to improve one's life."[2] Although a suicide attempt may seem like a peculiar way to improve one's life, we should not assume without further investigation that a suicide attempt is irrational or foolish. For adults, at least, a suicide attempt frequently is successful in bringing about an improved relationship with significant others. According to one psychiatrist, "[t]he suicidal act...usually arouses sufficient sympathy to bring about some change in the circumstances surrounding the person who makes the attempt."[3] Similarly, the authors of another study made the following observation: "We regard these 34 attempts as successful in the sense that desired changes in the life situation of the patient occurred as a consequence of the attempt."[4]

The foregoing research findings as to the motivation of suicide attempts and the responses which these attempts often elicit suggest the relevance of a game theory perspective. From this angle the suicide attempter is a player in a game, so desperate as to be willing to risk a highly unfavorable outcome (death) in order to obtain a favorable outcome (survival and transformed relationships with others, or solved problems). It becomes easier, then, to understand the efforts of so many attempters to bring about lifesaving intervention as well as the high survival rate among attempters. It is estimated that only about one of every eight or ten suicide attempts results in death.

Studies of the subsequent mortality rate among survivors of suicide attempts tend to confirm the view of attempters as persons who, for the most part, are not intent on dying. Only about 1% of all surviving attempters kill themselves within a year of the attempt. This is still quite a bit higher than the suicide rate in the general population, but far lower than would be anticipated if most attempters unambivalently wanted to die.

The long-range suicide rate among surviving attempters is somewhat higher. Follow-up studies lasting as long as 15 years suggest that eventually somewhere between five and 15 percent of surviving attempters will kill themselves. Not surprisingly, subsequent suicide may depend on the response to the initial attempt. Thus, the authors of one study "found consistently that recovery requires a major change in the life situation."[5] This, of course, is just what we would expect if most attempters prefer to live, and, at least in part, have used the suicide attempt in order to manipulate a relationship to better advantage. Those who are successful in doing this, and they seem to be the majority, do not attempt suicide again. Others, discovering after a period of time has elapsed that their lives have not improved or have deteriorated, may well attempt suicide again, perhaps with greater definiteness of purpose in bringing about death.

B Suicide Prevention behind the Veil of Ignorance

If most suicide attempters either do not want to die or change their minds within a very short time after an attempt, a posited "right to commit suicide" may be a weak basis for defending a policy of non-interference with suicide attempts. Were there no other pertinent considerations, the saving of the lives of the high proportion of attempters who, having been restrained, would then want to live and who would be grateful for having been saved[6] would seem to constitute adequate grounds for authorizing interference.[7] As is often the case, however, there are other considerations, such as our desire to remain free from erroneous or unnecessary interference. The attempt, then, must be to find a suicide prevention policy that will reconcile our goal of saving lives with the preservation of values we consider it important not to jeopardize.

Let us imagine that we are asked to agree upon a suicide prevention policy, given what is known about suicide but prevented by a "veil of ignorance"[8] from knowing who among us will attempt or commit suicide, who may mistakenly be identified or vindictively accused of being suicidal, who will have easy access to top-quality legal representation, and so on. We insist upon the presence of the veil to prevent persons from demanding conditions or provisions tailored in advance to meet their own individual contingencies. Thus, a man who is fairly certain that he never would be falsely identified as suicidal and therefore wrongly threatened with deprivation of liberty might be willing to sacrifice the interests of others in not being misidentified. Such a person, therefore, should not be allowed to formulate a policy taking that knowledge into account.

It seems clear that behind the veil of ignorance we would be willing to tolerate some degree of interference with suicide attempts. We would want to save the lives of those among us who would attempt suicide, but who research indicated did not desire the outcome of death, and who later would be grateful for having been rescued. Moreover, there often are times when we decide to do something on the spur of the moment that we later regret. When the consequences of impulsive action are as extreme as they are in the case of suicide, we might well want some form of intervention to compel us to reflect on whether we really want the choice we have made. Here the motivation for intervention is not that the attempter does not at the moment of the attempt want to die, but that after some consideration he may not want to do so. This later, more considered judgment is preferred over the impulsive one, perhaps because we think it more accurately represents his "true" wishes.

We might also reasonably want to be restrained against committing suicide when our judgment is clouded or distorted, as it might be through chemical processes affecting the functioning of the brain (toxic psychosis) or when a highly upsetting event (such as a death in the family) occurs.

While rationally we would be willing to authorize some measure of interference to prevent us from committing suicide under circumstances such as those mentioned above, we also would insist that a number of limitations on the extent and methods of interference with suicidal individuals be imposed, lest other values be jeopardized. Central among these would be the retention of the ultimate right to commit suicide for those who found the pain or distress of living intolerable, and for whom the desire to end life represented something more than momentary dejection or discouragement. This ultimate control over the decision whether to continue living is something we would be extremely loath to give up, lest we be forced to live in misery for a long time. Moreover, since we would recognize that distress is subjective, we would be reluctant, in making provision for the right to die, to permit others to pass on the rationality of our decision to end life.

As a further requirement, we unquestionably would insist on procedural and substantive safeguards designed to protect nonsuicidal individuals from wrongful intervention, mistaken or deliberate.[9] The more extensive the intervention, the more safeguards we would require. When the intervention is so drastic as to entail loss of liberty for an extended period, loss of some civil rights, loss of earnings, separation from family and friends and serious stigmatization, we would want to be careful indeed that only those who were actually suicidal should be the subjects of intervention.

A third concern would be that the intervention not be excessively painful, unpleasant or protracted, for, if it were, the human costs of prevention might well be thought to exceed its benefits.

This analysis suggests that the ideal suicide prevention policy is one that would: (1) save, through methods entailing minimal unpleasantness, the lives of as many as possible of those who do not wish to die; (2) interfere as little as possible with those who after some chance for consideration persist in wanting to die; and (3) afford maximum protection against interference with the liberty of those who pose no threat of suicide. This sug-

gested policy goes very far toward respecting individual choice, but, on the basis of a principle of retrospective gratitude, departs from the most extreme libertarian position to allow very limited paternalistic intervention. . . .

INTERFERENCE WITH A SUICIDE ATTEMPT

[We now consider a suicide prevention policy specified as] the "minimal" policy of interfering with a suicide attempt in progress or about to begin and providing medical assistance, where needed, to the attempter. The degree of interference here is quite minor; it might include, for example, removing a person from a building ledge from which he was about to leap, giving artificial respiration to a person found unconscious from gas inhalation, or lavaging the stomach of someone who has taken sleeping pills. Where necessary, because of medical considerations or for purposes of restraint, transportation to a hospital emergency room or detention facility would be authorized. The duration of intervention, however, would be limited; the time span required for the kind of intervention we have in mind would not exceed 24 hours, and might frequently be less.[10]

At the end of this brief period, restraint would no longer be authorized; persons wishing to go about their business would be free to do so. In particular, they would be free to resume their suicidal behavior. To prevent the minimal policy from escalating into more protracted restraint, it would be necessary to require a waiting period before intervention could be repeated.

The foregoing policy confers benefits and also entails costs. The major benefit is that it would save the lives of almost all suicide attempters. There is abundant testimony from psychiatrists experienced in the treatment of suicide attempters that survivors of an attempt rarely pose a danger of immediate suicide, even when opportunities for further attempts are not lacking. For this reason, the stringent time limit on intervention would entail a sacrifice of very few lives. This feature makes the policy especially attractive. Moreover, even the small number of subsequent suicides that will continue to occur need not necessarily be considered failures of the policy, since those persons will at least have been provided a chance for reconsideration.[11]

There are several disadvantages to this policy. Some small number of individuals will die who would have changed their minds had they been held for a longer period. Others, firmly committed to suicide, will be detained for a period of some hours. This may be annoying, perhaps extremely distressing. Nevertheless, there are reasons for not being too concerned with this small number of individuals. First, their distress will come to an end in a few hours; secondly, those concerned with avoiding this delay could simply choose a time, place and method unlikely to attract attention.[12]

To reduce some of this imposition, the state might even accommodate determined attempters by granting immunity from any interference to those who register their intention to commit suicide in advance, or by providing resources for painless suicide following a short waiting period so as to be confident that only those who wish to die kill themselves. Despite these provisions, however, some genuinely suicidal persons are likely to be subjected to distress, embarrassment and inconvenience because, contrary to plans, their suicide attempt has been interrupted.

A third class of individuals who may suffer from the minimal policy consists of those who are falsely identified as having been engaged in a suicide attempt or whose attempt would have had no serious consequences and who would not have gone on to a more serious attempt in the absence of intervention. These persons may incur inconvenience and some degree of stigmatization as the result of having been considered suicidal.

Nevertheless, the negative consequences of mistaken identification do not seem serious enough to constitute fatal objections to this proposal. An analogy to arrests for criminal law violations is instructive. Under the "probable cause" standard some innocent persons undoubtedly are wrongly arrested and charged. Though regrettable, the undeserved inconvenience and stigmatization are thought to be unavoidable consequences of law enforcement practices believed to be necessary to the public welfare. Our desire to minimize the unavoidable evil might, for example, lead to protection of the confidentiality of arrest records, but not to outright elimination of the power to arrest, absent an alternative procedure to handle the charging of individuals with crimes and the production of them at trial. The judgment is made that our interest in safety from crime is sufficient to warrant risking some interference with our activities through wrongful arrest.[13] On the other side of the coin, a person suspected of criminal activity cannot lawfully be taken into custody unless there is at least "probable cause" to believe that he committed the crime. Relaxation of this restriction might result in the taking into custody of some criminals who at present are free to con-

tinue preying on innocent victims, but we forfeit this potential benefit in order to remain free from arrest based on mere suspicion of involvement in criminal activity.

It is doubtful that coercive suicide prevention is as justifiable as coercive crime prevention; the social consequences of unpunished serious crime probably are much greater than those of unprevented suicide. Failing to attach legal sanctions to acts seriously harmful to the life of another, for example, may lead to vigilantism. Nevertheless, the considerable benefits to be obtained from minimal restraint of suicide attempters seem to us sufficient to justify the limited degree of interference proposed here, notwithstanding its costs for "truly" suicidal persons and for those who are not suicidal at all....

NOTES

1 Douglas, "The Absurd in Suicide," in *On the Nature of Suicide* 111, 117–18 (E. Shneidman ed. 1969).
2 Rubinstein, Moses & Lidz, "On Attempted Suicide," 79 *A.M.A. Archives of Neurology & Psychiatry* 103, 111(1958). Characteristically, the authors of this study found:

The patient was involved in a struggle with the persons important to him and sought a modification of their attitudes or a specific change in his relationships with them. After a crisis was reached in this struggle, the patient sought to effect these changes through a suicide attempt....Patients sometimes told of seeking such changes prior to their suicide attempt, of seeking them through the attempt, and by still other means afterward....

Id. at 109.
3 Weiss, "The Suicidal Patient," in *American Handbook of Psychiatry* 115, 121 (S. Arieto ed. 1966).
4 Rubinstein, Moses & Lidz, *supra*, at 105.
5 Moss & Hamilton, "Psychotherapy of the Suicidal Patient," in *Clues to Suicide* 99, 107 (E. Shneidman & N. Farberow eds. 1957).
6 J. Choron, *Suicide* 50 (1972), cites several studies from different countries in which 90% to 100% of rescued suicide attempters reported they were glad they had been saved.
7 Alan Dershowitz has called this line of reasoning the "Thank you, doctor" doctrine (private conversation with the author). The concept also is employed under the label "future-oriented consent" in Wexler,

"Therapeutic Justice," 57 *Minn. L. Rev.* 289, 330–32 (1972). We shall refer to the concept in this article as the principle of retrospective gratitude.

8 J. Rawls, *A Theory of Justice* 136–42 (1971).

9 Thus, in Litman & Farberow, "Emergency Evaluation of Suicidal Potential," in *The Psychology of Suicide* 259, 268 (E. Shneidman, N. Farberow, & R. Litman eds. 1970), an example is given of a woman who claimed that her husband was living "in a dream world" and wanted him committed on grounds that he was likely to kill himself. Upon investigation it turned out that he frequently lost much of his wages gambling. The woman wanted him committed so that she could use his money to straighten out their financial affairs. Sympathetic as we might be with her plight, we would want to provide protection against the use of suicide prevention commitment proceedings to advance goals having nothing to do with suicide prevention. Even where there is no deliberate attempt to deceive or to misuse statutory provisions, we still would need to be on guard against family members who are sincere but mistaken in their belief that a suicide attempt may be imminent.

10 As defined here, then, minimal interference includes simple restraint at the scene, arrest and removal from the scene and very short-term detainment. Although we consider these together as "minimal," it ultimately might prove useful to distinguish among them and perhaps permit only the least restrictive. These distinctions need not be discussed here.

11 This need not mean that we should be complacent about suicides, only that this particular coercive policy cannot be made to shoulder the burden of suicide prevention.

12 Ordinarily this should not be too difficult. A major exception might be individuals incarcerated in total institutions where suicide, though certainly not impossible, can be made much more difficult by intensive surveillance and deprivation of materials from which weapons can be constructed. I am indebted to Andrew von Hirsch for this observation.

13 On the other hand, we become much more alarmed at more extended pretrial detention, as its disruptive effects mount rapidly when its duration begins to exceed 24 hours. It is clear that, behind the veil of ignorance, we would never accept the class bias built into current pretrial release procedures.

The Refusal of Life-Sustaining Treatment

Consent, Coercion, and Conflicts of Rights
Ruth Macklin

A biographical sketch of Ruth Macklin is found on page 192.

Macklin focuses attention on the moral issues raised by the case of the Jehovah's Witness who desires to refuse a blood transfusion for religious reasons. In her analysis, the right to refuse blood transfusions may be defended not only by appeal to the right to exercise one's religious beliefs but also by appeal to the autonomy of the patient *qua* person, that is, to the individual's right to decide matters affecting his or her own life and death. In direct conflict with these rights, however, is the right of the doctor to do what correct medical practice dictates. Macklin argues that it is morally justifiable to administer blood transfusions to minor children against the religious objections of parents. It is also morally justifiable to administer

Reprinted with permission of the author and the publisher from *Perspectives in Biology and Medicine*, vol. 20, no. 3 (Spring 1977), pp. 360–371. Copyright © 1977 by the University of Chicago.

blood transfusions to *incompetent* adult patients. However, she insists, the only justification for compelling a competent adult Jehovah's Witness to accept blood transfusions is a paternalistic one, and such a paternalistic intervention is morally unjustified. Still, the doctor's right to do what correct medical practice dictates must be respected. "A patient can knowingly refuse treatment, but he cannot demand mistreatment."

Cases of conflict of rights are not infrequent in law and morality. A range of cases that has gained increasing prominence recently centers around the autonomy of persons and their right to make decisions in matters affecting their own life and death. This paper will focus on a particular case of conflict of rights: the case of Jehovah's Witnesses who refuse blood transfusions for religious reasons and the question of whether or not there exists a right to compel medical treatment. The Jehovah's Witnesses who refuse blood transfusions do not do so because they want to die: in most cases, however, they appear to believe that they will die if their blood is not transfused. Members of this sect are acting on what is generally believed to be a constitutionally guaranteed right: freedom of religion, which is said to include not only freedom of religious belief, but also the right to act on such beliefs.

This study will examine a cluster of moral issues surrounding the Jehovah's Witness case. Some pertain to minor children of Jehovah's Witness parents, while others concern adult Witnesses who refuse treatment for themselves. The focus will be on the case as a moral one rather than a legal one, although arguments employed in some of the legal cases will be invoked. This is an issue at the intersection of law and morality—one in which the courts themselves have rendered conflicting decisions and have looked to moral principles for guidance. As is usually the case in ethics, whatever the courts may have decided does not settle the moral dispute, but the arguments and issues invoked in legal disputes often mirror the ethical dimensions of the case. The conflict—in both law and morals—arises out of a religious prohibition against blood transfusions, a prohibition that rests on an interpretation of certain scriptural passages by the Jehovah's Witness sect.

THE RELIGIOUS BASIS FOR THE PROHIBITION OF BLOOD TRANSFUSIONS

The Witnesses' prohibition of blood transfusions derives from an interpretation of several Old Testament pas-

sages, chief among which is the following from Lev. 17:10–14:

> And whatsoever man there be of the house of Israel, or of the strangers that sojourn among you, that eateth any manner of blood: I will even set my face against that soul that eateth blood, and will cut him off from among his people. . . .

The question immediately arises, On what basis do the Jehovah's Witnesses construe intravenous blood transfusions as an instance of eating blood? Witnesses sometimes claim that the prohibition against transfusions arises out of a literal interpretation of the relevant biblical passages, but the interpretation in question seems anything but "literal." One explanation for this is as follows: "Since they have been prohibited by the Bible from eating blood, they steadfastly proclaim that intravenous transfusion has no bearing on the matter, as it basically makes no difference whether the blood enters by the vein or by the alimentary tract. In their widely quoted reference *Blood, Medicine, and the Law of God* they constantly refer to the medical printed matter which early in the 20th century declared that blood transfusions are nothing more than a source of nutrition by a shorter route than ordinary" [1, p. 539]. Whether based on a literal interpretation of the Bible or not, the Witnesses' prohibition against transfusions extends not only to whole blood, but also to any blood derivative, such as plasma and albumin (blood substitutes are, however, quite acceptable) [1, p. 539].

This brief account of the basis of the religious prohibition has not yet addressed the moral issues involved: but for the sake of completeness, let us note two additional features of the Jehovah's Witness view—features that bear directly on the moral conflict.

The first point concerns the Witnesses' belief about the consequences of violating the prohibition: Receiving blood transfusions is an unpardonable sin resulting in withdrawal of the opportunity to attain eternal life [2]. In particular, the transgression is punishable by being "cut off": "Since the Witnesses do not believe in eternal damnation, to be 'cut off' signifies losing one's opportunity to qualify for resurrection" [3, p. 75]. A second, related feature of the Witnesses' belief system is their view that man's life on earth is not important: "They fervently believe that they are only passing through and that the faithful who have not been corrupted nor polluted will attain eternal life in Heaven" [1, p. 539]. This belief is important in the structure of a moral argument that pits the value of preservation of life on earth against other values, for example, presumed eternal life in Heaven. Put another way, the Witnesses can argue that the duty to preserve or prolong human life is always overridden by their perceived duty to God, so in a case of conflict, duty to God dictates the right course of action.

THE ADULT JEHOVAH'S WITNESS PATIENT

Freedom to exercise one's religious beliefs is one important aspect of the moral and legal issues involved in these cases. But in addition to this specific constitutionally guaranteed right, there are other rights and moral values that would be relevant even if religious freedom were not at issue. Even in cases that do not involve religious freedom at all, the question of the right to compel medical treatment against a patient's wishes raises some knotty moral problems. The Jehovah's Witness case may prove instructive for the range of cases in which religious freedom is not at issue.

Just which rights or values are involved in the adult Jehovah's Witness case, and how do they conflict? We shall return later to the right to act on one's religious beliefs, but first let us look at other moral concepts that enter into Witnesses' moral defense. Chief among these is the notion of autonomy. Does the patient in a medical setting have the autonomy that we normally accord persons simply by virtue of their being human? Or does one's status as a *patient* deprive him of a measure of autonomy normally accorded him as a nonpatient *person*? Many medical practitioners tend to argue for decreased autonomy of patients, while some religious ethicists, a number of moral philosophers, and a small number of physicians defend autonomous decision making on the part of patients. So one clearly identifiable moral issue concerns the autonomy of a person who becomes a patient. Does he or she have the right to make decisions about the details of medical treatment and about whether some treatments are to be undertaken at all?

One may defend the Witnesses' right to refuse blood transfusions by appealing to the autonomy of the patient *qua* person solely on moral grounds, without even invoking First Amendment freedoms (i.e., freedom of religion).

The right of autonomous decision making on the part of the patient is in direct conflict with a right claimed on behalf of the treating physician: the "professional" right (duty, perhaps) of a doctor to do what correct medical practice dictates. As one writer notes: "In our society, medical treatment is a right which is guaranteed to every citizen, regardless of his religious tenets. But it is also the physician's inherent, albeit uncodified, right not to have constraints applied to a therapeutic program, which he regards as necessary for the patient's welfare or survival" [3, p. 73]. Unlike other sorts of cases involving refusal of medical treatment on religious grounds (notably, Christian Scientists' refusal to accept any medical treatment), Jehovah's Witnesses are opposed only to one specific treatment regimen: transfusion of whole blood or blood fractions. As a result, Witnesses visit doctors, voluntarily enter hospitals, and submit themselves to the usual range of treatments, with the singular exception of accepting transfusions. The question arises, then, Does the physician have a duty to do everything for a patient that is dictated by accepted medical practice? In a court case in 1965 (*United States v. George*, 33 LW 2518), the court argued that "the patient voluntarily submitted himself to and insisted on medical treatment. At the same time, he sought to dictate a course of treatment to his physician which amounted to malpractice. The court held that under these circumstances, a physician cannot be required to ignore the mandates of his own conscience, even in the name of the exercise of religious freedom. A patient can knowingly refuse treatment, but he cannot demand mistreatment" [3, p. 78].

The right or duty of a physician, as described here, does seem to be in direct conflict with both (1) the religious freedom of the Jehovah's Witness patient and (2) the autonomy of the patient as a person, or his right to decide on matters affecting his own life and death. The worth of human life and the duty to preserve it are usually viewed as paramount moral values in our culture. Since those arguing in favor of the right to compel medical treatment will invoke this important value in their defense, the moral dilemma has no clear solution.

It is worth noting briefly several additional moral issues involved in the adult Jehovah's Witness case. One is the issue of informed consent. Because of the refusal of

Jehovah's Witnesses to grant consent to transfuse themselves or their relatives (including minor children), physicians may not (morally or legally) act contrary to the patient's wishes. But a court order may be obtained authorizing the physician to transfuse the patient. What, then, is the status of the requirement for "informed consent" in medical matters if the patient's publicly expressed wishes can be overridden by a doctor who obtains a court order? A second relevant moral issue concerns the competency of the Jehovah's Witness patient to make the decision about transfusion at the time that decision needs to be made. Is a semicomatose person competent to make decisions? Is a person in excruciating pain competent? A person suffering from mild shock? Surely, an unconscious person is not. In this last case, and perhaps the preceding ones as well, someone other than the patient must make the decision to refuse transfusion for him. Perhaps the patient, with death as the consequence of refusing treatment, would abandon his religious tenet in favor of the desire to live. Ought a family member decide for the patient, when the patient is unable to decide for himself? There is, obviously, no easy solution to these moral dilemmas. Arguments that rest on sound moral principles can be constructed to support either view, and such arguments have been embodied in several legal cases in the past few years. We shall return to these considerations in the final section, but first we turn to the overlapping, yet somewhat different set of issues concerning minor children of Jehovah's Witnesses.

TRANSFUSING MINOR CHILDREN OF JEHOVAH'S WITNESSES

The moral principles involved in the case of minor children of Jehovah's Witnesses differ in some important respects from principles that enter into the case of adult Witnesses who refuse transfusions for themselves. It is worth noting that all legal cases in which the transfusion of minor children was at issue were decided in favor of transfusing the child, against the religious objections of the parents. In these cases, the arguments given by the courts are a mixture of citation of legal statutes and precedents and appeal to moral principles. In one case in Ohio the court argued as follows: "...While [parents] may, under certain circumstances, deprive [their child] of his liberty or his property, under no circumstances, with or without religious sanction, may they deprive him of his life!" [4, p. 131]. In this and other legal decisions,

the religious right of the parents is seen as secondary to the right to life and health on the part of the child....

It might be argued that Jehovah's Witness parents, in refusing permission for blood to be given to their child, are acting in accordance with their perceived duty to God, as dictated by their religion, and that this duty to God overrides whatever secular duties they may have to preserve the life and health of their child. Here it can only be replied that when an action done in accordance with perceived duties to God results in the likelihood of harm or death to another person (whether child or adult), then the duties to preserve life here on earth take precedence. The duties of a physician are to preserve and prolong life and to alleviate suffering. These duties are not in the least mitigated by considerations of God's will, the possibility of life after death, or a view that God at some later time rewards those who suffer here on earth. Freedom of religion does not include the right to act in a manner that will result in harm or death to others.

If the parents refuse to grant permission for blood to be given to their child when failure to give blood will result in death or severe harm to the child, their *prima facie* right to retain control over their child no longer exists. Whatever the parents' reasons for refusing to allow blood to be given, and whether the parents believe that the child will survive or not, the case sufficiently resembles that of child neglect (in respect to harm to the child): in the absence of fulfillment of their primary duties, it is morally justifiable to take control of the child away from parents and administer blood transfusions against the parents' wishes and contrary to their religious convictions.

RIGHTS AND THE CONFLICT OF RIGHTS

It is evident that the case of the adult Jehovah's Witness who refuses blood transfusions for himself is a good deal more complicated than that of minor children of Jehovah's Witness parents. The arguments—both moral and legal—in the case of children rest largely on the moral belief that no one has the right or authority to make life-threatening decisions for persons unable to make those decisions for themselves. If this analysis is sound, it supplies a principle for dealing with the case of the adult patient who is not in a position to state his wishes at the time the treatment is medically required. This principle is avowedly paternalistic but is intended to be applied in those cases where a measure of paternalism seems morally justifiable. To the extent that a person is unable or not fully competent to decide for himself at the time transfusion is needed, it seems appropriate for medical personnel to decide in favor of life-saving treatment. Whatever a person may have claimed prior to an emergency in which death is imminent, and regardless of what relatives may claim on his behalf, it is morally wrong for others to act in a manner that will probably result in his death.

The task of ascertaining a person's competence to make decisions for himself presents a myriad of problems, some of them moral, some epistemological, and some conceptual. These problems are no different, in principle, from the difficulty of ascertaining the competency of retarded persons, the mentally ill, aged senile persons, and others. This is not to suggest that no difficulty exists but, rather, that similar problems arise in many other sorts of cases where competency needs to be ascertained for moral or legal or practical reasons.

There are several recent court cases dealing with adult Jehovah's Witness patients. In some of these cases the court refused the request to transfuse the patient: in others, the court decided that transfusion was warranted, despite the religious objections. The case of *John F. Kennedy Memorial Hospital v. Heston* was one of those in which transfusion was ordered, contrary to the patient's religious convictions. But it is important to note that the patient was deemed incompetent to make the decision for herself at the time transfusion was needed. The judge who delivered the court's opinion stated:

> Delores Heston, age 22 and unmarried, was severely injured in an automobile accident. She was taken to the plaintiff hospital where it was determined that she would expire unless operated upon for a ruptured spleen and that if operated upon she would expire unless whole blood was administered. . . . Miss Heston insists she expressed her refusal to accept blood, but the evidence indicated she was in shock on admittance to the hospital and in the judgment of the attending physicians and nurses was then or soon became disoriented and incoherent. Her mother remained adamant in her opposition to a transfusion, and signed a release of liability for the hospital and medical personnel. Miss Heston did not execute a release; presumably she could not. Her father could not be located. [5, p. 671]

This case, then, fits the principle suggested above: To the extent that a person is unable or not fully competent to decide for himself at the time transfusion is needed, it

seems appropriate for medical personnel to decide in favor of life-saving treatment.

In another case, *In re Osborne*, the court decided against transfusion. But here it was ascertained that the patient was not impaired in his ability to make judgments, that he "understood the consequences of his decision, and had with full understanding executed a statement refusing the recommended transfusion and releasing the hospital from liability" [6, p. 373]. This decision might be defended, in a moral argument, by appealing to the notion of the autonomy of persons; the legal defense rests, however, on the constitutionally guaranteed freedom of religion. A footnote in the court's opinion in *Osborne* says: "No case has come to light where refusal of medical care was based on individual choice absent religious convictions." But whether based on the moral concept of autonomy, or on the legal and moral right to act on one's religious beliefs, the right of a person (whose competency has been ascertained) to refuse medical treatment must be viewed as a viable moral alternative. Such a right rests on the precept of individual liberty that protects persons of sound mind against paternalistic interference by others.

CONCLUSION

It seems apparent that the only justification that can be offered for the coercive act of administering a blood transfusion without a person's consent and against his will is a paternalistic one. I follow that characterization of paternalism put forth by Gerald Dworkin: "the interference with a person's liberty of action justified by reasons referring exclusively to the welfare, good, happiness, needs, interests or values of the person being coerced" [7, p. 65]. Now a person's life is involved in his welfare or good in the extreme—so much so, it might be argued, that it is not on a par with other things that contribute to one's welfare. Indeed, the existence of life is a necessary condition for there being any welfare, happiness, needs, interests, or values at all. Still, interference with a person's (presumably rational) decision to end his life or allow it to end presupposes a belief on the part of the interferer that he knows what is best for the person. This would, in fact, be the case if a Jehovah's Witness patient believed that he would not die if he were not transfused in cases where informed medical opinion predicts the reverse. But the Witness who accepts the high probability of his own death and still refuses transfusion does not disagree concerning matters of empirical fact with those who wish to interfere on his behalf. Dworkin identifies this as a value conflict, a case in which "a value such as health—or indeed life—may be overridden by competing values. Thus the problem with the [Jehovah's Witness] and blood transfusions. It may be more important for him to reject 'impure substances' than to go on living" [7, p. 78]. But Dworkin is wrong if he construes this as solely a question of conflict in values, and he is also mistaken in identifying one of the competing values as rejection of "impure substances." It is, rather, eternal life over against mortal life that the Jehovah's Witness is weighing, and rather than risk being "cut off" he opts to allow his mortal life to terminate.

It would appear, then, that beliefs about metaphysical matters of fact—as well as competing values—are involved in the Jehovah's Witness's decision. That such beliefs may be mistaken or ill founded is not sufficient warrant for paternalistic interference, unless it can be shown that persons who entertain such beliefs are irrational. But it would fly in the face of longstanding traditions and practices—especially in America—to deem persons irrational solely on the basis of religious convictions that differ from our own. If, however, the Witnesses are not to be judged irrational by virtue of their religious belief system, then the one clearly acceptable ground for paternalistic intervention is pulled out from under. Medical practitioners are sometimes criticized for acting in a paternalistic manner toward patients, so it is not surprising to see physicians advocate a course of action that overrides a patient's expressed wishes. But if the patient is deemed competent or rational (by whatever practical criteria are employed or ought to be adopted), then there is no warrant for interfering with his decisions, even those that affect his continued existence. Unless all decisions to end one's life (or allow it to terminate) are viewed as *ex hypothesi* irrational, interference with a person's liberty to choose in favor of what he believes to take precedence over continued mortal existence is an act of unjustified paternalism. Paternalism may be considered justifiable in cases where the agent is incompetent to make informed or rational judgments about his own welfare. The Jehovah's Witness who refuses a blood transfusion may be *mistaken* about what is in his long-range welfare, but he is not incompetent to make judgments based on his belief system. It is only if we decide that his particular set of religious beliefs constitutes good evidence for his overall irrationality that we are justified in interfering paternalistically with his liberty. While I am personally inclined to view such religious belief systems as irrational (because they are not warranted on the evidence), I do not thereby deem their

proponents irrational *in a general sense* for holding such beliefs. And this, it seems, is the correct way of looking at the case of adult Jehovah's Witnesses who are deemed mentally competent (according to the usual medical criteria) and yet who refuse blood transfusions. Only if we are prepared to accept paternalistic interference with the liberty of (otherwise) rational or competent adults in similar cases are we justified in transfusing these patients against their expressed wishes.

We cannot let the matter rest here, however, because of the problems this solution would pose for medical practice. It has been argued above that the physician has a "right not to have constraints applied to a therapeutic program, which he regards as necessary for the patient's welfare or survival"; and one court opinion stated that "a physician cannot be required to ignore the mandates of his own conscience, even in the name of the exercise of religious freedom. A patient can knowingly refuse treatment, but he cannot demand mistreatment." Jehovah's Witnesses who present themselves for treatment and who are judged rational or competent to give or withhold consent should be given the option of either (a) being treated in accordance with the dictates of accepted medical practice, including blood transfusion if necessary; or (b) refusing in advance any treatment in which transfusion is normally a necessary component or is likely to be required in the case at hand. Presenting these options to the patient preserves his decision-making autonomy while not requiring the physician to embark on a treatment that amounts to malpractice.

If it is objected that this proposed solution violates the precepts of accepted medical practice, I can only reply that those precepts embody a measure of paternalism that is unjustifiable when judged against a principle of individual liberty that mandates autonomy of decision making for rational adult persons. Moreover, the precepts of accepted medical practice have been known to change, varying with the introduction of new medical technology, transformations in social consciousness, and other alterations in the status quo. Not all patients who can be treated vigorously are so treated; one aspect of current debates focuses on the moral dilemmas surrounding patient autonomy—the sorts of problems addressed in this paper. Consistent with the decision-making autonomy accorded a patient who is deemed rational enough to offer informed consent is the right of a physician to refuse to be dictated to in matters of medical competence. Once treatment is undertaken, the judgment that a blood transfusion is necessary would seem to be a judgment requiring medical competence. The decision to undertake treatment at all in such cases is not a purely medical matter but might well be decided by a patient who has full knowledge of the consequences yet who insists nonetheless on what amounts to partial treatment or mistreatment by attending physicians.

I have argued that the autonomy of patients, as rational persons, ought to be respected. But this autonomy implies a responsibility for one's decision—a responsibility that entails acceptance of the consequences. And these consequences include the right of physicians to reject a treatment regimen proposed by the patient, which is contrary to sound medical practice. If, faced with this consequence, some Jehovah's Witnesses opt for treatment with transfusion rather than no treatment at all, so much the better for such cases of conflict of rights. Those Witnesses who remain steadfast in their refusal to accept transfusions are exercising their right of autonomous decision making in matters concerning their own welfare—in the words of Justice Louis Brandeis, "the right to be let alone." In a judicial opinion rendered in a case involving a Jehovah's Witness who refused transfusion, Justice Warren Burger recalled Brandeis's view as follows: "Nothing in [his] utterance suggests that Justice Brandeis thought an individual possessed these rights only as to *sensible* beliefs, *valid* thoughts, *reasonable* emotions, or *well-founded* sensations. I suggest he intended to include a great many foolish, unreasonable, and even absurd ideas which do not conform, such as refusing medical treatment even at great risk"[8]. The risks are indeed great in the cases we have been discussing. But the sorts of risks to health or life a person may take, in the interest of something he considers worth the risk, appear to know no bounds. If an adult agent is rational and competent to make decisions, the risks are his to take.

REFERENCES

1 I. G. Thomas, R. W. Edmark, and T. W. Jones. *Am. Surg.*, 34:538, 1968.
2 W. T. Fitts, Jr., and M. J. Orloff. *Surg. Gynecol. Obstet.*, 180:502, 1959.
3 D. C. Schechter. *Am. J. Surg.*, 116:73, 1968.
4 *In re* Clark, 185 N.E. 2d 128, 1962.
5 John F. Kennedy Memorial Hospital *v* Heston, 279 A. 2d 670, 1971.
6 *In re* Osborne, 294 A. 2d 372, 1972.
7 G. Dworkin. *Monist*, 56:64, 1972.
8 Application of President and Directors of Georgetown College, 331 F. 2n 1010 (D.C. Cir.), 1964.

The Least Worst Death
M. Pabst Battin

M. Pabst Battin is associate professor of philosophy at the University of Utah. She is the author of *Ethical Issues in Suicide* (1982) and the coeditor of *Suicide: The Philosophical Issues* (1980). Her published articles include "Manipulated Suicide," "Euthanasia," and "Exact Replication in the Visual Arts."

Battin analyzes the notion of a "natural death" and its relationship to the refusal of medical treatment. On her analysis, a dying patient who chooses to embrace a "natural death" usually has in mind "a painless, conscious, dignified, culminative slipping-away." Such a patient will then typically assert his or her right to refuse medical treatment, since this is the only legally protected mechanism available for a patient trying to achieve a "natural death." But often, Battin maintains, refusal of treatment brings about a sort of death very far from what the patient had in mind. In her view, the key to this dilemma is the *selective* refusal of treatment. With a physician in the role of "strategist of natural death," Battin argues, a patient can effectively achieve "the least worst death among those that could naturally occur."

Reprinted with permission of the author and the publisher from *Hastings Center Report*, vol. 13 (April 1983), pp. 13–16.

In recent years "right-to-die" movements have brought into the public consciousness something most physicians have long known: that in some hopeless medical conditions, heroic efforts to extend life may no longer be humane, and the physician must be prepared to allow the patient to die. Physician responses to patients' requests for "natural death" or "death with dignity" have been, in general, sensitive and compassionate. But the successes of the right-to-die movement have had a bitterly ironic result: institutional and legal protections for "natural death" have, in some cases, actually made it more painful to die.

There is just one legally protected mechanism for achieving natural death: refusal of medical treatment. It is available to both competent and incompetent patients. In the United States, the competent patient is legally entitled to refuse medical treatment of any sort on any personal or religious grounds, except perhaps where the interests of minor children are involved. A number of court cases, including *Quinlan, Saikewicz, Spring,* and *Eichner,*[1] have established precedent in the treatment of an incompetent patient for a proxy refusal by a family member or guardian. In addition, eleven states now have specific legislation protecting the physician from legal action for failure to render treatment when a competent patient has executed a directive to be followed after he is no longer competent. A durable power of attorney, executed by the competent patient in favor of a trusted relative or friend, is also used to determine treatment choices after incompetence occurs.

AN EARLIER BUT NOT EASIER DEATH

In the face of irreversible, terminal illness, a patient may wish to die sooner but "naturally," without artificial prolongation of any kind. By doing so, the patient may believe he is choosing a death that is, as a contributor to the *New England Journal of Medicine* has put it, "comfortable, decent, and peaceful";[2] "natural death," the patient may assume, means a death that is easier than a medically prolonged one.[3] That is why he is willing to undergo death earlier and that is why, he assumes, natural death is legally protected. But the patient may conceive of "natural death" as more than pain-free; he may assume that it will allow time for reviewing life and saying farewell to family and loved ones, for last rites or final words, for passing on hopes, wisdom, confessions, and blessings to the next generation. These ideas are of course heavily stereotyped; they are the product of literary and cultural traditions associated with conventional death-bed scenes, reinforced by movies, books, and news stories, religious models, and just plain wishful thinking. Even the very term "natural" may have stereotyped connotations for the patient: something close to nature, uncontrived, and appropriate. As a result of these notions, the patient often takes "natural death" to be a painless, conscious, dignified, culminative slipping-away.

Now consider what sorts of death actually occur under the rubric of "natural death." A patient suffers a cardiac arrest and is not resuscitated. Result: sudden unconsciousness, without pain, and death within a number of seconds. Or a patient has an infection that is not treated. Result: the unrestrained multiplication of micro-organisms, the production of toxins, interference with organ function, hypotension, and death. On the way there may be fever, delirium, rigor or shaking, and light-headedness; death usually takes one or two days, depending on the organism involved. If the kidneys fail and dialysis or transplant is not undertaken, the patient is generally more conscious, but experiences nausea, vomiting, gastrointestinal hemorrhage (evident in vomiting blood), inability to concentrate, neuromuscular irritability or twitching, and eventually convulsions. Dying may take from days to weeks, unless such circumstances as high potassium levels intervene. Refusal of amputation, although painless, is characterized by fever, chills, and foul-smelling tissues. Hypotension, characteristic of dehydration and many other states, is not painful but also not pleasant: the patient cannot sit up or get out of bed, has a dry mouth and thick tongue, and may find it difficult to talk. An untreated respiratory death involves conscious air hunger. This means gasping, an increased breathing rate, a panicked feeling of inability to get air in or out. Respiratory deaths may take only minutes; on the other hand, they may last for hours. If the patient refuses intravenous fluids, he may become dehydrated. If he refuses surgery for cancer, an organ may rupture. Refusal of treatment does not simply bring about death in a vacuum, so to speak; death always occurs from some specific cause.

Many patients who are dying in these ways are either comatose or heavily sedated. Such deaths do not allow for a period of conscious reflection at the end of life, nor do they permit farewell-saying, last rites, final words, or other features of the stereotypically "dignified" death.

Even less likely to match the patient's conception of natural death are those cases in which the patient is still conscious and competent, but meets a death that is quite different than he had bargained for. Consider the bowel cancer patient with widespread metastases and a very poor prognosis who—perhaps partly out of consideration for the emotional and financial resources of his family—refuses surgery to reduce or bypass the tumor. How, exactly, will he die? This patient is clearly within his legal rights in refusing surgery, but the physician knows what the outcome is very likely to be: obstruction of the intestinal tract will occur, the bowel wall will perforate, the abdomen will become distended, there will be intractible vomiting (perhaps with a fecal character to the emesis), and the tumor will erode into adjacent areas, causing increased pain, hemorrhage, and sepsis. Narcotic sedation and companion drugs may be partially effective in controlling pain, nausea, and vomiting, but this patient will *not* get the kind of death he thought he had bargained for. Yet, he was willing to shorten his life, to use the single legally protected mechanism—refusal of treatment—to achieve that "natural" death. Small wonder that many physicians are skeptical of the "gains" made by the popular movements supporting the right to die.

WHEN THE RIGHT TO DIE GOES WRONG

Several distinct factors contribute to the backfiring of the right-to-die cause. First, and perhaps the most obvious, the patient may misjudge his own situation in refusing treatment or in executing a natural-death directive: his refusal may be precipitous and ill informed, based more on fear than on a settled desire to die. Second, the physician's response to the patient's request for "death with dignity" may be insensitive, rigid, or even punitive (though in my experience most physicians respond with compassion and wisdom). Legal constraints may also make natural death more difficult than might be hoped: safeguards often render natural-death requests and directives cumbersome to execute, and in any case, in a litigation-conscious society, the physician will often take the most cautious route.

But most important in the apparent backfiring of the right-to-die movement is the underlying ambiguity in the very concept of "natural death." Patients tend to think of the character of the experience they expect to undergo—a death that is "comfortable, decent, peaceful"—but all the law protects is the refusal of medical procedures. Even lawmakers sometimes confuse the two. The California and Kansas natural-death laws claim to protect what they romantically describe as "the natural process of dying." North Carolina's statute says it protects the right to a "peaceful and natural" death. But since these laws actually protect only refusal of treatment, they can hardly guarantee a peaceful, easy death. Thus, we see a widening gulf between the intent of the law to protect the patient's final desires, and the outcomes if the law is actually followed. The physician is caught in between: he recognizes his patient's right to die peacefully, naturally, and with whatever dignity is possible, but foresees the unfortunate results that may come about when the patient exercises this right as the law permits.

Of course, if the symptoms or pain become unbearable the patient may change his mind. The patient who earlier wished not to be "hooked up on tubes" now begins to experience difficulty in breathing or swallowing, and finds that a tracheotomy will relieve his distress. The bowel cancer patient experiences severe discomfort from obstruction, and gives permission for decompression or reductive surgery after all. In some cases, the family may engineer the change of heart because they find dying too hard to watch. Health care personnel may view these reversals with satisfaction: "See," they may say, "he really wants to live after all." But such reversals cannot always be interpreted as a triumph of the will to live; they may also be an indication that refusing treatment makes dying too hard.

OPTIONS FOR AN EASIER DEATH

How can the physician honor the dying patient's wish for a peaceful, conscious, and culminative death? There is more than one option.

Such a death can come about whenever the patient is conscious and pain-free; he can reflect and, if family, clergy, or friends are summoned at the time, he will be able to communicate as he wishes. Given these conditions, death can be brought on in various direct ways. For instance, the physician can administer a lethal quantity of an appropriate drug. Or the patient on severe dietary restrictions can violate his diet: the kidney-failure patient, for instance, for whom high potassium levels are fatal, can simply overeat on avocados. These ways of producing death are, of course, active euthanasia, or assisted or unassisted suicide. For many patients, such a death would count as "natural" and would satisfy the expectations under which they had chosen to die rather than to continue an intolerable existence. But for many patients (and for many physicians as well) a death that involves deliberate killing is morally wrong. Such a patient could never assent to an actively caused death, and even though it might be physically calm, it could hardly be emotionally or psychologically peaceful. This is not to say that active euthanasia or assisted suicide are morally wrong, but rather that the force of some patients' moral views about them precludes using such practices to achieve the kind of death they want. Furthermore, many physicians are unwilling to shoulder the legal risk such practices may seem to involve.

But active killing aside, the physician can do much to grant the dying patient the humane death he has chosen by using the sole legally protected mechanism that safeguards the right to die: refusal of treatment. This mechanism need not always backfire. For in almost any terminal condition, death can occur in various ways, and there are many possible outcomes of the patient's present condition. The patient who is dying of emphysema could die of respiratory failure, but could also die of cardiac arrest or untreated pulmonary infection. The patient who is suffering from bowel cancer could die of peritonitis following rupture of the bowel, but could also die of dehydration, of pulmonary infection, of acid-base imbalance, of electrolyte deficiency, or of an arrhythmia.

As the poet Rilke observes, we have a tendency to associate a certain sort of end with a specific disease: it is the "official death" for that sort of illness. But there are many other ways of dying than the official death, and the physician can take advantage of these. Infection and cancer, for instance, are old friends: there is increased frequency of infection in the immuno-compromised host. Other secondary conditions, like dehydration or metabolic derangement, may set in. Of course certain conditions typically occur a little earlier, others a little later, in the ordinary course of a terminal disease, and some are a matter of chance. The crucial point is that certain conditions will produce a death that is more comfortable, more decent, more predictable, and more permitting of conscious and peaceful experience than others. Some are better, if the patient has to die at all, and some are worse. Which mode of death claims the patient depends in part on circumstance and in part on the physician's response to conditions that occur. What the patient who rejects active euthanasia or assisted suicide may realisti-

cally hope for is this: the least worst death among those that could naturally occur. Not all unavoidable surrenders need involve rout; in the face of inevitable death, the physician becomes strategist, the deviser of plans for how to meet death most favorably.

He does so, of course, at the request of the patient, or, if the patient is not competent, the patient's guardian or kin. Patient autonomy is crucial in the notion of natural death. The physician could of course produce death by simply failing to offer a particular treatment to the patient. But to fail to *offer* treatment that might prolong life, at least when this does not compromise limited or very expensive resources to which other patients have claims, would violate the most fundamental principles of medical practice; some patients do not want "natural death," regardless of the physical suffering or dependency that prolongation of life may entail.

A scenario in which natural death is accomplished by the patient's selective refusal of treatment has one major advantage over active euthanasia and assisted suicide: refusal of treatment is clearly permitted and protected by law. Unfortunately, however, most patients do not have the specialized medical knowledge to use this self-protective mechanism intelligently. Few are aware that some kinds of refusal of treatment will better serve their desires for a "natural death" than others. And few patients realize that refusal of treatment can be selective. Although many patients with life-threatening illness are receiving multiple kinds of therapy, from surgery to nutritional support, most assume that it is only the major procedures (like surgery) that can be refused. (This misconception is perhaps perpetuated by the standard practice of obtaining specific consent for major procedures, like surgery, but not for minor, ongoing ones.) Then, too, patients may be unable to distinguish therapeutic from palliative procedures. And they may not understand the interaction between one therapy and another. In short, most patients do not have enough medical knowledge to foresee the consequences of refusing treatment on a selective basis; it is this that the physician must supply.

It is already morally and legally recognized that informed consent to a procedure involves explicit disclosure, both about the risks and outcomes of the proposed procedure and about the risks and outcomes of alternative possible procedures. Some courts, as in *Quackenbush*,[4] have also recognized the patient's right to explicit disclosure about the outcomes of refusing the proposed treatment. But though it is crucial in making a genuinely informed decision, the patient's right to information about the risks and outcomes of alternative kinds of refusal has not yet been recognized. So, for instance, in order to make a genuinely informed choice, the bowel cancer patient with concomitant infection will need to know about the outcomes of each of the principal options: accepting both bowel surgery and antibiotics; accepting antibiotics but not surgery; accepting surgery but not antibiotics; or accepting neither. The case may of course be more complex, but the principle remains: To recognize the patient's right to autonomous choice in matters concerning the treatment of his own body, the physician must provide information about all the legal options open to him, not just information sufficient to choose between accepting or rejecting a single proposed procedure.

One caveat: It sometimes occurs that physicians disclose the dismal probable consequences of refusing treatment in order to coerce patients into accepting the treatment they propose. This may be particularly common in surgery that will result in ostomy of the bowel. The patient is given a graphic description of the impending abdominal catastrophe—impaction, rupture, distention, hemorrhage, sepsis, and death. He thus consents readily to the surgery proposed. The paternalistic physician may find this maneuver appropriate, particularly since ostomy surgery is often refused out of vanity, depression, or on fatalistic grounds. But the physician who frightens a patient into accepting a procedure by describing the awful consequences of refusal is not honoring the patient's right to informed, autonomous choice: he has not described the various choices the patient could make, but only the worst.

Supplying the knowledge a patient needs in order to choose the least worst death need not require enormous amounts of additional energy or time on the part of the physician; it can be incorporated into the usual informed consent disclosures. If the patient is unable to accommodate the medical details, or instructs the physician to do what he thinks is best, the physician may use his own judgment in ordering and refraining from ordering treatment. If the patient clearly prefers to accept less life in hopes of an easy death, the physician should act in a way that will allow the least worst death to occur. In principle, however, the competent patient, and the proxy deciders for an incompetent patient, are entitled to explicit disclosure about all the alternatives for medical care. Physicians in burn units are already experienced in telling patients with very severe burns, where survival is unprecedented, what the outcome is likely to be if aggressive treatment is undertaken or if it is not—death in both cases, but under quite different conditions. Their expertise in these delicate matters might be most useful here. Informed refusal is just as much the patient's right as informed consent.

The role of the physician as strategist of natural death may be even more crucial in longer-term degenerative illnesses, where both physician and patient have far more advance warning that the patient's condition will deteriorate, and far more opportunity to work together in determining the conditions of the ultimate death. Of course, the first interest in both physician and patient will be strategies for maximizing the good life left. Nevertheless, many patients with long-term, eventually terminal illnesses, like multiple sclerosis, Huntington's chorea, diabetes, or chronic renal failure, may educate themselves considerably about the expected courses of their illnesses, and may display a good deal of anxiety about the end stages. This is particularly true in hereditary conditions where the patient may have watched a parent or relative die of the disease. But it is precisely in these conditions that the physician's opportunity may be greatest for humane guidance in the unavoidable matter of dying. He can help the patient to understand what the long-term options are in refusing treatment while he is competent, or help him to execute a natural-death directive or durable power of attorney that spells out the particulars of treatment refusal after he becomes incompetent.

Of course, some diseases are complex and not easy to explain. Patients are not always capable of listening very well, especially to unattractive possibilities concerning their own ends. And physicians are sometimes reluctant to acknowledge that their efforts to sustain life will eventually fail. Providing such information may also seem to undermine whatever hope the physician can nourish in the patient. But the very fact that the patient's demise is still far in the future makes it possible for the physician to describe various scenarios of how that death could occur, and at the same time give the *patient* control over which of them will actually happen. Not all patients will choose the same strategies of ending, nor is there any reason that they should. What may count as the "least worst" death to one person may be the most feared form of death to another. The physician may be able to increase the patient's psychological comfort immensely by giving him a way of meeting an unavoidable death on his own terms.

In both acute and long-term terminal illnesses, the key to good strategy is flexibility in considering *all* the possibilities at hand. These alternatives need not include active euthanasia or suicide measures of any kind, direct or indirect. To take advantage of the best of the naturally occurring alternatives is not to cause the patient's death, which will happen anyway, but to guide him away from the usual, frequently worst, end.

In the current enthusiasm for "natural death" it is not patient autonomy that dismays physicians. What does dismay them is the way in which respect for patient autonomy can lead to cruel results. The cure for that dismay lies in the realization that the physician can contribute to the *genuine* honoring of the patient's autonomy and rights, assuring him of "natural death" in the way in which the patient understands it, and still remain within the confines of good medical practice and the law.

REFERENCES

1 *In re Quinlan*, 355 A. 2d 647 (N.J. 1976); *Superintendent of Belchertown v. Saikewicz*, 370 N.E. 2d 417 (Mass. 1977); *In re Spring*, Mass. App., 399 N.E. 2d 493; *In re Eichner*, 73 A.D. 2d 431 (2nd Dept. 1980).

2 S. S. Spencer, "'Code' or 'No Code': A Nonlegal Opinion," *New England Journal of Medicine* 300 (1979), 138–140.

3 See Dallas M. High's analysis of the various senses of the term "natural death" in ordinary language, in "Is 'Natural Death' an Illusion?" *Hastings Center Report*, August 1978, pp. 37–42.

4 *In re Quackenbush*, 156 N.J. Super. 282, 353 A. 2d 785 (1978).

Resuscitation Decisions for Hospitalized Patients

President's Commission for the Study of Ethical Problems in Medicine and Biomedical and Behavioral Research

A descriptive account of the President's Commission is found on page 92.

Emphasizing the importance of advance deliberation, the Commission provides an extensive analysis of the ethical considerations relevant to resuscitation decisions. In the view of the Commission, patient self-determination is the most important ethical consideration. Accordingly, the decision of a competent patient should ordinarily be accepted. But the Commission also recognizes another important ethical consideration—patient well-being. Will resuscitation, in the judgment of the physician, promote patient welfare? After rejecting the idea that it is also appropriate to consider the costs of resuscitation in arriving at resuscitation decisions, the Commission proposes an overall scheme to guide decision making, taking into account both the competent and the incompetent patient.

Resuscitation after a cardiac arrest involves a series of steps directed toward sustaining adequate circulation of oxygenated blood to vital organs while heartbeat is restored.

Efforts typically involve the use of cardiac massage or chest compression and the delivery of oxygen under compression through an endo-tracheal tube into the lungs. An electrocardiogram is connected

Reprinted from President's Commission for the Study of Ethical Problems in Medicine and Biomedical and Behavioral Research, *Deciding to Forego Life-Sustaining Treatment* (1983), chapter 7, pp. 234–236, 239–248.

to guide the resuscitation team.... Various plastic tubes are usually inserted intravenously to supply medications or stimulants directly to the heart. Such medications can also be supplied by direct injection into the heart.... A defibrillator may be used, applying electric shock to the heart to induce contractions. A pacemaker...may be fed through a large blood vessel directly to the heart's surface.... These procedures, to be effective, must be initiated with a minimum of delay.... Many of the procedures are obviously highly intrusive, and some are violent in nature. The defibrillator, for example, causes violent (and painful) muscle contractions which...may cause fracture of vertebrae or other bones.[1]

Though initially developed for otherwise healthy persons whose heartbeat and breathing failed following surgery or near-drowning, resuscitation procedures are now used with virtually everyone who has a cardiac arrest in a hospital. The initial success rate for in-hospital resuscitation is about one in three for all victims and two in three for patients hospitalized with irregularities of heart rhythm. Among patients who are successfully resuscitated, about one in three recovers enough to be discharged from the hospital eventually. Especially when used on the general hospital population, long-term success is fairly rare. In the past decade, health care providers have begun to express concern that resuscitation is being used too frequently and sometimes on patients it harms rather than benefits.

Special Characteristics of CPR

Cardiopulmonary resuscitation of hospitalized patients has certain special features that must be taken into account in both individual and institutional decision-making:

- Cardiac arrest occurs at some point in the dying process of every person, whatever the underlying cause of death. Hence the decision whether or not to attempt resuscitation is potentially relevant for all patients.
- Without a heartbeat, a person will die within a very few minutes (that is, heartbeat and breathing will both irreversibly cease).
- Once a patient's heart has stopped, any delay in resuscitation greatly reduces the efficacy of the effort. Hence a decision about whether to resuscitate ought to be made in advance.
- Although resuscitation grants a small number of patients both survival and recovery, attempts at it usually fail; even when they reestablish heartbeat, they can cause substantial morbidity.
- Clinical signs during resuscitation efforts do not reliably predict functional recovery of a patient. Thus it is difficult to apply the sorts of adjustment and reconsideration that other interventions receive to a decision to resuscitate. Usually, the full range of efforts has to be applied until it is clear whether heartbeat can be restored.
- The conjectural nature of advance deliberations about whether or not to resuscitate may make the discussions difficult for the patient, family, and health care professionals.

Policies on Order Not to Resuscitate

Pioneering policies on "No Code" orders ("code" being the shorthand term for the emergency summoning of a "resuscitation team" by the announcement of "Code Blue" over a hospital's public address system) or "DNR orders" (for "Do Not Resuscitate") were published by several hospitals in 1976.[2] The policies followed the recognition by professional organizations that nonresuscitation was appropriate when well-being would not be served by an attempt to reverse cardiac arrest....

ETHICAL CONSIDERATIONS

The Presumption Favoring Resuscitation

Resuscitation must be instituted immediately after cardiac arrest to have the best chance of success. Because its omission or delayed application is a grievous error when it should have been used to attempt to save a life, most hospitals now provide for the rapid assembling of a team of skilled resuscitation professionals at the bedside of any patient whose heart stops.

When there has been no advance deliberation, this presumption in favor of resuscitation is justified. Although the concern a few years ago was about overtreatment, some health care professionals are now worried about unwarranted undertreatment—a weakening of the presumption in favor of resuscitation. Very different presuppositions are involved when a physician feels a need to justify resuscitating as opposed to not resuscitating someone. In either case, however, the risks of an inappropriate decision with grave consequences for a patient are great if the issues are not properly addressed according to well-developed criteria. In order to avoid using resuscitation in circumstances when it would be appropriate to omit it, advance deliberation on the subject is indicated in most cases. As in all decisions in medicine, the basic issue should be what medical interventions, if any, serve a particular patient's interests and preferences best. When a person's interests or preferences cannot be known under the circumstances, a presumption to sustain the patient's life is warranted.

The Values at Stake

In considering the relative merits of a decision to resuscitate a patient, concerns arise from each of three value considerations—self-determination, well-being, and equity.

Self-determination   Patient self-determination is especially important in decisions for or against resuscitation. Such decisions require that the value of extending life—usually for brief periods and commonly under conditions of substantial disability and suffering—be weighed against that of an earlier death. Different patients will have markedly different needs and concerns at the end of their lives; having a few more hours, days, or even weeks of life under constrained conditions can be much less important to some people than to others. In decisions concerning competent patients, therefore, first importance should be accorded to patient self-determination, and the patient's own decision should be accepted.

This great weight accorded to competent patients' self-determination means that attending physicians have a duty to ascertain patients' preferences,[3] which involves informing each patient of the possible need for CPR and of the likely consequences (both beneficial and harmful) of either employing or foregoing it if the need arises. When cardiac arrest is considered a significant possibility for a competent patient, a DNR order should be entered in the patient's hospital chart only after the patient has decided that is what he or she wants. When resuscitation is a remote prospect, however, the physician need not raise the issue unless CPR is known to be a subject of particular concern to the patient or to be against the patient's wishes. Some patients in the final stages of a terminal illness would experience needless harm in a detailed discussion of resuscitation procedures and consequences.[4] In such cases, the physician might discuss the situation in more general terms, seeking to elicit the individual's general preferences concerning "vigorous" or "extraordinary" efforts and inviting any further questions he or she may have.[5]

Well-being   A second important ethical consideration is whether resuscitation will promote a patient's welfare. A physician's assessment of "benefit" to a patient incorporates both objective facts, based on the physician's evaluation of the patient's physical status before and following resuscitation, and subjective values, in considering whether resuscitation or nonresuscitation best serves the patient's own values and goals. In virtually all cases the attending physician is in a better position to evaluate the former, while a competent patient is best able to determine the relative value of alternative outcomes.

Even though decisions about resuscitation should recognize the importance of patients' self-determination it may sometimes be necessary to question patients' choices on the grounds of protecting well-being. First, a patient may be mistaken about the course of treatment that will actually achieve the end he or she desires. Even a competent patient may initially misunderstand the nature of alternative outcomes or their relationship to his or her values because of the complexity of the alternatives, the psychological barriers to understanding information, and so forth. Dissonance between the physician's and the patient's assessments of benefit point to the need for such steps as further discussion, reexamination of the patient's decisionmaking capacity, and reassessment of the physician's understanding of patient's goals and values; indeed, in some cases patients may even wish to evaluate their values and goals.

Second, decisions may have to be based on "well-being" because "self-determination" is not possible under the circumstances. Many patients for whom a decision not to resuscitate is indicated have inadequate decisional capacity, often due to their underlying illnesses. In these cases, providers and surrogates must assess whether resuscitation—like any other medical intervention—is or is not likely to benefit the patient. Of course, physicians face many of the same difficulties in deciding that patients do, and their attempts to assess "benefit" will not always lead to clear conclusions.

Equity   The Commission has concluded previously that "society has an ethical obligation to ensure equitable access to...an adequate level of care without excessive burdens."[6] Should resuscitation always be considered part of the "adequate level"? Resuscitation decisions are currently made with little regard to the costs incurred or to the manner in which costs are distributed, except when competent patients decide to include such considerations as a reflection of their own concern for family well-being or for distributional justice. The Commission heard from a number of people, however, who wondered if providers and others should consider whether the costs of resuscitation are warranted for those patients for whom survival is very unlikely and who would, in any case, suffer overwhelming disabilities and diseases.

To determine whether cardiac resuscitation is a component of care that all hospitalized patients should have access to, the predicted value of this procedure would have to be compared with other medical procedures that generate comparable expenses and burdens. It is the Commission's sense that, at the moment, resuscitation efforts usually provide benefits that justify their cost, and thus resuscitation services generally should continue to be provided when desired by a patient or an appropriate surrogate. When, in a particular case, an attempt to resuscitate would clearly be against the patient's stated wishes or best interests, then the reason for not resuscitating does not arise from concerns for equitable use of societal resources, though it may incidentally help conserve them.

Of course, a more refined analysis of whether particular cases or categories of cases should be excluded under the definition of "adequate care" might be attempted. A controversial step would be to attempt to eliminate resuscitations that, while advancing a patient's interests or in accord with a patient's preferences, sustained a very marginal existence at a very high cost.[7]

However, the negative consequences of trying to discern such categories in a workable way provide strong arguments against adopting such policies. Explicitly precluding resuscitation for some categories of patients would almost certainly be insensitive to their values, denigrating to their self-esteem, and distressing to health care professionals. Also, the uncertainties over prognosis with resuscitation for each individual patient would make it very difficult to write clear and workable categories. It is unlikely that the costs incurred by marginally beneficial resuscitation are so substantial that their reduction should be a higher priority than the reduction of other well-documented kinds of wasteful or expensive and marginally beneficial care.

GUIDANCE FOR DECISIONMAKING

Competent Patients

When a competent patient's preference about resuscitation and a physician's assessment of its probable benefits coincide, the decision should simply be in accord with that agreement (see Table 1). When a physician is unclear whether resuscitation would benefit a patient but a competent patient has a clear preference on the subject, the moral claim of autonomy supports acting in accord with the patient's preference. Self-determination also supports honoring a previously competent patient's instructions.

Some patients, although apparently competent, do not express a preference for one course over another. Such patients may not have reached a judgment in their own minds (saying, for example, merely, "whatever you think, Doc") or they may simply be unwilling to articulate a view one way or the other. Provided that the patient's unwillingness to declare a view at the moment does not reflect incompetence, the physician should not immediately ask family members to substitute their views for those of the patient, but should instead seek to involve family members in other useful ways (assuming

that the patient does not object to their participation), comparable to the roles sometimes played by clergy, nurses, and other professionals. First, the family may be able to facilitate communication between the hospital staff and the patient, making sure that the issues to be addressed have been understood and helping to overcome any barriers to understanding. Second, they may be able to help the patient to make his or her preferences known to the care giving professionals. Ideally, these efforts will lead the patient to express a preference for or against resuscitation.

Of course, it is necessary to have some operative policy while a patient is being encouraged to make a choice, and patients should be informed about what that will be. Until the person expresses a clear preference, the policy in effect should be based on the physician's assessment of benefit to the patient; when it is unclear whether an attempt at CPR would be beneficial, there should be a presumption in favor of trying resuscitation.

When physicians and patients disagree about resuscitation, further discussion is warranted. Each can explain the basis of his or her position and why the other person's judgment seems unwarranted or mistaken. In some cases, consultation with experts may be helpful to resolve doubts about the facts of the case. Together, such steps often produce agreement.

Although disagreement in no way implies that a patient is incompetent, it will often be appropriate for the physician, and perhaps consultants or an advisory committee, to reexamine this issue if discussion does not lead to agreement between patient and physician—and also for the physician to reexamine his or her own thinking and to talk with advisors about it. The serious consequences of the patient's choice—which may include severe disability if resuscitation is tried or death if it is foregone—demand that this process be carried out with care. Once the adequacy of the patient's decisionmaking capacity is confirmed, then the patient's preference should be honored on grounds of self-determination, especially since the choice touches such important subjective values.

If a physician finds the course of action preferred by a competent patient to be medically or morally unacceptable and is unwilling to participate in carrying out the choice, he or she should help the patient find another physician. Indeed, such a change should be explored even when the physician is prepared to carry out the patient's wishes despite an initial disagreement if the difference of opinion created barriers to a good relationship.

TABLE 1   Resuscitation (CPR) of Competent Patients—Physician's Assessment in Relation to Patient's Preference

Physician's assessment	Patient favors CPR*	No preference	Patient opposes CPR*
CPR would benefit patient	Try CPR	Try CPR	Do not try CPR; review decision**
Benefit of CPR unclear	Try CPR	Try CPR	Do not try CPR
CPR would not benefit patient	Try CPR; review decision**	Do not try CPR	Do not try CPR

*Based on an adequate understanding of the relevant information.
**Such a conflict calls for careful reexamination by both patient and physician. If neither the physician's assessment nor the patient's preference changes, then the competent patient's decision should be honored.

Incompetent Patients

Decisionmaking for incompetent patients parallels that for competent ones except that when a physician or surrogate decisionmaker believes that resuscitation is not likely to benefit the patient, there are some additional constraints (see Table 2). Whenever a surrogate and physician disagree, as when only one thinks that resuscitation is warranted, the case should receive careful review, initially through intrainstitutional consultation or ethics committees. Urgent situations, however, or disagreements that are not resolved in this way should go to court. During such proceedings, resuscitation should be attempted if cardiac arrest occurs.

The review entailed will vary. When a physician feels that there is no benefit, a surrogate may either concur after additional consultations or may find another physician, especially if a consulting physician disagrees with the doctor who initially attended the patient. When a surrogate opposes resuscitation that a physician feels is beneficial, discussing the reasons in an impartial setting may uncover erroneous presuppositions, misunderstandings, or self-interested motives and allow for a resolution that is in the patient's best interests. When a surrogate is ambivalent, confirmation of the expected value of resuscitation by a consultant may be persuasive; continued ambivalence may signal the need for a new surrogate. The hospital will have to be able to ensure that helpful and effective responses are provided for these various situations.

If a patient has no surrogate and orders against resuscitation are contemplated, at least a *de facto* surrogate should be designated. When the physician feels that the decision against resuscitation is quite uncontroversial, a consultation with another physician, professional staff consensus, or agreement from an institutionally designated patient advocate can provide suitable confirmation of the initial judgment. Decisions like these are made commonly and should be within the scope of medical practice rather than requiring judicial proceedings. Decisions that are more complex or uncertain should occasion more formal intrainstitutional review and sometimes judicial appointment of a guardian.

TABLE 2   Resuscitation (CPR) of Incompetent Patients—Physician's Assessment in Relation to Surrogate's Preference

Physician's assessment	Surrogate favors CPR*	No preference	Surrogate opposes CPR*
CPR would benefit patient	Try CPR	Try CPR	Try CPR until review of decision
Benefit of CPR unclear	Try CPR	Try CPR	Try CPR until review of decision
CPR would not benefit patient	Try CPR until review of decision	Try CPR until review of decision	Do not try CPR

*Based on an adequate understanding of the relevant information.

Judicial Oversight

As made clear throughout this Report, the Commission believes that decisionmaking about life-sustaining care is rarely improved by resort to courts. Although physicians might want court adjudication when they believe that a patient's decision against resuscitation is clearly and substantially against his or her interests, courts are unlikely to require people to submit to such an intrusive and painful therapy unless they conclude that the patient is incompetent. Some form of review mechanism within a hospital is generally more appropriate and desirable for such disagreements. The courts are sometimes the appropriate forum for serious, intractable disagreements between a patient's surrogate and physician, however. When intrainstitutional procedures have not led to agreement in such cases, judges may well have to decide between two differing accounts of a patient's interests.

NOTES

1 *In re Dinnerstein*, 380 N.E.2d 134, 135–36 (Mass. App. 1978).
2 Mitchell T. Rabkin, Gerald Gillerman, and Nancy R. Rice, *Orders Not to Resuscitate*, 295 NEW ENG. J MED. 364 (1976); Optimum Care for Hopelessly Ill Patients: A Report of the Critical Care Committee of the Massachusetts General Hospital, 295 NEW ENG. J. MED. 362 (1976)....
3 Although the attending physician bears the responsibility, often others among the care giving professionals, religious advisors, or family members are in a good or better position to discuss the issues and convey the information. This is to be encouraged, but the physician is still obliged to see that it is done well.
4 *See, e.g.,* "Such explanations to the patient, on the other hand, are thoughtless to the point of being cruel, unless the patient inquires, which he is extremely unlikely to do." Steven S. Spencer, *"Code" or "No Code": A Non Legal Opinion*, 300 NEW ENG. J. MED. 138, 139 (1979). *But see* "The physician and family often underestimate the patient's ability to handle this issue and participate in the decision." Steven H. Miles, Ronald E. Cranford, and Alvin L. Schultz, *The Do-Not-Resuscitate Order in a Teaching Hospital*, 96 ANNALS INT. MED. 660, 661 (1982).
5 "Sometimes it seems cruel and unnecessary. Other times it is just difficult, in the midst of what is usually a very emotional and difficult time, to get around to the question of whether you want us pumping on your chest when you die.... Having taken care of someone for some period of time has usually generated prior tacit, if not overt, understanding between the patient and me on these issues."

(Michael Van Scoy-Mosher, *An Oncologist's Case for No-Code Orders*, in A. Edward Doudera and J. Douglas Peters, eds., LEGAL AND ETHICAL ASPECTS OF TREATING CRITICALLY AND TERMINALLY ILL PATIENTS, AUPHA Press, Ann Arbor, Mich. (1982) at 16....)
6 President's Commission for the Study of Ethical Problems in Medicine and Biomedical and Behavioral Research, SECURING ACCESS TO HEALTH CARE, U.S. Government Printing Office, Washington (1983) at 4.
7 Resuscitation efforts themselves commonly cost over $1000 and usually entail substantial derivative costs in caring for the surviving patients who suffer side effects.

Treatment Decisions for Incompetent Adults

Identifying the Key Decisionmaker and Making the Decision
Hastings Center Project Group on the Termination of Treatment

The Hastings Center Project Group on the Termination of Treatment was a research group whose twenty permanent members included physicians, nurses, lawyers, philosophers, and health-care administrators. Susan M. Wolf, J.D., served as project director. The principal fruit of the group's work was the publication of *Guidelines on the Termination of Life-Sustaining*

Reprinted with permission of Indiana University Press from *Guidelines on the Termination of Life-Sustaining Treatment and the Care of the Dying* (1987), pp. 22–29, 135–137.

Treatment and the Care of the Dying. Some brief excerpts from this rather extensive document are reprinted here.

> The Project Group suggests procedures for the identification of surrogate decision makers and contrasts decision making when patients lack decision-making capacity with decision making when patients possess decision-making capacity. In a brief appendix on the relevance of patient age as a factor in decision making, the Project Group is especially concerned with the age factor as a problem for the surrogate decision maker.

IDENTIFYING THE KEY DECISIONMAKER

Many decisions about life-sustaining treatment will emerge quite naturally from [an appropriate discussion process]. Everyone involved may agree about the best course of action. However, when the patient has the capacity to decide about the treatment, it is the patient who is the key decisionmaker, with the power to give binding consent or refusal. When the patient lacks the capacity, the key decisionmaker is someone else, a surrogate. Accordingly, the responsible health care professional will identify the key decisionmaker by determining whether the patient lacks decisionmaking capacity. Section (a) below elaborates on assessing capacity.

When the patient lacks capacity, the health care professional will go on to identify a surrogate decisionmaker for the patient, as described below in Section (b). Sometimes there may not be a single surrogate; a number of family members and concerned others may be involved in the decisionmaking process. When that is the case, the responsible health care professional should discuss the treatment decision with these individuals in order to allow them to reach a conclusion on how to proceed. (See the standards for surrogate decisionmaking set forth in Section (c) under "Making the Decision." However, if the group cannot reach a consensus about the treatment decision, then it will be necessary to identify a single surrogate.

In specifying the key decisionmaker, we do not recommend isolating that person from others. The decisionmaker does not act alone. The responsible health care professional and often other members of the health care team, as well as family and concerned friends, are crucial to the decisionmaking process.

(a) Assessing Decisionmaking Capacity

A patient has the capacity to make the treatment decision when he or she can understand the relevant information, reflect on it in accordance with his or her values, and communicate with caregivers. A patient need not have decisionmaking capacity for all purposes in order to have the capacity to make the decision at hand. Some people have the capacity to make one choice but not another. Patients should be presumed to have the capacity to decide about treatment, unless it is determined that they lack it.

The responsible health care professional should ensure that the assessment of a patient's decisionmaking capacity is properly conducted. This is an important responsibility. It may require consultation with others. Health care institutions should develop policy on how to assess capacity within the institution, and might decide upon even more safeguards than these Guidelines recommend. The patient should be notified, whenever he or she might understand, that a surrogate will be exercising decisionmaking authority and that the patient or others can challenge the determination of lack of capacity.

Once the responsible health care professional determines that the patient lacks decisionmaking capacity, the professional should assess whether there are ways to restore capacity. In some cases, lack of capacity may have a reversible cause, such as overmedication, pain, dehydration, or metabolic abnormalities. The professional should attempt to restore the patient's capacity prior to decisionmaking if possible.

(b) Identifying a Surrogate

When the patient lacks decisionmaking capacity, he or she should participate in the treatment decision as fully as possible; someone else, though, must serve as the ultimate source of consent or refusal. The responsible health care professional should identify this surrogate decisionmaker in consultation with other members of the health care team.

In identifying a surrogate, the professional should first honor any surrogate choice the patient has made— whether by advance directive or other written or oral statement. The professional should also recognize the authority of a surrogate appointed by a court when the appointed surrogate's powers include medical decision-making. (If a court has appointed one such person, but the patient has designated someone else, the professional should seek legal advice to determine which is the appropriate surrogate—unless the two agree on a treatment decision so that deciding between them becomes unnecessary.) If the patient has made no choice and there is no court-appointed surrogate, then the goal is to find the person who is most involved with the patient and most knowledgeable about the patient's present and past feelings and preferences. Thus the responsible health care professional will usually identify one of the following as the surrogate:

1. the person designated by the patient through an advance directive or any other written or oral statement;

2. a court-appointed surrogate, if the treatment decision in question is within the scope of the surrogate's authority (although this paragraph should not be construed to recommend such appointment); or

3. if neither of the above exists, the patient's spouse, a son or daughter, a parent, a brother or sister, or a concerned friend (in no priority order), as long as the surrogate is an adult, *i.e.*, has reached the age of majority in that state—usually 18 or 21. Immediate family members should be notified of the designation of a surrogate with lesser or no kinship.

(c)   The Patient Who Lacks a Ready Surrogate

One of the most difficult problems in medical decision-making is to whom to turn when the patient lacks decision-making capacity but has no one available and willing to act as surrogate. Various unsatisfactory ways of dealing with this have arisen, including waiting until the patient's medical condition worsens into an emergency so that consent to treat is implied by law and no surrogate is needed, or having the health care professional unilaterally decide for the patient. The first compromises patient care by waiting for a crisis and allows no orderly consideration of a decision to forgo treatment. The second compromises patient autonomy by leaving the decision in the hands of a person who may not know the pa-

tient's values. It also raises reasonable public concern, because there is no review and accountability for the decision that is made.

No decisionmaking mechanism is widely available to find attentive surrogates for the many people without them. There is also as yet no consensus on the proper solution. Some institutions and states are experimenting with a variety of mechanisms. Possibilities include some or all of the following: An institution, community agency, or other concerned provider organization could create a "surrogates committee" to provide a surrogate decisionmaker for each patient without capacity who lacks one. The responsible health care professional or health care institution could petition for a court-appointed guardian with authority to make health care decisions for each person without capacity and without a surrogate, a process that is costly, time-consuming, and public, but protective of civil rights and of the patient's estate. The state could permit ombudsmen functioning in state programs to provide ongoing personal advocacy for patients without capacity and with no surrogates, or to provide oversight for surrogates generated by surrogates committees. States, counties, or cities could establish Public Fiduciaries (or Public Guardians) who would investigate cases of possible incapacity and recommend appropriate court orders, including orders to provide ongoing representation for those with no surrogate. Courts could name private corporations as guardians; the corporations could provide services to the incapacitated patient while limiting the burden to the patient's representative, and could be required to adhere to regulatory or court-mandated standards.

Some combination of these kinds of procedures could create a surrogate for each patient, and provide the protection of institutional and public review of the surrogate's decisions. Some of these procedures may, however, be cumbersome and time-consuming. Whatever mechanisms are developed, each patient without decisionmaking capacity should have someone acting as his or her surrogate. Once a surrogate is put in place for a patient who lacked one, the surrogate should adhere to the same procedures and standards as other surrogates.

Some maintain that this kind of surrogate, who is not a family member or concerned friend of the patient, but may instead be a stranger, should have more limited discretion than a family or friend surrogate and perhaps should be subject to closer review. No wide agreement exists on this, however, or on the standards and mechanisms that would be used to further confine the discretion of a "stranger surrogate." We recommend that surrogates appointed for patients who lack them at least be held to the standards applied to family or friend surrogates, the standards set forth in Section (c) under "Making the Decision." The fact that the surrogate may not know the patient well may play a part in others' evaluations of the surrogate.

To summarize our recommendations:

1. Appropriate mechanisms need to be developed to make decisions for patients without decisionmaking capacity who lack surrogates, and to review those decisions.

2. Each health care institution should adopt a written procedure for decisionmaking about life-sustaining treatment when a patient lacks capacity and has no surrogate.

3. Someone other than the patient's responsible health care professional should preferably act as surrogate, unless the patient has previously designated the professional to act as surrogate. Even when the professional is vigorously promoting the patient's well-being, it is important to have another person participating, whose primary function is to make choices as the patient would if he or she were able. If it is not possible for someone other than the responsible professional to act as surrogate, the professional should seek review of decisions to forgo life-sustaining treatment by the institutional ethics committee or other institutional mechanism for advising on ethical issues.

4. Some form of institutional review should be available for decisions about life-sustaining treatment for such patients, whether by a committee or by some other group or person within the institution.

MAKING THE DECISION

(a) The Patient with Decisionmaking Capacity

If the patient has decisionmaking capacity, then the patient is the ultimate judge of the benefits and burdens of a life-sustaining treatment, and whether the burdens outweigh the benefits. Individuals differ in what they see as a burden and a benefit, and in how they weigh the two against each other. To most people burdens include pain

or suffering, hardships imposed on their loved ones, and financial cost. Most regard as benefits improved functioning, the relief of pain or suffering, the opportunity to live longer, and the chance to engage in satisfying activities.

Patients will usually find that life-sustaining treatment offers more benefits than burdens. In those cases, the treatment should be used. Some patients—particularly if they are terminally ill or suffering from an illness or disabling condition that is severe and irreversible—may decide that the burdens of a particular treatment outweigh the benefits, and choose to forgo that treatment. That choice should be honored. The responsible health care professional, however, should first discuss with the patient why he or she prefers to forgo treatment. Exploring the decision together is an important part of the process. If the patient is experiencing pain or suffering that can be ameliorated, the professional should discuss the possibility of amelioration to then see whether the patient still prefers to forgo treatment. The professional should make sure that the patient has not decided to forgo life-sustaining treatment in order to obtain relief from pain or suffering that can be alleviated without forgoing life-sustaining treatment.

(b) The Patient Whose Capacity Is Fluctuating or Uncertain

Some patients neither clearly possess nor clearly lack decisionmaking capacity; their capacity is fluctuating or uncertain. If the patient, responsible health care professional, and likely surrogate agree on the treatment decision, then there is no need to clarify the patient's capacity. When they do not agree or when no likely surrogate is on hand, and it is possible to adjust conditions or to delay the decision until the patient has decisionmaking capacity, that is the optimal course; the Guidelines above for patients with capacity then apply. If that is not possible, the Guidelines below for patients without decisionmaking capacity should apply instead.

(c) The Patient Who Lacks Decisionmaking Capacity

When a patient lacks the capacity to make the treatment decision, so that a surrogate decisionmaker has decisionmaking authority instead, the surrogate should seek to choose as the patient would if he or she were able. Because the strength of the evidence of the patient's preferences will vary, the surrogate should apply one of the three different standards listed below. Whenever a surrogate can come to no clear view as to whether to forgo treatment, treatment should be administered; using the treatment on a trial basis with reevaluation after a set interval should be considered

1 Follow the patient's explicit directives.* Where a patient who had decisionmaking capacity at the time, has left written directions in an advance directive or another form, or clear oral directions, and these directions seem intended to cover the situation presented, the surrogate should follow the directions.

2 Or apply the patient's preferences and values.* If the patient has left no directions about the treatment in question, the surrogate should apply what is known about the patient's preferences and values, trying to choose as the patient would have wanted.

3 Or choose as a reasonable person in the patient's circumstances would.** If there is not enough known about the patient's directions, preferences, and values to make an individualized decision, the surrogate should choose so as to promote the patient's interests as they would probably be conceived by a reasonable person in the patient's circumstances, selecting from within the range of choices that reasonable people would make. In order to flesh out this standard, we suggest below the major considerations involved in applying it to some important categories of patients:

(i) *The patient who is terminally ill.* In applying the "reasonable person" standard to the terminally ill patient without decisionmaking capacity, the major considerations are usually whether forgoing treatment will allow the patient to avoid the burden of prolonged dying with pain or suffering, and whether the patient has the potential benefit of achieving some satisfaction if he or she survives longer.

(ii) *The patient who has an illness or disabling condition that is severe and irreversible.* In applying the "reasonable person" standard to the patient with an illness or disabling condition that is severe and irreversible and who lacks decisionmaking capacity, the major consideration is the following: Would a reasonable person in the patient's circumstance

probably prefer the termination of treatment because the patient's life is largely devoid of opportunities to achieve satisfaction, or full of pain or suffering with no corresponding benefits?

(iii) *The patient with irreversible loss of consciousness.* For the patient who has suffered an irreversible loss of consciousness, the major considerations in applying the "reasonable person" standard are somewhat different. Patients who are permanently unconscious are unaware of benefits or burdens. The only possible benefit to them of life-sustaining treatment is the possibility that the diagnosis of irreversible unconsciousness is wrong and they will regain consciousness. Accordingly, the major considerations are whether a reasonable person in the patient's circumstance would find that this benefit, as well as the benefits to the patient's family and concerned friends (such as satisfaction in caring for the patient and the meaningfulness of the patient's continued survival) are outweighed by the burdens on those loved ones (such as financial cost or emotional suffering).

(The above list in no way suggests that treatment should be forgone just because a person falls into one of these categories; nor does it mean that treatment may not be terminated for other patients.)...

APPENDIX ON AGE AS A FACTOR IN DECISIONMAKING

Regardless of their age, human beings who face decisions about life-sustaining treatment are uniquely vulnerable; they need special protections, respect, and consideration from others. Such persons are usually seriously ill, gravely burdened by the present circumstances of their existence, and dependent upon the good will of their family, friends, and caregivers. At such a time, stereotypes and social prejudices are particularly demeaning and dangerous; special caution must be taken to prevent these attitudes from influencing decisions to terminate treatment.

There is today no serious moral controversy about the notion that prejudice based on race, sex, religion, or ethnic origin should play no part in decisions about medical treatment. But what of age? Here disagreement and moral uncertainty remain widespread. Many have argued that the patient's age should be a factor in termination of treatment decisions. They usually maintain

---

*These are sometimes called a "substituted judgment" standard.

**This is sometimes called a "best interests" standard.

that age should weigh against aggressive treatment, although age-based considerations logically could also tilt the other way. This is a special concern because many patients who face decisions about life-sustaining treatment are elderly people, and demographic trends suggest that this will be increasingly the case.

Factoring age into decisionmaking...is worrisome mainly in the context of surrogate decisionmaking. No doubt adults with decisionmaking capacity often take their own age into consideration in decisions about life-sustaining treatment. Some may feel they are "too young to die," others may feel that they have "lived long enough." Either way, there seems to be nothing inherently objectionable about this when individuals are making decisions about their own treatment.

But matters are considerably more complex when a surrogate must weigh the benefits and burdens of medical treatment on another's behalf....[I]t is easy for surrogates, and indeed health care professionals, to project their own attitudes—here about aging—onto the patient in making decisions. Yet even when they avoid this, the question of the relevance of age remains, since there may be a reasonable and objective—and not simply a prejudicial—link between a person's age and how beneficial or burdensome life-sustaining treatment might be.

In coping with these difficult issues, the following distinctions may be helpful. First, it is important to distinguish between age and functional ability. The effects of disease and individual biological variations are such that an older patient may be stronger and have a better prognosis than a younger patient with essentially the same life-threatening condition. For this reason age is at best a crude and imprecise factor to use in assessing a given patient's prognosis and the benefits and burdens of a given treatment.

In surrogate decisionmaking, age should always give way to a more clinically precise and individualized assessment of the patient's underlying physiological status. Age *per se* is not a morally relevant factor in assessing the quality of extended life for an individual. An extra year of life at age 85, say, is not inherently either more or less meaningful or beneficial than an extra year of life at age 55 or even 25. These judgments must be individualized to each patient. To ignore the particular circumstances and values of the patient and to make judgments based on age alone are to fall prey to precisely the kind of dehumanizing age prejudice that ethical decisionmaking must avoid.

Second, considerations of age may have a different status and significance in policy decisions concerning the allocation of resources and the development of new technologies than they do in clinical decisions concerning the treatment of an individual patient. In clinical decisionmaking, individualized judgments and assessments are almost always possible; health care professionals and surrogates can and should look beyond age to functional ability and to the patient's values and circumstances. In matters of health policy and the allocation of scarce resources this is not the case. Policies often have to be made in terms of more general criteria and classifications. There may be reasons for using age as a yardstick in making policy choices and allocation decisions.

The Severely Demented, Minimally Functional Patient: An Ethical Analysis

John D. Arras

A biographical sketch of John D. Arras is found on page 115.

Arras is principally concerned with the dilemmas of surrogate decision making posed by a recurrent kind of case: Decisions about life-sustaining treatment have to be made for an elderly, severely demented patient, and the patient has left behind no significant advance directives. Focusing attention on a particular case of this description, Arras first explains why evidence is insufficient to establish a moral certitude, on the basis of a substituted judgment standard, that life-sustaining treatment should be withheld. He then explains some of the dif-

Reprinted with permission of the American Geriatrics Society and the author from *Journal of the American Geriatrics Society*, vol. 36 (1988), pp. 939–944.

ficulties entailed by an effort to apply the best-interests standard to the case under consideration. In the end, Arras argues that both the substituted judgment and best-interest tests entail an unrealistic standard of evidence. Accordingly, he endorses "a procedural solution" to the perceived difficulties of surrogate decision making. In his view, within specified limits, the decisions of trustworthy surrogates are to be implemented.

Mrs. Smith, an 85-year-old resident of a nursing home, was transferred to the hospital for treatment of pneumonia. Although she has responded well to antibiotic therapy, her overall condition and prognosis remain grim. For the past 3 years her mental state has been steadily deteriorating due to a series of strokes which have finally rendered her severely demented. She is now nonambulatory, incapable of sitting up in bed, and uncommunicative most of the time. When she does talk, her speech is completely incoherent and repetitive. Mrs. Smith shows no signs of recognizing or remembering her family and primary caregivers. The nurses in charge of her care assert that she appears to experience pleasure only when her hair is combed or her back rubbed.

During her recovery from the pneumonia, Mrs. Smith began to have problems with swallowing food. Following a precipitous decline in her caloric intake, her son and daughter (the only involved family members) consented to the placement of a nasogastric tube. Mrs. Smith continually pulled out the tube, however, and continues to resist efforts to reinsert it.

The health care team faces difficult choices regarding Mrs. Smith's care. Foremost among them is whether her physicians should surgically insert a gastrostomy tube in spite of her aversive behavior. Mrs. Smith has neither left behind a living will nor has she indicated to family or friends at the nursing home what her preferences would be regarding life-sustaining care in this sort of circumstance. Both her son and daughter have stated that she would nevertheless not have wanted a gastrostomy tube inserted and would, if she could presently decide, prefer an earlier death to being sustained indefinitely in the twilight of her minimally functional condition. In defense of this claim, they note that she has always been a very active, independent person who avoided doctors whenever possible.

PROBING THE PATIENT'S SUBJECTIVITY

The first order of business in deciding for incompetent patients is to inquire, whenever possible, what the patient would want were she presently able to communicate. In the absence of a designated proxy or living will that speaks with rare precision about which modes of treatment are to be forgone under which circumstances, this task is more difficult than many commentators and jurists would have us think. The case before us yields two distinct sources of revelation bearing on the patient's putative subjective wishes regarding the present decision. As we shall see, neither provides evidence sufficiently compelling for us to conclude with moral certitude that she would not allow the insertion of a G-tube.

Extrapolating from the Patient's Prior Values

First, we have the testimony of family members who claim that the patient's character traits of independence and aloofness from physicians point to the conclusion that she would not want to be sustained by a G-tube. Although this claim may well be *plausible* and at least *consistent* with Mrs. Smith's previously held attitudes and behaviors, it would require a great leap of both faith and logic to conclude that evidence of this sort *entails* a negative decision on life-sustaining treatment. As several commentators have pointed out, there is a great difference between the degree of respect owed to a patient's *actual choices*, even choices made prior to the advent of incompetency, and to his or her preferences or tastes.[1-4] It is one thing to have negative attitudes towards aggressive life support, but it is quite another to actually refuse it in your own case. By doing so, a person *commits* himself or herself to a particular course of action and it is this commitment, rather than mere attitudes or generalized preferences abstracted from the particular details of choosing situations, that commands especially stringent respect.

Even if someone's generalized views about life, dependency, and doctors deserved the status of right claims, which they do not, they usually do not yield unequivocal answers to treatment dilemmas. Supposing that Mrs. Smith was indeed fiercely independent and skeptical of the medical profession, does this necessarily mean that she would prefer death to her present "twilight state" sustained by tube feedings? Conversely, if Mrs. Smith were an exceptionally dependent sort of person who actively sought and followed the advice of physicians, would that mean that she would presently prefer an indefinite extension of her barely conscious existence to an early death? Although such character traits indisputibly have *some* evidentiary value, they appear to be compatible with a range of possible responses.[4] In Mrs. Smith's case, it is certainly *plausible* that she would decline the insertion of a G-tube, but that is not the only plausible interpretation. For all we know, she might have been content, were she miraculously lucid and communicative for an instant, to accede to the operation rather than go peacefully into that dark night. The question for Mrs. Smith's caregivers, then—and we shall explore this point more fully later on—is not whether her loved ones have provided a uniquely correct extrapolation of her previous values to her present situation, for in most cases that will simply be an unattainable goal; rather, the question is whether their plausible invocations of her values and character traits should be given the benefit of the doubt.

The Evidentiary Value of Aversive Behavior

Mrs. Smith has been constantly pulling out her nasogastric tube and waiving off the attentions of her caregivers. What are we to make of this behavior? In contrast to the patient's previous preferences and attitudes, which are ill-matched in their generality to the concreteness of the present situation, Mrs. Smith's aversive behavior at least has the advantage of being contemporaneous. She is extubating herself right here and now. According to Daniel Callahan,[5] a philosopher who generally sees no justification for terminating food and fluids in severely demented patients, such behavior constitutes a "clear signal" mandating withdrawal of the tube.

But a clear signal of what? It is crucial to remember at this juncture that Mrs. Smith is severely demented and completely incompetent. Even though her aversive behavior occurs in the present, it is the behavior of a woman who has completely lost her rational capacity. She cannot even recognize her family, let alone engage in sophisticated deliberations bearing on the respective benefits and burdens of continued tube feeding in her minimally functional state versus an earlier death. Aphasic but otherwise competent patients might be able to send clear signals under such circumstances, but not Mrs. Smith, whose behavior appears to be freighted with a variety of possible meanings.

It is possible that her tube-pulling represents a firm and fixed present desire to forgo aggressive life-sustaining treatments in favor of an early death. It is also possible that it signals some kind of deeply sedimented personal desire manifested in spite of her present incompetence. But it is equally possible that her aversive behavior is nothing more than an elemental reflex signalling only her transient irritation from the tube. Nasogastric tubes *are* bothersome and sometimes painful intrusions, and one need not entertain sophisticated benefit-burden calculations to wish merely to be rid of such noxious stimuli. Thus, the interpretive options range from deeply intentional options for death in the face of minimally functional existence to reflexes of an almost exclusively physiological nature.

Mrs. Smith's "signal" is thus anything but clear, and this is a significant fact for her caregivers to ponder. While aversive behavior expressive of deeply sedimented personal values should be accorded the same degree of respect allotted to general character traits and attitudes, aversive reflexes to unpleasant stimuli should command little, if any, deference from surrogate decision-makers. Small children extubate themselves all the time, but no one would view such actions as a "clear signal" of a wish to die. The real problem facing Mrs. Smith's physicians is that they have no reliable way of discerning the "real meaning" behind her ongoing resistance to feeding tubes. It would certainly help if Mrs. Smith had been known to shun tube feeding even while she was competent, for that would at least provide some plausible evidence connecting her presently aversive behavior to sedimented preferences. But in the absence of such a record, the meaning of her "rejection" remains profoundly unclear.

Given the inconclusiveness of this inquiry into the patient's previous attitudes and present behavior, her caregivers might reasonably shift their focus of attention away from the patient's elusive subjectivity and toward a more objective assessment of her "best interest."

THE BEST INTEREST STANDARD

In the absence of reliable indicators of the patient's actual or hypothetical preferences, courts and commentators recommend an inquiry into the best interests of the patient.[6,7] What course of action (or inaction) will bring about the best overall result for the patient? Rather than finding this "objective" path an easier route to the correct decision, caregivers attempting to apply such a test to the case of a severely demented, minimally functional patient such as Mrs. Smith will immediately confront a series of equally perplexing questions. What will be the actual impact of placing a G-tube on Mrs. Smith's well being? What definition of the good will ground their assessments of her best interests? And, given her low level of functioning, is it quite accurate even to describe Mrs. Smith as a full-fledged "person" with actual, discernable interests? Since these exceedingly difficult questions lack intuitively obvious answers, perhaps the best way to proceed is to examine categories of patients on either side of Mrs. Smith on the continuum of incompetency, categories that do yield fairly firm moral intuitions, and then attempt to locate a proper response to her case by means of "moral triangulation." Needless to say, the clarity and distinctness of these idealized categories often become somewhat blurred in real clinical situations, but there is still considerable theoretical value in discussing our responses to clear-cut cases.

Patients in Persistent Vegetative States

What if, instead of being minimally functional, Mrs. Smith were completely non-functional? (We shall call this hypothetical patient, Mrs. Jones.) What if, instead of slowly declining into a twilight of consciousness, she were to have experienced a protracted period of anoxia that consigned her to a persistently vegetative condition? Although still alive, Mrs. Jones would subsist on brainstem activity alone, her neo-cortex—the physical substratum of her capacity for consciousness—having been completely destroyed. She would thus persist in countless sleep-wake cycles, unable to connect with the world and with her past through conscious awareness, unable to plan or hope for better circumstances, unable even to perceive pleasure or pain. What rights, if any, would Mrs. Jones have, and what duties would be owed her by caregivers?

If we were to apply straightforwardly the best interests test to the case of Mrs. Jones, we would be hard pressed to discover actual interests that could be meaningfully imputed to her. Lacking consciousness, she lacks a conception of herself as a moral agent with real interests in continued life and in the pursuit of her own vision of the good. Lacking the ability to experience pleasure and pain, she cannot be physically benefitted or harmed.[8] Indeed, as several commentators have pointed out, her only remaining interest in staying alive is based on the miniscule possibility that she has been misdiagnosed and could possibly regain some degree of con-

sciousness in the future.[9] Apart from that slimmest of chances, she has no interests that might be assessed through a best interests test.

If we seek a solution to the problem of Mrs. Jones in an examination of her best interest, we discover the paradoxical result that her best interest will probably be served by further treatment. True, except for the possibility of misdiagnosis, she cannot be benefitted in any way by continued existence, but her lack of capacity for conscious experience renders her equally incapable of being harmed by further treatments and the extension of her life. Thus, we cannot say, as the best interest test would appear to require, that Mrs. Jones is being excessively burdened by her treatments or that she would be "better off dead." This result is indeed paradoxical, because if anyone's life need not be maintained, one would think that patients in persistently vegetative conditions must be at the top of the list.

Given the vanishingly small likelihood of misdiagnosis, especially after the passage of several weeks, I would argue that it is ethically appropriate to treat all PVS patients as though they had no interests either for or against treatment. Since continued medical interventions cannot realistically be thought to benefit them in any way, since caregivers cannot realistically be thought to have duties towards patients who cannot be helped or harmed, and since such treatments entail considerable costs—including the expenditure of huge sums of money, the time and energy of caregivers, and emotional strains on survivors—they may be ethically forgone.

The important lesson here is that although a rigorously patient-centered best interest test might be ethically appropriate in most cases involving incompetent patients, it cannot be meaningfully applied when the patient under consideration lacks all fundamentally human capacities. In cases such as this, a judgment in favor of nontreatment must be based, not on an objective weighing of benefits and burdens to the patient—for such patients are capable of neither benefit nor burden—but rather upon a judgment that the patient has ceased to be a "person" in any meaningful moral sense. Once this determination has been made, it is then ethically permissible to consider the financial and emotional impact of continued treatment upon other interested parties.[10] Certainly some families will, for religious or other personal reasons, continue to request life-sustaining treatments for their persistently vegetative relations; but others would be acting ethically to request the termination of all medical care, including artificially administered food and fluids.

Marginally Functional Patients

On the other side of Mrs. Smith are those patients who might usefully be described as "marginally functional." Mr. Black, for example, is a 90-year-old man presenting with rectal bleeding and suspected colon cancer who refuses a laparotomy to confirm the diagnosis. "I have lived a good-life," he says, "and I don't want any surgery." His daughter, to whom he appears very close, concurs with his decision. Although Mr. Black appears on the surface to be sufficiently competent to make this decision, subsequent examinations by liaison psychiatrists reveal a glaring absence of short term memory and significant confusion about his medical diagnosis and surroundings. He is described as "pleasantly demented."

Although patients like Mr. Black are strictly speaking incapable of rational decision-making most or all of the time, they differ from Mrs. Jones in their ability to reason, albeit rather poorly, in their ability to relate to other persons, and in their capacities to experience emotions, pain and pleasure. Notwithstanding their inability to make most health care decisions, these patients are clearly "persons" with a multitude of interests that can be advanced or frustrated by their caregivers. In spite of their deficits and relatively low quality of life, such moderately functional patients have every right to a patient-centered best interests analysis. While invasive, painful and risky surgery may or may not eventually be deemed to be in Mr. Black's best interests, his capacities for experiencing the world are sufficiently intact to rule out any thought of forgoing other sorts of life-sustaining therapies, such as artificial nutrition and hydration.

The Minimally Functional Patient

Returning now to the example of Mrs. Smith, we find her to fall squarely between the permanently vegetative and moderately functional patient. Like the totally nonfunctional, vegetative patient, she is so demented that she lacks most of the criteria of "moral personhood."[11] Unfortunately, she appears to have been reduced to a mere shell of her former self. She can no longer reason, communicate (except in the most rudimentary, reflexive manner), relate to her family, or experience manifestations of love. Indeed, it is doubtful that she can be accurately described as a self-conscious, moral agent whose identity through time is cemented by the bonds of memory. There is, in cases such as this

where the psychological glue of memory has given out, simply no enduring "self" there.[12] Formerly a self-conscious moral agent with a well-defined idea of good, hopes and plans for the future, Mrs. Smith has been reduced to a mere locus of transient sensations. As philosopher James Rachels[13] puts it, she continues to have biological life, but her *biographical* life has come to an end.

On the other hand, Mrs. Smith resembles Mr. Black at least in her possession of some conscious life, albeit on a very low level, and in her ability to experience pleasure, pain, and perhaps some rudimentary emotions. Although she is not a "person" in the strict sense, she does have some interests. Insofar as she is open to pleasure and pain, she has a definite interest in experiencing the former and avoiding the latter. How might a "best interests" test be applied to someone like Mrs. Smith?

Better Off Dead?   In order to justify the termination of food and fluids under a best interests test, decision-makers would have to show that the burdens of a patient's life with the proposed treatment would clearly and markedly outweigh whatever benefits she might derive from continued life.[7] In other words, they would have to show that the patient would be "better off dead."

The most influential formulation of this best interests test, the majority opinion in the *Conroy* case, requires not merely that the burdens of life clearly outweigh the benefits, but also that further treatment would be inhumane due to the presence of severe and uncontrollable pain.[7] The court's motivation in establishing such a strict standard is not hard to grasp. While people might disagree about the desirability of persisting in a minimally functional condition, severe and intractable pain is presumably something that just about everyone would prefer to avoid. It is this nearly universal sentiment that death would be preferable to a life of unmitigated pain and suffering that gives this test an air of "objectivity," as opposed to the subjectivity of tests based upon the patient's past preferences.

How then would this strict formula apply to Mrs. Smith? As we have seen, there isn't much to place in the "benefits" column. No longer able to take food by mouth or to interact meaningfully with her family and caregivers, it appears that Mrs. Smith experiences few pleasures apart from an occasional rub or combing. The only possible benefit to be derived from further treatment would appear to be the indefinite continuation of this twilight existence. And although the patient might conceivably derive some pleasure merely from lying in bed and dwelling in her alien world, it is highly doubtful that such a patient—bereft of memory, a sense of continuing selfhood, hopes and plans—could possibly have an interest in, or be benefitted by, *continued* existence.

Given Mrs. Smith's low level of existence, it is equally difficult to discern the burdens of continued treatment. To be sure, she will experience some degree of pain and discomfort from the surgical insertion of a G-tube, but this pain will not approximate the kind of prolonged, severe and intractable pain required by the *Conroy* best interests formula.

Another possible source of pain and suffering would be the forcible imposition of medical treatment against the wishes of the incompetent patient. Even incompetent patients can have strong preferences for or against treatment or diagnostic procedures, and even if these preferences are not well grounded in medical reality or in the patient's previously authentic value system, forcible treatment will often be experienced as a painful and humiliating violation. Although this kind of coercion need not be thought of as a violation of the patient's autonomy, which may have already been destroyed by dementia, the pain, humiliation, distrust and hostility it engenders must nevertheless be counted in any best interest calculation. In some cases, Mr. Black's for example, the negative consequences of forcing treatment may not be worth the gains.

In Mrs. Smith's case, however, the side effects of coercive treatment are likely to be nonexistent. As we have already seen, her aversive reaction to NG tube feeding could just as easily be ascribed to immediate physical discomfort as to some deep-seated desire to die through the refusal of life-sustaining treatment. Mrs. Smith is probably too demented at this point to have preferences about tube feedings or to acknowledge the forcible imposition of surgery over against her aversive behavior. It is highly unlikely, then, that she would experience the insertion of a G-tube as a violation of her wishes (no matter how distorted) or as a painful humiliation.

In the absence of any persistent and severe pain underlying her condition, it would appear highly doubtful that the burdens of Mrs. Smith's continued existence clearly and markedly outweigh the benefits, even when the benefits approach zero. A literal reading and application of the *Conroy* formula would thus lead to the conclusion that the G-tube should be surgically implanted and that she should be maintained indefinitely with artificial nutrition and hydration.

Limitations of the Best Interest Standard   Not everyone will be satisfied with this result. Those who believe that quality of life should never affect treatment decisions will no doubt applaud this conclusion, but others might well think that something important has been left out of our deliberations. Judge Handler,[7] the lone dissenter in *Conroy* identifies this missing factor as a legitimate concern for the patient's probable feelings about broader issues, such as privacy, dependency, dignity and bodily integrity. By focusing the entire best interests discussion upon the narrow issue of pain, we tend to reduce the patient from the full-fledged person that she once was to the status of a mere physical repository of pleasures and pains. Is this crudely hedonistic notion of the good an adequate or desirable measure of humane treatment decisions for minimally functional patients? Should we simply ignore the patient's probable responses to such abject dependency and daily violations of dignity?

Although Judge Handler's dissent eloquently pinpoints a major shortcoming of the *Conroy* best interests formula, it is problematical in its own right. Specifically, it is unclear how Judge Handler's concerns for these larger issues of privacy and dignity might be grafted onto the *Conroy* best interests formula. That test, let us recall, attempts to ascertain the *present* best interests of patients; it asks about the present and future benefits and burdens likely to be experienced by the patient. The obvious problem for Judge Handler's proposed enlargement of this formula is that severely demented, minimally functional patients like Mrs. Smith are presently incapable of experiencing what more functional patients would describe as insults to their privacy, dignity and physical integrity. Although it is quite possible that the formerly competent Mrs. Smith would have been appalled at the loss of dignity entailed by her present situation, the present Mrs. Smith knows nothing of dignitary insults or violations of privacy. She is so demented that she cannot be affected, one way or the other, by solicitude for her present responses to these larger, humanistic issues.

In order to vindicate Judge Handler's concerns, we will have to reintroduce them at the stage of our inquiry into the patient's prior preferences (ie, the substituted judgment test). Under that test, we would have to show that Mrs. Smith would have clearly viewed continued treatment under these circumstances as an indignity, and that she would have preferred an early death to the insertion of a G-tube. The problem with this move is that, as we have already seen, Mrs. Smith left behind neither a precise advance directive nor a pattern of analogous choices that clearly demonstrate what she would have wanted under present circumstances. Indeed, our earlier failure to provide this sort of clear evidence mandated our present effort to find a solution in terms of Mrs. Smith's best interests.

So we have come full circle. Our inability to satisfy a rigorous substituted judgment test required us to search for a solution in terms of Mrs. Smith's best interests. But the best interest test, at least as articulated in *Conroy*, led to an unacceptably narrow focus on pain that excluded important values. Mrs. Smith's present lack of capacity to appreciate such values finally led us back again to the substituted judgment test. Clearly, something has gone wrong here.

A PROCEDURAL SOLUTION

According to lawyer-bioethicist Nancy Rhoden,[4] the problem lies not in our inability to come up with better evidence of a patient's wishes or level of pain and suffering, but rather in the questions we are asking. She argues convincingly that both the substituted judgment and best interests tests set the standard of evidence far too high. By requiring *clear and convincing* evidence either that a patient's prior values would dictate the withdrawal of life-sustaining treatment or that the burdens of a patient's life outweigh the benefits, these tests establish a standard that cannot realistically be met by the kinds of evidence we are likely to have at our disposal. As we have seen, in the absence of a carefully drafted living will, a durable power of attorney, or severe and intractable pain, it will rarely be *clear* either that a patient would have refused treatment or that death is in her best interests. Given the usual evidentiary materials at hand, in most cases the best we can do is conclude that forgoing treatment is *probably* what the patient would have wanted, or that death is *likely* to be in the patient's best interest, although we will never know for sure in either case.

To be sure, there are some easy cases where a patient's best interests are clearly and perceptibly being violated. For example, greedy relatives might request the termination of treatment that could realistically return the patient to a good quality of life; or guilt-ridden relatives might press for full resuscitative measures on a moribund patient riddled with metastatic cancer. But

apart from such clear-cut cases of unmistakable under-treatment and overtreatment, most of the truly problematical cases (like Mrs. Smith's) fall into a vast gray area between these extremes where the patient's best interests will remain unclear and largely inscrutable. Our problem, then, is that we have been asking questions for which there exist, in most of the hard cases at least, no clearly correct answers.

Rhoden's solution, in which I concur, is to bypass this substantive impasse with a procedural solution. Taking her cue from the President's Commission report[6] addressed to the problem of severely impaired newborns, she argues that when a proposed course of action falls into the gray area of uncertainty, involved and well-intentioned family members should have discretion to decide as they see fit. Presumably, they will invoke precisely the same kinds of evidence bearing on the patient's value system, religious affiliation, quality of life, and the potential benefits and burdens of treatment, but they would not be held to a standard of evidence requiring that their choice be uniquely correct.

To be sure, many caring and well-meaning family members will also want to weigh the impact of continued treatment upon themselves and the family unit. Sometimes the ongoing provision of care and treatment to severely demented patients like Mrs. Smith can impose great burdens, both financial and emotional, upon families. I believe that such concerns are for the most part inevitable and that they often subtly color treatment decisions even when officially banished under the auspices of the usual ethical-legal standards. This is to be expected and should not give us grounds for concern so long as the case originally falls within the gray area of ethical ambiguity, and so long as the interests of family do not *clearly* violate the bests interests of the patient.

The correct question for us, then, is not whether forgoing treatment is clearly the right answer, but rather whether Mrs. Smith's case falls into the problematical gray area. If it does, then the decision of a trustworthy surrogate should prevail over objections from caregivers, unless the latter can show a clear violation of best interests. Since a case must exhibit considerable ethical ambiguity to fall into this gray zone in the first place, we should expect that well-meaning and ethically sensitive people will reach different conclusions about the care of such patients. The opinions of trustworthy surrogates should be given priority simply because they are usually in the best position to assess the prior wishes and best interests of incompetent patients, and because their familial and emotional bonding to patients usually gives them a greater claim than members of the health care team.[6]

What, then, are the boundaries of the gray area? When is a case sufficiently ambiguous to warrant our trust in surrogate decision-making? We can begin with a reassertion of the *Conroy* best interest formula. If a patient's capacity for benefitting from continued life appears to be eclipsed by the constant presence of severe and intractable pain, then the case falls either in the gray area or the clear-cut zone of nontreatment. I would add that this imbalance of burdens over benefits need not be conclusively proven by clear and convincing evidence. It should be sufficient merely for the surrogate to make a strong case that the burdens are disproportionate to the benefits. In Mrs. Smith's case, however, no such claim can be made.

In the absence of severe pain, we must ask whether the patient is genuinely capable of benefitting from continued existence. Does she recognize and interact with other persons, including her family and caregivers? Does she have a sufficiently intact self to conceive of the future and to care about what happens in it? If the answers to these questions are negative, even if the patient is capable of some rudimentary physical pleasures, I would argue that the patient has no real interest in continued life or the administration of life-sustaining treatments and thus falls squarely into the gray area.

Mrs. Smith fits this profile. She is so demented that she cannot recognize family or caregivers. Her memory is so depleted, and her sense of self so fractured, that she cannot be said to have genuinely human interests.

Since the boundaries of this morally ambiguous zone will inevitably correspond to the limits of societal toleration, it will often be helpful to ask what most reasonable people would want for themselves in this circumstance. Although this question is generally not allowed in more patient-centered inquiries into the patient's prior preferences or best interests, it should be allowable here, where we are merely trying to determine whether a case is sufficiently morally problematic to fit into the gray zone. If we ask the question with regard to Mrs. Smith, I think that the overwhelming majority of persons would say that they would rather die than continue to live in such a physically, emotionally and socially impoverished state.

Another useful clue is to ask how we would have responded to Mrs. Smith's death from lack of adequate nutrition had it occurred prior to the advent of artificial feeding. No doubt there would have been the inevitable sadness associated with the death of any human being, but there would have been no shock, no outrage, no sense of tragedy, nor even any feeling that death had deprived her of any real benefits. The predominant response to such a death would most likely have been relief, both for the sake of the patient and for her loved ones.

In such cases, the only apparent rationale for the imposition of life-sustaining technologies is that since they exist, they must be used. And the more they are used, the more pervasive their presence in hospital and long-term care facilities, the more their expanded use assumes the necessity of a moral imperative. But it is precisely here, in cases such as Mrs. Smith's, that we must pause to ask about the proper uses of such technologies. If they do nothing to further the real interests of patients, if all they do is to prolong the biological existence of patients whose biographical lives have long since come to an end, then biomedical technologies assume the status of idols—ie, inanimate objects worshipped by the human beings who created them, objects that return to dominate us rather than serving our purposes.

REFERENCES

1 Dworkin R: Autonomy and the Demented Self. Milbank Quarterly 64: supp. 2, 4–16, 1986
2 Buchanan A, Brock DW: Deciding for Others. Milbank Quarterly 64: supp. 2, 71, 1986
3 Dresser, R: Life, Death, and Incompetent Patients: Conceptual Infirmities and Hidden Values in the Law. Arizona Law Review 28: 376–379, 1986
4 Rhoden NK: Litigating Life and Death. Harvard Law Review 102, January 1989 (in press)
5 Callahan D: Setting Limits: Medical Goals in an Aging Society. New York, Simon & Schuster, 1987, p 192
6 President's Commission for the Study of Ethical Problems in Medicine and Biomedical and Behavioral Research: Deciding to Forego Life Sustaining Treatment, Washington, DC, U.S. Government Printing Office, 1983, p 134 ff
7 In re Conroy, 98 N.J. 321, 486 A.2d 1209 (1985)
8 Cranford RE: The Persistent Vegetative State: The Medical Reality (Getting the Facts Straight). Hastings Cent Rep 18:27–32, February/March 1988
9 Feinberg J: The Rights of Animals and Unborn Generations, *in* Rights, Justice, and the Bounds of Lib-

erty. Princeton, Princeton University Press, 1980, p 176–177

10 Arras JD: Quality of Life in Neonatal Ethics: Beyond Denial and Evasion, *in* Weil WB, Benjamin M, (eds): Ethical Issues at the Outset of Life. Boston, Blackwell, 1987, p 151–186

11 Engelhardt, HT: The Foundations of Bioethics. New York, Oxford University Press, 1986

12 Brock, DW: Justice and the Severely Demented Elderly. J Med Philos 13:1, Feb 73–99, 1988

13 Rachels J: The End of Life. New York, Oxford University Press, 1986

ANNOTATED BIBLIOGRAPHY: CHAPTER 6

Battin, M. Pabst: *Ethical Issues in Suicide* (Englewood Cliffs, N.J.: Prentice-Hall, 1982). In this very useful book, Battin provides a comprehensive discussion of the traditional arguments concerning suicide. She also suggests an analysis of the concept of rational suicide, discusses suicide intervention as well as suicide facilitation, and considers the notion of suicide as a right.

————, and David J. Mayo, eds.: *Suicide: The Philosophical Issues* (New York: St. Martin's Press, 1980). This valuable collection of articles includes material on the concept of suicide, the morality of suicide, and the rationality of suicide. There are also subsections entitled "Suicide and Psychiatry" and "Suicide, Law, and Rights."

Beauchamp, Tom L.: "Suicide and the Value of Life." In Tom Regan, ed., *Matters of Life and Death* (New York: Random House, 1980), pp. 67–108. In this long essay on the philosophical aspects of suicide, Beauchamp provides both a conceptual analysis of suicide and an evaluation of various moral views.

Beck, Robert N., and John B. Orr, eds.: *Ethical Choice: A Case Study Approach* (New York: Free Press, 1970). Section 2 of this work is entitled "Suicide" and conveniently reprints several classical sources on suicide: Seneca, St. Augustine, St. Thomas Aquinas, Hume, and Schopenhauer.

Cantor, Norman L.: *Legal Frontiers of Death and Dying* (Bloomington, Ind.: Indiana University Press, 1987). In an attempt both to clarify the state of the law and to critique it, Cantor presents an expansive discussion of life-sustaining treatment decisions.

Chell, Byron: "Competency: What It Is, What It Isn't, and Why It Matters." In John F. Monagle and David C. Thomasma, eds., *Medical Ethics: A Guide for Health Professionals* (Rockville, Md.: Aspen, 1988), pp. 99–110. Chell presents an analysis of competency and identifies a process for determining the competency of patients who refuse life-saving treatment for religious reasons.

Guidelines on the Termination of Life-Sustaining Treatment and the Care of the Dying: A Report by the Hastings Center (1987). This document first presents general guidelines on the decision-making process and then presents guidelines relevant to specific treatment modalities. Also included are guidelines on advance directives.

Jackson, David L., and Stuart Youngner: "Patient Autonomy and 'Death with Dignity': Some Clinical Caveats," *New England Journal of Medicine* 301 (August 23, 1979), pp. 404–408. The authors introduce a number of clinical case reports from a medical intensive care unit. Their principal point is that "superficial and automatic acquiescence to the concepts of patient autonomy and death with dignity" can lead to clinically inappropriate decisions.

Miller, Bruce L.: "Autonomy and the Refusal of Lifesaving Treatment," *Hastings Center Report* 11 (August 1981), pp. 22–28. Miller distinguishes four senses of autonomy in an effort to deal with refusal of lifesaving treatment cases that feature at least an apparent conflict between medical judgment and patient autonomy.

President's Commission for the Study of Ethical Problems in Medicine and Biomedical and Behavioral Research: *Deciding to Forego Life-Sustaining Treatment* (1983). This document is valuable in its entirety, but one chapter is especially noteworthy: Chapter 4 provides material on the determination of incapacity, surrogate decision making, and advance directives.

Schneiderman, Lawrence J., and Roger G. Spragg: "Ethical Decisions in Discontinuing Mechanical Ventilation," *New England Journal of Medicine* 318 (April 14, 1988), pp. 984–988. The authors attempt to clarify the ethical considerations involved in making decisions to discontinue mechanical ventilation, and they propose an overall decision-making scheme.

Szasz, Thomas: "The Case against Suicide Prevention," *American Psychologist* 41 (July 1986), pp. 806–812. Szasz argues that it is never justifiable to employ coercion in an effort to prevent an adult from committing suicide.

Tomlinson, Tom, and Howard Brody: "Ethics and Communication in Do-Not-Resuscitate Orders," *New England Journal of Medicine* 318 (January 7, 1988), pp. 43–46. The authors argue that is is important to distinguish among three distinct rationales for DNR orders: (1) no medical benefit; (2) poor quality of life before CPR; (3) poor quality of life after CPR. In their view, when "no medical benefit" is the rationale for a DNR order, the physician need not ascertain the patient's preferences.

Velasquez, Manuel G.: "Defining Suicide," *Issues in Law & Medicine* 3 (1987), pp. 37–51. Velasquez critiques some definitions of suicide as too broad, rejects others as too narrow, then advances his own proposal.

Wanzer, Sidney H., et al.: "The Physician's Responsibility toward Hopelessly Ill Patients," *New England Journal of Medicine* 310 (April 12, 1984), pp. 955–959. A group of ten physicians suggests a set of guidelines for the treatment of hopelessly ill (adult) patients. The patient's role in decision making is asserted as paramount, and aggressive treatment of the hopelessly ill patient is identified as inappropriate when it would "only prolong a difficult and uncomfortable process of dying." In an article of the same title, subtitled "A Second Look" in *NEJM* 320 (March 30, 1989), pp. 844–849, Wanzer et al. present an updated account.

Youngner, Stuart J.: "Do-Not-Resuscitate Orders: No Longer Secret, but Still a Problem," *Hastings Center Report* 17 (February 1987), pp. 24–33. Youngner argues for the importance of: (1) the improved documentation and specification of DNR orders; (2) the involvement of patient, family, and staff (including nurses) in DNR decisions; and (3) the regular (at least daily) review of a patient's DNR status. He also insists that DNR status does not entail medical or psychological abandonment.

CHAPTER 7

EUTHANASIA AND THE DEFINITION OF DEATH

INTRODUCTION

The moral justifiability of euthanasia is not a newly emerging issue, but it is an issue that is debated with a new intensity in contemporary times. Recent advances in biomedical technology have made it possible to prolong human life in ways undreamed of by past generations of medical practitioners. As a result, it is not unusual to find a person who has lived a long and useful life now permanently incapable of functioning in any recognizably human fashion. Biological life continues; but some find it tempting to say that human life, in any meaningful sense, has ceased. In one case the patient is in an irreversible coma, reduced to a vegetative existence. In another case the patient's personality has completely deteriorated. In still another case the patient alternates inescapably between excruciating pain and drug-induced stupor. In each of these cases, the quality of human life has deteriorated. There is no longer any capacity for creative employment, intellectual pursuit, or the cultivation of interpersonal relationships. In short, in each of these three cases life seems to have been rendered meaningless in the sense that the individual has lost all capacity for normal human satisfactions. In the first case there is simply no consciousness, which is a necessary condition for deriving satisfaction. In the second case consciousness has been dulled to such an extent that there is no longer any capacity for satisfaction. In the third case excruciating pain and sedation combine to undercut the possibility of satisfaction.

At the other end of the spectrum of life, we are confronted with the severely impaired newborn child. In some tragic cases, a child seems to have no significant potential for meaningful human life. For example, an anencephalic child, one born with a partial or total absence of the brain, has no prospect for human life as we know it. Biomedical technology is sometimes sufficient to sustain or at least temporarily prolong the life of a severely impaired newborn, depending on the particular nature of the child's medical condition, but one question commands attention. Is the child better off dead?

Religious people pray and nonreligious people hope that death will come quickly to themselves or to loved ones who are in the midst of terminal illnesses and forced to endure pain and/or indignity. The same attitudes often prevail in the face of tragically compromised new-borns. The prevalence of these attitudes seems to confirm the truth, however sad, that some human beings, by virtue of their medical condition, are better off dead. But if it is true that someone is better off dead, then mercy is on the side of death, and the issue of euthanasia comes to the fore. Euthanasia, in its various forms, is discussed in this chapter. Also discussed is a closely related topic—the definition of death.

The Moral Justifiability of Euthanasia

Discussions of the moral justifiability of euthanasia often involve reference to distinctions that are themselves controversial. Such distinctions include that between ordinary and extraordinary means of prolonging life, that between killing and allowing to die, and that between active and passive euthanasia. Indeed, the very concept of euthanasia is controversial. In accordance with what might be called the "narrow construal of euthanasia," euthanasia is equivalent to mercy *killing*. In this view, if a physician administers a lethal dose of a drug to a terminally ill patient (on grounds of mercy), this act is a paradigm of euthanasia. If, on the other hand, a physician *allows the patient to die* (e.g., by withholding or withdrawing a respirator), this does not count as euthanasia. In accordance with what might be called the "broad construal of euthanasia," the category of euthanasia encompasses both killing and allowing to die (on grounds of mercy). Those who adopt the broad construal of euthanasia often distinguish between active euthanasia (i.e., killing) and passive euthanasia (i.e., allowing to die). Although there seem to be clear cases of killing (e.g., the lethal dose) and clear cases of allowing to die (e.g., withholding or withdrawing a respirator), there are more troublesome cases as well. Suppose a physician administers pain medication with the knowledge that the patient's life will be shortened as a result. A case of killing? Suppose a physician withholds "ordinary means" of life support, whatever that might be. A case of allowing to die? Sometimes it is even said that *withdrawing* life-sustaining treatment is active ("pulling the plug!") in a way that *withholding* it is not, but it is implausible to think that there is an important moral difference between withdrawing and withholding life-sustaining treatment.

The historically important distinction between ordinary and extraordinary means of prolonging life is perhaps especially problematic. The idea that extraordinary means are not mandatory, whereas ordinary means are, has been embraced in many quarters. The language of "extraordinary means" is sometimes found in "living wills," judicial opinions, and codelike statements expressing principles of medical ethics. In addition, some philosophers continue to defend the moral importance of the distinction between ordinary and extraordinary means, but many contemporary commentators believe that the distinction is of no fundamental importance, even if ambiguities of meaning can be clearly resolved.

There is one further distinction, itself relatively uncontroversial, that plays an important role in discussions of euthanasia. *Voluntary* euthanasia proceeds with the (informed) consent of the person involved. *Involuntary* euthanasia proceeds without the consent of the person involved, when the person involved is *incapable* of (informed) consent. The possibility of involuntary euthanasia might arise, for example, in the case of a comatose adult.[1] The much discussed case of Karen Ann Quinlan is a case of this sort.[2] The possibility of involuntary euthanasia might also arise with regard to adults who have for any number of reasons (e.g., Alzheimer's disease) lost their decision-making capacity, and it might arise with regard to children. Indeed, a very prominent variety of involuntary euthanasia involves severely impaired newborns. When the voluntary/involuntary distinction is combined with the active/passive distinction, it is clear that four types of euthanasia can be generated: (1) active voluntary euthanasia, (2) passive voluntary euthanasia, (3) active involuntary euthanasia, and (4) passive involuntary euthanasia.

A very common view on the morality of euthanasia, so common that it might justifiably be termed the "standard view," may be explicated as follows: Withholding or withdrawing life-sustaining treatment is morally acceptable (under certain specifiable conditions), but mercy killing is never morally acceptable. Those who operate in accordance with the narrow conception of euthanasia would express the standard view by saying that withholding or withdrawing life-sustaining treatment can be morally acceptable, but *euthanasia* is never morally acceptable. Those who operate in accordance with the broad conception of euthanasia would express the standard view by saying that *passive euthanasia* is morally acceptable (under certain specifiable conditions), but *active euthanasia* is never morally acceptable. The standard view, especially as expressed in a 1973 formulation by the American Medical Association (AMA), is vigorously attacked by James Rachels in one of this chapter's readings. Thomas D. Sullivan accuses Rachels of misconstruing the sense behind the standard view. Sullivan offers a defense of the standard view. Rachels, in turn, criticizes Sullivan's reliance on the distinction between intentional and nonintentional terminations of life and the distinction between ordinary and extraordinary means of life support.

The withholding or withdrawing of life-sustaining treatment in the case of terminally ill patients is surely an established part of medical practice. Moreover, several religious traditions explicitly acknowledge the morality of this practice. In addition, it is widely believed that a patient has the moral (and legal) right to refuse any medical treatment, a right that would encompass the refusal of life-sustaining treatment. Thus, there is a substantial body of opinion, perhaps something close to a consensus view, maintaining the moral legitimacy of withholding or withdrawing life-sustaining treatment in the case of terminally ill patients. There is no such consensus view on the morality of *mercy killing*, which will be referred to here as "active euthanasia."

Those who argue for the moral legitimacy of active euthanasia emphasize considerations of humaneness. In the case of *voluntary* active euthanasia, the humanitarian appeal is often conjoined with an appeal to the primacy of individual autonomy. Thus the case for the morality of voluntary active euthanasia incorporates two basic arguments: (1) It is cruel and inhumane to refuse the plea of a terminally ill person that his or her life be mercifully ended in order to avoid future suffering and indignity. (2) Individual choice should be respected to the extent that it does not result in harm to others. Since no one is harmed by terminally ill patients' undergoing active euthanasia, a decision to have one's life ended in this fashion should be respected.

In defending the moral legitimacy of active euthanasia in this chapter, Rachels appeals directly to humanitarian considerations, but he also constructs an argument based on the Golden Rule. Typically, those who argue against the moral legitimacy of active euthanasia rest their case on one or both of the following strategies of argument: (1) They appeal to some "sanctity of life" principle to the effect that the intentional termination of (innocent) human life is always immoral. Sullivan advances this sort of argument in his defense of the standard view. (2) They advance a rule-utilitarian argument to the effect that any systematic acceptance of active euthanasia would lead to damaging consequences for society (e.g., via a lessening of respect for human life). This second sort of argument recurs in discussions of the legalization of active euthanasia.

Active Euthanasia and Social Policy

Should active euthanasia be legalized? If so, in what form or forms and with what safeguards? Although active euthanasia is presently illegal in all fifty states, proposals for its legalization have been recurrently advanced. Most commonly, it is the legalization of *voluntary* active euthanasia that has been proposed.

Two specific models for the legalization of voluntary active euthanasia are discussed in this chapter. One model is provided by a set of guidelines under which voluntary active euthanasia is presently permitted in the Netherlands. Another model is provided by the provisions of the "Humane and Dignified Death Act," a California legislative proposal. In one of this chapter's selections, Marcia Angell clarifies the difference between these two models. She also argues that the risk of abuse would be much greater in the proposed California legislation than it is in the Dutch system. In another selection in this chapter, Alex Ralph Demac constructs an overall case against the "Humane and Dignified Death Act." In the course of their discussions, both Angell and Demac refer to some of the standard arguments for and against the legalization of voluntary active euthanasia.

The Definition of Death

Two groups of patients are at the center of controversy in contemporary discussions of "the definition of death." In the first group are patients whose *entire* brain has irreversibly ceased functioning. They are irreversibly comatose, but cardiopulmonary function (heartbeat and respiration) is successfully maintained by a respirator and concomitant life-support systems. These patients are frequently identified as "brain-dead" or "whole-brain-dead." They will be referred to here as "brain-dead." In a second group of patients, brainstem function is sufficient to sustain heartbeat and respiration, but irreversible damage to "the higher brain," the cerebral cortex, is so severe that these patients are suspended in what is called a "persistent vegetative state" (PVS). Consciousness, and thus cognition, has been irreversibly lost. Are the patients in each of these groups alive or dead? In any case, what treatment is morally appropriate for patients in each group?

The traditional standard for the determination of death is the permanent absence of respiration and pulsation. According to this standard, "brain-dead" patients are alive so long as artificial life-support systems sustain cardiopulmonary functioning. In 1968, an ad hoc committee of the Harvard Medical School issued a report that is a frequent reference point in contemporary discussions of "the definition of death." In this report, the Ad Hoc Committee specified a set of tests for the identification of a permanently nonfunctioning (whole) brain—the condition of "brain-death." In the view of the Ad Hoc Committee, when this condition has been diagnosed, "death is to be declared and *then* the respirator turned off."[3] Thus, in essence, the Ad Hoc Committee advanced a new standard for the determination of death. A "brain-dead" patient is a dead patient, despite the fact that cardiopulmonary functioning is artificially sustained.

It is a matter of substantial import whether "brain-dead" patients are alive or dead. Taking the vital organs of these patients for transplantation purposes is morally unproblematic if they are dead, presuming of course that appropriate consent procedures have been followed. If they are alive, however, taking their vital organs could well be the cause of their death. There are also important implications in the context of passive euthanasia discussions. When a respirator is withdrawn from a "brain-dead" patient, how are we to conceptualize this action? If the patient is alive, then it is sensible to describe withdrawing the respirator as an act of passive euthanasia. But if the patient is already dead, we cannot say, in withdrawing the respirator, that we are allowing the patient to die; hence we cannot say that we are dealing with an act of passive euthanasia.

The substance of the Harvard proposal has achieved a significant measure of public acceptance. For example, the President's Commission for the Study of Ethical Problems in Medicine and Biomedical and Behavioral Research in its 1981 report, *Defining Death*, recommends the adoption by all states of the Uniform Determination of Death Act:

An individual who has sustained either (1) irreversible cessation of circulatory and respiratory functions, or (2) irreversible cessation of all functions of the entire brain, including the brain stem, is dead. A determination of death must be made in accordance with accepted medical standards.

Charles M. Culver and Bernard Gert, in one of this chapter's selections, define death as the permanent cessation of functioning of the *organism as a whole*. In their view, which is compatible with the substance of the Harvard proposal, a patient who has undergone a permanent loss of functioning of the entire brain is dead, but a patient in a persistent vegetative state is not dead, even though, as they say, the organism has ceased to be a person. Indeed, insisting that "we must not confuse the death of an organism which was a person with an organism's ceasing to be a person," Culver and Gert explicitly argue against a competing definition of death, according to which the permanent loss of consciousness and cognition is sufficient for death. By way of contrast, Daniel Wikler in this chapter is fundamentally sympathetic to a "higher-brain" or "neocortical" conception of death. In his view, widening the definition of death to include persistent vegetative state is an analytic move that is conceptually sound. Of course, as Wikler points out, if it is true that patients in persistent vegetative state are already dead, "then nothing that happens to them causes their death." In particular, the act of inducing cardiac arrest could no longer be conceptualized as an act of killing the patient, nor could it be conceptualized as active euthanasia. Similarly, since the patient is already dead, the removal of organs for transplantation could not sensibly be understood as an action tantamount to killing the patient.

Culver and Gert, committed to the more common view that the patient in persistent vegetative state is still alive, also consider the issue of what treatment is morally appropriate. Although they reject the notion of killing a PVS patient, they endorse allowing the patient to die by discontinuing all care, even "ordinary and routine care." Presumably the discontinuance of "ordinary and routine care" would include the withdrawal of nutrition and hydration—"food and water"—from the patient. But at this point we are confronted with a more generic question, one that has relevance to other classes of patients as well (e.g., severely impaired newborns). Is it ever morally appropriate to withhold nutrition and hydration from a patient?

Those who systematically oppose withholding nutrition and hydration often call attention to the symbolic significance of food and water—their intimate connection with notions of care and concern. They also typically argue that there is some sort of basic difference between the provision of food and water and the provision of other life-sustaining medical treatments. In one of this chapter's selections, however, Joanne Lynn and James F. Childress insist that there is no reason to apply a different standard to nutrition and hydration. In their view, artificial nutrition and hydration may be withheld whenever they do not offer the patient a net benefit.

The Treatment of Impaired Newborns

The selective nontreatment of severely impaired newborns, sometimes identified as the practice of passive (involuntary) euthanasia, is an issue that first made its way into the public consciousness in the early 1970s. In the 1980s, the issue gained an even higher profile. Media attention focused on a rash of "Baby Doe" cases, and the Reagan administration was conspicuous in its effort to activate the machinery of government via the introduction of "Baby Doe" regulations.[4] As a result, the practice of selective nontreatment of severely impaired newborns has been subjected to intense scrutiny, with regard to both its legality and its morality.

The central moral question with regard to the treatment of impaired newborns may be identified as follows: Under what conditions, if any, is it morally acceptable to allow a severely impaired newborn to die? Two other closely related issues are also worthy of mention. The first has to do with the procedural question: Who should make the decision to treat or not treat? It has sometimes been argued that the decision is a medical one, to be made by physicians. But the more common view is that the parents are the appropriate decision makers, as informed by consultation with physicians and (perhaps) as limited by boundaries set by society at large. In this regard, it is often suggested that hospital ethics committees be assigned the responsibility of reviewing decisions to treat or not treat severely impaired newborns. The second issue worthy of mention has to do with the moral legitimacy of active euthanasia. If it is morally acceptable to allow a severely impaired newborn to die, on grounds that the child is better off dead, then is it not also morally acceptable (perhaps morally preferable) to kill the child as painlessly as possible?

Broadly speaking, there are three different views on the moral acceptability of allowing severely impaired newborns to die.

(1) It is morally acceptable to allow a severely impaired newborn to die if and only if death would be in the infant's best interests, that is, if and only if the infant would be better off dead. Defenders of this view are firmly committed to so-called quality-of-life judgments, but they systematically reject the contention that the cost (emotional and/or financial) of caring for severely impaired newborns is a relevant factor in the decision to treat or not to treat. A very similar but somewhat less restrictive view would endorse allowing a severely impaired newborn to die if and only if there is no significant potential for a meaningful human existence. In one of this chapter's selections, the members of The Hastings Center Research Project on the Care of Imperiled Newborns argue for the primacy of the best-interests standard, but they also insist that in some cases a "relational potential" standard comes into play. According to this standard, treatment is optional for an infant who lacks the potential for human relationships.

(2) It is morally acceptable to allow a severely impaired newborn to die if at least one of the following conditions is satisfied: (*a*) there is no significant potential for a meaningful human existence; (*b*) the emotional and/or financial hardship of caring for the severely defective newborn child would constitute a grave burden for the family. It is the introduction of the cost factor that distinguishes view (2) from view (1). Defenders of this second view, such as H. Tristram Engelhardt, Jr., often emphasize that the newborn child does not have the status of personhood, thereby defending the legitimacy of the cost factor.

(3) It is never morally acceptable to allow a severely impaired newborn to die. Or, to put it more exactly, it would never be morally acceptable to withhold treatment from a severely impaired newborn unless it would be morally acceptable to withhold such treatment from a normal infant. Although there is no requirement to prolong the life of a *dying* infant, whatever medical treatment is considered appropriate for an otherwise normal infant must be provided for the seriously impaired newborn as well. For example, if antibiotics are indicated for an otherwise normal infant with pneumonia, then antibiotics may not be withheld in a case where pneumonia arises for an infant whose central nervous system is severely compromised. In this view, it is usually presumed that a newborn child has the status of personhood and, however severely impaired, has a right to life. Defenders of this view, such as John A. Robertson in one of this chapter's selections, often make arguments against the validity of quality-of-life judgments (as featured in both of the aforementioned views) as well as the validity of the cost factor (as featured exclusively in the second view).

T.A.M.

NOTES

1 As discussed in the Introduction to Chapter 6, it is often suggested that competent adults make a "living will" in order to express their wishes with regard to the treatment they would

desire, should they become incompetent. In this way, it is thought, individual autonomy is fostered, and others (e.g., physicians and family) can be relieved of the responsibility for making involuntary euthanasia decisions.

2 In the Quinlan case, Joseph Quinlan, the father of comatose 21-year-old Karen Ann Quinlan, sought to be appointed guardian of the person and property of his daughter. As guardian, he would then authorize the discontinuance of the mechanical respirator that was thought to be sustaining the vital life processes of his daughter. Judge Muir of the Superior Court of New Jersey decided against the request of Joseph Quinlan. *In re Quinlan*, 137 N. J. Super 227 (1975). Justice Hughes of the Supreme Court of New Jersey overturned the lower-court decision. *In re Quinlan*, 70 N. J. 10, 335 A. 2d 647 (1976). When the respirator was finally withdrawn, Karen Ann Quinlan proved capable of breathing on her own. She remained alive in a "persistent vegetative state" for a period of about ten years.

3 The Ad Hoc Committee of the Harvard Medical School to Examine the Definition of Brain Death, "A Definition of Irreversible Coma," *Journal of the American Medical Association* 205 (August 6, 1968), p. 338.

4 The so-called final Baby Doe rule was published by the Department of Health and Human Services on April 15, 1985. For one interpretation of this rule, see Thomas H. Murray, "The Final, Anticlimactic Rule on Baby Doe," *Hastings Center Report* 15 (June 1985), pp. 5–9. For an alternative interpretation, see John C. Moskop and Rita L. Saldanha, "The Baby Doe Rule: Still a Threat," *Hastings Center Report* 16 (April 1986), pp. 8–14.

The Morality of Active Euthanasia

Active and Passive Euthanasia
James Rachels

James Rachels is professor of philosophy at the University of Alabama in Birmingham. Specializing in ethics, he is the author of such articles as "Why Privacy Is Important," "On Moral Absolutism," and "Can Ethics Provide Answers?" He is also the author of *The Elements of Moral Philosophy* (1986) and *The End of Life: Euthanasia and Morality* (1986), and he is the editor of *Understanding Moral Philosophy* (1976).

Rachels identifies the standard (conventional) view on the morality of euthanasia as the doctrine that permits passive euthanasia but rejects active euthanasia. He then argues that the conventional doctrine may be challenged for four reasons. First of all, active euthanasia is in many cases more humane than passive euthanasia. Second, the conventional doctrine leads to decisions concerning life and death on irrelevant grounds. Third, the doctrine rests on a distinction between killing and letting die that itself has no moral importance. Fourth, the most common arguments in favor of the doctrine are invalid.

The distinction between active and passive euthanasia is thought to be crucial for medical ethics. The idea is that it is permissible, at least in some cases, to withhold treat-

Reprinted by permission from the *New England Journal of Medicine*, vol. 292, no. 2 (January 9, 1975), pp. 78–80.

ment and allow a patient to die, but it is never permissible to take any direct action designed to kill the patient. This doctrine seems to be accepted by most doctors, and it is endorsed in a statement adopted by the House of Delegates of the American Medical Association on December 4, 1973:

The intentional termination of the life of one human being by another—mercy killing—is contrary to that for which the medical profession stands and is contrary to the policy of the American Medical Association.

The cessation of the employment of extraordinary means to prolong the life of the body when there is irrefutable evidence that biological death is imminent is the decision of the patient and/or his immediate family. The advice and judgment of the physician should be freely available to the patient and/or his immediate family.

However, a strong case can be made against this doctrine. In what follows I will set out some of the relevant arguments, and urge doctors to reconsider their views on this matter.

To begin with a familiar type of situation, a patient who is dying of incurable cancer of the throat is in terrible pain, which can no longer be satisfactorily alleviated. He is certain to die within a few days, even if present treatment is continued, but he does not want to go on living for those days since the pain is unbearable. So he asks the doctor for an end to it, and his family joins in the request.

Suppose the doctor agrees to withhold treatment, as the conventional doctrine says he may. The justification for his doing so is that the patient is in terrible agony, and since he is going to die anyway, it would be wrong to prolong his suffering needlessly. But now notice this. If one simply withholds treatment, it may take the patient longer to die, and so he may suffer more than he would if more direct action were taken and a lethal injection given. This fact provides strong reason for thinking that, once the initial decision not to prolong his agony has been made, active euthanasia is actually preferable to passive euthanasia, rather than the reverse. To say otherwise is to endorse the option that leads to more suffering rather than less, and is contrary to the humanitarian impulse that prompts the decision not to prolong his life in the first place.

Part of my point is that the process of being "allowed to die" can be relatively slow and painful, whereas being given a lethal injection is relatively quick and painless. Let me give a different sort of example. In the United States about one in 600 babies is born with Down's syndrome. Most of these babies are otherwise healthy—that is, with only the usual pediatric care, they will proceed to an otherwise normal infancy. Some, however, are born with congenital defects such as intestinal obstructions that require operations if they are to live. Sometimes, the parents and the doctor will decide not to

operate, and let the infant die. Anthony Shaw describes what happens then:

> ...When surgery is denied [the doctor] must try to keep the infant from suffering while natural forces sap the baby's life away. As a surgeon whose natural inclination is to use the scalpel to fight off death, standing by and watching a salvageable baby die is the most emotionally exhausting experience I know. It is easy at a conference, in a theoretical discussion, to decide that such infants should be allowed to die. It is altogether different to stand by in the nursery and watch as dehydration and infection wither a tiny being over hours and days. This is a terrible ordeal for me and the hospital staff—much more so than for the parents who never set foot in the nursery.[1]

I can understand why some people are opposed to all euthanasia, and insist that such infants must be allowed to live. I think I can also understand why other people favor destroying these babies quickly and painlessly. But why should anyone favor letting "dehydration and infection wither a tiny being over hours and days"? The doctrine that says that a baby may be allowed to dehydrate and wither, but may not be given an injection that would end its life without suffering, seems so patently cruel as to require no further refutation. The strong language is not intended to offend, but only to put the point in the clearest possible way.

My second argument is that the conventional doctrine leads to decisions concerning life and death made on irrelevant grounds.

Consider again the case of the infants with Down's syndrome who need operations for congenital defects unrelated to the syndrome to live. Sometimes, there is no operation, and the baby dies, but when there is no such defect, the baby lives on. Now, an operation such as that to remove an intestinal obstruction is not prohibitively difficult. The reason why such operations are not performed in these cases is, clearly, that the child has Down's syndrome and the parents and doctor judge that because of that fact it is better for the child to die.

But notice that this situation is absurd, no matter what view one takes of the lives and potentials of such babies. If the life of such an infant is worth preserving, what does it matter if it needs a simple operation? Or, if one thinks it better that such a baby should not live on, what difference does it make that it happens to have an unobstructed intestinal tract? In either case, the matter of life and death is being decided on irrelevant grounds. It is the Down's syndrome, and not the intestines, that is the issue. The matter should be decided, if at all, on that basis, and not be allowed to depend on the essentially irrelevant question of whether the intestinal tract is blocked.

What makes this situation possible, of course, is the idea that when there is an intestinal blockage, one can "let the baby die," but when there is no such defect there is nothing that can be done, for one must not "kill" it. The fact that this idea leads to such results as deciding life or death on irrelevant grounds is another good reason why the doctrine should be rejected.

One reason why so many people think that there is an important moral difference between active and passive euthanasia is that they think killing someone is morally worse than letting someone die. But is it? Is killing, in itself, worse than letting die? To investigate this issue, two cases may be considered that are exactly alike except that one involves killing whereas the other involves letting someone die. Then, it can be asked whether this difference makes any difference to the moral assessments. It is important that the cases be exactly alike, except for this one difference, since otherwise one cannot be confident that it is this difference and not some other that accounts for any variation in the assessments of the two cases. So, let us consider this pair of cases:

In the first, Smith stands to gain a large inheritance if anything should happen to his six-year-old cousin. One evening while the child is taking his bath, Smith sneaks into the bathroom and drowns the child, and then arranges things so that it will look like an accident.

In the second, Jones also stands to gain if anything should happen to his six-year-old cousin. Like Smith, Jones sneaks in planning to drown the child in his bath. However, just as he enters the bathroom Jones sees the child slip and hit his head, and fall face down in the water. Jones is delighted; he stands by, ready to push the child's head back under if it is necessary, but it is not necessary. With only a little thrashing about, the child drowns all by himself, "accidentally," as Jones watches and does nothing.

Now Smith killed the child, whereas Jones "merely" let the child die. That is the only difference between them. Did either man behave better, from a moral point of view? If the difference between killing and letting die were in itself a morally important matter, one should say that Jones's behavior was less reprehensible than Smith's. But does one really want to say that? I think not. In the first place, both men acted from the same motive, personal gain, and both had exactly the same end in view when they acted. It may be inferred from Smith's conduct that he is a bad man, although

that judgment may be withdrawn or modified if certain further facts are learned about him—for example, that he is mentally deranged. But would not the very same thing be inferred about Jones from his conduct? And would not the same further considerations also be relevant to any modification of this judgment? Moreover, suppose Jones pleaded, in his own defense, "After all, I didn't do anything except just stand there and watch the child drown. I didn't kill him; I only let him die." Again, if letting die were in itself less bad than killing, this defense should have at least some weight. But it does not. Such a "defense" can only be regarded as a grotesque perversion of moral reasoning. Morally speaking, it is no defense at all.

Now, it may be pointed out, quite properly, that the cases of euthanasia with which doctors are concerned are not like this at all. They do not involve personal gain or the destruction of normal, healthy children. Doctors are concerned only with cases in which the patient's life is of no further use to him, or in which the patient's life has become or will soon become a terrible burden. However, the point is the same in these cases: the bare difference between killing and letting die does not, in itself, make a moral difference. If a doctor lets a patient die, for humane reasons, he is in the same moral position as if he had given the patient a lethal injection for humane reasons. If his decision was wrong—if, for example, the patient's illness was in fact curable—the decision would be equally regrettable no matter which method was used to carry it out. And if the doctor's decision was the right one, the method used is not in itself important.

The AMA policy statement isolates the crucial issue very well; the crucial issue is "the intentional termination of the life of one human being by another." But after identifying this issue, and forbidding "mercy killing," the statement goes on to deny that the cessation of treatment is the intentional termination of life. This is where the mistake comes in, for what is the cessation of treatment, in these circumstances, if it is not "the intentional termination of the life of one human being by another"? Of course it is exactly that, and if it were not, there would be no point to it.

Many people will find this judgment hard to accept. One reason, I think, is that it is very easy to conflate the question of whether killing is, in itself, worse than letting die, with the very different question of whether most actual cases of killing are more reprehensible than most actual cases of letting die. Most actual cases of killing are clearly terrible (think, for example, of all the murders reported in the newspapers), and one hears of such cases every day. On the other hand, one hardly ever hears of a case of letting die, except for the actions of doctors who are motivated by humanitarian reasons. So one learns to think of killing in a much worse light than of letting die. But this does not mean that there is something about killing that makes it in itself worse than letting die, for it is not the bare difference between killing and letting die that makes the difference in these cases. Rather, the other factors—the murderer's motive of personal gain, for example, contrasted with the doctor's humanitarian motivation—account for different reactions to the different cases.

I have argued that killing is not in itself any worse than letting die; if my contention is right, it follows that active euthanasia is not any worse than passive euthanasia. What arguments can be given on the other side? The most common, I believe, is the following:

"The important difference between active and passive euthanasia is that, in passive euthanasia, the doctor does not do anything to bring about the patient's death. The doctor does nothing, and the patient dies of whatever ills already afflict him. In active euthanasia, however, the doctor does something to bring about the patient's death: he kills him. The doctor who gives the patient with cancer a lethal injection has himself caused his patient's death; whereas if he merely ceases treatment, the cancer is the cause of the death."

A number of points need to be made here. The first is that it is not exactly correct to say that in passive euthanasia the doctor does nothing, for he does do one thing that is very important: he lets the patient die. "Letting someone die" is certainly different, in some respects, from other types of action—mainly in that it is a kind of action that one may perform by way of not performing certain other actions. For example, one may let a patient die by way of not giving medication, just as one may insult someone by way of not shaking his hand. But for any purpose of moral assessment, it is a type of action nonetheless. The decision to let a patient die is subject to moral appraisal in the same way that a decision to kill him would be subject to moral appraisal: it may be assessed as wise or unwise, compassionate or sadistic, right or wrong. If a doctor deliberately let a patient die who was suffering from a routinely curable illness, the doctor would certainly be to blame for what he had done, just as he would be to blame if he had needlessly killed the patient. Charges against him would then be appropriate. If so, it would be no defense at all for him to insist that he didn't "do anything." He would have done something very serious indeed, for he let his patient die.

Fixing the cause of death may be very important from a legal point of view, for it may determine whether criminal charges are brought against the doctor. But I do not think that this notion can be used to show a moral difference between active and passive euthanasia. The reason why it is considered bad to be the cause of someone's death is that death is regarded as a great evil—and so it is. However, if it has been decided that euthanasia—even passive euthanasia—is desirable in a given case, it has also been decided that in this instance death is no greater an evil than the patient's continued existence. And if this is true, the usual reason for not wanting to be the cause of someone's death simply does not apply.

Finally, doctors may think that all of this is only of academic interest—the sort of thing that philosophers may worry about but that has no practical bearing on their own work. After all, doctors must be concerned about the legal consequences of what they do, and active euthanasia is clearly forbidden by the law. But even so, doctors should also be concerned with the fact that the law is forcing upon them a moral doctrine that may well be indefensible, and has a considerable effect on their practices. Of course, most doctors are not now in the position of being coerced in this matter, for they do not regard themselves as merely going along with what the law requires. Rather, in statements such as the AMA policy statement that I have quoted, they are endorsing this doctrine as a central point of medical ethics. In that statement, active euthanasia is condemned not merely as illegal but as "contrary to that for which the medical profession stands," whereas passive euthanasia is approved. However, the preceding considerations suggest that there is really no moral difference between the two, considered in themselves (there may be important moral differences in some cases in their *consequences*, but, as I pointed out, these differences may make active euthanasia, and not passive euthanasia, the morally preferable option). So, whereas doctors may have to discriminate between active and passive euthanasia to satisfy the law, they should not do any more than that. In particular, they should not give the distinction any added authority and weight by writing it into official statements of medical ethics.

NOTE

1 Shaw A.: 'Doctor, Do We Have a Choice?' *The New York Times Magazine,* January 30, 1972, p. 54.

Active and Passive Euthanasia: An Impertinent Distinction?
Thomas D. Sullivan

Thomas D. Sullivan is professor of philosophy at the College of St. Thomas in St. Paul, Minnesota. He is the author of "Between Thoughts and Things: The Status of Meaning" and "Adequate Evidence for Religious Assent" and the coauthor of "Benevolence and Absolute Prohibitions." He is also the author of an article on abortion, "In Defense of Total Regard."

Sullivan, responding directly to Rachels, offers a defense of the standard (traditional) view on the morality of euthanasia. Sullivan charges Rachels with misconstruing the sense behind the traditional view. On Sullivan's analysis, the traditional view is not dependent on the distinction between killing and letting die. Rather, it simply forbids the *intentional* termination of life, whether by killing or letting die. The cessation of *extraordinary* means, he maintains, is morally permissible because, although death is foreseen, it need not be intended.

Because of recent advances in medical technology, it is today possible to save or prolong the lives of many persons who in an earlier era would have quickly perished. Unhappily, however, it often is impossible to do so without commiting the patient and his or her family to a future filled with sorrows. Modern methods of neurosurgery can successfully close the opening at the base of the spine of a baby born with severe myelomeningocoele, but do nothing to relieve the paralysis that afflicts it from the waist down or to remedy the patient's incontinence of stool and urine. Antibiotics and skin grafts can spare the life of a victim of severe and massive burns, but fail to eliminate the immobilizing contractions of arms and legs, the extreme pain, and the hideous disfigurement of the face. It is not surprising, therefore, that physicians and moralists in increasing number recommend that assistance should not be given to such patients, and that some have even begun to advocate the deliberate hastening of death by medical means, provided informed consent has been given by the appropriate parties.

The latter recommendation consciously and directly conflicts with what might be called the "traditional" view of the physician's role. The traditional view, as articulated, for example, by the House of Delegates of the American Medical Association in 1973, declared:

> The intentional termination of the life of one human being by another—mercy killing—is contrary to that for which

From *Human Life Review*, vol. III, no. 3 (Summer 1977), pp. 40–46. Reprinted with permission from The Human Life Foundation, Inc., 150 East 35th Street, New York, N.Y., 10016

the medical profession stands and is contrary to the policy of the American Medical Association.

> The cessation of the employment of extra-ordinary means to prolong the life of the body when there is irrefutable evidence that biological death is imminent is the decision of the patient and/or his immediate family. The advice and judgment of the physician should be freely available to the patient and/or his immediate family.

Basically this view involves two points: (1) that it is impermissible for the doctor or anyone else to terminate intentionally the life of a patient, but (2) that it is permissible in some cases to cease the employment of "extraordinary means" of preserving life, even though the death of the patient is a foreseeable consequence.

Does this position really make sense? Recent criticism charges that it does not. The heart of the complaint is that the traditional view arbitrarily rules out all cases of intentionally acting to terminate life, but permits what is in fact the moral equivalent, letting patients die. This accusation has been clearly articulated by James Rachels in a widely-read article that appeared in a recent issue of the *New England Journal of Medicine*, entitled "Active and Passive Euthanasia."[1] By "active euthanasia" Rachels seems to mean *doing something* to bring about patient's death, and by "passive euthanasia," not doing anything, i.e., just letting the patient die. Referring the A.M.A. statement, Rachels sees the traditional position as always forbidding active euthanasia, but permitting passive euthanasia. Yet, he argues, passive euthanasia may be in some cases morally indistinguishable from active euthanasia, and in other cases even worse

make his point he asks his readers to consider the case of a Down's syndrome baby with an intestinal obstruction that easily could be remedied through routine surgery. Rachels comments:

> I can understand why some people are opposed to all euthanasia and insist that such infants must be allowed to live. I think I can also understand why other people favor destroying these babies quickly and painlessly. But why should anyone favor letting "dehydration and infection wither a tiny being over hours and days"? The doctrine that says that a baby may be allowed to dehydrate and wither, but may not be given an injection that would end its life without suffering, seems so patently cruel as to require no further refutation.[2]

Rachels' point is that decisions such as the one he describes as "patently cruel" arise out of a misconceived moral distinction between active and passive euthanasia, which in turn rests upon a distinction between killing and letting die that itself has no moral importance.

> One reason why so many people think that there is an important difference between active and passive euthanasia is that they think killing someone is morally worse than letting someone die. But is it?...To investigate this issue two cases may be considered that are exactly alike except that one involves killing whereas the other involves letting someone die. Then, it can be asked whether this difference makes any difference to the moral assessments....
>
> In the first, Smith stands to gain a large inheritance if anything should happen to his six-year-old cousin. One evening while the child is taking his bath, Smith sneaks into the bathroom and drowns the child, and then arranges things so that it will look like an accident.
>
> In the second, Jones also stands to gain if anything should happen to his six-year-old cousin. Like Smith, Jones sneaks in planning to drown the child in his bath. However, just as he enters the bathroom Jones sees the child slip and hit his head, and fall face down in the water. Jones is delighted; he stands by, ready to push the child's head back under if it is necessary, but it is not necessary. With only a little thrashing about, the child drowns all by himself, "accidentally," as Jones watches and does nothing.[3]

Rachels observes that Smith killed the child, whereas Jones "merely" let the child die. If there's an important moral distinction between killing and letting die, then,

we should say that Jones' behavior from a moral point of view is less reprehensible than Smith's. But while the law might draw some distinctions here, it seems clear that the acts of Jones and Smith are not different in any important way, or, if there is a difference, Jones' action is even worse.

In essence, then, the objection to the position adopted by the A.M.A. of Rachels and those who argue like him is that it endorses a highly questionable moral distinction between killing and letting die, which, if accepted, leads to indefensible medical decisions. Nowhere does Rachels quite come out and say that he favors active euthanasia in some cases, but the implication is clear. Nearly everyone holds that it is sometimes pointless to prolong the process of dying and that in those cases it is morally permissible to let a patient die even though a few hours or days could be salvaged by procedures that would also increase the agonies of the dying. But if it is impossible to defend a general distinction between letting people die and acting to terminate their lives directly, then it would seem that active euthanasia also may be morally permissible.

Now what shall we make of all this? It *is* cruel to stand by and watch a Down's baby die an agonizing death when a simple operation would remove the intestinal obstruction, but to offer the excuse that in failing to operate we didn't *do* anything to bring about death is an example of moral evasiveness comparable to the excuse Jones would offer for his action of "merely" letting his cousin die. Furthermore, it is true that if someone is trying to bring about the death of another human being, then it makes little difference from the moral point of view if his purpose is achieved by action or by malevolent omission, as in the cases of Jones and Smith.

But if we acknowledge this, are we obliged to give up the traditional view expressed by the A.M.A. statement? Of course not. To begin with, we are hardly obliged to assume the Jones-like role Rachels assigns the defender of the traditional view. We have the option of operating on the Down's baby and saving its life. Rachels mentions that possibility only to hurry past it as if that is not what his opposition would do. But, of course, that is precisely the course of action most defenders of the traditional position would choose.

Secondly, while it may be that the reason some rather confused people give for upholding the traditional view is that they think killing someone is always worse than letting them die, nobody who gives the matter much thought puts it that way. Rather they say that killing someone is clearly morally worse than not killing

them, and killing them can be done by acting to bring about their death or by refusing ordinary means to keep them alive in order to bring about the same goal.

What I am suggesting is that Rachels' objections leave the position he sets out to criticize untouched. It is worth noting that the jargon of active and passive euthanasia—and it is jargon—does not appear in the resolution. Nor does the resolution state or imply the distinction Rachels attacks, a distinction that puts a moral premium on overt behavior—moving or not moving one's parts—while totally ignoring the intentions of the agent. That no such distinction is being drawn seems clear from the fact that the A.M.A. resolution speaks approvingly of ceasing to use extraordinary means in certain cases, and such withdrawals might easily involve bodily movement, for example unplugging an oxygen machine.

In addition to saddling his opposition with an indefensible distinction it doesn't make, Rachels proceeds to ignore one that it does make—one that is crucial to a just interpretation of the view. Recall the A.M.A. allows the withdrawal of what it calls extra-ordinary means of preserving life; clearly the contrast here is with ordinary means. Though in its short statement those expressions are not defined, the definition Paul Ramsey refers to as standard in his book, *The Patient as Person*, seems to fit.

> Ordinary means of preserving life are all medicines, treatments, and operations, which offer a reasonable hope of benefit for the patient and which can be obtained and used without excessive expense, pain, and other inconveniences.
>
> Extra-ordinary means of preserving life are all those medicines, treatments, and operations which cannot be obtained without excessive expense, pain, or other inconvenience, or which, if used, would not offer a reasonable hope of benefit.[4]

Now with this distinction in mind, we can see how the traditional view differs from the position Rachels mistakes for it. The traditional view is that the intentional termination of human life is impermissible, irrespective of whether this goal is brought about by action or inaction. Is the action or refraining *aimed at* producing a death? Is the termination of life *sought, chosen or planned*? Is the intention deadly? If so, the act or omission is wrong.

But we all know it is entirely possible that the unwillingness of a physician to use extra-ordinary means for preserving life may be prompted not by a determination to bring about death, but by other motives. For ex-

ample, he may realize that further treatment may offer little hope of reversing the dying process and/or be excruciating, as in the case when a massively necrotic bowel condition in a neonate is out of control. The doctor who does what he can to comfort the infant but does not submit it to further treatment or surgery may foresee that the decision will hasten death, but it certainly doesn't follow from that fact that he intends to bring about its death. It is, after all, entirely possible to foresee that something will come about as a result of one's conduct without intending the consequence or side effect. If I drive downtown, I can foresee that I'll wear out my tires a little, but I don't drive downtown with the intention of wearing out my tires. And if I choose to forego my exercises for a few days, I may think that as a result my physical condition will deteriorate a little, but I don't omit my exercise with a view to running myself down. And if you have to fill a position and select Green, who is better qualified for the post than her rival Brown, you needn't appoint Mrs. Green with the intention of hurting Mr. Brown, though you may foresee that Mr. Brown will feel hurt. And if a country extends its general education programs to its illiterate masses, it is predictable the suicide rate will go up, but even if the public officials are aware of this fact, it doesn't follow that they initiate the program with a view to making the suicide rate go up. In general, then, it is not the case that all the foreseeable consequences and side effects of our conduct are necessarily intended. And it is because the physician's withdrawal of extra-ordinary means can be otherwise motivated than by a desire to bring about the predictable death of the patient that such action cannot categorically be ruled out as wrong.

But the refusal to use ordinary means is an altogether different matter. After all, what is the point of refusing assistance which offers reasonable hope of benefit to the patient without involving excessive pain or other inconvenience? How could it be plausibly maintained that the refusal is not motivated by a desire to bring about the death of the patient? The traditional position, therefore, rules out not only direct actions to bring about death, such as giving a patient a lethal injection, but malevolent omissions as well, such as not providing minimum care for the newborn.

The reason the A.M.A. position sounds so silly when one listens to arguments such as Rachels' is that he slights the distinction between ordinary and extra-ordinary means and then drums on cases where *ordinary* means are refused. The impression is thereby conveyed that the traditional doctrine sanctions omissions that are morally indistinguishable in a substantive way from direct killings, but then incomprehensively refuses to permit quick and painless termination of life. If the traditional doctrine would approve of Jones' standing by with a grin on his face while his young cousin drowned in a tub, or letting a Down's baby wither and die when ordinary means are available to preserve its life, it would indeed be difficult to see how anyone could defend it. But so to conceive the traditional doctrine is simply to misunderstand it. It is not a doctrine that rests on some supposed distinction between "active" and "passive euthanasia," whatever those words are supposed to mean, nor on a distinction between moving and not moving our bodies. It is simply a prohibition against intentional killing, which includes both direct actions and malevolent omissions.

To summarize—the traditional position represented by the A.M.A. statement is not incoherent. It acknowledges, or more accurately, insists upon the fact that withholding ordinary means to sustain life may be tantamount to killing. The traditional position can be made to appear incoherent only by imposing upon it a crude idea of killing held by none of its more articulate advocates.

Thus the criticism of Rachels and other reformers, misapprehending its target, leaves the traditional position untouched. That position is simply a prohibition of murder. And it is good to remember, as C. S. Lewis, once pointed out:

No man, perhaps, ever at first described to himself the act he was about to do as Murder, or Adultery, or Fraud, or Treachery....And when he hears it so described by other men he is (in a way) sincerely shocked and surprised.

Those others 'don't understand.' If they knew what it had really been like for him, they would not use those crude 'stock' names. With a wink or a titter, or a cloud of muddy emotion, the thing has slipped into his will as something not very extraordinary, something of which, rightly understood in all of his peculiar circumstances, he may even feel proud.[5]

I fully realize that there are times when those who have the noble duty to tend the sick and the dying are deeply moved by the sufferings of their patients, especially of the very young and the very old, and desperately wish they could do more than comfort and companion them. Then, perhaps, it seems that universal moral principles are mere abstractions having little to do with the agony of the dying. But of course we do not see best when our eyes are filled with tears.

NOTES

1 *New England Journal of Medicine*, 292; 78–80. Jan. 9, 1975. [Reprinted, this volume, pp. 367–370.]
2 Ibid., pp. 78–79. [This volume, p. 368.]
3 Ibid., p. 79. [This volume, p. 369.]
4 Paul Ramsey, *The Patient As Person* (New Haven and London: Yale University Press, 1970), p. 122. Ramsey abbreviates the definition first given by Gerald Kelly, S.J., *Medico-Moral Problems* (St. Louis, Missouri: The Catholic Hospital Association, 1958), p. 129.
5 C. S. Lewis, *A Preface to Paradise Lost* (London and New York: Oxford University Press, 1970), p. 126.

More Impertinent Distinctions and a Defense of Active Euthanasia
James Rachels

A biographical sketch of James Rachels is found on p. 367.

This selection falls into two major sections. In the first major section, Rachels responds to Sullivan; in the second, he develops arguments in support of the moral justifiability of active euthanasia. Rachels makes a new departure in responding to Sullivan. He presents two additional arguments against the standard (traditional) view on the morality of euthanasia. Rachels

Reprinted from Thomas A. Mappes and Jane S. Zembaty, eds., *Biomedical Ethics* (New York: McGraw–Hill, 1981), pp.355–359. Copyright © 1978 by James Rachels. Also from Tom Regan, ed., *Matters of Life and Death: New Introductory Essays in Moral Philosophy*. Copyright © 1980 by Random House, Inc. Reprinted by permission of Random House, Inc.

contends, first, that the traditional view is mistaken because it depends on an indefensible distinction between intentional and nonintentional terminations of life. Next he contends that the traditional view is mistaken because it depends on an indefensible distinction between ordinary and extraordinary means of treatment. Rachels's defense of active euthanasia rests on two arguments—the argument from mercy and the argument from the Golden Rule.

Many thinkers, including almost all orthodox Catholics, believe that euthanasia is immoral. They oppose killing patients in any circumstances whatever. However, they think it is all right, in some special circumstances, to allow patients to die by withholding treatment. The American Medical Association's policy statement on mercy killing supports this traditional view. In my paper "Active and Passive Euthanasia"[1] I argued, against the traditional view, that there is in fact no moral difference between killing and letting die—if one is permissible, then so is the other.

Professor Sullivan[2] does not dispute my argument; instead he dismisses it as irrelevant. The traditional doctrine, he says, does not appeal to or depend on the distinction between killing and letting die. Therefore, arguments against that distinction "leave the traditional position untouched."

Is my argument really irrelevant? I don't see how it can be. As Sullivan himself points out,

> Nearly everyone holds that it is sometimes pointless to prolong the process of dying and that in those cases it is morally permissible to let a patient die even though a few hours or days could be salvaged by procedures that would also increase the agonies of the dying. But if it is impossible to defend a general distinction between letting people die and acting to terminate their lives directly, then it would seem that active euthanasia also may be morally permissible.(372)

But traditionalists like Professor Sullivan hold that active euthanasia—the direct killing of patients—is *not* morally permissible; so, if my argument is sound, their view must be mistaken. I cannot agree, then, that my argument "leaves the traditional position untouched."

However, I shall not press this point. Instead I shall present some further arguments against the traditional position, concentrating on those elements of the position which Professor Sullivan himself thinks most important. According to him, what is important is, first, that we should never *intentionally* terminate the life of a patient, either by action or omission, and second, that we may

cease or omit treatment of a patient, knowing that this will result in death, only if the means of treatment involved are *extraordinary*.

INTENTIONAL AND NONINTENTIONAL TERMINATION OF LIFE

We can, of course, distinguish between what a person does and the intention with which he does it. But what is the significance of this distinction for ethics?

> The traditional view [says Sullivan] is that the intentional termination of human life is impermissible, irrespective of whether this goal is brought about by action or inaction. Is the action or refraining *aimed at* producing a death? Is the termination of life *sought, chosen or planned*? Is the intention deadly? If so, the act or omission is wrong.(373)

Thus on the traditional view there is a very definite sort of moral relation between act and intention. An act which is otherwise permissible may become impermissible if it is accompanied by a bad intention. The intention makes the act wrong.

There is reason to think that this view of the relation between act and intention is mistaken. Consider the following example. Jack visits his sick and lonely grandmother, and entertains her for the afternoon. He loves her and his only intention is to cheer her up. Jill also visits the grandmother, and provides an afternoon's cheer. But Jill's concern is that the old lady will soon be making her will; Jill wants to be included among the heirs. Jack also knows that his visit might influence the making of the will, in his favor, but that is no part of his plan. Thus Jack and Jill do the very same thing—they both spend an afternoon cheering up their sick grandmother—and what they do may lead to the same consequences, namely influencing the will. But their intentions are quite different.

Jack's intention was honorable and Jill's was not. Could we say on that account that what Jack did was right, but what Jill did was wrong? No; for Jack and Jill did the very same thing, and if they did the same thing, we cannot say that one acted rightly and the other wrongly.[3] Consistency requires that we assess similar actions similarly. Thus if we are trying to evaluate their *actions*, we must say about one what we say about the other.

However, if we are trying to assess Jack's *character*, or Jill's, things are very different. Even though their actions were similar, Jack seems admirable for what he did, while Jill does not. What Jill did—comforting an elderly sick relative—was a morally good thing, but we would not think well of her for it since she was only scheming after the old lady's money. Jack, on the other hand, did a good thing *and* he did it with an admirable intention. Thus we think well, not only of what Jack did, but of Jack.

The traditional view, as presented by Professor Sullivan, says that the intention with which an act is done is relevant to determining whether the act is right. The example of Jack and Jill suggests that, on the contrary, the intention is not relevant to deciding whether the *act* is right or wrong, but instead it is relevant to assessing the character of the person who does the act, which is very different.

Now let us turn to an example that concerns more important matters of life and death. This example is adapted from one used by Sullivan himself (373). A massively necrotic bowel condition in a neonate is out of control. Dr. White realizes that further treatment offers little hope of reversing the dying process and will only increase the suffering; so, he does not submit the infant to further treatment—even though he knows that this decision will hasten death. However, Dr. White does not seek, choose, or plan that death, so it is not part of his intention that the baby dies.

Dr. Black is faced with a similar case. A massively necrotic bowel condition in a neonate is out of control. He realizes that further treatment offers little hope of saving the baby and will only increase its suffering. He decides that it is better for the baby to die a bit sooner than to go on suffering pointlessly; so, with the intention of letting the baby die, he ceases treatment.

According to the traditional position, Dr. White's action was acceptable, but Dr. Black acted wrongly. However, this assessment faces the same problem we encountered before. Dr. White and Dr. Black did *the very same thing*: their handling of the cases was identical. Both doctors ceased treatment, knowing that the baby would die sooner, and both did so because they regarded continued treatment as pointless, given the infants' prospects. So how could one's action be acceptable and the other's not? There was, of course, a subtle difference in their *attitudes* toward what they did. Dr. Black said to

himself, "I want this baby to die now, rather than later, so that it won't suffer more; so I won't continue the treatment." A defender of the traditional view might choose to condemn Dr. Black for this, and say that his character is defective (although I would not say that); but the traditionalist should not say that Dr. Black's *action* was wrong on that account, at least not if he wants to go on saying that Dr. White's action was right. A pure heart cannot make a wrong act right; neither can an impure heart make a right act wrong. As in the case of Jack and Jill, the intention is relevant, not to determining the rightness of actions, but to assessing the character of the people who act.

There is a general lesson to be learned here. The rightness or wrongness of an act is determined by the reasons for or against it. Suppose you are trying to decide, in this example, whether treatment should be continued. What are the reasons for and against this course of action? On the one hand, if treatment is ceased the baby will die very soon. On the other hand, the baby will die eventually anyway, even if treatment is continued. It has no chance of growing up. Moreover, if its life is prolonged, its suffering will be prolonged as well, and the medical resources used will be unavailable to others who would have a better chance of a satisfactory cure. In light of all this, you may well decide against continued treatment. But notice that there is no mention here of anybody's intentions. The intention you would have, if you decided to cease treatment, is not one of the things you need to consider. It is not among the reasons either for or against the action. That is why it is irrelevant to determining whether the action is right.

In short, a person's intention is relevant to an assessment of his character. The fact that a person intended so-and-so by his action may be a reason for thinking him a good or a bad person. But the intention is not relevant to determining whether the act itself is morally right. The rightness of the act must be decided on the basis of the objective reasons for or against it. It is permissible to let the baby die, in Sullivan's example, because of the facts about the baby's condition and its prospects—not because of anything having to do with anyone's intentions. Thus the traditional view is mistaken on this point.

ORDINARY AND EXTRAORDINARY MEANS OF TREATMENT

The American Medical Association policy statement says that life-sustaining treatment may sometimes be stopped if the means of treatment are "extraordinary"; the implication is that "ordinary" means of treatment may not be withheld. The distinction between ordinary and extraordinary treatments is crucial to orthodox Catholic thought in this area, and Professor Sullivan reemphasizes its importance: he says that, while a physician may sometimes rightly refuse to use extraordinary means to prolong life, "the refusal to use ordinary means is an altogether different matter."(373)

However, upon reflection it is clear that it is sometimes permissible to omit even very ordinary sorts of treatments.

> Suppose that a diabetic patient long accustomed to self-administration of insulin falls victim to terminal cancer, or suppose that a terminal cancer patient suddenly develops diabetes. Is he in the first case obliged to continue, and in the second case obliged to begin, insulin treatment and die painfully of cancer, or in either or both cases may the patient choose rather to pass into diabetic coma and an earlier death?... What of the conscious patient suffering from painful incurable disease who suddenly gets pneumonia? Or an old man slowly deteriorating who from simply being inactive and recumbent gets pneumonia: Are we to use antibiotics in a likely successful attack upon this disease which from time immemorial has been called "the old man's friend"?[4]

These examples are provided by Paul Ramsey, a leading theological ethicist. Even so conservative a thinker as Ramsey is sympathetic with the idea that, in such cases, life-prolonging treatment is not mandatory: the insulin and the antibiotics need not be used. Yet surely insulin and antibiotics are "ordinary" treatments by today's medical standards. They are common, easily administered, and cheap. There is nothing exotic about them. So it appears that the distinction between ordinary and extraordinary means does not have the significance traditionally attributed to it.

But what of the *definitions* of "ordinary" and "extraordinary" means which Sullivan provides? Quoting Ramsey, he says that

> Ordinary means of preserving life are all medicines, treatments, and operations, which offer a reasonable hope of benefit for the patient and which can be obtained and used without excessive expense, pain, and other inconveniences.
>
> Extra-ordinary means of preserving life are all those medicines, treatments, and operations which cannot be obtained without excessive expense, pain, or other inconvenience, or which, if used, would not offer a reasonable hope of benefit.(373)

Do these definitions provide us with a useful distinction—one that can be used in determining when a treatment is mandatory and when it is not?

The first thing to notice is the way the word "excessive" functions in these definitions. It is said that a treatment is extraordinary if it cannot be obtained without *excessive* expense or pain. But when is an expense "excessive"? Is a cost of $10,000 excessive? If it would save the life of a young woman and restore her to perfect health, $10,000 does not seem excessive. But if it would only prolong the life of Ramsey's cancer-stricken diabetic a short while, perhaps $10,000 is excessive. The point is not merely that what is excessive changes from case to case. The point is that what is excessive *depends on* whether it would be a good thing for the life in question to be prolonged.

Second, we should notice the use of the word "benefit" in the definitions. It is said that ordinary treatments offer a reasonable hope of *benefit* for the patient; and that treatments are extraordinary if they will not benefit the patient. But how do we tell if a treatment will benefit the patient? Remember that we are talking about life-prolonging treatments; the "benefit," if any, is the continuation of life. Whether continued life is a benefit depends on the details of the particular case. For a person with a painful terminal illness, a temporarily continued life may not be a benefit. For a person in irreversible coma, such as Karen Quinlan, continued biological existence is almost certainly not a benefit. On the other hand, for a person who can be cured and resume a normal life, life-sustaining treatment definitely is a benefit. Again, the point is that in order to decide whether life-sustaining treatment is a benefit we must *first* decide whether it would be a good thing for the life in question to be prolonged.

Therefore, these definitions do not mark out a distinction that can be used to help us decide when treatment may be omitted. We cannot by using the definitions identify which treatments are extraordinary, and then use that information to determine whether the treatment may be omitted. For the definitions require that we must *already* have decided the moral questions of life and death *before* we can answer the question of which treatments are extraordinary!

We are brought, then, to this conclusion about the distinction between ordinary and extraordinary means. If we apply the distinction in a straightforward, common-sense way, the traditional doctrine is false, for it is clear that it is sometimes permissible to omit ordinary treatments. On the other hand, if we define the terms as suggested by Ramsey and Sullivan, the distinction is useless in practical decision-making. In either case, the distinction provides no help in formulating an acceptable ethic of letting die.

To summarize what has been said so far, the distinction between killing and letting die has no moral importance; on that Professor Sullivan and I agree. He, however, contends that the distinctions between intentional and nonintentional termination of life, and ordinary and extraordinary means, must be at the heart of a correct moral view. I believe that the arguments given above refute this view. Those distinctions are no better than the first one. The traditional view is mistaken.

In my original paper I did not argue in favor of active euthanasia. I merely argued that active and passive euthanasia are equivalent: *if* one is acceptable, so is the other. However, Professor Sullivan correctly inferred that I do endorse active euthanasia. I believe that it is morally justified in some instances and that at least two strong arguments support this position. The first is the argument from mercy; the second is the argument from the golden rule.

THE ARGUMENT FROM MERCY

Preliminary Statement of the Argument

The single most powerful argument in support of euthanasia is the argument from mercy. It is also an exceptionally simple argument, at least in its main idea, which makes one uncomplicated point. Terminal patients sometimes suffer pain so horrible that it is beyond the comprehension of those who have not actually experienced it. Their suffering can be so terrible that we do not like even to read about it or think about it; we recoil even from the descriptions of such agony. The argument from mercy says: Euthanasia is justified because it provides an end to *that*.

The great Irish satirist Jonathan Swift took eight years to die, while, in the words of Joseph Fletcher, "His mind crumbled to pieces."[5] At times the pain in his blinded eyes was so intense he had to be restrained from tearing them out with his own hands. Knives and other potential instruments of suicide had to be kept from him. For the last three years of his life, he could do nothing but sit and drool; and when he finally died it was only after convulsions that lasted thirty-six hours.

Swift died in 1745. Since then, doctors have learned how to eliminate much of the pain that accompanies terminal illness, but the victory has been far from complete. So, here is a more modern example.

Stewart Alsop was a respected journalist who died in 1975 of a rare form of cancer. Before he died, he wrote movingly of his experiences as a terminal patient. Although he had not thought much about euthanasia before, he came to approve of it after rooming briefly with someone he called Jack:

The third night that I roomed with Jack in our tiny double room in the solid-tumor ward of the cancer clinic of the National Institutes of Health in Bethesda, Md., a terrible thought occurred to me.

Jack had a melanoma in his belly, a malignant solid tumor that the doctors guessed was about the size of a softball. The cancer had started a few months before with a small tumor in his left shoulder, and there had been several operations since. The doctors planned to remove the softball-sized tumor, but they knew Jack would soon die. The cancer had metastasized—it had spread beyond control.

Jack was good-looking, about 28, and brave. He was in constant pain, and his doctor had prescribed an intravenous shot of a synthetic opiate—a pain-killer, or analgesic—every four hours. His wife spent many of the daylight hours with him, and she would sit or lie on his bed and pat him all over, as one pats a child, only more methodically, and this seemed to help control the pain. But at night, when his pretty wife had left (wives cannot stay overnight at the NIH clinic) and darkness fell, the pain would attack without pity.

At the prescribed hour, a nurse would give Jack a shot of the synthetic analgesic, and this would control the pain for perhaps two hours or a bit more. Then he would begin to moan, or whimper, very low, as though he didn't want to wake me. Then he would begin to howl, like a dog.

When this happened, either he or I would ring for a nurse, and ask for a pain-killer. She would give him some codeine or the like by mouth, but it never did any real good—it affected him no more than half an aspirin might affect a man who had just broken his arm. Always the nurse would explain as encouragingly as she could that there was not long to go before the next intravenous shot—"Only about 50 minutes now." And always poor Jack's whimpers and howls would become more loud and frequent until at last the blessed relief came.

The third night of this routine, the terrible thought occurred to me: "If Jack were a dog," I thought, "what would be done with him?" The answer was obvious: the pound, and chloroform. No human being with a spark of pity could let a living thing suffer so, to no good end.[6]

The NIH clinic is, of course, one of the most modern and best-equipped hospitals we have. Jack's suffering was not the result of poor treatment in some backward rural facility; it was the inevitable product of his disease, which medical science was powerless to prevent.

I have quoted Alsop at length not for the sake of indulging in gory details but to give a clear idea of the kind of suffering we are talking about. We should not gloss over these facts with euphemistic language, or squeamishly avert our eyes from them. For only by keeping them firmly and vividly in mind can we appreciate the full force of the argument from mercy: If a person prefers—and even begs for—death as the only alternative to lingering on *in this kind of torment*, only to die anyway after a while, then surely it is not immoral to help this person die sooner. As Alsop put it, "No human being with a spark of pity could let a living thing suffer so, to no good end."

The Utilitarian Version of the Argument

In connection with this argument, the utilitarians should be mentioned. They argue that actions and social policies should be judged right or wrong *exclusively* according to whether they cause happiness or misery; and they argue that when judged by this standard, euthanasia turns out to be morally acceptable. The utilitarian argument may be elaborated as follows:

1. Any action or social policy is morally right if it serves to increase the amount of happiness in the world or to decrease the amount of misery. Conversely, an action or social policy is morally wrong if it serves to decrease happiness or to increase misery.

2. The policy of killing, at their own request, hopelessly ill patients who are suffering great pain, would decrease the amount of misery in the world. (An example could be Alsop's friend Jack.)

3. Therefore, such a policy would be morally right.

The first premise of this argument, (1), states the Principle of Utility, which is the basic utilitarian assumption. Today most philosophers think that this principle is wrong, because they think that the promotion of happiness and the avoidance of misery are not the *only* morally important things. Happiness, they say, is only one among many values that should be promoted: freedom, justice, and a respect for people's rights are also important. To take one example: People *might* be happier if there were no freedom of religion; for, if everyone adhered to the same religious beliefs, there would be greater harmony among people. There would be no unhappiness caused within families by Jewish girls marrying Catholic boys, and so forth. Moreover, if people were brainwashed well enough, no one would mind not having freedom of choice. Thus happiness would be increased. But, the argument continues, even if happiness *could* be increased this way, it would not be right to deny people freedom of religion, because people have a right to make their own choices. Therefore, the first premise of the utilitarian argument is unacceptable.

There is a related difficulty for utilitarianism, which connects more directly with the topic of euthanasia. Suppose a person is leading a miserable life—full of more unhappiness than happiness—but does *not* want to die. This person thinks that a miserable life is better than none at all. Now I assume that we would all agree that the person should not be killed; that would be plain, unjustifiable murder. Yet it *would* decrease the amount of misery in the world if we killed this person—it would lead to an increase in the balance of happiness over unhappiness—and so it is hard to see how, on strictly utilitarian grounds, it could be wrong. Again, the Principle of Utility seems to be an inadequate guide for determining right and wrong. So we are on shaky ground if we rely on *this* version of the argument from mercy for a defense of euthanasia.

Doing What Is in Everyone's Best Interests

Although the foregoing utilitarian argument is faulty, it is nevertheless based on a sound idea. For even if the promotion of happiness and avoidance of misery are not the *only* morally important things, they are still very important. So, when an action or social policy would decrease misery, that is *a* very strong reason in its favor. In the cases of voluntary euthanasia we are now considering, great suffering is eliminated, and since the patient requests it, there is no question of violating individual rights. That is why, regardless of the difficulties of the Principle of Utility, the utilitarian version of the argument still retains considerable force.

I want now to present a somewhat different version of the argument from mercy, which is inspired by utilitarianism but which avoids the difficulties of the foregoing version by not making the Principle of Utility a premise of the argument. I believe that the following argument is sound and proves that active euthanasia *can* be justified:

1. If an action promotes the best interests of *everyone* concerned, and violates *no one's* rights, then that action is morally acceptable.

2. In at least some cases, active euthanasia promotes the best interests of everyone concerned and violates no one's rights.

3. Therefore, in at least some cases active euthanasia is morally acceptable.

It would have been in everyone's best interests if active euthanasia had been employed in the case of Stewart Alsop's friend, Jack. First, and most important, it would have been in Jack's own interests, since it would have provided him with an easier, better death, without pain. (Who among us would choose Jack's death, if we had a choice, rather than a quick painless death?) Second, it would have been in the best interests of Jack's wife. Her misery, helplessly watching him suffer, must have been almost equal to his. Third, the hospital staff's best interests would have been served, since if Jack's dying had not been prolonged, they could have turned their attention to other patients whom they could have helped. Fourth, other patients would have benefited since medical resources would no longer have been used in the sad, pointless maintenance of Jack's physical existence. Finally, if Jack himself requested to be killed, the act would not have violated his rights. Considering all this, how can active euthanasia in this case be wrong? How can it be wrong to do an action that is merciful, that benefits everyone concerned, and that violates no one's rights?

THE ARGUMENT FROM THE GOLDEN RULE

"Do unto others as you would have them do unto you" is one of the oldest and most familiar moral maxims. Stated in just that way, it is not a very good maxim: Suppose a sexual pervert started treating others as he would like to be treated himself; we might not be happy with the results. Nevertheless, the basic idea behind the golden rule is a good one. The basic idea is that moral rules apply impartially to everyone alike; therefore, you cannot say that you are justified in treating someone else in a certain way unless you are willing to admit that that person would also be justified in treating *you* in that way if your positions were reversed.

Kant and the Golden Rule

The great German philosopher Immanuel Kant (1724–1804) incorporated the basic idea of the Golden Rule into his system of ethics. Kant argued that we should act only on rules that we are willing to have applied universally; that is, we should behave as we would be willing to have *everyone* behave. He held that there is one supreme principle of morality, which he called "the Categorical Imperative." The Categorical Imperative says:

> Act only according to that maxim by which you can at the same time will that it should become a universal law.[7]

Let us discuss what this means. When we are trying to decide whether we ought to do a certain action, we must first ask what general rule or principle we would be following if we did it. Then, we ask whether we would be willing for everyone to follow that rule, in similar circumstances. (This determines whether "the maxim of the act"—the rule we would be following—can be "willed" to be "a universal law.") If we would not be willing for the rule to be followed universally, then we should not follow it ourselves. Thus, if we are not willing for others to apply the rule to *us*, we ought not apply it to *them*.

In the eighteenth chapter of St. Matthew's gospel there is a story that perfectly illustrates this point. A man is owed money by another, who cannot pay, and so he has the debtor thrown into prison. But he himself owes money to the king and begs that *his* debt be forgiven. At first the king forgives the debt. However, when the king hears how this man has treated the one who owed him, he changes his mind and "delivers him unto the tormentors" until he can pay. The moral is clear: If you do not think that others should apply the rule "Don't forgive debts!" to *you*, then you should not apply it to others.

The application of all this to the question of euthanasia is fairly obvious. Each of us is going to die someday, although most of us do not know when or how. But suppose you were told that you would die in one of two ways, and you were asked to choose between them. First, you could die quietly, and without pain, from a fatal injection. Or second, you could choose to die of an affliction so painful that for several days before death you would be reduced to howling like a dog, with your family standing by helplessly, trying to comfort you, but going through its own psychological hell. It is hard to believe that any sane person, when confronted by these possibilities, would choose to have a rule applied that would force upon him or her the second option. And if we would not want such a rule, which excludes euthanasia, applied to us, then we should not apply such a rule to others.

Implications for Christians

There is a considerable irony here. Kant [himself] was personally opposed to active euthanasia, yet his own Categorical Imperative seems to sanction it. The larger irony, however, is for those in the Christian Church who have for centuries opposed active euthanasia. According to the New Testament accounts, Jesus himself promulgated the Golden Rule as the supreme moral principle— "This is the Law and the Prophets," he said. But if this is the supreme principle of morality, then how can active euthanasia be always wrong? If I would have it done to me, how can it be wrong for me to do likewise to others?

R. M. Hare has made this point with great force. A Christian as well as a leading contemporary moral philosopher, Hare has long argued that "universalizability" is one of the central characteristics of moral judgment. ('Universalizability' is the name he gives to the basic idea embodied in both the Golden Rule and the Categorical Imperative. It means that a moral judgment must conform to universal principles, which apply to everyone alike, if it is to be acceptable.) In an article called "Euthanasia: A Christian View," Hare argues that Christians, if they took Christ's teachings about the Golden Rule seriously, would not think that euthanasia is always wrong. He gives this (true) example:

> The driver of a petrol lorry [i.e., a gas truck] was in an accident in which his tanker overturned and immediately caught fire. He himself was trapped in the cab and could not be freed. He therefore besought the bystanders to kill him by hitting him on the head, so that he would not roast to death. I think that somebody did this, but I do not know what happened in court afterwards.
>
> Now will you please all ask yourselves, as I have many times asked myself, what you wish that men should

do to you if you were in the situation of that driver. I cannot believe that anybody who considered the matter seriously, as if he himself were going to be in that situation and had now to give instructions as to what rule the bystanders should follow, would say that the rule should be one ruling out euthanasia absolutely.[8]

We might note that *active* euthanasia is the only option here; the concept of passive euthanasia, in these circumstances, has no application....

Professor Sullivan finds my position pernicious. In his penultimate paragraph he says that the traditional doctrine "is simply a prohibition of murder," and that those of us who think otherwise are confused, teary-eyed sentimentalists. But the traditional doctrine is not that. It is a muddle of indefensible claims, backed by tradition but not by reason.

NOTES

1 "Active and Passive Euthanasia," *The New England Journal of Medicine*, vol. 292 (Jan. 9, 1975), pp. 78–80. [Reprinted, this volume, pp. 367–370.]
2 "Active and Passive Euthanasia: An Impertinent Distinction?" *The Human Life Review*, vol. III (1977), pp. 40–46. Parenthetical references in the text are to this article [as reprinted in this volume, pp. 371–374].
3 It might be objected that they did not "do the same thing," for Jill manipulated and deceived her grandmother, while Jack did not. If their actions are described in this way, then it may seem that "what Jill did" was wrong, while "what Jack did" was not. However, this description of what Jill did incorporates her intention into the description of the act. In the present context we must keep the act and the intention separate, in order to discuss the relation between them. If they *cannot* be held separate, then the traditional view makes no sense.
4 *The Patient as Person* (New Haven: Yale University Press, 1970), pp. 115–116.
5 *Morals and Medicine* (Boston: Beacon Press, 1960), p. 174.
6 "The Right to Die with Dignity," *Good Housekeeping*, August 1974, pp. 69, 130.
7 *Foundations of the Metaphysics of Morals*, p. 422.
8 *Philosophical Exchange* (Brockport, New York), II:I (Summer 1975), p. 45.

Active Euthanasia and Social Policy

Euthanasia
Marcia Angell

Marcia Angell, M.D., is executive editor of the *New England Journal of Medicine*. She has written editorials such as "Disease as a Reflection of the Psyche" and "Respecting the Autonomy of Competent Patients." Her other published articles include "Cost Containment and the Physician" and "Medicine: The Endangered Patient-Centered Ethic."

Angell identifies the conditions under which (active) euthanasia is permitted in the Netherlands and calls attention to two major differences between the Dutch guidelines and the provisions of a California legislative proposal, the "Humane and Dignified Death Act." After reviewing some of the standard arguments both for and against legalizing euthanasia, she argues that the risk of abuse would be much greater in the proposed California legislation than it is in the Dutch system.

Over the past decade the issue of whether it is ever permissible to withhold life-sustaining treatment has been debated by doctors and ethicists and in the courts and state legislatures. Gradually, a consensus has emerged that it is indeed permissible and even mandatory to withhold life-sustaining treatment under certain circumstances.[1-3] Now attention has begun to turn toward the issue of euthanasia. Euthanasia means purposely terminating the life of a patient to prevent further suffering, and it is illegal. Thus, it is different from withholding life-sustaining treatment. It is also different from administering a drug, such as morphine, that may hasten death but has another purpose. For many, the beginning of a debate about euthanasia is ominous—a step down a slippery slope leading to widespread disregard for the value of human life. For others, it signifies an opportunity to deal more humanely and rationally with prolonged meaningless suffering. My purpose here is to provide some background on this issue and to present arguments for and against euthanasia.

In the Netherlands, euthanasia officially remains a crime, punishable by up to 12 years in prison, but it is practiced fairly commonly and openly there, protected by a body of case law and by strong public support. Estimates are that 5000 to 8000 Dutch lives are ended by euthanasia each year.[4] The Dutch Medical Association in 1984 suggested guidelines for performing euthanasia,[5] and in 1985 a government-appointed Commission on

Reprinted by permission from the *New England Journal of Medicine*, vol. 319 (November 17, 1988), pp. 1348–1350.

Euthanasia issued a report[6] that in essence endorsed the guidelines and recommended a change in the criminal code to permit euthanasia. Although a change is unlikely during the tenure of the present government, it will almost certainly be an important issue in the next general election. The guidelines under which euthanasia is performed in the Netherlands are stringent. Four essential conditions must be met: (1) The patient must be competent. This requirement excludes many groups of patients for whom the question of withholding life-sustaining treatment has been most contentious in the United States—such as patients with advanced Alzheimer's disease, retarded patients, handicapped newborns, and patients, such as Karen Quinlan, who are in a persistent vegetative state. (2) The patient must request euthanasia voluntarily, consistently, and repeatedly over a reasonable time, and the request must be well documented. This requirement prevents euthanasia in response to an ill-considered or impulsive request. (3) The patient must be suffering intolerably, with no prospect of relief, although there needn't be a terminal disease. Thus, depression, for which there is treatment, would not be a reason for euthanasia, but amyotrophic lateral sclerosis might be. (4) Euthanasia must be performed by a physician in consultation with another physician not involved in the case; the usual method is to induce sleep with a barbiturate, followed by a lethal injection of curare.

In California this year, an unsuccessful effort was made to collect enough signatures on a petition to place a proposed law on the fall ballot that would legalize euthanasia.[7] This initiative was sponsored by Americans Against Human Suffering, the political arm of the Hemlock Society, an organization devoted to promoting the idea of appropriate euthanasia. In two important ways the provisions of the proposed law in California differed from the Dutch guidelines. First, they were more stringent than the Dutch guidelines in that they required a candidate for euthanasia to be terminally ill, with a life expectancy of less than six months with or without medical treatment. Second, they were more lax than the Dutch guidelines in that they permitted euthanasia by advance directive. A competent adult, healthy or not, could assign a durable power of attorney to authorize euthanasia if he became terminally ill and incompetent within seven years. Thus, unlike the situation in the Netherlands, euthanasia would be possible for incompetent as well as competent patients, provided they had once been competent; only children and those born mentally retarded would be excluded. Note that both the Dutch guidelines and the California proposal would preclude performing euthanasia at the sole discretion of a physician, as purportedly occurred in the case of Debbie.[8]

Most observers believe that the California initiative failed because of organizational problems, not voter sentiment. Public opinion polls have shown fairly consistently that about three fifths of the American public favor legalizing euthanasia under certain conditions (compared with about three quarters of the Dutch public).[9] Americans Against Human Suffering intends to repeat its effort to place the issue on the ballot in California in 1990 and also to make similar efforts in Washington, Oregon, and Florida.

What are the arguments for and against legalizing euthanasia? And where do doctors fit in? Arguments against euthanasia are more familiar than those for it. First, we have strong legal, religious, and cultural taboos against taking human life, almost regardless of the circumstances (wars, self-defense, and legal executions being the notable exceptions). These reflect the supreme value we place on human life, as well as a concern that any compromise of this position might lead to a general erosion of our respect for life. Thus, many would acknowledge that there may be circumstances in which euthanasia would be appropriate for an individual patient but would oppose it because it would tend to devalue life. Related to this argument is the fear that the devaluation would be selective, that euthanasia might occur too often among the weak and powerless in our society—

that is, among the very old, the poor, or the handicapped. Lessons learned from the Nazis fuel this fear.

There is also concern that euthanasia could be abused not only by society at large but by individuals. Inevitably, despite safeguards (even as stringent as those in the Netherlands), there must be some vagueness in any language permitting euthanasia. For example, how do we define intolerable suffering? Exactly what is a voluntary, repeated, and consistent request? This vagueness reflects the variations and subtleties of the circumstances as well as the inadequacies of language. However, it makes it easy to imagine the ne'er-do-well nephew persuading his rich old uncle to request euthanasia.

Finally, doctors have their own set of special concerns about euthanasia. Many of us believe that euthanasia is appropriate under certain conditions and that it should indeed be legalized, but that we should not perform it ourselves. According to this view, doctors should only extend life, never shorten it, and patients must be in no doubt about what our function is. A poll of doctors released June 2 by the University of Colorado at Denver Center for Health Ethics and Policy showed that three fifths of them favored legalizing euthanasia, but nearly half of those would not perform it themselves.

The principal argument in favor of euthanasia is that it is more humane than forcing a patient to continue a life of unmitigated suffering. According to this view, there is no moral difference under some circumstances between euthanasia and withholding life-sustaining treatment. In both situations, the purpose is a merciful death, and the only practical difference is that withholding life-sustaining treatment entails more suffering because it takes longer. Furthermore, it requires an element of happenstance, such as the development of pneumonia for which there is treatment that could be withheld. Proponents of euthanasia also argue that it furthers the principle of individual self-determination, and that this enhances rather than diminishes respect for human life. They believe that it is contradictory to permit patients to refuse life-sustaining treatment, while not honoring their request for euthanasia.

If euthanasia were permissible, the best way to minimize the possibility of abuse would be to limit its availability, as in the Netherlands, to competent patients who request it because of their current situation and not because of a hypothetical future one. This would mean denying euthanasia to incompetent patients, even with an advance directive, and would thus sharply limit its use. Nevertheless, such a limitation may be the price of preventing abuse. Furthermore, it could be argued that the suffering of incompetent patients, certainly those in a persistent vegetative state, is experienced more by their families than by themselves.

If euthanasia were legalized, doctors morally opposed to it should not, of course, be required to perform it. On the other hand, doctors who believe in the desirability of euthanasia under certain conditions, but who would refuse to perform it, raise a different issue. Can they appropriately excuse themselves from a difficult part of what they consider good patient care? Would they favor the creation of a profession especially dedicated to performing euthanasia (a problematic and, I think, unsavory prospect)?

Whatever their view of the morality and appropriateness of legalizing euthanasia and of performing it, doctors should be prepared for its emergence as an important issue in the years ahead and should be ready to debate it. Perhaps, also, those who favor legalizing euthanasia but would not perform it should rethink their position. Our ability to extend life through new technologies will certainly grow, and with it will grow the dilemmas created by the extension of intractable suffering.

REFERENCES

1 President's Commission for the Study of Ethical Problems in Medicine and Biomedical and Behavioral Research. Deciding to forego life-sustaining treatment: a report on the ethical, medical, and legal issues in treatment decisions. Washington, D.C.: Government Printing Office, 1983.

2 Annas GJ, Glantz LH. The right of elderly patients to refuse life-sustaining treatment. Milbank Q 1986; 64:Suppl 2:95–162.

3 Current Opinions of the Council on Ethical and Judicial Affairs of the AMA—1986. Withholding or withdrawing life-prolonging treatment. Chicago: American Medical Association, 1986.

4 Pence GE. Do not go slowly into that dark night: mercy killing in Holland. Am J Med 1988; 84:139–41.

5 Central Committee of the Royal Dutch Medical Association. Vision on euthanasia. Med Contact 1984; 39:990–8.

6 Final report of the Netherlands State Commission on Euthanasia: an English summary. Bioethics 1987; 1:163–74.

7 The Humane and Dignified Death Act. California Civil Code, Title 10.5.

8 It's over, Debbie. JAMA 1988; 259:272.

9 Roper Organization of New York City. The 1988 Roper poll on attitudes toward active voluntary euthanasia. Los Angeles: National Hemlock Society, 1988.

Thoughts on Physician-Assisted Suicide
Alex Ralph Demac

Alex Ralph Demac, M.D., is presently resident in psychiatry at Yale University School of Medicine. The article reprinted here was originally published while Demac was in medical school at the University of California, San Diego.

Demac argues against the "Humane and Dignified Death Act," a California legislative proposal that would legalize active euthanasia and physician-assisted suicide under specified conditions. First, he critiques the arguments made by The Hemlock Society and its president (Derek Humphrey) in support of the legislation. Second, he calls attention to a number of dangers inherent in the legalization of mercy killing. Third, he objects to the legislation on the grounds that it would have negative effects on physicians and their image.

From *The Western Journal of Medicine*, vol. 148 (February 1988), pp. 228–230. Reprinted by permission of *The Western Journal of Medicine* and the author.

We live in a society where the average person is unfamiliar and uncomfortable with death. Beginning with what many psychologists think is an innate block to realizing our own mortality, we go on to shield ourselves in every way possible from the occurrence of death. People die in institutions rather than in the home, and the opportunity to spend time with the dead person at the time of death and perhaps at the funeral home later are quite abbreviated compared to the days-long vigils over the dead of other times and other societies. Our culture emphasizes youth and shuns and ignores the aged, as if to banish from our minds the deterioration and demise for which we all are bound.

Many, if not most, people have never been present at the death of another. Certainly, as we get older and our friends and relatives die, the truth becomes more evident, but we are so conditioned to denial that the truth often is hard indeed to accept.

Into this setting come two organizations: the Hemlock Society and Americans Against Human Suffering. In euphemistic terms they call for "the right to self-deliverance," "voluntary active euthanasia," and "assisted suicide." In the boldest, clearest possible terms, what they seek is legalized mercy killing. The Americans Against Human Suffering organization is gathering signatures for a ballot initiative—the so-called Humane and Dignified Death Act (California Civil Code, Title 10.5) —that would make physician intervention to cause the death of a consenting, terminally ill patient a legally protected activity in the state of California. If its sponsors are successful, the act will be submitted to the voters in the form of a referendum.

Under the terms of the proposed initiative, any person certified by two physicians as being terminally ill and unlikely to live longer than six months would be entitled, upon the execution of a simple document, with witnesses, to immediate assistance from his or her physician in committing suicide. This would involve anything from writing a prescription for a lethal drug to "any medical procedure that will terminate the life of the qualified patient swiftly, painlessly, and humanely." The physician and any who help in this task would be immune from criminal, civil, or administrative liability. Any physician refusing to assist in the killing would be required to make arrangements for the transfer of the patient's care to another, more willing physician.

In his book, *Let Me Die Before I Wake*, Humphrey makes the case for this legislation simply, poignantly, and persuasively.[1] His argument is primarily one for patient autonomy and personal sovereignty. A terminally ill patient, he says, should have the right to choose the time and circumstances of his or her death. The patient should not have to suffer through a mental or physical decline, emotional and/or physical pain, and the additional expense of treatment if he or she does not want to. If there is no hope, why prolong suffering needlessly?

Patients in this position currently face a number of barriers to "self-deliverance." First, their behavior is legally and socially unsanctioned, so they must make their preparations furtively. Second, the most effective drugs for committing suicide are available only by prescription. People are, therefore, forced to go to great lengths to accumulate a lethal hoard of pharmaceuticals, and in many cases may have to use slower, less certain, and less comfortable drugs or choose other methods of suicide. Third, and perhaps most compelling, is the question of what happens to people who are physically or mentally unable to accomplish their own suicides and know no compassionate souls who will risk helping them. Are they to be abandoned to slow, lingering, painful, undignified, and expensive deaths?

In a series of case histories, Humphrey tells the stories of terminally ill people who accomplish suicide with the help of spouses, children, and friends. In each case the person dies happier, the friends and relatives feel good about their participation, and the last hours spent together are filled with a sense of love, serenity, and even triumph. Why not let all people who choose to die in this way do so without hindrance?

The answer to this question has less to do, I think, with how and when we let people die than it does with how and when we let people kill. Certainly, in my opinion, people who make up their minds to kill themselves have the moral right to do so. They may be considered foolish. They may be called inconsiderate to inflict emotional pain on those who value their lives and will mourn their passing. I think that it is their lives, and so long as they are discreet in choosing the time and method of suicide and attentive to the details, they should not have a problem. The real difficulty begins when they want someone to help them.

We live in a polis that rigidly limits the conditions under which one person may kill or help to kill another. Soldiers are allowed to kill enemies during military confrontations. Police and civilians are allowed to kill in self-defense. Certain criminals may be put to death as punishment for their crimes. All of these cases involve people whose lives have been devalued by virtue of their assuming evil roles relative to the commonweal. While a physician is permitted to hasten a patient's death by giving morphine, the killing is a by-product of pain relief rather than a stated goal.

The proposed legislation would therefore extend government's role in a significant new direction. It would be given the power and the responsibility to kill the "good guys," people who have not hurt anyone but have devalued their own lives based on their personal views of their lives and circumstances. What are the justifications, limitations, and dangers of such an expansion of power?

The Hemlock Society says that terminally ill people should not have to suffer, but why should anyone have to suffer? Suffering exists and abounds, not simply among the terminally ill. Should anyone who suffers be entitled to help in committing suicide? A possible response is that terminally ill people are unique in that they have no hope. Others have the possibility of relief, of a life after the suffering, but the terminally ill do not. It may, therefore, be argued that there is no reason to force the terminally ill to suffer through as long a period as six months before they finally die and are released.

There are, however, many who suffer great physical pain without hope of relief. For example, the severely handicapped or the severely and chronically ill have to suffer, with no prognosis for improvement. If the terminally ill should not be forced to suffer for six months, why should these people be forced to suffer for years? More to the point, what is the nature of this suffering? Under the proposed initiative, a person would be entitled to assisted death from the moment of being diagnosed as being six months from death, even if no significant deterioration or pain had yet occurred. A terminally ill patient, then, with little physical pain could demand help in committing suicide while a chronically handicapped but not terminally ill person with much more severe pain could not. It is, therefore, impossible to argue that the terminally ill suffer uniquely or are uniquely entitled to a particular form of relief. We must either refuse to grant them assisted suicide on demand or extend the right to others as well.

An important question to ask at this juncture is whether suicide is the only possible solution to the suffering of a terminally ill person. Many believe that it is not. If significant pain does exist, there is no reason why it cannot be palliated by the armamentarium of pain relievers, including morphine and neurosurgery, that are available. If pain is so terrible that death can provide the only relief, it is generally and increasingly recognized that physicians may increase the dosage of morphine until death is in fact effected. This is something the patients can discuss with their physicians in advance, so that they may be assured that they will not suffer unduly.

The Hemlock Society maintains that the terminally ill should not have to suffer the emotional distress and indignity of physical and mental deterioration and increasing dependence on others. Quality of life, however, is entirely subjective, and the hospice movement has shown that even severely debilitated patients can lead meaningful lives. The loss of youth and vitality is eventually suffered by everyone, if they live long enough. As Dyck has pointed out:

> If minimizing suffering is linked with killing, we have the unfortunate implication that killing is a quicker, more painless way to alleviate suffering than is the provision of companionship for the lonely and long-term care for those who are either dying or recuperating from illnesses.[2]

The Hemlock Society further states that terminally ill people should not have to receive pointless, expensive, life-prolonging treatment. This is certainly justified, and as living wills and the right to refuse treatment become institutionalized, as they increasingly are, this will not be a problem. Termination of treatment issues, however, should not be confused with termination of life by "assisted suicide."

While it is difficult for me to understand why death by mercy killing is necessary to ease the départure of a terminally ill person, I see a number of dangers inherent in its legalization. First and foremost, it is quite possible that a social and psychological climate would be created under which terminally ill people would be *expected* to exercise this option. A large amount of money, including a major portion of Medicare payments, is now spent on the care of the terminally ill and could instead be used for other things. Governor Richard Lamm of Colorado has spoken of the duty of the elderly to die. It would be easy for this attitude to be spread in the media to the point where it might act as a pressure on the terminally ill to opt for death by mercy killing. Families and physicians caring for the terminally ill might well be tempted to urge this option on a person to save themselves from the strain of such care.

Furthermore, because, as previously discussed, there is nothing qualitatively unique about the suffering of the terminally ill, it is likely that the right to death by mercy killing and the pressure to take that option would soon be extended to all chronically ill, elderly, and handicapped people. In fact, the underlying assumption of The Humane and Dignified Death Act, which is that poor quality of life is a justification for death, would put society on a slippery slope with no bottom in sight. It is easy to envision a time, especially during an economic depression or a war, when resources are scarce and anyone would be entitled to assisted suicide simply because they were dissatisfied with the quality of their lives. During such a time, a "reasonable person" rule might be applied to those not able to make a choice—the insane, the mentally retarded, or handicapped children—who might be put to death without having any say in the matter on the basis of their relatively poor quality of life.

A final question relating to assisted suicide is who should do the assisting. The Humane and Dignified Death Act calls for physicians to assume this role, but should they? Just as physicians do not participate in executions, they need not be involved in mercy killing. There could be certified thanatologists, or euthanasia societies could establish right-to-die clinics. If physicians are the killers, it arguably could effect a great change in their image and role. Certainly, if assisted suicide becomes a treatment option, all physicians will be required to mention it to their patients or be liable for not keeping their patients properly informed. The proposed legislation requires that a physician opposed to killing a patient must find that patient a physician who will. In this way the physician's complicity is coerced, and proper medical conduct is defined by those outside the profession. On the other hand, in this age of commercial medicine, one can readily imagine physicians competing with one another through advertisements on the basis of their euthanasia services. The image of physicians would thus change from being champions of life to angels of death.

The problem with laws is that often they provide a sledgehammer where a feather is needed. It is widely noted that there are instances when physicians have actively helped patients to die. The impulse is to enshrine this practice in law so that any patient may receive such help and no physician need fear a penalty for providing it. The problem is that this would make the practice easier and more commonplace than it should be and leave society open to the undesirable consequences mentioned.

A more sensible middle ground has been taken in the Netherlands. While they have not legalized physician-assisted suicide, authorities in that country have worked with the Royal Dutch Medical Association to determine criteria under which physicians may be permitted to help terminally ill patients to die. These include the stipulation that euthanasia will be carried out only if there is unbearable suffering that fails all pain-killing efforts. The goal, according to one Dutch practitioner, is to "prevent the deed's arising from mere subjective despair in an exhausted patient or from a doctor's proselytizing" (*The New York Times*, October 31, 1986, p. A4). Implicit is that such a decision should be arrived at by a physician and patient in the context of a long-standing and intimate physician-patient relationship. It is not a decision to be arrived at casually or between physicians and patients who are strangers to one another. Furthermore, cooperation by a physician or other party in such an act should not be coerced in any way.

While suicide in the face of death may be a dramatic assertion of self-determination and the legalization of such practice an affirmation of personal autonomy, we as a society are not ready for such a big step. At this time, we should move forward carefully, allowing the courts, the medical profession, and the public to monitor the situation as we go. The worst thing we could do is to pass a referendum whose provisions would be clumsily broad, and which, by the very nature of referendums, would be difficult to amend as its flaws became apparent.

REFERENCES

1 Humphrey D: Let Me Die Before I Wake, 4th Ed. Los Angeles, The National Hemlock Society, 1987
2 Dyck A: Beneficent euthanasia and benemortasia: Alternative views of mercy. *In* Kohl M (Ed): Beneficent Euthanasia. Buffalo, NY, Prometheus Books, 1975, pp. 121–122

The Definition of Death

Why "Update" Death?

President's Commission for the Study of Ethical Problems in Medicine and Biomedical and Behavioral Research

A descriptive account of the President's Commission is found on page 92.

In this selection, taken from the first chapter of its report, *Defining Death*, the Commission provides a compact account of both (1) the interrelationships of brain, heart, and lung functions and (2) the loss of brain functions. Emphasis is placed on the difference between "whole brain death" and a "persistent vegetative state" in which brainstem function persists. Although reference is made to the Commission's view that "the cessation of the vital functions of the entire brain [is] the only proper neurologic basis for declaring death," the analysis and argumentation the Commission presents in support of this view is found only in subsequent chapters of the report.

For most of the past several centuries, the medical determination of death was very close to the popular one. If a person fell unconscious or was found so, someone (often but not always a physician) would feel for the pulse, listen for breathing, hold a mirror before the nose to test for condensation, and look to see if the pupils were fixed. Although these criteria have been used to determine death since antiquity, they have not always been universally accepted.

DEVELOPING CONFIDENCE IN THE HEART-LUNG CRITERIA

In the eighteenth century, macabre tales of "corpses" reviving during funerals and exhumed skeletons found to have clawed at coffin lids led to widespread fear of premature burial. Coffins were developed with elaborate escape mechanisms and speaking tubes to the world above, mortuaries employed guards to monitor the newly dead for signs of life, and legislatures passed laws requiring a delay before burial....

...The invention of the stethoscope in the mid-nineteenth century enabled physicians to detect heartbeat with heightened sensitivity. The use of this instrument by a well-trained physician, together with other

Reprinted from President's Commission for the Study of Ethical Problems in Medicine and Biomedical and Behavioral Research, *Defining Death* (1981), pp. 13–20.

clinical measures, laid to rest public fears of premature burial. The twentieth century brought even more sophisticated technological means to determine death, particularly the electrocardiograph (EKG), which is more sensitive than the stethoscope in detecting cardiac functioning.

THE INTERRELATIONSHIPS OF BRAIN, HEART, AND LUNG FUNCTIONS

The brain has three general anatomic divisions: the cerebrum, with its outer shell called the cortex; the cerebellum; and the brainstem, composed of the midbrain, the pons, and the medulla oblongata. Traditionally, the cerebrum has been referred to as the "higher brain" because it has primary control of consciousness, thought, memory and feeling. The brainstem has been called the "lower brain," since it controls spontaneous, vegetative functions such as swallowing, yawning and sleep-wake cycles. It is important to note that these generalizations are not entirely accurate. Neuroscientists generally agree that such "higher brain" functions as cognition or consciousness probably are not mediated strictly by the cerebral cortex; rather, they probably result from complex interrelations between brainstem and cortex.

Respiration is controlled in the brainstem, particularly the medulla. Neural impulses originating in the respiratory centers of the medulla stimulate the diaphragm and intercostal muscles, which cause the lungs to fill with air. Ordinarily, these respiratory centers adjust the rate of breathing to maintain the correct levels of carbon dioxide and oxygen. In certain circumstances, such as heavy exercise, sighing, coughing or sneezing, other areas of the brain modulate the activities of the respiratory centers or even briefly take direct control of respiration.

Destruction of the brain's respiratory center stops respiration, which in turn deprives the heart of needed oxygen, causing it too to cease functioning. The traditional signs of life—respiration and heartbeat—disappear: the person is dead. The "vital signs" traditionally used in diagnosing death thus reflect the direct interdependence of respiration, circulation and the brain.

The artificial respirator and concomitant life-support systems have changed this simple picture. Normally, respiration ceases when the functions of the diaphragm and intercostal muscles are impaired. This results from direct injury to the muscles or (more commonly) because the neural impulses between the brain and these muscles are interrupted. However, an artificial respirator (also called a ventilator) can be used to compensate for the inability of the thoracic muscles to fill the lungs with air. Some of these machines use negative pressure to expand the chest wall (in which case they are called "iron lungs"); others use positive pressure to push air into the lungs. The respirators are equipped with devices to regulate the rate and depth of "breathing," which are normally controlled by the respiratory centers in the medulla. The machines cannot compensate entirely for the defective neural connections since they cannot regulate blood gas levels precisely. But, provided that the lungs themselves have not been extensively damaged, gas exchange can continue and appropriate levels of oxygen and carbon dioxide can be maintained in the circulating blood.

Unlike the respiratory system, which depends on the neural impulses from the brain, the heart can pump blood without external control. Impulses from brain centers modulate the inherent rate and force of the heartbeat but are not required for the heart to contract at a level of function that is ordinarily adequate. Thus, when artificial respiration provides adequate oxygenation and associated medical treatments regulate essential plasma components and blood pressure, an intact heart will continue to beat, despite loss of brain functions. At present, however, no machine can take over the functions of the heart except for a very limited time and in limited circumstances (e.g., a heart-lung machine used during surgery). Therefore, when a severe injury to

the heart or major blood vessels prevents the circulation of the crucial blood supply to the brain, the loss of brain functioning is inevitable because no oxygen reaches the brain.

LOSS OF VARIOUS BRAIN FUNCTIONS

The most frequent causes of irreversible loss of functions of the whole brain are: (1) direct trauma to the head, such as from a motor vehicle accident or a gunshot wound, (2) massive spontaneous hemorrhage into the brain as a result of ruptured aneurysm or complications of high blood pressure, and (3) anoxic damage from cardiac or respiratory arrest or severely reduced blood pressure.

Many of these severe injuries to the brain cause an accumulation of fluid and swelling in the brain tissue, a condition called cerebral edema. In severe cases of edema, the pressure within the closed cavity increases until it exceeds the systolic blood pressure, resulting in a total loss of blood flow to both the upper and lower portions of the brain. If deprived of blood flow for at least 10–15 minutes, the brain, including the brainstem, will completely cease functioning. Other pathophysiologic mechanisms also result in a progressive and, ultimately, complete cessation of intracranial circulation.

Once deprived of adequate supplies of oxygen and glucose, brain neurons will irreversibly lose all activity and ability to function. In adults, oxygen and/or glucose deprivation for more than a few minutes causes some neuron loss. Thus, even in the absence of direct trauma and edema, brain functions can be lost if circulation to the brain is impaired. If blood flow is cut off, brain tissues completely self-digest (autolyze) over the ensuing days.

When the brain lacks all functions, consciousness is, of course, lost. While some spinal reflexes often persist in such bodies (since circulation to the spine is separate from that of the brain), all reflexes controlled by the brainstem as well as cognitive, affective and integrating functions are absent. Respiration and circulation in these bodies may be generated by a ventilator together with intensive medical management. In adults who have experienced irreversible cessation of the functions of the entire brain, this mechanically generated functioning can continue only a limited time because the heart usually stops beating within two to ten days. (An infant or small child who has lost all brain functions will typically suffer cardiac arrest within several weeks, although respiration and heartbeat can sometimes be maintained even longer.)

Less severe injury to the brain can cause mild to profound damage to the cortex, lower cerebral structures, cerebellum, brainstem, or some combination thereof. The cerebrum, especially the cerebral cortex, is more easily injured by loss of blood flow or oxygen than is the brainstem. A 4–6 minute loss of blood flow—caused by, for example, cardiac arrest—typically damages the cerebral cortex permanently, while the relatively more resistant brainstem may continue to function.

When brainstem functions remain, but the major components of the cerebrum are irreversibly destroyed, the patient is in what is usually called a "persistent vegetative state" or "persistent noncognitive state." Such persons may exhibit spontaneous, involuntary movements such as yawns or facial grimaces, their eyes may be open and they may be capable of breathing without assistance. Without higher brain functions, however, any apparent wakefulness does not represent awareness of self or environment (thus, the condition is often described as "awake but unaware"). The case of Karen Ann Quinlan has made this condition familiar to the general public. With necessary medical and nursing care—including feeding through intravenous or nasogastric tubes, and antibiotics for recurrent pulmonary infections—such patients can survive months or years, often without a respirator. (The longest survival exceeded 37 years.)

CONCLUSION: THE NEED FOR RELIABLE POLICY

Medical interventions can often provide great benefit in avoiding *irreversible* harm to a patient's injured heart, lungs, or brain by carrying a patient through a period of acute need. These techniques have, however, thrown new light on the interrelationship of these crucial organ systems. This has created complex issues for public policy as well.

For medical and legal purposes, partial brain impairment must be distinguished from complete and irreversible loss of brain functions or "whole brain death." The President's Commission, as subsequent chapters explain more fully, regards the cessation of the vital functions of the entire brain—and not merely portions thereof, such as those responsible for cognitive functions—as the only proper neurologic basis for declaring death. This conclusion accords with the overwhelming consensus of medical and legal experts and the public.

Present attention to the "definition" of death is part of a process of development in social attitudes and legal rules stimulated by the unfolding of biomedical knowledge. In the nineteenth century increasing knowledge and practical skill made the public confident that death could be diagnosed reliably using cardiopulmonary criteria. The question now is whether, when medical intervention may be responsible for a patient's respiration and circulation, there are other equally reliable ways to diagnose death....

The Definition and Criterion of Death
Charles M. Culver and Bernard Gert

Charles M. Culver is professor of psychiatry and Elizabeth DeCamp McInerny Professor of Medical Ethics, Dartmouth Medical School. Bernard Gert is Stone Professor of Intellectual and Moral Philosophy, Dartmouth College, and adjunct professor of psychiatry, Dartmouth Medical School. Frequent collaborators, Culver and Gert are the coauthors of *Philosophy in Medicine: Conceptual and Ethical Issues in Medicine and Psychiatry* (1982) and of such articles as "The Justification of Paternalism" and "The Morality of Involuntary Hospitalization." Very prominent among Gert's other philosophical works is *The Moral Rules* (1970).

Culver and Gert consider it essential to distinguish among the *definition* of death, the *criterion* of death, and the *tests* of death. In discussing the definition of death, they begin by giving reasons why death must be considered an event rather than a process. They define death as the permanent cessation of functioning of the *organism as a whole*, and they argue against a competing definition according to which the permanent loss of consciousness and cognition is sufficient for death. In their view, patients who are in a chronic vegetative state are alive but are no longer persons, and it is morally justifiable to allow them to die by discontinuing even "ordinary and routine care." With regard to the *criterion* of death, Culver and Gert maintain that the correct criterion is the permanent loss of functioning of the entire brain, *not* the permanent loss of cardiopulmonary function. They conclude with a brief discussion of the appropriate *tests* of death.

Much of the confusion arising from the current brain death controversy is due to the failure to distinguish three distinct elements: (1) the definition of death; (2) the medical criterion for determining that death has occurred; and (3) the tests to prove that the criterion has been satisfied. We shall first define death in a way which makes its ordinary meaning explicit, then provide a criterion of death which fulfills this definition, and finally, indicate which tests have demonstrated perfect validity in determining that the criterion of death is satisfied.[1]

The definitions of death which appear in legal dictionaries and the new statutory definitions of death do not say what the layman actually means by death but merely set out the criteria by which physicians legally determine when death has occurred. *Death*, however, is not a technical term but a common term in everyday use. We believe that a proper understanding of the ordinary meaning of this word or concept must be developed before a medical criterion is chosen. We must decide what is ordinarily meant by death before physicians can decide how to measure it.

Agreement on the definition and criterion of death is literally a life-and-death matter. Whether a spontaneously breathing patient in a chronic vegetative state is classified as dead or alive depends on our understanding of the definition of death. Even given the definition, the status of a patient with a totally and permanently nonfunctioning brain who is being maintained on a ventilator depends on the criterion of death employed. Defining death is primarily a philosophical task; providing the criterion of death is primarily medical; and choosing the tests to prove that the criterion is satisfied is solely a medical matter.

THE DEFINITION OF DEATH

Death as a Process or an Event

It has been claimed that death is a process rather than an event (Morison, 1971). This claim is supported by the fact that a standard series of degenerative and destructive changes occurs in the tissues of an organism, usually following but sometimes preceding the irreversible cessation of spontaneous ventilation and circulation. These changes include: necrosis of brain cells, necrosis of other vital organ cells, cooling, rigor mortis, dependent lividity, and putrefaction. This process actually persists for years, even centuries, until the skeletal remains have disintegrated, and could even be viewed as beginning with the failure of certain organ systems during life. Because these changes occur in a fairly regular and ineluctable fashion, it is claimed that the stipulation of any particular point in this process as the moment of death is arbitrary.

The following argument, however, shows the theoretical inadequacy of any definition which makes death a process. If we regard death as a process, then either (1) the process starts when the person is still living, which confuses the process of death with the process of dying, for we all regard someone who is dying as not yet dead, or (2) the process of death starts when the person is no longer alive, which confuses the process of death with the process of disintegration. Death should be viewed not as a process but as the event that separates the process of dying from the process of disintegration.

On a practical level, regarding death as a process makes it impossible to declare the time of death with any precision. This is not a trivial issue. There are pressing medical, legal, social, and religious reasons to declare the time of death with some precision, including the interpretation of wills, burial times and procedures, mourning times, and decisions regarding the aggressiveness of medical support. There are no countervailing practical or theoretical reasons for regarding death as a process rather than an event in formulating a definition of death. We shall say that death occurs at some definite time, although this time may not always be specifiable with complete precision.

Choices for a Definition of Death

The definition of death must capture our ordinary use of the term, for *death*, as noted earlier, is a word used by everyone and is not primarily a medical or legal term. In this ordinary use, certain facts are assumed, and we shall assume them as well. Therefore we shall not apply our analysis to science fiction speculations, for example, about brains continuing to function independently of the rest of the organism (Gert, 1967, 1971). Thus we shall assume that all and only living organisms can die, that the living can be distinguished from the dead with very good reliability, and that the moment when an organism leaves the former state and enters the latter can be determined with a fairly high degree of precision. We shall regard death as permanent. We know that some people claim to have been dead for several minutes and then to have returned to life, but we regard this as only a dramatic way of saying that consciousness was temporarily lost (for example, because of a brief episode of cardiac arrest).

Although there are religious theories that death involves the soul leaving the body, we know that religious persons and secularists do not disagree in their ordinary application of the term *dead*. We acknowledge that the body can remain physically intact for some time after death and that some isolated parts of the organism may continue to function (for example, it is commonly believed that hair and nails continue to grow after death). We shall now present our definition of death and contrast it to a proposed alternative.

We define death as the permanent cessation of functioning of the organism as a whole. By the organism as a whole, we do not mean the whole organism, that is, the sum of its tissue and organ parts, but rather the highly complex interaction of its organ subsystems. The organism need not be whole or complete—it may have lost a limb or an organ (such as the spleen)—but it still remains an organism.

By the functioning of the organism as a whole, we mean the spontaneous and innate activities of integration of all or most subsystems (for example, neuroendocrine control) and at least limited response to the environment (for example, temperature change). However, it is not necessary that all of the subsystems be integrated. Individual subsystems may be replaced (for example, by pacemakers, ventilators, or pressors) without changing the status of the organism as a whole.

It is possible for individual subsystems to function for a time after the organism as a whole has permanently ceased to function. Spontaneous ventilation ceases either immediately after or just before the permanent cessation of functioning of the organism as a whole, but spontaneous circulation, with artificial ventilation, may persist for up to two weeks after the organism as a whole has ceased to function.

An example of an activity of the organism as a whole is temperature regulation. The control of this complex process is located in the hypothalamus and is important for normal maintenance of all cellular processes. It is lost when the organism as a whole has ceased to function.

Consciousness and cognition are sufficient to show the functioning of the organism as a whole in higher animals, but they are not necessary. Lower organisms never have consciousness and even when a higher organism is comatose, evidence of the functioning of the organism as a whole may still be evident, for example, in temperature regulation.

We believe that the permanent cessation of the functioning of the organism as a whole is what has traditionally been meant by death. This definition retains death as a biological occurrence which is not unique to human beings; the same definition applies to other higher animals. We believe that death is a biological phenomenon and should apply equally to related species. When we talk of the death of a human being, we mean the same thing as we do when we talk of the death of a dog or a cat. This is supported by our ordinary use of the term *death*, and by law and tradition. It is also in accord with social and religious practices and is not likely to be affected by future changes in technology.

An alternative definition of death as the irreversible loss of that which is essentially significant to the nature of man has been proposed by Veatch (1976). Though this definition initially seems very attractive, it does not state what we ordinarily mean when we speak of death. It is not regarded as self-contradictory to say that a person has lost that which is essentially significant to the nature of man, but is still alive. For example, we all acknowledge that permanently comatose patients in chronic vegetative states are sufficiently brain-damaged that they have irreversibly lost all that is essentially significant to the nature of man but we still consider them to be living (for example, Karen Ann Quinlan; see Beresford, 1977).

The patients described by Brierley and associates (1971) are also in this category. These patients had complete neocortical destruction with preservation of the brainstem and diencephalic (posterior brain) structures. They had isoelectric (flat) electroencephalograms (EEGs) (indicating neocortical death) and were permanently comatose, although they had normal spontaneous breathing and brainstem reflexes; they were essentially in a permanent, severe, chronic vegetative state (Jennett and Plum, 1972). They retained many of the vital functions of the organism as a whole, including neuroendocrine control (that is, homeostatic interrelationships between the brain and various hormonal glands) and spontaneous circulation and breathing.

This alternative definition actually states what it means to cease to be a person rather than what it means for that person to die. *Person* is not a biological concept but rather a concept defined in terms of certain kinds of abilities and qualities of awareness. It is inherently vague. Death is a biological concept. Thus in a literal sense, death can be applied directly only to biological organisms and not to persons. We do not object to the phrase "death of a person," but the phrase in common usage actually means the death of the organism which was the person. For example, one might overhear in the hospital wards, "The person in room 612 died last night." In this common usage, one is referring to the death of the organism which was a person. By our analysis, Veatch (1976) and others have used the phrase "death of a person" metaphorically, applying it to an organism which has ceased to be a person but has not died.

Without question, consciousness and cognition are essential human attributes. If they are lost, life has lost its meaning. A patient in a chronic vegetative state is usually regarded as living in only the most basic biological sense. But it is just this basic biological sense that we want to capture in our definition of death. We must not confuse the death of an organism which was a person with an organism's ceasing to be a person. We are immediately aware of the loss of personhood in these patients and are repulsed by the idea of continuing to treat them as if they were persons. But were we to consider these chronic vegetative patients as actually dead, serious problems would arise. First, a slippery slope condition would be introduced wherein the question could be asked: How much neocortical damage is necessary before we declare a patient dead? Surely patients in a chronic vegetative state, although usually not totally satisfying the tests for neocortical destruction, have permanently lost their consciousness and cognition. Then what about the somewhat less severely brain-damaged patient?

By considering permanent loss of consciousness and cognition as a criterion for ceasing to be a person and not for death of the organism as a whole, the slippery slope phenomenon is put where it belongs: not in the definition of death, but in the determination of possible grounds for nonvoluntary euthanasia, that is, providing possible grounds for killing the organism, or allowing it to die, in those instances in which the organism is no longer a person. The justification of nonvoluntary euthanasia must be kept strictly separate from the definition of death. Most of us would like our organism to die when we cease to be persons, but this should not be accomplished by blurring the distinctions between biological death and the loss of personhood.

When an organism ceases to be a person, that is, when it permanently loses all consciousness and cognition, then practical problems arise. How are we to treat this organism? (1) Should we treat it just as we treat a person, making every effort to keep it alive? (2) Should we cease caring for it, either in part or at all, and allow it to die? (3) Should we kill it?

In our view, an organism that is no longer a person has no claim to be treated as a person. But just as one treats a corpse with respect, even more so would one expect that such a living organism be treated with respect. This does not mean, however, that one should strive to keep the organism alive. No one benefits by doing this; on the contrary, given the care needed to keep such an organism alive, it seems an extravagant waste of both economic and human resources to attempt to do so. On the other hand, it seems unjustified to require anyone to actively kill it. Even though the organism is no longer a person, it still looks like a person, and unless there are overwhelming reasons for killing it, it seems best not to do anything that might weaken the prohibition against killing. This leaves the second alternative, discontinuing all care and allowing the patient to die. This can take either of two forms: discontinuing medical treatment or discontinuing all ordinary and routine care. The latter is the position we favor.

It is important to note that the patient will not suffer from lack of care, for since the patient is no longer a person this means that it has permanently lost all consciousness and cognition. Any patient who retains even the slightest capacity to suffer pain or discomfort of any kind remains a person and must be treated as such. We make this point to emphasize our position that only patients who have completely and permanently lost all consciousness and cognition should have all care discontinued. We believe that discontinuing all care and allowing the patient who is no longer a person to die is the preferred alternative, and the one that should be recommended to the legal guardian or next of kin as the course of action to be followed.

THE CRITERION OF DEATH

We have argued that the correct definition of death is permanent cessation of functioning of the organism as a whole. We will now inspect the two competing criteria of death: (1) the permanent loss of cardiopulmonary functioning and (2) the total and irreversible loss of functioning of the whole brain.

Characteristics of Optimum Criteria and Tests

Given that death is the permanent cessation of functioning of the organism as a whole, a criterion will yield a false-positive if it is satisfied, and yet it would still be possible for that organism to function as a whole. By far the most important requirement for a criterion of death is that it yield no false-positives.

A criterion of death, however, cannot have any exceptions; this is what enables it to serve as a legal definition of death. It is not sufficient that the criterion be correct 99.99 percent of the time. This means that not only can the criterion yield no false-positives, it can also yield no false-negatives. A criterion of death yields a false-negative if it is not satisfied and yet the organism as a whole has irreversibly ceased to function. Of course, one may sometimes determine death without using the criterion, but it can never be that the criterion is satisfied and yet the person is not dead, or that the criterion is not satisfied and the person is dead. This is why it is so easy to mistake a criterion for an ordinary definition; it is rather a kind of operational definition, and serves as part of the legal definition, but the real operational definition is provided by the tests which show whether or not the criterion is satisfied.

Permanent Loss of Cardiopulmonary Functioning

Permanent termination of heart and lung function has been used as a criterion of death throughout history. The ancients observed that all other bodily functions ceased shortly after cessation of these vital functions, and the irreversible process of bodily disintegration inevitably followed. Thus permanent loss of spontaneous cardiopulmonary function was found to predict permanent nonfunctioning of the organism as a whole. Further, if there were no permanent loss of spontaneous cardiopulmonary function, then the organism as a whole continued to function. Therefore permanent loss of cardiopulmonary function served as an adequate criterion of death.

Because of current ventilation/circulation technology, permanent loss of spontaneous cardiopulmonary functioning is no longer necessarily predictive of permanent nonfunctioning of the organism as a whole. Consider a conscious, talking patient who is unable to breathe because of suffering from poliomyelitis and who requires an iron lung (thus having permanent loss of spontaneous pulmonary function), who has also developed asystole (loss of spontaneous heartbeat) requiring a permanent pacemaker (thus having permanent loss of spontaneous cardiac function). It would be absurd to regard such a person as dead.

It might be proposed that it is not the permanent loss of *spontaneous* cardiopulmonary function that is the criterion of death, but rather the permanent loss of all cardiopulmonary function, whether spontaneous or artificially supported. But now that ventilation and circulation can be mechanically maintained, an organism with permanent loss of whole brain functioning can have permanently ceased to function as a whole days to weeks before the heart and lungs cease to function with artificial support. Thus this supposed criterion would not be satisfied, yet the person would be dead. The heart and lungs now seem to have no unique relationship to the functioning of the organism as a whole. Continued artificially supported cardiopulmonary function is no longer perfectly correlated with life, and permanent loss of spontaneous cardiopulmonary functioning is no longer perfectly correlated with death.

Total and Irreversible Loss of Whole Brain Functioning

The criterion for the cessation of functioning of the organism as a whole is the permanent loss of functioning of the entire brain. This criterion is perfectly correlated with the permanent cessation of functioning of the organism as a whole because it is the brain that is necessary for the functioning of the organism as a whole. It integrates, generates, interrelates, and controls complex bodily activities. A patient on a ventilator with a totally destroyed brain is merely a preparation of artificially maintained subsystems since the organism as a whole has ceased to function.

The brain generates the signal for breathing through brainstem ventilatory centers and aids in the control of circulation through brainstem blood pressure control centers. Destruction of the brain produces apnea (inability to breath) and generalized vasodilatation (opening of the peripheral blood vessels); in all cases, despite the most aggressive support, the adult heart stops within a week and that of the child within two weeks (Ingvar et al., 1978). Thus when the organism as a whole has ceased to function, the artificially supported vital subsystems quickly fail. Many other functions of the organism as a whole, including neuroendocrine control, temperature control, food-searching behaviors, and sexual activity, reside in the more primitive regions (hypothalamus, brainstem) of the brain. Thus total and irreversible loss of functioning of the whole brain and not merely the neocortex is required as the criterion for the permanent loss of the functioning of the organism as a whole.

Using permanent loss of functioning of the whole brain as the criterion for death of the organism as a whole is also consistent with tradition. Throughout history, whenever a physician was called to ascertain the occurrence of death, his examination included the following important signs indicative of permanent loss of functioning of the whole brain: unresponsivity, lack of spontaneous movements including breathing; and absence of pupillary light response. Only one important sign, lack of heartbeat, was not directly indicative of whole brain destruction. But since the heartbeat stops within several minutes of apnea, permanent absence of the vital signs is an important sign of permanent loss of whole brain functioning. Thus, in an important sense, permanent loss of whole brain functioning has always been the underlying criterion of death.

THE TESTS OF DEATH

Given the definition of death as the permanent cessation of functioning of the organism as a whole, and the criterion of death as the total and irreversible cessation of functioning of the whole brain, the next step is the examination of the available tests of death. The tests must

be such that they will never yield a false-positive result. Of secondary importance, they should produce few and relatively brief false-negatives.

Cessation of Heartbeat and Ventilation

The physical findings of permanent absence of heartbeat and respiration are the traditional tests of death. In the vast majority of deaths not complicated by artificial ventilation, these classic tests are still applicable. They show that the criterion of death has been satisfied since they always quickly produce permanent loss of functioning of the whole brain. However, when mechanical ventilation is being used, these tests lose most of their utility due to the production of numerous false-negatives for as long a time as one to two weeks, that is, death of the organism as a whole with still intact circulatory-ventilatory subsystems. Thus though the circulation-ventilation tests will suffice in most instances of death, if there is artificial maintenance of circulation or ventilation the special tests for permanent cessation of whole brain functioning will be needed.

Irreversible Cessation of Whole Brain Functioning

Numerous formalized sets of tests have been established to determine that the criterion of permanent loss of whole brain functioning has been met. These include, among others, tests described by the Harvard Medical School Ad Hoc Committee (Beecher, 1968) and the National Institutes of Health Collaborative Study of Cerebral Survival (1977). They have all been recently reviewed (Black, 1978; Molinari, 1978). What we call tests have sometimes been called "criteria," but it is important to distinguish these second-level criteria from the first-level criteria. While the first-level criteria must be for the death of the organism and must be understandable by the layman, the second-level criteria (tests) determine the permanent loss of functioning of the whole brain and need not be understandable by anyone except qualified clinicians. To avoid confusion, we prefer to use the designation "tests" for the second-level criteria.

All the proposed tests require total and permanent absence of all functioning of the brainstem and both hemispheres. They vary slightly from one set to another, but all require unresponsivity (deep coma), absent pupillary light reflexes, apnea (inability to breathe), and absent brainstem reflexes. They also require the absence of drug intoxication and low body temperature, and the newer sets require the demonstration that a lesion of the brain exists. Isoelectric (flat) EEGs are generally required, and tests disclosing the absence of cerebral blood flow are of confirmatory value (NIH Collaborative Study, 1977). All tests require the given loss of function to be present for a particular time interval, which in the case of the absence of cerebral blood flow may be as short as thirty minutes.

Current tests of irreversible loss of whole brain function may produce many false-negatives of a sort during the thirty-minute to twenty-four-hour interval between the successive neurologic examinations which the tests require. Certain sets of tests, particularly those requiring electrocerebral silence by EEG, may produce false-negatives if an EEG artifact is present and cannot confidently be distinguished from brain wave activity. Generally, a few brief false-negatives are tolerable and even inevitable, since tests must be delineated conservatively in order to eliminate any possibility of false-positives.

There are many studies which show perfect correlation between the loss of whole brain function tests of the Ad Hoc Committee of the Harvard Medical School and total brain necrosis at postmortem examination. Veith et al. (1977a) conclude that "the validity of the criteria [tests] must be considered to be established with as much certainty as is possible in biology or medicine" (p. 1652). Thus, when a physician ascertains that a patient satisfies the validated loss of whole brain function tests, he can be confident that the loss of whole brain functioning is permanent. Physicians should apply only tests which have been completely validated....

NOTE

1 This [article] is adapted in part from Bernat, Culver, and Gert (1981).

REFERENCES

American Bar Association. House of Delegates redefines death, urges redefinition of rape, and undoes the Houston amendments. *American Bar Association Journal*, 1975, *61*, 463–464.

Beecher, Henry K. A definition of irreversible coma: report of the Ad Hoc Committee of the Harvard Medical School to examine the definition of brain death. *Journal of the American Medical Association*, 1968, *205*, 337–340.

Beresford, H. Richard. The Quinlan decision: problems and legislative alternatives. *Annals of Neurology*, 1977, *2*, 74–81.

Bernat, James L., Culver, Charles M., and Gert, Bernard. On the definition and criterion of death. *Annals of Internal Medicine*, 1981, *94*, 389–394.

Black, Peter M. Brain death. *New England Journal of Medicine*, 1978, *299*, 338–344, 393–401.

Brierley, J.B., Adams, J.H., Graham, D.I., and Simpson, J.A. Neocortical death after cardiac arrest. *Lancet*, 1971, *2*, 560–565.

Capron, Alexander M., and Kass, Leon R. A statutory definition of the standards for determining human death: an appraisal and a proposal. *University of Pennsylvania Law Review*, 1972, *121*, 87–118.

Gert, Bernard. Can the brain have a pain? *Philosophy and Phenomenological Research*, 1967, *27*, 432–436.

Gert, Bernard. Personal identity and the body. *Dialogue*, 1971, *10*, 458–478.

Hastings Center Task Force on Death and Dying. Refinements in criteria for the determination of death: an appraisal. *Journal of the American Medical Association*, 1972, *221*, 48–53.

Ingvar, David H., Brun, Arne, Johansson, Lars, and Sammuelsson, Sven M. Survival after severe cerebral anoxia with destruction of the cerebral cortex: the apallic syndrome. *Annals of the New York Academy of Science*, 1978, *315*, 184–214.

Jennett, B., and Plum, F. Persistent vegetative state after brain damage. A syndrome in search of a name. *Lancet*, 1972, *1*, 734–737.

Jonas, Hans. *Philosophical Essays: From Ancient Creed to Technological Man*. Englewood Cliffs, N.J.: Prentice-Hall, 1974, pp. 134–140.

Law Reform Commission of Canada. *Criteria for the Determination of Death*. Ottawa: Law Reform Commission of Canada, 1979.

Molinari, Gaetano F. Review of clinical criteria of brain death. *Annals of the New York Academy of Science*, 1978, *315*, 62–69.

Morison, Robert S. Death: process or event? *Science*, 1971, *173*, 694–698.

NIH Collaborative Study of Cerebral Survival. An appraisal of the criteria of cerebral death: a summary statement. *Journal of the American Medical Association*, 1977, *237*, 982–986.

President's Commission for the Study of Ethical Problems in Medicine and Biomedical and Behavioral Research. *"Defining Death," a Report on the Medical, Legal and Ethical Issues in the Determination of Death. Washington, D.C., 1981.

Veatch, Robert M. Death, Dying and the Biological Revolution: Our Last Quest for Responsibility. New Haven, Conn.: Yale University Press, 1976.

Veith, Frank J., Fein, Jack M., Tendler, Moses D., Veatch, Robert M., Kleiman, Marc A., and Kalkines, George. Brain death I. A status report of medical and ethical considerations. Journal of the American Medical Association, 1977a, 238, 1651–1655.

Veith, Frank J., Fein, Jack M., Tendler, Moses D., Veatch, Robert M., Kleiman, Marc A., and Kalkines, George. Brain death II. A status report of legal considerations. Journal of the American Medical Association, 1977b, 238, 1744–1748.

The Definition of Death and Persistent Vegetative State
Daniel Wikler

Daniel Wikler is professor of medical ethics at the University of Wisconsin Medical School, Madison. He has also served on the staff of the President's Commission for the Study of Ethical Problems in Medicine and Biomedical and Behavioral Research. His many articles in biomedical ethics include "Paternalism and the Mildly Retarded," "Ought We Try to Save Aborted Fetuses?" and "Personal Responsibility for Illness."

Wikler directly confronts the possibility of redefining death (in accordance with a higher-brain conception) to include persistent vegetative state. He identifies a number of factors likely to hinder acceptance of such a redefinition, and he especially takes seriously the problem of clinical uncertainty in the diagnosis of PVS, and yet he is fundamentally sympathetic to the idea of redefinition. Wikler argues—primarily on the basis of an interesting thought experiment—that a redefinition of death to include PVS is conceptually sound. He also argues that such a definition offers us a notable strategic advantage.

There is [one] approach...that could resolve the treatment dilemmas regarding persistent vegetative state, short of requiring an outcome to...much larger debates: The definition of death could be changed to include permanent loss of sentience. Under such a definition, further treatment of vegetative patients would not be required of any facility or provider of health care, and except in unusual circumstances all "life" supports, including nutrition and hydration, would be withdrawn. If the revised statute followed the pattern of existing definitions of death, cessation of treatment would not even require an invocation of the patient's wishes.

There is a strategic advantage in this approach. The definition of death is a problem that has been resolved, and if it can be expanded to include persistent vegetative state, the latter might be removed from the arena of controversy. The law, however, should not rely solely on strategic considerations in defining death. A statute determines only the patient's legal status, but life and death are more than legal concepts. People are either alive or dead—or perhaps in-between—on ice floes and space ships far from the reach of any laws. Any law that made patients legally dead whom we would otherwise, for good reasons, deem alive would smack of expediency over principle.

But what kinds of grounds suffice to define death? One proposal is that they should be moral ones: the boundary from life to death is crossed at that time at which treatment should be discontinued. This claim, however, confuses the definition of death with its moral implications. Once death has occurred, treatment may cease, but these are distinct matters.

Reprinted with permission of the author and the publisher from Hastings Center Report, vol. 18 (February/March 1988), pp. 44–47.

The definition of death, then, needs to be settled on ground independent of legal and moral purposes. It is akin to a question of fact—is the patient still among us?—rather than one of action. Indeed, classifying those in persistent vegetative state as dead can serve as a *justification* for ending treatment, which it could not do, on pain of circularity, were the classification itself merely a treatment decision.

This methodological point needs emphasis, I believe, because any proposal to expand the definition of death to include persistent vegetative state will look like definitional gerrymandering to many people. To avoid the appearance of playing with words to avoid difficult moral choices, the argument for classifying vegetative patients as dead must be made convincing independently of the uses to which it would be put.[1]

While I believe that this case can be made, it will not be easy to present it to the public in a convincing way. It requires a substantial adjustment in our thinking about death, one that changes the focus from biological to psychological processes. Under both the traditional, cardiopulmonary definition and the newer whole-brain definition, death is identified as the moment of cessation of biological processes. The definitions differ over which biological processes constitute the organism's life: breathing and circulation, on the older definition, neural regulation of these processes according to the new. An expanded brain-death definition, meanwhile, would focus on those brain processes that sponsor consciousness and feeling. Once these brain functions have permanently ceased, the individual is dead.

Nothing in this definition (variously called "personal," "mental," or "cortical") implies that the patient's *body* dies when the higher brain functions cease. In this view, the *body* of the patient in persistent vegetative state is still alive, and could remain so, but the *patient* is not. This view admittedly has an air of paradox: we are our bodies, so how could we be dead while our bodies remained alive? Yet, this kind of thinking is not wholly unfamiliar. Tumor cells cultured in the laboratory are living remains of patients who have died of cancer; in the same way, the entire functioning body of the patient in persistent vegetative state is his living remains. Moreover, the traditional definitions of death also make a distinction between the patient's demise and his body's: the patient ceases to exist at the time of death, but his body does not. The new definition adds only that the patient's body not only exists but lives.

It may be intuitively difficult to accept that the entity in persistent vegetative state, still a living body, is not the patient. Or, even more to the point, that the body, in so many respects healthy, is dead in any but a metaphorical sense. Yet we have crossed this hurdle before: Patients who are "whole-brain-dead," qualifying under brain-death statutes adopted by most states, also breathe, circulate blood, digest, and carry out other life functions. To be sure, "cortically" dead patients are more intact, needing no respirators or constant attention, but what they *do* is not so different. The reeducation necessary to accept them as dead is not as great as that required under the redefinition we have already adopted.

In one respect, expanding the definition of death to include persistent vegetative state would be easier to absorb than the original brain-death formulation. Some, perhaps most, of the acceptance of whole-brain-death can be explained by the widespread belief that *it* meant permanent cessation of consciousness and the loss of qualities that make life worth living.[2] An expanded definition, then would catch up with the public's reason for accepting the old one.

Scholars will be less interested, however, in the chance for public acceptance than in whether an expanded definition is, in the appropriate sense, valid or correct—whether, that is, patients in persistent vegetative state *really are dead*. This is a complex philosophical issue that cannot be fully addressed here.[3] An argument can be made, however, that such a definition comports with educated common sense. Consider this thought experiment: a man is decapitated, and physicians are able to keep both the head and the body functioning more or less as normal. They cannot, however, reconnect them. Which is the patient?

The answer cannot be, "Both," for body and head may be widely separated in location. Nearly everyone able to choose one or the other will, I believe, choose the head. After decapitation, the head *is* the patient, and the conditions of its health and death are those of the patient as a whole. Losing a body through decapitation is considerably more distressing, in this story, than losing a limb, but it is not more threatening to one's identity. The body, meanwhile, continues to live. It is not the patient, and may survive the patient if the latter cannot be kept alive.

This is, very roughly, what happens in persistent vegetative state.[4] Though brain and body remain physically intact, they are functionally severed. Those parts of the brain that make consciousness and feeling possible are irreversibly lost, and the continued functioning of the body has no more significance in the patient's life than would, say, a kidney removed from his body and prospering for decades to come in the body of another. That the whole body (except for relevant parts of the brain) is involved rather than one organ is not a difference that makes a difference.

What bearing does such an outlandish thought experiment have on the real-world clinical and legal issue of brain death? It does not show that the expanded definition would be practical, or even desirable. But it does show that it is conceptually sound, and given the mental leap required to view as dead a patient whose body is fairly healthy, this is an essential accomplishment.[5]

Even so, a definition of death that included persistent vegetative state faces objections on several levels. It may be politically difficult, if only because the public may not yet have digested the recent expansion of the definition to include whole-brain-death. Moreover, no national movement exists to expand the definition, and key professional groups not only have abstained from calling for the change but show no sign of having been convinced of its value or appropriateness. The President's Commission, whose report endorsing a whole-brain definition prompted a slew of state statutes, acted only after acceptance of the idea by the medical profession and progressive judicial and legal opinion.

Clinical uncertainties present an equally important objection. A key factor in expanding the definition of death to include whole-brain-death was the certainty of diagnosis. An infallible procedure for diagnosing persistent vegetative state has yet to be produced. Near-total certainty of prognosis must be achieved before a higher-brain death statute can be considered. In this respect, the resolution of the moral dilemma awaits further development of medical technique.

Even were reliable tests available, the public would need reassurances. The widespread fascination with stories of people reviving after many years in "coma," often in the face of flat predictions to the contrary by physicians, proved troublesome even to the whole-brain definition of death. After several members of the President's Commission explained the whole-brain definition to the public on *Nightline*, the usually informed host segued to a story of a patient who had returned to consciousness from a prolonged vegetative period. That case clearly did not meet the conditions of the proposed brain-death criterion, and so had nothing to do with the Commission's proposal, but nevertheless was presented as an apparent counterexample.

The problems of redefining death to include persistent vegetative state, however, depend in the end upon the public's willingness to accept it. Since the public may not have a precise understanding of the last revision in the definition of death, widespread acceptance of a new definition is difficult to predict. Much depends on how the new definition is understood. One clue would come at the bedside, in the reactions of family members to being told that their apparently healthy loved one is to be pronounced dead: here the precedent is favorable. Family members encountering whole-brain-dead loved ones who breathe and maintain normal blood pressure and temperature, have come to accept their doctors' assurances that the patient is already dead.

Patients in persistent vegetative state, however, present more of a problem. The main reason is their relative independence from life-sustaining machinery: the signs of life, such as breathing, cannot be explained away as effects of life supports. Perhaps the most problematic aspect, however, is that a withdrawal of life supports cannot be relied upon to produce an immediate cessation of remaining life functions. After death would be pronounced, a living body remains, and its disposal is bound to raise questions.

...A definition of death that included persistent vegetative state would not avoid the problem of killing and letting die; it would reintroduce it at a new level. The living body of the patient pronounced dead will go on breathing unless it is killed or allowed to die. We must do one or the other, since burying a breathing body is unthinkable. How, then, would a re-redefinition of death be of any use in addressing the dilemmas associated with persistent vegetative state?

This question, like the problem of accurate diagnosis, was a source of confusion in the previous movement to redefine death. The relationship between (whole) brain death and the cessation of principal vital functions such as breathing and circulation (i.e., death traditionally defined) remains a source of uneasiness if not contradiction. Many doctors, and some authorities, would in unguarded moments speak of pronouncing death on a brain-dead patient, so that life supports could be removed and the patient "allowed to die." To some, the fact that brain-dead patients could not be kept "alive" for more than a few weeks even with intensive care was sufficient reason for accepting the new definition. Careful retraining of speech habits has been necessary to avoid this kind of phraseology.

Again, however, important precedents have been established by the first redefinition of death. If patients in persistent vegetative state are dead, then nothing that happens to them causes their death. Just as the public accepts the idea that brain-dead patients may have their vital organs removed—an action that could not possibly be maneuvered into the "letting die" category—so may they come to accept the administration of an agent that causes cardiac arrest to patients in persistent vegetative state. In both cases, the logic of redefinition of death ensures that the taboo on taking the life of a person does not apply.

In this way, a new revision of the definition of death resolves the dilemma of killing and letting die. It permits us to surmount the present, difficult stage of the evolution of clinical practice in which we hesitate to terminate what life resides in patients in persistent vegetative state but do permit an agonizing period of "dying" of starvation....

The strategy of widening the definition of death might seem to open the door to abuse, an ever-looser criterion that would deliver death sentences by meddling with the dictionary. But in fact this objection points to one of this strategy's strengths. The definition must comport with common usage and common sense, and these provide constraints on further stretching. Persistent vegetative state is not a vague concept; indeed, it could be expanded slightly to read "permanent cessation of consciousness and feeling" without losing precision. This (presumably) final step in redefining death, then, would include the permanently unconscious among those defined as dead, but would not affect the merely unhappy, confused, or disoriented. The mentally disabled were, in times past, victimized by euthanasia, but they cannot be threatened by the definition of death.

This advantage is also a limitation. Though a redefinition of death might resolve some of the problems associated with persistent vegetative state, it will be of no use in addressing the dilemmas of dying for patients in less fully debilitated conditions. It separates the *Quinlans* from the *Conroys* and is silent on the latter.

This outcome, however, may be for the best. Persistent vegetative state is not merely an advanced stage of dementia; it is amentia, an absence of everything for which people value existence. Its position as the limiting case on the continuum—the patient from whom all life has ebbed—is what justifies regarding it as death. The same cannot be said of lesser states of decline. We should expect differences in the value attached to these states, and there exists no consensus on the wider questions of control over dying. Disposition of patients in persistent vegetative state, then, may be a part of the general problem resolvable through the definition of death, leaving the broader, wider issues for the public debate they deserve.

REFERENCES

1 Much of the literature favorable to the wider definition of death fails, to its detriment, to recognize the importance of this requirement. David R. Smith's otherwise admirable article, "Legal Recognition of Neocortical Death," *Cornell Law Review* 71 (1986), pp. 850–88, for example, contends that in persistent vegetative state, "rightly viewed, human death has already occurred" (p. 872) but does not say why this is the "right" view.

2 Some of this confusion is documented in S. J. Youngner et al., "'Brain Death' and Organ Retrieval: A Cross-Sectional Survey of Knowledge and Concepts among Health Professionals," *JAMA* 261 (1989), pp. 2205–2210. See also D. Wikler and A. Weisbard, "Appropriate Confusion over Brain Death," *JAMA* 261 (1989), p. 2246.

My own unsystematic sampling during the past decade indicates that many doctors, most lawyers and nurses, and nearly all members of the public do not understand the "official" reasoning (i.e., in accord with the rationale given in the President's Commission report) behind the statutes. See *Defining Death*, President's Commission for the Study of Ethical Problems in Medicine and Biomedical and Behavioral Research, Washington D.C.: Government Printing Office, 1981.

3 The issues set out in Michael B. Green and Daniel Wikler, "Brain Death and Personal Identity," *Philosophy and Public Affairs* 9(2): Winter 1980, pp. 105–133; Daniel Wikler, "Conceptual Issues in the Definition of Death," *Theoretical Medicine* Vol. 5, 1984, 167–80; and Karen Gervais, *Redefining Death*, New Haven: Yale University Press, 1987.

4 Except that the brainstem remains intact. No precise analogy is possible because the part of the brain that sponsors consciousness is not anatomically distinct from that which keeps the vegetative body alive.

5 Those not convinced by this brief argument are referred to Green and Wikler, "Brain Death and Personal Identity."

Nutrition and Hydration

Must Patients Always Be Given Food and Water?
Joanne Lynn and James F. Childress

Joanne Lynn, M.D., is associate professor in the division of geriatric medicine at George Washington University. She has also served as assistant director on the staff of the President's Commission for the Study of Ethical Problems in Medicine and Biomedical and Behavioral Research, and she is the editor of *By No Extra-Ordinary Means* (1986). James F. Childress is Kyle Professor of Religious Studies and also professor of medical education at the University of Virginia. Widely published in biomedical ethics, he is the author of *Priorities in Biomedical Ethics* (1981) and *Who Should Decide?* (1982) and the coauthor of *Principles of Biomedical Ethics* (1979).

Lynn and Childress confront the following question: Is it ever permissible to withhold or withdraw nutrition and hydration from a patient? Their special concern is with decision making in the case of an incompetent patient. In their view, it is *not obligatory* to provide medical nutrition and hydration whenever (1) the treatment would be futile, (2) there is no possibility of patient benefit, or (3) the burden created by the treatment would be disproportionate to the benefit provided. After explicating these matters, Lynn and Childress identify and reject a number of arguments that could be directed against their position.

Many people die from the lack of food or water. For some, this lack is the result of poverty or famine, but for others it is the result of disease or deliberate decision. In the past, malnutrition and dehydration must have accompanied nearly every death that followed an illness of more than a few days. Most dying patients do not eat much on their own, and nothing could be done for them until the first flexible tubing for instilling food or other liquid into the stomach was developed about a hundred years ago. Even then, the procedure was so scarce, so costly in physician and nursing time, and so poorly tolerated that it was used only for patients who clearly could benefit. With the advent of more reliable and efficient procedures in the past few decades, these conditions can be corrected or ameliorated in nearly every patient who would otherwise be malnourished or dehydrated. In fact, intravenous lines and nasogastric tubes have become common images of hospital care.

Providing adequate nutrition and fluids is a high priority for most patients, both because they suffer di-

Reprinted with permission of the authors and the publisher from *Hastings Center Report*, vol. 13 (October 1983), pp. 17–21.

rectly from inadequacies and because these deficiencies hinder their ability to overcome other diseases. But are there some patients who need not receive these treatments? This question has become a prominent public policy issue in a number of recent cases. In May 1981, in Danville, Illinois, the parents and the physician of newborn conjoined twins with shared abdominal organs decided not to feed these children. Feeding and other treatments were given after court intervention, though a grand jury refused to indict the parents.[1] Later that year, two physicians in Los Angeles discontinued intravenous nutrition to a patient who had severe brain damage after an episode involving loss of oxygen following routine surgery. Murder charges were brought, but the hearing judge dismissed the charges at a preliminary hearing. On appeal, the charges were reinstated and remanded for trial.[2]

In April 1982, a Bloomington, Indiana, infant who had tracheoesophageal fistula and Down syndrome was not treated or fed, and he died after two courts ruled that the decision was proper but before all appeals could be heard.[3] When the federal government then moved to ensure that such infants would be fed in the future,[4] the Surgeon General, Dr. C. Everett Koop, initially stated that there is never adequate reason to deny nutrition and fluids to a newborn infant.

While these cases were before the public, the nephew of Claire Conroy, an elderly incompetent woman with several serious medical problems, petitioned a New Jersey court for authority to discontinue her nasogastric tube feedings. Although the intermediate appeals court has reversed the ruling,[5] the trial court held that he had this authority since the evidence indicated that the patient would not have wanted such treatment and that its value to her was doubtful.

In all these dramatic cases and in many more that go unnoticed, the decision is made to deliberately withhold food or fluid known to be necessary for the life of the patient. Such decisions are unsettling. There is now widespread consensus that sometimes a patient is best served by not undertaking or continuing certain treatments that would sustain life, especially if these entail substantial suffering. But food and water are so central to an array of human emotions that it is almost impossible to consider them with the same emotional detachment that one might feel toward a respirator or a dialysis machine.

Nevertheless, the question remains: should it ever be permissible to withhold or withdraw food and nutrition? The answer in any real case should acknowledge the psychological contiguity between feeding and loving and between nutritional satisfaction and emotional satisfaction. Yet this acknowledgment does not resolve the core question.

Some have held that it is intrinsically wrong not to feed another. The philosopher G.E.M. Anscombe contends: "For wilful starvation there can be no excuse. The same can't be said quite without qualification about failing to operate or to adopt some courses of treatment."[6] But the moral issues are more complex than Anscombe's comment suggests. Does correcting nutritional deficiencies always improve patients' well-being? What should be our reflective moral response to withholding or withdrawing nutrition? What moral principles are relevant to our reflections? What medical facts about ways of providing nutrition are relevant? And what policies should be adopted by the society, hospitals, and medical and other health care professionals?

In our effort to find answers to these questions, we will concentrate upon the care of patients who are incompetent to make choices for themselves. Patients who are competent to determine the course of their therapy may refuse any and all interventions proposed by others, as long as their refusals do not seriously harm or impose unfair burdens upon others. A competent patient's decision regarding whether or not to accept the provision of food and water by medical means such as tube feeding or intravenous alimentation is unlikely to raise questions of harm or burden to others.

What then should guide those who must decide about nutrition for a patient who cannot decide? As a start, consider the standard by which other medical decisions are made: one should decide as the incompetent person would have if he or she were competent, when that is possible to determine, and advance that person's interests in a more generalized sense when individual preferences cannot be known.

THE MEDICAL PROCEDURES

There is no reason to apply a different standard to feeding and hydration. Surely, when one inserts a feeding tube, or creates a gastrostomy opening, or inserts a needle into a vein, one intends to benefit the patient. Ideally, one should provide what the patient believes to be of benefit, but at least the effect should be beneficial in the opinions of surrogates and caregivers.

Thus, the question becomes: is it ever in the patient's interest to become malnourished and dehydrated, rather than to receive treatment? Posing the question so starkly points to our need to know what is entailed in treating these conditions and what benefits the treatments offer.

The medical interventions that provide food and fluids are of two basic types. First, liquids can be delivered by a tube that is inserted into a functioning gastrointestinal tract, most commonly through the nose and esophagus into the stomach or through a surgical incision in the abdominal wall and directly into the stomach. The liquids used can be specially prepared solutions of nutrients or a blenderized version of an ordinary diet. The nasogastric tube is cheap; it may lead to pneumonia and often annoys the patient and family, sometimes even requiring that the patient be restrained to prevent its removal.

Creating a gastrostomy is usually a simple surgical procedure, and, once the wound is healed, care is very simple. Since it is out of sight, it is aesthetically more acceptable and restraints are needed less often. Also, the gastrostomy creates no additional risk of pneumonia. However, while elimination of a nasogastric tube requires only removing the tube, a gastrostomy is fairly permanent, and can be closed only by surgery.

The second type of medical intervention is intravenous feeding and hydration, which also has two major forms. The ordinary hospital or peripheral IV, in which fluid is delivered directly to the bloodstream through a small needle, is useful only for temporary efforts to improve hydration and electrolyte concentrations. One cannot provide a balanced diet through the veins in the limbs: to do that requires a central line, or a special catheter placed into one of the major veins in the chest. The latter procedure is much more risky and vulnerable to infections and technical errors, and it is much more costly than any of the other procedures. Both forms of intravenous nutrition and hydration commonly require restraining the patient, cause minor infections and other ill effects, and are costly, especially since they ordinarily require the patient to be in a hospital.

None of these procedures, then, is ideal; each entails some distress, some medical limitations, and some costs. When may a procedure be foregone that might improve nutrition and hydration for a given patient? Only when the procedure and the resulting improvement in nutrition and hydration do not offer the patient a net benefit over what he or she would otherwise have faced.

Are there such circumstances? We believe that there are; but they are few and limited to the following three kinds of situations: 1. The procedures that would be required are so unlikely to achieve improved nutritional and fluid levels that they could be correctly considered futile; 2. The improvement in nutritional and fluid balance, though achievable, could be of no benefit to the patient; 3. The burdens of receiving the treatment may outweigh the benefit.

WHEN FOOD AND WATER MAY BE WITHHELD

Futile Treatment

Sometimes even providing "food and water" to a patient becomes a monumental task. Consider a patient with a severe clotting deficiency and a nearly total body burn. Gaining access to the central veins is likely to cause hemorrhage or infection, nasogastric tube placement may be quite painful, and there may be no skin to which to suture the stomach for a gastrostomy tube. Or consider a patient with severe congestive heart failure who develops cancer of the stomach with a fistula that delivers food from the stomach to the colon without passing through the intestine and being absorbed. Feeding the patient may be possible, but little is absorbed. Intravenous feed-

ing cannot be tolerated because the fluid would be too much for the weakened heart. Or consider the infant with infarction of all but a short segment of bowel. Again, the infant can be fed, but little if anything is absorbed. Intravenous methods can be used, but only for a short time (weeks or months) until their complications, including thrombosis, hemorrhage, infections, and malnutrition, cause death.

In these circumstances, the patient is going to die soon, no matter what is done. The ineffective efforts to provide nutrition and hydration may well directly cause suffering that offers no counterbalancing benefit for the patient. Although the procedures might be tried, especially if the competent patient wanted them or the incompetent patient's surrogate had reason to believe that this incompetent patient would have wanted them, they cannot be considered obligatory. To hold that a patient must be subjected to this predictably futile sort of intervention just because protein balance is negative or the blood serum is concentrated is to lose sight of the moral warrant for medical care and to reduce the patient to an array of measurable variables.

No Possibility of Benefit

Some patients can be reliably diagnosed to have permanently lost consciousness. This unusual group of patients includes those with anencephaly, persistent vegetative state, and some preterminal comas. In these cases, it is very difficult to discern how any medical intervention can benefit or harm the patient. These patients cannot and never will be able to experience any of the events occurring in the world or in their bodies. When the diagnosis is exceedingly clear, we sustain their lives vigorously mainly for their loved ones and the community at large.

While these considerations probably indicate that continued artificial feeding is best in most cases, there may be some cases in which the family and the caregivers are convinced that artificial feeding is offensive and unreasonable. In such cases, there seems to be no adequate reason to claim that withholding food and water violates any obligations that these parties or the general society have with regard to permanently unconscious patients. Thus, if the parents of an anencephalic infant or of a patient like Karen Quinlan in a persistent vegetative state feel strongly that no medical procedures should be applied to provide nutrition and hydration, and the caregivers are willing to comply, there should be no barrier in law or public policy to thwart the plan.[7]

Disproportionate Burden

The most difficult cases are those in which normal nutritional status or fluid balance could be restored, but only with a severe burden for the patient. In these cases, the treatment is futile in a broader sense—the patient will not actually benefit from the improved nutrition and hydration. A patient who is competent can decide the relative merits of the treatment being provided, knowing the probable consequences, and weighing the merits of life under various sets of constrained circumstances. But a surrogate decision maker for a patient who is incompetent to decide will have a difficult task. When the situation is irremediably ambiguous, erring on the side of continued life and improved nutrition and hydration seems the less grievous error. But are there situations that would warrant a determination that this patient, whose nutrition and hydration could surely be improved, is not thereby well served?

Though they are rare, we believe there are such cases. The treatments entailed are not benign. Their effects are far short of ideal. Furthermore, many of the patients most likely to have inadequate food and fluid intake are also likely to suffer the most serious side effects of these therapies.

Patients who are allowed to die without artificial hydration and nutrition may well die more comfortably than patients who receive conventional amounts of intravenous hydration.[8] Terminal pulmonary edema, nausea, and mental confusion are more likely when patients have been treated to maintain fluid and nutrition until close to the time of death.

Thus, those patients whose "need" for artificial nutrition and hydration arises only near the time of death may be harmed by its provision. It is not at all clear that they receive any benefit in having a slightly prolonged life, and it does seem reasonable to allow a surrogate to decide that, for this patient at this time, slight prolongation of life is not warranted if it involves measures that will probably increase the patient's suffering as he or she dies.

Even patients who might live much longer might not be well served by artificial means to provide fluid and food. Such patients might include those with fairly severe dementia for whom the restraints required could be a constant source of fear, discomfort, and struggle. For such a patient, sedation to tolerate the feeding mechanisms might preclude any of the pleasant experiences that might otherwise have been available. Thus, a decision not to intervene, except perhaps briefly to ascertain that there are no treatable causes, might allow such a patient to live out a shorter life with fair freedom of movement and freedom from fear, while a decision to maintain artificial nutrition and hydration might consign the patient to end his or her life in unremitting anguish. If this were the case a surrogate decision maker would seem to be well justified in refusing the treatment.

INAPPROPRIATE MORAL CONSTRAINTS

Four considerations are frequently proposed as moral constraints on foregoing medical feeding and hydration. We find none of these to dictate that artificial nutrition and hydration must always be provided.

The Obligation to Provide "Ordinary" Care

Debates about appropriate medical treatment are often couched in terms of "ordinary" and "extraordinary" means of treatment. Historically, this distinction emerged in the Roman Catholic tradition to differentiate optional treatment from treatment that was obligatory for medical professionals to offer and for patients to accept. These terms also appear in many secular contexts, such as court decisions and medical codes. The recent debates about ordinary and extraordinary means of treatment have been interminable and often unfruitful, in part because of a lack of clarity about what the terms mean. Do they represent the premises of an argument or the conclusion, and what features of a situation are relevant to the categorization as "ordinary" or "extraordinary"?

Several criteria have been implicit in debates about ordinary and extraordinary means of treatment; some of them may be relevant to determining whether and which treatments are obligatory and which are optional. Treatments have been distinguished according to their simplicity (simple/complex), their naturalness (natural/artificial), their customariness (usual/unusual), their invasiveness (noninvasive/invasive), their chance of success (reasonable chance/futile), their balance of benefits and burdens (proportionate/disproportionate), and their expense (inexpensive/costly). Each set of paired terms or phrases in the parentheses suggests a continuum: as the treatment moves from the first of the paired terms to the second, it is said to become less obligatory and more optional.

However, when these various criteria, widely used in discussions about medical treatment, are carefully examined, most of them are not morally relevant in distinguishing optional from obligatory medical treatments.

For example, if a rare, complex, artificial, and invasive treatment offers a patient a reasonable chance of nearly painless cure, then one would have to offer a substantial justification not to provide that treatment to an incompetent patient.

What matters, then, in determining whether to provide a treatment to an incompetent patient is not a prior determination that this treatment is "ordinary" per se, but rather a determination that this treatment is likely to provide this patient benefits that are sufficient to make it worthwhile to endure the burdens that accompany the treatment. To this end, some of the considerations listed above are relevant: whether a treatment is likely to succeed is an obvious example. But such considerations taken in isolation are not conclusive. Rather, the surrogate decision maker is obliged to assess the desirability to this patient of each of the options presented, including nontreatment. For most people at most times, this assessment would lead to a clear obligation to provide food and fluids.

But sometimes, as we have indicated, providing food and fluids through medical interventions may fail to benefit and may even harm some patients. Then the treatment cannot be said to be obligatory, no matter how usual and simple its provision may be. If "ordinary" and "extraordinary" are used to convey the conclusion about the obligation to treat, providing nutrition and fluids would have become, in these cases, "extraordinary." Since this phrasing is misleading, it is probably better to use "proportionate" and "disproportionate," as the Vatican now suggests,[9] or "obligatory" and "optional."

Obviously, providing nutrition and hydration may sometimes be necessary to keep patients comfortable while they are dying even though it may temporarily prolong their dying. In such cases, food and fluids constitute warranted palliative care. But in other cases, such as a patient in a deep and irreversible coma, nutrition and hydration do not appear to be needed or helpful, except perhaps to comfort the staff and family. And sometimes the interventions needed for nutrition and hydration are so burdensome that they are harmful and best not utilized.

The Obligation to Continue Treatments Once Started

Once having started a mode of treatment, many caregivers find it very difficult to discontinue it. While this strongly felt difference between the ease of withholding a treatment and the difficulty of withdrawing it provides a

psychological explanation of certain actions, it does not justify them. It sometimes even leads to a thoroughly irrational decision process. For example, in caring for a dying, comatose patient, many physicians apparently find it harder to stop a functioning peripheral IV than not to restart one that has infiltrated (that is, has broken through the blood vessel and is leaking fluid into surrounding tissue), especially if the only way to reestablish an IV would be to insert a central line into the heart or to do a cutdown (make an incision to gain access to the deep large blood vessels).

What factors might make withdrawing medical treatment morally worse than withholding it? Withdrawing a treatment seems to be an action, which, when it is likely to end in death, initially seems more serious than an omission that ends in death. However, this view is fraught with errors. Withdrawing is not always an act: failing to put the next infusion into a tube could be correctly described as an omission, for example. Even when withdrawing is an act, it may well be morally correct and even morally obligatory. Discontinuing intravenous lines in a patient now permanently unconscious in accord with that patient's well-informed advance directive would certainly be such a case. Furthermore, the caregiver's obligation to serve the patient's interests through both acts and omissions rules out the exculpation that accompanies omissions in the usual course of social life. An omission that is not warranted by the patient's interests is culpable.

Sometimes initiating a treatment creates expectations in the minds of caregivers, patients, and family that the treatment will be continued indefinitely or until the patient is cured. Such expectations may provide a reason to continue the treatment as a way to keep a promise. However, as with all promises, caregivers could be very careful when initiating a treatment to explain the indications for its discontinuation, and they could modify preconceptions with continuing reevaluation and education during treatment. Though all patients are entitled to expect the continuation of care in the patient's best interests, they are not and should not be entitled to the continuation of a particular mode of care.

Accepting the distinction between withholding and withdrawing medical treatment as morally significant also has a very unfortunate implication: caregivers may become unduly reluctant to begin some treatments precisely because they fear that they will be locked into continuing treatments that are no longer of value to the patient. For example, the physician who had been unwilling to stop the respirator while the infant, Andrew

Stinson, died over several months is reportedly "less eager to attach babies to respirators now."[10] But if it were easier to ignore malnutrition and dehydration and to withhold treatments for these problems than to discontinue the same treatments when they have become especially burdensome and insufficiently beneficial for this patient, then the incentives would be perverse. Once a treatment has been tried, it is often much clearer whether it is of value to this patient, and the decision to stop it can be made more reliably.

The same considerations should apply to starting as to stopping a treatment, and whatever assessment warrants withholding should also warrant withdrawing.

The Obligation to Avoid Being the Unambiguous Cause of Death

Many physicians will agree with all that we have said and still refuse to allow a choice to forego food and fluid because such a course seems to be a "death sentence." In this view death seems to be more certain from malnutrition and dehydration than from foregoing other forms of medical therapy. This implies that it is acceptable to act in ways that are likely to cause death, as in not operating on a gangrenous leg, only if there remains a chance that the patient will survive. This is a comforting formulation for caregivers, to be sure, since they can thereby avoid feeling the full weight of the responsibility for the time and manner of a patient's death. However, it is not a persuasive moral argument.

First, in appropriate cases discontinuing certain medical treatments is generally accepted despite the fact that death is as certain as with nonfeeding. Dialysis in a patient without kidney function or transfusions in a patient with severe aplastic anemia are obvious examples. The dying that awaits such patients often is not greatly different from dying of dehydration and malnutrition.

Second, the certainty of a generally undesirable outcome such as death is always relevant to a decision, but it does not foreclose the possibility that this course is better than others available to this patient. Ambiguity and uncertainty are so common in medical decision making that caregivers are tempted to use them in distancing themselves from direct responsibility. However, caregivers are in fact responsible for the time and manner of death for many patients. Their distaste for this fact should not constrain otherwise morally justified decisions.

The Obligation to Provide Symbolically Significant Treatment

One of the most common arguments for always providing nutrition and hydration is that it symbolizes, expresses, or conveys the essence of care and compassion. Some actions not only aim at goals, they also express values. Such expressive actions should not simply be viewed as means to ends; they should also be viewed in light of what they communicate. From this perspective food and water are not only goods that preserve life and provide comfort; they are also symbols of care and compassion. To withhold or withdraw them—to "starve" a patient—can never express or convey care.

Why is providing food and water a central symbol of care and compassion? Feeding is the first response of the community to the needs of newborns and remains a central mode of nurture and comfort. Eating is associated with social interchange and community, and providing food for someone else is a way to create and maintain bonds of sharing and expressing concern. Furthermore, even the relatively low levels of hunger and thirst that most people have experienced are decidedly uncomfortable, and the common image of severe malnutrition or dehydration is one of unremitting agony. Thus, people are rightly eager to provide food and water. Such provision is essential to minimally tolerable existence and a powerful symbol of our concern for each other.

However, *medical* nutrition and hydration, we have argued, may not always provide net benefits to patients. Medical procedures to provide nutrition and hydration are more similar to other medical procedures than to typical human ways of providing nutrition and hydration, for example, a sip of water. It should be possible to evaluate their benefits and burdens, as we evaluate any other medical procedure. Of course, if family, friends, and caregivers feel that such procedures affirm important values even when they do not benefit the patient, their feelings should not be ignored. We do not contend that there is an obligation to withhold or to withdraw such procedures (unless consideration of the patient's advance directives or current best interest unambiguously dictates that conclusion); we only contend that nutrition and hydration may be foregone in some cases.

The symbolic connection between care and nutrition or hydration adds useful caution to decision making. If decision makers worry over withholding or withdrawing medical nutrition and hydration, they may inquire more seriously into the circumstances that putatively justify their decisions. This is generally salutary for health care decision making. The critical inquiry may well yield the sad but justified conclusion that the patient will be served best by not using medical procedures to provide food and fluids.

A LIMITED CONCLUSION

Our conclusion—that patients or their surrogates, in close collaboration with their physicians and other caregivers and with careful assessment of the relevant information, can correctly decide to forego the provision of medical treatments intended to correct malnutrition and dehydration in some circumstances—is quite limited. Concentrating on incompetent patients, we have argued that in most cases such patients will be best served by providing nutrition and fluids. Thus, there should be a presumption in favor of providing nutrition and fluids as part of the broader presumption to provide means that prolong life. But this presumption may be rebutted in particular cases.

We do not have enough information to be able to determine with clarity and conviction whether withholding or withdrawing nutrition and hydration was justified in the cases that have occasioned public concern, though it seems likely that the Danville and Bloomington babies should have been fed and that Claire Conroy should not.

It is never sufficient to rule out "starvation" categorically. The question is whether the obligation to act in the patient's best interests was discharged by withholding or withdrawing particular medical treatments. All we have claimed is that nutrition and hydration by medical means need not always be provided. Sometimes they may not be in accord with the patient's wishes or interests. Medical nutrition and hydration do not appear to be distinguishable in any morally relevant way from other life-sustaining medical treatments that may on occasion be withheld or withdrawn.

NOTES

1 John A. Robertson, "Dilemma in Danville," *The Hastings Center Report* 11 (October 1981), 5–8.

2 T. Rohrlich, "2 Doctors Face Murder Charges in Patient's Death," L. A. *Times*, August 19, 1982, A-1; Jonathan Kirsch, "A Death at Kaiser Hospital," *California* 7 (1982), 79ff; Magistrate's findings, *California v. Barber and Nejdl*, No. A 925586, Los Angeles Mun. Ct. Cal., (March 9, 1983); Superior Court of California, County of Los Angeles, *California v. Barber and Nejdl*, No. AO 25586, tentative decision May 5, 1983.

3 *In re Infant Doe*, No. GU 8204-00 (Cir. Ct. Monroe County, Ind., April 12, 1982), writ of mandamus dismissed sub nom. *State ex rel. Infant Doe v. Baker*, No. 482 S140 (Indiana Supreme Ct. May 27, 1982).

4 Office of the Secretary, Department of Health and Human Services, "Nondiscrimination on the Basis of Handicap," *Federal Register* 48 (1983), 9630–32. [Interim final rule modifying 45 C.F.R. #84.61]. See Judge Gerhard Gesell's decision, *American Academy of Pediatrics v. Heckler*, No. 83-0774, U.S. District Court, D.C., April 24, 1983; and also George J. Annas, "Disconnecting the Baby Doe Hotline," *The Hastings Center Report* 13 (June 1983), 14–16.

5 *In re Claire C. Conroy*, Sup Ct NJ (Chancery Div-Essex Co. No. P-19083E) February 2, 1983; *In re Claire C. Conroy*, Sup Ct NJ (Appellate Div. No. 4-2483-82T1) July 8, 1983.

6 G. E. M. Anscombe, "Ethical Problems in the Management of Some Severely Handicapped Children: Commentary 2," *Journal of Medical Ethics* 7 (1981), 117–124, at 122.

7 The President's Commission for the Study of Ethical Problems in Medicine and Biomedical and Behavioral Research, *Deciding to Forego Life-Sustaining Treatment* (Washington, D. C.: Government Printing Office, 1982), pp. 171–96.

8 Joyce V. Zerwekh, "The Dehydration Question," *Nursing 83* (January 1983), 47–51, with comments by Judith R. Brown and Marion B. Dolan.

9 The Sacred Congregation for the Doctrine of the Faith, *Declaration on Euthanasia*, Vatican City, May 5, 1980.

10 Robert and Peggy Stinson, *The Long Dying of Baby Andrew* (Boston: Little, Brown and Company, 1983), p. 355.

The Treatment of Impaired Infants

Ethical Issues in Aiding the Death of Young Children
H. Tristram Engelhardt, Jr.

H. Tristram Engelhardt, Jr., M.D., Ph.D. (in philosophy), is professor of medicine and community medicine at Baylor College of Medicine. He is the editor of the *Journal of Medicine and Philosophy* and coeditor of a number of volumes called the *Philosophy and Medicine* series. Engelhardt is also the author of *The Foundations of Bioethics* (1986) and has published numerous articles on issues in biomedical ethics and the philosophy of medicine.

After reviewing the differences between the euthanasia of adults and the euthanasia of children, Engelhardt focuses attention on the status of children. In his view, young children are not persons in a strict sense. Rather, they are persons only in "a social sense," by virtue of their role in a family and society. Since young children "belong" to their parents, it is the parents who are the proper decision makers with regard to the treatment or nontreatment of severely impaired newborns. Engelhardt finds it morally acceptable to allow a severely impaired newborn to die when (1) it is unlikely that the child can attain a "good quality of life" (i.e., a developed personal life) and/or (2) it seems clear that providing continued care for the child would constitute a "severe burden" for the family. Engelhardt goes on to develop the concept of "the injury of continued existence," arguing that a child has a right not to have its life prolonged in those cases where life would be painful and futile. Thus, he maintains, allowing a severely impaired newborn to die (in some cases) is not only *morally acceptable* but indeed *morally demanded*. In concluding, Engelhardt briefly discusses the justifiability of active euthanasia of severely impaired newborns.

Euthanasia in the pediatric age group involves a constellation of issues that are materially different from those of adult euthanasia.[1] The difference lies in the somewhat obvious fact that infants and young children are not able to decide about their own futures and thus are not persons in the same sense that normal adults are. While adults usually decide their own fate, others decide on behalf of young children. Although one can argue that euthanasia is or should be a personal right, the sense of such an argument is obscure with respect to children. Young children do not have any personal rights, at least none that they can exercise on their own behalf with regard to the manner of their life and death. As a result, euthanasia of young children raises special questions concerning the standing of the rights of children, the status of parental rights, the obligations of adults to prevent the suffering of children, and the possible effects on society of allowing or expediting the death of seriously defective infants.

What I will refer to as the euthanasia of infants and young children might be termed by others infanticide, while some cases might be termed the withholding of extraordinary life-prolonging treatment.[2] One needs a term that will encompass both death that results from active intervention and death that ensues when one simply ceases further therapy.[3] In using such a term, one must recognize that death is often not directly but only obliquely intended. That is, one often intends only to treat no further, not actually to have death follow, even though one knows death will follow.[4]

Finally, one must realize that deaths as the result of withholding treatment constitute a significant proportion of neonatal deaths. For example, as high as 14 percent of children in one hospital have been identified as dying after a decision was made not to treat further, the presumption being that the children would have lived longer had treatment been offered.[5]

Even popular magazines have presented accounts of parental decisions not to pursue treatment.[6] These decisions often involve a choice between expensive treatment with little chance of achieving a full, normal life for the child and "letting nature take its course," with the child dying as a result of its defects. As this suggests, many of these problems are products of medical progress. Such children in the past would have died. The quandaries are in a sense an embarrassment of riches; now that one *can* treat such defective children, *must* one treat them? And, if one need not treat such defective children, may one expedite their death?

I will here briefly examine some of these issues. First, I will review differences that contrast the euthanasia of adults to euthanasia of children. Second, I will review the issue of the rights of parents and the status of children. Third, I will suggest a new notion, the concept of the "injury of continued existence," and draw out some of its implications with respect to a duty to prevent suffering. Finally, I will outline some important questions that remain unanswered even if the foregoing issues can be settled. In all, I hope more to display the issues involved in a difficult question than to advance a particular set of answers to particular dilemmas.

For the purpose of this paper, I will presume that adult euthanasia can be justified by an appeal to freedom. In the face of imminent death, one is usually choosing between a more painful and more protracted dying and a less painful or less protracted dying, in circumstances where either choice makes little difference with regard to the discharge of social duties and responsibilities. In the case of suicide, we might argue that, in general, social duties (for example, the duty to support one's family) restrain one from taking one's own life. But in the face of imminent death and in the presence of the pain and deterioration of a fatal disease, such duties are usually impossible to discharge and are thus rendered moot. One can, for example, picture an extreme case of an adult with a widely disseminated carcinoma, including metastases to the brain, who because of severe pain and debilitation is no longer capable of discharging any social duties. In these and similar circumstances, euthanasia becomes the issue of the right to control one's own body, even to the point of seeking assistance in suicide. Euthanasia is, as such, the issue of assisted suicide, the universalization of a maxim that all persons should be free, *in extremis*, to decide with regard to the circumstances of their death.

Further, the choice of positive euthanasia could be defended as the more rational choice: the choice of a less painful death and the affirmation of the value of a rational life. In so choosing, one would be acting to set limits to one's life in order not to live when pain and physical and mental deterioration make further rational life impossible. The choice to end one's life can be understood as a noncontradictory willing of a smaller set of states of existence for oneself, a set that would not include a painful death. As such, it would not involve a desire to destroy oneself. That is, adult euthanasia can be construed as an affirmation of the rationality and autonomy of the self.[7]

The remarks above focus on the active or positive euthanasia of adults. But they hold as well concerning what is often called passive or negative euthanasia, the refusal of life-prolonging therapy. In such cases, the patient's refusal of life-prolonging therapy is seen to be a right that derives from personal freedom, or at least from a zone of privacy into which there are no good grounds for social intervention.[8]

Again, none of these considerations apply directly to the euthanasia of young children, because they cannot participate in such decisions. Whatever else pediatric, in particular neonatal, euthanasia involves, it surely involves issues different from those of adult euthanasia. Since infants and small children cannot commit suicide, their right to assisted suicide is difficult to pose. The difference between the euthanasia of young children and that of adults resides in the difference between children and adults. The difference, in fact, raises the troublesome question of whether young children are persons, or at least whether they are persons in the sense in which adults are. Answering that question will resolve in part at least the right of others to decide whether a young child should live or die and whether he should receive life-prolonging treatment.

THE STATUS OF CHILDREN

Adults belong to themselves in the sense that they are rational and free and therefore responsible for their actions. Adults are *sui juris*. Young children, though, are neither self-possessed nor responsible. While adults exist in and for themselves, as self-directive and self-conscious beings, young children, especially newborn infants, exist for their families and those who love them. They are not, nor can they in any sense be, responsible for themselves. If being a person is to be a responsible agent, a bearer of rights and duties, children are not persons in a strict sense. They are, rather, persons in a social sense: others must act on their behalf and bear responsibility for them. They are, as it were, entities defined by their place in social roles (for example, mother-child, family-child) rather than beings that define themselves as persons, that is, in and through themselves. Young children live as persons in and through the care of those who are responsible for them, and those responsible for them exercise the children's rights on their behalf. In this sense children belong to families in ways that most adults do not. They exist in and through their family and society.

Treating young children with respect has, then, a sense different from treating adults with respect. One can respect neither a newborn infant's or very young child's wishes nor its freedom. In fact, a newborn infant or young child is more an entity that is valued highly because it will grow to be a person and because it plays a social role as if it were a person.[9] That is, a small child is treated as if it were a person in social roles such as mother-child and family-child relationships, though strictly speaking the child is in no way capable of claiming or being responsible for the rights imputed to it. All the rights and duties of the child are exercised and "held in trust" by others for a future time and for a person yet to develop.

Medical decisions to treat or not to treat a neonate or small child often turn on the probability and cost of achieving that future status—a developed personal life. The usual practice of letting anencephalic children (who congenitally lack all or most of the brain) die can be understood as a decision based on the absence of the possibility of achieving a personal life. The practice of refusing treatment to at least some children born with meningomyelocele can be justified through a similar, but more utilitarian, calculus. In the case of anencephalic children one might argue that care for them as persons is futile since they will never be persons. In the case of a child with meningomyelocele, one might argue that when the cost of cure would likely be very high and the probable lifestyle open to attainment very truncated, there is not a positive duty to make a large investment of money and suffering. One should note that the cost here must include not only financial costs but also the anxiety and suffering that prolonged and uncertain treatment of the child would cause the parents.

This further raises the issue of the scope of positive duties not only when there is no person present in a strict sense, but when the likelihood of a full human life is also very uncertain. Clinical and parental judgment may and should be guided by the expected lifestyle and the cost (in parental and societal pain and money) of its attainment. The decision about treatment, however, belongs properly to the parents because the child belongs to them in a sense that it does not belong to anyone else, even to itself. The care and raising of the child falls to the parents, and when considerable cost and little prospect of reasonable success are present, the parents may properly decide against life-prolonging treatment.

The physician's role is to present sufficient information in a usable form to the parents to aid them in making a decision. The accent is on the absence of a positive duty to treat in the presence of severe inconvenience (costs) to the parents; treatment that is very costly is not obligatory. What is suggested here is a general notion that there is never a duty to engage in extraordinary treatment and that "extraordinary" can be defined in terms of costs. This argument concerns children (1) whose future quality of life is likely to be seriously compromised and (2) whose present treatment would be very costly. The issue is that of the circumstances under which parents would not be obliged to take on severe burdens on behalf of their children or those circumstances under which society would not be so obliged. The argument should hold as well for those cases where the expected future life would surely be of normal quality, though its attainment would be extremely costly. The fact of little likelihood of success in attaining a normal life for the child makes decisions to do without treatment more plausible because the hope of success is even more remote and therefore the burden borne by parents or society becomes in that sense more extraordinary. But very high costs themselves could be a sufficient criterion, though in actual cases judgments in that regard would be very difficult when a normal life could be expected.[10]

The decisions in these matters correctly lie in the hands of the parents, because it is primarily in terms of the family that children exist and develop—until children become persons strictly, they are persons in virtue of their social roles. As long as parents do not unjustifiably neglect the humans in those roles so that the value and purpose of that role (that is, child) stands to be eroded (thus endangering other children), society need not intervene. In short, parents may decide for or against the treatment of their severely deformed children.

However, society has a right to intervene and protect children for whom parents refuse care (including treatment) when such care does not constitute a severe burden and when it is likely that the child could be brought to a good quality of life. Obviously, "severe burden" and "good quality of life" will be difficult to define and their meanings will vary, just as it is always difficult to say when grains of sand dropped on a table constitute a heap. At most, though, society need only intervene when the grains clearly do not constitute a heap, that is, when it is clear that the burden is light and the chance of a good quality of life for the child is high. A small child's dependence on his parents is so essential that society need intervene only when the absence of intervention would lead to the role "child" being undermined. Society must value mother-child and family-child relationships and should intervene only in cases where (1) neglect is unreasonable and therefore would undermine respect and care for children, or (2) where societal intervention would prevent children from suffering unnecessary pain.[11]

THE INJURY OF CONTINUED EXISTENCE

But there is another viewpoint that must be considered: that of the child or even the person that the child might become. It might be argued that the child has a right not to have its life prolonged. The idea that forcing existence on a child could be wrong is a difficult notion, which, if true, would serve to amplify the foregoing argument. Such an argument would allow the construal of the issue in terms of the perspective of the child, that is, in terms of a duty not to treat in circumstances where treatment would only prolong suffering. In particular, it would at least give a framework for a decision to stop treatment in cases where, though the costs of treatment are not high, the child's existence would be characterized by severe pain and deprivation.

A basis for speaking of continuing existence as an injury to the child is suggested by the proposed legal concept of "wrongful life." A number of suits have been initiated in the United States and in other countries on the grounds that life or existence itself is, under certain circumstances, a tort or injury to the living person.[12] Although thus far all such suits have ultimately failed, some have succeeded in their initial stages. Two examples may be instructive. In each case the ability to receive recompense for the injury (the tort) presupposed the existence of the individual, whose existence was itself the injury. In one case a suit was initiated on behalf of a child against his father alleging that his father's siring him out of wedlock was an injury to the child.[13] In another case a suit on behalf of a child born of an inmate of a state mental hospital impregnated by rape in that institution was brought against the state of New York.[14] The suit was brought on the grounds that being born with such historical antecedents was itself an injury for which recovery was due. Both cases presupposed that nonexistence would have been preferable to the conditions under which the person born was forced to live.

The suits for tort for wrongful life raise the issue not only of when it would be preferable not to have been born but also of when it would be *wrong* to cause a person to be born. This implies that someone should have judged that it would have been preferable for the child never to have had existence, never to have been in the position to judge that the particular circumstances of life were intolerable.[15] Further, it implies that the person's existence under those circumstances should have been prevented and that, not having been prevented, life was not a gift but an injury. The concept of tort for wrongful life raises an issue concerning the responsibility for giving another person existence, namely, the notion that giving life is not always necessarily a good and justifiable action. Instead, in certain circumstances, so it has been argued, one may have a duty *not* to give existence to another person. This concept involves the claim that certain qualities of life have a negative value, making life an injury, not a gift; it involves, in short, a concept of human accountability and responsibility for human life. It contrasts with the notion that life is a gift of God and thus similar to other "acts of God" (that is, events for which no man is accountable). The concept thus signals the fact that humans can now control reproduction and that where rational control is possible humans are accountable. That is, the expansion of human capabilities has resulted in an expansion of human responsibilities such that one must now decide when and under what circumstances persons will come into existence.

The concept of tort for wrongful life is transferable in part to the painfully compromised existence of children who can only have their life prolonged for a short, painful, and marginal existence. The concept suggests that allowing life to be prolonged under such circumstances would itself be an injury of the person whose painful and severely compromised existence would be made to continue. In fact, it suggests that there is a duty not to prolong life if it can be determined to have a substantial negative value for the person involved.[16] Such issues are moot in the case of adults, who can and should decide for themselves. But small children cannot make such a choice. For them it is an issue of justifying prolonging life under circumstances of painful and compromised existence. Or, put differently, such cases indicate the need to develop social canons to allow a decent death for children for whom the only possibility is protracted, painful suffering.

I do not mean to imply that one should develop a new basis for civil damages. In the field of medicine, the need is to recognize an ethical category, a concept of wrongful continuance of existence, not a new legal right. The concept of injury for continuance of existence, the proposed analogue of the concept of tort for wrongful life, presupposes that life can be of a negative value such that the medical maxim *primum non nocere* ("first do no harm") would require not sustaining life.[17]

The idea of responsibility for acts that sustain or prolong life is cardinal to the notion that one should not under certain circumstances further prolong the life of a child. Unlike adults, children cannot decide with regard to euthanasia (positive or negative), and if more than a utilitarian justification is sought, it must be sought in a duty not to inflict life on another person in circumstances where that life would be painful and futile. This position must rest on the facts that (1) medicine now can cause the prolongation of the life of seriously deformed children who in the past would have died young and that (2) it is not clear that life so prolonged is a good for the child. Further, the choice is made not on the basis of costs to the parents or to society but on the basis of the child's suffering and compromised existence.

The difficulty lies in determining what makes life not worth living for a child. Answers could never be clear. It seems reasonable, however, that the life of children with diseases that involve pain and no hope of survival should not be prolonged. In the case of Tay-Sachs disease (a disease marked by a progressive increase in spasticity and dementia usually leading to death at age three or four), one can hardly imagine that the terminal stages of spastic reaction to stimuli and great difficulty in swallowing are at all pleasant to the child (even insofar as it can only minimally perceive its circumstances). If such a child develops aspiration pneumonia and is treated, it can reasonably be said that to prolong its life is to inflict suffering. Other diseases give fairly clear portraits of lives not worth living: for example, Lesch-Nyhan disease, which is marked by mental retardation and compulsive self-mutilation.

The issue is more difficult in the case of children with diseases for whom the prospects for normal intelligence and a fair lifestyle do exist, but where these chances are remote and their realization expensive. Children born with meningomyelocele present this dilemma. Imagine, for example, a child that falls within Lorber's fifth category (an IQ of sixty or less, sometimes blind, subject to fits, and always incontinent). Such a child has little prospect of anything approaching a normal life, and there is a good chance of its dying even with treatment.[18] But such judgments are statistical. And if one does not treat such children, some will still survive and, as John

Freeman indicates, be worse off if not treated.[19] In such cases one is in a dilemma. If one always treats, one must justify extending the life of those who will ultimately die anyway and in the process subjecting them to the morbidity of multiple surgical procedures. How remote does the prospect of a good life have to be in order not to be worth great pain and expense?[20] It is probably best to decide, in the absence of a positive duty to treat, on the basis of the cost and suffering to parents and society. But, as Freeman argues, the prospect of prolonged or even increased suffering raises the issue of active euthanasia.[21]

If the child is not a person strictly, and if death is inevitable and expediting it would diminish the child's pain prior to death, then it would seem to follow that, all else being equal, a decision for active euthanasia would be permissible, even obligatory.[22] The difficulty lies with "all else being equal," for it is doubtful that active euthanasia could be established as a practice without eroding and endangering children generally, since, as John Lorber has pointed out, children cannot speak in their own behalf.[23] Thus, although there is no argument in principle against the active euthanasia of small children, there could be an argument against such practices based on questions of prudence. To put it another way, even though one might have a duty to hasten the death of a particular child, one's duty to protect children in general could override that first duty. The issue of active euthanasia turns in the end on whether it would have social consequences that refraining would not, on whether (1) it is possible to establish procedural safeguards for limited active euthanasia and (2) whether such practices would have a significant adverse effect on the treatment of small children in general. But since these are procedural issues dependent on sociological facts, they are not open to an answer within the confines of this article. In any event, the concept of the injury of continued existence provides a basis for the justification of the passive euthanasia of small children—a practice already widespread and somewhat established in our society—beyond the mere absence of a positive duty to treat.[24]

CONCLUSION

Though the lack of certainty concerning questions such as the prognosis of particular patients and the social consequence of active euthanasia of children prevents a clear answer to all the issues raised by the euthanasia of infants, it would seem that this much can be maintained: (1) Since children are not persons strictly but exist in and through their families, parents are the appropriate ones to decide whether or not to treat a deformed child when (*a*) there is not only little likelihood of full human life but also great likelihood of suffering if the life is prolonged, or (*b*) when the cost of prolonging life is very great. Such decisions must be made in consort with a physician who can accurately give estimates of cost and prognosis and who will be able to help the parents with the consequences of their decision. (2) It is reasonable to speak of a duty not to treat a small child when such treatment will only prolong a painful life or would in any event lead to a painful death. Though this does not by any means answer all the questions, it does point out an important fact—that medicine's duty is not always to prolong life doggedly but sometimes is quite the contrary.

NOTES

1 I am grateful to Laurence B. McCullough and James P. Morris for their critical discussion of this paper. They may be responsible for its virtues, but not for its shortcomings.

2 The concept of extraordinary treatment as it has been developed in Catholic moral theology is useful: treatment is extraordinary and therefore not obligatory if it involves great costs, pain, or inconvenience, and is a grave burden to oneself or others without a reasonable expectation that such treatment would be successful. See Gerald Kelly, S.J., *Medico-Moral Problems* (St. Louis: The Catholic Hospital Association Press, 1958), pp. 128–141. Difficulties are hidden in terms such as "great costs" and "reasonable expectation," as well as in terms such as "successful." Such ambiguity reflects the fact that precise operational definitions are not available. That is, the precise meaning of "great," "reasonable," and "successful" are inextricably bound to particular circumstances, especially particular societies.

3 I will use the term euthanasia in a broad sense to indicate a deliberately chosen course of action or inaction that is known at the time of decision to be such as will expedite death. This use of euthanasia will encompass not only positive or active euthanasia (acting in order to expedite death) and negative or passive euthanasia (refraining from action in order to expe-

dite death), but acting and refraining in the absence of a direct intention that death occur more quickly (that is, those cases that fall under the concept of double effect). See note 4.

4 But, both active and passive euthanasia can be appreciated in terms of the Catholic moral notion of double effect. When the doctrine of double effect is invoked, one is strictly not intending euthanasia, but rather one intends something else. That concept allows actions or omissions that lead to death (1) because it is licit not to prolong life *in extremis* (allowing death is not an intrinsic evil), (2) if death is not actually willed or actively sought (that is, the evil is not directly willed), (3) if that which is willed is a major good (for example, avoiding useless major expenditure of resources or serious pain), and (4) if the good is not achieved by means of the evil (for example, one does not will to save resources or diminish pain *by* the death). With regard to euthanasia the doctrine of double effect means that one need not expend major resources in an endeavor that will not bring health but only prolong dying and that one may use drugs that decrease pain but hasten death. See Richard McCormick, *Ambiguity in Moral Choice* (Milwaukee: Marquette University Press, 1973). I exclude the issue of double effect from my discussion because I am interested in those cases in which the good may follow directly from the evil—the death of the child. In part, though, the second section of this paper is concerned with the concept of proportionate good.

5 Raymond S. Duff and A. G. M. Campbell, "Moral and Ethical Dilemmas in the Special-Care Nursery," *The New England Journal of Medicine*, 289 (Oct. 25, 1973), pp. 890–894.

6 Roger Pell, "The Agonizing Decision of Joanne and Roger Pell," *Good Housekeeping* (January 1972), pp. 76–77, 131–135.

7 This somewhat Kantian argument is obviously made in opposition to Kant's position that suicide involves a default of one's duty to oneself "...to preserve his life simply because he is a person and must therefore recognize a duty to himself (and a strict one at that)," as well as a contradictory volition: "that man ought to have the authorization to withdraw himself from all obligation, that is, to be free to act as if no authorization at all were required for this withdrawal, involves a contradiction. To destroy the subject of morality in his own person is tantamount to obliterating from the world..." Immanuel Kant, *The Metaphysical Principles of Virtue: Part II of the Metaphysics of*

Morals, trans. James Ellington (Indianapolis: Bobbs-Merrill, 1964), p. 83; Akademie Edition, VI, 422–423.

8 Norman L. Cantor, "A Patient's Decision to Decline Life-Saving Medical Treatment: Bodily Integrity Versus the Preservation of Life," *Rutgers Law Review*, 26 (Winter 1972), p. 239.

9 By "young child" I mean either an infant or child so young as not yet to be able to participate, in any sense, in a decision. A precise operational definition of "young child" would clearly be difficult to develop. It is also not clear how one would bring older children into such decisions. See, for example, Milton Viederman. "Saying 'No' to Hemodialysis: Exploring Adaptation," and Daniel Burke, "Saying 'No' to Hemodialysis: An Acceptable Decision," both in *The Hastings Center Report*, 4 (September 1974), pp. 8–10, and John E. Schowalter, Julian B. Ferholt, and Nancy M. Mann, "The Adolescent Patient's Decision to Die," *Pediatrics*, 51 (January 1973), pp. 97–103.

10 An appeal to high costs alone is probably hidden in judgments based on statistics: even though there is a chance for a normal life for certain children with apparently severe cases of meningomyelocele, one is not obliged to treat since that chance is small, and the pursuit of that chance is very expensive. Cases of the costs being low but the expected suffering of the child being high will be discussed under the concept of the injury of continued existence. It should be noted that none of the arguments in this paper bear on cases where neither the cost nor the suffering of the child is considerable. Cases in this last category probably include, for example, children born with mongolism complicated only by duodenal atresia.

11 I have in mind here the issue of physicians, hospital administrators, or others being morally compelled to seek an injunction to force treatment of the child in the absence of parental consent. In these circumstances, the physician, who is usually best acquainted with the facts of the case, is the natural advocate of the child.

12 G. Tedeschi, "On Tort Liability for 'Wrongful Life,' " *Israel Law Review*, 1 (1966), p. 513.

13 Zepeda v. Zepeda: 41 Ill. App. 2d 240, 190 N.E. 2d 849 (1963).

14 Williams v. State of New York: 46 Misc. 2d 824, 260 N.Y.S. 2d 953 (Ct. Cl., 1965).

15 Torts: "Illegitimate Child Denied Recovery against Father for 'Wrongful Life,' " *Iowa Law Review*, 49 (1969), p. 1009.

16 It is one thing to have a conceptual definition of the injury of continued existence (for example, causing a person to continue to live under circumstances of severe pain and deprivation when there are no alternatives but death) and another to have an operational definition of that concept (that is, deciding what counts as such severe pain and deprivation). This article has focused on the first, not the second, issue.

17 H. Tristram Engelhardt, Jr., "Euthanasia and Children: The Injury of Continued Existence," *The Journal of Pediatrics*, 83 (July 1973), pp. 170–171.

18 John Lorber, "Results of Treatment of Myelomeningocele," *Developmental Medicine and Child Neurology*, 13 (1971), p. 286.

19 John M. Freeman, "The Shortsighted Treatment of Myelomeningocele: A Long-Term Case Report," *Pediatrics*, 53 (March 1974), pp. 311–313.

20 John M. Freeman, "To Treat or Not to Treat," *Practical Management of Meningomyelocele*, ed. John Freeman (Baltimore: University Park Press, 1974), p. 21.

21 John Lorber, "Selective Treatment of Myelomeningocele: To Treat or Not to Treat," *Pediatrics*, 53 (March 1974), pp. 307–308.

22 I am presupposing that no intrinsic moral distinctions exist in cases such as these, between acting and refraining, between omitting care in the hope that death will ensue (that is, rather than the child living to be even more defective) and acting to ensure that death will ensue rather than having the child live under painful and seriously compromised circumstances. For a good discussion of the distinction between acting and refraining, see Jonathan Bennett, "Whatever the Consequences," *Analysis*, 26 (January 1966), pp. 83–102; P. J. Fitzgerald, "Acting and Refraining," *Analysis*, 27 (March 1967), pp. 133–139; Daniel Dinello, "On Killing and Letting Die," *Analysis*, 31 (April 1971), pp. 83–86.

23 Lorber, "Selective Treatment of Myelomeningocele," p. 308.

24 Positive duties involve a greater constraint than negative duties. Hence it is often easier to establish a duty not to do something (not to treat further) than a duty to do something (to actively hasten death). Even allowing a new practice to be permitted (for example, active euthanasia) requires a greater attention to consequences than does establishing the absence of a

positive duty. For example, at common law there is no basis for action against a person who watches another drown without giving aid; this reflects the difficulty of establishing a positive duty.

Involuntary Euthanasia of Defective Newborns
John A. Robertson

John A. Robertson is professor of law at the School of Law, University of Texas at Austin. He is the author of *The Rights of the Critically Ill* (1983) and has published such articles as "Compensating Injured Research Subjects: The Law," "Medical Ethics in the Courtroom," and "Rights, Symbolism, and Public Policy in Fetal Tissue Transplants."

Robertson, in vivid contrast to Engelhardt, denies that the undesirable consequences of treating a severely impaired (defective) newborn can morally justify nontreatment. The consequentialist argument directly under attack by Robertson has two versions. One version is based on the suffering of the severely impaired newborn, whereas the other version is based on the suffering of others (principally the family but also health professionals and society as a whole). The first version of the consequentialist argument, identified by Robertson as the "quality-of-life argument," maintains that withholding treatment is morally justified because the severely impaired newborn is better off dead. Although Robertson insists that it is often false that death is a better fate than continued life for the severely impaired newborn, his fundamental objection to the quality-of-life argument stems from his reluctance to accept proxy assessments of quality-of-life. The second version of the consequentialist argument holds that withholding treatment is morally justified because of the emotional and financial burden falling on those who would have to provide the continued care for a severely impaired child. Robertson's central objection to this version of the consequentialist argument has to do with its utilitarian spirit, but he also argues that it is seldom plausible to think that the suffering of others is so grave as to outweigh the impaired newborn's interest in life.

One of the most perplexing dilemmas of modern medicine concerns whether "ordinary"[1] medical care justifiably can be withheld from defective newborns. Infants with malformations of the central nervous system[2] such as anencephaly,[3] hydrocephaly,[4] Down's syndrome,[5] spina bifida,[6] and myelomeningocele[7] often require routine surgical or medical attention[8] merely to stay alive. Until recent developments in surgery and pediat-

Reprinted with permission of the publisher from *Stanford Law Review*, vol 27 (January 1975), pp. 213–214; 251–261. Copyright © 1975 by the Board of Trustees of the Leland Stanford Junior University.

rics, these infants would have died of natural causes. Today with treatment many will survive for long periods, although some will be severely handicapped and limited in their potential for human satisfaction and interaction. Because in the case of some defective newborns, the chances are often slim that they will ever lead normal human lives, it is now common practice for parents to request, and for physicians to agree, not to treat such infants. Without treatment the infant usually dies....

If we reject the argument that defective newborns are not persons, the question remains whether circumstances exist in which the consequences of treatment as compared with nontreatment are so undesirable that the omission of care is justified....

...Many parents and physicians deeply committed to the loving care of the newborn think that treating severely defective infants causes more harm than good, thereby justifying the withholding of ordinary care. In their view the suffering and diminished quality of the child's life do not justify the social and economic costs of treatment. This claim has a growing commonsense appeal, but it assumes that the utility or quality of one's life can be measured and compared with other lives, and that health resources may legitimately be allocated to produce the greatest personal utility. This argument will now be analyzed from the perspective of the defective patient and others affected by his care.

A THE QUALITY OF THE DEFECTIVE INFANT'S LIFE

Comparisons of relative worth among persons, or between persons and other interests, raise moral and methodological issues that make any argument that relies on such comparisons extremely vulnerable. Thus the strongest claim for not treating the defective newborn is that treatment seriously harms the infant's own interests, whatever may be the effects on others. When maintaining his life involves great physical and psychosocial suffering for the patient, a reasonable person might conclude that such a life is not worth living. Presumably the patient, if fully informed and able to communicate, would agree. One then would be morally justified in withholding lifesaving treatment if such action served to advance the best interests of the patient.

Congenital malformations impair development in several ways that lead to the judgment that deformed retarded infants are "a burden to themselves."[9] One is the severe physical pain, much of it resulting from repeated surgery that defective infants will suffer. Defective children also are likely to develop other pathological features, leading to repeated fractures, dislocations, surgery, malfunctions, and other sources of pain. The shunt, for example, inserted to relieve hydrocephalus, a common problem in defective children, often becomes clogged, necessitating frequent surgical interventions.

Pain, however, may be intermittent and manageable with analgesics. Since many infants and adults experience great pain, and many defective infants do not, pain alone, if not totally unmanageable, does not sufficiently show that a life is so worthless that death is preferable. More important are the psychosocial deficits resulting from the child's handicaps. Many defective children never can walk even with prosthesis, never interact with normal children, never appreciate growth, adolescence, or the fulfillment of education and employment, and seldom are even able to care for themselves. In cases of severe retardation, they may be left with a vegetative existence in a crib, incapable of choice or the most minimal response to stimuli. Parents or others may reject them, and much of their time will be spent in hospitals, in surgery, or fighting the many illnesses that beset them. Can it be said that such a life is worth living?

There are two possible responses to the quality-of-life argument. One is to accept its premises but to question the degree of suffering in particular cases, and thus restrict the justification for death to the most extreme cases. The absence of opportunities for schooling, career, and interaction may be the fault of social attitudes and the failings of healthy persons, rather than a necessary result of congenital malformations. Psychosocial suffering occurs because healthy, normal persons reject or refuse to relate to the defective, or hurry them to poorly funded institutions. Most nonambulatory, mentally retarded persons can be trained for satisfying roles. One cannot assume that a nonproductive existence is necessarily unhappy: even social rejection and nonacceptance can be mitigated. Moreover, the psychosocial ills of the handicapped often do not differ in kind from those experienced by many persons. With training and care, growth, development, and a full range of experiences are possible for most people with physical and mental handicaps. Thus, the claim that death is a far better fate than life cannot in most cases be sustained.

This response, however, avoids meeting the quality-of-life argument on its strongest grounds. Even if many defective infants can experience growth, interaction, and most human satisfactions if nurtured, treated, and trained, some infants are so severely retarded or grossly deformed that their response to love and care, in fact their capacity to be conscious, is always minimal. Although mongoloid and nonambulatory spina bifida children may experience an existence we would hesitate to adjudge worse than death, the profoundly retarded, nonambulatory, blind, deaf infant who will spend his few years in the back-ward cribs of a state institution is clearly a different matter.

To repudiate the quality-of-life argument, therefore, requires a defense of treatment in even these extreme cases. Such a defense would question the validity of any surrogate or proxy judgments of the worth or quality of life when the wishes of the person in question cannot be ascertained. The essence of the quality-of-life argument is a proxy's judgment that no reasonable person can prefer the pain, suffering, and loneliness of, for example, life in a crib at an IQ level of 20, to an immediate, painless death.

But in what sense can the proxy validly conclude that a person with different wants, needs, and interests, if able to speak, would agree that such a life were worse than death? At the start one must be skeptical of the proxy's claim to objective disinterestedness. If the proxy is also the parent or physician, as has been the case in pediatric euthanasia, the impact of treatment on the proxy's interests, rather than solely on those of the child, may influence his assessment. But even if the proxy were truly neutral and committed only to caring for the child, the problem of egocentricity and knowing another's mind remains. Compared with the situation and life prospects of a "reasonable man," the child's potential quality of life indeed appears dim. Yet a standard based on healthy, ordinary development may be entirely inappropriate to this situation. One who has never known the pleasures of mental operation, ambulation, and social interaction surely does not suffer from their loss as much as one who has. While one who has known these capacities may prefer death to a life without them, we have no assurance that the handicapped person, with no point of comparison, would agree. Life, and life alone, whatever its limitations, might be of sufficient worth to him.

One should also be hesitant to accept proxy assessments of quality-of-life because the margin of error in such predictions may be very great. For instance, while one expert argues that by a purely clinical assessment he can accurately forecast the minimum degree of future handicap an individual will experience, such forecasting is not infallible, and risks denying care to infants whose disability might otherwise permit a reasonably acceptable quality-of-life. Thus given the problems in ascertaining another's wishes, the proxy's bias to personal or culturally relative interests, and the unreliability of predictive criteria, the quality-of-life argument is open to serious question. Its strongest appeal arises in the case of a grossly deformed, retarded, institutionalized child, or one with incessant unmanageable pain, where continued life is itself torture. But these cases are few, and cast doubt on the utility of any such judgment. Even if the

judgment occasionally may be defensible, the potential danger of quality-of-life assessments may be a compelling reason for rejecting this rationale for withholding treatment.

B THE SUFFERING OF OTHERS

In addition to the infant's own suffering, one who argues that the harm of treatment justifies violation of the defective infant's right to life usually relies on the psychological, social, and economic costs of maintaining his existence to family and society. In their view the minimal benefit of treatment to persons incapable of full social and physical development does not justify the burdens that care of the defective infant imposes on parents, siblings, health professionals, and other patients. Matson, a noted pediatric neurosurgeon, states:

> [I]t is the doctor's and the community's responsibility to provide [custodial] care and to minimize suffering; but, at the same time, it is also their responsibility not to prolong such individual, familial, and community suffering unnecessarily, and not to carry out multiple procedures and prolonged, expensive, acute hospitalization in an infant whose chance for acceptable growth and development is negligible.[10]

Such a frankly utilitarian argument raises problems. It assumes that because of the greatly curtailed orbit of his existence, the costs or suffering of others is greater than the benefit of life to the child. This judgment, however, requires a coherent way of measuring and comparing interpersonal utilities, a logical-practical problem that utilitarianism has never surmounted. But even if such comparisons could reliably show a net loss from treatment, the fact remains that the child must sacrifice his life to benefit others. If the life of one individual, however useless, may be sacrificed for the benefit of any person, however useful, or for the benefit of any number of persons, then we have acknowledged the principle that rational utility may justify any outcome. As many philosophers have demonstrated, utilitarianism can always permit the sacrifice of one life for other interests, given the appropriate arrangement of utilities on the balance sheet. In the absence of principled grounds for such a decision, the social equation involved in mandating direct, involuntary euthanasia becomes a difference of degree, not kind, and we reach the point where protection of life depends solely on social judgments of utility.

These objections may well be determinative. But if we temporarily bracket them and examine the extent to which care of the defective infant subjects others to suffering, the claim that inordinate suffering outweighs the infant's interest in life is rarely plausible. In this regard we must examine the impact of caring for defective infants on the family, health professions, and society-at-large.

The Family

The psychological impact and crisis created by birth of a defective infant is devastating. Not only is the mother denied the normal tension release from the stresses of pregnancy, but both parents feel a crushing blow to their dignity, self-esteem and self-confidence. In a very short time, they feel grief for the loss of the normal expected child, anger at fate, numbness, disgust, waves of helplessness, and disbelief. Most feel personal blame for the defect, or blame their spouse. Adding to the shock is fear that social position and mobility are permanently endangered. The transformation of a "joyously awaited experience into one of catastrophe and profound psychological threat"[11] often will reactivate unresolved maturational conflicts. The chances for social pathology—divorce, somatic complaints, nervous and mental disorders—increase and hard-won adjustment patterns may be permanently damaged.

The initial reactions of guilt, grief, anger, and loss, however, cannot be the true measure of family suffering caused by care of a defective infant, because these costs are present whether or not the parents choose treatment. Rather, the question is to what degree treatment imposes psychic and other costs greater than would occur if the child were not treated. The claim that care is more costly rests largely on the view that parents and family suffer inordinately from nurturing such a child.

Indeed, if the child is treated and accepted at home, difficult and demanding adjustments must be made. Parents must learn how to care for a disabled child, confront financial and psychological uncertainty, meet the needs of other siblings, and work through their own conflicting feelings. Mothering demands are greater than with a normal child, particularly if medical care and hospitalization are frequently required. Counseling or professional support may be nonexistent or difficult to obtain. Younger siblings may react with hostility and guilt, older with shame and anger. Often the normal feedback

of child growth that renders the turmoil of childrearing worthwhile develops more slowly or not at all. Family resources can be depleted (especially if medical care is needed), consumption patterns altered, or standards of living modified. Housing may have to be found closer to a hospital, and plans for further children changed. Finally, the anxieties, guilt, and grief present at birth may threaten to recur or become chronic.

Yet, although we must recognize the burdens and frustrations of raising a defective infant, it does not necessarily follow that these costs require nontreatment, or even institutionalization. Individual and group counseling can substantially alleviate anxiety, guilt, and frustration, and enable parents to cope with underlying conflicts triggered by the birth and the adaptations required. Counseling also can reduce psychological pressures on siblings, who can be taught to recognize and accept their own possibly hostile feelings and the difficult position of their parents. They may even be taught to help their parents care for the child.

The impact of increased financial costs also may vary. In families with high income or adequate health insurance, the financial costs are manageable. In others, state assistance may be available. If severe financial problems arise or pathological adjustments are likely, institutionalization, although undesirable for the child, remains an option. Finally, in many cases, the experience of living through a crisis is a deepening and enriching one, accelerating personality maturation, and giving one a new sensitivity to the needs of spouse, siblings, and others. As one parent of a defective child states: "In the last months I have come closer to people and can understand them more. I have met them more deeply. I did not know there were so many people with troubles in the world."[12]

Thus, while social attitudes regard the handicapped child as an unmitigated disaster, in reality the problem may not be insurmountable, and often may not differ from life's other vicissitudes. Suffering there is, but seldom is it so overwhelming or so imminent that the only alternative is death of the child.

Health Professionals

Physicians and nurses also suffer when parents give birth to a defective child, although, of course, not to the degree of the parents. To the obstetrician or general practitioner the defective birth may be a blow to his professional identity. He has the difficult task of informing the parents of the defects, explaining their causes, and dealing with the parents' resulting emotional shock. Often he feels guilty for failing to produce a normal baby. In addition, the parents may project anger or hostility on the physician, questioning his professional competence or seeking the services of other doctors. The physician also may feel that his expertise and training are misused when employed to maintain the life of an infant whose chances for a productive existence are so diminished. By neglecting other patients, he may feel that he is prolonging rather than alleviating suffering.

Nurses, too, suffer role strain from care of the defective newborn. Intensive-care-unit nurses may work with only one or two babies at a time. They face the daily ordeals of care—the progress and relapses—and often must deal with anxious parents who are themselves grieving or ambivalent toward the child. The situation may trigger a nurse's own ambivalence about death and mothering, in a context in which she is actively working to keep alive a child whose life prospects seem minimal.

Thus, the effects of care on physicians and nurses are not trivial, and must be intelligently confronted in medical education or in management of a pediatric unit. Yet to state them is to make clear that they can but weigh lightly in the decision of whether to treat a defective newborn. Compared with the situation of the parents, these burdens seem insignificant, are short term, and most likely do not evoke such profound emotions. In any case, these difficulties are hazards of the profession—caring for the sick and dying will always produce strain. Hence, on these grounds alone it is difficult to argue that a defective person may be denied the right to life.

Society

Care of the defective newborn also imposes societal costs, the utility of which is questioned when the infant's expected quality-of-life is so poor. Medical resources that can be used by infants with a better prognosis, or throughout the health-care system generally, are consumed in providing expensive surgical and intensive-care services to infants who may be severely retarded, never lead active lives, and die in a few months or years. Institutionalization imposes costs on taxpayers and reduces the resources available for those who might better benefit from it, while reducing further the quality of life experienced by the institutionalized defective.

One answer to these concerns is to question the impact of the costs of caring for defective newborns. Precise data showing the costs to taxpayers or the trade-offs

with health and other expenditures do not exist. Nor would ceasing to care for the defective necessarily lead to a reallocation within the health budget that would produce net savings in suffering or life; in fact, the released resources might not be reallocated for health at all. In any case, the trade-offs within the health budget may well be small. With advances in prenatal diagnosis of genetic disorders many deformed infants who would formerly require care will be aborted beforehand. Then, too, it is not clear that the most technical and expensive procedures always constitute the best treatment for certain malformations. When compared with the almost seven percent of the GNP now spent on health, the money in the defense budget, or tax revenues generally, the public resources required to keep defective newborns alive seem marginal, and arguably worth the commitment to life that such expenditures reinforce. Moreover, as the Supreme Court recently recognized,[13] conservation of the taxpayer's purse does not justify serious infringement of fundamental rights. Given legal and ethical norms against sacrificing the lives of nonconsenting others, and the imprecisions in diagnosis and prediction concerning the eventual outcomes of medical care, the social cost argument does not compel nontreatment of defective newborns....

NOTES

1 Few persons would argue that "extraordinary" care must be provided a defective newborn, or indeed, to any person. The difficult question, however, is to distinguish "ordinary" from "extraordinary" care....In this Article "ordinary" care refers to those medical and surgical procedures that would normally be applied in situations not involving physically or mentally handicapped persons.

2 The need for ordinary treatment will also arise with noncentral nervous system malformations such as malformations of the cardiovascular, respiratory, orogastrointestinal, urogenital, muscular and skeletal systems, as well as deformities of the eye, ear, face, endocrine glands, and skin. *See generally* J. Warkany, CONGENITAL MALFORMATIONS (1971). Often these defects will accompany central nervous system malformations. The medical-ethical dilemma discussed in this Article has arisen chiefly with regard to central nervous system problems, perhaps because the presence of such defects seriously affects intelli-

gence, social interaction, and the potential for development and growth, and will be discussed only in the context of the major central nervous system malformations. Parents of physically deformed infants with normal intelligence might face the same choice, but because of the child's capacity for development, pressure to withhold ordinary treatment will be less severe.

3 Anencephaly is partial or total absence of the brain. J. Warkany, *supra* note 2, at 189–99.

4 Hydrocephaly is characterized by an increase of free fluid in the cranial cavity which results in a marked enlargement of the head. *Id.* at 217. It is a symptom of many diverse disorders, and is associated with hereditary and chromosomal syndromes. *Id.* at 217–18. Warkany describes the symptoms as follows: "Bulging of the forehead, protrusion of the parietal areas and extension of the occipital region are characteristic changes.... The skin of the scalp is thin and stretched and its veins are dilated.... The head cannot be held up, and walking and talking are delayed. The legs are spastic, the tendon reflexes increased and convulsions may occur. Anorexia, vomiting and emaciation complicate severe cases. As a rule, hydrocephalic children are dull and lethargic. Blindness can develop, but hearing and the auditory memory may be good. Physical and mental development depend on several factors, such as rapidity of onset, intracranial pressure, compensatory growth of the head, nature of the basic malformations and progress or arrest of the process. Such variability makes the prognosis and evaluation of therapeutic measures difficult. Pressure on the hypothalamic area can cause obesity or precocious puberty in exceptional cases." *Id.* at 226–27.

5 Down's syndrome or mongolism is a chromosomal disorder producing mental retardation caused by the presence of 47 rather than 46 chromosomes in a patient's cells, and marked by a distinctively shaped head, neck, trunk, and abdomen. *Id.* at 311–12, 324. For summary of clinical and pathological characteristics, *see id.* at 324–31.

6 Spina bifida refers generally to midline defects of the osseous spine. The defect usually appears in the pos-

terior aspects of the vertebral canal, and may be marked by an external saccular protrusion (spina bifida cystica). *Id.* at 272. Spina bifida is often seriously involved with urinary tract deficiency, hydrocephaly, and may involve paralysis of the lower extremities. *Id.* at 286–88. While there are important differences between spina bifida, meningoceles, and myelomeningocele, the terms will be used interchangeably in discussing and evaluating the duty to treat.

7 The saccular enlargements of spina bifida cystica protruding through osseous defects of the vertebral column that contain anomalous meninges and spinal fluid but do not have neural elements affixed to their walls are called meningoceles. If the spinal cord or nerves are included in the formation of the sac, the anomaly is called myelomeningocele. *Id.* at 272. As with spina bifida, myelomeningocele may substantially interfere with locomotion, sphincter and bladder control, and may be accompanied by kyphoscoliosis and hydrocephaly leading to mental retardation. For a description of symptoms and treatment alternatives, *see* Lorber, *Results of Treatment of Myelomeningocele*, 13 DEVELOP. MED. & CHILD NEUROL. 279–303 (1971).

8 The infant might suffer from duodenal atresia and need surgery to connect the stomach to the intestine; or need an appendectomy; or antibiotics to fight pneumonia; or suffer from Respirator Distress Syndrome and need breathing assistance. In some cases the question is whether to begin or continue feeding.

9 Smith & Smith, *Selection for Treatment in Spina Bifida Cystica*, 4 BRIT. MED. J. 189, 195 (1973).

10 Matson, *Surgical Treatment of Myelomeningocele*, 42 PEDIATRICS 225, 226 (1968).

11 Goodman, *Continuing Treatment of Parents with Congenitally Defective Infants*, SOCIAL WORK, Vol. 9, No. I, at 92 (1964).

12 *Quoted in* Johns, *Family Reactions to the Birth of a Child with a Congenital Abnormality*, 26 OBSTET. GYNECOL. SURVEY 635, 637 (1971).

13 *Memorial Hosp. v. Maricopa County*, 415 U.S. 250 (1974).

Standards of Judgment for Treatment of Imperiled Newborns
Members of The Hastings Center Research Project on the Care of Imperiled Newborns

In 1984, The Hastings Center initiated a research project dedicated to the problem of determining appropriate care for imperiled newborns. Philosophers, physicians, nurses, and lawyers were among the many project participants, and Arthur L. Caplan served as project director. A brief excerpt from the 1987 project report is reprinted here.

Concerned with the problem of selective nontreatment, the project group members first reject two distinctive sanctity-of-life positions—"vitalism" and "the medical indications policy." They then endorse the employment of quality-of-life standards, with the provision that quality must be measured by reference to the infant's own well-being and not in terms of social utility. In their view, two distinctive quality-of-life standards are relevant to the problem of selective nontreatment. In most cases, the relevant standard is the best interest of the infant, which would allow (and in fact mandate) nontreatment only when continued life would be worse for the infant than an early death. In some cases, however, the relevant standard is that of "relational potential," which would make treatment optional for an infant who lacks the potential for human relationships.

As parents and clinicians evaluate specific strategies for responding to uncertainty, it is essential to ask how they should determine whether treatment is *ethically right* for a particular infant. The ethical questions can only be resolved by establishing reasonable standards of judgment against which to measure strategies and procedures.

"SANCTITY OF LIFE" STANDARDS

Many critics of the practice of selective nontreatment argue that we must concentrate on the *sanctity* of life. But what does it mean to base our decisions on the sanctity of each child's life? Does it mean that caregivers may *never* forgo treatment, or that they may do so only for the most catastrophically afflicted newborns? Without further specification, the "sanctity of life" standard remains a vague slogan, rather than a meaningful guide to decisionmaking.

Vitalism

The most extreme sanctity of life position would hold that "where there is life, there is hope," and that so long as a child continues to cling to life, he or she must be

Reprinted with permission of the publisher from *Hastings Center Report*, vol. 17 (December 1987), pp. 13–16.

treated. According to this view, which we shall call "vitalism," the mere presence of a heartbeat, respiration, or brain activity is a compelling reason to sustain all efforts to save the child's life. Only the moment of death relieves caregivers of their duty to treat. An adherent of this vitalist philosophy would accordingly hold that, except in cases where the child has been declared dead, all withholding and withdrawal of treatment is ethically wrong.

This most extreme sanctity of life position has few advocates. Its major flaw is that it would insist upon aggressive treatments even for those children who are deemed to be in the process of dying. If responsible physicians have concluded that a particular child cannot be saved, that he will soon die, then it seems pointless and cruel to continue to treat the child with medical interventions that are by no means benign. By insisting on treatment even in such hopeless cases, the vitalist can justly be accused of worshipping an abstraction, "life," rather than focusing on the concrete good of the patient. As theologian Paul Ramsey has cogently argued, the appropriate response to a dying patient is not the futile imposition of painful medical treatments, but rather kind and respectful *care* designed to ease the child's passing.

The Medical Indications Policy

A more reasonable sanctity of life position has been proposed by Paul Ramsey and adopted (with some modifications) in various versions of the Department of Health and Human Services so-called "Baby Doe Rules." According to this standard, each child possesses equal dignity and intrinsic worth (i.e. "sanctity") and therefore no child should be denied life-sustaining medical treatments simply on the basis of his or her "handicap" or future quality of life. Such treatments must be provided to all infants, except (1) when the infant is judged to be in the process of dying, or (2) when the contemplated treatment is itself deemed to be "medically contraindicated." As Ramsey puts it, *treatments* may be compared in order to see which will be medically beneficial for a child, but abnormal *children* may not be compared with normal children in order to determine who shall live.

This policy is supported by two complementary ethical principles. First, the "nondiscrimination principle" states that children with impairments may not be selected for nontreatment solely on the basis of their "handicapping condition." If an otherwise normal child would receive a certain treatment—for example, surgery to repair an intestinal blockage—then a child with an abnormality must receive like treatment. Failure to do so discriminates unfairly against the child with impairments.

Second, the "medical benefit principle" states that caregivers are obliged to provide any and all treatments deemed, according to "reasonable medical judgment," to be "medically beneficial" to the patient. This means that if a certain medical or surgical procedure would be likely to bring about its intended result of avoiding infection or some other fatal consequence, then it must be provided to the child.

Although this medical indications policy was obviously well intended, insofar as it attempted to prevent instances of *unjust* discrimination against newborns with impairments, we believe that it is an overly rigid and inappropriate guide to decisionmaking. The first problem is that the nondiscrimination principle would have decisionmakers ignore, not just relatively mild handicaps of the sort encountered in most children with spina bifida and Down syndrome, but also impairments that are genuinely catastrophic.

Consider, for example, the child suffering from severe birth asphyxia who also happens to have a grave heart defect. Although surgeons would be willing to operate to fix the heart of an otherwise normal infant, the fact that this particular infant will never be sufficiently conscious to interact with his environment would appear to be a factor that the child's caretakers might permissi-

bly take into consideration. Should the child be subjected to major and painful cardiac surgery only so that he might subsist in a permanently unconscious state? Even though treatment might be withheld from such a grievously afflicted infant "solely on the basis of his handicap," such a decision would in no way count as *unjust* discrimination precisely because the child's handicap is so severe that he can no longer meaningfully be compared to an "otherwise normal" infant.

The second problem with the medical indications policy lies in its "medical benefit" principle. Although this principle works well in many cases—for example, mild to moderate spina bifida—it does so because we think that the treatment confers a benefit, not merely upon the child's spine, but rather upon the whole child.

QUALITY OF LIFE STANDARDS

Although we conclude that quality of life judgments are ethically proper, and indeed inevitable, a great deal of care must be given to specifying why quality of life matters and what qualitative conditions might justify the denial of treatment. Merely invoking the phrase "quality of life" will get us no farther than invocations of the "sanctity of life."

The phrase "quality of life," as used in medical contexts, is ambiguous and frequently misunderstood. It is sometimes used to denote the social worth of an individual, the value that individual has for society. According to this interpretation, a person's quality of life is determined by utilitarian criteria, measured by balancing the burdens and benefits to others, especially family members. It is this meaning of the phrase that gives rise to the greatest worries about undertreatment of newborns with impairments.

This interpretation of quality of life has been defended on the grounds that external circumstances are crucially important in the outlook for certain newborns and because of the increased stress families undergo in raising children with disabilities. Despite the recognition that these external factors play a role in parental attitudes toward treatment, the consensus of this report is that "quality of life" should refer to the present or future characteristics of the infant, judged by standards of the infant's own well-being and not in terms of social utility.

Another way of understanding "quality of life" is as measured against a norm of "acceptable" life. Yet it is often noted that what would not be acceptable to some people, for themselves, is clearly acceptable to others. A danger lies in drawing the line too high, thereby ruling as "unacceptable" the life of a person with multiple handicaps or with mild-to-moderate mental retardation. When quality-of-life assessments are made for newborns with impairments, caution must be exercised to avoid this pitfall.

An example of drawing the line of "acceptable" life too high is "the ability to work or marry," a factor cited by the British pediatrician, John Lorber. An example of a very low standard is permanent coma, a criterion appearing in the 1984 Child Abuse Amendments. This threshold is so low as to be noncontroversial.

A subset of the quality of life standard and an alternative to a medical indications policy is the standard known as the "best interest of the child." Traditionally, this standard has been employed by courts in making child custody determinations and other decisions involving placement of an infant or child.

Unlike the medical indications policy, the "best interest" standard does incorporate quality of life considerations. This standard holds that infants should be treated with life-sustaining therapy except when (1) the infant is dying, (2) treatment is medically contraindicated (the two exceptions built into the medical indications policy), and (3) continued life would be worse for the infant than an early death. The third condition opens the door to quality of life considerations, but requires that such considerations be viewed from the infant's point of view. That is, certain states of being, marked by severe and intractable pain and suffering, can be viewed as worse than death. Thus, according to the best interest standard, there is room to consider the possibility that an infant's best interest can lie in withholding or withdrawing medical treatments, resulting in death.

Care must be taken, however, not to employ a standard based on the sensibilities of unimpaired adults; for example, one in which adult decision-makers judge, from their own perspective, that they would not want to live a life with mental or physical disabilities. An infant-centered quality of life standard should be as objective as possible, in an attempt to determine whether continued life would be a benefit, from the child's point of view. An impaired child does not have the luxury of comparing his life to a "normal" existence; for such a child, it is a question of life with impairments versus no life at all.

The greatest merit of the best interest standard lies precisely in its child-centeredness. This focus on the individual child will aid decisionmakers in avoiding the twin evils of overtreatment, sanctioned by the medical indications policy, and undertreatment, which might result from allowing negative consequences for the family or society to determine what treatment is appropriate for the infant.

Although we believe the best interest of the infant should remain the primary standard for decisionmaking on behalf of newborns with impairments, it has limits. In addition to the undeniable problem of vagueness, there is the further question of the applicability of this standard to some of the most troubling dilemmas in the neonatal nursery. As one critic has noted about the standard suggested in the President's Commission report, *Deciding to Forego Life-Sustaining Treatment*:

> The fact that the child-based best-interest standard would mandate treatment even in the face of a prognosis bereft of any distinctly human potentiality reveals a feature of that standard that has so far gone unnoticed. In such extreme cases, the best-interest standard tends to view the absence of pain as the only morally relevant consideration. No matter that the infant is doomed to a life of very short duration, and lacks the capacity for any distinctly human development or activity; so long as the child does not experience any severe burdens, interpreted from her point of view, the fact that she can anticipate no distinctly human benefits is of no moral consequence.

In an article published in 1974, Father Richard McCormick explained and defended a quality of life viewpoint that differs from the best interest standard. Noting that modern medicine can keep almost anyone alive, he posed the question: "Granted that we can easily save the life, what kind of life are we saving?" McCormick admits this is a quality of life judgment, and holds that we must face the possibility of answering this question when it arises.

McCormick's guideline is "the potential for human relationships associated with the infant's condition." Translated into the language of "best interests," an individual who lacks any present capacity or future potential for human relationships can be said to have no interests at all, except perhaps to be free from pain and discomfort.

Our conclusion is that there is a need for two different standards embodying relational potential considerations. The prevailing "best interest" notion presupposes that all infants have interests, but for some, the burdens of continued life can outweigh the benefits. The alternative "relational potential" standard focuses on the potential of the individual for human relationships, and presumes that some severely neurologically impaired children cannot be said to have interests to which a best interest standard might apply. In employing these two standards, decisionmakers should first determine whether the best interest standard applies to the case at hand. For the large majority of infants this standard is applicable, and should be used to determine whether life-sustaining treatment should be administered. However, if an infant is so severely neurologically impaired as to render the best interest standard inapplicable, then the alternative standard, lack of potential for human relationships, becomes the relevant criterion, placing decisionmaking within the realm of parental discretion.

When the best interest standard is applicable, because the infant's best interest can be determined, decisionmakers are obligated either to institute or to forgo life-sustaining treatment. In contrast, the relational potential standard is nonobligatory: it permits the withholding or withdrawing of therapy from infants who lack the potential for human relationships, but it does not require that treatment be forgone. Continued treatment would not benefit such infants, but neither would it harm them. An example might be an infant born with trisomy 13. Most such infants do not survive beyond the first year of life, are severely or profoundly mentally retarded, and have multiple malformations. Their chances of being able to experience human interactions are minimal. Unlike the best interest standard, which is infant-centered, the relational potential standard allows the interests of others—e.g., family or society—to weigh in the decision about whether to treat....

ANNOTATED BIBLIOGRAPHY: CHAPTER 7

Beauchamp, Tom L.: "A Reply to Rachels on Active and Passive Euthanasia." In Tom L. Beauchamp and Seymour Perlin, eds., *Ethical Issues in Death and Dying* (Englewood Cliffs, N.J.: Prentice-Hall, 1978), pp. 246–258. Beauchamp suggests that rule-utilitarian considerations can provide a basis for defending the moral significance of the distinction between active and passive euthanasia.

Cranford, Ronald E.: "The Persistent Vegetative State: The Medical Reality (Getting the Facts Straight)," *Hastings Center Report* 18 (February/March 1988), pp. 27–32. Cranford clarifies the medical facts about persistent vegetative state and distinguishes a number of neurologic conditions that may be confused with it.

Downing, A. B., ed.: *Euthanasia and the Right to Death: The Case for Voluntary Euthanasia* (New York: Humanities Press; London: Peter Owen, 1969). Two articles are especially notable in this collection of material on euthanasia. In "The Principle of Euthanasia," Antony Flew constructs "a general moral case for the establishment of a legal right" to voluntary (active) euthanasia. In a very well known article, "Euthanasia Legislation: Some Non-Religious Objections," Yale Kamisar argues against the legalization of voluntary (active) euthanasia.

Fleishman, Alan R., and Thomas H. Murray: "Ethics Committees for Infants Doe?" *Hastings Center Report* 13 (December 1983), pp. 5–9. The authors recommend the establishment of hospital ethics committees for the purpose of reviewing nontreatment decisions for seriously ill newborns. They provide an overall sketch of how such committees might function.

Gustafson, James M.: "Mongolism, Parental Desires, and the Right to Life," *Perspectives in Biology and Medicine* 16 (Summer 1973), pp. 529–557. Gustafson provides a thorough discussion and ethical analysis of a case in which a Down's syndrome infant, suffering from an intestinal blockage, was allowed to die. Gustafson emphasizes that a Down's syndrome child has some significant potential for a satisfying life and suggests that the infant should have been saved.

"Imperiled Newborns." Report of The Hastings Center Research Project on the Care of Imperiled Newborns. *Hastings Center Report* 17 (December 1987), pp. 5–32. This report is organized in seven sections and provides a wealth of factual information, conceptual clarification, and ethical analysis.

Kohl, Marvin, ed.: *Beneficent Euthanasia* (Buffalo, N.Y.: Prometheus Books, 1975). This anthology includes a number of helpful articles on the moral aspects of euthanasia. Also included are articles that provide statements of various religious positions on euthanasia. Other articles address the medical and legal aspects of euthanasia.

Lynn, Joanne, ed.: *By No Extraordinary Means: The Choice to Forgo Life-Sustaining Food and Water* (Bloomington, Ind.: Indiana University Press, 1986). This anthology provides a wide range of material on the issue of forgoing artificial nutrition and hydration.

McCormick, Richard A.: "To Save or Let Die: The Dilemma of Modern Medicine," *Journal of the American Medical Association* 229 (July 8, 1974), pp. 172–176. In dealing with the problem of selective nontreatment of severely impaired newborns, McCormick argues that infants having no significant potential for human relationships may be allowed to die.

May, William E., et al.: "Feeding and Hydrating the Permanently Unconscious and Other Vulnerable Persons," *Issues in Law and Medicine* 3 (Winter 1987), pp. 203–217. A group of ten authors argues that it is morally wrong to withhold or withdraw artificial nutrition and hydration from the permanently unconscious or from those who are seriously debilitated but nondying.

"Mercy, Murder, and Morality: Perspectives on Euthanasia," *Hastings Center Report* 19 (January/February 1989), Special Supplement, pp. 1–32. This supplement contains nine articles on various aspects of (active) euthanasia. Especially noteworthy is an article by Daniel Callahan, "Can We Return Death to Disease?" Callahan argues against the morality of active euthanasia and defends the coherence and importance of the distinction between killing and allowing to die.

President's Commission for the Study of Ethical Problems in Medicine and Biomedical and Behavioral Research: *Deciding to Forego Life-Sustaining Treatment* (1983). This document is valuable in its entirety, but two chapters are especially noteworthy. Chapter 5 deals with patients who have permanently lost consciousness but are not "brain-dead," and Chapter 6 deals with seriously ill newborns.

————: *Defining Death* (1981). In this document, the Commission provides an overall account of its deliberations leading to the recommendation that the Uniform Determination of Death Act be adopted in each of the states.

Rachels, James: "Euthanasia." In Tom Regan, ed., *Matters of Life and Death* (New York: Random House, 1980), pp. 28–66. In this long essay, Rachels evaluates (1) arguments for and against the morality of active euthanasia and (2) arguments for and against legalizing it. He concludes that active euthanasia is morally acceptable and that it ought to be legalized.

Sherlock, Richard: "Selective Non-Treatment of Defective Newborns: A Critique," *Ethics in Science & Medicine* 7 (1980), pp. 111–117. Sherlock contends, against those who advocate nontreatment of newborns whose life "is not worth living anyway," that no one has succeeded in specifying reasonable, nonarbitrary criteria for the identification of such lives.

Steinbock, Bonnie, ed.: *Killing and Letting Die* (Englewood Cliffs, N.J.: Prentice-Hall, 1980). This anthology provides a wealth of material on the killing/letting die distinction.

Trammell, Richard L.: "Euthanasia and the Law," *Journal of Social Philosophy* 9 (January 1978), pp. 14–18. Trammell contends that the legalization of voluntary positive (i.e., active) euthanasia would probably not "result in overall positive utility for the class of people eligible to choose." He emphasizes the unwelcome pressures that would be created by legalization.

Weir, Robert F.: *Selective Nontreatment of Handicapped Newborns: Moral Dilemmas in Neonatal Medicine* (New York: Oxford University Press, 1984). Weir surveys and critically analyzes a wide range of views (advanced by various pediatricians, attorneys, and ethicists) on the subject of selective nontreatment. He then presents and defends an overall policy for the guidance of decision making in this area.

Zaner, Richard M.: *Death: Beyond Whole-Brain Criteria* (Dordrecht: Kluwer Academic Publishers, 1988). Most of the authors in this collection of material defend a "higher-brain" conception of death. Of particular interest are an essay by Robert M. Veatch and an essay by Edward T. Bartlett and Stuart J. Youngner.

CHAPTER 8

ABORTION AND MATERNAL/FETAL CONFLICTS

INTRODUCTION

The first object of concern in this chapter is the issue of the ethical (moral) acceptability of abortion. Some attention is then given to the social policy aspects of abortion, especially in conjunction with developments in the U.S. Supreme Court. Finally, several ethical problems associated with maternal/fetal conflicts are identified and explored.

Abortion: The Ethical Issue

Discussions of the ethical acceptability of abortion often take for granted (1) an awareness of the various kinds of reasons that may be given for having an abortion and (2) a minimal sort of acquaintance with the biological development of a human fetus.

Reasons for Abortion   Why would a woman have an abortion? The following catalog, not meant to provide an exhaustive survey, is sufficient to indicate that there is a wide range of potential reasons for abortion. (*a*) In certain extreme cases, if the fetus is allowed to develop normally and come to term, the mother herself will die. (*b*) In other cases it is not the mother's life but her health, physical or mental, that will be severely endangered if the pregnancy is allowed to continue. (*c*) There are also cases in which the pregnancy will probably, or surely, produce a severely impaired child,[1] and (*d*) there are others in which the pregnancy is the result of rape or incest.[2] (*e*) There are instances in which the mother is unmarried and there will be the social stigma of illegitimacy. (*f*) There are other instances in which having a child, or having another child, will be an unbearable financial burden. (*g*) Certainly common, and perhaps most common of all, are those instances in which having a child will interfere with the happiness of the woman, or the joint happiness of the parents, or even the joint happiness of a family unit that already includes children. Here there are almost endless possibilities. The woman may desire a professional career. A couple may be content and happy together and feel their relationship would be damaged by the intrusion of a child. Parents may have older children and not feel up to raising another child, and so forth.

The Biological Development of a Human Fetus   During the course of a human pregnancy, in the nine-month period from conception to birth, the product of conception undergoes a continual process of change and development. *Conception* takes place when a male germ cell (the spermatozoon) combines with a female germ cell (the ovum), resulting in a single cell (the single-cell zygote), which embodies the full genetic code, twenty-three pairs of chromosomes. The single-cell zygote soon begins a process of cellular division. The resultant multi-cell zygote, while continuing to grow and beginning to take shape, proceeds to move through the fallopian tube and then to undergo gradual *implantation* at the uterine wall. The unborn entity is formally designated a zygote up until the time that implantation is complete, almost two weeks after conception. Thereafter, until the end of the eighth week, roughly the point at which brain waves can be detected, the unborn entity is formally designated an *embryo*. It is in this embryonic period that organ systems and other human characteristics begin to undergo noticeable development. From the end of the eighth week until birth, the unborn entity is formally designated a *fetus*. (The term "fetus," however, is commonly used as a general term to designate the unborn entity, whatever its stage of development.) Two other points in the development of the fetus are especially noteworthy as relevant to discussions of abortion, but these points are usually identified by reference to gestational age as calculated not from conception but from the first day of the woman's last menstrual period. Accordingly, somewhere between the twelfth and the sixteenth week there usually occurs *quickening*, the point at which the mother begins to feel the movements of the fetus. And somewhere in the neighborhood of the twenty-fourth week, *viability* becomes a realistic possibility. Viability is the point at which the fetus is capable of surviving outside the womb.

With the facts of fetal development in view, it may be helpful to indicate the various medical techniques of abortion. Early (first trimester) abortions were at one time performed by *dilatation and curettage* (D&C) but are now commonly performed by *uterine aspiration*, also called "suction curettage." The D&C features the stretching (dilatation) of the cervix and the scraping (curettage) of the inner walls of the uterus. Uterine aspiration simply involves sucking the fetus out of the uterus by means of a tube connected to a suction pump. Later abortions require *dilatation and evacuation* (D&E), *induction techniques*, or *hysterotomy*. In the D&E, which is the abortion procedure commonly used in the early stages of the second trimester, a forceps is used to dismember the fetus within the uterus; the fetal remains are then withdrawn through the cervix. In one commonly employed induction technique, a saline solution injected into the amniotic cavity induces labor, thus expelling the fetus. Another induction technique employs prostaglandins (hormonelike substances) to induce labor. Hysterotomy—in essence a miniature cesarean section—is a major surgical procedure and is uncommonly employed in the United States.

A brief discussion of fetal development together with a cursory survey of various reasons for abortion has prepared the way for a formulation of the ethical issue of abortion in its broadest terms. *Up to what point of fetal development, if any, and for what reasons, if any, is abortion ethically acceptable?* Some hold that abortion is *never* ethically acceptable, or at most is acceptable only where abortion is necessary to save the life of the mother. This view is frequently termed the *conservative* view on abortion. Others hold that abortion is *always* ethically acceptable—at any point of fetal development and for any of the standard reasons. This view is frequently termed the *liberal* view on abortion. Still others are anxious to defend more *moderate* views, holding that abortion is ethically acceptable up to a certain point of fetal development *and/or* holding that some reasons provide a sufficient justification for abortion whereas others do not.

The Conservative View and the Liberal View

The *moral status* of the fetus has been a pivotal issue in discussions of the ethical acceptability of abortion. The concept of moral status is commonly explicated in terms of rights. On this construal, to say that a fetus has moral status is to say that the fetus has rights. What kind of rights, if any, does the fetus have? Does it have the same rights as more visible humans, and thus *full moral status*, as conservatives typically contend? Does it have no rights, and thus *no (significant) moral status*, as liberals typically contend? (Or perhaps, as some moderates argue, does the fetus have a subsidiary or *partial moral status*, however this is to be conceptualized?) If the fetus has no rights, the liberal is prone to argue, then it does not have any more right to life than a piece of tissue such as an appendix, and an abortion is no more morally objectionable than an appendectomy. If the fetus has the same rights as any other human being, the conservative is prone to argue, then it has the same right to life as the latter, and an abortion, except perhaps when the mother's life is endangered, is as morally objectionable as any other murder.

Discussions of the moral status of the fetus often refer directly to the biological development of the fetus and pose the question: At what point in the continuous development of the fetus do we have a human life? In the context of such discussions, "human" implies full moral status, "nonhuman" implies no (significant) moral status, and any notion of partial moral status is systematically excluded. To distinguish the human from the nonhuman, to "draw the line," and to do so in a nonarbitrary way, is the central matter of concern. The *conservative* on abortion typically holds that the line must be drawn at conception. Usually the conservative argues that conception is the only point at which the line can be nonarbitrarily drawn. Against attempts to draw the line at points such as implantation, quickening, viability, or birth, considerations of continuity in the development of the fetus are pressed. The conservative is sometimes said to employ "slippery slope arguments," that is, to argue that a line cannot be securely drawn anywhere along the path of fetal development. It is said that the line will inescapably slide back to the point of conception in order to find objective support. John T. Noonan argues in this fashion, at least in part, as he provides a defense of the conservative view in one of the selections in this chapter.

With regard to "drawing the line," the *liberal* typically contends that the fetus remains nonhuman even in its most advanced stages of development. The liberal, of course, does not mean to deny that a fetus is biologically a human fetus. Rather the claim is that the fetus is not human in any morally significant sense, that is, the fetus has no (significant) moral status. This point is often made in terms of the concept of personhood. Mary Anne Warren, who defends the liberal view on abortion in one of this chapter's selections, argues that the fetus is not a person. She also contends that the fetus bears so little resemblance to a person that it cannot be said to have a significant right to life. It is important to notice that, as Warren analyzes the concept of personhood, even a newborn baby is not a person. This conclusion, as might be expected, prompts Warren to a consideration of the moral justifiability of infanticide, an issue closely related to the problem of abortion.

Although the conservative view on abortion is most commonly predicated upon the straightforward contention that the fetus is a person from conception, there are at least two other lines of argument that have been advanced in its defense. One conservative, advancing what might be labeled "the presumption argument," writes:

> In being willing to kill the embryo, we accept responsibility for killing what we must admit *may* be a person. There is some reason to believe it is—namely the *fact* that it is a living, human individual and the inconclusiveness of arguments that try to exclude it from the protected circle of personhood.
> *To be willing to kill what for all we know could be a person is to be willing to kill it if it is a person.* And since we cannot absolutely settle if it is a person except by a metaphysical postulate, for

all practical purposes we must hold that to be willing to kill the embryo is to be willing to kill a person.[3]

In accordance with this line of argument, although it may not be possible to conclusively show that the fetus is a person from conception, we must presume that it is. Another line of argument that has been advanced by some conservatives emphasizes the potential rather than the actual personhood of the fetus. Even if the fetus is not a person, it is said, there can be no doubt that it is a potential person. Accordingly, by virtue of its potential personhood, the fetus must be accorded a right to life. Mary Anne Warren, in response to this line of argument, argues that the potential personhood of the fetus provides no basis for the claim that it has a significant right to life.

Moderate Views

The conservative and liberal views, as explicated, constitute two extreme poles on the spectrum of ethical views of abortion. Each of the extreme views is marked by a formal simplicity. The conservative proclaims abortion to be immoral, irrespective of the stage of fetal development and irrespective of alleged justifying reasons. The one exception, admitted by some conservatives, is the case in which abortion is necessary to save the life of the mother.[4] The liberal proclaims abortion to be morally acceptable, irrespective of the stage of fetal development.[5] Moreover, there is no need to draw distinctions between those reasons that are sufficient to justify abortion and those that are not. No justification is needed. The moderate, in vivid contrast to both the conservative and the liberal, is unwilling to sweepingly condemn or condone abortion. Some abortions are morally justifiable; some are morally objectionable. In some moderate views, the stage of fetal development is a relevant factor in the assessment of the moral acceptability of abortion. In other moderate views, the alleged justifying reason is a relevant factor in the assessment of the moral acceptability of abortion. In still other moderate views, both the stage of fetal development and the alleged justifying reason are relevant factors in the assessment of the moral acceptability of abortion.

Moderate views have been developed in accordance with the following clearly identifiable strategies:

1 **Moderation of the Conservative View** One strategy for generating a moderate view presumes the typical conservative contention that the fetus has full moral status from conception. What is denied, however, is that we must conclude to the moral impermissibility of abortion in *all* cases. In one of this chapter's readings, Jane English attempts to moderate the conservative view in just this way. She argues that certain abortion cases may be assimilated to cases of self-defense. Thus, for English, on the presumption that the fetus from conception has full moral status, some reasons are sufficient to justify abortion whereas others are not.

2 **Moderation of the Liberal View** A second strategy for generating a moderate view presumes the liberal contention that the fetus has no (significant) moral status even in the latest stages of pregnancy. What is denied, however, is that we must conclude to the moral permissibility of abortion in *all* cases. It might be said, in accordance with this line of thought, that abortion, even though it does not violate the rights of the fetus (which is presumed to have no rights), remains ethically problematic because of the negative social consequences of the practice of abortion. Such an argument seems especially forceful in the later stages of pregnancy, when the fetus increasingly resembles a newborn infant. It is argued that very late abortions have a brutalizing effect on those involved and, in various ways, lead to the breakdown of attitudes associated with respect for human life. Jane English, in an effort to moderate the liberal view, advances an argument of this general type. Even if the fetus is not a person, she

holds, it is gradually becoming increasingly personlike. Appealing to a "coherence of attitudes," she argues that abortion in the later stages of pregnancy demands more weighty justifying reasons than it does in the earlier stages.

3 Moderation in "Drawing the Line" A third strategy for generating a moderate view, in fact a whole range of moderate views, is associated with "drawing the line" discussions. Whereas the conservative typically draws the line between human (full moral status) and nonhuman (no moral status) at conception and the liberal typically draws that same line at birth (or sometime thereafter), a moderate view may be generated by drawing the line somewhere between these two extremes. For example, one might draw the line at implantation, at the point where brain activity begins, at quickening, at viability, and so forth. Whereas drawing the line at implantation would tend to generate a rather "conservative" moderate view, drawing the line at viability would tend to generate a rather "liberal" moderate view. Wherever the line is drawn, it is the burden of any such moderate view to show that the point specified is a nonarbitrary one. Once such a point has been specified, however, it might be argued that abortion is ethically acceptable before that point and ethically unacceptable after that point. Or further stipulations may be added in accordance with strategies (1) and (2) above.

4 Moderation in the Assignment of Moral Status A fourth strategy for generating a moderate view is dependent upon assigning the fetus some sort of subsidiary or *partial moral status*, an approach taken by Daniel Callahan in one of this chapter's readings. It would seem that anyone who defends a moderate view based on the concept of partial moral status must first of all face the problem of explicating the nature of such partial moral status. Second, and closely related, there is the problem of showing how the interests of those with partial moral status are to be weighed against the interests of those with full moral status.

Abortion and Social Policy

In the United States, the Supreme Court's decision in *Roe v. Wade* (1973) has been the focal point of the social policy debate over abortion. This case had the effect, for all practical purposes, of legalizing "abortion-on-request." The Court held that it was unconstitutional for a state to have laws prohibiting the abortion of a previable fetus. According to the Court, a woman has a constitutionally guaranteed right to decide to terminate a pregnancy (prior to viability), although a state, for reasons related to maternal health, may restrict the manner and circumstances in which abortions are performed subsequent to the end of the first trimester. The reasoning underlying the Court's holding in *Roe* can be found in the majority opinion reprinted in this chapter.

Since the action of the Court in *Roe* had the practical effect of establishing a woman's legal right to choose whether or not to abort, it was enthusiastically received by "right-to-choose" forces. On the other hand, "right-to-life" forces, committed to the conservative view on the morality of abortion, vehemently denounced the Court for "legalizing murder." In response to *Roe*, right-to-life forces adopted a number of political strategies. The most significant of these strategies will be discussed here.

Right-to-life forces originally worked for the enactment of a constitutional amendment directly overruling *Roe*. The proposed "Human Life Amendment"—declaring the personhood of the fetus—was calculated to achieve the legal prohibition of abortion, allowing an exception only for abortions necessary to save the life of a pregnant woman. Right-to-life support also emerged for the idea of a constitutional amendment allowing Congress and/or each state to decide whether to restrict abortion. (If this sort of amendment were enacted, it would undoubtedly have the effect of prohibiting abortion or at least severely restricting it in a number of states.) Right-to-choose forces reacted in strong opposition to these proposed constitutional amendments. In their view, any effort to achieve the legal prohibition of abortion represents an illicit attempt by one group (conservatives on abortion) to impose their moral views on those who have different views. Thus, to some extent the justifiability of restrictive abortion laws is bound up with a much broader question: Is it justifiable to employ the law in an effort to "enforce morality"? (Cf. the discussion of the principle of legal moralism in Chapter 1.)

In 1980, right-to-life forces were notably successful in achieving a more limited political aim, the cutoff of Medicaid funding for abortion. Medicaid is a social program designed to provide public funds to pay for the medical care of impoverished people. At issue in *Harris v. McRae*, decided by the Supreme Court in 1980, was the constitutionality of the so-called Hyde Amendment, legislation that had passed Congress with vigorous right-to-life support. The Hyde Amendment, in the version considered by the Court, restricted federal Medicaid funding to (1) cases in which the mother's life is endangered and (2) cases of rape and incest. The Court, in a five-to-four decision, upheld the constitutionality of the Hyde Amendment. According to the Court, a woman's right to an abortion does not entail *the right to have society fund the abortion*. But if there is no constitutional obstacle to the cutoff of Medicaid funding for abortion, it must still be asked if society's refusal to fund the abortions of poor women is an ethically sound social policy. Considerations of social justice are often pressed by those who argue that it is not.

In the wake of *Roe*, right-to-life forces made recurrent efforts to secure the passage of statutes designed (in various ways) to place obstacles in the path of women seeking an abortion. In *Akron v. Akron Center for Reproductive Health* (1983), the Supreme Court considered the constitutionality of a local ordinance of this sort. The most important provisions of the ordinance were: (1) the requirement that any abortion subsequent to the first trimester be performed in a hospital (as opposed to a clinic); (2) the requirement that the attending physician (as opposed to other trained personnel) personally inform the patient of a host of particulars concerning fetal development, the emotional and physical risks of abortion, etc., "in order to insure...truly informed consent"; and (3) the requirement that a physician not perform an abortion until 24 hours after a consent form had been signed by the pregnant woman. In a six-to-three decision, the Court reaffirmed *Roe v. Wade* and declared each of the ordinance's provisions unconstitutional. The Court called attention to the additional financial burdens created by provisions (1) and (3) in invalidating them. Although endorsing the importance of informed consent, the Court emphasized two problems related to provision (2). First, "the information required is designed not to inform the woman's consent but rather to persuade her to withhold it altogether." Second, a physician may legitimately delegate the counseling task to another qualified individual.

With the decision of the Supreme Court in *Webster v. Reproductive Health Services* (1989), right-to-life forces celebrated a dramatic victory. Two crucial provisions of a Missouri statute were upheld. One provision bans the use of *public* facilities and *public* employees in the performance of abortions. Another requires physicians to perform tests to determine the viability of any fetus believed to be 20 weeks or older. In essence, *Webster* represents for right-to-life forces the first benefits of a long-term strategy to undermine *Roe v. Wade* by controlling (through the political process) the appointment of new Supreme Court justices. From the perspective of right-to-choose forces, of course, the *Webster* decision is a deeply disturbing one, since it seems to indicate the present Court's willingness to retreat from *Roe*. The opinion of Chief Justice William H. Rehnquist in *Webster* is reprinted in this chapter.

Maternal/Fetal Conflicts

If a pregnant woman has made the decision to carry her fetus to term (i.e., if she has ruled out the possibility of an abortion), does she have a moral obligation to conduct her life so as to maximize the possibility that her child will be born healthy? Clearly, maternal behavior can have a negative impact on the well-being of a developing fetus. For example, the following maternal behaviors are thought to create some likelihood of fetal harm: (1) maintaining an unhealthy diet, (2) smoking, (3) excessive consumption of alcohol, (4) recreational drug use. Moreover, if a pregnant women suffers from certain medical conditions, additional complications arise. For example, if a diabetic women does not exercise tight control over her blood sugar, it is likely that her fetus will be negatively affected.

If a woman should be prepared to endure inconvenience and life-style modification during pregnancy, should she also be prepared to accept invasive medical procedures in the name of fetal well-being? If physicians tell her that a cesarean delivery is medically indicated for her child, is she morally obliged to undergo the pain and risks associated with the procedure? If physicians tell her that her fetus is suffering from a medical condition that can be treated in utero, is she morally obliged to undergo a procedure that would be identified as "fetal therapy"? Surely it makes a difference how well-established and efficacious a certain medical procedure is, how risky it is for the mother, and how necessary it would seem to be for the fetus. But suppose, in a certain case, that physicians form the view that a woman is acting in a morally irresponsible manner. If educational efforts fail to elicit a woman's consent to a medical procedure considered necessary for the well-being of her fetus, is persuasion in order? If efforts to persuade also fail, is coercion in order?

In one of this chapter's selections, Thomas H. Murray maintains that a pregnant woman has a moral duty to avoid harming her "not-yet-born child," but he emphasizes that this duty must be balanced against a multitude of other moral considerations, all of which have a rightful place within the overall moral context of her life. He also considers the dilemma faced by physicians who believe that a pregnant women is failing to act in the best interests of her fetus. With regard to social policy in the area of maternal/fetal conflicts, Murray expresses strong reservations about the employment of coercion against a pregnant woman. In this chapter's final selection, Lawrence J. Nelson and Nancy Milliken argue even more strongly against coercive intervention. In their view, physicians may rightly attempt to persuade pregnant women to act in the name of fetal welfare, but pregnant women should never be compelled to undergo any form of medical treatment or behavior change.

T.A.M.

NOTES

1 The first subsection of Chapter 9 provides an extensive discussion of prenatal diagnosis and selective abortion.
2 The expression "therapeutic abortion" suggests abortion for medical reasons. Accordingly, abortions corresponding to (a), (b), and (c) are usually said to be therapeutic. More problematically, abortions corresponding to (d) have often been identified as therapeutic. Perhaps it is presumed that pregnancies resulting from rape or incest are traumatic, thus a threat to mental health. Or perhaps calling such an abortion "therapeutic" is just a way of indicating that it is thought to be justifiable.
3 Germain Grisez, *Abortion: The Myths, the Realities, and the Arguments* (New York: Corpus Books, 1970), p. 306.
4 One especially prominent conservative view is associated with the Roman Catholic Church. In accordance with Catholic moral teaching, the *direct* killing of innocent human life is forbidden. Hence, abortion is forbidden. Even if the mother's life is in danger, perhaps because her heart or kidney function is inadequate, abortion is impermissible. In two special

cases, however, procedures resulting in the death of the fetus are allowable. In the case of an ectopic pregnancy, where the developing fetus is lodged in the fallopian tube, the fallopian tube may be removed. In the case of a pregnant woman with a cancerous uterus, the cancerous uterus may be removed. In these cases, the death of the fetus is construed as *indirect* killing, the foreseen but unintended by-product of a surgical procedure designed to protect the life of the mother. As the exchange between James Rachels and Thomas D. Sullivan in Chapter 7 makes clear, the distinction between direct and indirect killing is a controversial one. Sullivan relies on the distinction between intentional and nonintentional terminations of life whereas Rachels contends that the distinction has no moral significance. If, however, the distinction between direct and indirect killing is a defensible one, it might still be suggested that the distinction is not rightly applied in the Roman Catholic view of abortion. For example, some critics contend that abortion may be construed as indirect killing, indeed an allowable form of indirect killing, in at least all cases where it is necessary to save the life of the mother. For one helpful exposition and critical analysis of the Roman Catholic position on abortion, see Daniel Callahan, *Abortion: Law, Choice and Morality* (New York: Macmillan, 1970), chap. 12, pp. 409–447.

5 In considering the liberal contention that abortions are morally acceptable irrespective of the stage of fetal development, we should take note of an ambiguity in the concept of abortion. Does "abortion" refer merely to the termination of a pregnancy in the sense of detaching the fetus from the mother, or does "abortion" entail the death of the fetus as well? Whereas the abortion of a *previable* fetus entails its death, the "abortion" of a *viable* fetus, by means of hysterotomy (a miniature cesarean section), does not entail the death of the fetus and would seem to be tantamount to the birth of a baby. With regard to the "abortion" of a *viable* fetus, liberals can defend the woman's right to detach the fetus from her body without contending that the woman has the right to insist on the death of the child.

The Morality of Abortion

An Almost Absolute Value in History
John T. Noonan, Jr.

John T. Noonan, Jr., formerly professor of law at the University of California, Berkeley, is judge, U.S. Court of Appeals, Ninth Circuit, California. His research interests extend beyond matters of law to philosophical and theological issues, and his intellectual allegiance in this regard is with the Roman Catholic tradition. Among his books are *Contraception: A History of Its Treatment by the Catholic Theologians and Canonists* (1965), *Persons and Masks of the Law* (1976), and *A Private Choice: Abortion in America in the Seventies* (1979).

Noonan, defending the conservative view on abortion, immediately raises the question of how to determine the *humanity* of a being. In an updated version of the traditional theological view he contends that, if a being is conceived by human parents and thereby has a human genetic code, then that being is a *human being*. Conception is the point at which the nonhuman becomes the human. Noonan argues that other alleged criteria of humanity are inadequate. He also argues, primarily through an analysis of probabilities, that his own criterion of humanity is objectively based and nonarbitrary. Finally, Noonan contends, once the humanity of the fetus is recognized, we must judge abortion morally wrong, except in those rare cases where the mother's life is in danger.

The most fundamental question involved in the long history of thought on abortion is: How do you determine the humanity of a being? To phrase the question that way is to put in comprehensive humanistic terms what the theologians either dealt with as an explicitly theological question under the heading of "ensoulment" or dealt with implicitly in their treatment of abortion. The Christian position as it originated did not depend on a narrow theological or philosophical concept. It had no relation to theories of infant baptism. It appealed to no special theory of instantaneous ensoulment. It took the world's view on ensoulment as that view changed from Aristotle to Zacchia. There was, indeed, theological influence affecting the theory of ensoulment finally adopted, and, of course, ensoulment itself was a theological concept, so that the position was always explained in theological terms. But the theological notion of ensoulment could easily be translated into humanistic language by substituting "human" for "rational soul"; the problem of knowing when a man is a man is common to theology and humanism.

If one steps outside the specific categories used by the theologians, the answer they gave can be analyzed as a refusal to discriminate among human beings on the basis of their varying potentialities. Once conceived, the being was recognized as man because he had man's potential. The criterion for humanity, thus, was simple and all-embracing: if you are conceived by human parents, you are human.

The strength of this position may be tested by a review of some of the other distinctions offered in the contemporary controversy over legalizing abortion. Perhaps the most popular distinction is in terms of viability. Before an age of so many months, the fetus is not viable, that is, it cannot be removed from the mother's womb and live apart from her. To that extent, the life of the fetus is absolutely dependent on the life of the mother. This dependence is made the basis of denying recognition to its humanity.

There are difficulties with this distinction. One is that the perfection of artificial incubation may make the fetus viable at any time: it may be removed and artificially sustained. Experiments with animals already show that such a procedure is possible. This hypothetical extreme case relates to an actual difficulty: there is considerable elasticity to the idea of viability. Mere length of life is not an exact measure. The viability of the fetus depends on the extent of its anatomical and functional development. The weight and length of the fetus are better guides to the state of its development than age, but weight and length vary. Moreover, different racial groups have different ages at which their fetuses are viable. Some evidence, for example, suggests that Negro fetuses mature more quickly than white fetuses. If viability is the norm, the standard would vary with race and with many individual circumstances.

The most important objection to this approach is that dependence is not ended by viability. The fetus is still absolutely dependent on someone's care in order to continue existence; indeed a child of one or three or even five years of age is absolutely dependent on another's care for existence; uncared for, the older fetus or the younger child will die as surely as the early fetus detached from the mother. The unsubstantial lessening in dependence at viability does not seem to signify any special acquisition of humanity.

A second distinction has been attempted in terms of experience. A being who has had experience, has lived and suffered, who possesses memories, is more human than one who has not. Humanity depends on formation by experience. The fetus is thus "unformed" in the most basic human sense.

This distinction is not serviceable for the embryo which is already experiencing and reacting. The embryo is responsive to touch after eight weeks and at least at that point is experiencing. At an earlier stage the zygote is certainly alive and responding to its environment. The distinction may also be challenged by the rare case where aphasia has erased adult memory: has it erased humanity? More fundamentally, this distinction leaves even the older fetus or the younger child to be treated as an unformed inhuman thing. Finally, it is not clear why experience as such confers humanity. It could be argued that certain central experiences such as loving or learning are necessary to make a man human. But then human beings who have failed to love or to learn might be excluded from the class called man.

A third distinction is made by appeal to the sentiments of adults. If a fetus dies, the grief of the parents is not the grief they would have for a living child. The fetus is an unnamed "it" till birth, and is not perceived as personality until at least the fourth month of existence when movements in the womb manifest a vigorous presence demanding joyful recognition by the parents.

Yet feeling is notoriously an unsure guide to the humanity of others. Many groups of humans have had difficulty in feeling that persons of another tongue, color, religion, sex, are as human as they. Apart from reactions to alien groups, we mourn the loss of a ten-year-old boy more than the loss of his one-day-old brother or his 90-year-old grandfather. The difference felt and the grief expressed vary with the potentialities extinguished, or the experience wiped out; they do not seem to point to any substantial difference in the humanity of baby, boy, or grandfather.

Distinctions are also made in terms of sensation by the parents. The embryo is felt within the womb only after about the fourth month. The embryo is seen only at birth. What can be neither seen nor felt is different from what is tangible. If the fetus cannot be seen or touched at all, it cannot be perceived as man.

Yet experience shows that sight is even more untrustworthy than feeling in determining humanity. By sight, color became an appropriate index for saying who was a man, and the evil of racial discrimination was given foundation. Nor can touch provide the test: a being confined by sickness, "out of touch" with others, does not thereby seem to lose his humanity. To the extent that touch still has appeal as a criterion, it appears to be a survival of the old English idea of "quickening"—a possible mistranslation of the Latin *animatus* used in the canon law. To that extent touch as a criterion seems to be dependent on the Aristotelian notion of ensoulment, and to fail when this notion is discarded.

Finally, a distinction is sought in social visibility. The fetus is not socially perceived as human. It cannot communicate with others. Thus, both subjectively and objectively, it is not a member of society. As moral rules are rules for the behavior of members of society to each other, they cannot be made for behavior toward what is not yet a member. Excluded from the society of men, the fetus is excluded from the humanity of men.

By force of the argument from the consequences, this distinction is to be rejected. It is more subtle than that founded on an appeal to physical sensation, but it is equally dangerous in its implications. If humanity depends on social recognition, individuals or whole groups may be dehumanized by being denied any status in their society. Such a fate is fictionally portrayed in *1984* and has actually been the lot of many men in many societies.

In the Roman empire, for example, condemnation to slavery meant the practical denial of most human rights; in the Chinese Communist world, landlords have been classified as enemies of the people and so treated as nonpersons by the state. Humanity does not depend on social recognition, though often the failure of society to recognize the prisoner, the alien, the heterodox as human has led to the destruction of human beings. Anyone conceived by a man and a woman is human. Recognition of this condition by society follows a real event in the objective order, however imperfect and halting the recognition. Any attempt to limit humanity to exclude some group runs the risk of furnishing authority and precedent for excluding other groups in the name of the consciousness or perception of the controlling group in the society.

A philosopher may reject the appeal to the humanity of the fetus because he views "humanity" as a secular view of the soul and because he doubts the existence of anything real and objective which can be identified as humanity. One answer to such a philosopher is to ask how he reasons about moral questions without supposing that there is a sense in which he and the others of whom he speaks are human. Whatever group is taken as the society which determines who may be killed is thereby taken as human. A second answer is to ask if he does not believe that there is a right and wrong way of deciding moral questions. If there is such a difference, experience may be appealed to: to decide who is human on the basis of the sentiment of a given society has led to consequences which rational men would characterize as monstrous.

The rejection of the attempted distinctions based on viability and visibility, experience and feeling, may be buttressed by the following considerations: Moral judgments often rest on distinctions, but if the distinctions are not to appear arbitrary fiat, they should relate to some real difference in probabilities. There is a kind of continuity in all life, but the earlier stages of the elements of human life possess tiny probabilities of development. Consider for example, the spermatozoa in any normal ejaculate: There are about 200,000,000 in any single ejaculate, of which one has a chance of developing into a zygote. Consider the oocytes which may become ova: there are 100,000 to 1,000,000 oocytes in a female infant, of which a maximum of 390 are ovulated. But once spermatozoon and ovum meet and the conceptus is formed, such studies as have been made show that roughly in only 20 percent of the cases will spontaneous abortion occur. In other words, the chances are about 4 out of 5 that this new being will develop. At this stage in the life of the being there is a sharp shift in probabilities, an immense jump in potentialities. To make a distinction between the rights of spermatozoa and the rights of the fertilized ovum is to respond to an enormous shift in possibilities. For about twenty days after conception the egg may split to form twins or combine with another egg to form a chimera, but the probability of either event happening is very small.

It may be asked, What does a change in biological probabilities have to do with establishing humanity? The argument from probabilities is not aimed at establishing humanity but at establishing an objective discontinuity which may be taken into account in moral discourse. As life itself is a matter of probabilities, as most moral reasoning is an estimate of probabilities, so it seems in accord with the structure of reality and the nature of moral thought to found a moral judgment on the change in probabilities at conception. The appeal to probabilities is the most commonsensical of arguments, to a greater or smaller degree all of us base our actions on probabilities, and in morals, as in law, prudence and negligence are often measured by the account one has taken of the probabilities. If the chance is 200,000,000 to 1 that the movement in the bushes into which you shoot is a man's, I doubt if many persons would hold you careless in shooting; but if the chances are 4 out of 5 that the movement is a human being's, few would acquit you of blame. Would the argument be different if only one out of ten children conceived came to term? Of course this argument would be different. This argument is an appeal to probabilities that actually exist, not to any and all states of affairs which may be imagined.

The probabilities as they do exist do not show the humanity of the embryo in the sense of a demonstration in logic any more than the probabilities of the movement in the bush being a man demonstrate beyond all doubt that the being is a man. The appeal is a "buttressing" consideration, showing the plausibility of the standard adopted. The argument focuses on the decisional factor in any moral judgment and assumes that part of the business of a moralist is drawing lines. One evidence of the nonarbitrary character of the line drawn is the difference of probabilities on either side of it. If a spermatozoon is destroyed, one destroys a being which had a chance of far less than 1 in 200 million of developing into a reasoning being, possessed of the genetic code, a heart and other organs, and capable of pain. If a fetus is destroyed, one destroys a being already possessed of the genetic code, organs, and sensitivity to pain, and one which had an 80 percent chance of developing further into a baby outside the womb who, in time, would reason.

The positive argument for conception as the decisive moment of humanization is that at conception the new being receives the genetic code. It is this genetic information which determines his characteristics, which is the biological carrier of the possibility of human wisdom, which makes him a self-evolving being. A being with a human genetic code is man.

This review of current controversy over the humanity of the fetus emphasizes what a fundamental question the theologians resolved in asserting the inviolability of the fetus. To regard the fetus as possessed of equal rights with other humans was not, however, to decide every case where abortion might be employed. It did decide the case where the argument was that the fetus should be aborted for its own good. To say a being was human was to say it had a destiny to decide for itself which could not be taken from it by another man's decision. But human beings with equal rights often come in conflict with each other, and some decision must be made as to whose claims are to prevail. Cases of conflict involving the fetus are different only in two respects: the total inability of the fetus to speak for itself and the fact that the right of the fetus regularly at stake is the right to life itself.

The approach taken by the theologians to these conflicts was articulated in terms of "direct" and "indirect." Again, to look at what they were doing from outside their categories, they may be said to have been drawing lines or "balancing values." "Direct" and "indirect" are spatial metaphors; "line-drawing" is another. "To weigh" or "to balance" values is a metaphor of a more complicated mathematical sort hinting at the process which goes on in moral judgments. All the metaphors suggest that, in the moral judgments made, comparisons were necessary, that no value completely controlled. The principle of double effect was no doctrine fallen from heaven, but a method of analysis appropriate where two relative values were being compared. In Catholic moral theology, as it developed, life even of the innocent was not taken as an absolute. Judgments on acts affecting life issued from a process of weighing. In the weighing, the fetus was always given a value greater than zero, always a value separate and independent from its parents. This valuation was crucial and fundamental in all Christian thought on the subject and marked it off from any approach which considered that only the parents' interests needed to be considered.

Even with the fetus weighed as human, one interest could be weighed as equal or superior: that of the mother in her own life. The casuists between 1450 and 1895 were willing to weigh this interest as superior. Since 1895, that interest was given decisive weight only in the two special cases of the cancerous uterus and the ectopic pregnancy. In both of these cases the fetus itself had little chance of survival even if the abortion were not performed. As the balance was once struck in favor of the mother whenever her life was endangered, it could be so struck again. The balance reached between 1895 and 1930 attempted prudentially and pastorally to forestall a multitude of exceptions for interests less than life.

The perception of the humanity of the fetus and the weighing of fetal rights against other human rights constituted the work of the moral analysts. But what spirit animated their abstract judgments? For the Christian community it was the injunction of Scripture to love your neighbor as yourself. The fetus as human was a neighbor; his life had parity with one's own. The commandment gave life to what otherwise would have been only rational calculation.

The commandment could be put in humanistic as well as theological terms: Do not injure your fellow man without reason. In these terms, once the humanity of the fetus is perceived, abortion is never right except in self-defense. When life must be taken to save life, reason alone cannot say that a mother must prefer a child's life to her own. With this exception, now of great rarity, abortion violates the rational humanist tenet of the equality of human lives.

For Christians the commandment to love had received a special imprint in that the exemplar proposed of love was the love of the Lord for his disciples. In the light given by this example, self-sacrifice carried to the point of death seemed in the extreme situations not without meaning. In the less extreme cases, preference for one's own interest to the life of another seemed to express cruelty or selfishness irreconcilable with the demands of love.

On the Moral and Legal Status of Abortion
Mary Anne Warren

Mary Anne Warren is associate professor of philosophy at San Francisco State University. Among her published articles are "Secondary Sexism and Quota Hiring," "Do Potential People Have Moral Rights?" and "Is Androgyny the Answer to Sexual Stereotyping?" She is also the author of *The Nature of Woman: An Encyclopedia and Guide to the Literature* (1980) and *Gendercide: The Implications of Sex Selection* (1985).

Warren, defending the liberal view of abortion, promptly distinguishes two senses of the term "human": (1) One is *human in the genetic sense* when one is a member of the biological species *Homo sapiens*. (2) One is *human in the moral sense* when one is a full-fledged member of the moral community. Warren attacks the presupposition underlying Noonan's argument against abortion—that the fetus is human in the moral sense. She contends that the moral community, the set of beings with full and equal moral rights, consists of all and only people (persons). (Thus she takes the concept of personhood to be equivalent to the concept of humanity in the moral sense.) After analyzing the concept of person, she concludes that a fetus is so unlike a person as to have no significant right to life. Nor, she argues, does the fetus's *potential* for being a person provide us any basis for ascribing to it any significant right to life. It follows, she contends, that a woman's right to obtain an abortion is absolute. Abortion is morally justified at any stage of fetal development. It also follows, she contends, that no legislation against abortion can be justified on the grounds of protecting the rights of the fetus. In a concluding postscript, Warren briefly assesses the moral justifiability of infanticide.

Reprinted by permission from vol. 57, no. 1, of *The Monist*, LaSalle, Illinois 61301. "Postscript on Infanticide" reprinted with permission of the author from *The Problem of Abortion*, second edition, edited by Joel Feinberg (Belmont, Calif.: Wadsworth, 1984).

The question which we must answer in order to produce a satisfactory solution to the problem of the moral status of abortion is this: How are we to define the moral community, the set of beings with full and equal moral rights, such that we can decide whether a human fetus is a member of this community or not? What sort of entity, exactly, has the inalienable rights to life, liberty, and the pursuit of happiness? Jefferson attributed these rights to all *men*, and it may or may not be fair to suggest that he intended to attribute them *only* to men. Perhaps he ought to have attributed them to all human beings. If so, then we arrive, first, at Noonan's problem of defining what makes a being human, and, second, at the equally vital question which Noonan does not consider, namely, What reason is there for identifying the moral community with the set of all human beings, in whatever way we have chosen to define that term?

1   ON THE DEFINITION OF "HUMAN"

One reason why this vital second question is so frequently overlooked in the debate over the moral status of abortion is that the term 'human' has two distinct, but not often distinguished, senses. This fact results in a slide of meaning, which serves to conceal the fallaciousness of the traditional argument that since (1) it is wrong to kill innocent human beings, and (2) fetuses are innocent human beings, then (3) it is wrong to kill fetuses. For if 'human' is used in the same sense in both (1) and (2) then, whichever of the two senses is meant, one of these premises is question-begging. And if it is used in two different senses then of course the conclusion doesn't follow.

Thus, (1) is a self-evident moral truth,[1] and avoids begging the question about abortion, only if 'human being' is used to mean something like 'a full-fledged member of the moral community.' (It may or may not also be meant to refer exclusively to members of the species *Homo sapiens*.) We may call this the *moral* sense of 'human.' It is not to be confused with what we will call the *genetic* sense, i.e., the sense in which *any* member of the species is a human being, and no member of any other species could be. If (1) is acceptable only if the moral sense is intended, (2) is non-question-begging only if what is intended is the genetic sense.

In "Deciding Who is Human," Noonan argues for the classification of fetuses with human beings by pointing to the presence of the full genetic code, and the potential capacity for rational thought.[2] It is clear that what

he needs to show, for his version of the traditional argument to be valid, is that fetuses are human in the moral sense, the sense in which it is analytically true that all human beings have full moral rights. But, in the absence of any argument showing that whatever is genetically human is also morally human, and he gives none, nothing more than genetic humanity can be demonstrated by the presence of the human genetic code. And, as we will see, the *potential* capacity for rational thought can at most show that an entity has the potential for *becoming* human in the moral sense.

2   DEFINING THE MORAL COMMUNITY

Can it be established that genetic humanity is sufficient for moral humanity? I think that there are very good reasons for not defining the moral community in this way. I would like to suggest an alternative way of defining the moral community, which I will argue for only to the extent of explaining why it is, or should be, self-evident. The suggestion is simply that the moral community consists of all and only *people*, rather than all and only human beings,[3] and probably the best way of demonstrating its self-evidence is by considering the concept of personhood, to see what sorts of entity are and are not persons, and what the decision that a being is or is not a person implies about its moral rights.

What characteristics entitle an entity to be considered a person? This is obviously not the place to attempt a complete analysis of the concept of personhood, but we do not need such a fully adequate analysis just to determine whether and why a fetus is or isn't a person. All we need is a rough and approximate list of the most basic criteria of personhood, and some idea of which, or how many, of these an entity must satisfy in order to properly be considered a person.

In searching for such criteria, it is useful to look beyond the set of people with whom we are acquainted, and ask how we would decide whether a totally alien being was a person or not. (For we have no right to assume that genetic humanity is necessary for personhood.) Image a space traveler who lands on an unknown planet and encounters a race of beings utterly unlike any he has ever seen or heard of. If he wants to be sure of behaving morally toward these beings, he has to somehow decide whether they are people, and hence have full moral rights, or whether they are the sort of thing which he need not feel guilty about treating as, for example, a source of food.

How should he go about making this decision? If he has some anthropological background, he might look for such things as religion, art, and the manufacturing of tools, weapons, or shelters, since these factors have been used to distinguish our human from our prehuman ancestors, in what seems to be closer to the moral than the genetic sense of 'human.' And no doubt he would be right to consider the presence of such factors as good evidence that the alien beings were people, and morally human. It would, however, be overly anthropocentric of him to take the absence of these things as adequate evidence that they were not, since we can imagine people who have progressed beyond, or evolved without ever developing, these cultural characteristics.

I suggest that the traits which are most central to the concept of personhood, or humanity in the moral sense, are, very roughly, the following:

1. Consciousness (of objects and events external and/or internal to the being), and in particular the capacity to feel pain;

2. Reasoning (the *developed* capacity to solve new and relatively complex problems);

3. Self-motivated activity (activity which is relatively independent of either genetic or direct external control);

4. The capacity to communicate, by whatever means, messages of an indefinite variety of types, that is, not just with an indefinite number of possible contents, but on indefinitely many possible topics;

5. The presence of self-concepts, and self-awareness, either individual or racial, or both.

Admittedly, there are to apt to be a great many problems involved in formulating precise definitions of these criteria, let alone in developing universally valid behavioral criteria for deciding when they apply. But I will assume that both we and our explorer know approximately what (1)–(5) mean, and that he is also able to determine whether or not they apply. How, then, should he use his findings to decide whether or not the alien beings are people? We needn't suppose that an entity must have *all* of these attributes to be properly considered a person; (1) and (2) alone may well be sufficient for personhood, and quite probably (1)–(3) are sufficient. Neither do we need to insist that any one of these criteria

is *necessary* for personhood, although once again (1) and (2) look like fairly good candidates for necessary conditions, as does (3), if 'activity' is construed so as to include the activity of reasoning.

All we need to claim, to demonstrate that a fetus is not a person, is that any being which satisfies *none* of (1)–(5) is certainly not a person. I consider this claim to be so obvious that I think anyone who denied it, and claimed that a being which satisfied none of (1)–(5) was a person all the same, would thereby demonstrate that he had no notion at all of what a person is—perhaps because he had confused the concept of a person with that of genetic humanity. If the opponents of abortion were to deny the appropriateness of these five criteria, I do not know what further arguments would convince them. We would probably have to admit that our conceptual schemes were indeed irreconcilably different, and that our dispute could not be settled objectively.

I do not expect this to happen, however, since I think that the concept of a person is one which is very nearly universal (to people), and that it is common to both proabortionists and antiabortionists, even though neither group has fully realized the relevance of this concept to the resolution of their dispute. Furthermore, I think that on reflection even the antiabortionists ought to agree not only that (1)–(5) are central to the concept of personhood, but also that it is a part of this concept that all and only people have full moral rights. The concept of a person is in part a moral concept; once we have admitted that x is a person we have recognized, even if we have not agreed to respect, x's right to be treated as a member of the moral community. It is true that the claim that x is a *human being* is more commonly voiced as part of an appeal to treat x decently than is the claim that x is a person, but this is either because 'human being' is here used in the sense which implies personhood, or because the genetic and moral sense of 'human' have been confused.

Now if (1)–(5) are indeed the primary criteria of personhood, then it is clear that genetic humanity is neither necessary nor sufficient for establishing that an entity is a person. Some human beings are not people, and there may well be people who are not human beings. A man or woman whose consciousness has been permanently obliterated but who remains alive is a human being which is no longer a person; defective human beings, with no appreciable mental capacity, are not and presumably never will be people; and a fetus is a human being which is not yet a person, and which therefore cannot coherently be said to have full moral rights. Citizens of the next century should be prepared to recognize highly advanced, self-aware robots or computers, should such be developed, and intelligent inhabitants of other worlds, should such be found, as people in the fullest sense, and to respect their moral rights. But to ascribe full moral rights to an entity which is not a person is as absurd as to ascribe moral obligations and responsibilities to such an entity.

3 FETAL DEVELOPMENT AND THE RIGHT TO LIFE

Two problems arise in the application of these suggestions for the definition of the moral community to the determination of the precise moral status of a human fetus. Given that the paradigm example of a person is a normal adult human being, then (1) How like this paradigm, in particular how far advanced since conception, does a human being need to be before it begins to have a right to life by virtue, not of being fully a person as of yet, but of being *like* a person? and (2) To what extent, if any, does the fact that a fetus has the *potential* for becoming a person endow it with some of the same rights? Each of these questions requires some comment.

In answering the first question, we need not attempt a detailed consideration of the moral rights of organisms which are not developed enough, aware enough, intelligent enough, etc., to be considered people, but which resemble people in some respects. It does seem reasonable to suggest that the more like a person, in the relevant respects, a being is, the stronger is the case for regarding it as having a right to life, and indeed the stronger its right to life is. Thus we ought to take seriously the suggestion that, insofar as "the human individual develops biologically in a continuous fashion...the rights of a human person might develop in the same way."[4] But we must keep in mind that the attributes which are relevant in determining whether or not an entity is enough like a person to be regarded as having some of the same moral rights are no different from those which are relevant to determining whether or not it is fully a person—i.e., are no different from (1)–(5)— and that being genetically human, or having recognizable human facial and other physical features, or detectable brain activity, or the capacity to survive outside the uterus, are simply not among these relevant attributes.

Thus it is clear that even though a seven- or eight-month fetus has features which make it apt to arouse in us almost the same powerful protective instinct as is commonly aroused by a small infant, nevertheless it is not significantly more personlike than is a very small embryo. It is *somewhat* more personlike; it can apparently feel and respond to pain, and it may even have a rudimentary form of consciousness, insofar as its brain is quite active. Nevertheless, it seems safe to say that it is not fully conscious, in the way that an infant of a few months is, and that it cannot reason, or communicate messages of indefinitely many sorts, does not engage in self-motivated activity, and has no self-awareness. Thus, in the *relevant* respects, a fetus, even a fully developed one, is considerably less personlike than is the average mature mammal, indeed the average fish. And I think that a rational person must conclude that if the right to life of a fetus is to be based upon its resemblance to a person, then it cannot be said to have any more right to life than, let us say, a newborn guppy (which also seems to be capable of feeling pain), and that a right of that magnitude could never override a woman's right to obtain an abortion, at any stage of her pregnancy.

There may, of course, be other arguments in favor of placing legal limits upon the stage of pregnancy in which an abortion may be performed. Given the relative safety of the new techniques of artificially inducing labor during the third trimester, the danger to the woman's life or health is no longer such an argument. Neither is the fact that people tend to respond to the thought of abortion in the later stages of pregnancy with emotional repulsion, since mere emotional responses cannot take the place of moral reasoning in determining what ought to be permitted. Nor, finally, is the frequently heard argument that legalizing abortion, especially late in the pregnancy, may erode the level of respect for human life, leading, perhaps, to an increase in unjustified euthanasia and other crimes. For this threat, if it is a threat, can be better met by educating people to the kinds of moral distinctions which we are making here than by limiting access to abortion (which limitation may, in its disregard for the rights of women, be just as damaging to the level of respect for human rights).

Thus, since the fact that even a fully developed fetus is not personlike enough to have any significant right to life on the basis of its personlikeness shows that no legal restrictions upon the stage of pregnancy in which an abortion may be performed can be justified on the grounds that we should protect the rights of the older fetus; and since there is no other apparent justification for such restrictions, we may conclude that they are entirely unjustified. Whether or not it would be *indecent* (whatever that means) for a women in her seventh month to obtain an abortion just to avoid having to postpone a trip to Europe, it would not, in itself, be *immoral*, and therefore it ought to be permitted.

4 POTENTIAL PERSONHOOD AND THE RIGHT TO LIFE

We have seen that a fetus does not resemble a person in any way which can support the claim that it has even some of the same rights. But what about its *potential*, the fact that if nurtured and allowed to develop naturally it will very probably become a person? Doesn't that alone give it at least some right to life? It is hard to deny that the fact that an entity is a potential person is a strong prima facie reason for not destroying it; but we need not conclude from this that a potential person has a right to life, by virtue of that potential. It may be that our feeling that it is better, other things being equal, not to destroy a potential person is better explained by the fact that potential people are still (felt to be) an invaluable resource, not to be lightly squandered. Surely, if every speck of dust were a potential person, we would be much less apt to conclude that every potential person has a right to become actual.

Still, we do not need to insist that a potential person has no right to life whatever. There may well be something immoral, and not just imprudent, about wantonly destroying potential people, when doing so isn't necessary to protect anyone's rights. But even if a potential person does have some prima facie right to life, such a right could not possibly outweigh the right of a woman to obtain an abortion, since the rights of any actual person invariably outweigh those of any potential person, whenever the two conflict. Since this may not be immediately obvious in the case of a human fetus, let us look at another case.

Suppose that our space explorer falls into the hands of an alien culture, whose scientists decide to create a few hundred thousand or more human beings, by breaking his body into its component cells, and using these to create fully developed human beings, with, of course, his genetic code. We may imagine that each of these newly created men will have all of the original man's abilities, skills, knowledge, and so on, and also have an individual self-concept, in short that each of them will be a bona fide (though hardly unique) person. Imagine that the whole project will take only seconds, and that its chances of success are extremely high, and that our explorer knows all of this, and also knows that these people

will be treated fairly. I maintain that in such a situation he would have every right to escape if he could, and thus to deprive all of these potential people of their potential lives; for his right to life outweighs all of theirs together, in spite of the fact that they are all genetically human, all innocent, and all have a very high probability of becoming people very soon, if only he refrains from acting.

Indeed, I think he would have a right to escape even if it were not his life which the alien scientists planned to take, but only a year of his freedom, or, indeed, only a day. Nor would he be obligated to stay if he had gotten captured (thus bringing all these people-potentials into existence) because of his own carelessness, or even if he had done so deliberately, knowing the consequences. Regardless of how he got captured, he is not morally obligated to remain in captivity for *any* period of time for the sake of permitting any number of potential people to come into actuality, so great is the margin by which one actual person's right to liberty outweighs whatever right to life even a hundred thousand potential people have. And it seems reasonable to conclude that the rights of a woman will outweigh by a similar margin whatever right to life a fetus may have by virtue of its potential personhood.

Thus, neither a fetus's resemblance to a person, nor its potential for becoming a person provides any basis whatever for the claim that it has any significant right to life. Consequently, a woman's right to protect her health, happiness, freedom, and even her life,[5] by terminating an unwanted pregnancy, will always override whatever right to life it may be appropriate to ascribe to a fetus, even a fully developed one. And thus, in the absence of any overwhelming social need for every possible child, the laws which restrict the right to obtain an abortion, or limit the period of pregnancy during which an abortion may be performed, are a wholly unjustified violation of a woman's most basic moral and constitutional rights.[6]

POSTSCRIPT ON INFANTICIDE, FEBRUARY 26, 1982

One of the most troubling objections to the argument presented in this article is that it may appear to justify not only abortion but infanticide as well. A newborn infant is not a great deal more personlike than a nine-month fetus, and thus it might seem that if late-term abortion is sometimes justified, then infanticide must also be sometimes justified. Yet most people consider that infanticide is a form of murder, and thus never justified.

While it is important to appreciate the emotional force of this objection, its logical force is far less than it may seem at first glance. There are many reasons why infanticide is much more difficult to justify than abortion, even though if my argument is correct neither constitutes the killing of a person. In this country, and in this period of history, the deliberate killing of viable newborns is virtually never justified. This is in part because neonates are so very *close* to being persons that to kill them requires a very strong moral justification—as does the killing of dolphins, whales, chimpanzees, and other highly personlike creatures. It is certainly wrong to kill such beings just for the sake of convenience, or financial profit, or "sport."

Another reason why infanticide is usually wrong, in our society, is that if the newborn's parents do not want it, or are unable to care for it, there are (in most cases) people who are able and eager to adopt it and to provide a good home for it. Many people wait years for the opportunity to adopt a child, and some are unable to do so even though there is every reason to believe that they would be good parents. The needless destruction of a viable infant inevitably deprives some person or persons of a source of great pleasure and satisfaction, perhaps severely impoverishing their lives. Furthermore, even if an infant is considered to be unadoptable (e.g., because of some extremely severe mental or physical handicap) it is still wrong in most cases to kill it. For most of us value the lives of infants, and would prefer to pay taxes to support orphanages and state institutions for the handicapped rather than to allow unwanted infants to be killed. So long as most people feel this way, and so long as our society can afford to provide care for infants which are unwanted or which have special needs that preclude home care, it is wrong to destroy any infant which has a chance of living a reasonably satisfactory life.

If these arguments show that infanticide is wrong, at least in this society, then why don't they also show that late-term abortion is wrong? After all, third trimester fetuses are also highly personlike, and many people value them and would much prefer that they be preserved; even at some cost to themselves. As a potential source of pleasure to some family, a viable fetus is just as valuable as a viable infant. But there is an obvious and crucial difference between the two cases: once the infant is born, its continued life cannot (except, perhaps, in very exceptional cases) pose any serious threat to the woman's life or health, since she is free to put it up for adoption, or, where this is impossible, to place it in a state-supported institution. While she might prefer that it die, rather than being raised by others, it is not clear that such a preference would constitute a right on her part. True, she may suffer greatly from the knowledge that her child will be thrown into the lottery of the adoption system, and that she will be unable to ensure its well-being, or even to know whether it is healthy, happy, doing well in school, etc.: for the law generally does not permit natural parents to remain in contact with their children, once they are adopted by another family. But there are surely better ways of dealing with these problems than by permitting infanticide in such cases. (It might help, for instance, if the natural parents of adopted children could at least receive some information about their progress, without necessarily being informed of the identity of the adopting family.)

In contrast, a pregnant woman's right to protect her own life and health clearly outweighs other people's desire that the fetus be preserved—just as, when a person's life or limb is threatened by some wild animal, and when the threat cannot be removed without killing the animal, the person's right to self-protection outweighs the desires of those who would prefer that the animal not be harmed. Thus, while the moment of birth may not mark any sharp discontinuity in the degree to which an infant possesses a right to life, it does mark the end of the mother's absolute right to determine its fate. Indeed, if and when a late-term abortion could be safely performed without killing the fetus, she would have no absolute right to insist on its death (e.g., if others wish to adopt it or pay for its care), for the same reason that she does not have a right to insist that a viable infant be killed.

It remains true that according to my argument neither abortion nor the killing of neonates is properly considered a form of murder. Perhaps it is understandable that the law should classify infanticide as murder or homicide, since there is no other existing legal category which adequately or conveniently expresses the force of our society's disapproval of this action. But the moral distinction remains, and it has several important consequences.

In the first place, it implies that when an infant is born into a society which—unlike ours—is so impoverished that it simply cannot care for it adequately without endangering the survival of existing persons, killing it or allowing it to die is not necessarily wrong—provided that there is no *other* society which is willing and able to provide such care. Most human societies, from those at the hunting and gathering stage of economic development to the highly civilized Greeks and Romans, have permitted the practice of infanticide under such unfortunate circumstances, and I would argue that it shows a serious lack of understanding to condemn them as morally backward for this reason alone.

In the second place, the argument implies that when an infant is born with such severe physical anomalies that its life would predictably be a very short and/or very miserable one, even with the most heroic of medical treatment, and where its parents do not choose to bear the often crushing emotional, financial and other burdens attendant upon the artificial prolongation of such a tragic life, it is not morally wrong to cease or withhold treatment, thus allowing the infant a painless death. It is wrong (and sometimes a form of murder) to practice involuntary euthanasia on persons, since they have the right to decide for themselves whether or not they wish to continue to live. But terminally ill neonates cannot make this decision for themselves, and thus it is incumbent upon responsible persons to make the decision for them, as best they can. The mistaken belief that infanticide is always tantamount to murder is responsible for a great deal of unnecessary suffering, not just on the part of infants which are made to endure needlessly prolonged and painful deaths, but also on the part of parents, nurses, and other involved persons, who must watch infants suffering needlessly, helpless to end that suffering in the most humane way.

I am well aware that these conclusions, however modest and reasonable they may seem to some people, strike other people as morally monstrous, and that some people might even prefer to abandon their previous support for women's right to abortion rather than accept a theory which leads to such conclusions about infanticide. But all that these facts show is that abortion is not an isolated moral issue; to fully understand the moral status of abortion we may have to reconsider other moral issues as well, issues not just about infanticide and euthanasia, but also about the moral rights of women and of nonhuman animals. It is a philosopher's task to criticize mistaken beliefs which stand in the way of moral understanding, even when—perhaps especially when—those beliefs are popular and widespread. The belief that moral strictures against killing should apply equally to *all* genetically human entities, and *only* to genetically human entities, is such an error. The overcoming of this error will undoubtedly require long and often painful struggle; but it must be done.

NOTES

1 Of course, the principle that it is (always) wrong to kill innocent human beings is in need of many other modifications, e.g., that it may be permissible to do so to save a greater number of other innocent human beings, but we may safely ignore these complications here.

2 John Noonan, "Deciding Who is Human," *Natural Law Forum*, 13 (1968), 135.

3 From here on, we will use 'human' to mean genetically human, since the moral sense seems closely connected to, and perhaps derived from, the assumption that genetic humanity is sufficient for membership in the moral community.

4 Thomas L. Hayes, "A Biological View," *Commonweal*, 85 (March 17, 1967), 677–78; quoted by Daniel Callahan, in *Abortion: Law, Choice and Morality* (London: Macmillan & Co., 1970).

5 That is, insofar as the death rate, for the woman, is higher for childbirth than for early abortion.

6 My thanks to the following people, who were kind enough to read and criticize an earlier version of this paper: Herbert Gold, Gene Glass, Anne Lauterbach, Judith Thomson, Mary Mothersill, and Timothy Binkley.

Abortion Decisions: Personal Morality
Daniel Callahan

Daniel Callahan, a philosopher, has been since 1969 the director of The Hastings Center. He has also been executive editor of *The Commonweal* (1961–1968). His numerous publications reflect an enduring concern with issues in biomedical ethics. He is, for example, the author of *Setting Limits: Medical Goals in an Aging Society* (1987) and the coeditor of *Ethical Issues in Human Genetics* (1973) and *Abortion: Understanding Differences* (1984).

Callahan defends one kind of moderate view on the problem of the ethical acceptability of abortion. On the issue of the moral status of the fetus, he steers a middle course. He rejects the "tissue" theory, the view that the fetus has negligible moral status, on the grounds that such a theory is out of tune with both the biological evidence and a respect for the sanctity of human life. On the other hand, he contends that the fetus does not qualify as a person and thus rejects the view that the fetus has full moral status. His contention that the fetus is nevertheless an "important and valuable form of human life" can be understood as implying that the fetus has some kind of *partial* moral status. In Callahan's view, a respect for the sanctity of human life should incline every woman to a strong initial (moral) bias against abortion. Yet, he argues, since a woman has duties to herself, her family, and her society, there may be circumstances in which such duties would override the prima facie duty not to abort.

...To press the problem to a finer point, what ought [women] to think about as they try to work out their own views on abortion?

Only a few suggestions will be made here, taking the form of arguing for an ethic of personal responsibility which tries, in the process of decision-making, to make itself aware of a number of things. The biological evidence should be considered, just as the problem of methodology must be considered; the philosophical assumptions implicit in different uses of the word "human" need to be considered; a philosophical theory of biological analysis is required; the social consequences of different kinds of analyses and different meanings of the word "human" should be thought through; consistency of meaning and use should be sought to avoid *ad hoc* and arbitrary solutions.

It is my own conviction that the "developmental school" offers the most helpful and illuminating approach to the problem of the beginning of human life, avoiding, on the one hand, a too narrow genetic criterion of human life and, on the other, a too broad and socially

dangerous social definition of the "human." Yet the kinds of problems which appear in any attempt to decide upon the beginning of life suggest that no one position can be either proved or disproved from biological evidence alone. It becomes a question of trying to do justice to the evidence while, at the same time, realizing that how the evidence is approached and used will be a function of one's way of looking at reality, one's moral policy, the values and rights one believes need balancing, and the type of questions one thinks need to be asked. At the very least, however, the genetic evidence for the uniqueness of zygotes and embryos (a uniqueness of a different kind than that of the uniqueness of sperm and ova), their potentiality for development into a human person, their early development of human characteristics, their genetic and organic distinctness from the organism of the mother, appear to rule out a treatment even of zygotes, much less the more developed stages of the conceptus, as mere pieces of "tissue," of no human significance or value. The "tissue" theory of the significance of the conceptus can only be made plausible by a systematic disregard of the biological evidence. Moreover, though one may conclude that a conceptus is only potential human life, in the process of continually actualizing its potential through growth and development, a respect for the sanctity of life, with its bias in favor even of undeveloped life, is enough to make the taking of such life a moral problem. There is a choice to be made and it is a moral choice....

It is possible to imagine a huge number of situations where a woman could, in good and sensitive conscience, choose abortion as a moral solution to her personal or social difficulties. But, at the very least, the bounds of morality are overstepped when either through a systematic intellectual negligence or a willful choosing of that moral solution most personally convenient, personal choice is deliberately made easy and problem-free....

...Abortion is *one* way to solve the problem of an unwanted or hazardous pregnancy (physically, psychologically, economically or socially), but it is rarely the only way, at least in affluent societies (I would be considerably less certain about making the same statement about poor societies). Even in the most extreme cases—rape, incest, psychosis, for instance—alternatives will usually be available and different choices, open. It is not necessarily the end of every woman's chance for a happy, meaningful life to bear an illegitimate child. It is not necessarily the automatic destruction of a family to have a seriously defective child born into it. It is not necessarily the ruination of every family living in overcrowded housing to have still another child. It is not inevitable that every immature woman would become even more so if she bore a child or another child. It is not inevitable that a gravely handicapped child can hope for nothing from life. It is not inevitable that every unwanted child is doomed to misery. It is not written in the essence of things, as a fixed law of human nature, that a woman cannot come to accept, love and be a good mother to a child who was initially unwanted. Nor is it a fixed law that she could not come to cherish a grossly deformed child. Naturally, these are only generalizations. The point is only that human beings are as a rule flexible, capable of doing more than they sometimes think they can, able to surmount serious dangers and challenges, able to grow and mature, able to transform inauspicious beginnings into satisfactory conclusions. Everything in life, even in procreative and family life, is not fixed in advance; the future is never wholly unalterable....

Assuming...that most women would seek a broader ethical horizon than that of their exclusively personal self-interest, what might they think about when faced with an abortion decision? A respect for the sanctity of human life should, I believe, incline them toward a general and strong bias against abortion. Abortion is an act of killing, the violent, direct destruction of potential human life, already in the process of development. That fact should not be disguised, or glossed over by euphemism and circumlocution. It is not the destruction of a human person—for at no stage of its development does the conceptus fulfill the definition of a person, which implies a developed capacity for reasoning, willing, desiring and relating to others—but it is the destruction of an important and valuable form of human life. Its value and its potentiality are not dependent upon the attitude of the woman toward it; it grows by its own biological dynamism and has a genetic and morphological potential distinct from that of the woman. It has its own distinctive and individual future. If contraception and abortion are both seen as forms of birth limitation, they are distinctly different acts; the former precludes the possibility of a conceptus being formed, while the latter stops a conceptus already in existence from developing. The bias implied by the principle of the sanctity of human life is toward the protection of all forms of human life, especially, in ordinary circumstances, the protection of the right to life. That right should be accorded even to doubtful life; its existence should not be wholly dependent upon the personal self-interest of the woman.

Yet she has her own rights as well, and her own set of responsibilities to those around her; that is why she may have to choose abortion. In extreme situations of overpopulation, she may also have a responsibility for the survival of the species or of a people. In many circumstances, then, a decision in favor of abortion—one which overrides the right to life of that potential human being she carries within—can be a responsible moral decision, worthy neither of the condemnation of others nor of self-condemnation. But the bias of the principle of the sanctity of life is against a routine, unthinking employment of abortion; it bends over backwards not to take life and gives the benefit of the doubt to life. It does not seek to diminish the range of responsibility toward life—potential or actual—but to extend it. It does not seek the narrowest definition of life, but the widest and the richest. It is mindful of individual possibility, on the one hand, and of a destructive human tendency, on the other, to exclude from the category of "the human" or deny rights to those beings whose existence is or could prove burdensome to others....

...Moral seriousness presupposes one is concerned with the protection and furthering of life. This means that, out of respect for human life, one bends over backwards not to eliminate human life, not to desensitize oneself to the meaning and value of potential life, not to seek definitions of the "human" which serve one's self-interest only. A desire to respect human life in all of its forms means, therefore, that one voluntarily imposes upon oneself a pressure against the taking of life; that one demands of oneself serious reasons for doing so, even in the case of a very early embryo; that one use not only the mind but also the imagination when a decision is being made; that one seeks not to evade the moral issues but to face them; that one searches out the alternatives and conscientiously entertains them before turning to abortion. A bias in favor of the sanctity of human life in all of its forms would include a bias against abortion on the part of women; it would be the last rather than the first choice when unwanted pregnancies occurred. It would be an act to be avoided if at all possible.

A bias of this kind, voluntarily imposed by a woman upon herself, would not trap her; for it is also part of a respect for the dignity of life to leave the way open for an abortion when other reasonable choices are not available. For she also has duties toward herself, her family and her society. There can be good reasons for taking the life even of a very late fetus; once that also is seen and seen as a counterpoise in particular cases to the general bias against the taking of potential life, the way is open to choose abortion. The bias of the moral policy implies the need for moral rules which seek to preserve life. But, as a policy which leaves room for choice—rather than entailing a fixed set of rules—it is open to flexible interpretation when the circumstances point to the wisdom of taking exception to the normal ordering of the rules in particular cases. Yet, in that case, one is not genuinely taking exception to the rules. More accurately, one would be deciding that, for the preservation or furtherance of other values or rights—species-right, person-rights—a choice in favor of abortion would be serving the sanctity of life. That there would be, in that case, conflict between rights, with one set of rights set aside (reluctantly) to serve another set, goes without saying. A subversion of the principle occurs when it is made out that there is no conflict and thus nothing to decide.

Abortion and the Concept of a Person
Jane English

Jane English was a philosopher whose life came to a tragic end, at the age of 31, in a 1978 mountain climbing accident on the Matterhorn. She had taught at the University of North Carolina, Chapel Hill, and had published such articles as "Justice between Generations" and "Sex Equality in Sports." She was also the editor of *Sex Equality* (1977).

English begins by arguing that one of the central issues in the abortion debate, whether a fetus is a person, cannot be decisively resolved. However, she contends, whether we presume that the fetus is or is not a person, we must arrive at a moderate stance on the problem of abortion. In an effort to moderate the *conservative* view, English argues that it is unwarranted to conclude, from the presumption that the fetus is a person, that abortion is always morally impermissible. Reasoning on the basis of a self-defense model, she finds abortion morally permissible in many cases. In an effort to moderate the *liberal* view, English argues that it is unwarranted to conclude, from the presumption that the fetus is not a person, that abortion is always morally permissible. Even if the fetus is not a person, she argues, the similarity between a fetus and a baby is sufficient to make abortion problematic in the later stages of pregnancy.

Reprinted from vol. 5, no. 2 (October 1975), of the *Canadian Journal of Philosophy*, by permission of the Canadian Association for Publishing in Philosophy.

The abortion debate rages on. Yet the two most popular positions seem to be clearly mistaken. Conservatives maintain that a human life begins at conception and that therefore abortion must be wrong because it is murder. But not all killings of humans are murders. Most notably, self defense may justify even the killing of an innocent person.

Liberals, on the other hand, are just as mistaken in their argument that since a fetus does not become a person until birth, a woman may do whatever she pleases in and to her own body. First, you cannot do as you please with your own body if it affects other people adversely.[1] Second, if a fetus is not a person, that does not imply that you can do to it anything you wish. Animals, for example, are not persons, yet to kill or torture them for no reason at all is wrong.

At the center of the storm has been the issue of just when it is between ovulation and adulthood that a person appears on the scene. Conservatives draw the line at conception, liberals at birth. In this paper I first examine our concept of a person and conclude that no single criterion can capture the concept of a person and no sharp line can be drawn. Next I argue that if a fetus is a person, abortion is still justifiable in many cases; and if a fetus is not a person, killing it is still wrong in many cases. To a large extent, these two solutions are in agreement. I conclude that our concept of a person cannot and need not bear the weight that the abortion controversy has thrust upon it.

I

The several factions in the abortion argument have drawn battle lines around various proposed criteria for determining what is and what is not a person. For example, Mary Anne Warren[2] lists five features (capacities for reasoning, self-awareness, complex communication, etc.) as her criteria for personhood and argues for the permissibility of abortion because a fetus falls outside this concept. Baruch Brody[3] uses brain waves. Michael Tooley[4] picks having-a-concept-of-self as his criterion and concludes that infanticide and abortion are justifiable, while the killing of adult animals is not. On the other side, Paul Ramsey[5] claims a certain gene structure is the defining characteristic. John Noonan[6] prefers conceived-of-humans and presents counterexamples to various other candidate criteria. For instance, he argues against viability as the criterion because the newborn and infirm would then be non-persons, since they cannot

live without the aid of others. He rejects any criterion that calls upon the sorts of sentiments a being can evoke in adults on the grounds that this would allow us to exclude other races as non-persons if we could just view them sufficiently unsentimentally.

These approaches are typical: foes of abortion propose sufficient conditions for personhood which fetuses satisfy, while friends of abortion counter with necessary conditions for personhood which fetuses lack. But these both presuppose that the concept of a person can be captured in a strait jacket of necessary and/or sufficient conditions.[7] Rather, "person" is a cluster of features, of which rationality, having a self concept and being conceived of humans are only part.

What is typical of persons? Within our concept of a person we include, first, certain biological factors: descended from humans, having a certain genetic makeup, having a head, hands, arms, eyes, capable of locomotion, breathing, eating, sleeping. There are psychological factors: sentience, perception, having a concept of self and of one's own interests and desires, the ability to use tools, the ability to use language or symbol systems, the ability to joke, to be angry, to doubt. There are rationality factors: the ability to reason and draw conclusions, the ability to generalize and to learn from past experience, the ability to sacrifice present interests for greater gains in the future. There are social factors: the ability to work in groups and respond to peer pressures, the ability to recognize and consider as valuable the interests of others, seeing oneself as one among "other minds," the ability to sympathize, encourage, love, the ability to evoke from others the responses of sympathy, encouragement, love, the ability to work with others for mutual advantage. Then there are legal factors: being subject to the law and protected by it, having the ability to sue and enter contracts, being counted in the census, having a name and citizenship, the ability to own property, inherit, and so forth.

Now the point is not that this list is incomplete, or that you can find counterinstances to each of its points. People typically exhibit rationality, for instance, but someone who was irrational would not thereby fail to qualify as a person. On the other hand, something could exhibit the majority of these features and still fail to be a person, as an advanced robot might. There is no single core of necessary and sufficient features which we can draw upon with the assurance that they constitute what really makes a person; there are only features that are more or less typical.

This is not to say that no necessary or sufficient conditions can be given. Being alive is a necessary condition

for being a person, and being a U.S. Senator is sufficient. But rather than falling inside a sufficient condition
or outside a necessary one, a fetus lies in the penumbra
region where our concept of a person is not so simple.
For this reason I think a conclusive answer to the question whether a fetus is a person is unattainable.

Here we might note a family of simple fallacies that
proceed by stating a necessary condition for personhood
and showing that a fetus has that characteristic. This is a
form of the fallacy of affirming the consequent. For example, some have mistakenly reasoned from the premise
that a fetus is human (after all, it is a human fetus rather
than, say, a canine fetus), to the conclusion that it is *a*
human. Adding an equivocation on "being," we get the
fallacious argument that since a fetus is something both
living and human, it is a human being.

Nonetheless, it does seem clear that a fetus has very
few of the above family of characteristics, whereas a
newborn baby exhibits a much larger proportion of
them—and a two-year-old has even more. Note that one
traditional anti-abortion argument has centered on
pointing out the many ways in which a fetus resembles a
baby. They emphasize its development ("It already has
ten fingers...") without mentioning its dissimilarities to
adults (it still has gills and a tail). They also try to evoke
the sort of sympathy on our part that we only feel toward
other persons ("Never to laugh...or feel the sun-
shine?"). This all seems to be a relevant way to argue,
since its purpose is to persuade us that a fetus satisfies so
many of the important features on the list that it ought
to be treated as a person. Also note that a fetus near the
time of birth satisfies many more of these factors than a
fetus in the early months of development. This could
provide reason for making distinctions among the different stages of pregnancy, as the U.S. Supreme Court has
done.[8]

Historically, the time at which a person has been
said to come into existence has varied widely. Muslims
date personhood from fourteen days after conception.
Some medievals followed Aristotle in placing ensoulment at forty days after conception for a male fetus and
eighty days for a female fetus.[9] In European common
law since the Seventeenth Century, abortion was considered the killing of a person only after quickening, the
time when a pregnant woman first feels the fetus move
on its own. Nor is this variety of opinions surprising. Biologically, a human being develops gradually. We
shouldn't expect there to be any specific time or sharp
dividing point when a person appears on the scene.

For these reasons I believe our concept of a person
is not sharp or decisive enough to bear the weight of a
solution to the abortion controversy. To use it to solve
that problem is to clarify *obscurum per obscurius*.

II

Next let us consider what follows if a fetus is a person
after all. Judith Jarvis Thomson's landmark article, "A
Defense of Abortion,"[10] correctly points out that some
additional argumentation is needed at this point in the
conservative argument to bridge the gap between the
premise that a fetus is an innocent person and the conclusion that killing it is always wrong. To arrive at this
conclusion, we would need the additional premise that
killing an innocent person is always wrong. But killing
an innocent person is sometimes permissible, most notably in self defense. Some examples may help draw out
our intuitions or ordinary judgments about self defense.

Suppose a mad scientist, for instance, hypnotized
innocent people to jump out of the bushes and attack innocent passers-by with knives. If you are so attacked, we
agree you have a right to kill the attacker in self defense,
if killing him is the only way to protect your life or to
save yourself from serious injury. It does not seem to
matter here that the attacker is not malicious but himself
an innocent pawn, for your killing of him is not done in
a spirit of retribution but only in self defense.

How severe an injury may you inflict in self defense? In part this depends upon the severity of the injury to be avoided: you may not shoot someone merely
to avoid having your clothes torn. This might lead one to
the mistaken conclusion that the defense may only equal
the threatened injury in severity; that to avoid death you
may kill, but to avoid a black eye you may only inflict a
black eye or the equivalent. Rather, our laws and customs seem to say that you may create an injury somewhat, but not enormously, greater than the injury to be
avoided. To fend off an attack whose outcome would be
as serious as rape, a severe beating or the loss of a finger,
you may shoot; to avoid having your clothes torn, you
may blacken an eye.

Aside from this, the injury you may inflict should
only be the minimum necessary to deter or incapacitate
the attacker. Even if you know he intends to kill you,
you are not justified in shooting him if you could equally
well save yourself by the simple expedient of running
away. Self defense is for the purpose of avoiding harms
rather than equalizing harms.

Some cases of pregnancy present a parallel situation. Though the fetus is itself innocent, it may pose a

threat to the pregnant woman's well-being, life prospects or health, mental or physical. If the pregnancy presents a slight threat to her interests, it seems self defense cannot justify abortion. But if the threat is on a par with a serious beating or the loss of a finger, she may kill the fetus that poses such a threat, even if it is an innocent person. If a lesser harm to the fetus could have the same defensive effect, killing it would not be justified. It is unfortunate that the only way to free the woman from the pregnancy entails the death of the fetus (except in very late stages of pregnancy). Thus a self defense model supports Thomson's point that the woman has a right only to be freed from the fetus, not a right to demand its death.[11]

The self defense model is most helpful when we take the pregnant woman's point of view. In the pre-Thomson literature, abortion is often framed as a question for a third party; do you, a doctor, have a right to choose between the life of the woman and that of the fetus? Some have claimed that if you were a passer-by who witnessed a struggle between the innocent hypnotized attacker and his equally innocent victim, you would have no reason to kill either in defense of the other. They have concluded that the self defense model implies that a woman may attempt to abort herself, but that a doctor should not assist her. I think the position of the third party is somewhat more complex. We do feel some inclination to intervene on behalf of the victim rather than the attacker, other things equal. But if both parties are innocent, other factors come into consideration. You would rush to the aid of your husband whether he was attacker or attackee. If a hypnotized famous violinist were attacking a skid row bum, we would try to save the individual who is of more value to society. These considerations would tend to support abortion in some cases.

But suppose you are a frail senior citizen who wishes to avoid being knifed by one of these innocent hypnotics, so you have hired a bodyguard to accompany you. If you are attacked, it is clear we believe that the bodyguard, acting as your agent, has a right to kill the attacker to save you from a serious beating. Your rights of self defense are transferred to your agent. I suggest that we should similarly view the doctor as the pregnant woman's agent in carrying out a defense she is physically incapable of accomplishing herself.

Thanks to modern technology, the cases are rare in which a pregnancy poses as clear a threat to a woman's bodily health as an attacker brandishing a switchblade. How does self defense fare when more subtle, complex and long-range harms are involved?

To consider a somewhat fanciful example, suppose you are a highly trained surgeon when you are kidnapped by the hypnotic attacker. He says he does not intend to harm you but to take you back to the mad scientist who, it turns out, plans to hypnotize you to have a permanent mental block against all your knowledge of medicine. This would automatically destroy your career which would in turn have a serious adverse impact on your family, your personal relationships and your happiness. It seems to me that if the only way you can avoid this outcome is to shoot the innocent attacker, you are justified in so doing. You are defending yourself from a drastic injury to your life prospects. I think it is no exaggeration to claim that unwanted pregnancies (most obviously among teenagers) often have such adverse life-long consequences as the surgeon's loss of livelihood.

Several parallels arise between various views on abortion and the self defense model. Let's suppose further that these hypnotized attackers only operate at night, so that it is well known that they can be avoided completely by the considerable inconvenience of never leaving your house after dark. One view is that since you could stay home at night, therefore if you go out and are selected by one of these hypnotized people, you have no right to defend yourself. This parallels the view that abstinence is the only acceptable way to avoid pregnancy. Others might hold that you ought to take along some defense such as Mace which will deter the hypnotized person without killing him, but that if this defense fails, you are obliged to submit to the resulting injury, no matter how severe it is. This parallels the view that contraception is all right but abortion is always wrong, even in cases of contraceptive failure.

A third view is that you may kill the hypnotized person only if he will actually kill you, but not if he will only injure you. This is like the position that abortion is permissible only if it is required to save a woman's life. Finally we have the view that it is all right to kill the attacker, even if only to avoid a very slight inconvenience to yourself and even if you knowingly walked down the very street where all these incidents have been taking place without taking along any Mace or protective escort. If we assume that a fetus is a person, this is the analogue of the view that abortion is always justifiable, "on demand."

The self defense model allows us to see an important difference that exists between abortion and infanticide, even if a fetus is a person from conception. Many have argued that the only way to justify abortion without justifying infanticide would be to find some characteristic of personhood that is acquired at birth. Michael Tooley, for one, claims infanticide is justifiable because the really significant characteristics of person are acquired some time after birth. But all such approaches look to characteristics of the developing human and ignore the relation between the fetus and the woman. What if, after birth, the presence of an infant or the need to support it posed a grave threat to the woman's sanity or life prospects? She could escape this threat by the simple expedient of running away. So a solution that does not entail the death of the infant is available. Before birth, such solutions are not available because of the biological dependence of the fetus on the woman. Birth is the crucial point not because of any characteristics the fetus gains, but because after birth the woman can defend herself by a means less drastic than killing the infant. Hence self defense can be used to justify abortion without necessarily thereby justifying infanticide.

III

On the other hand, supposing a fetus is not after all a person, would abortion always be morally permissible? Some opponents of abortion seem worried that if a fetus is not a full-fledged person, then we are justified in treating it in any way at all. However, this does not follow. Non-persons do get some consideration in our moral code, though of course they do not have the same rights as persons have (and in general they do not have moral responsibilities), and though their interests may be overridden by the interests of persons. Still, we cannot treat them in any way at all.

Treatment of animals is a case in point. It is wrong to torture dogs for fun or to kill wild birds for no reason at all. It is wrong Period, even though dogs and birds do not have the same rights persons do. However, few people think it is wrong to use dogs as experimental animals, causing them considerable suffering in some cases, provided that the resulting research will probably bring discoveries of great benefit to people. And most of us think it all right to kill birds for food or to protect our crops. People's rights are different from the consideration we give to animals, then, for it is wrong to experiment on people, even if others might later benefit a great deal as a result of their suffering. You might volunteer to be a subject, but this would be supererogatory; you certainly have a right to refuse to be a medical guinea pig.

But how do we decide what you may or may not do to non-persons? This is a difficult problem, one for which I believe no adequate account exists. You do not want to say, for instance, that torturing dogs is all right whenever the sum of its effects on people is good—when it doesn't warp the sensibilities of the torturer so much that he mistreats people. If that were the case, it would be all right to torture dogs if you did it in private, or if the torturer lived on a desert island or died soon afterward, so that his actions had no effect on people. This is an inadequate account, because whatever moral consideration animals get, it has to be indefeasible, too. It will have to be a general proscription of certain actions, not merely a weighing of the impact on people on a case-by-case basis.

Rather, we need to distinguish two levels on which consequences of actions can be taken into account in moral reasoning. The traditional objections to Utilitarianism focus on the fact that it operates solely on the first level, taking all the consequences into account in particular cases only. Thus Utilitarianism is open to "desert island" and "lifeboat" counterexamples because these cases are rigged to make the consequences of actions severely limited.

Rawls' theory could be described as a teleological sort of theory, but with teleology operating on a higher level.[12] In choosing the principles to regulate society from the original position, his hypothetical choosers make their decision on the basis of the total consequences of various systems. Furthermore, they are constrained to choose a general set of rules which people can readily learn and apply. An ethical theory must operate by generating a set of sympathies and attitudes toward others which reinforces the functioning of that set of moral principles. Our prohibition against killing people operates by means of certain moral sentiments including sympathy, compassion and guilt. But if these attitudes are to form a coherent set, they carry us further: we tend to perform supererogatory actions, and we tend to feel similar compassion toward person-like non-persons.

It is crucial that psychological facts play a role here. Our psychological constitution makes it the case that for our ethical theory to work, it must prohibit certain treatment of non-persons which are significantly person-like. If our moral rules allowed people to treat some person-like non-persons in ways we do not want people to be treated, this would undermine the system of sympathies and attitudes that makes the ethical system work. For this reason, we would choose in the original position to make mistreatment of some sorts of animals wrong in general (not just wrong in the cases with public impact), even though animals are not themselves parties in the original position. Thus it makes sense that it is those animals whose appearance and behavior are most like those of people that get the most consideration in our moral scheme.

It is because of "coherence of attitudes," I think, that the similarity of a fetus to a baby is very significant. A fetus one week before birth is so much like a newborn baby in our psychological space that we cannot allow any cavalier treatment of the former while expecting full sympathy and nurturative support for the latter. Thus, I think that anti-abortion forces are indeed giving their strongest arguments when they point to the similarities between a fetus and a baby, and when they try to evoke our emotional attachment to and sympathy for the fetus. An early horror story from New York about nurses who were expected to alternate between caring for six-week premature infants and disposing of viable 24-week aborted fetuses is just that—a horror story. These beings are so much alike that no one can be asked to draw a distinction and treat them so very differently.

Remember, however, that in the early weeks after conception, a fetus is very much unlike a person. It is hard to develop these feelings for a set of genes which doesn't yet have a head, hands, beating heart, response to touch or the ability to move by itself. Thus it seems to me that the alleged "slippery slope" between conception and birth is not so very slippery. In the early stages of pregnancy, abortion can hardly be compared to murder for psychological reasons, but in the latest stages it is psychologically akin to murder.

Another source of similarity is the bodily continuity between fetus and adult. Bodies play a surprisingly central role in our attitudes toward persons. One has only to think of the philosophical literature on how far physical identity suffices for personal identity or Wittgenstein's remark that the best picture of the human soul is the human body. Even after death, when all agree the body is no longer a person, we still observe elaborate customs of respect for the human body; like people who torture dogs, necrophiliacs are not to be trusted with people.[13] So it is appropriate that we show respect to a fetus as the body continuous with the body of a person. This is a degree of resemblance to persons that animals cannot rival.

Michael Tooley also utilizes a parallel with animals. He claims that it is always permissible to drown newborn kittens and draws conclusions about infanticide.[14] But it is only permissible to drown kittens when their survival would cause some hardship. Perhaps it would be a burden to feed and house six more cats or to find other homes for them. The alternative of letting them starve produces even more suffering than the drowning. Since the kittens get their rights second-hand, so to speak, *via* the need for coherence in our attitudes, their interests are often overridden by the interests of full-fledged persons. But if their survival would be no inconvenience to people at all, then it is wrong to drown them, *contra* Tooley.

Tooley's conclusions about abortion are wrong for the same reason. Even if the fetus is not a person, abortion is not always permissible, because of the resemblance of a fetus to a person. I agree with Thomson that it would be wrong for a woman who is seven months pregnant to have an abortion just to avoid having to postpone a trip to Europe. In the early months of pregnancy when the fetus hardly resembles a baby at all, then, abortion is permissible whenever it is in the interests of the pregnant woman or her family. The reasons would only need to outweigh the pain and inconvenience of the abortion itself. In the middle months, when the fetus comes to resemble a person, abortion would be justifiable only when the continuation of the pregnancy or the birth of the child would cause harms—physical, psychological, economic or social—to the woman. In the late months of pregnancy, even on our current assumption that a fetus is not a person, abortion seems to be wrong except to save a woman from significant injury or death.

The Supreme Court has recognized similar gradations in the alleged slippery slope stretching between conception and birth. To this point, the present paper has been a discussion of the moral status of abortion only, not its legal status. In view of the great physical, financial and sometimes psychological costs of abortion, perhaps the legal arrangement most compatible with the proposed moral solution would be the absence of restrictions, that is, so-called abortion "on demand."

So I conclude, first, that application of our concept of a person will not suffice to settle the abortion issue. After all, the biological development of a human being is gradual. Second, whether a fetus is a person or not, abortion is justifiable early in pregnancy to avoid modest harms and seldom justifiable late in pregnancy except to avoid significant injury or death.[15]

NOTES

1 We also have paternalistic laws which keep us from harming our own bodies even when no one else is affected. Ironically, anti-abortion laws were originally

designed to protect pregnant women from a dangerous but tempting procedure.

2 Mary Anne Warren, "On the Moral and Legal Status of Abortion," *Monist* 57 (1973), p. 55.

3 Baruch Brody, "Fetal Humanity and the Theory of Essentialism," in Robert Baker and Frederick Elliston (eds.), *Philosophy and Sex* (Buffalo, N.Y., 1975).

4 Michael Tooley, "Abortion and Infanticide," *Philosophy and Public Affairs* 2 (1971).

5 Paul Ramsey, "The Morality of Abortion," in James Rachels, ed., *Moral Problems* (New York, 1971).

6 John Noonan, "Abortion and the Catholic Church: A Summary History," *Natural Law Forum* 12 (1967), pp. 125–131.

7 Wittgenstein has argued against the possibility of so capturing the concept of a game, *Philosophical Investigations* (New York, 1958), § 66–71.

8 Not because the fetus is partly a person and so has some of the rights of persons, but rather because of the rights of person-like non-persons. This I discuss in part III below.

9 Aristotle himself was concerned, however, with the different question of when the soul takes form. For historical data, see Jimmye Kimmey, "How the Abortion Laws Happened," *Ms.* 1 (April, 1973), pp. 48ff, and John Noonan, *loc. cit.*

10 J. J. Thomson, "A Defense of Abortion," *Philosophy and Public Affairs* 1 (1971).

11 *Ibid.*, p. 52.

12 John Rawls, *A Theory of Justice* (Cambridge, Mass., 1971), § 3–4.

13 On the other hand, if they can be trusted with people, then our moral customs are mistaken. It all depends on the facts of psychology.

14 *Op. cit.*, pp. 40, 60–61.

15 I am deeply indebted to Larry Crocker and Arthur Kuflik for their constructive comments.

Abortion and Social Policy

Majority Opinion in *Roe v. Wade*
Justice Harry Blackmun

Harry Blackmun, associate justice of the United States Supreme Court, is a graduate of Harvard Law School. After some fifteen years in private practice he became legal counsel to the Mayo Clinic (1950–1959). Justice Blackmun also served as United States circuit judge (1959–1970) before his appointment in 1970 to the Supreme Court.

In this case, a pregnant single woman, suing under the fictitious name of Jane Roe, challenged the constitutionality of the existing Texas criminal abortion law. According to the Texas Penal Code, the performance of an abortion, except to save the life of the mother, constituted a crime that was punishable by a prison sentence of two to five years. At the time this case was finally resolved by the Supreme Court, abortion legislation varied widely from state to state. Some states, principally New York, had already legalized abortion on demand. Most other states, however, had legalized various forms of therapeutic abortion but had retained some measure of restrictive abortion legislation.

Justice Blackmun, writing an opinion concurred in by six other justices, argues that a woman's decision to terminate a pregnancy is encompassed by a *right to privacy*—but only up to a certain point in the development of the fetus. As the right to privacy is not an absolute right, it must yield at some point to the state's legitimate interests. Justice Blackmun contends that the state has a legitimate interest in protecting the health of the mother and that this interest becomes compelling at approximately the end of the first trimester in the development of

United States Supreme Court; January 22, 1973. 410 U.S. 113, 93 S.Ct. 705.

the fetus. He also contends that the state has a legitimate interest in protecting potential life and that this interest becomes compelling at the point of viability.

It is... apparent that at common law, at the time of the adoption of our Constitution, and throughout the major portion of the 19th century, abortion was viewed with less disfavor than under most American statutes currently in effect. Phrasing it another way, a woman enjoyed a substantially broader right to terminate a pregnancy than she does in most States today. At least with respect to the early stage of pregnancy, and very possibly without such a limitation, the opportunity to make this choice was present in this country well into the 19th century. Even later, the law continued for some time to treat less punitively an abortion procured in early pregnancy....

Three reasons have been advanced to explain historically the enactment of criminal abortion laws in the 19th century and to justify their continued existence.

It has been argued occasionally that these laws were the product of a Victorian social concern to discourage illicit sexual conduct. Texas, however, does not advance this justification in the present case, and it appears that no court or commentator has taken the argument seriously....

A second reason is concerned with abortion as a medical procedure. When most criminal abortion laws were first enacted, the procedure was a hazardous one for the woman. This was particularly true prior to the development of antisepsis. Antiseptic techniques, of course, were based on discoveries by Lister, Pasteur, and others first announced in 1867, but were not generally accepted and employed until about the turn of the century. Abortion mortality was high. Even after 1900, and perhaps until as late as the development of antibiotics in the 1940's, standard modern techniques such as dilation and curettage were not nearly so safe as they are today. Thus it has been argued that a State's real concern in enacting a criminal abortion law was to protect the pregnant woman, that is, to restrain her from submitting to a procedure that placed her life in serious jeopardy.

Modern medical techniques have altered this situation. Appellants and various *amici* refer to medical data indicating that abortion in early pregnancy, that is, prior to the end of first trimester, although not without its risk, is now relatively safe. Mortality rates for women undergoing early abortions, where the procedure is le-

gal, appear to be as low as or lower than the rates for normal childbirth. Consequently, any interest of the State in protecting the woman from an inherently hazardous procedure, except when it would be equally dangerous for her to forego it, has largely disappeared. Of course, important state interests in the area of health and medical standards do remain. The State has a legitimate interest in seeing to it that abortion, like any other medical procedure, is performed under circumstances that insure maximum safety for the patient. This interest obviously extends at least to the performing physician and his staff, to the facilities involved, to the availability of after-care, and to adequate provision for any complication or emergency that might arise. The prevalence of high mortality rates at illegal "abortion mills" strengthens, rather than weakens, the State's interest in regulating the conditions under which abortions are performed. Moreover, the risk to the woman increases as her pregnancy continues. Thus the State retains a definite interest in protecting the woman's own health and safety when an abortion is performed at a late stage of pregnancy.

The third reason is the State's interest—some phrase it in terms of duty—in protecting prenatal life. Some of the argument for this justification rests on the theory that a new human life is present from the moment of conception. The State's interest and general obligation to protect life then extends, it is argued, to prenatal life. Only when the life of the pregnant mother herself is at stake, balanced against the life she carries within her, should the interest of the embryo or fetus not prevail. Logically, of course, a legitimate state interest in this area need not stand or fall on acceptance of the belief that life begins at conception or at some other point prior to live birth. In assessing the State's interest, recognition may be given to the less rigid claim that as long as at least *potential* life is involved, the State may assert interests beyond the protection of the pregnant woman alone.

Parties challenging state abortion laws have sharply disputed in some courts the contention that a purpose of these laws, when enacted, was to protect prenatal life. Pointing to the absence of legislative history to support the contention, they claim that most state laws were designed solely to protect the woman. Because medical advances have lessened this concern, at least with respect to abortion in early pregnancy, they argue that with respect to such abortions the laws can no longer be justified by any state interest. There is some scholarly support for this view of original purpose. The few state courts called upon to interpret their laws in the late 19th and early 20th centuries did focus on the State's interest in protecting the woman's health rather than in preserving the embryo and fetus....

The Constitution does not explicitly mention any right of privacy. In a line of decisions, however, going back perhaps as far as *Union Pacific R. Co. v. Botsford* (1891), the Court has recognized that a right of personal privacy, or a guarantee of certain areas or zones of privacy, does exist under the constitution. In varying contexts the Court or individual Justices have indeed found at least the roots of that right in the First Amendment, ...in the Fourth and Fifth Amendments...in the penumbras of the Bill of Rights...in the Ninth Amendment ...or in the concept of liberty guaranteed by the first section of the Fourteenth Amendment....These decisions make it clear that only personal rights that can be deemed "fundamental" or "implicit in the concept of ordered liberty,"...are included in this guarantee of personal privacy. They also make it clear that the right has some extension to activities relating to marriage,... procreation,...contraception,...family relationships, ... and child rearing and education,...

This right of privacy, whether it be founded in the Fourteenth Amendment's concept of personal liberty and restrictions upon state action, as we feel it is, or, as the District Court determined, in the Ninth Amendment's reservation of rights to the people, is broad enough to encompass a woman's decision whether or not to terminate her pregnancy....

...[A]ppellants and some *amici* argue that the woman's right is absolute and that she is entitled to terminate her pregnancy at whatever time, in whatever way, and for whatever reason she alone chooses. With this we do not agree. Appellants' arguments that Texas either has no valid interest at all in regulating the abortion decision, or no interest strong enough to support any limitation upon the woman's sole determination, is unpersuasive. The Court's decisions recognizing a right of privacy also acknowledge that some state regulation in areas protected by that right is appropriate. As noted above, a state may properly assert important interests in safe-guarding health, in maintaining medical standards, and in protecting potential life. At some point in pregnancy, these respective interests become sufficiently compelling to sustain regulation of the factors that gov-

ern the abortion decision. The privacy right involved, therefore, cannot be said to be absolute....

We therefore conclude that the right of personal privacy includes the abortion decision, but that this right is not unqualified and must be considered against important state interests in regulation.

We note that those federal and state courts that have recently considered abortion law challenges have reached the same conclusion....

Although the results are divided, most of these courts have agreed that the right of privacy, however based, is broad enough to cover the abortion decision; that the right, nonetheless, is not absolute and is subject to some limitations; and that at some point the state interests as to protection of health, medical standards, and prenatal life, become dominant. We agree with this approach....

The appellee and certain *amici* argue that the fetus is a "person" within the language and meaning of the Fourteenth Amendment. In support of this they outline at length and in detail the well-known facts of fetal development. If this suggestion of personhood is established, the appellant's case, of course, collapses, for the fetus' right to life is then guaranteed specifically by the Amendment. The appellant conceded as much on reargument. On the other hand, the appellee conceded on reargument that no case could be cited that holds that a fetus is a person within the meaning of the Fourteenth Amendment....

All this, together with our observation, *supra*, that throughout the major portion of the 19th century prevailing legal abortion practices were far freer than they are today, persuades us that the word "person," as used in the Fourteenth Amendment, does not include the unborn....Indeed, our decision in *United States v. Vuitch* (1971) inferentially is to the same effect, for we there would not have indulged in statutory interpretation favorable to abortion in specified circumstances if the necessary consequence was the termination of life entitled to Fourteenth Amendment protection.

...As we have intimated above, it is reasonable and appropriate for a State to decide that at some point in time another interest, that of health of the mother or that of potential human life, becomes significantly involved. The woman's privacy is no longer sole and any right of privacy she possesses must be measured accordingly.

Texas urges that, apart from the Fourteenth Amendment, life begins at conception and is present throughout pregnancy, and that, therefore, the State has a compelling interest in protecting that life from and after conception. We need not resolve the difficult question of when life begins. When those trained in the respective disciplines of medicine, philosophy, and theology are unable to arrive at any consensus, the judiciary, at this point in the development of man's knowledge, is not in a position to speculate as to the answer.

It should be sufficient to note briefly the wide divergence of thinking on this most sensitive and difficult question. There has always been strong support for the view that life does not begin until live birth. This was the belief of the Stoics. It appears to be the predominant, though not the unanimous, attitude of the Jewish faith. It may be taken to represent also the position of a large segment of the Protestant community, insofar as that can be ascertained; organized groups that have taken a formal position on the abortion issue have generally regarded abortion as a matter for the conscience of the individual and her family. As we have noted, the common law found greater significance in quickening. Physicians and their scientific colleagues have regarded that event with less interest and have tended to focus either upon conception or upon live birth or upon the interim point at which the fetus becomes "viable," that is, potentially able to live outside the mother's womb, albeit with artificial aid. Viability is usually placed at about seven months (28 weeks) but may occur earlier, even at 24 weeks....

In areas other than criminal abortion the law has been reluctant to endorse any theory that life, as we recognize it, begins before live birth or to accord legal rights to the unborn except in narrowly defined situations and except when the rights are contingent upon live birth....In short, the unborn have never been recognized in the law as persons in the whole sense.

In view of all this, we do not agree that, by adopting one theory of life, Texas may override the rights of the pregnant woman that are at stake. We repeat, however, that the State does have an important and legitimate interest in preserving and protecting the health of the pregnant woman, whether she be a resident of the State or a nonresident who seeks medical consultation and treatment there, and that it has still *another* important and legitimate interest in protecting the potentiality of human life. These interests are separate and distinct. Each grows in substantiality as the woman approaches term and, at a point during pregnancy, each becomes "compelling."

With respect to the State's important and legitimate interest in the health of the mother, the "compelling"

point, in the light of present medical knowledge, is at approximately the end of the first trimester. This is so because of the now established medical fact...that until the end of the first trimester mortality in abortion is less than mortality in normal childbirth. It follows that, from and after this point, a State may regulate the abortion procedure to the extent that the regulation reasonably relates to the preservation and protection of maternal health. Examples of permissible state regulation in this area are requirements as to the qualifications of the person who is to perform the abortion; as to the licensure of that person; as to the facility in which the procedure is to be performed, that is, whether it must be a hospital or may be a clinic or some other place of less-than-hospital status; as to the licensing of the facility; and the like.

This means, on the other hand, that, for the period of pregnancy prior to this "compelling" point, the attending physician, in consultation with his patient, is free to determine, without regulation by the State, that in his medical judgment the patient's pregnancy should be terminated. If that decision is reached, the judgment may be effectuated by an abortion free of interference by the State.

With respect to the State's important and legitimate interest in potential life, the "compelling" point is at viability. This is so because the fetus then presumably has the capability of meaningful life outside the mother's womb. State regulation protective of fetal life after viability thus has both logical and biological justifications. If the State is interested in protecting fetal life after viability, it may go so far as to proscribe abortion during that period except when it is necessary to preserve the life or health of the mother....

To summarize and repeat:

1 A state criminal abortion statute of the current Texas type, that excepts from criminality only a *life saving* procedure on behalf of the mother, without regard to pregnancy stage and without recognition of the other interests involved, is violative of the Due Process Clause of the Fourteenth Amendment.

  a For the stage prior to approximately the end of the first trimester, the abortion decision and its effectuation must be left to the medical judgment of the pregnant woman's attending physician.

  b For the stage subsequent to approximately the end of the first trimester, the State, in promoting its interest in the health of the mother, may, if it chooses, regulate the abortion procedure in ways that are reasonably related to maternal health.

c   For the stage subsequent to viability the State, in promoting its interest in the potentiality of human life, may, if it chooses, regulate, and even proscribe, abortion except where it is necessary, in appropriate medical judgment, for the preservation of the life or health of the mother.

2   The State may define the term "physician," as it has been employed [here], to mean only a physician currently licensed by the State, and may proscribe any abortion by a person who is not a physician as so defined.

...The decision leaves the State free to place increasing restrictions on abortion as the period of pregnancy lengthens, so long as those restrictions are tailored to the recognized state interests. The decision vindicates the right of the physician to administer medical treatment according to his professional judgment up to the points where important state interests provide compelling justifications for intervention. Up to those points the abortion decision in all its aspects is inherently, and primarily, a medical decision, and basic responsibility for it must rest with the physician. If an individual practitioner abuses the privilege of exercising proper medical judgment, the usual remedies, judicial and intraprofessional, are available....

Opinion in *Webster v. Reproductive Health Services*
Justice William H. Rehnquist

William H. Rehnquist, chief justice of the U.S. Supreme Court, is a graduate of Stanford University Law School. In 1969, after spending a number of years in private practice, he became assistant attorney general, Office of Legal Counsel, U.S. Department of Justice. He was appointed to the Supreme Court in 1972 and became chief justice of the Court in 1986.

At issue in this case is the constitutionality of certain provisions of a Missouri statute designed to place restrictions on abortion. Of special importance are provisions banning the use of *public* facilities and *public* employees in the performance of abortions and a provision requiring physicians to perform tests to determine the viability of any fetus believed to be 20 weeks or older.

In announcing the judgment of a bitterly divided Court, Chief Justice Rehnquist argues that just as it is constitutionally acceptable for a state to refuse to fund abortions directly (e.g., through Medicaid), it is constitutionally acceptable for a state to prohibit the use of public facilities and employees in the performance of abortions. In upholding the constitutionality of the viability-testing provision, he maintains that this provision "permissibly furthers" the state's interest in protecting potential human life. Chief Justice Rehnquist also argues that the present case does not call for a reexamination of *Roe v. Wade*, but he makes very clear his view that the *Roe* trimester framework is both "unsound in principle and unworkable in practice."

This appeal concerns the constitutionality of a Missouri statute regulating the performance of abortions. The

United States Supreme Court. 109 S.Ct. 3040 (1989).

United States Court of Appeals for the Eighth Circuit struck down several provisions of the statute on the ground that they violated this Court's decision in *Roe v. Wade* (1973) and cases following it. We noted probable jurisdiction and now reverse.

I

In June 1986, the Governor of Missouri signed into law Missouri Senate Committee Substitute for House Bill No. 1596 (hereinafter Act or statute), which amended existing state law concerning unborn children and abortions. The Act consisted of 20 provisions, 5 of which are now before the Court. The first provision, or preamble, contains "findings" by the state legislature that "[t]he life of each human being begins at conception," and that "unborn children have protectable interests in life, health, and well-being." The Act further requires that all Missouri laws be interpreted to provide unborn children with the same rights enjoyed by other persons, subject to the Federal Constitution and this Court's precedents. Among its other provisions, the Act requires that, prior to performing an abortion on any woman whom a physician has reason to believe is 20 or more weeks pregnant, the physician ascertain whether the fetus is viable by performing "such medical examinations and tests as are necessary to make a finding of the gestational age, weight, and lung maturity of the unborn child." The Act also prohibits the use of public employees and facilities to perform or assist abortions not necessary to save the mother's life, and it prohibits the use of public funds, employees, or facilities for the purpose of "encouraging or counseling" a woman to have an abortion not necessary to save her life.

In July 1986, five health professionals employed by the State and two nonprofit corporations brought this class action in the United States District Court for the Western District of Missouri to challenge the constitutionality of the Missouri statute. Plaintiffs, appellees in this Court, sought declaratory and injunctive relief on the ground that certain statutory provisions violated the First, Fourth, Ninth, and Fourteenth Amendments to the Federal Constitution....

Plaintiffs filed this suit "on their own behalf and on behalf of the entire class consisting of facilities and Missouri licensed physicians or other health care professionals offering abortion services or pregnancy counseling and on behalf of the entire class of pregnant females seeking abortion services or pregnancy counseling within the State of Missouri." The two nonprofit corporations are Reproductive Health Services, which offers family planning and gynecological services to the public, including abortion services up to 22 weeks "gestational age,"* and Planned Parenthood of Kansas City, which provides abortion services up to 14 weeks gestational age....

Several weeks after the complaint was filed, the District Court temporarily restrained enforcement of several provisions of the Act....

The Court of Appeals for the Eighth Circuit affirmed, with one exception not relevant to this appeal. The Court of Appeals determined that Missouri's declaration that life begins at conception was "simply an impermissible state adoption of a theory of when life begins to justify its abortion regulations." Relying on *Colautti v. Franklin* (1979), it further held that the requirement that physicians perform viability tests was an unconstitutional legislative intrusion on a matter of medical skill and judgment. The Court of Appeals invalidated Missouri's prohibition on the use of public facilities and employees to perform or assist abortions not necessary to save the mother's life. It distinguished our decisions in *Harris* v. *McRae* (1980) and *Maher* v. *Roe* (1977), on the ground that "'[t]here is a fundamental difference between providing direct funding to effect the abortion decision and allowing staff physicians to perform abortions at an existing publicly owned hospital.'" The Court of Appeals struck down the provision prohibiting the use of public funds for "encouraging or counseling" women to have nontherapeutic abortions, for the reason that this provision was both overly vague and inconsistent with the right to an abortion enunciated in *Roe* v. *Wade*....

II

Decision of this case requires us to address four sections of the Missouri Act: (a) the preamble; (b) the prohibition on the use of public facilities or employees to perform abortions; (c) the prohibition on public funding of abortion counseling; and (d) the requirement that physicians conduct viability tests prior to performing abortions. We address these *seriatim*.

A

The Act's preamble, as noted, sets forth "findings" by the Missouri legislature that "[t]he life of each human being begins at conception," and that "[u]nborn children have protectable interests in life, health, and well-being." The Act then mandates that state laws be interpreted to provide unborn children with "all the rights, privileges, and immunities available to other persons,

---

*The Act defines "gestational age" as the "length of pregnancy as measured from the first day of the woman's last menstrual period."

citizens, and residents of this state," subject to the Constitution and this Court's precedents. In invalidating the preamble, the Court of Appeals relied on this Court's dictum that "'a State may not adopt one theory of when life begins to justify its regulation of abortions.' " It rejected Missouri's claim that the preamble was "abortion-neutral," and "merely determine[d] when life begins in a nonabortion context, a traditional state prerogative." The court thought that "[t]he only plausible inference" from the fact that "every remaining section of the bill save one regulates the performance of abortions" was that "the state intended its abortion regulations to be understood against the backdrop of its theory of life."

The State contends that the preamble itself is precatory and imposes no substantive restrictions on abortions....

...Certainly the preamble does not by its terms regulate abortion or any other aspect of appellees' medical practice. The Court has emphasized that *Roe* v. *Wade* "implies no limitation on the authority of a State to make a value judgment favoring childbirth over abortion." The preamble can be read simply to express that sort of value judgment.

We think the extent to which the preamble's language might be used to interpret other state statutes or regulations is something that only the courts of Missouri can definitively decide.... It will be time enough for federal courts to address the meaning of the preamble should it be applied to restrict the activities of appellees in some concrete way.... We therefore need not pass on the constitutionality of the Act's preamble.

B

Section 188.210 provides that "[i]t shall be unlawful for any public employee within the scope of his employment to perform or assist an abortion, not necessary to save the life of the mother," while § 188.215 makes it "unlawful for any public facility to be used for the purpose of performing or assisting an abortion not necessary to save the life of the mother." The Court of Appeals held that these provisions contravened this Court's abortion decisions. We take the contrary view.

As we said earlier this Term..., "our cases have recognized that the Due Process Clauses generally confer no affirmative right to governmental aid, even where such aid may be necessary to secure life, liberty, or property interests of which the government itself may not deprive the individual." In *Maher* v. *Roe, supra,* the Court

upheld a Connecticut welfare regulation under which Medicaid recipients received payments for medical services related to childbirth, but not for nontherapeutic abortions. The Court rejected the claim that this unequal subsidization of childbirth and abortion was impermissible under *Roe* v. *Wade.* As the Court put it:

> "The Connecticut regulation before us is different in kind from the laws invalidated in our previous abortion decisions. The Connecticut regulation places no obstacles—absolute or otherwise—in the pregnant woman's path to an abortion. An indigent woman who desires an abortion suffers no disadvantage as a consequence of Connecticut's decision to fund childbirth; she continues as before to be dependent on private sources for the service she desires. The State may have made childbirth a more attractive alternative, thereby influencing the woman's decision, but it has imposed no restriction on access to abortions that was not already there. The indigency that may make it difficult—and in some cases, perhaps, impossible—for some women to have abortions is neither created nor in any way affected by the Connecticut regulation."

Relying on *Maher,* the Court in *Poelker* v. *Doe* (1977) held that the city of St. Louis committed "no constitutional violation...in electing, as a policy choice, to provide publicly financed hospital services for childbirth without providing corresponding services for nontherapeutic abortions."

More recently, in *Harris* v. *McRae* (1980), the Court upheld "the most restrictive version of the Hyde Amendment," which withheld from States federal funds under the Medicaid program to reimburse the costs of abortions, "'except where the life of the mother would be endangered if the fetus were carried to term.' " As in *Maher* and *Poelker,* the Court required only a showing that Congress' authorization of "reimbursement for medically necessary services generally, but not for certain medically necessary abortions" was rationally related to the legitimate governmental goal of encouraging childbirth.

The Court of Appeals distinguished these cases on the ground that "[t]o prevent access to a public facility does more than demonstrate a political choice in favor of childbirth; it clearly narrows and in some cases forecloses the availability of abortion to women." The court reasoned that the ban on the use of public facilities "could prevent a woman's chosen doctor from performing an abortion because of his unprivileged status at other hospitals or because a private hospital adopted a similar anti-abortion stance." It also thought that "[s]uch a rule could increase the cost of obtaining an abortion and delay the timing of it as well."

We think that this analysis is much like that which we rejected in *Maher, Poelker,* and *McRae.* As in those cases, the State's decision here to use public facilities and staff to encourage childbirth over abortion "places no governmental obstacle in the path of a woman who chooses to terminate her pregnancy." Just as Congress' refusal to fund abortions in *McRae* left "an indigent woman with at least the same range of choice in deciding whether to obtain a medically necessary abortion as she would have had if Congress had chosen to subsidize no health care costs at all," Missouri's refusal to allow public employees to perform abortions in public hospitals leaves a pregnant woman with the same choices as if the State had chosen not to operate any public hospitals at all. The challenged provisions only restrict a woman's ability to obtain an abortion to the extent that she chooses to use a physician affiliated with a public hospital. This circumstance is more easily remedied, and thus considerably less burdensome, than indigency, which "may make it difficult—and in some cases, perhaps, impossible—for some women to have abortions" without public funding. Having held that the State's refusal to fund abortions does not violate *Roe* v. *Wade,* it strains logic to reach a contrary result for the use of public facilities and employees. If the State may "make a value judgment favoring childbirth over abortion and... implement that judgment by the allocation of public funds," surely it may do so through the allocation of other public resources, such as hospitals and medical staff....

...Thus we uphold the Act's restrictions on the use of public employees and facilities for the performance or assistance of nontherapeutic abortions.

C

The Missouri Act contains three provisions relating to "encouraging or counseling a woman to have an abortion not necessary to save her life." Section 188.205 states that no public funds can be used for this purpose; § 188.210 states that public employees cannot, within the scope of their employment, engage in such speech; and § 188.215 forbids such speech in public facilities. The Court of Appeals did not consider § 188.205 separately from §§ 188.210 and 188.215. It held that all three of these provisions were unconstitutionally vague, and that

"the ban on using public funds, employees, and facilities to encourage or counsel a woman to have an abortion is an unacceptable infringement of the woman's fourteenth amendment right to choose an abortion after receiving the medical information necessary to exercise the right knowingly and intelligently."

Missouri has chosen only to appeal the Court of Appeals' invalidation of the public funding provision, § 188.205. A threshold question is whether this provision reaches primary conduct, or whether it is simply an instruction to the State's fiscal officers not to allocate funds for abortion counseling. We accept, for purposes of decision, the State's claim that § 188.205 "is not directed at the conduct of any physician or health care provider, private or public," but "is directed solely at those persons responsible for expending public funds."

Appellees contend that they are not "adversely" affected under the State's interpretation of § 188.205, and therefore that there is no longer a case or controversy before us on this question....A majority of the Court agrees with appellees that the controversy over § 188.205 is now moot....

D

Section 188.029 of the Missouri Act provides:

"Before a physician performs an abortion on a woman he has reason to believe is carrying an unborn child of twenty or more weeks gestational age, the physician shall first determine if the unborn child is viable by using and exercising that degree of care, skill, and proficiency commonly exercised by the ordinarily skillful, careful, and prudent physician engaged in similar practice under the same or similar conditions. In making this determination of viability, the physician shall perform or cause to be performed such medical examinations and tests as are necessary to make a finding of the gestational age, weight, and lung maturity of the unborn child and shall enter such findings and determination of viability in the medical record of the mother."

As with the preamble, the parties disagree over the meaning of this statutory provision. The State emphasizes the language of the first sentence, which speaks in terms of the physician's determination of viability being made by the standards of ordinary skill in the medical profession. Appellees stress the language of the second sentence, which prescribes such "tests as are necessary" to make a finding of gestational age, fetal weight, and lung maturity.

The Court of Appeals read § 188.029 as requiring that after 20 weeks "doctors *must* perform tests to find gestational age, fetal weight and lung maturity." The court indicated that the tests needed to determine fetal weight at 20 weeks are "unreliable and inaccurate" and would add $125 to $250 to the cost of an abortion. It also stated that "amniocentesis, the only method available to determine lung maturity, is contrary to accepted medical practice until 28–30 weeks of gestation, expensive, and imposes significant health risks for both the pregnant woman and the fetus."

We must first determine the meaning of § 188.029 under Missouri law. Our usual practice is to defer to the lower court's construction of a state statute, but we believe the Court of Appeals has "fallen into plain error" in this case. "'In expounding a statute, we must not be guided by a single sentence or member of a sentence, but look to the provisions of the whole law, and to its object and policy.' " The Court of Appeals' interpretation also runs "afoul of the well-established principle that statutes will be interpreted to avoid constitutional difficulties."

We think the viability-testing provision makes sense only if the second sentence is read to require only those tests that are useful to making subsidiary findings as to viability. If we construe this provision to require a physician to perform those tests needed to make the three specified findings *in all circumstances*, including when the physician's reasonable professional judgment indicates that the tests would be irrelevant to determining viability or even dangerous to the mother and the fetus, the second sentence of § 188.029 would conflict with the first sentence's *requirement* that a physician apply his reasonable professional skill and judgment. It would also be incongruous to read this provision, especially the word "necessary," to require the performance of tests irrelevant to the expressed statutory purpose of determining viability. It thus seems clear to us that the Court of Appeals' construction of § 188.029 violates well-accepted canons of statutory interpretation used in the Missouri courts....

The viability-testing provision of the Missouri Act is concerned with promoting the State's interest in potential human life rather than in maternal health. Section 188.029 creates what is essentially a presumption of viability at 20 weeks, which the physician must rebut with tests indicating that the fetus is not viable prior to performing an abortion. It also directs the physician's determination as to viability by specifying consideration, if

feasible, of gestational age, fetal weight, and lung capacity. The District Court found that "the medical evidence is uncontradicted that a 20-week fetus is *not* viable," and that "23½ to 24 weeks gestation is the earliest point in pregnancy where a reasonable possibility of viability exists." But it also found that there may be a 4-week error in estimating gestational age, which supports testing at 20 weeks.

In *Roe* v. *Wade*, the Court recognized that the State has "important and legitimate" interests in protecting maternal health and in the potentiality of human life. During the second trimester, the State "may, if it chooses, regulate the abortion procedure in ways that are reasonably related to maternal health." After viability, when the State's interest in potential human life was held to become compelling, the State "may, if it chooses, regulate, and even proscribe, abortion except where it is necessary, in appropriate medical judgment, for the preservation of the life or health of the mother."

In *Colautti* v. *Franklin, supra,* upon which appellees rely, the Court held that a Pennsylvania statute regulating the standard of care to be used by a physician performing an abortion of a possibly viable fetus was void for vagueness. But in the course of reaching that conclusion, the Court reaffirmed its earlier statement in *Planned Parenthood of Central Missouri* v. *Danforth* (1976), that "'the determination of whether a particular fetus is viable is, and must be, a matter for the judgement of the responsible attending physician.' " The dissent ignores the statement in *Colautti* that "neither the legislature nor the courts may proclaim one of the elements entering into the ascertainment of viability—be it weeks of gestation or fetal weight or any other single factor—as the determinant of when the State has a compelling interest in the life or health of the fetus." To the extent that § 188.029 regulates the method for determining viability, it undoubtedly does superimpose state regulation on the medical determination of whether a particular fetus is viable. The Court of Appeals and the District Court thought it unconstitutional for this reason. To the extent that the viability tests increase the cost of what are in fact second-trimester abortions, their validity may also be questioned under *Akron* v. *Akron Center for Reproductive Health* (1983), where the Court held that a requirement that second trimester abortions must be performed in hospitals was invalid because it substantially increased the expense of those procedures.

We think that the doubt cast upon the Missouri statute by these cases is not so much a flaw in the statute as it is a reflection of the fact that the rigid trimester analysis of the course of a pregnancy enunciated in *Roe* has resulted in subsequent cases like *Colautti* and *Akron* making constitutional law in this area a virtual Procrustean bed. Statutes specifying elements of informed consent to be provided abortion patients, for example, were invalidated if they were thought to "structur[e] ...the dialogue between the woman and her physician." *Thornburgh* v. *American College of Obstetricians and Gynecologists* (1986). As the dissenters in *Thornburgh* pointed out, such a statute would have been sustained under any traditional standard of judicial review, or for any other surgical procedure except abortion.

Stare decisis is a cornerstone of our legal system, but it has less power in constitutional cases, where, save for constitutional amendments, this Court is the only body able to make needed changes. We have not refrained from reconsideration of a prior construction of the Constitution that has proved "unsound in principle and unworkable in practice." We think the *Roe* trimester framework falls into that category.

In the first place, the rigid *Roe* framework is hardly consistent with the notion of a Constitution cast in general terms, as ours is, and usually speaking in general principles, as ours does. The key elements of the *Roe* framework—trimesters and viability—are not found in the text of the Constitution or in any place else one would expect to find a constitutional principle. Since the bounds of the inquiry are essentially indeterminate, the result has been a web of legal rules that have become increasingly intricate, resembling a code of regulations rather than a body of constitutional doctrine. As JUSTICE WHITE has put it, the trimester framework has left this Court to serve as the country's "*ex officio* medical board with powers to approve or disapprove medical and operative practices and standards throughout the United States."

In the second place, we do not see why the State's interest in protecting potential human life should come into existence only at the point of viability, and that there should therefore be a rigid line allowing state regulation after viability but prohibiting it before viability. The dissenters in *Thornburgh*, writing in the context of the *Roe* trimester analysis, would have recognized this fact by positing against the "fundamental right" recognized in *Roe* the State's "compelling interest" in protecting potential human life throughout pregnancy....

The tests that § 188.029 requires the physician to perform are designed to determine viability. The State here has chosen viability as the point at which its interest in potential human life must be safeguarded. It is true that the tests in question increase the expense of abor-

tion, and regulate the discretion of the physician in determining the viability of the fetus. Since the tests will undoubtedly show in many cases that the fetus is not viable, the tests will have been performed for what were in fact second-trimester abortions. But we are satisfied that the requirement of these tests permissibly furthers the State's interest in protecting potential human life, and we therefore believe § 188.029 to be constitutional.

The dissent takes us to task for our failure to join in a "great issues" debate as to whether the Constitution includes an "unenumerated" general right to privacy as recognized in cases such as *Griswold* v. *Connecticut* (1965) and *Roe*. But *Griswold* v. *Connecticut*, unlike *Roe*, did not purport to adopt a whole framework, complete with detailed rules and distinctions, to govern the cases in which the asserted liberty interest would apply. As such, it was far different from the opinion, if not the holding, of *Roe* v. *Wade*, which sought to establish a constitutional framework for judging state regulation of abortion during the entire term of pregnancy. That framework sought to deal with areas of medical practice traditionally subject to state regulation, and it sought to balance once and for all by reference only to the calendar the claims of the State to protect the fetus as a form of human life against the claims of a woman to decide for herself whether or not to abort a fetus she was carrying. The experience of the Court in applying *Roe* v. *Wade* in later cases suggests to us that there is wisdom in not unnecessarily attempting to elaborate the abstract differences between a "fundamental right" to abortion, as the Court described it in *Akron*, a "limited fundamental constitutional right," which JUSTICE BLACKMUN's dissent today treats *Roe* as having established, or a liberty interest protected by the Due Process Clause, which we believe it to be. The Missouri testing requirement here is reasonably designed to ensure that abortions are not performed where the fetus is viable—an end which all concede is legitimate—and that is sufficient to sustain its constitutionality.

The dissent also accuses us, *inter alia*, of cowardice and illegitimacy in dealing with "the most politically divisive domestic legal issue of our time." There is no doubt that our holding today will allow some governmental regulation of abortion that would have been prohibited under the language of cases such as *Colautti* v. *Franklin* and *Akron* v. *Akron Center for Reproductive Health, Inc., supra*. But the goal of constitutional adjudication is surely not to remove inexorably "politically divisive" issues from the ambit of the legislative process, whereby the people through their elected representatives deal with matters of concern to them. The goal of constitutional adjudication is to hold true the balance between that which the Constitution puts beyond the reach of the democratic process and that which it does not. We think we have done that today. The dissent's suggestion that legislative bodies, in a Nation where more than half of our population is women, will treat our decision today as an invitation to enact abortion regulation reminiscent of the dark ages not only misreads our views but does scant justice to those who serve in such bodies and the people who elect them.

III

Both appellants and the United States as *Amicus Curiae* have urged that we overrule our decision in *Roe* v.

Wade. The facts of the present case, however, differ from those at issue in *Roe*. Here, Missouri has determined that viability is the point at which its interest in potential human life must be safeguarded. In *Roe*, on the other hand, the Texas statute criminalized the performance of *all* abortions, except when the mother's life was at stake. This case therefore affords us no occasion to revisit the holding of *Roe*, which was that the Texas statute unconstitutionally infringed the right to an abortion derived from the Due Process Clause, and we leave it undisturbed. To the extent indicated in our opinion, we would modify and narrow *Roe* and succeeding cases.

Because none of the challenged provisions of the Missouri Act properly before us conflict with the Constitution, the judgment of the Court of Appeals is *Reversed*.

Maternal/Fetal Conflicts

Moral Obligations to the Not-Yet Born: The Fetus as Patient
Thomas H. Murray

Thomas H. Murray is director, Center for Biomedical Ethics, Case Western Reserve University. He is the coeditor of *Feeling Good and Doing Better: Ethics and Nontherapeutic Drug Use* (1984) and *Which Babies Shall Live?* (1985). His published articles include "The Final Anticlimactic Rule on Baby Doe" and "Genetic Screening in the Workplace: Ethical Issues."

Murray distinguishes between fetuses who will be aborted and fetuses who will be brought to live birth. He calls the latter "not-yet-born" children and argues that we have moral obligations to them. In his view, even if it is morally permissible to abort a fetus prior to viability, it does not follow that it is permissible to harm a not-yet-born child prior to viability; the timing of harm is morally irrelevant. In exploring the scope and magnitude of a woman's obligation to avoid harming a not-yet-born child, Murray warns against losing track of the overall moral context of a woman's life. In typical cases, he argues, a woman's duty to avoid harming her not-yet-born child must be balanced against a multitude of other moral considerations. Murray also provides a brief analysis of an obstetrician's duty to ensure that the fetus-patient is being protected. With regard to public policy, he maintains that "the state must be very cautious in using its power to enforce particular notions of maternal duties."

The health of the not-yet-born child—the fetus intended to be brought to live birth—periodically emerges as a subject of concern. From dramatic interventions such as

Reprinted with permission of the author and the publisher from *Clinics in Perinatology*, vol. 14 (June 1987), pp. 329–343.

fetal surgery through drugs and special diets on to efforts to get pregnant women to abstain from alcohol and tobacco or to bar them from workplaces possibly toxic to developing fetuses, there has been a recent surge of ideas on how to prevent, ameliorate, or remedy damage to the not-yet-born.

Many things might be done *with,* *by* or *to* a pregnant woman to benefit her not-yet-born child. They range from the most physically intrusive to the least, from the most technologically sophisticated to mundane efforts at education and persuasion, from those with clearly established benefit to the fetus to those of highly uncertain benefit. The ethical issues raised by interventions of all kinds designed to aid a fetus share essential features. Once some form of fetal surgery becomes established, the case of a woman who refuses it will raise many of the same moral questions as that of a woman whose alcoholism threatens her fetus's health to a point where incarceration or institutionalization are being considered. Although different in several respects, both of the cases require asking how far the state—and physicians as agents of the state—ought to go in coercively intervening in the life of a woman in order to benefit her fetus. And both presume at least a tentative answer to a difficult ethical question: What is the moral status of a fetus?

To answer such a question sensibly and with a modicum of wisdom is our ultimate goal. A burgeoning literature on fetal therapies, fetal surgery, fetal rights, and maternal-fetal conflicts has enlivened the argument. While technologically sophisticated interventions like fetal surgery are receiving the most attention, they will probably be relevant to only a minute proportion of all pregnancies. Yet most of the ethical questions raised by fetal surgery are equally pertinent to a host of other, less glamorous means to the same end. Some sample questions include the following:

> How far should we go in getting diabetic women to manage their disease during pregnancy?: Should we inform them of the consequences to their fetus? Should we try to persuade them gently? Browbeat them? If they refuse to cooperate should we initiate civil or criminal proceedings to try and coerce them? Should we try to institutionalize them as has been done in some cases of drug addicted mothers, and then perhaps strip them of their children once they are born?
>
> What about a mother suspected of using drugs—legal or illegal—that might deleteriously affect the fetus? What of the mother who smokes or drinks? How hard do we try to discourage her smoking or drinking during pregnancy? If she continues to do either or both heavily, at what point if any do we move beyond persuasion to coercion?
>
> If we think that low levels of a potentially embryotoxic or fetotoxic substance are present in a workplace, should all pregnant women be kept out? What about "potentially pregnant," that is, nonsterile women? Many

United States companies have "Fetal Protection Policies" that do just that.[25]

KEY ISSUES

Given the present, chaotic state of the debate over fundamental issues of ethics, law, and public policy regarding the fetus, offering simple answers to questions such as the ones just asked would require ignoring even more important questions. It is more valuable in the long run to clarify some of the fundamental issues now. Five are discussed in this article.

1. Whether there are any moral duties to a fetus.

2. Whether viability affects those duties.

3. How the concept of duties to a fetus is frequently misused.

4. What pitfalls must be avoided in moving from moral judgments to public policy.

5. The importance of the social and historical context of the current debate.

DO WE HAVE MORAL DUTIES TO A FETUS?

The moral status of those fetuses who will never be born alive is problematic. Right-to-life advocates claim that even the fertilized ovum is a person, entitled to all the protections and respect due every person. Many other people, including many of those with qualms about abortion, believe that the fetus, especially in its early stages of development, has a lesser moral stature than adults, infants, or even late-term fetuses. No consensus exists on such fetuses. Fortunately, we can discuss the fetus as patient without becoming bogged down in the mire of the abortion debate. All we need is a simple distinction between those fetuses destined to be brought to live birth, and those who will not know extrauterine life.

The Not-Yet-Born Child

The situation is quite different for fetuses who will be born alive. A few theorists argue that the fetus, or even the infant and young child, has no moral status, or else an inferior one.[24] Some writers, while not directly addressing the question, argue that whatever moral claims the fetus might have are always secondary to those of the woman in whose body the fetus lies.[2] Nonetheless, there is good reason to believe that we have moral obligations to the fetus destined to be born, who we will call the not-yet-born child to distinguish it from both the already-born child and from the fetus who will not be born alive. Further, this view has considerable popular support, as evidenced by the efforts aimed at preserving fetal health through antenatal medical care, public health education of pregnant women, and the like.

The Timing of a Harm Is Irrelevant

Imagine two different cases. In the first, a man assaults a woman with the intention of inflicting grave harm on her fetus. He succeeds, causing permanent, irreparable—but not fatal—damage to the fetus's spinal cord, resulting in paralysis. In the second case, all the circumstances are identical, except that the man attacks an infant rather than a fetus, with the same result—permanent, irreparable paralysis. Was the first act any less wrong than the second? In both cases, lifelong harm was done to humans who, whatever your beliefs about when personhood begins, would eventually cross that line and attain full moral status.

My thesis, in short, is that the timing of a harm, in itself, is not morally relevant. An act resulting in harm to a not-yet-born person (who will eventually be a full-fledged person according to everyone's moral theory) is as great a harm as if it were done later. The morally relevant factors are the usual ones: the actor's intentions; excuses; mitigating circumstances; and so on. In practice, a fetus is rarely harmed intentionally; typically, harm to a fetus occurs as a result of intentional or unintentional harm to its mother. The lack of intention to harm then is what affects our judgment about the wrongness of the act, and not the fact that it was a not-yet-born person who was harmed. We would judge unintended harm to a child or adult in a similar manner. The debate over the ethics of abortion aside, then, we can talk sensibly and without inherent contradiction about moral duties to the fetus destined to become a person—to the not-yet-born person. There will be duties to avoid harm, and there may be duties to render aid.

We can discuss moral duties to not-yet-born persons without becoming hopelessly trapped in the abortion debate. Before moving on to discuss the scope of our duties to the fetus, we need to consider whether viability affects these duties.

THE MORAL RELEVANCE OF VIABILITY

Viability is, at best, a slippery concept. For one thing it is a moving front. As our ability to save younger and smaller newborns improves, the so-called age of viability is reached earlier. Physicians frequently use viability as a statistical concept: the age at which some unspecified percentage of newborns will survive. Sometimes the concept is used with reference to specific infants. We could describe survival possibilities as a probabilistic function of weight or gestational age. For example, the BW or GA 10 would be the birthweight or gestational age at which 10 per cent of infants survive. The GA 50 would be the level at which 50 per cent live, and so on. These numbers would change as our ability to save these infants changes.

Viability and Abortion

The central question is whether our moral obligations to the fetus change as a function of viability. Viability as a determinant of our duties to a fetus was given great importance by its inclusion in the well-known Supreme Court abortion decision, *Roe v. Wade*.[19] The complex ruling says in its summary: "For the stage subsequent to viability, the State in promoting its interest in the potentiality of human life may, if it chooses, regulate, and even proscribe, abortion except where it is necessary, in appropriate medical judgment, for the preservation of the life or health of the mother."[19]

Viability serves as a threshhold in *Roe v. Wade*. Even though the Court uses the ambiguous phrase "potentiality of human life," behind their decision must lie some notion of the fetus growing in legal and presumably moral stature as it approaches term. Otherwise, there would be no justification for linking the State's interest in protecting that potential life with viability which, at the time of that decision (1973), roughly coincided with the end of the second trimester for most fetuses.

Attempting to uncover the moral reasoning underlying a legal decision can be perilous because one may simply be wrong and because it may encourage the unfortunate tendency to see moral disapproval as a sufficient reason for taking legal action, something we will take up later. Bearing that caution in mind, we nonetheless must try to determine what moral ideas underlie the legal reasoning in *Roe v. Wade*. The court appears to believe that, prior to viability, whatever claim the fetus may have not to be killed is outweighed by a woman's right to choose whether or not to bear and give birth to a child, with all that those activities bring in their wake. After viability, the fetus's increasing nearness to actual rather than merely potential life strengthens its moral claim against being killed to the point where it overrides the mother's right to choose not to bear a child, though not so far as to force her to risk her own life in doing so.

Viability Is Irrelevent for Nonfatal Harms

In other words, for the problem of deciding whether a woman can abort her fetus, it may be important to know what the fetus's moral status is *at that particular moment*: whether or not it is a person or how close it is to becoming a full-fledged person may be important in this context. In stark contrast, the fetus's moral standing at that moment in its development is not relevant to judging our duties to avoid or avert nonfatal harms, since, as far as we know, the fetus will some day be a full person, and the timing of such nonlethal harms is not pertinent to determining their wrongfulness. Interestingly, the law itself seems to agree.

Until 1946, a child injured prenatally then born alive but impaired rarely found a court willing to sustain a suit for damages. But in that year began what Prosser, who wrote the standard reference work on tort law, called "the most spectacular abrupt reversal of a well settled rule in the whole history of the law of torts. The child, provided that he is born alive, is permitted to maintain an action for the consequences of prenatal injuries, and if he dies of such injuries after birth an action will lie for his wrongful death."[16] Prosser believed that the earlier denials of claims on behalf of children injured while they were still fetuses were based on invalid reasoning, and he approved of the reversal.

With the concept of prenatal injuries established as a valid one, does it matter whether the fetus was viable at the time of injury? Some courts have required that the fetus have been viable, or at least "quickened" at the time of injury.[16] But many courts have rejected viability as a relevant factor in determining whether the born child may recover for prenatal injury.[9] One critic of the concept of fetal rights says pointedly: "[V]iability is a meaningless distinction in the fetal rights context because the state's interest in the health of its future citi-

zens is equally strong throughout pregnancy."[8] Prosser himself says: "[c]ertainly the [previable] infant may be no less injured; and all logic is in favor of ignoring the stage at which it occurs." Acknowledging that proving injury early in pregnancy might be difficult, he concludes "[t]his, however, goes to proof rather than principle; and if, as is undoubtedly the case there are injuries as to which reliable medical proof is possible, it makes no sense to deny recovery on any such arbitrary basis."[16] The moral principle, that is, does not depend on the arbitrary criterion of viability.

While most cases have focused on recovering damages for harms already done, a number of recent cases attempt to prevent harm by affecting the pregnant woman's behavior, even to the point of outright coercion....[F]orced caesarean cases...are one sort of example.[23] In another case (reported by a newspaper) a physician accused a woman, seven months pregnant, of endangering her fetus's development by abusing drugs. The woman was ordered to enter a drug rehabilitation program and undergo regular urinalyses until the child was born.[21] Whether this is a reasonable response to the problem is the subject of the next section.

MISUSING THE IDEA OF DUTIES TO A FETUS

A recurrent theme in this essay is the danger of making moral judgments or public policy without sufficient regard for context. Just this sort of misuse of the concept of duties to a fetus occurs with unsettling frequency.

The Dangers of Oversimplifying Moral Decisions

The moral world we inhabit is one marked by a multiplicity of interests and duties. We are certainly entitled to give good moral weight to our own interests. Then there are duties to those with whom we have special relationships, relationships that prescribe even strenuous moral duties in certain domains. Finally, we have duties to "strangers"—those with whom no special moral relationship exists. Most significant moral decisions have implications for many of these interests and relationships simultaneously. For example, a woman who must decide whether to place her fetus at risk of harm by working in a factory with low levels of a suspected fetotoxin must weigh her own interests in having a job with the psychological and material benefits that may bring against the risks imposed on herself as well as her fetus. She must also consider possible benefits to her fetus that the job makes possible, such as improved nutrition for herself and prenatal care facilitated by health insurance. Then there may be others dependent on her working: a spouse, other children, perhaps elderly parents. When we portray the ethical dimensions of her decision as beginning and ending with the question of whether or not she has duties to avoid exposing her fetus to risks, we rip such a complex decision out of its moral, as well as its social and political, context. Yet, this is commonly done. Or, not much better, the woman's "right" to do whatever she desires is counterposed to the fetus's right to protection from harm. Once the problem is framed this way, giving a nuanced answer becomes impossible. A more complex view of the moral life, one that encompasses a multiplicity of legitimate moral concerns, of interests and duties, of roles and relationships, allows us to frame the question in a way that can be answered, if not more easily, at least more satisfactorily.

Warnings of Fearful Consequences

In a clash of rights, complex issues can become stripped of their nuances and turned into simplistic all-or-none contests. On either extreme, we can imagine bleak consequences. If, on the one hand, we give pre-eminence to the fetus's right to avoid being harmed, then must pregnant women structure every detail of their lives in order to avoid all suspected risks to their not-yet-born-child? Such an attitude appears to have influenced some companies to adopt so-called "Fetal Protection Policies," or FPPs, that deny employment opportunities to women.[25] Fears of what would happen should fetal rights gain the upper hand generate a litany of nightmarish possibilities:

> A woman could be held civilly or criminally liable for fetal injuries caused by accidents resulting from maternal negligence, such as automobile or household accidents. She could also be held liable for any behavior during her pregnancy having potentially adverse effects on her fetus, including failure to eat properly, using prescription, nonprescription and illegal drugs, smoking, drinking alcohol, exposing herself to infectious disease or to any workplace hazards, engaging in immoderate exercise or sexual intercourse, residing at high altitudes for prolonged periods, or using a general anesthetic or drugs to induce rapid labor during delivery. If the current trend in fetal rights continues, pregnant women would live in constant fear

that any accident or "error" in judgment could be deemed "unacceptable" and become the basis for a criminal prosecution by the state or a civil suit...[8]

On the other hand, if we give full sway to the woman's right to control her body, can we even level moral criticism against a case such as the one of a woman who at 40 weeks gestation, in labor with abruptio placenta with fetal distress, refused a caesarean section? After the infant was delivered stillborn, she explained to a nurse that "the death of the fetus solved complicated personal problems."[12] The language of rights in conflict may not permit us to give full and weighty consideration to a host of factors that we believe are important in making moral judgments. Examining relationships, legitimate interests, and duties may give us a more adequate picture of the moral choices people face.

Obligations to the Not-Yet-Born Are Not All or None

Take, for example, the case of the woman who must decide whether to accept a job that might pose some risk to her fetus. Let us suppose that she intends to bring the child to birth, so we do not have to worry about the ethics of abortion. As far as we know, this is a not-yet-born child; therefore the woman has some obligation to avoid harming it while it is still a fetus. What is the scope and intensity of this obligation? Must she refuse the job?

Because of the link between most discussions of the fetus's moral status and abortion, there is an unfortunate tendency to think of our obligations to the fetus as all-or-none. But there are other creatures dependent on us, to whom we have obligations, but where those duties do not unequivocally overwhelm all other considerations—our children for example. We certainly have a duty to do what is reasonable to protect our young children from harm. That requires keeping them from known and probable dangers. But we are not required to sacrifice everything else to this task. We should teach them not to play in busy streets, and offer them a protected play-area. But must we build crash-proof barriers around their playground, strong enough to stop a cement truck run wild? Obviously not. That would be beyond "reasonable" responsibility. Anytime we take them in a car, there is a risk of injury or death. Responsible parents should provide a secure carseat for their infant or toddler. But we are not forbidden from going for a drive, even though no matter how carefully we drive there is always the distinct possibility of an accident.

What is it that makes certain risks reasonable, and others the kind that responsible parents would not take? The probability of harm and its severity should it occur are certainly relevant. Also significant is the importance of the purpose for which the risk is run and the avoidability of the risk. If we want the children to see their grandparents, a long car ride may be unavoidable. And exposing our child to the considerable risks of cytotoxic drugs is clearly justifiable if and only if our purpose is to treat them for cancer.

My purpose here is to put us on more familiar ground than the exotic situations in which questions of fetal status typically arise. Two points come out of the discussion. First, whatever moral duties we might have to a fetus—a not-yet-born child—they may equal but not exceed our duties to already-born children. The circumstances of a fetus's physical enclosure within and link to its mother's body confuses many discussions. This linkage may mean that a broader range of actions might affect the fetus, and the facts of the case will be accordingly affected. But the same moral considerations apply equally to both the not-yet-born and the already-born—considerations such as intentions, probability and severity of risk, and duties to others. Second, duties to the not-yet-born, like duties to the already-born, are usually just one of many factors to be considered in judging the moral acceptability of an act.

Another advantage of discussing our obligations to the not-yet-born and already-born together is that it enables us to talk about fathers and not just mothers. To the extent that cultural blinders distort our view of a mother's responsibility to her fetus, then looking at a case with comparable morally relevant features, but one that asks about a father's responsibility to his child, may restore some moral clarity.

A Father–Child Analogy

Take the plausible case of a man who lost his job in the oil fields of west Texas. He has two children counting on him for support; his wife is also out of work. An offer comes of a job in a petrochemical plant near Houston. Taking that job will mean moving his family to a part of Texas crawling with petrochemical complexes where toxic releases into the air, ground, and water are not unknown, and where the risk of cancer is somewhat, though not drastically, higher than in their current community. There are a number of good reasons to take the job. He will be able to afford better food, clothing, and housing for his family and himself. Being unemployed

threatens his sense of self-worth, which depresses him and incidentally also makes him a less thoughtful parent and spouse. Like most unemployed Americans, when he lost his job he also lost his health insurance; the new job will assure better access to health care for himself and his family. Perhaps the schools are better in the new community. Suppose he accepts the job even though he knows and regrets the increased risk that will mean for his children. Decisions such as this are all-things-considered choices: by their nature they involve weighing and balancing many things. Would we say that this man's choice was immoral? That he should not have exposed his children to the slightly increased risk of cancer whatever else was involved? It would make better sense to say that he made a responsible, morally defensible decision, even if we share his regret about the increased risk to which his children as well as his wife and himself will be exposed.

How was this man's decision any different from that of a woman who chooses to accept a job, knowing that her fetus will be exposed to some low but nonetheless increased risk of harm because of exposures there? Perhaps she too is without health insurance. Perhaps having a job is important to her sense of self-worth. Perhaps there are other children and a spouse at home who are dependent on her. The fact that she carries a fetus within her, a not-yet-born child, that she has moral duties to protect that fetus from harm, and that the workplace increases slightly the probability of harm does not make her decision immoral. Exactly the same considerations were relevant to the man's decision. To the extent that the morally relevant factors are comparable—and in this case they might well be identical—the decisions are equally justified. And if the circumstances vary, at least we know the kinds of morally significant considerations that will influence our judgments.[15] Whether it is a man or a woman is not relevant. Nor, I have argued, does it matter whether it is a not-yet-born or already-born child.

FROM ETHICAL JUDGMENTS TO PUBLIC POLICY

We do not ban all conduct we regard as morally suspect, nor do we compel people to carry out every moral duty. Many things are left to personal conscience, to moral suasion, or to social pressure. For good reasons, including moral ones, we are reluctant to allow the state to force its view of correct conduct on individuals unless the harm to be avoided is grave, especially when doing so requires coercion, bodily invasion, or incarceration. These means are among the most repugnant and are reserved for extreme circumstances. If we conclude then that a woman morally ought to quit smoking during pregnancy, moderate or eliminate her consumption of alcohol, and do likewise with caffeine, this does not automatically justify heavy-handed state intervention to assure that she does these things. Some wrongs are minimally so. The state should not exercise its often great power on such things. Sometimes the effort to correct a wrong itself creates new moral problems. The moral and other costs of enforcement may outweigh the good that might be done.

The fetus becomes a "patient" when its welfare becomes the physician's concern. The obstetrician caring for a mother and not-yet-born child has two patients. In much the way that a pediatrician advises parents about their newborn's diet, monitors the infant's health, and prescribes needed medication or other therapeutic interventions, an obstetrician routinely does the same for the mother and the fetus-patient. How extensive is the obstetrician's duty to assure that the fetus-patient's welfare is being protected?

The "Child-as-Maximum" Principle

One useful guideline might be called the "child-as-maximum" principle. The principle says that our obligations to ensure the fetus's welfare can equal but not exceed our obligations to a born child. If a pediatrician would not be obliged to do more than try to persuade parents to do a certain thing—say observe a special diet—then under conditions of comparable burdens and benefits, obstetricians cannot be obliged to do more to protect a fetus, although they may be required to do less.

One inescapable difference between the obstetrician's and the pediatrician's case is of course that the former's second patient, the fetus, is encased in the body of the first patient, the mother. All interventions directed at the fetus literally must go through its mother. The burdens created, therefore, generally will be much greater, as will be the potential for morally wronging one person in the effort to aid another. This is why the child-as-maximum principle emphasizes that our duties to a born child constitute an upper-bound for our duties to a not-yet-born child rather than a strict equivalence. A drug that might benefit a fetus but that will be harmful to the mother can be refused. That same drug for that same being, now born, should probably be adminis-

tered. The pediatrician in the latter instance is justified in pushing harder for consent from the parents than was the obstetrician.

A Variety of Needs, a Range of Interventions

One study shows that women who smoke a pack of cirarettes or more a day have babies on average about 180 gm smaller at birth than women who do not smoke. The same study found that women who drank twenty or more beers per month sacrificed roughly 100 gm of birthweight, while those who consumed 300 or more grams of caffeine daily (three or four cups of coffee or seven cola beverages) had babies 40 to 50 gm smaller on average.[11] What should physicians do? When the risks are small, we usually employ education and persuasion. That is the typical and appropriate response to maternal smoking, diet, nutritional supplements, and the like. These anchor one end of a continuum of possible "interventions." We can move to stronger measures, such as New York City has done, by requiring that signs be posted in public places serving alcohol warning pregnant women that alcohol may endanger their fetus's health. This is a public policy that relies as much on shame as on the educative effect of the signs.

Beyond this is a broad range of more traditionally "medical" interventions: managing maternal diabetes in pregnancy[4]; placing women with PKU on low-phenylalanine diets when they wish to become pregnant[18]; treating fetal methylmelonic acidemia by giving Vitamin B-12 to the mother[20]; treating congenital hypothyroidism by injections into the amniotic fluid[26]; drug therapy for fetal ventricular tachycardia,[10] and other possibilities.

There are surgical routes as well. In addition to the familiar exchange transfusions for erythroblastosis fetalis, a variety of still-experimental fetal surgeries are under development. They include procedures responding to urinary tract obstruction,[5] ventriculomegaly,[1] diaphragmatic hernia,[7] and hematopoietic stem cell transplantation for severe immunologic deficiencies.[22] (The law and ethics of fetal surgery have been amply discussed elsewhere.[3, 14, 17])

Our ethical analysis of any proposed interventions to benefit a fetus intended to be brought to birth should include at least the following considerations:

1. How certain is the benefit to the fetus? (Is the intervention experimental? Is it well-established? Does it carry substantial risks to the fetus?)

2. How great are the benefits? (Will a successful intervention make a large or small difference in the fetus's prognosis?)

3. How intrusive, coercive, or harmful will it be to the mother?

4. Will anything be lost or gained by waiting until after the child is born?

Even if we are convinced that the mother has a moral responsibility to agree to the intervention, the question of how far we should go in attempting to persuade or coerce her raises an entirely new set of issues at the intersection of ethics and public policy. Once we move to the level of policy, political and historical considerations become very important. At this point, a brief look at another era's concern for the health of the not-yet-born is appropriate.

ALCOHOL AND "RACE-DECAY" IN EDWARDIAN ENGLAND

This is not the first time that parental behavior has been held responsible for harm to the not-yet-born or the already-born. The oldest prenatal health advice of which I am aware is in the Old Testament. In Judges 13:7 the mother of Samson is told "Behold, thou shalt conceive and bear a son: and drink no wine or strong drink."

Many women today are fearful and suspicious of the movement towards ascribing moral status to the fetus. For women who aspire to compete in the economic marketplace on an equal footing with men, those fears and suspicions have substantial historical validity. Past social movements to protect helpless infants and not-yet-born children have had something less than pure and altruistic motives. One illuminating example comes from England at the turn of the century—the Edwardian era.

In the first decade of this century, England found itself losing its empire abroad and awash with immigrants at home: immigrants, moreover, whose children were more likely to survive infancy than their British neighbors. A number of laypeople and physicians believed they understood the problem—alcohol. A campaign to arouse public ire against parents who drank flourished in the first decade of the 1900s. While it was directed largely against women who drank, men came in for their share of the blame as well. Indeed, one highly influential Swiss study reported that 78 per cent of women unable to breastfeed had fathers who drank heavily. But for the most part, women were faulted.

In 1906, a British physician wrote:

Undoubtedly much of the high infant mortality is due to alcoholism, and conditions directly...or indirectly arising from this morbid condition. The widespread prevalence of alcoholism among women, especially during the reproductive period of life, is one of the most important factors making for racial-decay.[6]

"Race-decay" is but one of many dubious reasons given for worrying about women and drink. George Sims, a prominent journalist of the time, had a related concern: "What can be the future of our Empire, if on a falling birth rate 120,000 infants continue to die annually in the first year of their lives...![6] And he knew the cause: "Bad motherhood is the first great cause of our appalling infant mortality."[6] No less an examplar of success than Andrew Carnegie, the American industrialist, pointed to the drunken worker as a central threat to British productivity.[6]

For the most part, this was a campaign waged by the upper classes, including a number of male physicians, against working class women. They were not doing their national duty by outreproducing the immigrants—Jews, Italians, Scots, and Irish. Theophilus Hyslop, a physician active in the anti-drink movement, referred to immigrants derogatorily and declared that if the British worker would give up alcohol, he could "drive the foreigner from our midst."[6]

Perhaps Dr. Robert Jones best expressed the sentiment feared by contemporary women: "Women are now the companions of men in...industrial pursuits, and the freedom to work on equal terms with men has caused ...the same depressing physical and mental influences ..., for which stimulants offer a temporary relief."[6] Women, that is, as vessels of reproduction, as the assurers of racial integrity, as the saviors of the empire, as the protectors of the innocent must be made to look after their offspring, and not be contaminated in the labor marketplace.

Many women understand any contemporary movement emphasizing their biologic role as bearers of children to be a threat to their economic liberty and equality—"fetal rights" being no exception. The need to control reproduction so that they could compete in the job market emerged as a major theme among pro-choice activists in Kristin Luker's study of anti- and pro-abortion activists. Conversely, having and raising children were crucial sources of self-value for many who worked against abortion.[13] Because it focuses attention on women's reproductive capacities, it is not surprising that the trend toward regarding the fetus as a patient has evoked concern and controversy. And with the long history of efforts to keep women in roles defined by and in the interests of men, it is no less surprising that women regard the current trend with suspicion. Legitimate concerns for fetal rights can also be carried along by other, questionable, motives and may carry with them other destructive social consequences.

CONCLUSIONS

Five points emerge from this analysis. First, we can discuss moral duties to the fetus destined to be born—to the not-yet-born child—without logical contradiction and without becoming hopelessly mired in debate over abortion.

Second, whether the fetus is viable may be regarded as morally significant in the context of abortion decisions, but it is not directly relevant to our duties to not-yet-born children. This is so because of the irrelevance of the timing of a harm.

Third, that we do have moral duties to fetuses, viable and previable alike, may not have the horrendous consequences for women that is typically thought. Our common error has been to focus exclusively on a pregnant woman's duty to avoid harming her fetus, without regard for the multitude of other moral considerations she ought to include in her decision. A more complex and adequate view of the moral life understands that in such decisions a host of factors may be relevant such as promises made, the woman's own interests, her obligations to other family members, and the welfare of her not-yet-born child. Seeing the mother's moral relationship to the fetus as morally analogous to a father's relationship to his child will help avoid oversimplification.

Fourth, establishing that women have moral duties to their not-yet-born children does not justify automatically coercive public policies to force them to fulfill those obligations. Again, the analogy to fathers and children may be helpful. The state must be very cautious in using its power to enforce particular notions of maternal duties. Effective enforcement might necessitate forcible invasion of a woman's body or prolonged incarceration. These are usually "last resorts" used only under very restricted circumstances. We must be careful to assure that

they are not used more casually against pregnant women.

Fifth, women have ample reason to be suspicious of the growing tendency to focus on the welfare of the fetus-as-patient and, by implication, on the woman's role as bearer of children. Historically, movements allegedly directed toward aiding fetuses and children have often been motivated as much by other, less praiseworthy concerns, including racism, and especially by men's fear of women's political, social, and economic equality.

Rather than arguing over "fetal rights," let us use the less heated language of moral obligations to not-yet-born children. We must not oversimplify complex moral decisions, especially our tendency to focus on a pregnant woman's obligations to her not-yet-born child as the *only* morally important factor in her decisions. We would not tolerate such oversimplification when discussing parents' duties toward their children, and we must not tolerate it in the difficult decisions we now face regarding the welfare of the not-yet-born. History provides forceful reminders of the dangers of thinking of women as mere "vessels of reproduction." Finally, we must continue the work of clarifying our obligations toward both the fetus destined to be born and the mother who retains her full moral individuality and interests, and in whose body that developing person exists for a time.

REFERENCES

1 Clewell WH, Meier PR, Manchester DK, et al: Ventriculomegaly: Evaluation and management. Sem Perinatol 9:98–102, 1985

2 Engelhardt HT: The Foundations of Bioethics. New York, Oxford, 1986

3 Fletcher JC: Ethical considerations in and beyond experimental fetal therapy. Sem Perinatol 9:130–135, 1985

4 Gabbe SG: Management of diabetes mellitus in pregnancy. Am J Obstet Gynecol 153:824–827, 1985

5 Golbus MS, Filly RA, Callen PW, et al: Fetal urinary tract obstruction: Management and selection for treatment. Sem Perinatol 9:91–97, 1985

6 Gutzke DW: "The cry of the children": The Edwardian medical campaign against maternal drinking. Br J Addiction 79:71–84, 1984

7 Harrison MR, Adzick NS, Nakayama DK, et al: Fetal diaphragmatic hernia: Fatal but fixable. Sem Perinatol 9:103–112, 1985

8 Johnsen DE: The creation of fetal rights: Conflicts with women's constitutional rights to liberty, privacy, and equal protection. Yale Law J 95:599–625, 1986

9 Keeton WP, Dobbs D, Keeton R, et al: Prosser and Keeton on the Law of Torts. Edition 5. Mineola, NY, West Publishing Co, 1984

10 Kleinman CS, Copel JA, Weinstein EM, et al: In utero diagnosis and treatment of fetal supraventricular tachycardia. Sem Perinatol 9:113–129, 1985

11 Kuzma JW, Sokol RJ: Maternal drinking behavior and decreased intrauterine growth. Alcohol Clin Exp Res 6:396–402, 1982

12 Leiberman JR, Mazor M, Chaim W, et al: The fetal right to live. Obstet Gynecol 53:515–517, 1979

13 Luker K: Abortion and the Politics of Motherhood. University of California, Berkeley, 1984

14 Murray TH: Ethical issues in fetal surgery. Bull Am Col Surg 70(6):6–10, 1985

15 Murray TH: Who do fetal protection policies really protect? Tech Rev 88(7):12–13, 20, 1985

16 Prosser WL: Handbook of the Law of Torts. Edition 3. St Paul, MN, West Publishing Co, 1964

17 Robertson JA: Legal issues in fetal therapy. Sem Perinatol 9:136–142, 1985

18 Robertson JA, Schulman JD: PKU women and pregnancy: The limits of reproductive autonomy. Unpublished manuscript

19 Roe v Wade. 410 U.S. 113, 1973

20 Schulman JD: Prenatal treatment of biochemical disorders. Sem Perinatol 9:75–78, 1985

21 Shaw MW: Conditional prospective rights of the fetus. J Leg Med 5:63–116, 1984

22 Simpson TJ, Golbus MS: In utero fetal hematopoietic stem cell transplantation. Sem Perinatol 9:68–74, 1985

23 Strong C: Ethical conflicts between mother and fetus in obstetrics. Clin Perinatol 14:313–327, 1987.

24 Tooley M: Abortion and Infanticide. New York, Oxford University Press, 1983

25 US Congress, Office of Technology Assessment: Reproductive Health Hazards in the Workplace. US Government Printing Office: Washington, DC, 1985

26 Weiner S, Scharf JF, Bolognese PJ, et al: Antenatal diagnosis and treatment of fetal goiter. J Reprod Med 24:39–42, 1980

Compelled Medical Treatment of Pregnant Women: Life, Liberty, and Law in Conflict

Lawrence J. Nelson and Nancy Milliken

Lawrence J. Nelson, Ph.D. (in philosophy), J.D., is a full-time bioethics consultant in private practice. In this capacity, he is associated with the Bioethics Consultation Group, Berkeley, California. Among his many articles are "The Baby Doe Regulations," "AIDS Confidentiality: An Ethical Dilemma," and "How Should Ethics Committees Treat Advance Directives?" Nancy Milliken, M.D., is assistant professor, department of obstetrics, gynecology, and the reproductive sciences, University of California, San Francisco. She is the coauthor of several articles, including "Symposium: Ethical Dilemmas of Infertility" and "AIDS: The Ethics of an Epidemic."

Nelson and Milliken consider the dilemma that arises for physicians when a pregnant woman rejects medical treatment that is thought to be in the best interests of her fetus. Although the authors believe that physicians are justified in attempting to persuade such a woman to accept treatment, they are systematically opposed to any form of coercive intervention, even in cases where intervention would seem to present both great benefit for the fetus and low risk for the woman. In their view, there are strong policy reasons against compelling

Reprinted with permission of the authors and the publisher from *Journal of the American Medical Association*, vol. 259 (February 19, 1988), pp. 1060–1066. Copyright © 1988, American Medical Association.

pregnant women to undergo any form of medical treatment or behavior change. Although Nelson and Milliken recognize that a pregnant woman (who does not intend to abort) has "an affirmative ethical obligation to accept reasonable, nonexperimental medical treatment for the sake of her fetus," they maintain that there is no sound basis for the legal enforcement of this ethical obligation.

As recently stated by the ethics committee of the American College of Obstetricians and Gynecologists, the maternal-fetal relationship is a "unique one" as it involves "two patients with access to one through the other."[1] In no other situation is the physician faced with one patient literally inside the body of another patient. Conceptually, the medical care of each can be approached independently, but practically, neither can be treated without affecting the other. Because of this unique relationship, conflicts between the interests of the woman and the fetus can arise if the former refuses treatment recommended for the benefit of the latter (eg, refusing cesarean section for documented fetal distress and anoxia) or if she is unwilling or unable to change behaviors that potentially could harm her fetus, such as smoking, consuming alcohol, eating inadequately, or engaging in certain job-related or recreational activities.

Kolder et al[2] recently documented a substantial number of court-ordered obstetric procedures performed despite a woman's refusal of treatment considered necessary to preserve the life or health of the fetus. As the survey included only obstetricians directing fellowship and residency programs in maternal-fetal medicine, there certainly are instances of compelled treatment not included in their report. Other recent reports seem to confirm this.[3–5] Perhaps most important, the report by Kolder et al documented that almost half of the fellowship directors thought that judicial force should be used to impose treatment thought to be lifesaving, including surgery, on unconsenting pregnant women for the sake of the fetus. Court-ordered obstetric treatment raises a host of fundamental ethical and legal questions for physicians, pregnant women, and society—questions that have not been adequately explored in the medical literature.

In this article, we will first discuss the ethical basis of the physician-patient relationship during pregnancy and present our perspective on the ethical reconciliation of maternal-fetal conflict. . . . Finally, we will present the policy reasons why neither the medical profession nor society should support judicially compelled treatment of pregnant women. We conclude that the pregnant woman's ethical obligation to care for her fetus should not be legally enforced.

OBSTETRICS, ETHICS, AND THE PHYSICIAN-PATIENT RELATIONSHIP

As a result of the rapid development of obstetric knowledge and technology, the physician's relationship to the fetus has changed dramatically. In part because the fetus has become the subject of many direct medical interventions, it has emerged as the obstetrician's second patient. The preface to the most recent edition of *Williams Textbook of Obstetrics* reflects this view: "Quality of life for the mother and her infant is our most important concern. Happily, we live and work in an era in which the fetus is established as our second patient with many rights and privileges comparable to those previously achieved only after birth."[6] Although this excerpt is not a description of a fetus' legal rights, it does suggest that obstetricians commonly conceptualize the fetus as a patient to whom they owe ethical duties as they would to any other patient.

The fetus has not become a patient in its own right because the goal of obstetrics has changed; that goal has always been the birth of a healthy baby to a healthy mother. Rather, medicine's means to achieve this goal have changed significantly during the past few decades. Formerly, the physician was able to treat only the mother and had to assume that in maintaining her health, the health of the fetus would be enhanced. The fetus itself was largely beyond the diagnostic and therapeutic reach of the physician. Advances in knowledge of fetal physiology and the development of new technology have enabled physicians to see the fetus in detail with ultrasound, to assess its condition with amniocentesis and fetal heart rate monitoring, and to operate on it in utero. In short, medicine's enhanced ability to treat the fetus directly has profoundly affected, perhaps even created, physicians' perception of the fetus as a separate patient. Such a perception is reinforced by clinical experience of the fetus as a technically interesting and challenging patient.

One might infer from the foregoing that it is only the new emphasis on the fetus as patient that determines the physician's ethical obligation to promote its well-being. This is not true. The physician's obligation to promote fetal health is firmly rooted in his or her ethical obligations to the pregnant woman. In seeking prenatal care, a pregnant woman is at least implicitly demonstrating that she has freely chosen to pursue a successful pregnancy. Regardless of an individual physician's conceptualization of the fetus as a separate patient, he or she is required to monitor the fetus and recommend appropriate treatment in accordance with the standard of care because of the woman's choice to bring her pregnancy to term. The failure to do so would be both ethically wrong and medical malpractice. Therefore, the fetus does not need to be seen as a second or separate obstetric patient to create a duty on the part of a physician to render it excellent care.

While the physician's relationship to the fetus has undergone significant expansion and qualitative change, the physician's relationship to a pregnant woman has a venerable history. The pregnant woman who presents for prenatal care is clearly the obstetrician's patient. Their interaction is governed by the fiduciary nature of any physician-patient relationship in which an individual patient voluntarily entrusts the physician with her medical concerns, and the physician reciprocates with the skillful application of medical knowledge to serve the patient's interests faithfully. The ethical principle of beneficence requires a physician to implement the therapy that best promotes the patient's health while minimizing potential harm. In the context of obstetrics, the physician has the responsibility to monitor the health of both the woman and the fetus and to advocate treatment intended to enhance the health of both.

In addition to the principle of beneficence, the physician is ethically obliged to recognize the principle of respect for individual autonomy. In keeping with this latter principle, all adult patients traditionally are deemed to have the right to accept or reject medical recommendations based on their personal priorities and values,[7] a right respected and protected by the law.[8–11] Like other adults, a pregnant woman must make decisions about medical care within the broader context of her life. Her responsibility to her fetus will sometimes be weighed against responsibilities to her children, husband, and others with whom she has a special relationship. Her decisions also may be influenced by a religious faith or commitments to strongly held personal values, and she may not always agree with her physician's advice.

Usually it is frustrating for physicians when patients do not follow their advice. Often it is painful when the patient's medically foolish decision results in serious damage or death. Perhaps nowhere are the physician's frustration and pain with a patient's noncompliance more excruciating than in obstetrics, where the decisions of the pregnant woman affect not only her own health but also that of her fetus. However, these feelings alone do not ethically justify ignoring or circumventing a pregnant woman's refusal to follow medical advice.

Because she is an autonomous adult, a competent pregnant woman has the same prerogative as other adults to control her own life and what will happen to her body. In addition, because conceiving and bearing a child is a highly personal and private matter, others (including physicians) should be very reluctant to substitute their value judgments in such a matter for those of the woman herself. Therefore, due to respect for an individual's autonomy and privacy, physicians should recognize and honor a competent pregnant woman's informed decision to reject medical advice about her care.

This view surely can be criticized for ignoring the value of the fetus as a being with interests separate from those of its mother. Factually, a fetus is a human life with a distinct genetic constitution that develops and possesses an organ system distinct from its mother's. However, the ethical evaluation of fetal life varies dramatically within our society. Some contend that a fertilized human ovum is a human life with the same rights as any live-born man or woman.[12] Others see the fetus as at most a potential human life that receives the protection of the ethical principle forbidding harm to persons only after it lives outside of the mother's body. Still others have claimed that a fetus achieves protectable ethical status at quickening or when it reaches the point of viability.[4] A more recent view argues that the fetus gains ethical status when it has developed neurologically to the point where it has consciousness.[13] Not only is there a lack of agreement on how to value fetal life, particularly when it comes into conflict with the interests of the mother, but this disagreement is violently expressed both literally in abortion clinic bombings and figuratively in slogan slinging on both sides of the issue.

In light of this seemingly intractable controversy, it is arbitrary for a physician to resolve maternal-fetal conflict by claiming that his or her ethical evaluation of the fetus is the "right" one while the woman's is "wrong."

When there is such profound disagreement, we believe that the ethically preferable course of action is to leave the determination of the weight of the fetus' interests to the mother in conflict situations. Nonetheless, it is certainly ethically permissible (perhaps even mandatory) for a physician to try to persuade a pregnant woman refusing medically indicated treatment to change her mind. Neither patient autonomy nor the doctrine of informed consent requires physicians to accept patient refusal passively and without inquiry, protest, or argument. However, the purposeful use of threats or deception to "convince" a patient to change her mind is ethically unacceptable....

MEDICAL AND SOCIAL POLICY

In our view, there is no compelling ethical or legal justification for requiring competent pregnant women to undergo medical treatment against their will. Others disagree and advocate the use of coercion against pregnant women in certain situations.[17–19] Commenting on the Kolder study, Annas[20] detected the beginning of an alliance between physicians and the courts to force pregnant women to accept medical treatment for the sake of their fetuses. Before such an alliance becomes entrenched, its assumptions, its terms, and what its operation would entail must be carefully examined.

The most plausible case for compelling a pregnant woman to undergo treatment for the sake of her fetus can be made in those situations when either the failure to provide the indicated treatment puts the fetus at great risk of serious physical harm or the treatment promises to be of significant benefit to the fetus, and the risks of the treatment itself to the mother and fetus are low or minimal. For example, Chervenak and McCullough[18] have proposed guidelines that would permit fetal diagnosis and treatment, presumably even against the mother's wishes, when "the risks [of treatment] to the fetus are minimal, the potential benefit to the fetus is substantial, and the risks to the woman are those she should reasonably accept on behalf of the fetus." In short, forced maternal treatment would be sanctioned if treatment presented substantial benefit to the fetus and low risk to the mother. This is a simple, appealing, and reasonable-sounding proposal until one tries to define its terms or apply it to clinical situations.

It is extremely difficult to identify clearly the clinical situations in which the failure to provide treatment poses a risk of harm to the fetus serious enough to warrant forcible intervention. Would only the certainty of fetal demise without intervention warrant compelled treatment, or would the risk of fetal harm be sufficient? If the risk of harm would be the relevant criterion, the degree of severity of harm sufficient to justify the undeniably serious act of forcing treatment on an unconsenting adult woman would have to be identified. The standard could be articulated as "serious harm," "grave harm," or "significant harm." However phrased, such a standard is ripe for idiosyncratic and arbitrary interpretation. Forcing women to undergo medical treatment against their wills is too weighty a matter to be left to the vagaries of personal interpretation by physicians and judges. Moreover, such an inherently vague standard contains the risk of unequal treatment of women in similar medical situations.

Attempts to devise precise criteria encounter the problem of medical uncertainty. In many obstetric situations, the medical knowledge may not be available to make the correct diagnosis or to describe accurately the likelihood of occurrence of fetal harm.[5, 15] For example, abnormalities on the fetal heart rate tracing may not be indicative of true fetal distress or predictive of fetal damage in the absence of medical intervention. As Kolder et al[2] rightly noted, while physicians are quick to embrace uncertainty as a justification for their errors, they are less quick to recognize its effect on patient self-determination. Furthermore, reported cases of court-ordered cesarean sections in which the woman delivered vaginally without incident despite medical predictions that she could not do so[5, 21, 22] illustrate that if physicians' medical recommendations are legally enforceable, they will be allowed to be wrong, while the women involved will never be allowed to be right or wrong. As Elias and Annas[15] have observed, "It seems wrong to say that patients have the right to be wrong in all cases except pregnancy."

In addition to these difficult problems in identifying the fetal risk that would purportedly justify a decision to force medical treatment on a woman, there are similar problems in judging what constitutes an "acceptable" level of risk of harm to the mother. Using Chervenak and McCullough's term, one can justifiably be puzzled about the ability to identify those risks that a woman should "reasonably" accept for the benefit of her fetus. This formulation also fails to mention who is to decide what is "reasonable" in this context, a substantial problem given the elasticity of the term. What is one person's "serious harm" could well be "minor" to another person.

Furthermore, whoever makes this judgment will invariably have to make tricky assessments regarding maternal factors that may significantly increase the risk of the proposed intervention. For example, there is an undeniably greater risk of morbidity and mortality associated with cesarean delivery as compared with vaginal delivery.[6] These risks may significantly increase in the presence of maternal thrombocytopenia, a recent myocardial infarction, or pulmonary conditions that would complicate the administration of general anesthesia, which might be necessary in an emergency. We suggest that no one has the wisdom or ethical authority to declare what is an "acceptable" or "reasonable" risk for a woman to take if she herself is unwilling to face it.

In addition, some women refuse treatment for religious reasons.[14] For example, pregnant Jehovah's Witnesses have been known to refuse blood transfusions.[10, 16, 23] To force such a woman to receive blood may, in her own mind, expose her to eternal damnation as well as cause her to suffer psychological stress or rejection within her earthly community. It is important to distinguish between this situation and the routine practice of having neonates or children receive transfusions over the religious objections of their parents. A live-born child can be given a transfusion without forcibly invading the mother's body, although it does "invade" her wishes, while a transfusion done for the sake of the fetus must necessarily invade the mother's body and ignore her wishes.

Because our society values bodily integrity highly, the "geographical" difference between a live-born child and a fetus is a very significant one. Our society and its legal system go to great lengths to protect the right of persons to preserve their bodily integrity.[4] For example, the legal system does not force persons to donate organs involuntarily to others, even if they are relatives in desperate need. In *McFall vs Shimp*, a man terminally ill with aplastic anemia sued to compel his cousin to donate bone marrow in a late effort to save his life.[24] The judge refused to compel the donation and stated that legal compulsion of such a bodily intrusion, even though it entailed little risk of harm, "would change every concept and principle upon which our society is founded."[24] Another judge refused to order a woman to undergo a cesarean section after acknowledging that he lacked the right to force her to donate an organ to a child of hers, even if that child were dying.[25]

Furthermore, our society refuses to force the donation of organs or tissue from cadavers to benefit or save the lives of the thousands in need of them. (The American Council on Transplantation estimates that of more than 23,000 potential cadaver organ donors available yearly, only 3000 [about 13%] actually become donors.) We see no good reason why pregnant women should be treated with less respect than corpses. In fact, it seems bizarre that many persons should die for want of a vital organ that could be taken from a corpse, while a living pregnant woman can be forced to undergo major surgery that exposes her to a not insubstantial risk of harm or death.

A policy that would permit the courts or the police to intervene in the activities of pregnant women that arguably placed their fetuses at some risk of harm must be considered in light of its potential effectiveness and what its enforcement would require. Every action a pregnant woman takes has a potential impact on her fetus, including the simplest and most common activities of daily living: eating, drinking, sexual intercourse, and physical activity (whether too much in the case of a woman at risk of preterm labor or too little in the case of women with clearly excessive weight gain). In addition, women may expose their fetuses to potential harm when they work, due to occupational hazards. Consequently, an effective public policy designed to prevent fetal harm would require extensive monitoring of and possible interference with each of these activities. This would entail an unprecedented social intrusion into the homes and private lives of pregnant women and their families.

The only plausible justification for a policy with such tremendous impact on the lives and civil liberties of pregnant women would be overwhelming need. However, it is far from clear that such need exists. Common clinical experience shows that it is an unusual woman who does not do everything within reason for the best interests of her fetus. In fact, clinicians are often impressed with the medical risks and lifestyle restrictions voluntarily assumed by pregnant women to ensure a good outcome for their pregnancies. In short, situations in which fetuses may die or be born damaged as a direct result of maternal behavior are likely to be rare.[15] This being so, the price of intervention to women's liberty and privacy seems too high.

We recognize that the behavior of women who are abusers of alcohol or drugs poses significant potential for fetal harm. However, there are solid reasons to doubt that a system of legal punishment or intervention would decrease the incidence of this behavior, as it is usually an addiction over which these women have little control. If anything, a system of legal coercion and punishment might drive these women away from the prenatal care that they and their fetuses especially need.

The enactment of a public policy that would compel women to avoid certain behaviors for the sake of the fetus would also drastically change the nature of the physician–pregnant woman relationship. While many physicians probably can recall a case in which they might have welcomed legal sanction to force a pregnant woman to prevent fetal harm, they may underestimate the impact of such a precedent on their relationship to all patients. The relationship between a physician and a pregnant woman would become much less one of a partnership dedicated to a common goal and more a relationship of adversaries, like police officer and criminal suspect. The ability of a pregnant woman and her physician to negotiate a better course of care when the optimal course is not chosen by the patient would become severely compromised if she could be forced to do whatever the physician recommended.[15] In addition, some pregnant women undoubtedly would refrain from seeking prenatal care or lie about their behaviors or symptoms if they knew their physicians could use the truth to force treatment on them. This, of course, would severely restrict physicians' ability to diagnose correctly and treat adequately both pregnant women and their fetuses.

The philosophical question confronting society is whether it wishes to enforce a policy that would entail on an unprecedented scale serious invasions of a woman's privacy, restriction of her civil liberties, and interference with her religious and personal beliefs. In a secular society such as ours that embraces no particular moral point of view and that attempts to encompass groups with widely divergent views on how persons should live their own lives, individuals are required to forgo "the temptation to impose by state force [their] own view of proper private morality."[26] Given the heated and intractable controversy surrounding the ethical evaluation of the fetus and the well-established interests of all adult persons in bodily integrity and self-determination, we conclude that the decision of a competent pregnant woman to forgo medical treatment likely to benefit her fetus should remain hers, even if others see her choice as unethical.

CONCLUSION

There are many troublesome questions surrounding the use of judicial force to compel pregnant women to un-

dergo medical treatment or behavior change for the benefit of their fetuses. We believe that it is unwise, in the last analysis, to recognize fetal rights that would create an adversarial relationship between a pregnant woman and her fetus. Incompleteness of medical knowledge and the unavoidable uncertainty of medical diagnostic and therapeutic techniques make it impossible to define a clear, precise, and accurate medical model on which society could base a fair and uniformly applied legal policy that would sanction the use of force against pregnant women. There is also insufficient reason to undermine the ethical principle of patient autonomy and the legal right to self-determination and bodily integrity for a subset of our society, namely, pregnant women.

Ultimately, it is not feasible to determine in a just and fair manner which actions or inactions of a pregnant woman should warrant interventions as drastic as involuntary treatment or surgery. It is also not possible to enforce such a policy effectively without extensive and probably distasteful intrusion into the private lives of pregnant women and their families. Furthermore, it is speculative at best whether these changes would cause improvement in the relationship between prenatal care givers and pregnant women and in the effectiveness of prenatal care. We suspect it would in fact do quite the contrary.

We conclude that a pregnant woman who does not intend to have a legal abortion has an affirmative ethical obligation to accept reasonable, nonexperimental medical treatment for the sake of her fetus and to behave otherwise in a manner intended to benefit and not harm her fetus. This obligation is rooted in her unique and significant influence on the health and development of the human entity she voluntarily carries, an entity that will ultimately develop into a person with human rights. Nevertheless, we do not believe that this ethical obligation should be legally enforced. The attempt to do so would not itself be ethical, practically effective, or advantageous for society or the individual. In fact, such legal enforcement would create more harm than it could prevent. Thus, the interventionist "solution" to the problem of maternal-fetal conflict is worse than the original problem.

Finally, we endorse the goal of enhancing fetal health. Physicians will play an essential role in achieving this goal by fulfilling their ethical obligations to pregnant women. This will include monitoring the health of pregnant women and their fetuses and recommending treatment to maximize the prospects of both. While physicians have an ethical obligation to respect the decisions of an informed, competent pregnant woman, they may ethically be an advocate for the fetus when the pregnant woman is making her choices. This advocacy may include the use of persuasion to try to influence the woman to do the "right" thing, but not the use of threats, lies, or physical force. Because most prenatal care relationships between physicians and pregnant women last several months, there is an opportunity to anticipate conflicts and spend additional time to ensure that a pregnant woman's fears or misinformation, which may prevent her from doing what is best for her pregnancy, can be addressed and corrected.

If society and the medical profession are truly interested in enhancing fetal health, their efforts should be directed toward increasing the availability and quality of voluntary prenatal care for all pregnant women and the availability of drug and alcohol rehabilitation programs and other social services for those pregnant women who need them and discouraging physicians from running to the courthouse for an order forcing a woman to accept treatment she does not want. John Stuart Mill has said, "Mankind are greater gainers by suffering each other to live as seems good to themselves, than by compelling each to live as seems good to the rest."[27] We agree: society will, in the end, gain far more by allowing each pregnant woman to live as seems good to her, rather than by compelling each to live as seems good to the rest of us.

ACKNOWLEDGMENT

The preparation on this article was assisted in part by a grant from the Robert Wood Johnson Foundation, Princeton, NJ. The opinions expressed herein are those of the authors and do not necessarily represent the views of the Foundation.

REFERENCES

1 Gianelli DM: ACOG issues guidelines on maternal, fetal rights. *American Medical News*, Aug 28, 1987, p 7.
2 Kolder VE, Gallagher J, Parsons MT: Court-ordered obstetrical interventions. *N Engl J Med* 1987; 316:1192–1196.
3 Gallagher J: Prenatal invasions and interventions: What's wrong with fetal rights. *Harv Women's Law J* 1987;10:9–58.
4 Nelson LJ, Buggy BP, Weil CJ: Forced medical treatment of pregnant women: 'Compelling each to live as seems good to the rest.' *Hastings Law J* 1986;37:703–763.
5 Rhoden N: The judge in the delivery room: The emergence of court-ordered cesareans. *Calif Law Rev* 1986;74:1951–2030.
6 Pritchard JA, MacDonald PC, Gant NF: *Williams Obstetrics*. East Norwalk, Conn, Appleton-Century-Crofts, 1985, pp xi, 867–871.
7 Jonsen AR, Siegler M, Winslade WJ: *Clinical Ethics*. New York, Macmillan Publishing Co Inc, 1986, pp 47–51.
8 *Bouvia vs Superior Court*, 179 Cal App 3d 1127 (Cal App 1986).
9 *Bartling vs Superior Court*, 163 Cal App 3d 186 (Cal App 1984).
10 *Mercy Hospital vs Jackson*, 510 A 2d 562 (Md 1986).
11 *Satz vs Perlmutter*, 379 So 2d 359 (Fla 1980).
12 Congregation for the Doctrine of the Faith: *Instruction on Respect for Human Life in Its Origin and on the Dignity of Procreation*. Vatican City, Vatican Polyglot Press, 1987.
13 Gertler GB: Brain birth: A proposal for defining when a fetus is entitled to human life status. *South Calif Law Rev* 1986;59:1061–1078.
14 *Jefferson vs Griffin Spalding County Hospital Authority*, 274 SE 2d 457 (Ga 1981).
15 Elias E, Annas GJ: *Reproductive Genetics and the Law*. Chicago, Year Book Medical Publishers Inc, 1987, pp 118–120, 253–262.
16 *Raleigh Fitkin–Paul Morgan Memorial Hospital vs Anderson*, 201 A 2d 537 (NJ 1964), cert denied, 377 US 984.
17 Robertson JA: Legal issues in fetal therapy. *Semin Perinatol* 1985;9:136–142.
18 Chervenak FA, McCullough LB: Perinatal ethics: A practical analysis of obligations to mother and fetus. *Obstet Gynecol* 1985;66:442–446.
19 Mathieu D: Respecting liberty and preventing harm: Limits of state intervention in prenatal choice. *Harv J Law Public Policy* 1985;8:19–52.
20 Annas GJ: Protecting the liberty of pregnant patients. *N Engl J Med* 1987;316:1213–1214.
21 *In re Baby Jeffries*, No. 14004 (Jackson Cty P Ct Mich, May 24, 1982).

22 Fletcher JC: Ethical considerations in and beyond experimental fetal therapy. *Semin Perinatol* 1985; 9:130–135.

23 *In re Application of Jamaica Hospital*, 491 NYS 2d 898 (NY Sup Ct 1985).

24 *McFall vs Shimp*, No. 78-17711 (C P Allegheny Cty Penn, July 26, 1978).

25 Unpublished opinion, No. 84-7-50006-D (Super Ct Benton Cty Wash, April 20, 1984).

26 Engelhardt HT Jr: Introduction, in Bondeson W, Engelhardt HT, Spicker S, et al (eds): *Abortion and the Status of the Fetus*. Dordrecht, the Netherlands, D Reidel Publishing Co, 1983, pp xi-xxxii.

27 Mill JS: On liberty, in Warnock M (ed): *Utilitarianism and Other Writings*. New York, World Publishers, 1962, pp 126–250.

ANNOTATED BIBLIOGRAPHY: CHAPTER 8

Armstrong, Robert L.: "The Right to Life," *Journal of Social Philosophy* 8 (January 1977), pp 13–19. Armstrong develops an interesting and somewhat distinctive moderate view on the morality of abortion. Although fetuses are not actual persons, he contends, they may be said to have a right to life on the basis of their potential personhood, but *only* if they have what he calls "real or serious" potentiality.

Brody, Baruch: "On the Humanity of the Foetus." In Robert L. Perkins, ed., *Abortion: Pro and Con* (Cambridge, Mass.: Schenkman, 1974), pp. 69–90. Brody critically examines the various proposals for "drawing the line" on the humanity of the fetus, ultimately suggesting that the most defensible view would draw the line at the point where fetal brain activity begins.

Chervenak, Frank A., and Laurence B. McCullough: "Perinatal Ethics: A Practical Method of Analysis of Obligations to Mother and Fetus," *Obstetrics & Gynecology* 66 (September 1985), pp. 442–446. The authors present an overall framework for analyzing moral conflicts in the practice of obstetrics. They suggest that it may sometimes be appropriate to compel a woman to accept fetal therapy.

Engelhardt, H. Tristram, Jr.: "The Ontology of Abortion," *Ethics* 84 (April 1974), pp. 217–234. Engelhardt focuses attention on the issue of "whether or to what extent the fetus is a person." He argues that, strictly speaking, a human person is not present until the later stages of infancy. However, he finds the point of viability significant in that, with viability, an infant can play the social role of "child" and thus be treated "as if it were a person."

Feinberg, Joel: "Abortion." In Tom Regan, ed., *Matters of Life and Death* (New York: Random House, 1980), pp. 183–217. In this long essay, Feinberg analyzes the strengths and weaknesses of alternative views about the moral status of the fetus. He also considers the extent to which abortion is morally justifiable *if* it is granted that the fetus is a person.

———, ed.: *The Problem of Abortion*, 2nd ed. (Belmont, Calif.: Wadsworth, 1984). This excellent anthology features a wide range of articles on the moral justifiability of abortion.

Fleischman, Alan R., and Ruth Macklin: "Fetal Therapy: Ethical Considerations, Potential Conflicts." In William B. Weil, Jr. and Martin Benjamin, eds., *Ethical Issues at the Outset of Life* (Boston: Blackwell Scientific Publications, 1987), pp. 121–138. The authors examine the ethical dilemmas associated with various kinds of fetal therapy. They suggest resolutions that accord with their adherence to a consequentialist scheme of ethical analysis.

Humber, James M.: "Abortion: The Avoidable Moral Dilemma," *Journal of Value Inquiry* 9 (Winter 1975), pp. 282–302. Humber, defending the conservative view on the morality of abortion, examines and rejects what he identifies as the major defenses of abortion. He al contends that proabortion arguments are typically so poor that they can only be viewed as "after-the-fact-rationalizations."

Johnsen, Dawn: "A New Threat to Pregnant Women's Autonomy," *Hastings Center Report* 17 (August 1987), pp. 33–40. Johnsen argues that the power of the state should not be used to coerce pregnant women to behave in ways considered to be best for their fetuses. In her view, the assertion of "fetal rights" against a pregnant woman is not an effective way of promoting a healthy fetal environment.

Langerak, Edward A.: "Abortion: Listening to the Middle," *Hastings Center Report* 9 (October 1979), pp. 24–28. Langerak suggests a theoretical framework for a moderate view that incorporates two "widely shared beliefs": (1) that there is something about the fetus *itself* that makes abortion morally problematic and (2) that late abortions are significantly more problematic than early abortions.

Rhoden, Nancy K.: "The New Neonatal Dilemma: Live Births from Late Abortions." *Georgetown Law Journal* 72 (June 1984), pp. 1451–1509. Rhoden reviews the various medical techniques employed for second-trimester abortions and considers the dilemma that arises when a late second-trimester abortion results in live birth. She also discusses the future of second-trimester abortions in the light of technological developments and constitutional considerations.

Ross, Steven L.: "Abortion and the Death of the Fetus," *Philosophy and Public Affairs* 11 (Summer 1982), pp. 232–245. Ross draws a distinction between abortion as the termination of pregnancy and abortion as the termination of the life of the fetus. He proceeds to defend abortion in the latter sense, insisting that it is justifiable for a woman to desire not only the termination of pregnancy but also the death of the fetus.

Strong, Carson: "Ethical Conflicts between Mother and Fetus in Obstetrics." *Clinics in Perinatology* 14 (June 1987), pp. 313–327. Strong argues that it is sometimes ethical for physicians to override the decision of a pregnant woman who refuses treatment needed for the fetus. He considers in particular the maternal/fetal conflict that arises in conjunction with cesarean deliveries.

Sumner, L. W.: "Toward a Credible View of Abortion," *Canadian Journal of Philosophy* 4 (September 1974), pp. 163–181. Rejecting both the conservative and liberal views on the morality of abortion, Sumner develops a "more credible, because more moderate, alternative." Following a developmental approach, he holds that the moral status of the fetus increases as the fetus develops.

Thomson, Judith Jarvis: "A Defense of Abortion," *Philosophy and Public Affairs* 1 (Fall 1971), pp. 47–66. In this widely discussed article, Thomson attempts to "moderate the conservative view." For the sake of argument, she grants the premise that the fetus (from conception) is a person. Still, she argues, under certain conditions abortion remains morally permissible.

Tooley, Michael: *Abortion and Infanticide* (New York: Oxford, 1983). In this long book, Tooley defends the liberal view on the morality of abortion. He insists that the question of the morality of abortion cannot be satisfactorily resolved "in isolation from the questions of the morality of infanticide and of the killing of nonhuman animals."

CHAPTER 9

GENETICS AND HUMAN REPRODUCTION

INTRODUCTION

With the rapid advance of knowledge and techniques in human genetics and the biology of human reproduction, a number of complex and troubling ethical issues have arisen. This chapter is designed to address some of the most important of these issues.

Genetic Disease and the Language of Genetics

Tay-Sachs disease is one prominent example of a genetic disease. This disease, which most commonly affects Jewish children of Eastern European heritage, is characterized by progressive neurological degeneration and death in early childhood. Although a child afflicted with Tay-Sachs disease has the disease by virtue of his or her genetic inheritance, the child's parents do not have the disease. (Those afflicted with Tay-Sachs disease do not survive to reproduce.) The parents are "carriers." Tay-Sachs carriers are those persons who have one normal gene and one variant or defective gene (the Tay-Sachs gene) at the same location on paired chromosomes. The Tay-Sachs gene is a *recessive* gene. When it is paired with a normal gene, as is the case with the carrier, the normal gene is dominant. As a result, the carrier does not manifest the disease. However, if a child inherits the Tay-Sachs gene from both parents, then the child will be afflicted with Tay-Sachs disease.

Since Tay-Sachs disease is traceable to a recessive gene, it is said to be a recessive disease. Moreover, it is said to be an *autosomal* recessive disease, where the word "autosomal" simply indicates that the defective genes are located on some pair of chromosomes other than the sex chromosomes. Further, in the language of genetics, Tay-Sachs carriers are said to be in the *heterozygous* state, whereas a child afflicted with Tay-Sachs disease is said to be in the *homozygous* state, with regard to the Tay-Sachs gene. Carriers, having the Tay-Sachs gene paired with a different (normal) gene, are heterozygous with regard to the Tay-Sachs gene. The afflicted child, having two identical Tay-Sachs genes, is homozygous with regard to the

481

Tay-Sachs gene. The carrier is sometimes termed a "heterozygote," the afflicted child a "homozygote."

According to the laws of heredity, when two cariers of a trait associated with an autosomal recessive disease produce offspring, there is one chance in four (25 percent) that their child will be afflicted with the genetic disease in question. There are two chances in four (50 percent) that their child will be, like them, a carrier. Finally, there is one chance in four (25 percent) that their child will be free both of the disease and of the carrier status.

The genetic disease usually called "sickle-cell anemia" is, like Tay-Sachs disease, a well-known autosomal recessive disease. Most commonly affecting blacks, sickle-cell anemia is characterized by acute attacks of abdominal pain and exhibits a range of severity. It is estimated that 10–12 percent of blacks in the United States carry the sickle-cell trait. As is typical of autosomal recessive diseases, if two carriers of the sickle-cell trait produce offspring, there is one chance in four (25 percent) that their child will be afflicted with sickle-cell anemia.

Cystic fibrosis provides one further example of an autosomal recessive disease. In the United States, since about 1 in 20 Caucasians carries the cystic fibrosis gene, about 1 in 400 Caucasian couples will be a carrier-carrier pairing, and thus be at risk (1 chance in 4) of producing offspring with the disease. Most victims of cystic fibrosis do not survive their teenage years. The disease is primarily characterized by a disfunction of the exocrine glands. This disfunction results in abnormal amounts of mucus that can obstruct organ passages and produce intense pulmonary and digestive distress.

Huntington's chorea provides a leading example of a genetic disease in the category of autosomal *dominant* diseases. Typically, the symptoms of Huntington's chorea emerge only in the prime of life, between the ages of 35 and 50. It is characterized by mental and physical deterioration, leading to death within a period of several years. The defective gene responsible for Huntington's chorea is a dominant one. If a person has the defective gene, that person will eventually fall victim to the disease. Moreover, there is one chance in two (50 percent) that the person carrying the defective gene will pass it on to each of his or her children.

In contrast to *autosomal* genetic diseases, some genetic diseases are linked to mutant genes located on the sex chromosomes. Prominent among the genetic diseases in this latter category are the so-called X-linked diseases. Hemophilia, a well-known disease characterized by uncontrollabe bleeding, is a leading example of an X-linked disease. Of the forty-six chromosomes that constitute the normal complement of genetic material in human beings, there are two sex chromosomes. A female has two X chromosomes and a male has one X and one Y chromosome. In human reproduction, if the sperm fertilizing the egg provides an X chromosome, the child will be female. If the sperm fertilizing the egg provides a Y chromosome, the child will be male. (The egg always provides an X chromosome.) Now, hemophilia is a *recessive* X-linked disease. A female, therefore, will have the disease of hemophilia only if she has the mutant gene on both of her X chromosomes. If a female has one normal gene and one mutant gene, however, she will be a carrier. Since a male has only one X chromosome, if he has the mutant gene associated with hemophilia, he will have the disease. On the assumption that a female carrier mates with a male who is free of the disease, there is no risk that their female children will have the disease. Female children will inherit a normal gene from their father and thus themselves be free of the disease, although there is one chance in two (50 percent) that they will inherit their mother's mutant gene and be, like her, a carrier. In contrast, there is one chance in two (50 percent) that male children will have the disease of hemophilia.

Prenatal Diagnosis and Selective Abortion

A number of techniques are presently employed for the detection of chromosomal abnormalities, many genetic diseases, and certain serious anatomical abnormalities in the fetus *in utero*. Among these techniques, amniocentesis and chorionic villi sampling are the most prominent, although ultrasound is also of great importance. Ultrasound is a noninvasive technique that produces a visual representation of the developing fetus and thereby allows the detection of many anatomical abnormalities.

In amniocentesis, a needle is inserted through a pregnant woman's abdomen, and a sample of the amniotic fluid surrounding the fetus is withdrawn. Because there are fetal cells in the amniotic fluid, a continually increasing number of genetic diseases in the fetus can be detected through biochemical studies and recombinant DNA techniques. Also detectable, via chromosomal analysis, are conditions associated with an abnormal number of chromosomes or an abnormal arrangement of chromosomes. Down's syndrome, for example, is associated with the presence of an extra chromosome, namely, three instead of two number 21 chromosomes. Amniocentesis can also be employed for the detection of neural-tube defects (anencephaly and spina bifida). In this case, a positive diagnosis rests on the presence of increased levels of alpha-fetoprotein in the amniotic fluid.

Amniocentesis, first introduced in the late 1960s, has achieved wide acceptance among physicians as a relatively low-risk medical procedure. However, it is not ordinarily performed prior to 14 to 16 weeks' gestation, and selective abortion must await the results of diagnostic testing, usually available around the twentieth week. Since second-trimester abortions are in many ways more problematic than first-trimester abortions, a procedure capable of combining the prenatal diagnostic value of amniocentesis with the possibility of first-trimester abortion is much to be preferred, assuming of course that risk factors are within acceptable limits. Chorionic villi sampling (CVS), a procedure developed in Europe and first introduced in the United States in 1983, has now emerged as a clear alternative to amniocentesis in the detection of genetic diseases and chromosomal abnormalities. In CVS, a procedure that can be performed in the first trimester, a small amount of tissue is extracted from the placenta. At the present time, it is thought that CVS is largely comparable to amniocentesis in terms of risk factors (e.g., possibility of miscarriage or possibility of maternal infection).

Since prenatal diagnosis is ordinarily undertaken with an eye toward selective abortion, the practice of prenatal diagnosis clearly confronts us with one particular aspect of the more general problem of abortion, as discussed in Chapter 8. (There is also a close link with the problem of the treatment of impaired newborns, as discussed in Chapter 7.) Is the practice of selective abortion, on grounds of genetic defect, ethically acceptable? Leon R. Kass, in one of this chapter's selections, abstracts from the problem of abortion in general and raises some ethical difficulties for the practice of selective (genetic) abortion. In another selection in this chapter, Eric T. Juengst provides a far-ranging discussion of the ethics of prenatal diagnosis. He argues that prenatal diagnosis is a defensible medical practice despite any misgivings that might arise about the practice of selective abortion on grounds of genetic defect. Juengst rejects, however, the employment of prenatal diagnosis for purposes of sex selection.

Morality and Reproductive Risk

One important ethical issue associated with human genetics has to do with the morality of reproduction under circumstances of genetic risk. In one of this chapter's selections, L. M. Purdy argues that it is surely morally wrong to reproduce in those cases where there is high risk of serious genetic disease. If it is justifiable to maintain that there is a moral obligation of the sort that Purdy outlines, we may find outselves once more faced with the problem of prenatal diagnosis and selective abortion. Clearly, in those cases (e.g., Tay-Sachs disease, sickle-cell anemia, cystic fibrosis) where prenatal diagnosis is available, abortion offers a means of sidestepping the risk of serious genetic disease.

Purdy considers in detail the case of Huntington's chorea. A special complication of this autosomal dominant disease is that its victims reach a reproductive age well before the time at which symptoms of the disease emerge. If no presymptomatic test were available—as was uniformly the case when Purdy's article was written—a potential parent with the knowledge that he or she is at 50 percent risk for Huntington's chorea would be confronted with a difficult dilemma. If the deleterious gene is in fact present, there is a 50 percent chance that it will be inherited by any offspring. In such circumstances, since there is a high risk (25 percent) of serious genetic disease, Purdy argues that reproduction is immoral. But recent developments have somewhat eased the dilemma of reproduction that has heretofore confronted a person at risk for Huntington's chorea. Consequent to the discovery in 1983 of a "marker" for the Huntington's chorea gene, both a presymptomatic test and a prenatal diagnostic test have been developed. However, these tests suffer from two basic limitations. First, an informative result can be produced only when several family members are available and willing to produce DNA samples. Second, because there is only a .96 correlation between the marker DNA and the deleterious gene, there is always at least a 4 perent chance that the test will produce an incorrect result. When the Huntington's chorea gene itself is discovered, and this is confidently expected in the near future, both a presymptomatic test and a prenatal diagnostic test will be free of the above limitations. With the availability of such tests, Purdy would presumably require the employment of one or both as a condition of responsible reproduction for those whose offspring are at risk for Huntington's chorea.

Closely associated with the issue of the morality of reproduction under circumstances of genetic risk is another ethical issue, the justifiability of the use of coercive measures to achieve social control over individual reproductive decisions. It is one thing to say that certain reproductive choices are immoral and quite another to say that coercive measures for the control of reproductive choices are justified. Such coercive controls as compulsory sterilization and mandatory amniocentesis followed by forced abortion are widely rejected as invasive of fundamental rights. Mandatory screening programs for the identification of carriers, while surely less intrusive than other coercive measures, are also widely opposed as unjustifiable. Those who argue in support of coercive measures sometimes introduce claims, difficult to assess, about the dangers of uncontrolled reproduction leading to a deterioration of the human gene pool. Thus proposals for coercive measures often reflect a "negative eugenics" rationale.[1] Such proposals are rejected by those who maintain that there is no clear and present danger of genetic deterioration.[2]

Reproductive Technologies and the Treatment of Infertility

Human reproduction, as it naturally occurs, is characterized by sexual intercourse, tubal fertilization, implantation in the uterus, and subsequent *in utero* gestation. The expression "reproductive technologies" can be understood as applicable to an array of technical procedures that would replace the various steps in the natural process of reproduction, to a lesser or greater extent.

Artificial insemination is a procedure that replaces sexual intercourse as a means of achieving tubal fertilization. Artificial insemination has long been available, primarily as a means of overcoming infertility on the part of a male, usually a husband. It is sometimes possible that the husband's infertility may be overcome by AIH, artificial insemination with the sperm of the *husband*. More often, the couple must turn to AID, artificial insemination with the sperm of a *donor*. AID has also been employed when it has been established that the husband carries a mutant gene that would place a couple's offspring at genetic risk. Moreover, it has been suggested, most prominently in the work of the well-known geneticist Hermann J. Muller, that AID be voluntarily employed as a way of achieving the aims of positive eugenics.[3] Muller recommended the formation of sperm banks, which would collect and store the sperm of men judged to be "outstanding" in various ways. His idea was that an "enlightened" couple who desired a child would have recourse to one of these banks in order to arrange for the wife's artificial insemination. Another controversial use of AID is its employment by unmarried women. Probably even more controversial is the employment of artificial insemination within the context of a "surrogate motherhood arrangement." In the most typical case, a wife's infertility motivates a couple to seek out a so-called "surrogate mother." The surrogate agrees to be artificially inseminated with the husband's sperm, in order to bear a child for the couple.

In vitro fertilization (IVF) literally means fertilization "in glass." The sperm of a husband (or a donor) is united, in a laboratory, with the ovum of a wife (or a donor). Whereas artificial insemination is a technically simple procedure, *in vitro* fertilization followed by embryo transfer (to the uterus for implantation) is a system of reproductive technology that features a high degree of technical sophistication. The first documented "test tube baby," Louise Brown, was born in England in July 1978. Her birth was the culmination of years of collaboration between a gynecologist, Patrick Steptoe, and an embryologist, Robert Edwards. This pioneering team developed methods for obtaining mature eggs from a woman's ovaries (via a minor surgical procedure called a laparoscopy), effectively fertilizing eggs in the laboratory, cultivating them to the eight-cell stage, and then transferring a developing embryo to the uterus for implantation.

Reproductive centers throughout the United States now provide *in vitro* procedures for the treatment of infertility. Although success rates continue to be somewhat unimpressive, it is expected that they will improve as techniques are further refined. An important development in this regard is the achievement of the first frozen embryo birth by an Australian team in 1984. Since it is now also possible, with the use of fertility drugs, to harvest a crop of mature eggs (perhaps ten or so) from a woman's ovaries, embryos frozen at the eight-cell stage can be thawed over a period of several months in an effort to achieve a successful implantation. Of course, the freezing of embryos is a technique that seems to suggest a number of ominous possibilities. But the freezing of unfertilized eggs, which at face value seems preferable to the freezing of embryos, has proven to be technically more difficult.

In vitro fertilization followed by embryo transfer is a system of reproductive technology that replaces not only sexual intercourse but also tubal fertilization in the natural process of reproduction. But consider also the future possibility of dispensing with implantation and *in utero* gestation as well. There seems to be no theoretical obstacle to totally artificial gestation, which would take place within the confines of an artificial womb. If *ectogenesis*, the process of artificial gestation, becomes a reality, then the combination of *in vitro* fertilization and ectogenesis would provide us with a system of reproductive technology in which each element in the natural process of reproduction has been effectively replaced. At the present time, however, *in vitro* fertilization (accompanied by embryo transfer) is seen primarily as a means of overcoming female infertility, especially infertility due to obstruction of the fallopian tubes.

One important spinoff of IVF technology is a procedure known as GIFT, that is, gamete intrafallopian transfer. In this procedure, eggs are obtained as they would be for IVF, but instead of fertilization *in vitro*, the eggs are placed together with sperm in the fallopian tube (or tubes) where it is hoped that fertilization will take place *in vivo* (i.e., in the living situation). Although there is some risk of ectopic pregnancy in GIFT, the success rates for this procedure seem to be slightly higher than the success rates for IVF in combination with embryo transfer.

In contrast to a woman whose infertility can be traced to fallopian-tube obstruction, consider a woman whose ovaries are either absent or nonfunctional. Since she has no ova, she cannot produce genetic offspring. If her uterus is functional, however, there is no biological obstacle to her bearing a child. Let us suppose that she very much wants to bear a child that is her husband's genetic offspring. Her problem can be addressed by some form of *egg donation*, and there are three major possibilities to consider.[4] (1) *In vitro* fertilization of a donor egg with the husband's sperm, followed by embryo transfer to the wife. (2) Artificial insemination of an egg donor with the husband's sperm, producing *in vivo* fertilization; nonsurgical removal of the embryo via lavage (a washing out) of the donor's uterus; recovery of the embryo and transfer to the uterus of the wife.[5] (3) Transfer of a donor egg together with the husband's sperm to the wife's fallopian tube, thus employing GIFT in an effort to achieve tubal fertilization and subsequent implantation. Since both (1) and (2), in contrast to (3), entail embryo transfers that involve a donated egg, the expressions "surrogate embryo transfer" and "prenatal adoption" are sometimes used to describe them.

In the case just discussed, a woman has a functional uterus but nonfunctional ovaries. Consider now the converse case: a woman has functional ovaries but a nonfunctional uterus. Perhaps she has had a hysterectomy. She is capable of becoming, in a manner of speaking, the *genetic* but not the *gestational* mother of a child. Now, suppose that she and her husband desire a child "of their own." This situation gives rise to the possibility of a surrogate motherhood arrangement somewhat different than the kind predicated upon artificial insemination. In this case, *in vitro* fertilization could be employed to fertilize the wife's egg with the husband's sperm. The embryo could then be transferred to the uterus of a surrogate who would agree to bear the child for the couple.

One other proposed scheme of reproductive technology is based on cloning, a form of asexual reproduction. Many scientists believe that the techniques necessary for successful human cloning will be available in the not-too-distant future. Accordingly, the following sequence of events can be imagined: A mature human egg will be obtained from a woman and enucleated in a laboratory—that is, the nucleus of the egg cell will be removed. Meanwhile, a body cell from a donor (who might be anyone including the woman who has provided the egg) will be obtained and enucleated. The resultant nucleus, which contains the donor's heretofore unique genotype, will undergo a process calculated to activate its dormant genes and then be inserted into the egg cell. From this point, the renucleated egg will develop in the way that a newly fertilized egg ordinarily develops. Implantation (not necessarily into the uterus of the woman from whom the original egg was obtained) and subsequent *in utero* gestation will then lead to the birth of a human "clone." In contrast to offspring resulting from sexual reproduction, where the resultant genotype is the result of contributions by two parents, the "clone" will have the same genotype as his or her "parent."

Reproductive Technologies: Ethical Concerns

To what extent, if at all, is it ethically acceptable to employ the various reproductive technologies just discussed? A host of ethical concerns have been expressed about these technologies, and a brief survey of the most prominent of these concerns should prove helpful.

Most of the ethical opposition to artificial insemination derives from religious views. AID especially has been attacked on the grounds that it illicitly separates procreation from the marriage relationship. Inasmuch as AID introduces a third party (the sperm donor) into a marriage relationship, it has been called a form of adultery. Even AIH, which cannot be accused of separating procreation from the marriage relationship, has not uniformly escaped attack. Some religious ethicists have gone so far as to contend that procreation is morally illicit whenever it is not the product of personal lovemaking. Although these sorts of objections frequently recur in discussions of *in vitro* fertilization, the various forms of egg donation, and cloning, they seem to have little force for those who do not share the basic worldview from which they proceed.

In one of this chapter's selections, Herbert T. Krimmel argues that it is wrong for a person to create a child with the intention of abdicating parental responsibility for it. The argument is meant to apply both to egg donation and sperm donation. Krimmel also objects to an unmarried woman's resorting to AID, on the grounds that it is unfair to intentionally deprive a child of a father. But his primary concern is to develop the case against surrogate motherhood. In another selection in this chapter, John A. Robertson contends that surrogate motherhood is an ethically acceptable practice. Since the Krimmel-Robertson exchange serves very effectively to introduce the many strands of argument in the continuing debate over surrogate motherhood, no further discussion of this controversial practice will be provided here.

Some of the ethical opposition to *in vitro* fertilization is based on the perceived "unnaturalness" of the procedure. Closely related is the charge that the procedure depersonalizes or dehumanizes procreation. Other opponents of *in vitro* fertilization have argued that we must abstain from any intervention that inflicts unknown risks on developing offspring. Another recurrent argument against *in vitro* fertilization is that its acceptance by society will lead to the acceptance of more and more objectionable developments in reproductive technology.

In addition to arguments advanced in support of a wholesale rejection of *in vitro* fertilization, a number of concerns having a more limited scope can be identified. Some commentators have been quite willing to endorse the employment of *in vitro* fertilization and embryo transfer within the framework of a marital relationship but find any third-party involvement, such as egg donation or surrogate motherhood, objectionable. Other critics object primarily to a frequent concomitant of *in vitro* procedures, the discarding of embryos considered unneeded or unsuitable for implantation. (Those who consider even an early embryo a person are especially vocal on this score.) Although the practice of freezing embryos offers a partial solution to the problem of surplus embryos, some would argue that, in this case, the "solution" creates more problems than it solves.

Two readings in this chapter focus directly on the ethics of IVF. In providing an overall defense of IVF, Peter Singer rejects many of the standard arguments against it. He also contends that there is no ethical problem with freezing *early* embryos, discarding them, or using them for research purposes. Susan Sherwin, in a very different spirit, works out a critique of IVF within the framework of feminist ethics. From a feminist point of view, she maintains, IVF is morally problematic for a number of closely related reasons. Although there is a diversity of views in the feminist community about the ethics of IVF, many feminists believe that the availability of IVF (and other reproductive technologies) is at best a mixed blessing for women.

In terms of ethical acceptability, cloning would seem to be the most problematic of all the reproductive technologies. Whereas the fundamental value of the other reproductive technologies under discussion can be located in the relief of infertility, the connection between cloning and the relief of infertility is more tenuous. Related to this consideration is the argument that cloning is the reproductive technology most likely to be misused, to the detriment of society. Of course, the stock charges against reproductive technology—that it is "unnatural" and depersonalizes reproduction—are also raised against cloning. But probably the most important arguments against cloning are those that emphasize psychological and social difficulties associated with a clone's manner of origin and lack of genetic uniqueness. One other noteworthy argument calls attention to the biological danger that would attend widespread cloning. Widespread cloning would have the effect of limiting the variety of genotypes in the species and thus limit species adaptability in the face of changing circumstances.

Genetic Engineering

An important distinction underlies many discussions of the ethics of genetic engineering (intervention). In *therapeutic* genetic engineering, the intervention is directed at the cure of disease. In *nontherapeutic* genetic engineering, the intervention is directed at the enhancement of human capabilities (e.g., memory). In this chapter's final reading, H. J. J. Leenen argues that there is no fundamental difference between therapeutic genetic engineering and more conventional therapeutic interventions. Thus he believes that the prospect of therapeutic genetic engineering does not raise any unique moral problems. However, he firmly rejects any employment of nontherapeutic genetic engineering. A contrasting view on the ethics of nontherapeutic genetic engineering can be found in a brief discussion at the end of the selection by Singer on the ethics of IVF.

It may be possible in the forseeable future to cure genetic diseases (e.g., cystic fibrosis) by direct genetic manipulation of somatic cells. Is there any reason from an ethical point of view that somatic-cell gene therapy should not be developed and employed? A commonly heard complaint against any form of direct genetic manipulation is that it places human beings in the role of "playing God." A related worry can be phrased in the form of a "slippery slope" argument: The acceptance of somatic-cell gene therapy will lead to the acceptance of more and more objectionable forms of genetic intervention. Despite these concerns, most ethicists would concur with Leenen's judgment that somatic-cell gene therapy is ethically acceptable. As for germ-line genetic therapy, which Leenen also endorses, there is more significant disagreement among ethicists. In germ-line genetic therapy, since intervention involves sperm, ova, or embryos, the resultant changes would be passed on to future generations.

T.A.M.

NOTES

1 Roughly, positive eugenics aims at enhancing the genetic heritage of the species, whereas negative eugenics aims at preventing deterioration of the gene pool.
2 This view is defended by Marc Lappé, "Moral Obligations and the Fallacies of 'Genetic Control,'" *Theological Studies* 33 (September 1972), pp. 411–427.
3 See, for example, Hermann J. Muller, "Means and Aims in Human Genetic Betterment," in T. M. Sonneborn, ed., *The Control of Human Heredity and Evolution* (New York: Macmillan, 1965), pp. 100–122.
4 Some form of egg donation might also be considered when a woman's own ova would place her offspring at risk for genetic disease.
5 To date, the success rates for this technique have not been impressive. There is also a risk of unwanted pregnancy on the part of the donor, because lavage might fail to wash out the embryo.

Reproductive Risk, Prenatal Diagnosis, and Selective Abortion

Genetic Diseases: Can Having Children Be Immoral?
L. M. Purdy

L. M. Purdy is associate professor of philosophy at Wells College (Aurora, N.Y.). She has also taught at Cornell University, where she was postdoctoral associate in the Program on Science, Technology, and Society. Specializing in ethics and political philosophy, she has published articles such as "In Defense of Hiring Apparently Less Qualified Women" and "Nature and Nurture: A False Dichotomy?"

Purdy argues that it is morally wrong to reproduce under some circumstances of genetic risk, most clearly in cases where there is high risk of serious genetic disease. Much of her analysis focuses on Huntington's chorea, which she considers a clear case of high-risk, serious genetic disease. To support her basic thesis, Purdy advances and defends the following set of claims. (1) We have an obligation to try to provide every child with a "normal opportunity for health"; (2) In acting on this obligation, we do not do wrong in preventing the existence of possible children; (3) Where there is high risk of serious genetic disease, this obligation overrides the generally recognized right to reproduce. Proceeding on the assumption that victims of Huntington's chorea lead worse than average lives, Purdy maintains that it is morally wrong for those at risk of passing on this disease to reproduce.

I   INTRODUCTION

Suppose you know that there is a fifty percent chance you have Huntington's chorea, even though you are still free of symptoms, and that if you do have it, each of your children has a fifty percent chance of having it also.

Should you now have children?

There is always some possibility that a pregnancy will result in a diseased or handicapped child. But certain persons run a higher than average risk of producing such a child. Genetic counselors are increasingly able to calculate the probability that certain problems will occur; this means that more people can find out whether they are in danger of creating unhealthy offspring *before* the birth of a child.

Since this kind of knowledge is available, we ought to use it wisely. I want in this paper to defend the thesis that it is wrong to reproduce when we know there is a high risk of transmitting a serious disease or defect. My argument for this claim is in three parts. The first is that we should try to provide every child with a normal opportunity for health; the second is that in the course of doing this it is not wrong to prevent possible children from existing. The third is that this duty may require us to refrain from childbearing.[1]

One methodological point must be made. I am investigating a problem in biomedical ethics: this is a philosophical enterprise. But the conclusion has practical importance since individuals do face the choice I examine. This raises a question: what relation ought the outcome of this inquiry bear to social policy?[2] It may be held that a person's reproductive life should not be interfered with. Perhaps this is a reasonable position, but it does not follow from it that it is never wrong for an individual to have children or that we should not try to determine when this is the case. All that does follow is that we may not coerce persons with regard to childbearing. Evaluation of this last claim is a separate issue which cannot be handled here.

I want to deal with this issue concretely. The reason for this is that, otherwise, discussion is apt to be vague and inconclusive. An additional reason is that it will serve to make us appreciate the magnitude of the difficulties faced by diseased or handicapped individuals. Thus it will be helpful to consider a specific disease. For this purpose I have chosen Huntington's chorea.[3]

II   HUNTINGTON'S CHOREA: COURSE AND RISK

Let us now look at Huntington's chorea. First we will consider the course of the disease, then its inheritance pattern.

The symptoms of Huntington's chorea usually begin between the ages of thirty and fifty, but young children can also be affected. It happens this way:

> Onset is insidious. Personality changes (obstinancy, moodiness, lack of initiative) frequently antedate or accompany the involuntary choreic movements. These usually appear first in the face, neck, and arms, and are jerky, irregular, and stretching in character. Contractions of the facial muscles result in grimaces; those of the respiratory muscles, lips, and tongue lead to hesitating, explosive speech. Irregular movements of the trunk are present; the gait is shuffling and dancing. Tendon reflexes are increased.... Some patients display a fatuous euphoria; others are spiteful, irascible, destructive, and violent. Paranoid reactions are common. Poverty of thought and impairment of attention, memory, and judgment occur. As the disease progresses, walking becomes impossible, swallowing difficult, and dementia profound. Suicide is not uncommon.[4]

The illness lasts about fifteen years, terminating in death.

Who gets Huntington's chorea? It is an autosomal dominant disease; this means it is caused by a single mutant gene located on a non-sex chromosome. It is passed from one generation to the next via affected individuals. When one has the disease, whether one has symptoms and thus knows one has it or not, there is a fifty percent chance that each child will have it also. If one has escaped it then there is no risk to one's children.[5]

How serious is this risk? For geneticists, a ten percent risk is high.[6] But not every high risk is unacceptable: this depends on what is at stake.

There are two separate evaluations in any judgment about a given risk. The first measures the gravity of the worst possible result; the second perceives a given risk as great or small. As for the first, in medicine as elsewhere, people may regard the same result quite differently:

> ...The subjective attitude to the disease or lesion itself may be quite at variance with what informed medical opinion may regard as a realistic appraisal. Relatively minor limb defects with cosmetic over-tones are examples here. On the other hand, some patients regard with equanimity genetic lesions which are of major medical importance.[7]

For devastating diseases like Huntington's chorea, this part of the judgment should be unproblematic: no one could want a loved one to suffer so.

There may be considerable disagreement, however, about whether a given probability is big or little. Individuals vary a good deal in their attitude toward this aspect of risk.[8] This suggests that it would be difficult to define the "right" attitude to a particular risk in many circumstances. Nevertheless, there are good grounds for arguing in favor of a conservative approach here. For it is reasonable to take special precautions to avoid very bad consequences, even if the risk is small. But the possible consequences here *are* very bad: a child who may inherit Huntington's chorea is a child with a much larger than average chance of being subjected to severe and prolonged suffering. Even if the child does not have the disease, it may anticipate and fear it, and anticipating an evil, as we all know, may be worse than experiencing it. In addition, if a parent loses the gamble, his child will suffer the consequences. But it is one thing to take a high risk for oneself; to submit someone else to it without his consent is another.

I think that these points indicate that the morality of procreation in situations like this demands further study. I propose to do this by looking first at the position

of the possible child, then at that of the potential parent.[9]

III REPRODUCTION: THE POSSIBLE CHILD'S POSITION

The first task in treating the problem from the child's point of view is to find a way of referring to possible future offspring without seeming to confer some sort of morally significant existence upon them. I will call children who might be born in the future but who are not now conceived "possible" children, offspring, individuals, or persons. I stipulate that this term implies nothing about their moral standing.

The second task is to decide what claims about children or possible children are relevant to the morality of childbearing in the circumstances being considered. There are, I think, two such claims. One is that we ought to provide every child with at least a normal opportunity for a good life. The other is that we do not harm possible children if we prevent them from existing. Let us consider both these matters in turn.

A Opportunity for a Good Life

Accepting the claim that we ought to try to provide for every child a normal opportunity for a good life involves two basic problems: justification and practical application.

Justification of the claim could be derived fairly straightforwardly from either utilitarian or contractarian theories of justice, I think, although a proper discussion would be too lengthy to include here. Of prime importance in any such discussion would be the judgment that to neglect this duty would be to create unnecessary unhappiness or unfair disadvantage for some persons.

The attempt to apply the claim that we should try to provide a normal opportunity for a good life leads to a couple of difficulties. One is knowing what it requires of us. Another is defining "normal opportunity." Let us tackle the latter problem first.

Conceptions of "normal opportunity" vary among societies and also within them: *de rigueur* in some circles are private music lessons and trips to Europe, while in others providing eight years of schooling is a major sacrifice. But there is no need to consider this complication since we are here concerned only with health as a prerequisite for normal opportunity. Thus we can retreat to the more limited claim that every parent should try to ensure normal health for his child. It might be thought that even this moderate claim is unsatisfactory since in some places debilitating conditions are the norm. One could circumvent this objection by saying that parents ought to try to provide for their children health normal for that culture, even though it may be inadequate if measured by some outside standard. This conservative position would still justify efforts to avoid the birth of children at risk for Huntington's chorea and other serious genetic diseases.

But then what does this stand require of us: is sacrifice entailed by the duty to try to provide normal health for our children? The most plausible answer seems to be that as the danger of serious disability increases, the greater the sacrifice demanded of the potential parent. This means it would be more justifiable to recommend that an individual refrain from childbearing if he risks passing on spina bifida than if he risks passing on webbed feet. Working out all the details of such a schema would clearly be a difficult matter; I do not think it would be impossible to set up workable guidelines, though.

Assuming a rough theoretical framework of this sort, the next question we must ask is whether Huntington's chorea substantially impairs an individual's opportunity for a good life.

People appear to have different opinions about the plight of such persons. Optimists argue that a child born into a family afflicted with Huntington's chorea has a reasonable chance of living a satisfactory life. After all, there is a fifty percent chance it will escape the disease if a parent has already manifested it, and a still greater chance if this is not so. Even if it does have the illness, it will probably enjoy thirty years of healthy life before symptoms appear; and, perhaps, it may not find the disease destructive. Optimists can list diseased or handicapped persons who have lived fruitful lives. They can also find individuals who seem genuinely glad to be alive. One is Rick Donohue, a sufferer from the Joseph family disease: "You know, if my mom hadn't had me, I wouldn't be here for the life I have had. So there is a good possibility I will have children."[10] Optimists therefore conclude that it would be a shame if these persons had not lived.

Pessimists concede these truths, but they take a less sanguine view of them. They think a fifty percent risk of serious disease like Huntington's chorea appallingly high. They suspect that a child born into an afflicted family is liable to spend its youth in dreadful anticipation and fear of the disease. They expect that the disease,

if it appears, will be perceived as a tragic and painful end to a blighted life. They point out that Rick Donohue is still young and has not yet experienced the full horror of his sickness.

Empirical research is clearly needed to resolve this dispute: we need much more information about the psychology and life history of sufferers and potential sufferers. Until we have it we cannot know whether the optimist or the pessimist has a better case; definitive judgment must therefore be suspended. In the meantime, however, common sense suggests that the pessimist has the edge.

If some diseased persons do turn out to have a worse than average life there appears to be a case against further childbearing in afflicted families. To support this claim two more judgments are necessary, however. The first is that it is not wrong to refrain from childbearing. The second is that asking individuals to so refrain is less of a sacrifice than might be thought.[11] I will examine each of these judgments.

B   The Morality of Preventing the Birth of Possible Persons

Before going on to look at reasons why it would not be wrong to prevent the birth of possible persons, let me try to clarify the picture a bit. To understand the claim it must be kept in mind that we are considering a prospective situation here, not a retrospective one: we are trying to rank the desirability of various alternative future states of affairs. One possible future state is this: a world where nobody is at risk for Huntington's chorea except as a result of random mutation. This state has been achieved by sons and daughters of persons afflicted with Huntington's chorea ceasing to reproduce. This means that an indeterminate number of children who might have been born were not born. These possible children can be divided into two categories: those who would have been miserable and those who would have lived good lives. To prevent the existence of members of the first category it was necessary to prevent the existence of all. Whether or not this is a good state of affairs depends on the morality of the means and the end. The end, preventing the existence of miserable beings, is surely good; I will argue that preventing the birth of possible persons is not intrinsically wrong. Hence this state of affairs is a morally good one.

Why then is it not in itself wrong to prevent the birth of possible persons? It is not wrong because there seems to be no reason to believe that possible individuals are either deprived or injured if they do not exist. They are not deprived because to be deprived in a morally significant sense one must be able to have experiences. But possible persons do not exist. Since they do not exist, they cannot have experiences. Another way to make this point is to say that each of us might not have been born, although most of us are glad we were. But this does not mean that it makes sense to say that we would have been deprived of something had we not been born. For if we had not been born, we would not exist, and there would be nobody to be deprived of anything. To assert the contrary is to imagine that we are looking at a world in which we do not exist. But this is not the way it would be: there would be nobody to look.

The contention that it is wrong to prevent possible persons from existing because they have a right to exist appears to be equally baseless. The most fundamental objection to this view is that there is no reason to ascribe rights to entities which do not exist. It is one thing to say that as-yet-nonexistent persons will have certain rights if and when they exist: this claim is plausible if made with an eye toward preserving social and environmental goods.[12] But what justification could there be for the claim that nonexistent beings have a right to exist?

Even if one conceded that there was a presumption in favor of letting some nonexistent beings exist, stronger claims could surely override it.[13] For one thing, it would be unfair not to recognize the prior claim of already existing children who are not being properly cared for. One might also argue that it is simply wrong to prevent persons who might have existed from doing so. But this implies that contraception and population control are also wrong.

It is therefore reasonable to maintain that because possible persons have no right to exist, they are not injured if not created. Even if they had that right, it could rather easily be overridden by counterclaims. Hence, since possible persons are neither deprived nor injured if not conceived, it is not wrong to prevent their existence.

C   Conclusion of Part III

At the beginning of Part III I said that two claims are relevant to the morality of childbearing in the circumstances being considered. The first is that we ought to provide every child with at least a normal opportunity for a good life. The second is that we do not deprive or injure possible persons if we prevent their existence.

I suggested that the first claim could be derived from currently accepted theories of justice: a healthy

body is generally necessary for happiness and it is also a prerequisite for a fair chance at a good life in our competitive world. Thus it is right to try to ensure that each child is healthy.

I argued, with regard to the second claim, that we do not deprive or injure possible persons if we fail to create them. They cannot be deprived of anything because they do not exist and hence cannot have experiences. They cannot be injured because only an entity with a right to exist could be injured if prevented from existing; but there are no good grounds for believing that they are such entities.

From the conjunction of these two claims I conclude that it is right to try to ensure that a child is healthy even if by doing so we preclude the existence of certain possible persons. Thus it is right for individuals to prevent the birth of children at risk for Huntington's chorea by avoiding parenthood. The next question is whether it is seriously wrong *not* to avoid parenthood.

IV   REPRODUCTION: THE POTENTIAL PARENT'S SITUATION

I have so far argued that if choreics live substantially worse lives than average, then it is right for afflicted families to cease reproduction. But this conflicts with the generally recognized freedom to procreate and so it does not automatically follow that family members ought not to have children. How can we decide whether the duty to try to provide normal health for one's child should take precedence over the right to reproduce?

This is essentially the same question I asked earlier: how much must one sacrifice to try to ensure that one's offspring is healthy? In answer to this I suggested that the greater the danger of serious disability, the more justifiable considerable sacrifice is.

Now asking someone who wants a child to refrain from procreation seems to be asking for a large sacrifice. It may, in fact, appear to be too large to demand of anyone. Yet I think it can be shown that it is not as great as it initially seems.

Why do people want children? There are probably many reasons, but I suspect that the following include some of the most common. One set of reasons has to do with the gratification to be derived from a happy family life—love, companionship, watching a child grow, helping mold it into a good person, sharing its pains and triumphs. Another set of reasons centers about the parents as individuals—validation of their place within a genetically continuous family line, the conception of children as a source of immortality, being surrounded by replicas of themselves.

Are there alternative ways of satisfying these desires? Adoption or technological means provide ways to satisfy most of the desires pertaining to family life without passing on specific genetic defects. Artificial insemination by donor is already available; implantation of donor ova is likely within a few years. Still another option will exist if cloning becomes a reality. In the meantime, we might permit women to conceive and bear babies for those who do not want to do so themselves.[14] But the desire to extend the genetic line, the desire for immortality, and the desire for children that physically resemble one cannot be met by these methods.

Many individuals probably feel these latter desires strongly. This creates a genuine conflict for persons at risk for transmitting serious genetic diseases like Huntington's chorea. The situation seems especially unfair because, unlike normal people, through no fault of their own, doing something they badly want to do may greatly harm others.

But if my common sense assumption that they are in grave danger of harming others is true, then it is imperative to scrutinize their options carefully. On the one hand, they can have children: they satisfy their desires but risk eventual crippling illness and death for their offspring. On the other, they can remain childless or seek nonstandard ways of creating a family: they have some unfulfilled desires, but they avoid risking harm to their children.

I think it is clear which of these two alternatives is best. For the desires which must remain unsatisfied if they forgo normal procreation are less than admirable. To see the genetic line continued entails a sinister legacy of illness and death; the desire for immortality cannot really be satisfied by reproduction anyway; and the desire for children that physically resemble one is narcissistic and its fulfillment cannot be guaranteed even by normal reproduction. Hence the only defense of these desires is that people do in fact feel them.

Now, I am inclined to accept William James' dictum regarding desires: "Take any demand, however slight, which any creature, however weak, may make. Ought it not, for its own sole sake be satisfied? If not, prove why not."[15] Thus I judge a world where more desires are satisfied to be better than one in which fewer are. But not all desires should be regarded as legitimate, since, as James suggests, there may be good reasons why these ought to be disregarded. The fact that their fulfillment will seriously harm others is surely such a reason. And I believe that the circumstances I have described are a clear example of the sort of case where a desire must be judged illegitimate, at least until it can be shown

that sufferers from serious genetic diseases like Huntington's chorea do not live considerably worse than average lives. Therefore, I think it is wrong for individuals in this predicament to reproduce.

V CONCLUSION

Let me recapitulate. At the beginning of this paper I asked whether it is wrong for those who risk transmitting severe genetic disease like Huntington's chorea to have "blood" children. Some despair of reaching an answer to this question.[16] But I think such pessimism is not wholly warranted, and that if generally accepted would lead to much unnecessary harm. It is true that in many cases it is difficult to know what ought to be done. But this does not mean that we should throw up our hands and espouse a completely laissez-faire approach: philosophers can help by probing the central issues and trying to find guidelines for action.

Naturally there is no way to derive an answer to this kind of problem by deductive argument from self-evident premises, for it must depend on a complicated interplay of facts and moral judgments. My preliminary exploration of Huntington's chorea is of this nature. In the course of the discussion I suggested that, if it is true that sufferers live substantially worse lives than do normal persons, those who might transmit it should not have any children. This conclusion is supported by the judgments that we ought to try to provide for every child a normal opportunity for a good life, that possible individuals are not harmed if not conceived, and that it is sometimes less justifiable for persons to exercise their right to procreate than one might think.

I want to stress, in conclusion, that my argument is incomplete. To investigate fully even a single disease, like Huntington's chorea, empirical research on the lives of members of afflicted families is necessary. Then, after developing further the themes touched upon here, evaluation of the probable consequences of different policies on society and on future generations is needed. Until the results of a complete study are available, my argument could serve best as a reason for persons at risk for transmitting Huntington's chorea and similar diseases to put off having children. Perhaps this paper will stimulate such inquiry.

NOTES

1 There are a series of cases ranging from low risk of mild disease or handicap to high risk of serious dis-

ease or handicap. It would be difficult to decide where the duty to refrain from procreation becomes compelling. My point here is that there are some clear cases.

I'd like to thank Lawrence Davis and Sidney Siskin for their helpful comments on an earlier version of this paper.

2 This issue is one which must be faced most urgently by genetic counselors. The proper role of the genetic counselor with regard to such decisions has been the subject of much debate. The dominant view seems to be that espoused by Lytt Gardner who maintains that it is unethical for a counselor to make ethical judgments about what his clients ought to do. ("Counseling in Genetics," *Early Diagnosis of Human Genetic Defects: Scientific & Ethical Considerations*, ed. Maureen Harris, [H.E.W. Publication No. (NIH) 72–25; Fogarty Center Proceedings No. 6]; p. 192.) Typically this view is unsupported by an argument. For other views see Bentley Glass, "Human Heredity and Ethical Problems" *Perspectives in Biology & Medicine*, Vol. 15 (winter '72) 237–53, esp. 242–52; Marc Lappé, "The Genetic Counselor Responsible to Whom?" *Hastings Center Report*, Vol. 1, No. 2 (Sept. '71) 6–8; E. C. Fraser, "Genetic Counseling" *Am. J. of Human Genetics* 26: 636–659, 1974.

3 I have chosen Huntington's chorea because it seems to me to be one of the clearest cases of high risk serious genetic disease known to the public, despite the fact that it does not usually manifest itself until the prime of life. The latter entails two further facts. First an individual of reproductive age may not know whether he has the disease; he therefore does not know the risk of passing on the disease. Secondly, an affected person may have a substantial number of years of healthy life before it shows itself. I do not think that this factor materially changes my case, however. Even if an individual does not in fact risk passing the disease to his children, *he cannot know that this is true*. And even thirty years of healthy life may well be seriously shadowed by anticipation and fear of the disease. Thus the fact that the disease develops late does not diminish its horror. If it could be shown that these factors could be adequately circumvented, my claim that there is a *class* of genetic disease of such severity that it would be wrong to risk passing them on would not be undermined.

It might also be thought that Huntington's chorea is insufficiently common to merit such attention. But, depending on reproductive patterns, the disease

could become a good deal more widespread. Consider the fact that in 1916 nine hundred and sixty-two cases could be traced from six seventeenth-century arrivals in America. (Gordon Rattray Taylor, *The Biological Time Bomb*, [New York, 1968], p. 176.) But more importantly, even if the disease did not spread, it would still be seriously wrong, I think, to inflict it unnecessarily on *any* members of new generations. Finally, it should be kept in mind that I am using Huntington's chorea as an example of the sort of disease we should try to eradicate. Thus the arguments presented here would be relevant to a wide range of genetic diseases.

4 *The Merck Manual* (Rahway, N.J.: Merck, 1972), p. 1346.

5 Hymie Gordon, "Genetic Counseling," *JAMA*, Vol. 217 No. 9 (August 30, 1971), 1217.

6 Charles Smith, Susan Holloway, and Alan E. H. Emery, "Individuals at Risk in Families—Genetic Disease," *J. of Medical Genetics*, 8(1971), 453. See also Townes in *Genetic Counseling*, ed. Daniel Bergsma, *Birth Defects Original Article Series*, Vol. VI, No. 1 (May 1970).

7 J. H. Pearn, "Patients' Subjective Interpretation of Risks Offered in Genetic Counseling," *Journal of Medical Genetics*, 10 (1973), 131.

8 Pearn, p. 132.

9 There are many important and interesting points that might be raised with respect to future generations and present society. There is no space to deal with them here, although I strongly suspect that conclusions regarding them would support my judgment that it is wrong for those who risk transmitting certain diseases to reproduce—for some discussion of future generations, see Gerald Leach, *The Biocrats*, (Middlesex, England: Penguin Books, 1972), p. 150; M. P. Golding, "Obligations to Future Generations," *Monist* 56 (Jan. 1972) 84–99; Gordon Rattray Taylor, *The Biological Time Bomb* (New York, 1968), esp. p. 176. For some discussions of society, see Daniel Callahan, "The Meaning and Significance of Genetic Disease: Philosophical Perspectives," *Ethical Issues in Human Genetics*, ed. Bruce Hilton et al. (New York, 1973), p. 87ff.; John Fletcher, "The Brink: The Parent-Child Bond in the Genetic Revolution," *Theological Studies* 33 (Sept. '72) 457–485; Glass (supra 2ᵃ); Marc Lappé, "Human Genetics," Annals of the *New York Academy of Sciences*, Vol. 26 (May 18, 1973) 152–59; Marc Lappé, "Moral Obligations and the Fallacies of 'Genetic Control,'"

Theological Studies Vol. 33, No. 3 (Sept '72), 411–427; Martin P. Golding, "Ethical Issues in Biological Engineering," *UCLA Law Review* Vol. 15: 267 (1968) 443–479; L. C. Dunn, *Heredity and Evolution in Human Populations* (Cambridge, Mass., 1959), p. 145; Robert S. Morison in *Ethical Issues in Human Genetics*, ed. Bruce Hilton et al. (New York, 1973), p. 208.

10 *The New York Times*, September 30, 1975, p. 1., col. 6. The Joseph family disease is similar to Huntington's chorea except that symptoms start appearing in the twenties. Rick Donohue is in his early twenties.

11 There may be a price for the individuals who refrain from having children. We will be looking at the situation from their point of view shortly.

12 This is in fact the basis for certain parental duties. An example is the maternal duty to obtain proper nutrition before and during pregnancy, for this is necessary if the child is to have normal health when it is born.

13 One might argue that as many persons as possible should exist so that they may enjoy life.

14 Some thinkers have qualms about the use of some or all of these methods. They have so far failed to show why they are immoral, although, naturally, much careful study will be required before they could be unqualifiedly recommended. See, for example, Richard Hull, "Genetic Engineering: Comment on Headings," *The Humanist*, Vol. 32 (Sept./Oct. 1972), 13.

15 *Essays in Pragmatism*, ed. A. Castell (New York, 1948), p. 73.

16 For example, see Leach, p. 138. One of the ways the dilemma described by Leach could be lessened would be if society emphasized those aspects of family life not dependent on "blood" relationships and downplayed those that are.

Implications of Prenatal Diagnosis for the Human Right to Life
Leon R. Kass

Leon R. Kass, a biologist as well as a medical doctor, is professor in the College, University of Chicago. He is the author of *Toward a More Natural Science: Biology and Human Affairs* (1985). Among the more prominent of his many articles on issues in biomedical ethics are "Regarding the End of Medicine and the Pursuit of Health," "Making Babies—The New Biology and the 'Old' Morality," and "The New Biology: What Price Relieving Man's Estate?"

Setting aside a discussion of the moral problem of abortion in general, Kass focuses on some of the ethical difficulties associated with the abortion of fetuses known by amniocentesis to be genetically defective. He maintains that the practice of *genetic* abortion, inasmuch as it involves a qualitative assessment of fetuses, represents a threat to the "radical moral equality of all human beings." As a result of the practice of genetic abortion, Kass suggests, we will be inclined to take a more negative view of those who are genetically defective or otherwise "abnormal." Thus we will be inclined to treat them in a second-class manner. Moreover, he contends, to commit ourselves to the practice of genetic abortion is to reflect acceptance of a very dangerous principle, that "defectives should not be born."

It is especially fitting on this occasion to begin by acknowledging how privileged I feel and how pleased I am to be a participant in this symposium. I suspect that I am not alone among the assembled in considering myself

Reprinted by permission of the author and Plenum Publishing Corporation from *Ethical Issues in Human Genetics*, edited by Bruce Hilton et al., 1973.

fortunate to be here. For I was conceived after antibiotics yet before amniocentesis, late enough to have benefited from medicine's ability to prevent and control fatal infectious diseases, yet early enough to have escaped from medicine's ability to prevent me from living to suffer from my genetic diseases. To be sure, my genetic vices are, as far as I know them, rather modest, taken individually—myopia, asthma and other allergies, bilateral forefoot adduction, bowleggedness, loquaciousness, and pessimism, plus some four to eight as yet undiagnosed recessive lethal genes in the heterozygous condition—but, taken together, and if diagnosable prenatally, I might never have made it.

Just as I am happy to be here, so am I unhappy with what I shall have to say. Little did I realize when I first conceived the topic, "Implications of Prenatal Diagnosis for the Human Right to Life," what a painful and difficult labor it would lead to. More than once while this paper was gestating, I considered obtaining permission to abort it, on the grounds that, by prenatal diagnosis, I knew it to be defective. My lawyer told me that I was legally in the clear, but my conscience reminded me that I had made a commitment to deliver myself of this paper, flawed or not. Next time, I shall practice better contraception.

Any discussion of the ethical issues of genetic counseling and prenatal diagnosis is unavoidably haunted by a ghost called the morality of abortion. This ghost I shall not vex. More precisely, I shall not vex the reader by telling ghost stories. However, I would be neither surprised nor disappointed if my discussion of an admittedly related matter, the ethics of aborting the genetically defective, summons that hovering spirit to the reader's mind. For the morality of abortion is a matter not easily laid to rest, recent efforts to do so notwithstanding. A vote by the legislature of the State of New York can indeed legitimatize the disposal of fetuses, but not of the moral questions. But though the questions remain, there is likely to be little new that can be said about them, and certainly not by me.

Yet before leaving the general question of abortion, let me pause to drop some anchors for the discussion that follows. Despite great differences of opinion both as to what to think and how to reason about abortion, nearly everyone agrees that abortion is a moral issue.[1] What does this mean? Formally, it means that a woman seeking or refusing an abortion can expect to be asked to justify her action. And we can expect that she should be able to give reasons for her choice other than "I like it" or "I don't like it." Substantively, it means that, in the absence of good reasons for intervention, there is some presumption in favor of allowing the pregnancy to continue once it has begun. A common way of expressing this presumption is to say that "the fetus has a right to continued life."[2] In this context, disagreement concerning the moral permissibility of abortion concerns what rights (or interests or needs), and whose, override (take precedence over, or outweigh) this fetal "right." Even

most of the "opponents" of abortion agree that the mother's right to live takes precedence, and that abortion to save her life is permissible, perhaps obligatory. Some believe that a woman's right to determine the number and spacing of her children takes precedence, while yet others argue that the need to curb population growth is, at least at this time, overriding.

Hopefully, this brief analysis of what it means to say that abortion is a moral issue is sufficient to establish two points. First, that the fetus is a living thing with some moral claim on us not to do it violence, and therefore, second, that justification must be given for destroying it.

Turning now from the general questions of the ethics of abortion, I wish to focus on the special ethical issues raised by the abortion of "defective" fetuses (so-called "abortion for fetal indications"). I shall consider only the cleanest cases, those cases where well-characterized genetic diseases are diagnosed with a high degree of certainty by means of amniocentesis, in order to sidestep the added moral dilemmas posed when the diagnosis is suspected or possible, but unconfirmed. However, many of the questions I shall discuss could also be raised about cases where genetic analysis gives only a statistical prediction about the genotype of the fetus, and also about cases where the defect has an infectious or chemical rather than a genetic cause (e.g., rubella, thalidomide).

My first and possibly most difficult task is to show that there is anything left to discuss once we have agreed not to discuss the morality of abortion in general. There is a sense in which abortion for genetic defect is, after abortion to save the life of the mother, perhaps the most defensible kind of abortion. Certainly, it is a serious and not a frivolous reason for abortion, defended by its proponents in sober and rational speech—unlike justifications based upon the false notion that a fetus is a mere part of a woman's body, to be used and abused at her pleasure. Standing behind genetic abortion are serious and well-intentioned people, with reasonable ends in view: the prevention of genetic diseases, the elimination of suffering in families, the preservation of precious financial and medical resources, the protection of our genetic heritage. No profiteers, no sex-ploiters, no racists. No arguments about the connection of abortion with promiscuity and licentiousness, no perjured testimony about the mental health of the mother, no arguments about the seriousness of the population problem. In short, clear objective data, a worthy cause, decent men and women. If abortion, what better reason for it?

Yet if genetic abortion is but a happily wagging tail on the dog of abortion, it is simultaneously the nose of a camel protruding under a rather different tent. Precisely because the quality of the fetus is central to the decision to abort, the practice of genetic abortion has implications which go beyond those raised by abortion in general. What may be at stake here is the belief in the radical moral equality of all human beings, the belief that all human beings possess equally and independent of merit certain fundamental rights, one among which is, of course, the right to life.

To be sure, the belief that fundamental human rights belong equally to all human beings has been but an ideal, never realized, often ignored, sometimes shamelessly. Yet it has been perhaps the most powerful moral idea at work in the world for at least two centuries. It is this idea and ideal that animates most of the current political and social criticism around the globe. It is ironic that we should acquire the power to detect and eliminate the genetically unequal at a time when we have finally succeeded in removing much of the stigma and disgrace previously attached to victims of congenital illness, in providing them with improved care and support, and in preventing, by means of education, feelings of guilt on the part of their parents. One might even wonder whether the development of amniocentesis and prenatal diagnosis may represent a backlash against these same humanitarian and egalitarian tendencies in the practice of medicine, which, by helping to sustain to the age of reproduction persons with genetic disease has itself contributed to the increasing incidence of genetic disease, and with it, to increased pressures for genetic screening, genetic counseling, and genetic abortion.

No doubt our humanitarian and egalitarian principles and practices have caused us some new difficulties, but if we mean to weaken or turn our backs on them, we should do so consciously and thoughtfully. If, as I believe, the idea and practice of genetic abortion points in that direction, we should make ourselves aware of it....

GENETIC ABORTION AND THE LIVING DEFECTIVE

The practice of abortion of the genetically defective will no doubt affect our view of and our behavior toward those abnormals who escape the net of detection and abortion. A child with Down's syndrome or with hemophilia or with muscular dystrophy born at a time when most of his (potential) fellow sufferers were destroyed prenatally is liable to be looked upon by the community as one unfit to be alive, as a second-class (or even lower) human type. He may be seen as a person who need not have been, and who would not have been, if only someone had gotten to him in time.

The parents of such children are also likely to treat them differently, especially if the mother would have wished but failed to get an amniocentesis because of ignorance, poverty, or distance from the testing station, or if the prenatal diagnosis was in error. In such cases, parents are especially likely to resent the child. They may be disinclined to give it the kind of care they might have before the advent of amniocentesis and genetic abortion, rationalizing that a second-class specimen is not entitled to first-class treatment. If pressed to do so, say by physicians, the parents might refuse, and the courts may become involved. This has already begun to happen.

In Maryland, parents of a child with Down's syndrome refused permission to have the child operated on for an intestinal obstruction present at birth. The physicians and the hospital sought an injunction to require the parents to allow surgery. The judge ruled in favor of the parents, despite what I understand to be the weight of precedent to the contrary, on the grounds that the child was Mongoloid, that is, had the child been "normal," the decision would have gone the other way. Although the decision was not appealed to and hence not affirmed by a higher court, we can see through the prism of this case the possibility that the new powers of human genetics will strip the blindfold from the lady of justice and will make official the dangerous doctrine that some men are more equal than others.

The abnormal child may also feel resentful. A child with Down's syndrome or Tay-Sachs disease will probably never know or care, but what about a child with hemophilia or with Turner's syndrome? In the past decade, with medical knowledge and power over the prenatal child increasing and with parental authority over the postnatal child decreasing, we have seen the appearance of a new type of legal action, suits for wrongful life. Children have brought suit against their parents (and others) seeking to recover damages for physical and social handicaps inextricably tied to their birth (e.g., congenital deformities, congenital syphilis, illegitimacy). In some of the American cases, the courts have recognized the justice of the child's claim (that he was injured due to parental negligence), although they have so far refused to award damages, due to policy considerations. In other countries, e.g., in Germany, judgments with compensation have gone for the plaintiffs. With the spread of amniocentesis and genetic abortion, we can only expect such cases to increase. And here it will be the soft-hearted rather than the hard-hearted judges who will establish the doctrine of second-class human beings, out of compassion for the mutants who escaped the traps set out for them.

It may be argued that I am dealing with a problem which, even if it is real, will affect very few people. It may be suggested that very few will escape the traps once we have set them properly and widely, once people are informed about amniocentesis, once the power to detect prenatally grows to its full capacity, and once our "superstitious" opposition to abortion dies out or is extirpated. But in order even to come close to this vision of success, amniocentesis will have to become part of every pregnancy—either by making it mandatory, like the test for syphilis, or by making it "routine medical practice," like the Pap smear. Leaving aside the other problems with universal amniocentesis, we could expect that the problem for the few who escape is likely to be even worse precisely because they will be few.

The point, however, should be generalized. How will we come to view and act toward the many "abnormals" that will remain among us—the retarded, the crippled, the senile, the deformed, and the true mutants—once we embark on a program to root out genetic abnormality? For it must be remembered that we shall always have abnormals—some who escape detection or whose disease is undetectable *in utero*, others as a result of new mutations, birth injuries, accidents, maltreatment, or disease—who will require our care and protection. The existence of "defectives" cannot be fully prevented, not even by totalitarian breeding and weeding programs. Is it not likely that our principle with respect to these people will change from "We try harder" to "Why accept second best?" The idea of "the unwanted because abnormal child" may become a self-fulfilling prophecy, whose consequences may be worse than those of the abnormality itself.

GENETIC AND OTHER DEFECTIVES

The mention of other abnormals points to a second danger of the practice of genetic abortion. Genetic abortion may come to be seen not so much as the prevention of genetic disease, but as the prevention of birth of defective or abnormal children—and, in a way, understandably so. For in the case of what other diseases does preventive medicine consist in the elimination of the patient-at-risk? Moreover, the very language used to discuss genetic disease leads us to the easy but wrong conclusion that the afflicted fetus or person is rather than has a disease. True, one is partly defined by his genotype, but only partly. A person is more than his disease. And yet we slide easily from the language of possession to the language of identity, from "He has hemophilia" to "He is a hemophiliac," from "She has diabetes" through "She is diabetic" to "She is a diabetic," from "The fetus has Down's syndrome" to "The fetus is a Down's." This way of speaking supports the belief that it is defective persons (or potential persons) that are being eliminated, rather than diseases.

If this is so, then it becomes simply accidental that the defect has a genetic cause. Surely, it is only because of the high regard for medicine and science, and for the accuracy of genetic diagnosis, that genotypic defectives are likely to be the first to go. But once the principle, "Defectives should not be born," is established, grounds other than cytological and biochemical may very well be sought. Even ignoring racialists and others equally misguided—of course, they cannot be ignored—we should know that there are social scientists, for example, who believe that one can predict with a high degree of accuracy how a child will turn out from a careful, systematic study of the socio-economic and psycho-dynamic environment into which he is born and in which he grows up. They might press for the prevention of socio-psychological disease, even of "criminality," by means of prenatal environmental diagnosis and abortion. I have heard rumor that a crude, unscientific form of eliminating potential "phenotypic defectives" is already being practiced in some cities, in that submission to abortion is allegedly being made a condition for the receipt of welfare payments. "Defectives should not be born" is a principle without limits. We can ill-afford to have it established.

Up to this point, I have been discussing the possible implications of the practice of genetic abortion for our belief in and adherence to the idea that, at least in fundamental human matters such as life and liberty, all men are to be considered as equals, that for these matters we should ignore as irrelevant the real qualitative differences amongst men, however important these differences may be for other purposes. Those who are concerned about abortion fear that the permissible time of eliminating the unwanted will be moved forward along the time continuum, against newborns, infants, and children. Similarly, I suggest that we should be concerned lest the attack on gross genetic inequality in fetuses be advanced along the continuum of quality and into the later stages of life.

I am not engaged in predicting the future; I am not saying that amniocentesis and genetic abortion will lead down the road to Nazi Germany. Rather, I am suggesting that the principles underlying genetic abortion simultaneously justify many futher steps down that road. The point was very well made by Abraham Lincoln:

> If A can prove, however conclusively, that he may, of right, enslave B—Why may not B snatch the same argument and prove equally, that he may enslave A?
>
> You say A is white, and B is black. It is color, then; the lighter having the right to enslave the darker? Take care. By this rule, you are to be slave to the first man you meet with a fairer skin than your own.
>
> You do not mean color exactly? You mean the whites are intellectually the superiors of the blacks, and, therefore have the right to enslave them? Take care again. By this rule, you are to be slave to the first man you meet with an intellect superior to your own.
>
> But, say you, it is a question of interest; and, if you can make it your interest, you have the right to enslave another. Very well. And if he can make it his interest, he has the right to enslave you.[3]

Perhaps I have exaggerated the dangers; perhaps we will not abandon our inexplicable preference for generous humanitarianism over consistency. But we should indeed be cautious and move slowly as we give serious consideration to the question "What price the perfect baby?"[4] . . .

NOTES

1 This strikes me as by far the most important inference to be drawn from the fact that men in different times and cultures have answered the abortion question differently. Seen in this light, the differing and changing answers themselves suggest that it is a question not easily put under, at least not for very long.

2 Other ways include: one should not do violence to living or growing things; life is sacred; respect nature; fetal life has value; refrain from taking innocent life; protect and preserve life. As some have pointed out, the terms chosen are of different weight, and would require reasons of different weight to tip the balance in favor of abortion. My choice of the "rights" terminology is not meant to beg the questions of whether such rights really exist, or of where they come from. However, the notion of a "fetal right to life" presents only a little more difficulty in this regard than does the notion of a "human right to life," since the former does not depend on a claim that the human fetus is already "human." In my sense of terms "right" and "life," we might even say that a dog or fetal dog has a "right to life," and that it would be cruel and immoral for a man to go around performing abortions even on dogs for no good reason.

3 Lincoln, A. (1854). In *The Collected Works of Abraham Lincoln*, R. P. Basler, editor. New Brunswick, New Jersey, Rutgers University Press, Vol. II, p. 222.

4 For a discussion of the possible biological rather than moral price of attempts to prevent the birth of defective children see Motulsky, A. G., G. R. Fraser, and J. Felsenstein (1971). In Symposium on Intra-uterine Diagnosis, D. Bergsma, editor. *Birth Defects: Original Article Series*, Vol. 7, No. 5. Also see Neel, J. (1972). In *Early Diagnosis of Human Genetic Defects: Scientific and Ethical Considerations*, M. Harris, editor. Washington, D.C., U.S. Government Printing Office, pp. 366–380.

Prenatal Diagnosis and the Ethics of Uncertainty
Eric T. Juengst

A biographical sketch of Eric T. Juengst is found on page 301.

Juengst begins with an account of the moral uncertainty attending prenatal diagnosis as a medical practice. Since prenatal diagnosis is closely associated with the practice of selective abortion, a moral tension can be seen between prenatal diagnosis and the therapeutic imper-

Excerpted from *Medical Ethics: A Guide for Health Professionals* by J.F. Monagle and D.C. Thomasma (eds.), pp. 12–25, with permission of Aspen Publishers, Inc., © 1988.

ative of the medical profession. And yet, Juengst argues, the provision of information is itself a legitimate purpose of prenatal diagnosis, and the primary obligation of the genetic counselor is not to the fetus but to the parents. In Juengst's view, then, prenatal diagnosis is an acceptable medical practice because it is a tool for helping parents to make their own reproductive choices. Juengst also considers two kinds of cases in which the counseling model of prenatal diagnosis comes into direct conflict with therapeutic concern for the fetus. Although he believes that there is a principled basis upon which to deny access to prenatal diagnosis purely for purposes of gender identification, he argues that access to prenatal diagnosis should not be denied to parents who are seeking information regarding a fetal defect that would be amenable to effective treatment after birth.

There are now a number of techniques relevant to the diagnosis of diseases and defects *in utero*.[1] Some, like fetal biopsy techniques, are informative, but relatively invasive.[2] Others, like maternal serum screening for fetal proteins, are less risky, but also less revealing.[3] This [essay] concentrates on two techniques that occupy the middle ground: amniocentesis and chorionic villi sampling. In amniocentesis, a needle is inserted through the mother's abdominal and uterine walls into the amniotic sac to withdraw fluid containing fetal amniocytes.[4] Chorionic villi sampling involves passing a catheter vaginally into the uterus to aspirate a sample of fetal tissue from the developing placenta.[5] Both kinds of fetal tissue are then available for analysis by a growing number of cytological, biochemical, and molecular tests....[6]

SELECTIVE ABORTION AND THE THERAPEUTIC IMPERATIVE

In most discussions about allocating a medical technology, the purpose of the technology is unproblematic. Most technologies provide some preventive or therapeutic benefit for patients with particular needs, and the problem is deciding how to distribute that benefit. One of the interesting features of the discussion of amniocentesis, however, has been the persistence of the question as to its purpose. Given that the risks of the procedure are low, what are the benefits it offers and are they legitimate ones for health care professionals to provide?

Implicit in the early use of amniocentesis prior to abortion seemed to be a belief that the prevention of harm by the selective abortion of diseased fetuses was the primary benefit to be gained from amniocentesis. Much of the ethical discussion has centered on the merits of this view and its implications for the appropriateness of amniocentesis as a medical practice.

Concern over the legitimacy of the practice is usually based on the recognition that, in the absence of more effective uses for the knowledge it produces, selective abortion is the primary practical intention behind performing an amniocentesis.[7] Critics find the practice unacceptable because they claim that selective abortion is an ethically inappropriate medical response to the diagnosis of fetal disease. Many of the arguments for this position reflect particular philosophical and theological views on the status of the fetus as a person and the moral rights to life and equal protection that it might possess.[8] As such, they are arguments against selective abortion as a general social practice and, to the extent that they are persuasive, indict amniocentesis indirectly.

However, there are also concerns about selective abortion as a *medical* practice, quite aside from the question of its social acceptability. Some argue that for health care professionals, it is irrelevant whether the fetal subject of an amniocentesis is a person or possesses rights. As long as the fetus is a legitimate *patient*, it falls within the scope of the practitioners' professional obligations and enjoys the benefits of their protection.[9]

One of the practices that the professional ethics of medicine has traditionally prohibited is the killing of patients, either for their own benefit or for the benefit of others.[10] Commentators point out that if the fetus is the patient in prenatal diagnosis, it is misleading to call the sequelae of positive diagnoses "therapeutic abortions" or to justify them in terms of the "prevention of harm." Fetal patients are selectively aborted precisely because they have been diagnosed as already suffering from incurable harms. Selective abortion on these grounds is neither therapeutic nor preventive; they say: it is simply a form of euthanasia.[11] As a result, some wonder whether amniocentesis might be an unacceptable practice for health care practitioners simply by the internal moral standards for their profession.

These concerns have been addressed in several ways. Some agree that selective abortion is not an ethically attractive response to the diagnosis of fetal disease, but they assert that it is also not the only possible response. They claim that in fact the intended purpose of amniocentesis is "the treatment and eventual cure of disease in the fetus or infant."[12] It is only because prenatal treatment has not yet caught up to diagnosis that selective abortion is a "sad, negative alternative."[13] An NIH consensus conference task force on antenatal diagnosis summarized this approach when it wrote,

> Thus, the techniques of prenatal diagnosis are not, except in very few instances, associated with any medical therapies for the alleviation of the diagnosed disorder. Many leaders in the development of this technology recognize this is unsatisfactory. They affirm that studies of the etiology of genetic and hereditary disorders are of the greatest importance and that, based on knowledge of etiology, therapeutic measures must be developed. Thus, prenatal diagnosis, while presently most often associated with the choice of abortion, is not inextricably linked to abortion: it may provide information leading to the planning for the birth of a defective infant and it has the potential for the better understanding of, and therapeutic interventions in, the disease state.[14]

In trying to establish an appropriate therapeutic purpose for amniocentesis, this argument looks both toward the past and the future. It points to the rationale behind the technology's development and to the promise of its eventual uses. These appeals are persuasive as far as they go. But even if the original intentions were laudably therapeutic, the proponents recognize that "realistically, for generations to come, the power to diagnose fetal disease will outstrip the power to treat with effective therapies."[15] While the prospects of future treatments might justify the use of prenatal diagnosis in *research* efforts designed to shorten that lag, how do they help in addressing the critics' concerns about turning to the "sad, negative alternative" as a regular practice in the clinical setting?

A second response to these concerns is to agree that (for the time being) selective abortion is the principal clinical option after amniocentesis, but then to argue that abortion is sometimes morally justified. Again, the consensus of the NIH task force:

> In addition, there is something profoundly troubling about allowing the birth of an infant who is known in advance to suffer from some serious disease or defect. While the prevention of that suffering is attained in this case by eliminating the potential sufferer rather than the cause of the suffering, many would consider it an act of mercy. Because the fetus holds so uncertain a place in the moral community, many (among them many who are deeply devoted to fetal wellbeing) consider that "act of mercy" to fall in quite a different moral category than a similar act performed on an already born human being of whatever age.[16]

As this quotation indicates, those who argue this way must distinguish the merciful killing of fetal patients, which they support, from active euthanasia in the clinical setting, which they condemn. Again, an array of philosophical views about the ontological status of the fetus and its membership in "the moral community" can be drawn upon to make this distinction.[17] But the hallmark of those views, as of their counterparts among critics of abortion, is the extent and intensity of scholarly disagreement over their merits. By contrast, the resources of traditional professional medical ethics are fairly sparse on these matters and cannot provide much guidance on the relevant distinction without appealing to one or another of these background views.

For the practitioner trying to decide how best to use amniocentesis, this dispute over the purpose of prenatal diagnosis creates a genuine problem of moral uncertainty. Is selective abortion an ethically appropriate response to fetal disease or not? Our cultural resources on the question are almost too rich, offering a perplexing variety of moral guidance, all of it equally controversial. The specific ethical resources of the profession, on the other hand, do not seem to provide enough guidance to definitively respond to the concerns. There are approaches to dealing with moral uncertainty, however, and in the next section one is outlined that allows practitioners to get beyond the moral quandary of selective abortion to the clinical business of prenatal diagnosis.

Before turning to that approach, there are two points about the moral quandary that are important to make. First, note that one of the primary clinical advantages of chorionic villi sampling is its capacity for circumventing some of that uncertainty. Unlike amniocentesis, chorionic villi sampling is performed during the first trimester of pregnancy, and the tissue samples it yields are immediately ready for laboratory analysis.[18] By allowing a diagnosis to be made much earlier in gestation, this technique allows the question of abortion to arise during a period in which the spontaneous abortion rate for defective fetuses is high and the philosophical status of the fetus, both as person and patient, is more tenuous than later.

It is also important to notice the source of the uncertainty over prenatal diagnosis as a medical practice. Both the concerns and their responses were framed against the basic clinical imperative to treat and cure disease. All the arguments so far have assumed that, for a diagnostic tool to have a legitimate medical purpose, it should be used to help benefit the victim of the diseases it uncovers. When prenatal diagnosis is understood in terms of this therapeutic imperative, the discussion naturally focuses on how the information it yields can help alleviate the suffering of the afflicted fetus. This perspective makes the asymmetry between our abilities to diagnose and treat the fetus morally troubling and prompts the discussion of whether selective abortion is an acceptable way to balance the therapeutic scales. Our uncertainty on that score is what creates most of the moral tension that accompanies the practice of prenatal diagnosis.

As strong as that tension is, however, it has not paralyzed the conscientious medical use of prenatal diagnosis. That is largely because the practice of prenatal diagnosis is also informed by another moral point of view, one which *does* provide the practitioner with a way to address this problem of uncertainty.

UNCERTAINTY AND THE ETHICS OF REPRODUCTIVE COUNSELING

There is [an] important argument in defense of amniocentesis that was not mentioned with the others above, even though all are usually raised together. Proponents almost always stress that, in addition to its therapeutic goals, "we regard the provision of information as an important and legitimate purpose of prenatal diagnosis" independent of whether that information is used on behalf of the fetus.[19] One statement of this position is as follows:

> The desired and intended result of prenatal diagnosis is information about the presence or absence of a possible disease or defect in the fetus. In practice, the test results are negative in more than 96 percent of amniocentesis cases, providing these families with many months of relief from anxiety.... When diagnosis of the presence of disease or defect is made, parents and physicians use that information to make choices about subsequent action.... Ethical considerations make it imperative to separate the fact of a positive diagnosis from the choice about subsequent ac-

tion. What parents and physicians decide to do is not automatically dictated by the diagnosis, but ought to be shaped by their ethical and social views.... These guidelines were developed in a moral framework favoring the protection of individual choice and the autonomy of parents, even when we disagree with their course of action.[20]

Notice that this approach defines the aim of performing an amniocentesis in terms of the parents' problems, not the fetus's. Prenatal diagnosis is, in essence, an adjunct to a form of psychological counseling: It provides information that practitioners can use to alleviate the parents' anxieties during pregnancy and to help them work through difficult reproductive decisions.[21]

This obviously reflects an important shift in the orientation of the discussion. Again, the discussion thus far has been informed, and limited, by the traditional ethics of clinical medicine. This shift reflects the influence of another professional tradition relevant to the practice of prenatal diagnosis: that of the genetic counselor. As the last lines of the passage above suggest, the ethical resources this tradition can contribute to the discussion have some important implications for the practitioner's response to the moral uncertainties of the practice.

The first important feature of this tradition is its relocation of the practitioner's primary professional obligations. As the purpose of amniocentesis shifts from helping the fetus to helping its parents, the latter become the practitioner's primary focus. The ethics of genetic counseling has traditionally been clear about the implications of this therapeutic shift for a counselor's professional commitments: "Counselors may find themselves pulled by an allegiance to the unborn child—whose well-being is, after all, the ultimate object of their concern as well as the motivating interest of the parents. As understandable as this concern may be, in the end it must give way to the duty owed to the counselee—the parents."[22]

The second important feature of this tradition is its substantive vision of the duties that the practitioner owes to the counselee. Along with duties to benefit and protect their patients, the ethics of clinical medicine commits physicians to the ideal of a physician-patient relationship marked by shared decision making.[23] In genetic counseling, the key to that relationship has been taken to be the practitioner's duty to respect patients' reproductive choices. Modern genetic counselors are especially careful not to impose their own values on their clients in the decision-making process. The goal of their practice is to improve their patients' abilities to cope with their reproductive experiences in their own terms. Thus, while counselors provide information, facilitate decision making, and make recommendations, they fully accept the obligation not to interfere with the reproductive decisions their clients make after counseling.[24]

In part, this ethical orientation has historical roots in the reaction of postwar clinical geneticists to the excesses of their eugenic predecessors. However, it also reflects an important strategy for dealing with the moral uncertainties of the reproductive decisions that genetic counselors help their clients make.[25] This strategy assumes that where moral uncertainty is high—either because of a paucity of ethical guidance or a variety of equally defensible views—practitioners may accept conscientious decisions favoring either side of an issue. Moreover, since reproductive issues in general and abortion issues in particular are among the most highly controverted and culturally colored moral issues, professionals engaged in helping people make reproductive decisions have a special obligation to respect their patients' considered judgments about these issues.[26]

This strategy seems to stand behind defenses of prenatal diagnosis like the one mounted in the last passage quoted above. References to the "ethical considerations" that allow practitioners to divorce the propriety of their diagnostic interventions from what happens as a result and to the "moral framework" favoring parental autonomy "even when we disagree with their course of action" allude to the view that, in the face of a plurality of moral positions on abortion, practitioners should bracket their own uncertainties and focus on enhancing the parents' ability to make autonomous and conscientious reproductive decisions. Prenatal diagnosis is an acceptable medical practice, then, as a tool for helping parents to make those choices.

In the practice of prenatal diagnosis, this counseling model usually operates simultaneously with a therapeutic concern for the fetus. This is an effective combination in most cases, since the practitioner's respect for parental choice coincides with his or her obligations to the fetus. However, some of the more vivid ethical problems the practitioner faces are created in the rare cases in which these points of view diverge....In particular, what is the range of reproductive choices the practitioner may facilitate through prenatal diagnosis when those choices conflict with his or her therapeutic obligations to the fetus?

Two kinds of cases that are especially important for today's practitioner are requests for prenatal diagnosis for sex selection and curable diseases. These kinds of cases pose limited, though real, problems for the practice of amniocentesis. The ease and efficacy of techniques like chorionic villi sampling, however, suggests that they will become increasingly common in the future.

PRENATAL DIAGNOSIS FOR SEX SELECTION

Is prenatal diagnosis performed in order to determine the gender of the fetus an acceptable practice in the absence of sex-linked genetic risks? Although this question has been faced by practitioners of amniocentesis, the maternal risks of late abortions and the experience of pregnancy past quickening have often been enough to dissuade candidates from the practice without having to deny them access to amniocentesis.[27] The main clinical promise of chorionic villi sampling, however, is precisely that it avoids those barriers to selective abortion by allowing diagnosis early in gestation.[28] This makes it physically and emotionally easier for the mother to have an abortion, and there is also greater uncertainty about the moral status of the fetus early in gestation, making an abortion easier to justify....

Most commentators have been critical of sex selection, even if they would not ban it. For example, in an important report on social issues in genetic screening, the President's Commission for the Study of Ethical Problems in Medicine and Biomedical and Behavioral Research states,

> Despite the strong reasons for not precluding individuals from having access to genetic services on the basis of what they may do with the information, society may sometimes be warranted in discouraging certain uses. A striking example would be the use of prenatal diagnosis solely to determine the sex of the fetus and to abort a fetus of the unwanted sex.[29]

The commission summarized the four most prominent arguments why, beyond the question of scarce resources, prenatal diagnosis for sex selection is an inappropriate use of the technology. The first three arguments impugn the motives of parents who would make such a request. First, such a request is often likely to be based on sexist thinking. Unlike selective abortion for defective fetuses, discrimination based on sheer prejudice against one gender is something that can be fairly confidently condemned as immoral. Second, the fact that parents are concerned enough to abort a child of the "wrong" sex raises questions about whether they are approaching the enterprise of having children responsibly or whether they are laboring under expectations that will end up working to the detriment of their children. Finally, the commission noted that "taken to an extreme, this attitude treats a child as an artifact and the reproductive process as a chance to design and produce human beings according to parental standards of excellence."[30]

Of course, these arguments rest on factual claims that may not be true for all parents who request prenatal diagnosis for sex selection. Thus, we cannot be sure, from the outset, that every request is a case of irrational sexism, nor can we determine how successfully prospective parents will raise their children or even what the final consequences of the practice would be on our cultural attitudes towards reproduction.[31] A thirty-year-old mother of three boys who would like a girl may have quite good reasons for her choice. In the face of uncertainty about the parents' motives, some argue, the practitioner should not deny them the benefit of the doubt.

These uncertainties do suggest that blanket policies against releasing sex information on request might be unjustified. But the commission also presented a fourth argument that is based less on uncertain empirical facts. The commission argued that

> although every reproductive decision based on information gained from genetic screening involves the conscious acceptance of certain characteristics and the rejection of others, a distinction can be made between seeking genetic information in order to correct or avoid unambiguous disabilities, or to improve the well-being of the fetus, and seeking such information merely to satisfy parental preferences that are not only idiosyncratic but also unrelated to the good of the fetus. Although in some cases it will be difficult to draw a clear line between these two types of interventions, sex selection appears to fall in the latter class.[32]

This argument returns to the issue of using the prenatal diagnosis for guidance, and in the process it integrates the two moral contexts of the practice—the genetic counselor's and the fetal therapist's—in an interesting way. In essence, it says that the purpose of the practice is to provide information relevant to making a *special subset* of reproductive decisions: decisions that revolve around the health of the fetus. Although the counselor's stress on the importance of parental autonomy

would keep those decisions in the parents' hands, the therapist's focus on the medical problems of the fetus tends to limit the range of decisions the practice can serve to ones made in response to those problems. Since gender is not a pathological problem, requests for assistance in making gender-based reproductive decisions can be appropriately denied.

This response goes beyond simply combining the two ethical frameworks for prenatal diagnosis and using one or the other as the need arises. Its effect is to integrate the perspectives, so that prenatal diagnosis remains recognizably a medical practice (addressing the health problems of the fetus), but a practice that focuses primarily on helping parents make reproductive decisions in the light of those problems. This integrated framework allows practitioners to show why women at risk for fetal defects are appropriate candidates for prenatal diagnosis even in the absence of effective treatment and women at risk for carrying a fetus of a certain gender are not.

PRENATAL DIAGNOSIS FOR A TREATABLE DEFECT

The second kind of access question raises problems even within the context of the integrated approach of the President's Commission. The clinical advantages of chorionic villi sampling, together with the expanding ability to diagnose genetic disorders at the molecular level, will mean increasing numbers of genetic diseases will be detectable *in utero*. Geneticists promise that with chorionic villi sampling, "prodigious opportunities exist for the first-trimester diagnosis of many different genetic disorders as long as the safety and accuracy are first assured. It is expected that all chromosomal abnormalities, biochemical genetic disorders whose enzymatic deficiencies have been characterized in cell culture, and all disorders in which the gene defect has been delineated will be detectable."[33] Of course, this will increase the *range* of detectable health-related fetal conditions as well as the number. As this happens, questions will become more frequent about the diagnosis of relatively minor conditions or of conditions like Huntington's disease or Alzheimer's disease that will not affect the fetus until much later in life.[34] Similarly, as more correlations are drawn between specific genetic markers and dispositions toward psychiatric conditions like depression, practitioners may face requests for testing for these markers. All of these questions will create tension between the practitioner's commitment to parental autonomy and his or her concern for fetal welfare. Perhaps most difficult will be requests for prenatal diagnosis for diseases for which there is effective therapy. Once the appropriate techniques are available, how should the practitioner respond to requests for prenatal diagnosis for a disease (e.g., phenylketonuria [PKU]) that is eminently treatable after birth?[35]

Here the two moral traditions that guide the practitioner seem at loggerheads. On one hand, the practitioner is committed to using chorionic villi sampling to provide the parents with the information they need in order to make reproductive decisions that concern fetal health. On the other hand, from the purely therapeutic point of view, the important benefits the practitioner can provide to the fetus make the obligation to do so in this case seem very strong. The conflict between the two perspectives generates conceptual uncertainty over who should be understood to be the primary patient. Usually, it is enough simply to accept, or reject, both parties as one's patients. Cases of treatable fetal problems, however, raise the necessity of arriving at some conclusion about the relative priority of the patients, even within the context of an integrated moral perspective that identifies them.[36]

A case can be made for placing the parents first, even in these hard cases. The argument starts with the merits of the genetic counselor's approach to the cultural and ethical complexities of reproductive decision making. Fetuses are patients only within the context of their parents' reproductive plans. These plans will be the starting point in all the cases a practitioner faces, as long as the presenting parents are not brain dead, comatose, or otherwise incapable of making reproductive choices. And parents' reproductive choices, as genetic counselors recognize, will be influenced by serious considerations that go well beyond the practitioner's ability to assess. Moreover, there are also significant risks in giving priority to the welfare of the fetus when it can be enhanced. These are primarily social risks, concerned with the consequences of such a move for the "right of privacy" by which reproductive choices have been traditionally protected.

To give priority to the therapeutic imperative in these cases would be to assume that it is an unacceptable medical practice to selectively abort a fetus that can be successfully treated for its condition. On this view, for example, requests for prenatal diagnosis for PKU may be legitimately denied if they are made with the intent to abort affected fetuses. However, to subordinate parental autonomy to fetal welfare in the way required to deny

prenatal diagnosis for PKU would also provide justification for an unacceptably large range of other limitations on parental decision making.

For example, practitioners might withhold the information that a fetus had PKU if they knew the parents would use that information to abort the fetus. Agreeing to treatment of the disease could be made a condition for the prenatal diagnosis. Moreover, if it is the fetal PKU victim's status as a *treatable patient* that justifies the restriction on parental access to prenatal diagnosis, would not a fetus which is prenatally treatable for other diseases merit similar protections? That is, might not clinics be justified in giving access only to parents committed to proceeding with prenatal therapies where they are available? In effect, limiting access to prenatal diagnosis would be a mirror image of the required-abortion policy. As the number of fetal treatments increased, the range of disorders for which selective abortion would no longer be held appropriate would grow, effectively limiting parental reproductive choice.[37]

Whether these developments would actually occur, of course, is uncertain. The point of the argument is not that giving priority to the therapeutic imperative would place us on some inevitable "slippery slope." The point is that doing so would by itself place us at the bottom of the slope—by providing the justification for all these coercive practices. On the other hand, giving priority to the parents' autonomy respects the context of the diagnostic intervention in the parents' reproductive decision making and protects the traditional moral privacy of those decisions. As the President's Commission stated,

> Nowhere is the need for freedom to pursue divergent conceptions of the good more deeply felt than in decisions concerning reproduction. It would be a cruel irony if technological advances undertaken in the name of providing information to expand the range of individual choices resulted in unanticipated social pressures to pursue a particular course of action."[38]

CONCLUSIONS

The moral framework that will guide the practice of prenatal diagnosis as a mature medical technology is still emerging. Its foundations are in the ethical traditions of clinical medicine and genetic counseling, with their complementary imperatives to enhance fetal welfare and facilitate parental choice. During the discussions of the safety and purpose of amniocentesis that shaped the youth of prenatal diagnosis, these two traditions could often be used interchangeably in establishing the legitimate boundaries of the practice. As the next generation of diagnostic techniques raises new moral, conceptual, and social uncertainties, the relationship between these two traditions will become increasingly crucial to the moral stability of the practice. Different approaches to integrating the professional obligations that each tradition stresses will produce divergent responses to the hard questions of access and eligibility that practitioners of prenatal diagnosis will increasingly face. One approach, designed with the new uncertainties in view, would try to improve the fit between these traditions in two steps. First, it would rely on medicine's therapeutic imperative to limit the range of appropriately diagnosed conditions to those relevant to the medical welfare of the fetus. But within that clinical sphere, it would reaffirm the commitment of the practitioner, as counselor, to enhance the parent's autonomy to make reproductive and therapeutic decisions in light of the information prenatal diagnosis can provide.

NOTES

1 Michael Harrison, Mitchell Golbus, and Roy Filly, eds., *The Unborn Patient: Prenatal Diagnosis and Treatment* (New York: Grune & Stratton, 1984); National Institute of Child Health and Human Development, *Antenatal Diagnosis: Report of a Consensus Development Conference*, NIH Publication no. 79–1973 (Bethesda, Md.: National Institutes of Health, 1979).

2 Harrison, Golbus, and Filly, *The Unborn Patient*, 125–39.

3 National Institute of Child Health and Human Development, *Antenatal Diagnosis*, 118–28.

4 Ibid., 33.

5 G. Simoni et al., "Diagnostic Application of First Trimester Trophoblast Sampling in 100 Pregnancies," *Human Genetics* 66 (1984): 252–259; C. H. Rodeck and J. M. Morsman, "First Trimester Chorion Biopsy," *British Medical Bulletin* 39 (1983): 338.

6 Frank Chervenak, Glenn Isaacson, and Maurice Mahoney, "Advances in the Diagnosis of Fetal Defects," *NEJM* 315 (1986): 305–7.

7 Jerome Lejeune, "On the Nature of Man," *American Journal of Human Genetics* 22 (1970): 121–28.

8 Leon Kass, "Implications of Prenatal Diagnosis for the Human Right to Life," in *Ethical Issues in Human Genetics*, ed. Bruce Hilton et al. (New York: Plenum Press, 1973), 185–99; Karen Lebacqz, "Prenatal Diagnosis and Selective Abortion," *Linacre Quarterly* 40 (1973): 109–27; Carol Tauer, "Personhood and Human Embryos and Fetuses," *Journal of Medicine and Philosophy* 10 (1985): 253–66.

9 Cf. Harrison, Golbus, and Filly, *The Unborn Patient*, 1–9; Roger Shinn, "The Fetus as Patient," in *Genetics and the Law III*, ed. A. Milunsky and G. Annas (New York: Plenum Press, 1985).

10 George Gruman, Sissela Bok, and Robert Veatch, "Death, Dying and Euthanasia," *The Encyclopedia of Bioethics*, ed. Warren Reich (New York: Macmillan, 1978).

11 Paul Ramsey, "Reference Points in Deciding about Abortion," in *The Morality of Abortion*, ed. John Noonan (Cambridge, Mass.: Harvard University Press, 1970).

12 Tabitha Powledge and John Fletcher, "Guidelines for the Ethical, Social and Legal Issues in Prenatal Diagnosis," *New England Journal of Medicine* 300 (1979): 170.

13 John Fletcher and Albert Jonsen, "Ethical Considerations," in *The Unborn Patient*.

14 National Institute of Child Health and Human Development, *Antenatal Diagnosis*, I–182, 3.

15 Fletcher and Jonsen, "Ethical Considerations," 166.

16 National Institute of Child Health and Human Development, *Antenatal Diagnosis*, I–192.

17 Cf. William Bondeson et al., eds., *Abortion and the Status of the Fetus* (Boston: D. Reidel, 1983).

18 Aubrey Milunski, "Prenatal Diagnosis: New Tools, New Problems," in *Genetics and the Law III*, 336–37.

19 Powledge and Fletcher, "Guidelines," 171.

20 Ibid., 170.

21 Thus, genetic counselors write that, far from simply "diagnosing" medical problems: "When the genetic counselor attempts to help the counselees reach appropriate health and reproductive decisions, he/she will probably use the same techniques that many psychotherapists would use under similar circumstances—clarification of motivations and beliefs, an examination of alternatives, with their pros and cons, a presentation of options not considered in the counselee's thinking, an identification and labeling of facts and fantasies, challenges to unrealistic beliefs, and so on. In other words, assisting counselees to make realistic personal decisions, a major goal of genetic counseling, perhaps more than any other function, requires that the counselor employ the skills of

the psychotherapist" (Seymour Kessler, "The Psychological Paradigm Shift in Genetic Counseling," *Social Biology* 27 ([1980]): 167–85).

22 Alexander Capron, "Automony, Confidentiality and Quality Care in Genetic Counseling," in *Genetic Counseling: Facts, Values, and Norms*, Birth Defects: Original Article Series, vol. 15, no. 2, ed. Alexander Capron et al. (New York: Alan R. Liss, 1979), 334.

23 Cf. President's Commission for the Study of Ethics in Medicine and Biomedical and Behavioral Research, *Making Health Care Decisions: The Ethical and Legal Implications of Informed Consent in the Patient-Practitioner Relationship* (Washington, D.C.: GPO, 1982), 36.

24 Cf. Alex Capron et al., eds. *Genetic Counseling: Facts, Values and Norms* Birth Defects Original Article Series, vol. 15, no. 2 (New York: Alan R. Liss, 1979).

25 James R. Sorenson, "Biomedical Innovation, Uncertainty, and Doctor-Patient Interaction," *Journal of Health and Social Behavior* 15 (1974): 366–74.

26 Thus, writers sensitive to the moral nuances of language have begun saying "intrauterine" instead of "prenatal" diagnosis to accommodate the focus on the parent and the possibility that the intervention may not precede a birth at all. Cf. LeRoy Walters, "Ethical Issues in Intrauterine Diagnosis and Therapy," *Fetal Therapy* 1 (1986): 32–37.

27 Haig Kazazian, "Prenatal Diagnosis for Sex Choice: A Medical View," *Hastings Center Report* 10 (1980): 17–18.

28 Milunsky, "Prenatal Diagnosis," 337.

29 President's Commission, *Screening and Counseling*, 56.

30 Ibid., 57.

31 John Fletcher, "Ethics and Amniocentesis for Fetal Sex Identification," *New England Journal of Medicine* 301 (1979): 550–53; Mary Ann Warren, "The Ethics of Sex Preselection," in *Biomedical Ethics Reviews 1985*, ed. James Humber and Robert Almeder (Clifton, N.J.: Humana Press, 1985), 73–93.

32 President's Commission, *Screening and Counseling*, 58.

33 Milunsky, "Prenatal Diagnosis," 338.

34 John Fletcher, "Ethical Issues in Genetic Screening and Antenatal Diagnosis," *Clinical Obstetrics and Gynecology* 24 (1981): 1156.

35 Neil Holtzman, "Ethical Issues in the Prenatal Diagnosis of Phenylketonuria," *Pediatrics* 74 (1984): 424–27.

36 Frederick Schauer, "Slippery Slopes," *Harvard Law Review* 50 (1985): 361–383.

37 As is currently happening in other places: Cf. Lawrence J. Nelson, Brian Buggy, and Carol Weil, "Forced Medical Treatment of Pregnant Women," *Hastings Law Journal* 37 (1986): 703–65; Richard Hull, James Nelson, and L. A. Gartner, "Ethical Issues in Prenatal Therapies," in *Biomedical Ethics Review: 1984*, ed. J. Humber and R. Almeder (Clifton, N.J.: Humana Press, 1984).

38 President's Commission, *Screening and Counseling*, 56.

Surrogate Motherhood

Surrogate Mothers: Not So Novel After All
John A. Robertson

A biographical sketch of John A. Robertson is found on page 415.

Robertson focuses attention on the most typical kind of surrogate mother arrangement, whereby a woman (the surrogate) contracts with a married couple to be artificially inseminated with the husband's sperm in order to bear a child for the couple. He analyzes the potential benefits and harms of surrogate motherhood and maintains that the practice is ethically acceptable. Because surrogate motherhood deliberately separates *biological* from *social* parentage, Robertson recognizes the risk of psychosocial harm to the offspring as a serious concern. But problems on this score, he contends, are no more serious than those associated with well-

Reprinted with permission of the author and the publisher from *Hastings Center Report*, vol. 13 (October 1983), pp. 28–34.

established practices such as ordinary adoption and AID. Against the view that it is wrong for a surrogate to use the reproductive process for selfish ends, Robertson contends that "the mere presence of selfish motives does not render reproduction immoral, as long as it is carried out in a way that respects the child's interests." With regard to public policy, he argues that the state may justifiably regulate but not block surrogate motherhood arrangements.

All reproduction is collaborative, for no man or woman reproduces alone. Yet the provision of sperm, egg, or uterus through artificial insemination, embryo transfer, and surrogate mothering makes reproduction collaborative in another way. A third person provides a genetic or gestational factor not present in ordinary paired reproduction. As these practices grow, we must confront the ethical issues raised and their implications for public policy.

Collaborative reproduction allows some persons who otherwise might remain childless to produce healthy children. However, its deliberate separation of genetic, gestational, and social parentage is troublesome. The offspring and participants may be harmed, and there is a risk of confusing family lineage and personal identity. In addition, the techniques intentionally manipulate a natural process that many persons want free of technical intervention. Yet many well-accepted practices, including adoption, artificial insemination by donor (AID), and blended families (families where children of different marriages are raised together) intentionally separate biologic and social parenting, and have become an accepted thread in the social fabric. Should all collaborative techniques be similarly treated? When, if ever, are they ethical? Should the law prohibit, encourage, or regulate them, or should the practice be left to private actors? Surrogate motherhood—the controversial practice by which a woman agrees to bear a child conceived by artificial insemination and to relinquish it at birth to others for rearing—illustrates the legal and ethical issues arising in collaborative reproduction generally.

HOW SURROGATE MOTHERING WORKS

For a fee of $5,000–10,000 a broker (usually a lawyer) will put an infertile couple (or less often, a single man) in contact with women whom he has recruited and screened who are willing to serve as surrogates. If the parties strike a deal, they will sign a contract in which the surrogate agrees to be artificially inseminated (usually by a physician) with the husband's sperm, to bear the child, and then at or soon after birth to relinquish all parental rights and transfer physical custody of the child to the couple for adoption by the wife. Typically the contract has provisions dealing with prenatal screening, abortion, and other aspects of the surrogate's conduct during pregnancy, as well as her consent to relinquish the child at birth. The husband and wife agree to pay medical expenses related to the pregnancy, to take custody of the child, and to place approximately $10,000 in escrow to be paid to the surrogate when the child is transferred. The lawyer will also prepare papers establishing the husband's paternity, terminating the surrogate's rights, and legalizing the adoption.

AN ALTERNATIVE TO AGENCY ADOPTIONS

Infertile couples who are seeking surrogates hire attorneys and sign contracts with women recruited through newspaper ads. The practice at present probably involves at most a few hundred persons. But repeated attention on *Sixty Minutes* and the *Phil Donahue Show* and in the popular press is likely to engender more demand, for thousands of infertile couples might find surrogate mothers the answer to their reproductive needs. What began as an enterprise involving a few lawyers and doctors in Michigan, Kentucky, and California is now a national phenomenon. There are surrogate mother centers in Maryland, Arizona, and several other states, and even a surrogate mother newsletter.

Surrogate mother arrangements occur within a tradition of family law that gives the gestational mother (and her spouse, if any) rearing rights and obligations. (However, the presumption that the husband is the father can be challenged, and a husband's obligations to his wife's child by AID will usually require his consent.)[1] Although no state has legislation directly on the subject of surrogate motherhood, independently arranged adoptions are lawful in most states. It is no crime to agree to bear a child for another, and then relinquish it for adoption. However, paying the mother a fee for adoption beyond medical expenses is a crime in some states, and in others will prevent the adoption from being approved.[2] Whether termination and transfer of parenting rights will be legally recognized depends on the state. Some states, like Hawaii and Florida, ask few questions and approve independent adoptions very quickly. Others, like Michigan and Kentucky, won't allow surrogate mothers to terminate and assign rearing rights to another if a fee has been paid, or even allow a paternity determination in favor of the sperm donor. The enforceability of surrogate contracts has also not been tested, and it is safe to assume that some jurisdictions will not enforce them. Legislation clarifying many of these questions has been proposed in several states, but has not yet been enacted.

Even this brief discussion highlights an important fact about surrogate motherhood and other collaborative reproductive techniques. They operate as an alternative to the nonmarket, agency system of allocating children for adoption, which has contributed to long queues for distributing healthy white babies. This form of independent adoption is controlled by the parties, planned before conception, involves a genetic link with one parent, and enables both the father and mother of the adopted child to be selected in advance.

Understood in these terms, the term "surrogate mother," which means substitute mother, is a misnomer. The natural mother, who contributes egg and uterus, is not so much a substitute mother as a substitute spouse who carries a child for a man whose wife is infertile. Indeed, it is the adoptive mother who is the surrogate mother for the child, since she parents a child borne by another. What, if anything, is wrong with this arrangement? Let us look more closely at its benefits and harms before discussing public policy.

ALL THE PARTIES CAN BENEFIT

Reproduction through surrogate mothering is a deviation from our cultural norms of reproduction, and to many persons it seems immoral or wrong. But surrogate mothering may be a good for the parties involved.

Surrogate contracts meet the desire of a husband and wife to rear a healthy child, and more particularly, a child with one partner's genes. The need could arise because the wife has an autosomal dominant or sex-linked genetic disorder, such as hemophilia. More likely, she is infertile and the couple feels a strong need to have children. For many infertile couples the inability to conceive is a major personal problem causing marital conflict and

filling both partners with anguish and self-doubt. It may also involve multiple medical work-ups and possibly even surgery. If the husband and wife have sought to adopt a child, they may have been told either that they do not qualify or to join the queue of couples waiting several years for agency adoptions (the wait has grown longer due to birth control, abortion, and the greater willingness of unwed mothers to keep their children[3]). For couples exhausted and frustrated by these efforts, the surrogate arrangement seems a godsend. While the intense desire to have a child often appears selfish, we must not lose sight of the deep-seated psychosocial and biological roots of the desire to generate children.[4]

The arrangement may also benefit the surrogate. Usually women undergo pregnancy and childbirth because they want to rear children. But some women want to have the experience of bearing and birthing a child without the obligation to rear. Philip Parker, a Michigan psychiatrist who has interviewed over 275 surrogate applicants, finds that the decision to be a surrogate springs from several motives.[5] Most women willing to be surrogates have already had children, and many are married. They choose the surrogate role primarily because the fee provides a better economic opportunity than alternative occupations, but also because they enjoy being pregnant and the respect and attention that it draws. The surrogate experience may also be a way to master, through reliving, guilt they feel from past pregnancies that ended in abortion or adoption. Some surrogates may also feel pleased, as organ donors do, that they have given the "gift of life" to another couple.[6]

The child born of a surrogate arrangement also benefits. Indeed, but for the surrogate contract, this child would not have been born at all. Unlike the ordinary agency or independent adoption, where a child is already conceived or brought to term, the conception of this child occurs solely as a result of the surrogate agreement. Thus even if the child does suffer identity problems, as adopted children often do because they are not able to know their mothers, this child has benefited, or at least has not been wronged, for without the surrogate arrangement, she would not have been born at all.[7]

BUT PROBLEMS EXIST TOO

Surrogate mothering is also troublesome. Many people think that it is wrong for a woman to conceive and bear a child that she does not intend to raise, particularly if she receives a fee for her services. There are potential costs to the surrogate and her family, the adoptive couple, the child, and even society at large from satisfying the generative needs of infertile couples in this way.

The couple must be willing to spend about $20,000–25,000, depending on lawyers' fees and the supply of and demand for surrogate mothers. (While this price tag makes the surrogate contract a consumption item for the middle classes, it is not unjust to poor couples, for it does not leave them worse off than they were.) The couple must also be prepared to experience, along with the adjustment and demands of becoming parents, the stress and anxiety of participating in a novel social relationship that many still consider immoral or deviant. What do they tell their friends or family? What do they tell the child? Will the child have contact with the mother? What is the couple's relationship with the surrogate and her family during the pregnancy and after? Without established patterns for handling these questions, the parties may experience confusion, frustration, and embarrassment.

A major source of uncertainty and stress is likely to be the surrogate herself. In most cases she will be a stranger, and may never even meet the couple. The lack of a preexisting relation between the couple and surrogate and the possibility that they live far apart enhance the possibility of mistrust. Is the surrogate taking care of herself? Is she having sex with others during her fertile period? Will she contact the child afterwards? What if she demands more money to relinquish the child? To allay these anxieties, the couple could try to establish a relationship of trust with the surrogate, yet such a relationship creates reciprocal rights and duties and might create demands for an undesired relationship after the birth. Even good lawyering that specifies every contingency in the contract is unlikely to allay uncertainty and anxiety about the surrogate's trustworthiness.

The surrogate may also find the experience less satisfying than she envisioned. Conceiving the child may require insemination efforts over several months at inconvenient locations. The pregnancy and birth may entail more pain, unpleasant side effects, and disruption than she expected. The couple may be more intrusive or more aloof than she wishes. As the pregnancy advances and the birth nears, the surrogate may find it increasingly difficult to remain detached by thinking of the child as "theirs" rather than "hers." Relinquishing the baby after birth may be considerably more disheartening and disappointing than she anticipated. Even if informed of this possibility in advance, she may be distressed for several weeks with feelings of loss, depression, and sleep distrubance.[8] She may feel angry at the couple for cutting off all contact with her once the baby is delivered, and guilty at giving up her child. Finally, she will have to face the loss of all contact with "her" child. As the reality of her situation dawns, she may regret not having bargained harder for access to "her baby."

As with the couple, the surrogate's experience will vary with the expectations, needs, and personalities of the parties, the course of the pregnancy, and an advance understanding of the problems that can arise. The surrogate should have a lawyer to protect her interests. Often, however, the couple's lawyer will end up advising the surrogate. Although he has recruited the surrogate, he is paid by and represents the couple. By disclosing his conflicting interest, he satisfies legal ethics, but he may not serve the interests of the surrogate as well as independent counsel.

HARMS TO THE CHILD

Unlike embryo transfer, gene therapy, and other manipulative techniques (some of which are collaborative), surrogate arrangements do not pose the risk of physical harm to the offspring. But there is the risk of psychosocial harm. Surrogate mothering, like adoption and artificial insemination by donor (AID), deliberately separates genetic and gestational from social parentage. The mother who begets, bears, and births does not parent. This separation can pose a problem for the child who discovers it. Like adopted and AID children, the child may be strongly motivated to learn the absent parent's identity and to establish a relationship, in this case with the mother and her family. Inability to make that connection, especially inability to learn who the mother is, may affect the child's self-esteem, create feelings of rootlessness, and leave the child thinking that he had been rejected due to some personal fault.[9] While this is a serious concern, the situation is tolerated when it arises with AID and adoptive children. Intentional conception for adoption—the essence of surrogate mothering—poses no different issue.

The child can also be harmed if the adoptive husband and wife are not fit parents. After all, a willingness to spend substantial money to fulfill a desire to rear children is no guarantee of good parenting. But then neither is reproduction by paired mates who wish intensely to have a child. The nonbiologic parent may resent or reject the child, but the same possibility exists with adoption, AID, or ordinary reproduction.

There is also the fear, articulated by such commentators as Leon Kass and Paul Ramsey,[10] that collaborative reproduction confuses the lineage of children and destroys the meaning of family as we know it. In surrogate mothering, as with ovum or womb donors, the genetic and gestational mother does not rear the child, though the biologic father does. What implications does this hold for the family and the child's lineage?

The separation of the child from the genetic or biologic parent in surrogate mothering is hardly unique. It arises with adoption, but surrogate arrangements are more closely akin to AID or blended families, where at least one parent has a blood-tie to the child and the child will know at least one genetic parent. He may, as adopted children often do, have intense desires to learn his biologic mother's identity and seek contact with her and her family. Failure to connect with biologic roots may cause suffering. But the fact that adoption through surrogate mother contracts is planned before conception does not increase the chance of identity confusion, lowered self-esteem, or the blurring of lineage that occurs with adoption or AID.

The greatest chance of confusing family lines arises if the child and couple establish relations with the surrogate and the surrogate's family. If that unlikely event occurs, questions about the child's relations with the surrogate's spouse, parents, and other children can arise. But these issues are not unique. Indeed, they are increasingly common with the growth of blended families. Surrogate mothering in a few instances may lead to a new variation on blended families, but its threat to the family is trivial compared to the rapid changes in family structure now occurring for social, economic, and demographic reasons.

In many cases surrogate motherhood and other forms of collaborative reproduction may shore up, rather than undermine, the traditional family by enabling couples who would otherwise be childless to have children. The practice of employing others to assist in child rearing—including wet-nurses, neonatal ICU nurses, day-care workers, and babysitters—is widely accepted. We also tolerate assistance in the form of sperm sales and donation of egg and gestation (adoption). Surrogate mothering is another method of assisting people to undertake child rearing, and thus serves the purposes of the marital union. It is hard to see how its planned nature obstructs that contribution.

USING BIRTH FOR SELFISH ENDS

A basic fear about the new reproductive technologies is that they manipulate a natural physiologic process in-

volved in the creation of human life. When one considers the potential power that resides in our ability to manipulate the genes of embryos, the charges of playing God or arrogantly tampering with nature and the resulting dark Huxleyian vision of genetically engineered babies decanted from bottles are not surprising. While *Brave New World* is the standard text for this fear, the 1982 film *Bladerunner* also evokes it. Trycorp., a genetic engineering corporation, manufactures "replicants," who resemble human beings in most respects, including their ability to remember their childhoods, but who are programmed to die in four years. In portraying the replicants' struggle for long life and full human status, the film raises a host of ethical issues relevant to gene manipulation, from the meaning of personhood to the duties we have in "fabricating" people to make them as whole and healthy as possible.

Such fears, however, are not a sufficient reason to stop splicing genes or relieving infertility through external fertilization.[11] In any event they have no application to surrogate mothering, which does not alter genes or even manipulate the embryo. The only technological aid is a syringe to inseminate and a thermometer to determine when ovulation occurs. Although embryo manipulation would occur if the surrogate received the fertilized egg of another woman, the qualms about surrogate mothering stem less from its potential for technical manipulation, and more from its attitude toward the body and mother-child relations. Mothers bear and give up children for adoption rather frequently when the conception is unplanned. But here the mother conceives the child for that purpose, deliberately using her body for a fee to serve the needs of others. It is the cold willingness to use her body as a baby-making machine and deny the mother-child gestational bond that bothers. (Ironically, the natural bond may turn out to be deeper and stronger than the surrogate imagined.)

Since the transfer of rearing duties from the natural gestational mother to others is widely accepted, the unwillingness of the surrogate mother to rear her child cannot in itself be wrong. As long as she transfers rearing responsibility to capable parents, she is not acting irresponsibly. Still, some persons assert that it is wrong to use the reproductive process for ends other than the good of the child.[12] But the mere presence of selfish motives does not render reproduction immoral, as long as it is carried out in a way that respects the child's interests. Otherwise most pregnancies and births would be immoral, for people have children to serve individual ends as well as the good of the child. In terms of instrumentalism, surrogate mothering cannot be distinguished from most other reproductive situations, whether AID, adoption, or simply planning a child to experience the pleasures of parenthood.

In this vein the problems that can arise when a defective child is born are cited as proof of the immorality of surrogate mothering. The fear is that neither the contracting couple nor the surrogate will want the defective child. In one recent case (*New York Times*, January 28, 1983, p. 18) a dispute arose when none of the parties wanted to take a child born with microcephaly, a condition related to mental retardation. The contracting man claimed on the basis of blood typing that the baby was not his, and thus he was not obligated under the contract to take it, or to pay the surrogate's fee. It turned out that [the] surrogate had borne her husband's child, for she had unwittingly become pregnant by him before being artificially inseminated by the contracting man. The surrogate and her husband eventually assumed responsibility for the child.

An excessively instrumental and callous approach to reproduction when a less than perfect baby is born is not unique to surrogate mothering. Similar reactions can occur whenever married couples have a defective child, as the Baby Doe controversy, which involved the passive euthanasia of a child with Down syndrome, indicates. All surrogate mothering is not wrong because in some instances a handicapped child will be rejected. Nor is it clear that this reaction is more likely in surrogate mothering than in conventional births for it reflects common attitudes toward handicapped newborns as much as alienation in the surrogate arrangement.

As with most situations, "how" something is done is more important than the mere fact of doing it. The morality of surrogate mothering thus depends on how the duties and responsibilities of the role are carried out, rather than on the mere fact that a couple produces a child with the aid of a collaborator. Depending on the circumstances, a surrogate mother can be praised as a benefactor to a suffering couple (the money is hardly adequate compensation) or condemned as a callous user of offspring to further her selfish ends. The view that one takes of her actions will also influence the role one wants the law to play.

WHAT SHOULD THE STATE'S ROLE BE?

What stance should public policy and the law take toward surrogate mothering? As with all collaborative reproduction, a range of choices exists, from prohibition and regulation to active encouragement.

However, there may be constitutional limits to the state's power to restrict collaborative reproduction. The right not to procreate, through contraception and abortion, is now firmly established.[13] A likely implication of these cases, supported by rulings in other cases, is that married persons (and possibly single persons) have a right to bear, beget, birth, and parent children by natural coital means using such technological aids (microsurgery and in vitro fertilization, for example) as are medically available. It should follow that married persons also have a right to engage in noncoital, collaborative reproduction, at least where natural reproduction is not possible. The right of a couple to raise a child should not depend on their luck in the natural lottery, if they can obtain the missing factor of reproduction from others.[14]

If a married couple's right to procreative autonomy includes the right to contract with consenting collaborators, then the state will have a heavy burden of justification for infringing that right. The risks to surrogate, couple, and child do not seem sufficiently compelling to meet this burden, for they are no different from the harms of adoption and AID. Nor will it suffice to point to a communal feeling that such uses of the body are—aside from the consequences—immoral. Moral distaste alone does not justify interference with a fundamental right.

Although surrogate mothering is not now criminal, this discussion is not purely hypothetical. The ban in Michigan and several other states on paying fees for adoption beyond medical expenses has the same effect as an outright prohibition, for few surrogates will volunteer for altruistic reasons alone. A ban on fees is not necessary to protect the surrogate mother from coercion or exploitation, or to protect the child from abuse, the two objectives behind passage of those laws. Unlike the pregnant unmarried woman who "sells" her child, the surrogate has made a considered, knowing choice, often with the assistance of counsel, before becoming pregnant. She may of course choose to be a surrogate for financial reasons, but offering money to do unpleasant tasks is not in itself coercive.

Nor does the child's welfare support a ban on fees, for the risk is no greater than in natural paired reproduction that the parents will be unfit or abuse the child. The specter of slavery, which some opposed to surrogate mothering have raised, is unwarranted. It is quibbling to question whether the couple is "buying" a child or the mother's personal services. Quite clearly, the couple is buying the right to rear a child by paying the mother to beget and bear one for that very purpose. But the purchasers do not buy the right to treat the child or surrogate as a commodity or property. Child abuse and neglect laws still apply, with criminal and civil sanctions available for mistreatment.

The main concern with fees rests on moral and aesthetic grounds. An affront to moral sensibility arises over paying money for a traditionally noncommercial, intimate function. Even though blood and sperm are sold, and miners, professional athletes, and petrochemical workers sell some of their health and vitality, some persons think it wrong for women to bear children for money, in much the same way that paying money for sex or body organs is considered wrong. Every society excludes some exchanges from the marketplace on moral grounds. But the state's power to block exchanges that interfere with the exercise of a fundamental right is limited. Since blocking this exchange stops infertile couples from reproducing and rearing the husband's child, a harm greater than moral distaste is necessary to justify it.

Although the state cannot block collaborative reproductive exchanges on moral grounds, it need not subsidize or encourage surrogate contracts. One could argue that allowing the parties to a surrogate contract to use the courts to terminate parental rights, certify paternity, and legalize adoption is a subsidy and therefore not required of the state. Similarly, a state's refusal to enforce surrogate contracts as a matter of public policy could be taken as a refusal to subsidize rather than as interference with the right to reproduce. But given the state's monopoly of those functions and the impact its denial will have on the ability of infertile couples to find reproductive collaborators, it is more plausible to view the refusal to certify and effectuate surrogate contracts as an infringement of the right to procreate. Denying an adoption because it was agreed upon in advance for a fee interferes with the couple's procreative autonomy as much as any criminal penalty for paying a fee to or contracting with a collaborator. (The crucial distinction between interfering with and not encouraging the exercise of a right has been overlooked by the Michigan and Kentucky courts that have held constitutional the refusal to allow adoptions or paternity determinations where a fee has been paid to the surrogate mother. This error makes these cases highly questionable precedents.[15])

A conclusion that surrogate contracts must be *enforced*, however, does not require that they be specifically carried out in all instances. As long as damage remedies remain, there is no constitutional right to specific performance. For example, a court need not enjoin the surrogate who changes her mind about abortion or relinquishing the child once it is born. A surrogate who wants to breach the contract by abortion should pay damages, but not be ordered to continue the pregnancy, because of the difficulty in enforcing or monitoring the order. (Whether damages are a practical alternative in such cases will depend on the surrogate's economic situation, or whether bonding or insurance to assure her contractual obligation is possible.) On the other hand, a court could reasonably order the surrogate after birth to relinquish the child. Whether such an order should issue will depend on whether the surrogate's interest in keeping the child is deemed greater than the couple's interest in rearing (assuming that both are fit parents). A commitment to freedom of contract and the rights of parties to arrange collaborative reproduction would favor the adoptive couple, while sympathy for the gestational bond between mother and child would favor the mother. If the mother prevailed, the couple should still have other remedies, including visitation rights for the father, restitution of the surrogate's fee and other expenses, and perhaps money damages as well.

The constitutional status of a married couple's procreative choice shields collaborative arrangements from interference on moral grounds alone, but not from all regulation. While the parties may assign the rearing rights according to contract, the state need not leave the entire transaction to the vagaries of the private sector. Regulation to minimize harm and assure knowing choices would be permissible, as long as the regulation is reasonably related to promoting these goals.

For example, the state could set minimum standards for surrogate brokers, set age and health qualifications for surrogates, and structure the transaction to assure voluntary, knowing choices. The state could also define and allocate responsibilities among the parties to protect the best interests of the offspring—for example, refusing to protect the surrogate's anonymity, requiring that the contracting couple assume responsibility for a defective child, or even transferring custody to another if threats to the child's welfare justify such a move....

ACKNOWLEDGMENTS

The author gratefully acknowledges the comments of Rebecca Dresser, Mark Frankel, Inga Markovits, Philip Parker, Bruce Russel, John Sampson, and Ted Schneyer on earlier drafts.

REFERENCES

1 People v. Sorenson, 68 Cal. 2d 280, 437 P.2d 495; Walter Wadlington, "Artificial Insemination: The Dangers of a Poorly Kept Secret," *Northwestern Law Review* 64 (1970), 777.

2 See, for example, Michigan Statutes Annotated, 27.3178 (555.54)(555.69) (1980).

3 William Landes and Eleanor Posner, "The Economics of the Baby Shortage," *Journal of Legal Studies* 7 (1978), 323.

4 See Erik Erikson, *The Life Cycle Completed* (New York: Norton, 1980), pp. 122–124.

5 Philip Parker, "Surrogate Mother's Motivations: Initial Findings," *American Journal of Psychiatry* 140:1 (January 1983), 117–118; Philip Parker, "The Psychology of Surrogate Motherhood: A Preliminary Report of a Longitudinal Pilot Study" (unpublished). See also Dava Sobel, "Surrogate Mothers: Why Women Volunteer," *New York Times*, June 25, 1981, p. 18.

6 Mark Frankel, "Surrogate Motherhood: An Ethical Perspective," pp. 1–2. (Paper presented at Wayne State Symposium on Surrogate Motherhood, Nov. 20, 1982.)

7 See John Robertson, "In Vitro Conception and Harm to the Unborn," *Hastings Center Report* 8 (October 1978), 13–14; Michael Bayles, "Harm to the Unconceived," *Philosophy and Public Affairs* 5 (1976), 295.

8 A small, uncontrolled study found these effects to last some four to six weeks. Statement of Nancy Reame, R. N. at Wayne State University, Symposium on Surrogate Motherhood, Nov. 20, 1982.

9 Betty Jane Lifton, *Twice Born: Memoirs of an Adopted Daughter* (New York: Penguin, 1977); L. Dusky, "Brave New Babies," *Newsweek*, Dec. 6, 1982, p. 30.

10 Leon Kass, "Making Babies—the New Biology and the Old Morality," *The Public Interest* 26 (1972), 18; "Making Babies Revisited," *The Public Interest* 54 (1979), 32; Paul Ramsey, *Fabricated Man: The Ethics of Genetic Control* (New Haven: Yale University Press, 1970).

11 The President's Commission for the Study of Ethical Problems in Medicine and Biomedical and Behavioral Research, *Splicing Life: The Social and Ethical Issues of Genetic Engineering with Human Beings* (Washington, D.C., 1982), pp. 53–60.

12 Herbert Krimmel, Testimony before California Assembly Committee on Judiciary, Surrogate Parenting Contracts (November 14, 1982), pp. 89–96.

13 Griswold v. Connecticut, 381 U.S. 479 (1964); Eisenstadt v. Baird, 405 U.S. 438 (1972); Roe v. Wade, 410 U.S. 113 (1973); Planned Parenthood v. Danforth, 428 U.S. 52 (1976); Bellotti v. Baird, 443 U.S. 622 (1979); Carey v. Population Services International, 431 U.S. 678 (1977).

14 Although this article does not address the right of single persons to contract with others for reproductive purposes, it should be noted that the right of married persons to engage in collaborative reproduction does not entail a similar right for unmarried persons. For a more detailed exposition of the arguments for the reproductive rights of married and single persons, see John Robertson, "Procreative Liberty and the Control of Conception, Pregnancy and Childbirth," *Virginia Law Review* 69 (April 1983), 405, 418–420.

15 See Doe v. Kelley, 106 Mich. App. 164, 307 N.W. 2d 438 (1981). Syrkowski v. Appleyard, 9 Family Law Rptr. 2348 (April 5, 1983); In re Baby Girl, 9 Family Law Rptr. 2348 (March 8, 1983).

The Case against Surrogate Parenting
Herbert T. Krimmel

Herbert T. Krimmel is professor of law at Southwestern University School of Law, Los Angeles. His areas of specialization include jurisprudence and bioethics, and he is the coauthor of "Abortion and Human Life: A Christian Perspective" and "Abortion: An Inspection into the Nature of Human Life and Potential Consequences of Legalizing its Destruction."

Reprinted with permission of the author and the publisher from *Hastings Center Report*, vol. 13 (October 1983), pp. 35–39.

In Krimmel's view, it is fundamentally wrong to separate the decision to create a child from the decision to parent it. He does not object to the surrogate mother's role as host for a developing child, but he maintains that it is unethical for her to create a child (via the provision of an ovum) with the intention of abdicating all parental responsibilities. (For analogous reasons, he considers the donation of sperm in AID to be unethical.) "The procreator should desire the child for its own sake, and not as a means to attaining some other end." If surrogate motherhood arrangements are accepted by society, he maintains, there is a great danger that we will come to view children as commodities. He also argues that acceptance of surrogate motherhood arrangements would have other negative social consequences, most notably an increased stress upon the family structure. But his opposition to the legalization of surrogate motherhood arrangements is based first and foremost on his conviction that it is morally wrong for a person "to create a child, not because she desired it, but because it could be useful to her."

Is it ethical for someone to create a human life with the intention of giving it up? This seems to be the primary question for both surrogate mother arrangements and artificial insemination by donor (AID), since in both situations a person who is providing germinal material does so only upon assurance that someone else will assume full responsibility for the child he or she helps to create.

THE ETHICAL ISSUE

In analyzing the ethics of surrogate mother arrangements, it is helpful to begin by examining the roles the surrogate mother performs. First, she acts as a procreator in providing an ovum to be fertilized. Second, after her ovum has been fertilized by the sperm of the man who wishes to parent the child, she acts as host to the fetus, providing nurture and protection while the newly conceived individual develops.

I see no insurmountable moral objections to the functions the mother performs in this second role as host. Her actions are analogous to those of a foster mother or of a wet-nurse who cares for a child when the natural mother cannot or does not do so. Using a surrogate mother as a host for the fetus when the biological mother cannot bear the child is no more morally objectionable than employing others to help educate, train, or otherwise care for a child. Except in extremes, where the parent relinquishes or delegates responsibilities for a child for trivial reasons, the practice would not seem to raise a serious moral issue.

I would argue, however, that the first role that the surrogate mother performs—providing germinal material to be fertilized—does pose a major ethical problem.

The surrogate mother provides her ovum, and enters into a surrogate mother arrangement, with the clear understanding that she is to avoid responsibility for the life she creates. Surrogate mother arrangements are designed to separate in the mind of the surrogate mother the decision to create a child from the decision to have and raise that child. The cause of this dissociation is some other benefit she will receive, most often money.[1] In other words, her desire to create a child is born of some motive other than the desire to be a parent. This separation of the decision to create a child from the decision to parent it is ethically suspect. The child is conceived not because he is wanted by his biological mother, but because he can be useful to someone else. He is conceived in order to be given away.

At their deepest level, surrogate mother arrangements involve a change in motive for creating children: from a desire to have them for their own sake, to a desire to have them because they can provide some other benefit. The surrogate mother creates a child with the intention to abdicate parental responsibilities. Can we view this as ethical? My answer is no. I will explain why by analyzing various situations in which surrogate mother arrangements might be used.

WHY MOTIVE MATTERS

Let's begin with the single parent. A single woman might use AID, or a single man might use a surrogate mother arrangement, if she or he wanted a child but did not want to be burdened with a spouse.[2] Either practice would intentionally deprive the child of a mother or a father. This, I assert, is fundamentally unfair to the child.

Those who disagree might point to divorce or to the death of a parent as situations in which a child is deprived of one parent and must rely solely or primarily upon the other. The comparison, however, is inapt. After divorce or the death of a parent, a child may find herself with a single parent due to circumstances that were unfortunate, unintended, and undesired. But when surrogate mother arrangements are used by a single parent, depriving the child of a second parent is one of the intended and desired effects. It is one thing to ask how to make the best of a bad situation when it is thrust upon a person. It is different altogether to ask whether one may intentionally set out to achieve the same result. The morality of identical results (for example, killings) will oftentimes differ depending upon whether the situation is invited by, or involuntarily thrust upon, the actor. Legal distinctions following and based upon this ethical distinction are abundant. The law of self-defense provides a notable example.[3]

Since a woman can get pregnant if she wishes whether or not she is married, and since there is little that society can do to prevent women from creating children even if their intention is to deprive the children of a father, why should we be so concerned about single men using surrogate mother arrangements if they too want a child but not a spouse? To say that women can intentionally plan to be unwed mothers is not to condone the practice. Besides, society will hold the father liable in a paternity action if he can be found and identified, which indicates some social concern that people should not be able to abdicate the responsibilities that they incur in generating children. Otherwise, why do we condemn the proverbial sailor with a pregnant girlfriend in every port?

In many surrogate mother arrangements, of course, the surrogate mother will not be transferring custody of the child to a single man, but to a couple: the child's biological father and a stepmother, his wife. What are the ethics of surrogate mother arrangements when the child is taken into a two-parent family? Again, surrogate mother arrangements and AID pose similar ethical questions: The surrogate mother transfers her parental responsibilities to the wife of the biological father, while with AID the sperm donor relinquishes his interest in the child to the husband of the biological mother. In both cases the child is created with the intention of transferring the responsibility for its care to a new set of parents. The surrogate mother situation is more dramatic than AID since the transfer occurs after the child is born, while in the case of AID the transfer takes place at the time of the insemination. Nevertheless, the ethical point is the same: creating children for the purpose of transferring them. For a surrogate mother the question remains: Is it ethical to create a child for the purpose of transferring it to the wife of the biological father?

At first blush this looks to be little different from the typical adoption, for what is an adoption other than a transfer of responsibility from one set of parents to another? The analogy is misleading, however, for two reasons. First, it is difficult to imagine anyone conceiving children for the purpose of putting them up for adoption. And, if such a bizarre event were to occur, I doubt that we would look upon it with moral approval. Most adoptions arise either because an undesired conception is brought to term, or because the parents wanted to have the child, but find that they are unable to provide for it because of some unfortunate circumstances that develop after conception.

Second, even if surrogate mother arrangements were to be classified as a type of adoption, not all offerings of children for adoption are necessarily moral. For example, would it be moral for parents to offer their three-year-old for adoption because they are bored with the child? Would it be moral for a couple to offer for adoption their newborn female baby because they wanted a boy?

Therefore, even though surrogate mother arrangements may in some superficial ways be likened to adoption, one must still ask whether it is ethical to separate the decision to create children from the desire to have them. I would answer no. The procreator should desire the child for its own sake, and not as a means to attaining some other end. Even though one of the ends may be stated altruistically as an attempt to bring happiness to an infertile couple, the child is still being used by the surrogate. She creates it not because she desires it, but because she desires something from it.

To sanction the use and treatment of human beings as means to the achievement of other goals instead of as ends in themselves is to accept an ethic with a tragic past, and to establish a precedent with a dangerous future. Already the press has reported the decision of one couple to conceive a child for the purpose of using it as a bone marrow donor for its sibling (*Los Angeles Times*, April 17, 1979, p. I–2). And the bioethics literature contains articles seriously considering whether we should clone human beings to serve as an inventory of spare parts for organ transplants[4] and articles that foresee the use of comatose human beings as self-replenishing blood banks and manufacturing plants for human hormones.[5]

How far our society is willing to proceed down this road is uncertain, but it is clear that the first step to all these practices is the acceptance of the same principle that the Nazis attempted to use to justify their medical experiments at the Nuremberg War Crimes Trials: that human beings may be used as means to the achievement of other goals, and need not be treated as ends in themselves.[6]

But why, it might be asked, is it so terrible if the surrogate mother does not desire the child for its own sake, when under the proposed surrogate mother arrangements there will be a couple eagerly desiring to have the child and to be its parents? That this argument may not be entirely accurate will be illustrated in the following section, but the basic reply is that creating a child without desiring it fundamentally changes the way we look at children—instead of viewing them as unique individual personalities to be desired in their own right, we may come to view them as commodities or items of manufacture to be desired because of their utility. A recent newspaper account describes the business of an agency that matches surrogate mothers with barren couples as follows:

> Its first product is due for delivery today. Twelve others are on the way and an additional 20 have been ordered. The "company" is Surrogate Mothering Ltd. and the "product" is babies.[7]

The dangers of this view are best illustrated by examining what might go wrong in a surrogate mother arrangement, and most important, by viewing how the various parties to the contract may react to the disappointment.

WHAT MIGHT GO WRONG

Ninety-nine percent of the surrogate mother arrangements may work out just fine: the child will be born normal, and the adopting parents (that is, the biological father and his wife) will want it. But, what happens when, unforeseeably, the child is born deformed? Since many defects cannot be discovered prenatally by amniocentesis or other means, the situation is bound to arise.[8] Similarly, consider what would happen if the biological father were to die before the birth of the child. Or if the "child" turns out to be twins or triplets. Each of these instances poses an inevitable situation where the adopting parents may be unhappy with the prospect of getting the child or children. Although legislation can mandate that the adopting parents take the child or children in whatever condition they come or whatever the situation, provided the surrogate mother has abided by all the contractual provisions of the surrogate mother arrangement, the important point for our discussion is the attitude that the surrogate mother or the adopting parent might have. Consider the example of the deformed child.

When I participated in the Surrogate Parent Foundation's inaugural symposium in November 1981, I was struck by the attitude of both the surrogate mothers and the adopting parents to these problems. The adopting parents worried, "Do we have to take such a child?" and the surrogate mothers said in response, "Well, we don't want to be stuck with it." Clearly, both groups were anxious not [to] be responsible for the "undesirable child" born of the surrogate mother arrangement. What does this portend?

It is human nature that when one pays money, one expects value. Things that one pays for have a way of being seen as commodities. Unavoidable in surrogate mother arrangements are questions such as: "Did I get a good one?" We see similar behavior with respect to the adoption of children: comparatively speaking, there is no shortage of black, Mexican-American, mentally retarded, or older children seeking homes; the shortage is in attractive, intelligent-looking Caucasian babies.[9] Similarly, surrogate mother arrangements involve more than just the desire to have a child. The desire is for a certain type of child.

But, it may be objected, don't all parents voice these same concerns in the normal course of having children? Not exactly. No one doubts or minimizes the pain and disappointment parents feel when they learn that their child is born with some genetic or congenital birth defect. But this is different from the surrogate mother situation, where neither the surrogate mother nor the adopting parents may feel responsible, and both sides may feel that they have a legitimate excuse not to assume responsibility for the child. The surrogate mother might blame the biological father for having "defective sperm," as the adopting parents might blame the surrogate mother for a "defective ovum" or for improper care of the fetus during pregnancy. The adopting parents desire a normal child, not *this* child in any condition, and the surrogate mother doesn't want it in any event. So both sides will feel threatened by the birth of an "undesirable child." Like bruised fruit in the produce bin of a supermarket, this child is likely to become an object of avoidance.

Certainly, in the natural course of having children a mother may doubt whether she wants a child if the father has died before its birth; parents may shy away from a defective infant, or be distressed at the thought of multiple births. Nevertheless, I believe they are more likely to accept these contingencies as a matter of fate. I do not think this is the case with surrogate mother arrangements. After all, in the surrogate mother arrangement the adopting parents can blame someone outside the marital relationship. The surrogate mother has been hosting this child all along, and she is delivering it. It certainly *looks* far more like a commodity than the child that arrives in the natural course within the family unit.

A DANGEROUS AGENDA

Another social problem, which arises out of the first, is the fear that surrogate mother arrangements will fall prey to eugenic concerns.[10] Surrogate mother contracts typically have clauses requiring genetic tests of the fetus and stating that the surrogate mother must have an abortion (or keep the child herself) if the child does not pass these tests.[11]

In the last decade we have witnessed a renaissance of interest in eugenics. This, coupled with advances in biomedical technology, has created a host of abuses and new moral problems. For example, genetic counseling clinics now face a dilemma: amniocentesis, the same procedure that identifies whether a fetus suffers from certain genetic defects, also discloses the sex of a fetus. Genetic counseling clinics have reported that even when the fetus is normal, a disproportionate number of mothers abort female children.[12] Aborting normal fetuses simply because the prospective parents desire children of a certain sex is one result of viewing children as commodities. The recent scandal at the Repository for Germinal Choice, the so-called "Nobel Sperm Bank," provides another chilling example. Their first "customer" was, unbeknownst to the staff, a woman who "had lost custody of two other children because they were abused in an effort to 'make them smart.' "[13] Of course, these and similar evils may occur whether or not surrogate mother arrangements are allowed by law. But to the extent that they promote the view of children as commodities, these arrangements contribute to these problems. There is nothing wrong with striving for betterment, as long as it does not result in intolerance to that which is not perfect. But I fear that the latter attitude will become prevalent.

Sanctioning surrogate mother arrangements can also exert pressures upon the family structure. First, as was noted earlier, there is nothing technically to prevent the use of surrogate mother arrangements by single males desiring to become parents. Indeed, single females can already do this with AID or even without it. But even if legislation were to limit the use of the surrogate mother arrangement to infertile couples, other pressures would occur: namely the intrusion of a third adult into the marital community.[14] I do not think that society is ready to accept either single parenting or quasi-adulterous arrangements as normal.

Another stress on the family structure arises within the family of the surrogate mother. When the child is surrendered to the adopting parents it is removed not only from the surrogate mother, but also from her family. They too have interests to be considered. Do not the siblings of that child have an interest in the fact that their little baby brother has been "given" away?[15] One woman, the mother of a medical student who had often donated sperm for artificial insemination, expressed her feelings to me eloquently. She asked, "I wonder how many grandchildren I have that I have never seen and never been able to hold or cuddle."

Intrafamily tensions can also be expected to result in the family of the adopting parents due to the asymmetry of relationship the adopting parents will have toward the child. The adopting mother has no biological relationship to the child, whereas the adopting father is also the child's biological father. Won't this unequal biological claim on the child be used as a wedge in child-rearing arguments? Can't we imagine the father saying, "Well, he is my son, not yours"? What if the couple eventually gets divorced? Should custody in a subsequent divorce between the adopting mother and the biological father be treated simply as a normal child custody dispute? Or should the biological relationship between father and child weigh more heavily? These questions do not arise in typical adoption situations since both parents are equally unrelated biologically to the child. Indeed, in adoption there is symmetry. The surrogate mother situation is more analogous to second marriages, where the children of one party by a prior marriage are adopted by the new spouse. Since asymmetry in second marriage situations causes problems, we can anticipate similar difficulties arising from surrogate mother arrangements.

There is also the worry that the offspring of a surrogate mother arrangement will be deprived of important information about his or her heritage. This also happens with adopted children or children conceived by AID,[16] who lack information about their biological parents, which could be important to them medically. Another less popularly recognized problem is the danger of half-sibling marriages,[17] where the child of the surrogate mother unwittingly falls in love with a half sister or brother. The only way to avoid these problems is to dispense with the confidentiality of parental records; however, the natural parents may not always want their identity disclosed.

The legalization of surrogate mother arrangements may also put undue pressure upon poor women to use their bodies in this way to support themselves and their families. Analogous problems have arisen in the past with the use of paid blood donors.[18] And occasionally the press reports someone desperate enough to offer to sell an eye or some other organ.[19] I believe that certain things should be viewed as too important to be sold as commodities, and I hope that we have advanced from the time when parents raised children for profitable labor, or found themselves forced to sell their children.

While many of the social dilemmas I have outlined here have their analogies in other present-day occurrences such as divorced families or in adoption, every addition is hurtful. Legalizing surrogate mother arrangements will increase the frequency of these problems, and put more stress on our society's shared moral values.[20]

[CONCLUSION]

An infertile couple might prefer to raise a child with a biological relationship to the husband, rather than to raise an adopted child who has no biological relationship to either the husband or the wife. But does the marginal increase in joy that they might therefore experience outweigh the potential pain that they, or the child conceived in such arrangements, or others might suffer? Does their preference outweigh the social costs and problems that the legalization of surrogate mothering might well engender? I honestly do not know. I don't even know on what hypothetical scale such interests could be weighed and balanced. But even if we could weigh such interests, and even if personal preference outweighed the costs, I still would not be able to say that we could justify achieving those ends by these means; that ethically it would be permissible for a person to create a child, not because she desired it, but because it could be useful to her....

REFERENCES

1 See Philip J. Parker, "Motivation of Surrogate Mothers: Initial Findings," *American Journal of Psychiatry* 140:1 (January 1983), 117–18; see also Doe V. Kelley, Circuit Court of Wayne County Michigan (1980) reported in 1980 Rep. on Human Reproduction and Law II-A-1.

2 See, e.g., C. M. v. C. C., 152 N.J. Supp. 160, 377 A.2d 821 (1977); "Why She Went to 'Nobel Sperm Bank' for Child," *Los Angeles Herald Examiner*, Aug. 6, 1982, p. A9; "Womb for Rent," *Los Angeles Herald Examiner*, Sept. 21, 1981, p. A3.

3 See also Richard McCormick, "Reproductive Technologies: Ethical Issues" in *Encyclopedia of Bioethics*, edited by Walter Reich, Vol. 4 (New York: The Free Press, 1978) pp. 1454, 1459; Robert Snowden and G. D. Mitchell, *The Artificial Family* (London: George Allen & Unwin, 1981), p. 71.

4 See, e.g., Alexander Peters, "The Brave New World: Can the Law Bring Order within Traditional Concepts of Due Process?" *Suffolk Law Review* 4 (1970), 894, 901–02; Roderic Gorney, "The New Biology and the Future of Man," *UCLA Law Review* 15 (1968), 273, 302; J. G. Castel, "Legal Implications of Biomedical Science and Technology in the Twenty-First Century," *Canadian Bar Review* 51 (1973), 119, 127.

5 See Harry Nelson, "Maintaining Dead to Serve as Blood Makers Proposed: Logical, Sociologist Says," *Los Angeles Times*, February 26, 1974, p. II-1; Hans Jonas, "Against the Stream: Comments on the Definition and Redefinition of Death," in *Philosophical Essays: From Ancient Creed to Technological Man* (Chicago: University of Chicago Press, 1974), pp. 132–40.

6 See Leo Alexander, "Medical Science under Dictatorship," *New England Journal of Medicine* 241:2 (1949), 39; United States v. Brandt, Trial of the Major War Criminals, International Military Tribunal: Nuremberg, 14 November 1945–1 October 1946.

7 Bob Dvorchak, "Surrogate Mothers: Pregnant Idea Now a Pregnant Business," *Los Angeles Herald Examiner*, December 27, 1983, p. A1.

8 "Surrogate's Baby Born with Deformities Rejected by All," *Los Angeles Times*, January 22, 1983, p. I-17; "Man Who Hired Surrogate Did Not Father Ailing Baby," *Los Angeles Herald Examiner*, February 3, 1983, p. A6.

9 See, e.g., Adoption in America, Hearing before the Subcommittee on Aging, Family and Human Ser-

vices of the Senate Committee on Labor and Human Resources, 97th Congress. 1st Session (1981), p. 3 (comments of Senator Jeremiah Denton) and pp. 16–17 (statement of Warren Master, Acting Commissioner of Administration for Children, Youth and Families, HHS).

10 Cf. "Discussion: Moral, Social and Ethical Issues," in *Laws and Ethics of A.I.D. and Embryo Transfer* (1973) (comments of Himmelweit); reprinted in Michael Shapiro and Roy Spece, *Bioethics and Law* (St. Paul: West Publishing Company, 1981), p. 548.

11 See, e.g., Lane (Newsday), "Womb for Rent," *Tucson Citizen* (Weekender), June 7, 1980, p. 3; Susan Lewis, "Baby Bartering? Surrogate Mothers Pose Issues for Lawyers, Courts," *The Los Angeles Daily Journal*, April 20, 1981; see also Elaine Markoutsas, "Women Who Have Babies for Other Women," *Good Housekeeping* 96 (April 1981), 104.

12 See Morton A. Stenchever, "An Abuse of Prenatal Diagnosis," *Journal of the American Medical Association* 221 (1972), 408; Charles Westoff and Ronald R. Rindfus, "Sex Preselection in the United States: Some Implications," *Science* 184 (1974), 633, 636; see also Phyllis Battelle, "Is It a Boy or a Girl"? *Los Angeles Herald Examiner*, Oct. 8, 1981, p. A17.

13 "2 Children Taken from Sperm Bank Mother," *Los Angeles Times*, July 14, 1982; p. I-3; "The Sperm Bank Scandal," *Newsweek* 24 (July 26, 1982).

14 See Helmut Thielicke, *The Ethics of Sex*, John W. Doberstein, trans. (New York: Harper & Row, 1964).

15 According to one newspaper account, when a surrogate mother informed her nine-year-old daughter that the new baby would be given away, the daughter replied, "Oh good. If it's a girl we can keep it and give Jeffrey [her two-year-old half brother] away." "Womb for Rent," *Los Angeles Herald Examiner*, Sept. 21, 1981, p. A3.

16 See, e.g., Lorraine Dusky, "Brave New Babies?" *Newsweek* 30 (December 6, 1982). Also testimony of Suzanne Rubin before the California Assembly Committee on Judiciary, Surrogate Parenting Contracts, Assembly Publication No. 962, pp. 72–75 (November 19, 1982).

17 This has posed an increasing problem for children conceived through AID. See, e.g., Martin Curie-Cohen et al., "Current Practice of Artificial Insemination by Donor in the United States," *New England Journal of Medicine* 300 (1979), 585–89.

18 See, e.g., Richard M. Titmuss, *The Gift Relationship: From Human Blood to Social Policy* (New York: Random House, 1971).

19 See, e.g., "Man Desperate for Funds: Eye for Sale at $35,000," *Los Angeles Times*, February 1, 1975, p. II-1; "100 Answer Man's Ad for New Kidney," *Los Angeles Times*, September 12, 1974, p. I-4.

20 See generally Guido Calabresi, "Reflections on Medical Experimentation in Humans," *Daedalus* 98 (1969), 387–93; also see Michael Shapiro and Roy Spece, "On Being 'Unprincipled on Principle': The Limits of Decision Making 'On the Merits,' " in *Bioethics and Law*, pp. 67–71.

Baby M
Bonnie Steinbock

Bonnie Steinbock is associate professor of philosophy at the State University of New York at Albany. She is the editor of *Killing and Letting Die* (1980). Her published articles include "The Intentional Termination of Life," "Prenatal Wrongful Death," and "Drunk Driving."

Steinbock describes the custody battle that emerged in a well-known New Jersey case when surrogate mother Mary Beth Whitehead decided that she wanted to keep a child who, by contractual agreement, was to be given over at birth to a married couple (the Sterns). Although a lower court originally upheld the validity of the surrogacy contract and awarded custody to

From "Surrogate Motherhood as Prenatal Adoption," in *Law, Medicine and Health Care*, vol. 16 (Spring 1988), pp. 44–47. Reprinted with permission of the publisher (American Society of Law and Medicine).

the Sterns, the New Jersey Supreme Court in a precedent-setting judgment ruled that surrogacy contracts are invalid and unenforceable. However, the higher court upheld the custody decision of the lower court as being in Baby M's best interest, although it also ruled that Whitehead was the legal mother and thereby entitled to visitation rights. Steinbock herself endorses the custody decision on the basis of the best-interests test, but she argues that the awarding of visitation rights to Whitehead is incompatible with the best interests of the child.

Mary Beth Whitehead, a married mother of two, agreed to be inseminated with the sperm of William Stern and to give up the child to him for a fee of $10,000. The baby (whom Ms. Whitehead named Sara, and the Sterns named Melissa) was born on March 27, 1986. Three days later, Ms. Whitehead took her home from the hospital and turned her over to the Sterns.

Then Ms. Whitehead changed her mind. She went to the Sterns' home, distraught, and pleaded to have the baby temporarily. Afraid that she would kill herself, the Sterns agreed. The next week, Ms. Whitehead informed the Sterns that she had decided to keep the child, and threatened to leave the country if court action was taken.

At that point, the situation deteriorated into a cross between the Keystone Kops and Nazi stormtroopers. Accompanied by five policemen, the Sterns went to the Whitehead residence armed with a court order giving them temporary custody of the child. Ms. Whitehead managed to slip the baby out of a window to her husband, and the following morning the Whiteheads fled with the child to Florida, where Ms. Whitehead's parents lived. During the next three months, the Whiteheads lived in roughly twenty different hotels, motels, and homes to avoid apprehension. From time to time, Ms. Whitehead telephoned Mr. Stern to discuss the matter: he taped these conversations on advice of counsel. Ms. Whitehead threatened to kill herself, to kill the child, and to falsely accuse Mr. Stern of sexually molesting her older daughter.

At the end of July 1986, while Ms. Whitehead was hospitalized with a kidney infection, Florida police raided her mother's home, knocking her down, and seized the child. Baby M was placed in the custody of Mr. Stern, and the Whiteheads returned to New Jersey, where they attempted to regain custody. After a long and emotional court battle, Judge Harvey R. Sorkow ruled on March 31, 1987, that the surrogacy contract was valid, and that specific performance was justified in the best interests of the child. Immediately after reading his decision, he called the Sterns into his chambers so

that Mr. Stern's wife, Dr. Elizabeth Stern, could legally adopt the child.

This outcome was unexpected and unprecedented. Most commentators had thought that a court would be unlikely to order a reluctant surrogate to give up an infant merely on the basis of a contract.[1] Indeed, if Ms. Whitehead had never surrendered the child to the Sterns, but had simply taken her home and kept her there, the outcome undoubtedly would have been different. It is also likely that Ms. Whitehead's failure to obey the initial custody order angered Judge Sorkow, and affected his decision.

The decision was appealed to the New Jersey Supreme Court, which issued its decision on February 3, 1988. Writing for a unanimous court, Chief Justice Wilentz reversed the lower court's ruling that the surrogacy contract was valid. The court held that a surrogacy contract that provides money for the surrogate mother, and that includes her irrevocable agreement to surrender her child at birth, is invalid and unenforceable. Since the contract was invalid, Ms. Whitehead did not relinquish, nor were there any other grounds for terminating, her parental rights. Therefore, the adoption of Baby M by Dr. Stern was improperly granted, and Ms. Whitehead remains the child's legal mother.

The court further held that the issue of custody is determined solely by the child's best interests, and it agreed with the lower court that it was in Melissa's best interests to remain with the Sterns. However, Ms. Whitehead, as Baby M's legal as well as natural mother, is entitled to have her own interest in visitation considered. The determination of what kind of visitation rights should be granted to her, and under what conditions, was remanded to the trial court.

The distressing details of this case have led many people to reject surrogacy altogether. Do we really want police officers wrenching infants from their mothers' arms, and prolonged custody battles when surrogates find they are unable to surrender their children, as agreed? Advocates of surrogacy say that to reject the practice wholesale, because of one unfortunate instance, is an example of a "hard case" making bad policy. Opponents reply that it is entirely reasonable to focus on the worst potential outcomes when deciding public policy. Everyone can agree on at least one thing: this particular case seems to have been mismanaged from start to finish, and could serve as a manual of how not to arrange a surrogate birth.

First, it is now clear that Mary Beth Whitehead was not a suitable candidate for surrogate motherhood. Her ambivalence about giving up the child was recognized early on, although this information was not passed on to the Sterns.[2] Second, she had contact with the baby after birth, which is usually avoided in "successful" cases. Typically, the adoptive mother is actively involved in the pregnancy, often serving as the pregnant woman's coach in labor. At birth, the baby is given to the adoptive, not the biological mother. The joy of the adoptive parents in holding their child serves both to promote their bonding and to lessen the pain of separation of the biological mother.

At Ms. Whitehead's request, no one at the hospital was aware of the surrogacy arrangement. She and her husband appeared as the proud parents of "Sara Elizabeth Whitehead," the name on her birth certificate. Ms. Whitehead held her baby, nursed her, and took her home from the hospital—just as she would have done in a normal pregnancy and birth. Not surprisingly, she thought of Sara as her child, and she fought with every weapon at her disposal, honorable and dishonorable, to prevent her being taken away. She can hardly be blamed for doing so.[3]

Why did Dr. Stern, who supposedly had a very good relation with Ms. Whitehead before the birth, not act as her labor coach? One possibility is that Ms. Whitehead, ambivalent about giving up her baby, did not want Dr. Stern involved. At her request, the Sterns' visits to the hospital to see the newborn baby were unobtrusive. It is also possible that Dr. Stern was ambivalent about having a child. The original idea of hiring a surrogate was not hers, but her husband's. It was Mr. Stern who felt a "compelling" need to have a child related to him by blood, having lost all his relatives to the Nazis.

Furthermore, Dr. Stern was not infertile, as was stated in the surrogacy agreement. Rather, in 1979 she was diagnosed by two eye specialists as suffering from optic neuritis, which meant that she "probably" had multiple sclerosis. (This was confirmed by all four experts who testified.) Normal conception was ruled out by the Sterns in late 1982, when a medical colleague told

Dr. Stern that his wife, a victim of multiple sclerosis, had suffered a temporary paralysis during pregnancy. "We decided the risk wasn't worth it," Mr. Stern said.[4]

Ms. Whitehead's lawyer, Harold J. Cassidy, dismissed the suggestion that Dr. Stern's "mildest case" of multiple sclerosis determined the Sterns' decision to seek a surrogate. He noted that she was not even treated for multiple sclerosis until after the Baby M dispute had started. "It's almost as though it's an afterthought," he said.[5]

Judge Sorkow deemed the decision to avoid conception "medically reasonable and understandable." The Supreme Court did not go so far, noting that Dr. Stern's "anxiety appears to have exceeded the actual risk, which current medical authorities assess as minimal."[6] Nonetheless, the court acknowledged that her anxiety, including fears that pregnancy might precipitate blindness and paraplegia, was "quite real." Certainly, even a woman who wants a child very much may reasonably wish to avoid becoming blind and paralyzed as a result of pregnancy. Yet is it believable that a woman who really wanted a child would decide against pregnancy *solely* on the basis of *someone else's* medical experience? Would she not consult at least one specialist on her *own* medical condition before deciding it wasn't worth the risk? The conclusion that she was at best ambivalent about bearing a child seems irresistible.

This possibility conjures up many people's worst fears about surrogacy: that prosperous women, who do not want to interrupt their careers, will use poor and educationally disadvantaged women to bear their children....[But the] issue here is psychological: what kind of mother is Dr. Stern likely to be? If she is unwilling to undergo pregnancy, with its discomforts, inconveniences, and risks, will she be willing to make the considerable sacrifices that good parenting requires? Ms. Whitehead's ability to be a good mother was repeatedly questioned during the trial. She was portrayed as immature, untruthful, hysterical, overly identified with her children, and prone to smothering their independence. Even if all this is true—and I think that Ms. Whitehead's inadequacies were exaggerated—Dr. Stern may not be such a prize either. The choice for Baby M may have been between a highly strung, emotional, overinvolved mother, and a remote, detached, even cold one.[7]

The assessment of Ms. Whitehead's ability to be a good mother was biased by the middle-class prejudices of the judge and of the mental health officials who testified. Ms. Whitehead left school at fifteen, and is not conversant with the latest theories on child rearing: she made the egregious error of giving Sara teddy bears to play with, instead of the more "age-appropriate," expert-approved pans and spoons. She proved to be a total failure at patty-cake. If this is evidence of parental inadequacy, we're all in danger of losing our children.

The Supreme Court felt that Ms. Whitehead was "rather harshly judged" and acknowledged the possibility that the trial court was wrong in its initial award of custody. Nevertheless, it affirmed Judge Sorkow's decision to allow the Sterns to retain custody, as being in Melissa's best interests. George Annas disagrees with the "best interests" approach. He points out that Judge Sorkow awarded temporary custody of Baby M to the Sterns in May 1986, without giving the Whiteheads notice or an opportunity to obtain legal representation. That was a serious wrong and injustice to the Whiteheads. To allow the Sterns to keep the child compounds the original unfairness: "justice requires that reasonable consideration be given to returning Baby M to the permanent custody of the Whiteheads."[8]

But a child is not a possession, to be returned to the rightful owner. It is not fairness to all parties that should determine a child's fate, but what is best for her. As Chief Justice Wilentz rightly stated, "The child's interests come first: we will not punish it for judicial errors, assuming any were made."[9]

Subsequent events have substantiated the claim that giving custody to the Sterns was in Melissa's best interests. After losing custody, Ms. Whitehead, whose husband had undergone a vasectomy, became pregnant by another man. She divorced her husband and married Dean R. Gould last November. These developments indicate that the Whiteheads were not able to offer a stable home, although the argument can be made that their marriage might have survived if not for the strains introduced by the court battle and the loss of Baby M. But even if Judge Sorkow had no reason to prefer the Sterns to the Whiteheads back in May 1986, he was still right to give the Sterns custody in March 1987. To take her away then, at nearly eighteen months of age, from the only parents she had ever known would have been disruptive, cruel, and unfair to her.

Annas' preference for a just solution is premised partly on his belief that there *is* no "best interest" solution to this "tragic custody case." I take it that he means that however custody is resolved, Baby M is the loser. Either way, she will be deprived of one parent. However, a best-interests solution is not a perfect solution. It is simply the solution that is on balance best for the child, given the realities of the situation. Applying this standard, Judge Sorkow was right to give the Sterns cus-

tody, and the Supreme Court was right to uphold the decision.

The best-interests argument is based on the assumption that Mr. Stern has at least a *prima facie* claim to Baby M. We certainly would not consider allowing a stranger who kidnapped a baby and managed to elude the police for a year to retain custody on the grounds that he was providing a good home to a child who had known no other parent. However, the Baby M case is not analogous. First, Mr. Stern is Baby M's biological father and, as such, has at least some claim to raise her, which no non-parental kidnapper has. Second, Mary Beth Whitehead *agreed* to give him their baby. Unlike the miller's daughter in *Rumpelstiltskin*, the fairy tale to which the Baby M case is sometimes compared, she was not forced into the agreement. Because both Mary Beth Whitehead and Mr. Stern have *prima facie* claims to Baby M, the decision as to who should raise her should be based on her present best interests. Therefore we must, regretfully, tolerate the injustice to Ms. Whitehead, and try to avoid such problems in the future.

It is unfortunate that the court did not decide the issue of visitation on the same basis as custody. By declaring Ms. Whitehead-Gould the legal mother, and maintaining that she is entitled to visitation, the court has prolonged the fight over Baby M. It is hard to see how this can be in her best interests. This is no ordinary divorce case, where the child has a relation with both parents that it is desirable to maintain. As Mr. Stern said at the start of the court hearing to determine visitation, "Melissa has a right to grow and be happy and not be torn between two parents."[10]

The court's decision was well-meaning but internally inconsistent. Out of concern for the best interests of the child, it granted the Sterns custody. At the same time, by holding Ms. Whitehead-Gould to be the legal mother, with visitation rights, it precluded precisely what is most in Melissa's interest, a resolution of the situation. Further, the decision leaves open the distressing possibility that a Baby M situation could happen again. Legislative efforts should be directed toward ensuring that this worst-case scenario never occurs.

REFERENCES

1 See, for example, "Surrogate Motherhood Agreements: Contemporary Legal Aspects of a Biblical Notion," *University of Richmond Law Review*, 16 (1982): 470; "Surrogate Mothers: The Legal Issues," *American Journal of Law & Medicine*, 7 (1981): 338,

and Angela Holder, *Legal Issues in Pediatrics and Adolescent Medicine* (New Haven: Yale University Press, 1985), 8: "Where a surrogate mother decides that she does not want to give the baby up for adoption, as has already happened, *it is clear that no court will enforce a contract entered into before the child was born* in which she agreed to surrender her baby for adoption." Emphasis added.

2 Had the Sterns been informed of the psychologist's concerns as to Ms. Whitehead's suitability to be a surrogate, they might have ended the arrangement, costing the Infertility Center its fee. As Chief Justice Wilentz said, "It is apparent that the profit motive got the better of the Infertility Center." In the matter of Baby M, Supreme Court of New Jersey, A-39, at 45.

3 "[W]e think it is expecting something well beyond normal human capabilities to suggest that this mother should have parted with her newly born infant without a struggle.... We...cannot conceive of any other case where a perfectly fit mother was expected to surrender her newly born infant, perhaps forever, and was then told she was a bad mother because she did not." Id.: 79.

4 "Father Recalls Surrogate Was 'Perfect,'" *New York Times*, Jan. 6, 1987, B2.

5 Id.

6 In the matter of Baby M, supra note 2, at 8.

7 This possibility was suggested to me by Susan Vermazen.

8 George Annas, "Baby M: Babies (and Justice) for Sale," *Hastings Center Report*, 17, no. 3 (1987): 15.

9 In the matter of Baby M, supra note 2, at 75.

10 "Anger and Anguish at Baby M Visitation Hearing," *New York Times*, March 29, 1988, 17.

Reproductive Technologies

Creating Embryos
Peter Singer

Peter Singer is professor of philosophy and director, Centre for Human Bioethics, at Monash University, Victoria, Australia. He is the author of such books as *Animal Liberation* (1975) and *Practical Ethics* (1980). He is the coauthor of *Should the Baby Live?* (1985) and the editor of *Applied Ethics* (1986).

Singer identifies seven distinct objections that have been made to the use of *in vitro* fertilization (IVF) even in the "simple case"—a case in which a married couple is infertile, only eggs and sperm provided by the couple are involved, and all resulting embryos are transferred to the uterus of the wife. He takes some of these objections more seriously than others but ultimately concludes that none should "count against going ahead" with IVF in the simple case. Singer then considers a number of variations on the simple case, and he identifies the moral status of the embryo as an underlying issue of great importance. In his view, early embryos have no moral status because they are incapable of feeling pain or pleasure. Accordingly, he finds no ethical problem with freezing early embryos, discarding them, or using them for research purposes. Singer concludes with a brief discussion of future possibilities associated with IVF technology. In particular, he considers genetic engineering.

The treatment of human embryos became a matter of public controversy in July 1978. That month saw the birth of Louise Brown, the first human being to have developed from an embryo which at some point in its existence was outside a human body. This marked the beginning of what can properly be called a revolution in human reproduction. The point is not that *in vitro* fertilization (the technique used to make possible the birth of Louise Brown) is itself so extraordinary. On the contrary, *in vitro* fertilization, or IVF, can be seen as simply a way of overcoming certain forms of infertility, such as blocked fallopian tubes. In this sense, IVF is no more revolutionary than a microsurgical operation to remove the blockage in the tubes. But IVF is revolutionary because it brings the embryo out of the human body. Once the embryo is in the open, human beings can observe it, manipulate it, and make life-or-death decisions about it. These possibilities make IVF, and its future applications, a subject of the utmost moral importance.

Consider what has already happened, all within the first decade after Brown. Women who do not produce eggs have been given eggs by other women who do; they have then given birth to babies to whom they are genetically entirely unrelated (1).

Embryos have been frozen in liquid nitrogen, stored for more than a year, thawed, and then transferred to women who have given birth to normal children. In one case, two "twins"—that is, children conceived from eggs produced by a single ovulatory cycle—were born 16 months apart. Another case illustrated the pitfalls of embryo freezing: two embryos, in storage in a Melbourne laboratory, were orphaned when their parents were killed in a plane crash, apparently leaving no instructions regarding the disposition of their embryos (1).

Scientists have begun to speculate on the medical purposes to which embryos might be put. Dr. Robert Edwards, the scientist who, together with Patrick Steptoe, made it possible for Louise Brown to be born, has suggested that if embryos could be grown for about 17 days, we could take from them developing blood cells which would have the potential to overcome such fatal diseases as sickle cell anemia and perhaps leukemia (2).

There was a time when our ethical codes could slowly adapt to changing circumstances. Those days are gone. We have to decide, right now, whether the moral status of embryos is such that it is wrong to freeze them or experiment upon them. We have also to make an immediate decision on whether there is any objection to allowing some women to carry and bring to birth embryos to which they have no genetic link. We have, at most, until the end of the century to decide how to handle new technologies for selecting and manipulating embryos, technologies that will force us to ask which human qualities are most desirable. We must start by acquainting ourselves with the new techniques and deciding which of them should form part of the society in which we live.

IVF: THE SIMPLE CASE

The so-called simple case of IVF is that in which a married, infertile couple use an egg taken from the wife and sperm taken from the husband, and all embryos created are inserted into the womb of the wife. This case allows us to consider the ethics of IVF in itself, without the complications of the many other issues that can arise in different circumstances. Then we can go on to look at these complications separately.

The Technique

The technique itself is now well known and is fast becoming a routine part of infertility treatment in many countries. The infertile woman is given a hormone treatment to induce her ovaries to produce more than one egg in her next cycle. Her hormone levels are carefully monitored to detect the precise moment at which the eggs are ripening. At this time the eggs are removed. This is usually done by laparoscopy, a minor operation in which a fine tube is inserted into the woman's abdomen and the egg is sucked out up the tube. A laparoscope, a kind of periscope illuminated by fiber optics, is also inserted into the abdomen so that the surgeon can locate the place where the ripe egg is to be found. Instead of laparoscopy, some IVF teams are now using ultrasound techniques, which eliminate the need for a general anesthetic.

Once the eggs have been collected they are placed in culture in small glass dishes known as petri dishes, not in test tubes despite the popular label of "test-tube babies." Sperm is then obtained from the male partner by means of masturbation and placed with the egg. Fertilization follows in at least 80 percent of the ripe eggs. The resulting embryos are allowed to cleave once or twice and are usually transferred to the woman some 48 to 72 hours after fertilization. The actual transfer is done via the vagina and is a simple procedure.

It is after the transfer, when the embryo is back in the uterus and beyond the scrutiny of medical science, that things are most likely to go wrong. Even with the most experienced IVF teams, the majority of embryos transferred fail to implant in the uterus. One pregnancy for every five transfers is currently considered to be a good working average for a competent IVF team. Many of the newer teams fail to achieve anything like this rate. Nevertheless, there are so many units around the world now practicing IVF that thousands of babies have been produced as a result of the technique. IVF has ceased to be experimental and is now a routine, if still "last resort" method of treating some forms of infertility.

Objections to the Simple Case

There is some opposition to IVF even in the simple case. The most frequently heard objections are as follows:

1. IVF is unnatural.

2. IVF is risky for the offspring.

3. IVF separates the procreative and the conjugal aspects of marriage and so damages the marital relationship.

4. IVF is illicit because it involves masturbation.

5. Adoption is a better solution to the problem of childlessness.

6. IVF is an expensive luxury and the resources would be better spent elsewhere.

7. IVF allows increased male control over reproduction and hence threatens the status of women in the community.

We can deal swiftly with the first four of these objections. If we were to reject medical advances on the grounds that they are "unnatural" we would be rejecting modern medicine as a whole, for the very purpose of the medical enterprise is to resist the ravages of nature which would otherwise shorten our lives and make them much less pleasant. If anything is in accordance with the nature of our species, it is the application of our intelligence to overcome adverse situations in which we find ourselves. The application of IVF to infertile couples is a classic example of this application of human intelligence.

The claim that IVF is risky for the offspring is one that was argued with great force before IVF became a widely used technique. It is sufficient to note that the re-

sults of IVF so far have happily refuted these fears. The most recent Australian figures, for example, based on 934 births, indicate that the rate of abnormality was 2.7%, which is very close to the national average of 1.5%. When we take into account the greater average age of women seeking IVF, as compared with the childbearing population as a whole, it does not seem that the *in vitro* technique itself adds to the risk of an abnormal offspring. This view is reinforced by the fact that the abnormalities were all ones that arise with the ordinary method of reproduction; there have been no new "monsters" produced by IVF (3). Perhaps we still cannot claim with statistical certainty that the risk of defect is no higher with IVF than with the more common method of conception; but if the risk is higher at all, it would appear to be only very slightly higher, and still within limits which may be considered acceptable.

The third and fourth objections have been urged by spokesmen for certain religious groups, but they are difficult to defend outside the confines of particular religions. Few infertile couples will take seriously the view that their marital relationship will be damaged if they use the technique which offers them the best chance of having their own child. It is in any case extraordinarily paternalistic for anyone else to tell a couple that they should not use IVF because it will harm their marriage. That, surely, is for them to decide.

The objection to masturbation comes from a similar source and can be even more swiftly dismissed. Religious prohibitions on masturbation are taboos from past times which even religious spokesmen are beginning to consider outdated. Moreover, even if one could defend a prohibition on masturbation for sexual pleasure—perhaps on the (very tenuous) ground that sexual activity is wrong unless it is directed either toward procreation or toward the strengthening of the bond between marriage partners—it would be absurd to extend a prohibition with that kind of rationale to a case in which masturbation is being used in the context of a marriage and precisely in order to make reproduction possible. (The fact that some religions do persist in regarding masturbation as wrong, even in these circumstances, is indicative of the folly of an ethical system based on absolute rules, irrespective of the circumstances in which those rules are being applied, or the consequences of their application.)

Overpopulation and the Allocation of Resources

The next two objections, however, deserve more careful consideration. In an overpopulated world in which there are so many children who cannot be properly fed and cared for, there is something incongruous about using all the ingenuity of modern medicine to create more children. And similarly, when there are so many deaths caused by preventable diseases, is there not something wrong with the priorities which lead us to develop expensive techniques for overcoming the relatively less serious problem of infertility?

These objections are sound to the following extent: in an ideal world we would find loving families for unwanted children before we created additional children; and in an ideal world we would clear up all the preventable ill-health and malnutrition-related diseases before we went on to tackle the problem of infertility. But is it appropriate to ask, of IVF alone, whether it can stand the test of measurement against what we would do in an ideal world? In an ideal world, none of us would consume more than our fair share of resources. We would not drive expensive cars while others die for the lack of drugs costing a few cents. We would not eat a diet rich in wastefully produced animal products while others cannot get enough to nourish their bodies. We cannot demand more of infertile couples than we are ready to demand of ourselves. If fertile couples are free to have large families of their own, rather than adopt destitute children from overseas, infertile couples must also be free to do what they can to have their own families. In both cases, overseas adoption, or perhaps the adoption of local children who are unwanted because of some impairment, should be considered; but if we are not going to make this compulsory in the former case, it should not be made compulsory in the latter.

There is a further question: to what extent do infertile couples have a right to assistance from community medical resources? Again, however, we must not single out IVF for harsher treatment than we give to other medical techniques. If tubal surgery is available and covered by one's health insurance, or is offered as part of a national health scheme, then why should IVF be treated any differently? And if infertile couples can get free or subsidized psychiatry to help them overcome the psychological problems of infertility, there is something absurd about denying them free or subsidized treatment which could overcome the root of the problem, rather than the symptoms. By today's standards, after all, IVF is not an inordinately expensive medical technique; and there is no country, as far as I know, which limits its provision of free or subsidized health care to those cases in which the patient's life is in danger. Once we extend medical care to cover cases of injury, incapacity, and psychological distress, IVF has a strong claim to be included among the range of free or subsidized treatments available.

The Effect on Women

The final objection is one that has come from some feminists. In a recently published collection of essays by women titled *Test-Tube Women: What Future for Motherhood?*, several contributors are suspicious of the new reproductive technology. None is more hostile than Robyn Rowland, an Australian sociologist, who writes:

> Ultimately the new technology will be used for the benefit of men and to the detriment of women. Although technology itself is not always a negative development, the real question has always been—who controls it? Biological technology is in the hands of men (4).

And Rowland concludes with a warning as dire as any uttered by the most conservative opponents of IVF:

> What may be happening is the last battle in the long war of men against women. Women's position is most precarious...we may find ourselves without a product of any kind with which to bargain. For the history of "mankind" women have been seen in terms of their value as child-bearers. We have to ask, if that last power is taken and controlled by men, what role is envisaged for women in the new world? Will women become obsolete? Will we be fighting to retain or reclaim the right to bear children—has patriarchy conned us once again? I urge you sisters to be vigilant (4).

I can see little basis for such claims. For a start, women have figured quite prominently in the leading IVF teams in Britain, Australia, and the United States: Jean Purdy was an early colleague of Edwards and Steptoe in the research that led to the birth of Louise Brown; Linda Mohr has directed the development of embryo freezing at the Queen Victoria Medical Centre in Melbourne; and in the United States Georgeanna Jones and Joyce Vargyas have played leading roles in the groundbreaking clinics in Norfolk, Virginia, and at the University of Southern California, respectively. It seems odd for a feminist to neglect the contributions these women have made.

Even if one were to grant, however, that the technology remains predominantly in male hands, it has to be remembered that it was developed in response to the needs of infertile couples. From interviews I have conducted and meetings I have attended, my impression is that while both partners are often very concerned about their childlessness, in those cases in which one partner is more distressed than the other by this situation, that partner is usually the woman. Feminists usually accept that this is so, attributing it to the power of social conditioning in a patriarchal society; but the origin of the strong female desire for children is not really what is in question here. The question is: in what sense is the new technology an instrument of male domination over women? If it is true that the technology was developed at least as much in response to the needs of women as in response to the needs of men, then it is hard to see why a feminist should condemn it.

It might be objected that whatever the origins of IVF and no matter how benign it may be when used to help infertile couples, the further development of techniques such as ectogenesis—the growth of the embryo from conception totally outside the body, in an artificial womb—will reduce the status of women. Again, it is not easy to see why this should be so. Ectogenesis will, if it is ever successful, provide a choice for women. Shulamith Firestone argued several years ago in her influential feminist work *The Dialectic of Sex* (5) that this choice will remove the fundamental biological barrier to complete equality. Hence Firestone welcomed the prospect of ectogenesis and condemned the low priority given by our male-dominated society to research in this area.

Firestone's view is surely more in line with the drive to sexual equality than the position taken by Rowland. If we argue that to break the link between women and childbearing would be to undermine the status of women in our society, what are we saying about the ability of women to obtain true equality in other spheres of life? I am not so pessimistic about the abilities of women to achieve equality with men across the broad range of human endeavor. For that reason I think women will be helped, rather than harmed, by the development of a technology which makes it possible for them to have children without being pregnant. As Nancy Breeze, a very differently inclined contributor to the same collection of essays, puts it:

> Two thousand years of morning sickness and stretch marks have not resulted in liberation for women or children. If you should run into a Petri dish, it could turn out to be your best friend. So rock it; don't knock it! (6)

So to sum up this discussion of the ethics of the simple case of IVF: the ethical objections urged against IVF under these conditions are not strong. They should not count against going ahead with IVF when it is the best way of overcoming infertility and when the infertile couple are not prepared to consider adoption as a means of overcoming their problem. There is, admittedly, a serious question about how much of the national health budget should be allocated to this area. But then, there are serious questions about the allocation of resources in other areas of medicine as well.

IVF: OTHER CASES

IVF can be used in circumstances that differ from those of the simple case in the following respects:

1. The couple may not be legally married; or there may be no couple at all, the patient being a single woman.

2. The couple may not be infertile but may wish to use IVF for some other reason, for instance because the woman carries a genetic defect.

3. The sperm, or the egg, or both, may come from another person, not from the couple themselves.

4. Some of the embryos created may not be inserted into the womb of the wife; instead they may be frozen and stored for later use, or donated to others, or used for research, or simply discarded.

All of these variations on the simple case raise potentially difficult issues. I say "potentially difficult" because in some cases the difficulties arise only once we consider the more extreme instances. For instance, there are no good grounds for discriminating against couples who are not legally married but have a long-standing de facto relationship; on the other hand one would need to consider more carefully whether to allow a single woman to make use of IVF. It is true that single fertile women are entirely free to procreate as irresponsibly as they like; yet the doctor who assists an infertile woman to do the same must take some care that the child in whose creation he or she is assisting will grow up in circumstances that are compatible with a good start in life. A single mother may well be able to provide such circumstances, but it is at least appropriate for the doctor to make some inquiries before going ahead.

IVF for fertile couples when the woman carries a serious genetic defect is scarcely problematic; if we would allow artificial insemination when the man has a similar defect, we should also allow IVF when the woman is the carrier. Here too, however, there is a question about how far we should go. What if the defect is a very minor one? What if there is no defect at all, but the woman wants a donor egg from a friend whose intelligence or beauty she considers superior to her own? A California sperm bank is already offering selected women the sperm of Nobel Prize-winning scientists. It is only a matter of time before eggs are offered in the same manner. Nevertheless it seems clear that as long as IVF is in short supply, those who are infertile or who carry a serious genetic defect should have the first claim upon it. (The issue of genetic selection itself will be touched upon in the final section of this [essay].)

The use of donor sperm, eggs, and embryos raises further questions. There is a precedent in the use of donor sperm in artificial insemination. The lesson that has been learned here is that there is a great need for counseling the couple because there may be psychological problems when one parent is not the genetic parent of the child. There is also the question of whether the child is to be told of her or his genetic origins. Many adopted persons now consider that they have a right to full information about their genetic parents. There is a strong case for saying that the same applies to people born as a result of the use of donor sperm or eggs, and that nonidentifying data about the donor should be released to the parents, with a view to the child being informed at a later stage.

The most controversial of these issues is that of the moral status of the embryo; this is the question at stake when we consider whether to create more embryos than we are willing to put back into the womb at one time. Disposing of the embryos, or using them for research purposes, runs counter to the view held by some that the embryo is a human being with the same right to life as any other human being. Even embryo freezing does little to placate those who take this view, since on present indications the chances of a frozen embryo surviving to become a living child are not high. But, religious doctrines apart, is it plausible to hold that the embryo has a right to life? The moral status of the embryo is perhaps the most fundamental of all the moral issues raised by the reproduction revolution. Many people believe it to be an insoluble philosophical problem, one on which we just have to take our stand, more or less arbitrarily, without hope of persuading those of a different view. I believe,

on the contrary, that the issue is amenable to rational discussion. . . .

THE MORAL STATUS OF THE EMBRYO

. . . [A]ttempts to argue that the early embryo has a right to life [can be shown to be inadequate]. It remains only to say something positive about when in its development the embryo may acquire rights.

The answer must depend on the actual characteristics of the embryo. The minimal characteristic which is needed to give the embryo a claim to consideration is sentience, or the capacity to feel pain or pleasure. Until the embryo reaches that point, there is nothing we can do to the embryo which causes harm to *it*. We can, of course, damage it in such a way as to cause harm to the person it will become, if it lives, but if it never becomes a person, the embryo has not been harmed, because its total lack of awareness means that it can have no interest in becoming a person.

Once an embryo may be capable of feeling pain, there is a clear case for very strict controls over the experimentation which can be done with it. At this point the embryo ranks, morally, with other creatures who are conscious but not self-conscious. Many nonhuman animals come into this category, and in my view they have often been unjustifiably made to suffer in scientific research. We should have stringent controls over research to ensure that this cannot happen to embryos, just as we should have stringent controls to ensure that it cannot happen to animals.

Practical Implications of the Moral Status of Embryos

The conclusion to draw from this is that as long as the parents give their consent, there is no ethical objection to discarding a very early embryo. If the early embryo can be used for significant research, so much the better. What is crucial is that the embryo not be kept beyond the point at which it has formed a brain and a nervous system, and might be capable of suffering. Two government committees—the Warnock Committee in Britain (7) and the Waller Committee in Victoria, Australia (8) —have recently recommended that research on embryos should be allowed, but only up to 14 days after fertilization. This is the period at which the so-called "primitive streak," the first indication of the development of a nervous system, begins to form, and up to this stage there is certainly no possibility of the embryo feeling anything at all. In fact, the 14-day limit is unnecessarily conservative. A limit of, say, 28 days would still be very much on the safe side of the best estimates of when the embryo may be able to feel pain; but such a limit would, in contrast to the 14-day limit, allow research on embryos at the stage at which some of the more specialized cells have begun to form. As we saw earlier, this research would, according to Robert Edwards, have the potential to cure such terrible diseases as sickle cell anemia and leukemia (2).

As for freezing the embryo with a view to later implantation, the question here is essentially one of risk. If freezing carries no special risk of abnormality, there seems to be nothing objectionable about it. With embryo freezing, this appears to be the case. The ethical objections some people have to freezing embryos has led to the suggestion that it would be better to freeze eggs (7); for this and other reasons there has been a considerable research effort directed at freezing eggs. Human eggs are more difficult to freeze than human embryos, and until recently it had not proved possible to freeze them in a manner which allowed fertilization after thawing. In December 1985, however, an IVF team at Flinders University, in Adelaide, South Australia, announced that it had succeeded in obtaining a pregnancy from an egg which had been frozen and thawed before being fertilized (9). The technique used involved stripping away a protective outer layer from the egg, so that it would take up a chemical which would protect it during the freezing process. This technique does overcome the ethical problems some find in freezing embryos, but it does so at the cost of introducing a new potential cause of risk to the offspring, the risk that the chemicals absorbed by the egg may have some harmful effect (10). Whether or not this risk proves to be a real one, from the point of view of ethics, one may doubt whether the risk is worth running, if the primary reason for running it is to avoid objections, which we have now seen to be ill-founded, to the freezing of embryos.

Going beyond the simple case does bring us into a more ethically controversial area, but there is no overall case against applying IVF outside the restricted ambit of the simple case. The essential point is to consider each additional step carefully before it is taken. Some steps will prove unwise, but others will be beneficial and not open to any well-grounded objections.

THE FUTURE OF THE REPRODUCTION REVOLUTION

What lies ahead? IVF has opened the door to a wide range of further possibilities. In the near future we shall have to consider which of these possibilities to pursue, and which to reject. Here are some of the possibilities:

1. A surrogate could bear a child for another couple; the child would be the genetic child of the other couple, and would be returned to the genetic parents after birth. The genetic parents might be unable to conceive in the normal way, or they might simply find the surrogate arrangement more convenient. The surrogate might be paid for her services, or—in the case of otherwise infertile couples—she may have more altruistic motives.

2. Embryos may be used in order to provide "spare parts" for people who through accident or illness need some kind of transplant. It has been suggested that embryonic tissue could restore nerve function to paraplegics. Embryos might be grown to the point at which the organs begin to form, and then the organs could be separated and grown in culture until they were large enough to be used.

3. Several embryos could be produced, and some of their genetic characteristics identified; the one considered most desirable could then be implanted, and the remainder discarded; alternatively it will eventually be possible to modify the genetic properties of an embryo so as to eliminate defects and to build in desirable genetic qualities....

The proposal that embryos be used for "spare parts" has already caused howls of protest from those who regard embryos as having the same rights as normal human beings. [This view, however,] cannot be defended by rational argument. As long as there are adequate safeguards to ensure that the embryo is at all times incapable of suffering in any way, it is difficult to find sound ethical reason against this proposal—and it is obvious that the possible benefits are considerable.

Of all the possible applications of IVF, however, it is genetic selection and genetic engineering which raise the most far-reaching questions. Should we tinker with the human genetic pool? If so, in what way? Here I will limit myself to pointing out that we already tinker with the genetic pool when we offer genetic counseling, amniocentesis, and abortion to those who are at special risk of producing genetically defective offspring. And this is nothing new, at least insofar as its impact on the genetic pool is concerned: other societies have practiced infanticide to the same end, and of course in the past, even if one tried to rear the defective child, in most cases nature used its own brutal methods to ensure that the genes were eliminated from the gene pool.

So genetic engineering differs only in its techniques from what is now going on, and has gone on for a long time. But this difference is a significant one, because the new techniques are so much more powerful, and because they would, in principle, allow us to select for desirable traits as well as to select against undesirable ones. Many fear that these techniques will place too much power in the hands of governments, who will not be able to resist the temptation of designing future generations to be docile and to vote for the governing party at every election.

The fear that genetic engineering will produce the ultimate in entrenched dictatorship is exaggerated. Most political leaders want quick results, and it would take at least 18 years for genetic engineering to have any effect at the polls. If we have succeeded in keeping our freedom in the age of television and state education, we should be able to cling to it in the age of genetic engineering as well.

But should we allow positive modifications, as distinct from the elimination of defects, at all? In time we might come to accept the desirability of positive modifications. One reason for accepting this is that, looking around us, there is reason to think that natural selection has left ample room for improvement. Another reason is that the distinction between eliminating a defect and making a positive modification is a difficult one to draw. If we learn how to eliminate a wide range of defects which predispose us to common diseases, we will have created an abnormally healthy person. If we learn how to affect intelligence, should we stop short at eliminating mental ability below the above-average range? If we

eliminate abnormally depressive personalities, would it be wrong to try to produce people who tend to be a little more cheerful than most of us are now? If we eliminate tendencies toward criminal violence, might we not build just a little more kindness into the human constitution? If the risks of such an enterprise are great, so too are the potential rewards for us all.

REFERENCES

1 Singer P, Wells D. Making babies. New York: Scribner's, 1985.
2 Edwards RG. Paper presented at the Fourth World Congress on IVF. Melbourne, Australia, Nov 22, 1985.
3 Abstract. Proceedings of the Fifth Scientific Meeting of the Fertility Society of Australia, Adelaide, Dec. 2–6, 1986.
4 Rowland R. Reproductive technologies: the final solution to the woman question? In: Arditti R, Klein RD, Minden S, eds, Test-tube women: what future for motherhood? London: Pandora, 1984.
5 Firestone S. The dialectic of sex. New York: Bantam, 1971.
6 Breeze N. Who is going to rock the petri dish? In: Arditti R, Klein RD, Minden S, eds, Test-tube women: what future for motherhood? London: Pandora, 1984.
7 Warnock M (Chairperson). Report of the Committee of Inquiry into Human Fertilisation and Embryology. London: Her Majesty's Stationery Office, 1984, p 66.
8 Waller L (Chairman). Victorian Government Committee to Consider the Social, Ethical and Legal Issues Arising from In Vitro Fertilization. Report on the disposition of embryos produced by in vitro fertilization. Melbourne: Victorian Government Printer, 1984, p 47.
9 The Australian, Dec 19, 1985.
10 Trounson A. Paper presented at the Fourth World Congress on IVF, Melbourne, Australia, Nov 22, 1985.

Feminist Ethics and In Vitro Fertilization
Susan Sherwin

Susan Sherwin is associate professor of philosophy at Dalhousie University, Halifax, Nova Scotia. She is coeditor of *Moral Problems in Medicine* (1976; 2d ed., 1983). Her published articles include "The Concept of a Person in the Context of Abortion," "A Feminist Approach to Ethics," and "Feminist Ethics and Medical Ethics: Two Different Approaches to Contextual Ethics."

Sherwin outlines the nature of feminist ethics and provides a critique of *in vitro* fertilization (IVF) within that theoretical framework. From a feminist point of view, she maintains, IVF is morally problematic for a number of closely related reasons, including the following: (1) Although the desires of infertile couples for access to IVF are understandable and worthy of sympathetic regard, such desires themselves emerge from social arrangements and cultural values that are deeply oppressive to women. (2) IVF technology gives the appearance of providing women with increased reproductive freedom but in reality threatens women with a significant decrease of reproductive freedom. Sherwin also insists that those who find themselves in moral opposition to IVF have a responsibility to support medical and social developments that would reduce the perceived need of couples for IVF.

Many authors from all traditions consider it necessary to ask why it is that some couples seek [IVF] technology so desperately. Why is it so important to so many people to produce their 'own' child? On this question, theorists in the analytic tradition seem to shift to previously rejected ground and suggest that this is a natural, or at least a proper, desire. Englehardt, for example, says, 'The use of technology in the fashioning of children is integral to the goal of rendering the world congenial to persons.'[1] Bayles more cautiously observes that 'A desire to beget for its own sake... is probably irrational'; nonetheless, he immediately concludes, 'these techniques for fulfilling that desire have been found ethically permissible.'[2] R. G. Edwards and David Sharpe state the case most strongly: 'the desire to have children must be among the most basic of human instincts, and denying it can lead to considerable psychological and social difficulties.'[3] Interestingly, although the recent pronouncement of the Catholic Church assumes that 'the desire for a child is natural,'[4] it denies that a couple has a right to a child: 'The child is not an object to which one has a right.'[5]

Reprinted with permission of the author and the publisher from *Canadian Journal of Philosophy*, Supplementary Volume 13 (1987), pp. 276–284.

Here, I believe, it becomes clear why we need a deeper sort of feminist analysis. We must look at the sort of social arrangements and cultural values that underlie the drive to assume such risks for the sake of biological parenthood. We find that the capitalism, racism, sexism, and elitism of our culture have combined to create a set of attitudes which views children as commodities whose value is derived from their possession of parental chromosomes. Children are valued as privatized commodities, reflecting the virility and heredity of their parents. They are also viewed as the responsibility of their parents and are not seen as the social treasure and burden that they are. Parents must tend their needs on pain of prosecution, and, in return, they get to keep complete control over them. Other adults are inhibited from having warm, stable interactions with the children of others—it is as suspect to try to hug and talk regularly with a child who is not one's own as it is to fondle and hang longingly about a car or a bicycle which belongs to someone else—so those who wish to know children well often find they must have their own.

Women are persuaded that their most important purpose in life is to bear and raise children; they are told repeatedly that their life is incomplete, that they are lacking in fulfillment if they do not have children. And, in fact, many women do face a barren existence without children. Few women have access to meaningful, satisfying jobs. Most do not find themselves in the centre of the romantic personal relationships which the culture pretends is the norm for heterosexual couples. And they have been socialized to be fearful of close friendships with others—they are taught to distrust other women, and to avoid the danger of friendship with men other than their husbands. Children remain the one hope for real intimacy and for the sense of accomplishment which comes from doing work one judges to be valuable.

To be sure, children can provide that sense of self worth, although for many women (and probably for all mothers at some times) motherhood is not the romanticized satisfaction they are led to expect. But there is something very wrong with a culture where childrearing is the only outlet available to most women in which to pursue fulfillment. Moreover, there is something wrong with the ownership theory of children that keeps other adults at a distance from children. There ought to be a variety of close relationships possible between children and adults so that we all recognize that we have a stake in the well-being of the young, and we all benefit from contact with their view of the world.

In such a world, it would not be necessary to spend the huge sums on designer children which IVF requires while millions of other children starve to death each year. Adults who enjoyed children could be involved in caring for them whether or not they produced them biologically. And, if the institution of marriage survives, women and men would marry because they wished to share their lives together, not because the men needed someone to produce heirs for them and women needed financial support for their children. That would be a world in which we might have reproductive freedom of choice. The world we now live in has so limited women's options and self-esteem, it is legitimate to question the freedom behind women's demand for this technology, for it may well be largely a reflection of constraining social perspectives.

Nonetheless, I must acknowledge that some couples today genuinely mourn their incapacity to produce children without IVF and there are very significant and unique joys which can be found in producing and raising one's own children which are not accessible to persons in infertile relationships. We must sympathize with these people. None of us shall live to see the implementation of the ideal cultural values outlined above which would make the demand for IVF less severe. It is with real con-

cern that some feminists suggest that the personal wishes of couples with fertility difficulties may not be compatible with the overall interests of women and children.

Feminist thought, then, helps us to focus on different dimensions of the problem then do other sorts of approaches. But, with this perspective, we still have difficulty in reaching a final conclusion on whether to encourage, tolerate, modify, or restrict this sort of reproductive technology. I suggest that we turn to the developing theories of feminist ethics for guidance in resolving this question.[6]

In my view, a feminist ethics is a moral theory that focusses on relations among persons as well as on individuals. It has as a model an inter-connected social fabric, rather than the familiar one of isolated, independent atoms; and it gives primacy to bonds among people rather than to rights to independence. It is a theory that focusses on concrete situations and persons and not on free-floating abstract actions.[7] Although many details have yet to be worked out, we can see some of its implications in particular problem areas such as this.

It is a theory that is explicitly conscious of the social, political, and economic relations that exist among persons; in particular, as a feminist theory, it attends to the implications of actions or policies on the status of women. Hence, it is necessary to ask questions from the perspective of feminist ethics in addition to those which are normally asked from the perspective of mainstream ethical theories. We must view issues such as this one in the context of the social and political realities in which they arise, and resist the attempt to evaluate actions or practices in isolation (as traditional responses in biomedical ethics often do). Thus, we cannot just address the question of IVF per se without asking how IVF contributes to general patterns of women's oppression. As Kathryn Pyne Addelson has argued about abortion,[8] a feminist perspective raises questions that are inadmissable within the traditional ethical frameworks, and yet, for women in a patriarchal society, they are value questions of greater urgency. In particular, a feminist ethics, in contrast to other approaches in biomedical ethics, would take seriously the concerns just reviewed which are part of the debate in the feminist literature.

A feminist ethics would also include components of theories that have been developed as 'feminine ethics,' as sketched out by the empirical work of Carol Gilligan.[9] (The best example of such a theory is the work of Nel Noddings in her influential book *Caring*.)[10] In other words, it would be a theory that gives primacy to inter-personal relationships and woman-centered values such as nurturing, empathy, and co-operation. Hence, in the case of IVF, we must care for the women and men who are so despairing about their infertility as to want to spend the vast sums and risk the associated physical and emotional costs of the treatment, in pursuit of 'their own children.' That is, we should, in Noddings' terms, see their reality as our own and address their very real sense of loss. In so doing, however, we must also consider the implications of this sort of solution to their difficulty. While meeting the perceived desires of some women—desires which are problematic in themselves, since they are so compatible with the values of a culture deeply op-pressive to women—this technology threatens to further entrench those values which are responsible for that op-pression. A larger vision suggests that the technology of-fered may, in reality, reduce women's freedom and, if so, it should be avoided.

A feminist ethics will not support a wholly negative response, however, for that would not address our obli-gation to care for those suffering from infertility; it is the responsibility of those who oppose further implementa-tion of this technology to work towards the changes in the social arrangements that will lead to a reduction of the sense of need for this sort of solution. On the medi-cal front, research and treatment ought to be stepped up to reduce the rates of peral sepsis and gonorrhea which often result in tubal blockage, more attention should be directed at the causes and possible cures for male infer-tility, and we should pursue techniques that will permit safe reversible sterilization providing women with better alternatives to tubal ligation as a means of fertility con-trol; these sorts of technology would increase the control of many women over their own fertility and would be compatible with feminist objectives. On the social front, we must continue the social pressure to change the status of women and children in our society from that of breeder and possession respectively; hence, we must de-velop a vision of society as community where all partic-ipants are valued members, regardless of age or gender. And we must challenge the notion that having one's wife produce a child with his own genes is sufficient cause for the wives of men with low sperm counts to be expected to undergo the physical and emotional assault such tech-nology involves.

Further, a feminist ethics will attend to the nature of the relationships among those concerned. Annette Baier has eloquently argued for the importance of devel-oping an ethics of trust,[11] and I believe a feminist ethics

must address the question of the degree of trust appro-priate to the relationships involved. Feminists have noted that women have little reason to trust the medical specialists who offer to respond to their reproductive de-sires, for, commonly women's interests have not come first from the medical point of view.[12] In fact, it is accu-rate to perceive feminist attacks on reproductive technol-ogy as expressions of the lack of trust feminists have in those who control the technology. Few feminists object to reproductive technology per se; rather they express concern about who controls it and how it can be used to further exploit women. The problem with reproductive technology is that it concentrates power in reproductive matters in the hands of those who are not directly in-volved in the actual bearing and rearing of the child; i.e., in men who relate to their clients in a technical, profes-sional, authoritarian manner. It is a further step in the medicalization of pregnancy and birth which, in North America, is marked by relationships between pregnant women and their doctors which are very different from the traditional relationships between pregnant women and midwives. The latter relationships fostered an atmo-sphere of mutual trust which is impossible to replicate in hospital deliveries today. In fact, current approaches to pregnancy, labour, and birth tend to view the mother as a threat to the fetus who must be coerced to comply with medical procedures designed to ensure delivery of healthy babies at whatever cost necessary to the mother. Frequently, the fetus-mother relationship is medically characterized as adversarial and the physicians choose to foster a sense of alienation and passivity in the role they permit the mother. However well IVF may serve the in-terests of the few women with access to it, it more clearly serves the interests (be they commercial, professional, scholarly, or purely patriarchal) of those who control it.

Questions such as these are a puzzle to those en-gaged in the traditional approaches to ethics, for they al-ways urge us to separate the question of evaluating the morality of various forms of reproductive technology in themselves, from questions about particular uses of that technology. From the perspective of a feminist ethics, however, no such distinction can be meaningfully made. Reproductive technology is not an abstract activity, it is an activity done in particular contexts and it is those con-texts which must be addressed.

Feminist concerns [make] clear the difficulties we have with some of our traditional ethical concepts; hence, feminist ethics directs us to rethink our basic eth-ical notions. Autonomy, or freedom of choice, is not a matter to be determined in isolated instances, as is commonly assumed in many approaches to applied ethics. Rather it is a matter that involves reflection on one's whole life situation. The freedom of choice feminists appeal to in the abortion situation is freedom to define one's status as childbearer, given the social, economic, and political significance of reproduction for women. A feminist perspective permits us to understand that reproductive freedom includes control of one's sexuality, protection against coerced sterilization (or iatrogenic sterilization, e.g. as caused by the Dalkon Shield), and the existence of a social and economic network of support for the children we may choose to bear. It is the freedom to redefine our roles in society according to our concerns and needs as women.

In contrast, the consumer freedom to purchase technology, allowed only to a few couples of the privileged classes (in traditionally approved relationships), seems to entrench further the patriarchal notions of woman's role as childbearer and of heterosexual monogamy as the only acceptable intimate relationship. In other words, this sort of choice does not seem to foster autonomy for women on the broad scale. IVF is a practice which seems to reinforce sexist, classist, and often racist assumptions of our culture; therefore, on our revised understanding of freedom, the contribution of this technology to the general autonomy of women is largely negative.

We can now see the advantage of a feminist ethics over mainstream ethical theories, for a feminist analysis explicitly accepts the need for a political component to our understanding of ethical issues. In this, it differs from traditional ethical theories and it also differs from a simply feminine ethics approach, such as the one Noddings offers, for Noddings seems to rely on individual relations exclusively and is deeply suspicious of political alliances as potential threats to the pure relation of caring. Yet, a full understanding of both the threat of IVF, and the alternative action necessary should we decide to reject IVF, is possible only if it includes a political dimension reflecting on the role of women in society.

From the point of view of feminist ethics, the primary question to consider is whether this and other forms of reproductive technology threaten to reinforce the lack of autonomy which women now experience in our culture—even as they appear, in the short run, to be increasing freedom. We must recognize that the interconnections among the social forces oppressive to women underlie feminists' mistrust of this technology which advertises itself as increasing women's autonomy.[13]

The political perspective which directs us to look at how this technology fits in with general patterns of treatment for women is not readily accessible to traditional moral theories, for it involves categories of concern not accounted for in those theories—e.g. the complexity of issues which makes it inappropriate to study them in isolation from one another, the role of oppression in shaping individual desires, and potential differences in moral status which are connected with differences in treatment.

It is the set of connections constituting women's continued oppression in our society which inspires feminists to resurrect the old slippery slope arguments to warn against IVF. We must recognize that women's existing lack of control in reproductive matters begins the debate on a pretty steep incline. Technology with the potential to further remove control of reproduction from women makes the slope very slippery indeed. This new technology, though offered under the guise of increasing reproductive freedom, threatens to result, in fact, in a significant decrease in freedom, especially since it is a technology that will always include the active involvement of designated specialists and will not ever be a private matter for the couple or women concerned.

Ethics ought not to direct us to evaluate individual cases without also looking at the implications of our decisions from a wide perspective. My argument is that a theory of feminist ethics provides that wider perspective, for its different sort of methodology is sensitive to both the personal and the social dimensions of issues. For that reason, I believe it is the only ethical perspective suitable for evaluating issues of this sort.

NOTES

1 H. Tristram Englehardt, *The Foundations of Bioethics* (Oxford: Oxford University Press 1986), 239

2 Michael Bayles, *Reproductive Ethics* (Englewood Cliffs, NJ: Prentice-Hall 1984) 31

3 Robert G. Edwards and David J. Sharpe, 'Social Values and Research in Human Embryology,' *Nature* 231 (May 14, 1971), 87

4 Joseph Card Ratzinger and Alberto Bovone, 'Instruction on Respect for Human Life in its Origin and on the Dignity of Procreation: Replies to Certain Questions of the Day' (Vatican City: Vatican Polyglot Press 1987), 33

5 Ibid., 34

6 Many authors are now working on an understanding of what feminist ethics entail. Among the Canadian papers I am familiar with, are Kathryn Morgan's 'Women and Moral Madness,' Sheila Mullett's 'Only Connect: The Place of Self-Knowledge in Ethics,' both in this volume, and Leslie Wilson's 'Is a Feminine Ethics Enough?' *Atlantis* (forthcoming).

7 Susan Sherwin, 'A Feminist Approach to Ethics,' *Dalhousie Review* 64, 4 (Winter 1984–85) 704–13

8 Kathryn Pyne Addelson, 'Moral Revolution,' in Marilyn Pearsall, ed., *Women and Values* (Belmont, CA: Wadsworth 1986), 291–309

9 Carol Gilligan, *In a Different Voice* (Cambridge, MA: Harvard University Press 1982)

10 Nel Noddings, *Caring* (Berkeley: University of California Press 1984)

11 Annette Baier, 'What Do Women Want in a Moral Theory?' *Nous* 19 (March 1985) 53–64, and 'Trust and Antitrust,' *Ethics* 96 (January 1986) 231–60

12 Linda Williams presents this position particularly clearly in her invaluable work 'But What Will They Mean for Women? Feminist Concerns about the New Reproductive Technologies,' No. 6 in the *Feminist Perspective* Series, CRIAW.

13 Marilyn Frye vividly describes the phenomenon of inter-relatedness which supports sexist oppression by appeal to the metaphor of a bird cage composed of thin wires, each relatively harmless in itself, but, collectively, the wires constitute an overwhelming barrier to the inhabitant of the cage. Marilyn Frye, *The Politics of Reality: Essays in Feminist Theory* (Trumansburg, NY: The Crossing Press 1983), 4–7

Ethical Aspects of Surrogate Embryo Transfer
LeRoy Walters

A biographical sketch of LeRoy Walters is found on page 162.

The first human births resulting from surrogate embryo transfer (SET), following both *in vitro* and *in vivo* fertilization, occurred in late 1983 and early 1984, respectively. As these achievements were unfolding, Walters wrote this essay, in which he proposes a framework for ethical assessment. Mindful of the great value of anti-infertility techniques for those who suffer from involuntary infertility, he endorses the use of such a technique "provided that its benefits are not outweighed by safety considerations and social consequences." In accordance with this underlying framework of evaluation, Walters then provides an initial analysis of the safety considerations and social consequences relevant to the employment of SET.

The article by Hodgen published in this issue of *The Journal* [JAMA, Oct. 28, 1983, 2167–2171] suggests that some infertile women who cannot produce fertilizable ova may one day be able to bear children. Such women may have ovaries that are functionally deficient in a critical respect, or they may lack ovaries entirely. For these women, bearing a child that is genetically "their own" is a physical impossibility.

Any new technique that helps to reduce involuntary infertility is to be welcomed, provided that its benefits are not outweighed by safety considerations and social consequences. The present moment, when surrogate embryo transfer (SET) is being tested in primates and initially attempted in humans[1-3] seems the appropriate time to inventory the ethical issues that the clinical use of this new technique may raise.

Safety considerations in SET and accompanying techniques concern three biologic individuals—the oocyte or embryo donor, the embryo itself, and the embryo recipient. The risk factors vary somewhat, depending on whether SET is employed in conjunction with in vitro or in vivo fertilization. With SET after in vitro fertilization, the physical risks of the procedures to embryo and recipient are for the most part comparable with the risks of in vitro fertilization and embryo transfer without donation. Surrogate embryo transfer after in vivo fertilization may involve less risk to the early embryo than in vitro fertilization and embryo transfer, with or without donation, because the in vivo technique substantially reduces the time during which the early embryo is exposed to an artificial, extrauterine environment. Conversely, with SET after in vivo fertilization, the embryo recipient may be at slightly greater risk of acquiring an infection from the donor via the transfer procedure.

The physical risk differential is most striking in the case of the donor. An oocyte donor must undergo inhalation or conduction anesthesia during the oocyte recovery process. Therefore, it seems unlikely that most women would volunteer to undergo oocyte recovery merely for donation purposes, except under extraordinary circumstances. Much more likely is the scenario in which an oocyte has already been harvested for the woman's own in vitro fertilization and is not needed, thereby becoming available for donation. In contrast, with SET after in vivo fertilization, the physical risks to the donor—in this case, an *embryo* donor—are greatly reduced, but some hazards remain. Most important are the potential risks of uterine lavage—and, in the future, of possible superovulation—to the embryo donor. In veterinary medicine similar nonsurgical techniques have been employed successfully to recover bovine and equine embryos without apparent ill effect, although the non-human donors are either anesthesized or sedated.[4,5] Hodgen does note that an ectopic pregnancy occurred in one of the female monkey donors and suggests that the tubal pregnancy may have been an unintended result of retrograde uterine lavage. Hodgen's recommendation that human embryo donors be carefully monitored for possible ectopic pregnancy seems eminently reasonable. A further possibility is that a normal uterine pregnancy may ensue if the lavage procedure fails to retrieve all embryos from the donor's uterus. The embryo donor would then confront a decision about the continuation of an unexpected pregnancy.

The social consequences of a new biomedical technique cannot be predicted in great detail or with total accuracy. However, at least three general arenas of potential social impact for SET can be identified: (1) the family unit, (2) the medical care provision system, and (3) the commercial sphere. Surrogate embryo transfer necessarily involves the introduction of a third party into the relationship between a man and a woman, who will

usually be husband and wife. If the woman cannot produce fertilizable ova and if the couple wishes to bear and/or raise children, the members of the couple have no alternative but to select some kind of adoptive procedure. Their three primary options are the adoption of an already born child who is not genetically related to them, the employment of a surrogate mother who would perhaps be inseminated with the husband's sperm, or SET. Of these alternatives, SET most closely approximates the usual process of human reproduction. Both members of the couple are directly involved in the pregnancy, the man through providing semen and the woman through carrying the pregnancy to term and giving birth to the child. In addition, with SET the couple, particularly the woman, has greater control over the physiological environment of the developing fetus and embryo than in either postnatal adoption or surrogate-motherhood arrangements. The embryo recipient herself can determine what work schedule to follow, how much to rest, what foods and drugs to ingest, and whether to smoke cigarettes or drink alcoholic beverages.

Because the embryo or oocyte donor's involvement in SET is temporally limited, preimplantation adoption through SET will quite probably involve fewer psychological and legal complications than surrogate motherhood and subsequent adoption.[6,7] However, as in the case of surrogate motherhood, the adopting parents know little about the overall health status of the adopted embryo and child to be—far less than parents adopting a newborn infant know. If, after SET, an adopted embryo is delivered as a handicapped newborn, the adopting parents may tend to blame the donor for the infant's defects or even to reject the child. The recent controversy surrounding a handicapped child born to a surrogate mother in Michigan indicates that these possibilities are not merely theoretical (*The New York Times*, Jan. 23, 1983, p. 19).

Even if the neonate born after SET is normal, the adopting family and the health professionals involved will face several generic questions of disclosure and confidentiality that are similar to those raised by artificial insemination by donor and more traditional modes of adoption. For example, will the identity of the donor female be disclosed to the recipient couple, or vice versa? And will the resulting child be told that he or she was adopted before implantation? If so, will the child perhaps be interested in learning more about his or her biologic roots?

In short, preimplantation adoption through SET should be less disruptive to the family unit than surrogate-motherhood arrangements. The impact of

SET on the adopting family will probably be comparable with that of artificial insemination by donor or postnatal adoption; it may in fact be less because SET allows both members of the adopting couple to be biologically involved in either the initiation or sustenance of the pregnancy.

The possible impact of SET on the medical care provision system is more difficult to anticipate. A major concern is that SET may join in vitro fertilization as a high-technology anti-infertility technique available only to those able to afford a major expense. Private health insurers have been notably cautious in reimbursing the costs of in vitro fertilization, and state and federal medical assistance programs have made infertility treatment a low or nonexistent priority. According to a recent study published by the National Center for Health Statistics, there are 4.3 million currently married women in the United States aged 15 to 44 years who experience impaired fecundity. Of these, 47.3%, or more than 2 million women, want to bear a first child (840,000), a second child (641,000), or an additional child (556,000) but are prevented by infertility problems from doing so.[8] This situation requires both a national recognition of the devastating impact that involuntary infertility can have on the lives of the couples involved and a public policy on infertility treatment that is more in accord with that recognition.

A final potential social impact of SET is commercial and should be considered merely speculative. If semen donors are paid for their "donations," it is at least conceivable that oocyte or embryo donors, who undergo greater risk, will request equal treatment. Therefore, a group of professional donors could develop among women to parallel the already existing group of professional semen donors among men. Moreover, commercial oocyte or embryo banks (analogous to existing commercial sperm banks) could employ cryopreservation techniques like those recently reported from Australia (*Washington Post*, May 3, 1983, p. A14) to store donated oocytes or embryos until appropriate recipients are found.

The introduction of a commercial dimension into the transfer of human blood, germ cells, or organs between people has occasioned vigorous debate.[9-11] Strenuous opposition would be likely to greet any proposal to establish a commercial human-embryo bank on the ground that the sale of human embryos for adoption is more like the (prohibited) sale of infants for adoption than the (permitted) selling of human semen or blood.

At the very least, society may want to require that all prospective germ-cell or embryo donors receive careful screening, including karyotyping and pedigree analysis.

In summary, SET may provide a means for overcoming the involuntary infertility of a new group of patients. The safety of the technique for oocyte or embryo donors should be closely monitored, and its potential social impact on the family unit, the medical care provision system, and the commercial sphere should—even at this early stage of human application—be carefully assessed.

NOTES

1 Buster, J. E., Bustillo, M., Thornycroft, I., et al.: Non-surgical transfer of an in-vivo fertilised donated ovum to an infertility patient. *Lancet* 1983; 1:816–817.

2 Trounson, A., Leeton, J., Besanko, M., et al.: Pregnancy established in an infertile patient after transfer of a donated embryo fertilised in vitro. *Br Med J* 1983; 286:835–838.

3 Steptoe, P., Edwards, R. G., Trounson, A., et al.: Pregnancy in an infertile patient after transfer of an embryo fertilised in vitro. *Br Med J* 1983; 286:1351–1352.

4 Rowe, R. F., Del Campo, M. R., Critser, M. S., et al.: Embryo transfer in cattle: Nonsurgical collection techniques. *Am J Vet Res* 1980; 41:106–108.

5 Imel, K. J., Squires, E. L., Elsden, R. P., et al.: Collection and transfer of equine embryos. *J Am Vet Med Assoc* 1981; 179:987–991.

6 Ethical issues in surrogate motherhood. *ACOG Newsletter* 1983; 27:3, 11–12.

7 Parker, P. J.: Motivation of surrogate mothers: Initial findings. *Am J Psychiatry* 1983; 140:117–118.

8 Mosher, W. D., Pratt, W. F.: Reproductive impairments among married couples: United States, *Vital and Health Statistics*, series 23, data from the national survey of family growth; No. 11. National Center for Health Statistics, December 1982, pp. 13, 32.

9 Titmuss, R.: *The Gift Relationship: From Human Blood to Social Policy*. New York, Pantheon Books Inc., 1971.

10 Arrow, K. J.: Gifts and exchanges. *Philosophy Public Affairs* 1972; 1:343–362.

11 Curie-Cohen, M., Luttrell, L., Shapiro, S.: Current practice of artificial insemination by donor in the United States. *N Engl J Med* 1979; 300:585–590.

Genetic Engineering

Genetic Manipulation with Human Beings
H. J. J. Leenen

H. J. J. Leenen is professor of social medicine and health law, University of Amsterdam, The Netherlands. His published articles include "The Definition of Euthanasia," "Patient's Rights in Europe," and "Selection of Patients: an Insoluble Dilemma."

Leenen distinguishes between therapeutic and nontherapeutic genetic engineering. He endorses the employment of therapeutic genetic manipulation, both in the case of somatic-cell therapy and in the case of germ-line therapy, but he rejects the employment of nontherapeutic genetic engineering, whether it be "eugenic" or "enhancement" in its orientation. In Leenen's view, nontherapeutic genetic engineering is both dangerous and unfair to future generations.

The science of genetics is developing very rapidly. For a long time it has been possible to examine people's genetic constitution and to give genetic counselling. Everybody wants healthy offspring, and if they are at risk for having children with a congenital disease, people want to know this so they can decide whether or not to have children. Recent developments in medical science have made prenatal diagnosis possible. This new development can lead parents to decide on abortion of a defective fetus. In the 1970s a kind of revolution took place in genetics. In particular, the invention of DNA recombination caused a lot of confusion and fear among the lay public. This resulted in a unique phenomenon, viz. a self-imposed moratorium on DNA recombination in 1972. Uncertainties and unknown risks made the scientific community decide to stop all experiments. This moratorium was lifted after risk assessment and the introduction of safety measures. The continuation of DNA and other genetic research did not put an end to the debate on the ethical and legal aspects of genetic manipulation with human cells [1].

This ethical and legal debate pertains not only to the permissibility of genetic research and its risks, but also to the applications in human beings. Although the boundaries between experimentation and application are not always very clear, the main issue is whether manipulation with human cells, and especially germ line cells, should be allowed. Like many new scientific developments, genetics has a positive and a negative side. The risks are evident, but at the same time genetics can con-

tribute to the solution of human and social problems. The weight attached to each of the different aspects in the ethical and legal discussion largely determines the course it takes. At the beginning of any such discussion the negative aspects are often overstressed and fear of the unknown prevails. It takes some time to balance the various aspects of a problem. Questions as to the permissibility of genetic manipulation that will affect future generations are of a special kind. Does the living generation have duties to future generations, and is it entitled to make decisions about these future generations?

The ethical debate on this problem is in danger of becoming too absolute. The evolution of mankind consists of a series of human decisions about the generations to come. The more modern science succeeds in strengthening its grip on nature, the more mankind will take its future in its own hands. Consequently, human responsibility for its own future has increased and become more complex. That is one of the reasons why the role of ethics and law has grown. Increasing responsibility requires increasingly explicit values and standards. Moreover, the human race has always genetically influenced its own development, for example by the choice of partners in procreation and by laws on consanguinity. But other factors, such as the treatment of diseases, abortion, and artificial insemination by donors have also influenced the development of the human race. We have always made decisions that will affect future generations; other means of influencing the human race are education and the social development of society. It is evident that human evolution is affected not only by biological factors, but also by the social and physical environment. Human body length, for instance, depends not only on genetic condi-

Reprinted with permission from *Medicine and Law*, vol. 7 (1988), pp. 73–79. © Springer-Verlag 1988.

tions but also on nutritional and economic status. Physical environmental factors leave their imprint on human development. Some can even endanger heredity (e.g. radiation). So, at first sight, it is not clear why experimentation with and application of genetic techniques should not be allowed. Moreover, genetic manipulation may result in curing diseases of a genetic nature, which has never been possible by human intervention. This constitutes a strong argument in favor of genetic engineering with human cells.

The formulation of standards for genetic manipulation involves a great many problems. The main problem is that modern genetic research is still in the early stages. Therefore, little can be said about the development of future research and of the possible applications of its results on human beings. As a consequence it must be expected that norms drawn up today will need readjustment in the future. Callahan [2] proposed the introduction of the "imagination principle" in ethics. Some problems may be foreseen by extrapolation of what is known today, but the future can be imagined only to a limited extent. Evaluation of the development of science in the last 50 years reveals that many new inventions had never been envisioned and were the result of an accumulation of knowledge or of unexpected discoveries. It must be assumed that science will take unexpected directions and that new inventions will be made. So it can be taken for granted that ethics and health law will be confronted with new challenges.

In my opinion, one overriding standard is that the science of genetics with human cells has to remain within human boundaries. This is indeed a very general guideline. But nevertheless, it follows from this that the creation of animal-human creatures and of plant-human combinations is inadmissible. This is not to say that the same holds for hybrids, which cannot develop. When scientists transgress the boundaries of what is human, they place themselves outside human society.

This immediately raises the question of the meaning of the notion "human." This debate has been going on as long as humankind has existed and will probably go on forever. Interpretation of the word human has changed over time. Slavery was accepted earlier, but it is now considered unethical and illegal, and certain ways of treating people which were considered acceptable in the Middle Ages are now regarded as torture. But although the interpretation of the term has changed and will change again, nowadays there is largely consensus about it. This is reflected, for instance, in the formulation of human rights and the continual elaboration of the matters covered by these. It is to be expected that as science develops and human responsibility grows, this elaboration will go on and new human rights will be established.

Genetic experimentation and the application of its results to human beings have been discussed intensively in the last decade. As a result of this discussion some values and standards have been agreed upon. For the ethical and legal assessment several types of genetic manipulation have to be distinguished. The main distinction is the one between therapeutic and non-therapeutic genetic engineering. The therapeutic group contains somatic cell therapy and germ line gene therapy. Somatic cell therapy aims at correcting genetic defects in patients' somatic cells. Such corrections are restricted to the patients who are treated and are not transferred to their offspring. This is not true of germ line gene therapy: the insertion of a gene in a germ line cell to correct a disorder would result in correction of the disorder in the offspring too. Anderson [3] has suggested a subdivision of non-therapeutic genetic engineering into eugenic and enhancement genetic engineering, the second of which would involve insertion of a gene in an attempt to enhance a known characteristic; for instance an additional growth hormone gene might be placed into a normal child. Eugenic genetic engineering attempts to alter or improve complex human traits, each of which is coded by a large number of genes, e.g. personality, intelligence, character, formation of body organs.

THERAPEUTIC MANIPULATION

With reference to therapeutic genetic engineering, I am of the opinion that it is ethically and legally admissible. Curing a disease by gene therapy on somatic cells is ethically and legally no different from other types of therapy. Why should medication, surgery and invasive medical interventions be allowed and genetic therapy not? Some argue that gene therapy should only be applied in severe disorders and when conventional therapy would not suffice. I do not see the relevance of these limitations. Why not use the most effective treatment? Professional standards should determine which therapy is best. Of course, all requirements of that standard have to be met. As long as the gene therapy is in an experimental stage, experiments have to be carried out under the regulations concerning experiments on human beings. This implies, among other things, that previous research and experiments on animals must have revealed how a gene can be directed towards the cells causing the disorder, what risks are involved, and what effects insertion of the gene will have. The experiments have to be approved by an ethical committee, and the rules on patient's rights, e.g. informed consent, must be obeyed.

The same holds for germ line therapy. However, some are of the opinion that, because germ line cells are transferred to the offspring, different standards apply. It must be admitted that somatic cell genetic therapy concerns only the individual treated and is therefore a matter of personal self-determination whilst germ line therapy involves decisions affecting self-determination of any future offspring. But on the other hand, parents often take decisions about their children's health, and about that of fetuses in the case of treatment during pregnancy. And in the situation where the child has not yet been born and is therefore not able to make a decision about germ line therapy why not assume that future offspring will agree with elimination of a disease? There is no basis for the assumption that offspring want to be born ill. The fact that only the living can decide on germ line gene therapy supports the conclusion that it is justifiable to expect that future children would wish for germ line therapy. It is reasonable to recognize the responsibility a present generation has towards a future one for eliminating disease by germ line genetic therapy.

Does this imply that every decision comes under this responsibility? It could be argued that because of the difference between somatic cell therapy and germ line therapy, the restriction to severe genetic disorders for which no sufficient conventional therapy is available, which was rejected for somatic cell therapy, should apply in the case of germ line therapy. In this context, the arguments for such a restriction carry more weight because the intervention affects others. But at the same time, when therapy is at stake, why should prevention of a disease and of suffering that would be caused to the offspring by conventional treatment be rated lower than transmission of the disease followed by administration of a conventional treatment?

As to experiments on human beings, germ line therapy involves particular problems. Such experiments are difficult to assess, because the effects must be studied over several generations. It is arguable whether the results of animal experiments apply to human generation studies. Moreover, the same questions arise as have been discussed with reference to somatic cell therapy, i.e. how to direct the genes towards the cells that have to be cured, what the effects of the gene insertion will be, and what risks are involved. Experimental germ line therapy should also be carried out with strict adherence to the regulations for experiments on human beings.

NON-THERAPEUTIC ENGINEERING

What holds for therapeutic interventions does not hold for non-therapeutic genetic engineering. There is a solid ethical and legal basis for therapeutic measures, and even for assumptions about the wishes of a future generation. The elimination of suffering and disease justifies decision-making on its behalf. The situation is different in the case of enhancement and eugenic genetic engineering, where decisions made by the living on the basis of their values and standards fundamentally affect self-determination of the offspring. A firm ethical basis, with which future generations may be assumed to agree, is lacking for enhancement and eugenic procedures. At this point we enter fully into the discussion about what constitutes a human being. Because we know that our views on the definition of human have been developed over time and that this development will go on in the future, the present generation should avoid using genetic engineering to impose its own ideas about personality, intelligence, character traits, talents and the like on future generations. It may be argued that education has a similar effect, but reality shows that unlike genetic engineering, education leaves a considerable amount of freedom for decisions to be made on the basis of values that differ from those of parents and teachers. Such freedom does not exist when traits and talents are built into the reproductive cells. In the last case influences other than genetically determined ones will also play a role, and individuals who are identically programmed genetically will develop differently because of differences in time and environment and differences resulting from their own decisions, but this does not alter the determination of genetically built-in traits and talents in the development of the human being. Moreover, especially with eugenics it will be difficult, and perhaps even impossible, to reverse the effects. Enhancement genetic engineering and eugenics relieve future generations of a responsibility to which they are entitled in the evolution of humankind according to the succession of generations. We must not go gene-shopping for future generations. We could even limit and endanger the development of the human race, because the long-term consequences of our biological decisions are by definition out of our reach and we would cut off possibilities which are essential for future generations to survive.

Prohibition of non-therapeutic genetic engineering does not put an end to ethical and other problems. One of the first problems concerns equality. People are very unequal as a result of the natural lottery, and by heredity some are genetically more gifted than others. The more gifted have better chances in life. If we can do something to upgrade the possibilities for the less well off, why should they be denied this? But apart from the argument that society needs diversity, the risks of enhancement genetic engineering and eugenetics are evident. In weighing duties in this respect, equity in the distribution of social goods and social justice must prevail over genetic engineering. A second problem pertains to enhancement genetic engineering. It may be debatable in certain cases whether enhancement engineering would be therapeutic or not. This discussion is analogous to the debate on the nature of plastic surgery for improvement of the human figure or traits. Some, for instance, will describe plastic surgery on the female breast because the appearance of the patient's bosom distresses her and administration of growth hormone to a normal child who is unusually small, as forms of therapy. Others refute this view, as I am inclined myself. It would make the borderline between therapeutic and other types of genetic engineering very unclear. We might point out that some people undoubtedly suffer because they have no musical talent. The labelling of types of enhancement as therapy would actually obliterate the borderline between gene therapy versus enhancement and eugenic engineering and between curing a disease and improving a normal, healthy person.

Anderson [3] is of the opinion that enhancement genetic engineering could be justified on the grounds of preventive medicine. An example is the insertion of genes which would lower the cholesterol level and consequently decrease the risk of heart attacks. It cannot be denied that this would not be the same as curing a disease or a therapy, but there is some similarity with therapy, because the procedure would aim at the elimination of a known risk factor for a disease. But as discussed above, if we crossed the borderline to non-therapeutic genetic engineering we should have a lot of problems. From prevention as a general notion to eugenics is only a small step. Then why not prevent socially less well accepted traits? Perhaps a differentiation between prevention and the elimination of obvious risk factors should be considered. The discussion on prevention and enhancement genetic engineering has not yet come to an end.

SOCIETAL ASPECTS

Another important issue in ethics and health law concerning genetic engineering is the problem of societal responsibility versus individual self-determination and personal decisions about one's own offspring. For the purposes of this discussion it has to be stressed that genetic engineering of all four types is a public matter. The public has to be informed about what is going on and what the ethical and legal issues are. Genetic engineering is open to misunderstanding and can evoke public fear. Information will help people to see facts as they really are. The rejection of certain types of genetic engineering, i.e., enhancement and eugenics, also has to be publicly discussed. The same is true for germ line genetic therapy.

The danger of infringements of self-determination and individual freedom results partly from the development of genetic therapy as a rather economical method of eliminating diseases. Society could then exercise pressure on the individual to undergo such a treatment, to avoid incurring the costs that go with other forms of cure and care. Insurance companies and social security institutions could increase this pressure by paying only for the genetic treatment. Even the government could become involved in this process. In the case of germ line therapy, this encroachment on individual self-determination could become even more pronounced. The prevention of the birth of any children with severe disorders could develop into an argument for interfering with the freedom of choice in whether or not to have children. In this case fundamental values and legal principles would be at stake. In a situation where gene therapy led to social or even legal pressure on people and deprived them of the right to make their own decisions about medical treatment and procreation, the advantages of gene therapy would eventually result in a severe loss of human values and freedom.

REFERENCES

1 President's Commission for the Study of Ethical Problems in Medicine and Biomedical and Behavioral Research (1982) Splicing life: a report on the social and ethical issues of genetic engineering with human beings. U.S. Government Printing Office, Washington DC

2 Callahan D (1976) Ethical responsibility in science in the face of uncertain consequences. Ann NY Acad Sci 265:1–10

3 Anderson W (1985) Human gene therapy: scientific and ethical considerations. J Med Phil 3:275–291

ANNOTATED BIBLIOGRAPHY: CHAPTER 9

Bayles, Michael D.: *Reproductive Ethics* (Englewood Cliffs, N.J.: Prentice-Hall, 1984). Chapter 1 of this book includes sections on AID, surrogate motherhood, and IVF. Chapter 2 includes sections on sex preselection, carrier screening, and prenatal diagnosis.

Boone, C. Keith: "Bad Axioms in Genetic Engineering," *Hastings Center Report* 18 (August/ September 1988), pp. 9–13. Boone warns against reliance on simplistic axioms (e.g., we must not "play God" or "interfere with nature") in making ethical judgments in the area of genetic engineering. He emphasizes the need for balanced judgment and attempts to identify in the case of each simplistic axiom a partial truth wrongly represented as the whole truth.

Chadwick, Ruth F.: "Cloning," *Philosophy* 57 (April 1982), pp. 201–210. Chadwick contends, on utilitarian grounds, that cloning could be morally justified in some circumstances.

Glover, Jonathan: *What Sort of People Should There Be?* (New York: Penguin Books, 1984). Part One of this book (pp. 23–56) deals with genetic engineering. Glover argues in defense of using genetic engineering to enhance desirable human characteristics.

Holmes, Helen Bequaert: "In Vitro Fertilization: Reflections on the State of the Art," *Birth* 15 (September 1988), pp. 134–145. Holmes provides an account of the various steps in the current clinical practice of IVF and embryo transfer. She calls attention to a wide array of risks, clinical problems, and ethical issues.

———— et al., eds.: *The Custom-Made Child? Women-Centered Perspectives* (Clifton, N.J.: Humana, 1981). The material in this volume derives from a 1979 conference. There are subsections on prenatal diagnosis, sex preselection, and "manipulative reproductive technologies."

Hull, Richard T., ed.: *Ethical Issues in the New Reproductive Technologies* (Belmont, Calif.: Wadsworth, 1990). This anthology provides useful material on artificial insemination, IVF, and surrogate motherhood.

Humber, James M., and Robert F. Almeder, eds.: *Biomedical Ethics Reviews 1983* (Clifton, N.J.: Humana, 1983). Section II of this book (pp. 45–90) contains two long articles on surrogate motherhood. In "Surrogate Gestation: Law and Morality," Theodore M. Benditt concludes that "there is not much of a legal case or moral case" against surrogate gestation. In an exploratory essay, "Surrogate Motherhood: The Ethical Implications," Lisa H. Newton identifies and discusses five areas of moral concern.

Kass, Leon R.: "New Beginning in Life." In Michael Hamilton, ed., *The New Genetics and the Future of Man* (Grand Rapids, Mich.: Eerdmans, 1972), pp. 15–63. Kass raises a number of ethical objections to both IVF and cloning. His principal objections to such reproductive technologies are that (1) the experiments necessary for their development cannot be done in an ethically acceptable way, (2) they are prone to misuse, (3) their acceptance will lead to the acceptance of other undesirable developments, and (4) their employment amounts to "voluntary dehumanization," through the depersonalization of procreation. In addition, against cloning he emphasizes problems of identity and individuality. A largely parallel article by Kass is called "Making Babies: The New Biology and the 'Old' Morality," *The Public Interest* 26 (Winter 1972), pp. 18–56.

Law, Medicine & Health Care 16 (Spring/Summer 1988). This special issue is entirely dedicated to surrogate motherhood. Articles are organized under the headings of (1) civil liberties, (2) ethics, and (3) women's autonomy. Material is also provided on the case of Baby M.

McCormick, Richard A.: "Reproductive Technologies: Ethical Issues," *Encyclopedia of Bioethics* (1978), vol. 4, pp. 1454–1464. McCormick reviews the ethical issues associated with artificial insemination, IVF, and cloning. In an extensive discussion of artificial insemination, he makes clear the views of various religious ethicists.

Overall, Christine: *Ethics and Human Reproduction: A Feminist Analysis* (Boston: Allen & Unwin, 1987). Overall embraces a feminist perspective on reproductive ethics and contrasts a feminist approach with nonfeminist and antifeminist approaches. Chapter 2 deals with sex preselection, Chapter 6 deals with surrogate motherhood, and Chapter 7 deals with artificial reproduction.

President's Commission for the Study of Ethical Problems in Medicine and Biomedical and Behavioral Research: *Screening and Counseling for Genetic Conditions* (1983). In this report, the commission provides a helpful review of "the evolution and status of genetic services," then considers "ethical and legal implications." Explicit conclusions and recommendations are also announced.

————: *Splicing Life: The Social and Ethical Issues of Genetic Engineering with Human Beings* (1982). This report presents useful factual material and offers an overall social and ethical assessment of genetic engineering with human beings. The commission focuses first on concerns about "playing God" and then considers concerns about consequences.

Purdy, Laura M.: "Surrogate Mothering: Exploitation or Empowerment?" *Bioethics* 3 (January 1989), pp. 18–34. Purdy argues against the view that surrogate mothering is necessarily immoral. She acknowledges the danger that surrogate mothering could deepen the exploitation of women but also insists that surrogacy has the potential to empower women.

Rothman, Barbara Katz: *The Tentative Pregnancy: Prenatal Diagnosis and the Future of Motherhood* (New York: Viking Penguin, 1986). Rothman raises a host of concerns about the social impact of prenatal diagnosis.

Tiefel, Hans O.: "Human *In Vitro* Fertilization: A Conservative View," *Journal of the American Medical Association* 247 (June 18, 1982), pp. 3235–3242. Tiefel contends that "the decisive objection to clinical uses of [IVF] lies in the possible and even likely risk of greater than normal harm to offspring." He also argues that nonclinical (purely experimental) uses of IVF are morally unjustifiable, because such uses fail to accord due respect to human embryos.

Warren, Mary Anne: "IVF and Women's Interests: An Analysis of Feminist Concerns," *Bioethics* 2 (January 1988), pp. 37–57. Warren argues that, although IVF (and other reproductive technologies) "pose some significant dangers for women, it would be wrong to conclude that women's interests demand an end to IVF and other reproductive research." In an effort to guard against a possible negative impact on the interests of women, she insists that IVF is not an adequate overall societal response to the problem of involuntary infertility.

Wertz, Dorothy C., and John C. Fletcher: "Ethics and Medical Genetics in the United States: A National Survey," *American Journal of Medical Genetics* 29 (April 1988), pp. 815–827. The authors report the results of an empirical study of the attitudes of geneticists. They summarize fourteen clinical problems and three screening situations involving a moral choice.

————: "Fatal Knowledge? Prenatal Diagnosis and Sex Selection," *Hastings Center Report* 19 (May/June 1989), pp. 21–27. The authors argue against the employment of prenatal diagnosis for the purpose of sex selection.

CHAPTER 10

SOCIAL JUSTICE AND HEALTH-CARE POLICY

INTRODUCTION

In 1986 the United States spent 10.9 percent of its gross national product on health care. The money invested in health care was not the result of some overall, well-designed health-care policy, but the cumulative effect of decisions made by individuals, employers, hospitals, insurance companies, and local, state, and federal governments. Items paid for were as commonplace as aspirins and appendectomies and as technologically advanced as kidney and lung transplants. At the same time, not all the medical needs of people were met because of factors as diverse as poverty, a shortage of organ donors, the dearth of physicians in certain areas, and inadequate funding for medical and basic research. The escalating cost of health care and the promise of continuing expensive technological advances in medicine, on the one hand, and the inequitable distribution of medical resources, on the other, give a special sense of urgency to the questions currently being asked in our society regarding the funding and provision of health care. This chapter addresses a few of these questions and explores some of the central moral issues involved.

Justice, Rights, and Societal Obligations

Many of the readings in this chapter maintain that society has a moral obligation to make it possible for people to meet at least some of their medical needs and that it is part of the legitimate function of government to ensure some measure of access to medical care for all who need it. Does society have a moral obligation to ensure that everyone in society has access to at least some level of health care? If yes, what is the extent of the obligation? For example, should society ensure that everyone who needs and wants even the most sophisticated and specialized hospital care should have access to it? To every possible life-extending therapy? To only rudimentary care? And just what is the appropriate role of government in regard to funding and providing health care? Answering these kinds of questions requires (1) an understanding of various conceptions of justice as well as other possible grounds for establishing societal obligations regarding health care and (2) an understanding of the difference between the *public funding* and *public delivery* of health care.

Justice, Liberty, Equality, and the Right to Health Care   Three conceptions of justice are dominant in contemporary social-political theory: libertarian, socialist, and liberal. Two moral ideals, liberty and equality, are of key importance. A *libertarian* conception of justice holds liberty to be the ultimate moral ideal; a *socialist* conception of justice takes social equality to be the ultimate moral ideal; and a *liberal* conception of justice tries to combine both equality and liberty into one ultimate moral ideal.

The Libertarian Conception of Justice   On a libertarian view, individuals have certain moral rights to life, liberty, and property, which any just society must recognize and respect. These are conceived as negative rights, or rights of noninterference: If *A* has a right to *X*, no one should prevent *A* from pursuing *X* or deprive *A* of *X*, since *A* is entitled to it. (The distinction between negative and positive rights is discussed in Chapter 1.) According to a libertarian, the sole function of government is to protect the individual's life, liberty, and property against force and fraud. Everything else in society is a matter of individual responsibility, decision, and action. Providing for the welfare of those who cannot or will not provide for themselves is not a morally justifiable function of government. To make such provisions, the government would have to take from some against their will in order to give to others. This is perceived as an unjustifiable limitation on individual liberty. Individuals own their own bodies and, there-fore, the labor they exert. It follows, for the libertarian, that individuals have the right to what-ever income or wealth their labor can earn in a free marketplace, and no one has the right to take part of that income to provide health care for others.

The Socialist Conception of Justice   A direct challenge to libertarians comes from those who defend a socialist conception of justice. Although socialist views differ in many respects, one common element is a commitment to social equality and to government or collective mea-sures furthering that equality. Since social equality is the ultimate ideal, limitations on indi-vidual liberty that are necessary to promote equality are seen as justified. Socialists attack the libertarian views on the primacy of liberty in at least two ways. First, they offer defenses of their ideal of social equality. These take various forms and will not concern us here. Second, they point out the meaninglessness of rights of noninterference to those who lack adequate food, health care, and so forth. For those who lack the money to buy food and health care needed to sustain life, the libertarian right to life is an empty sham. The rights of liberty, such as the right to freely exchange goods, are a joke to those who cannot exercise such rights be-cause of economic considerations. Where libertarians stress freedom from government inter-ference, socialists stress the government's obligation to promote the welfare of its citizens by ensuring that their most important needs are met. Where libertarians stress *negative rights*, so-cialists stress *positive rights*. Where libertarians criticize socialism for the limitations it imposes on liberty, socialists criticize libertarianism for allowing gross inequalities among those who are "equally human."

The Liberal Conception of Justice   The liberal rejects the libertarian conception of justice since it fails to include what liberals perceive as a fundamental moral concern. Any purported conception of justice that fails to incorporate the requirement that those who have more than enough must help those in need is morally unacceptable. Like the socialist, the liberal recog-nizes the extent to which economic coercion in an industrial society actually limits the exercise of negative rights by those lacking economic power. Unlike the socialist, the liberal sees some of the negative rights of the libertarian as extremely important, but advocates institutions that will function to ensure certain basic liberties (e.g., freedom of speech) and yet provide for the basic needs of the disadvantaged members of society. Liberals are not opposed to all social and economic inequalities, but they disagree concerning both the morally acceptable extent of those inequalities and their correct justification. A utilitarian committed to a liberal position, for example, might hold that inequalities are justified to the extent that allowing them maximizes the total amount of good in society. A different approach is taken by an important contemporary philosopher, John Rawls, who maintains that the only justified inequalities in the distribution of primary social goods (e.g., income, opportunities) are those that will benefit everyone in society, especially the least advantaged.[1] The concern here is not with the total amount of good in a society but with the good of the least advantaged.

Theories of Justice and a Right to Health Care   What, if anything can be inferred from the above theories of justice regarding the existence of a moral right to health care? In one of this chapter's readings, Allen Buchanan asks this question in regard to both a libertarian and a liberal theory of justice. After discussing the libertarian approach as exemplified in the work of Robert M. Nozick, Buchanan points out that for the libertarian, there is no moral right to health care and no societal obligation to provide it. Citing Rawls's views as an example of a liberal position, Buchanan explains Rawls's central principles of justice before speculating about their implications regarding what constitutes justice in health care. According to Buchanan, the implications of Rawls's theory for a right to health care are far from clear.

Buchanan also discusses the stance that a utilitarian might take in regard to justice in general and a right to health care in particular. Clearly, he has in mind the perspective of a rule-utilitarian. (As noted in Chapter 1, unlike act-utilitarianism, rule-utilitarianism might be able to provide an adequate theoretical foundation for individual rights.) On a rule-utilitarian account, the correct conception of justice and of related moral rights is the one whose application maximizes the net amount of good in society. Buchanan examines some of the implications of a utilitarian approach for both a right to health care and for the scope of any such right. He notes that disagreement among utilitarians in regard to these implications is often due to disagreements about the empirical evidence that must be considered in order to determine which approach to health-care rights will maximize utility. Buchanan does not discuss the socialist position on justice. In another reading in this chapter, however, Kai Nielsen, although not explicitly arguing from a socialist position, does argue for a moral right to health care based on a conception of justice whose fundamental principle is the principle of moral equality. As Nielsen states this principle, it asserts that the life of everyone matters and matters equally. On Nielsen's account, if a society is committed to moral equality, open and free medical treatment of the same quality and extent must be available to everyone.

Beneficence, Health-Care Needs, and Societal Obligations   Some arguments advanced in support of a societal obligation to provide health care do not involve attempts to establish a right to health care. Rather, they appeal to considerations of beneficence in conjunction with considerations of the special nature of health-care needs. This strategy is adopted in one of this chapter's readings by the President's Commission for the Study of Ethical Problems in Medicine and Biomedical and Behavioral Research. The Commission asserts that society has an obligation to ensure that each of its members has access to adequate care without being subject to excessive burdens. This contention is based on (1) the special moral significance of some forms of health care; (2) the fact that many health-care needs are beyond individuals' control and, therefore, undeserved; and (3) the implausibility of expecting everyone to be able to meet their health-care needs using their own resources when these needs are so unpredictable, costly, and unevenly distributed among people. Unlike Nielsen, the Commission does not hold that the same quality and extent of care must be available to everyone in society. Rather they defend the view that society has an obligation to ensure that everyone has access to an adequate level of care. In their view, this is consistent with the existence of a two-tier system of medical care—one in which everyone is ensured access to at least some level of care, and those who are better off can purchase additional services should they wish to do so.

Government Role in Health-Care Delivery: Public Funding versus Public Provision   What part should the government in a just society play in the *delivery* of health-care services? To better understand this question it is useful to compare the health-care delivery systems in the United States and Britain.[2]

Britain   The British system is primarily a system of *public medical care*. In Britain, the entire hospital system is owned and operated by the government, which pays for about 95 percent of the nation's health-care costs. Most of the remaining 5 percent comes from private health insurance. Eighty percent of the health-care budget goes for hospital and community care. Services covered include both inpatient and outpatient treatment for acute and chronic illness (which includes mental handicaps and mental illness), prevention services, and community nursing. The remaining 20 percent of the budget is spent on general medical and dental practitioner care as well as on drugs and various medical appliances. To have access to this system of health care, individuals need only to sign up with a general practitioner, as 97 percent of the population has done. Specialists are seen only on the recommendation of the general practioner who has overall charge of the patient's care.

General practitioners, who comprise nearly one-half of all doctors in active practice, are paid an annual income by the government. The size of each practitioner's income is determined by the number of patients on his or her list and not by the times the physician sees a patient. A fee-for-service arrangement is unusual within the public health-care system, although a few procedures performed by physicians (e.g., immunizations) are paid for on that basis. Specialists, called consultants, are hospital employees and receive an annual salary that does not depend on the number of patients they see. If they wish, they may supplement their income by caring for private patients, but many choose not to engage in private practice at all. An independent pay review body, set up by the government, determines doctors' salaries after considering evidence from various sources, including the medical profession. Dentists, unlike general practitioners, are paid on a fee-for-service basis. Here, too, however, the fee is decided by negotiation with the government. Pharmacists are paid according to a schedule negotiated with the government, and prescription drugs are available for a small fee.

There is a small private sector in medicine, as noted earlier, which is currently growing. People who wish to do so can use this private sector. In addition, it is possible to carry a limited type of supplementary health insurance. This is carried by a small number of people.

United States   The United States system is primarily a system of *private medical care*. Most general hospitals are owned by nonprofit corporations, which are sponsored by both sectarian groups and private citizens, although the number of investor-owned, for-profit hospitals continues to increase significantly. Mental hospitals are run primarily by individual states. Some hospitals, especially those giving long-term care, are operated by some grouping of federal, state, and local governments. Most physicians are in private practice. This is true of general practitioners as well as specialists, including those affiliated with hospitals. Most physicians own or rent their equipment and their offices, singly or in groups. Dentists are in the same situation. Most physicians and dentists are paid on a fee-for-service basis—so much per office visit, so much per test, and so forth. There are salaried physicians, of course, who work for various organizations including health maintenance organizations (HMOs) which provide care on a prepaid rather than a fee-for-service basis.

A large percentage of the United States population has some form of private health insurance. In many cases this is paid largely or partly by employers' contributions. Federal funds provide government-financed insurance to people over 65 (Medicare) and to those below a certain income level (Medicaid). In addition, special groups, such as veterans or those suffering from specific diseases, such as cancer or tuberculosis, are directly cared for in hospitals operated by the government. Veterans' hospitals, for example, are operated by the federal government; other hospitals are supported by federal, state, and local funds. In 1986, about 85 percent of the United States population was covered by private or public health insurance. However, about 37 million Americans were neither eligible for Medicare or Medicaid nor covered by private health insurance. Although Medicare and Medicaid benefits are funded by public funds, they do not primarily involve the public provision of health care. Those covered use the same system of private medical care described above. Furthermore, when some members of Congress argued several years ago for some forms of compulsory health insurance, they were advocating neither the public funding of insurance coverage nor a system of public medical care. On their proposals, part of the funding for this insurance would have come from employee-employer contributions. The government would have paid for insurance coverage for those who were not covered by employee-employer contributions as well as for coverage for catastrophic illnesses for everyone.

Public or Private Care?   These two examples illustrate the difference between the *public financing of private medical care* (e.g., Medicare in the United States) and the *public offering of medical care* (e.g., the socialized system in Britain). Those who argue that society has an obligation to make it possible for everyone to meet all or some of their health-care needs are not necessarily arguing for a socialized system of medicine. They may simply be arguing for the public financing or partial financing of health care. (The President's Commission, for example, advocates a limited role for government even in regard to the funding of care.) One question that cannot be ignored, however, is whether a socialized system of medical care is morally preferable to a private one. In this chapter, Nielsen argues that a system based on a commitment to moral equality would have to take medicine out of the private sector altogether and place both the ownership and control of medicine in the public sector.

Macroallocation Decisions and the Problem of Rationing

In our society, policy decisions about the allocation of health-care resources are made every day by Congress, state legislatures, health organizations, private foundations, health insurance companies, and federal, state, and local agencies. The allocation decisions made by these kinds of groups about health-care expenditures and the distribution of health-care resources are usually called "macroallocation decisions." They are contrasted with "microallocation decisions," those made by particular hospital staffs and individual physicians about the allocation of available health-care resources.

Two of the most important questions raised concerning macroallocation decisions are the following: (1) How much of our total economic resources should go for health care? (2) How should this total be divided among specific areas, such as biomedical research, preventive measures, "crisis care," and the production of new equipment used in treatment and diagnosis? In respect to (1), further questions must be asked about the importance of health care vis-à-vis other goods. For example, current biomedical technology is making it possible to save and prolong lives that could not have been saved before. Is the value of prolonging these lives so great that we should adopt public policies that encourage prolongation no matter what it costs? Should other social goods, such as education, for example, receive less funding in order to prolong individual lives as long as possible? Answers here require decisions about what values society ought to encourage and about the kind of life most worth living. In respect to (2), questions must be answered regarding both the correct method for making macroallocation decisions and the values that should guide those decisions. Daniel Callahan, in a reading in this chapter, deals with some of these questions as he argues for the need to ration medical care.

Like the President's Commission, Callahan holds that society should provide a guaranteed level of care for every member of society. However, Callahan points out that the need to provide an adequate minimum for all would seem to require an expansion of health-care expenditures. At the same time, health-care costs and the proportion of the gross national product devoted to health-care costs are constantly escalating. Callahan argues that to provide a guaranteed minimum level of care to all, as well as to effectively control costs, we must set firm upper limits on what we provide. In his account, Callahan distinguishes between allocation and rationing. Allocation decisions are related to the first question above and involve the relative weight given to various goods (e.g., health care vis-à-vis education) in the distribution of social resources. Rationing decisions are related to the second question and deal with choices within a particular category concerning the relative weight to be given to competing needs. For example, when public funds are involved, should the funding of prenatal care take precedence over the funding of heart transplants?

Rationing and the Elderly   If Callahan is correct and it is necessary to ration health care, what are the morally appropriate criteria to use? One suggested criterion that has recently become the subject of increasing debate is age. Callahan, who in a second reading in this chapter advocates age-based rationing, points out that in 1986 those over 65 consumed 31 percent of the total of 450 billion dollars spent on health care in the United States. Demographers predict that by the year 2040, 21 percent of the United States population will be over 65 and will consume 45 percent of all health-care expenditures. In light of such projections, it is not surprising that the use of advanced age as a criterion for denying certain kinds of medical care is being proposed and defended. Three other articles in this chapter discuss age-based rationing—those by James F. Childress, Amitai Etzioni, and Robert M. Veatch. Childress grants that in principle, under ideal conditions, age-based rationing can be consistent with both the requirements of justice and the more general requirements of morality. However, he points out various problems for any attempt to ration health care on the basis of age under the conditions actually existing in our society. Etzioni condemns age-based rationing and argues specifically against Callahan's proposals. Veatch discusses utilitarian and justice-based arguments advanced by other writers in regard to age-based rationing. He concludes that it may be possible to establish fair and reasonable social policies that exclude the elderly from some types of medical care.

Microallocation Decisions

Physicians and hospital staffs must often make decisions about the allocation of scarce medical resources, such as artificial and natural organs. When there are too many medically qualified candidates for some medical procedure, the choice among candidates must be made on the basis of some nonmedical criteria. The central ethical question raised concerning the microallocation of scarce health-care resources is the following: When there are too many medically needy candidates for a scarce lifesaving medical resource, what criteria should be used to choose among the candidates?

The procedure that focused both popular and philosophical attention on the ethical problems raised by microallocation decisions was the method of kidney dialysis. In the 1960s and early 1970s, the scarcity of artificial kidney machines, which "wash the blood" of patients who have to be connected to them at regular intervals, forced hospitals to limit access to the procedure to a very small percentage of those needing treatment. With dialysis, the patients could not only stay alive, but even live normal lives within limits. Without dialysis, they died. Selection committees, composed of doctors and community leaders, set up their own moral criteria for choosing among competing applicants. In 1972 Congress made a macroallocation decision to fund kidney dialysis for almost everyone who needed it. This decision has, for the most part, eliminated the need for microallocation decisions about kidney dialysis. But several articles written by ethicists prior to the congressional ruling, including the article by Nicholas P. Rescher in this chapter, reveal the moral difficulties involved in the microallocation of any scarce lifesaving resource.

Basing his reasoning partially on utilitarian considerations, Rescher argues for the adoption of a complex set of criteria of selection; these include such social-value considerations as potential social contributions. Rescher's approach is not completely utilitarian, however, since he maintains that equity requires the consideration of past services even in the event that these considerations cannot be justified on utilitarian grounds. In another reading in this chapter, George J. Annas considers and contrasts four major approaches to microallocation decisions. He condemns the use of social-worth criteria and advocates a combination of approaches in the interest of fairness and equality as well as efficiency.

Policy Decisions and Individual Responsibility for Health

It is obvious from the discussion in this introduction that our society is faced with some difficult decisions in regard to the provision and funding of health care. What has not been considered thus far, however, is individual responsibility for health and the related notion that those whose health problems result from their irresponsibly engaging in risk-running behavior should pay a greater share of their health-care costs—either by paying a greater share of the taxes used for medical resources or by paying higher insurance premiums. More and more evidence supports the contention that one of the most important factors in maintaining good health is individual life-style. Heavy smoking, for example, is linked with cancer; heavy drinking with cirrhosis of the liver; obesity and inadequate exercise with cardiovascular and other diseases. In view of this, should smokers, alcohol consumers, and others indulging in high-risk behavior pay additional taxes on products such as alcohol in order to provide additional money for medical resources?

Answering this question involves complex empirical, conceptual, and ethical considerations. Relevant *empirical* questions include, for example: Do the extra medical costs necessitated by some high-risk behavior, such as heavy smoking, place a greater financial burden on society than the financial costs to society (e.g., to the social security system) of supporting octogenarians and septuagenarians whose lives may have been prolonged by healthy habits? Relevant *conceptual* issues include determining the appropriate criteria for distinguishing voluntary from involuntary high-risk behavior. Relevant *moral* issues include determining what constitutes fairness in the distribution of society's burdens and benefits. In this chapter's final reading, Robert M. Veatch examines some of the central empirical, conceptual, and moral issues raised by our growing realization of the link between individual life-styles and the need for medical care.

NOTES

1 John Rawls, *A Theory of Justice* (Cambridge, Mass.: Harvard, 1970). Philosophers disagree about the correct conclusions to be drawn from Rawls's theory in regard to the distribution of medical care. See, for example, Ronald M. Green, "Health Care and Justice in Contract Theory Perspective," in Robert M. Veatch and Roy Branson, eds., *Ethics and Health Policy*

(Cambridge, Mass.: Ballinger, 1976), pp. 111–126; and Norman Daniels, "Health Care Needs and Distributive Justice" in *Philosophy and Public Affairs* 10 (Spring 1981), pp. 146–179.

2 This section's descriptions of the British and U.S. systems are based, in part, on material in Howard H. Hiatt, *America's Health in the Balance: Choice or Chance* (New York: Harper and Row, 1987).

Justice, Rights, and Societal Obligations

Justice: A Philosophical Review
Allen Buchanan

Allen Buchanan is professor of philosophy at the University of Arizona. His areas of specialization are political philosopohy, ethics, and medical ethics. Buchanan is the author of *Marx and Justice: The Radical Critique of Liberalism* (1982) and *Ethics, Efficiency, and the Market* (1982). His published articles include "Medical Paternalism."

Buchanan begins by setting out three theoretical approaches to justice: (1) a utilitarian approach; (2) Rawls's theory of justice as fairness; and (3) Nozick's libertarian theory. He confronts each position with several questions about health care. These questions deal with a right to health care, the relative importance of health care or health-care needs vis-à-vis other goods or needs, the relative importance of various forms of health care, and the compatibility of our current health-care system with the demands of justice. Buchanan concludes that none of the three theoretical approaches provides unambiguous answers to all the questions raised and that the application of each depends on numerous unavailable empirical premises. This leaves a great deal of work to be done in developing an account of justice in health care.

INTRODUCTION

The past decade has seen the burgeoning of bioethics and the resurgence of theorizing about justice. Yet until now these two developments have not been as mutually enriching as one might have hoped. Bioethicists have tended to concentrate on micro issues (moral problems of individual or small group decisionmaking), ignoring fundamental moral questions about the macro structure within which the micro issues arise. Theorists of justice have advanced very general principles but have typically neglected to show how they can illuminate the particular problems we face in health care and other urgent areas.

Micro problems do not exist in an institutional vacuum. The parents of a severely impaired newborn and

From *Justice and Health Care*, edited by Earl Shelp, pp. 3–21: Copyright © 1981 by D. Reidel Publishing Company, Dordrecht, Holland. Reprinted by permission of Kluwer Academic Publishers.

the attending neonatologist are faced with the decision of whether to treat the infant aggressively or to allow it to die because neonatal intensive care units now exist which make it possible to preserve the lives of infants who previously would have died. Neonatal intensive care units exist because certain policy decisions have been made which allocated certain social resources to the development of technology for sustaining defective newborns rather than for preventing birth defects. Limiting moral inquiry to the micro issues supports an unreasoned conservatism by failing to examine the health care institutions within which micro problems arise and by not investigating the larger array of institutions of which the health care sector is only one part. Since not only particular actions but also policies and institutions may be just or unjust, serious theorizing about justice forces us to expand the narrow focus of the micro approach by raising fundamental queries about the background social, economic, and political institutions from which micro problems emerge.

On the other hand, the attention to individual cases which dominates contemporary bioethics can provide a much needed concrete focus for refining and assessing competing theories of justice. The adequacy or inadequacy of a moral theory cannot be determined by inspecting the principles which constitute it. Instead, rational assessment requires an on-going process in which general principles are revised and refined through confrontation with the rich complexity of our considered judgments about particular cases, while our judgments about particular cases are gradually structured and modified by our provisional acceptance of general principles. Since our considered judgments about particular cases may often be more sensitive and sure than our assessments of abstract principles, careful attention to accurately described, concrete moral situations is essential for theorizing about justice.

Further, it is not just that the problems of bioethics provide one class of test cases for theories of justice among others: the problems of bioethics are among the most difficult and pressing issues with which a theory of justice must cope. It appears, then, that the continued development of both bioethics and of theorizing about justice in general requires us to explore the problems of justice in health care. In this essay I hope to contribute to that enterprise by first providing a sketch of three major theories of justice and by then attempting to ascertain some of their implications for moral problems in health care.

THEORIES OF JUSTICE

Utilitarianism

Utilitarianism purports to be a comprehensive moral theory, of which a utilitarian theory of justice is only one part. There are two main types of comprehensive utilitarian theory: Act and Rule Utilitarianism. Act Utilitarianism defines rightness with respect to particular acts: an act is right if and only if it maximizes utility. Rule Utilitarianism defines rights with respect to rules of action and makes the rightness of particular acts depend upon the rules under which those acts fall. A rule is right if and only if general compliance with that rule (or with a set of rules of which it is an element) maximizes utility, and a particular action is right if and only if it falls under such a rule.

Both Act and Rule Utilitarianism may be versions of either Classic or Average Utilitarianism. Classic Utilitarianism defines the rightness of acts or rules as maximization of *aggregate* utility; Average Utilitarianism defines rightness as maximization of utility *per capita*. The aggregate utility produced by an act or by general compliance with a rule is the sum of the utility produced for each individual affected. Average utility is the aggregate utility divided by the number of individuals affected. 'Utility' is defined as pleasure, satisfaction, happiness, or as the realization of preferences, as the latter are revealed through individuals' choices.

The distinction between Act and Rule Utilitarianism is important for a utilitarian theory of justice, since the latter must include an account of when *institutions* are just. Thus, institutional rules may maximize utility even though those rules do not direct individuals as individuals or as occupants of institutional positions to maximize utility in a case by case fashion. For example, it may be that a judicial system which maximizes utility will do so by including rules which prohibit judges from deciding a case according to their estimates of what would maximize utility in that particular case. Thus the utilitarian justification of a particular action or decision may not be that it maximizes utility, but rather that it falls under some rule of an institution or set of institutions which maximizes utility.[1]

Some utilitarians, such as John Stuart Mill, hold that principles of justice are the most basic moral principles because the utility of adherence to them is especially great. According to this view, utilitarian principles of justice are those utilitarian moral principles which are of such importance that they may be *enforced*, if necessary. Some utilitarians, including Mill perhaps, also hold that among the utilitarian principles of justice are principles specifying individual rights, whether the latter are thought of as enforceable claims which take precedence over appeals to what would maximize utility in the particular case. Indeed, some contemporary rights theorists such as Ronald Dworkin define a (justified) right claim as one which takes precedence over mere appeals to what would maximize utility.

A utilitarian moral theory, then, can include rights principles which themselves prohibit appeals to utility maximization, so long as the justification of those principles is that they are part of an institutional system which maximizes utility. In cases where two or more rights principles conflict, considerations of utility may be invoked to determine which rights principles are to be given priority. Utilitarianism is incompatible with rights only if rights exclude appeals to utility maximization at all levels of justification, including the most basic institutional level. Rights founded ultimately on considerations of utility may be called *derivative*, to distinguish them from rights in the *strict* sense.

Utilitarianism is the most influential version of teleological moral theory. A moral theory is teleological if and only if it defines the good independently of the right and defines the right as that which maximizes the good. Utilitarianism defines the good as happiness (satisfaction, etc.), independently of any account of what is morally right, and then defines the right as that which maximizes the good (either in the particular case or at the institutional level). A moral theory is *deontological* if and only if it is not a teleological theory, i.e., if and only if it either does not define the good independently of the right or does not define the right as that which maximizes the good. Both the second and third theories of justice we shall consider are deontological theories.

John Rawls's Theory: Justice as Fairness

In *A Theory of Justice* Rawls pursues two main goals. The first is to set out a small but powerful set of principles of justice which underlie and explain the considered moral judgments we make about particular actions, policies, laws, and institutions. The second is to offer a theory of justice superior to Utilitarianism. These two goals are intimately related for Rawls because he believes that the theory which does a better job of supporting and accounting for our considered judgments is the better theory, other things being equal. The principles of justice Rawls offers are as follows:

1. The principle of greatest equal liberty:
   Each person is to have an equal right to the most extensive system of equal basic liberties compatible with a similar system of liberty for all ([6], pp. 60, 201–205).

2. The principle of equality of fair opportunity:
   Offices and positions are to be open to all under conditions of equality of fair opportunity—persons with similar abilities and skills are to have equal access to offices and positions.([6], pp. 60, 73, 83–89).[2]

3. The difference principle:
   Social and economic institutions are to be arranged so as to benefit maximally the worst off ([6], pp. 60, 75–83).[3]

The basic liberties referred to in (1) include freedom of speech, freedom of conscience, freedom from arbitrary arrest, the right to hold personal property, and freedom of political participation (the right to vote, to run for office, etc.).

Since the demands of these principles may conflict, some way of ordering them is needed. According to Rawls, (1) is *lexically prior* to (2) and (2) is *lexically prior* to (3). A principle 'P' is lexically prior to a principle 'Q' if and only if we are first to satisfy all the requirements of 'P' before going on to satisfy the requirements of 'Q.' Lexical priority allows no trade-offs between the demands of conflicting principles: the lexically prior principle takes absolute priority.

Rawls notes that "many kinds of things are said to be just or unjust: not only laws, institutions, and social systems, but also particular actions...decisions, judgments and imputations...." ([6], p. 7). But he insists that the primary subject of justice is the *basic structure* of society because it exerts a pervasive and profound influence on individuals' life prospects. The basic structure is the entire set of major political, legal, economic, and social institutions. In our society the basic structure includes the Constitution, private ownership of the means of production, competitive markets, and the monogamous family. The basic structure plays a large role in distributing the burdens and benefits of cooperation among members of society.

If the primary subject of justice is the basic structure, then the primary problem of justice is to formulate and justify a set of principles which a just basic structure must satisfy. These principles will specify how the basic structure is to distribute prospects of what Rawls calls *primary goods*. They include the basic liberties (listed above under (2)), as well as powers, authority, opportunities, income, and wealth. Rawls says that primary goods are things that every rational person is presumed to want, because they normally have a use, whatever a person's rational plan of life ([6], p. 62). Principle (1) regulates the distribution of prospects of basic liberties; (2) regulates the distribution of prospects of powers and authority, so far as these are attached to institutional offices and positions, and (3) regulates the distribution of prospects of the other primary goods, including wealth and income. Though the first and second principles require equality, the difference principle allows inequalities so long as the total system of institutions of which they are a part maximizes the prospects of the worst off to the primary goods in question.

Rawls advances three distinct types of justification for his principles of justice. Two appeal to our considered judgments, while the third is based on what he calls the Kantian interpretation of his theory.

The first type of justification rests on the idea, mentioned earlier, that if a set of principles provides the best account of our considered judgments about what is just or unjust, then that is a reason for accepting those principles. A set of principles accounts for our judgments only if those judgments can be derived from the principles, granted the relevant facts for their application.

Rawls's second type of justification maintains that if a set of principles would be chosen under conditions which, according to our considered judgments, are appropriate conditions for choosing principles of justice, then this is a reason for accepting those principles. The second type of justification includes three parts: (1) A set of conditions for choosing principles of justice must be specified. Rawls labels the complete set of conditions the 'original position.' (2) It must be shown that the conditions specified are (according to our considered judgments) the appropriate conditions of choice. (3) It must be shown that Rawls's principles are indeed the principles which would be chosen under those conditions.

Rawls construes the choice of principles of justice as an ideal social contract. "The principles of justice for the basic structure of society are the principles that free and rational persons...would accept in an initial situation of equality as defining the fundamental terms of their association" ([6], p. 11). The idea of a social contract has several advantages. First, it allows us to view principles of justice as the object of a *rational collective choice*. Second, the idea of *contractual obligation* is used to emphasize that the choice expresses a basic commitment and that the principles agreed on may be rightly enforced. Third, the idea of a contract as a *voluntary agreement* which set terms for mutual advantage suggests that the principles of justice should be "such as to draw forth the willing cooperation" ([6], p. 15) of all members of society, including those who are worse off.

The most important elements of the original position for our purposes are a) the characterization of the parties to the contract as individuals who desire to pursue their own life plans effectively and who "have a highest-order interest in how...their interests...are shaped and regulated by social institutions" ([8], p. 64); b) the 'veil of ignorance,' which is a constraint on the information the parties are able to utilize in choosing principles of justice; and c) the requirement that the principles are to be chosen on the assumption that they will be complied with by all (the universalizability condition) ([6], p. 132).

The parties are characterized as desiring to maximize their shares of primary goods, because these goods enable one to implement effectively the widest range of life plans and because at least some of them, such as freedom of speech and of conscience, facilitate one's freedom to choose and revise one's life plan or conception of the good. The parties are to choose "from behind a veil of ignorance" so that information about their own particular characteristics or social positions will not lead to bias in the choice of principles. Thus they are described as not knowing their race, sex, socioeconomic, or political status, or even the nature of their particular conceptions of the good. The informational restriction also helps to insure that the principles chosen will not place avoidable restrictions on the individual's freedom to choose and revise his or her life plan.[4]

Though Rawls offers several arguments to show that his principles would be chosen in the original position, the most striking is the maximum argument. According to this argument, the rational strategy in the original position is to choose that set of principles whose implementation will maximize the minimum share of primary goods which one can receive as a member of society, and principles (1), (2), and (3) will insure the greatest minimal share. Rawls's claim is that because these principles protect one's basic liberties and opportunities and insure an adequate minimum of goods such as wealth and income (even if one should turn out to be among the worst off) the rational thing is to choose them, rather than to gamble with one's life prospects by opting for alternative principles. In particular, Rawls contends that it would be irrational to reject his principles and allow one's life prospect to be determined by what would maximize utility, since utility maximization might allow severe deprivation or even slavery for some, so long as this contributed sufficiently to the welfare of others.

Rawls raises an important question about this second mode of justification when he notes that this original position is purely hypothetical. Granted that the agreement is never actually entered into, why should we regard the principles as binding? The answer, according to Rawls, is that we do in fact accept the conditions embodied in the original position ([6], p. 21). The following qualification, which Rawls adds immediately after claiming that the conditions which constitute the original position are appropriate for the choice of principles of justice according to our considered judgments, introduces his third type of justification: "Or if we do not [accept the conditions of the original position as appropriate for choosing principles of justice] *then perhaps we can be persuaded to do so by the philosophical* reflections" (emphasis added [6], p. 21). In the Kantian interpretation section of *A Theory of Justice*, Rawls sketches a certain kind of philosophical justification for the conditions which make up the orignial position (based on Kant's conception of the 'noumenal self' or autonomous agent).

For Kant an autonomous agent's will is determined by rational principles and rational principles are those which can serve as principles for all rational beings, not just for this or that agent, depending upon whether or not he has some particular desire which other rational beings may not have. Rawls invites us to think of the original position as the perspective from which autonomous agents see the world. The original position provides a "procedural interpretation" of Kant's idea of a Realm of Ends or community of "free and equal rational beings." We express our nature as autonomous agents when we act from principles that would be chosen in conditions which reflect that nature ([6], p. 252).

Rawls concludes that, when persons such as you and I accept those principles that would be chosen in the original position, we express our nature as autonomous agents, i.e., we act autonomously. There are three main grounds for this thesis, corresponding to the three features of the original position cited earlier. First, since the veil of ignorance excludes information about any particular desires which a rational agent may or may not have, the choice of principles is not determined by any particular desire. Second, since the parties strive to maximize their share of primary goods, and since primary goods are attractive to them because they facilitate freedom in choosing and revising life plans and because they are flexible means not tied to any particular ends, this is another respect in which their choice is not determined by particular desires. Third, the original position includes the requirement that they will be principles of rational agents in general and not just for agents who happen to have this or that particular desire.

In the *Foundation of the Metaphysics of Morals* Kant advances a moral philosophy which identifies autonomy with rationality [4]. Hence for Kant the question "Why should one express our nature as autonomous agents?" is answered by the thesis that rationality requires it. Thus *if* Rawls's third type of justification succeeds in showing that we best express our autonomy when we accept those principles in the belief that they would be chosen from the original position, and *if* Kant's identification of autonomy with rationality is successful, the result will be a justification of Rawls's principles which is distinct from both the first and second modes of justification. So far as this third type of justification does not make the acceptance of Rawls's principles hinge on whether the princi-

ples themselves or the conditions from which they would be chosen match our considered judgments, it is not directly vulnerable either to the charge that Rawls has misconstrued our considered judgments or that congruence with considered judgments, like the appeal to mere consensus, has no justificatory force.

It is important to see that Rawls understands his principles of justice as principles which generate *rights* in what I have called the strict sense. Claims based upon the three principles are to take precedence over considerations of utility and the principles themselves are not justified on the grounds that a basic structure which satisfies them will maximize utility. Moreover, Rawls's theory is not a teleological theory of any kind because it does not define the right as that which maximizes the good, where the good is defined independently of the right. Instead it is perhaps the most influential current instance of a deontological theory.

Nozick's Libertarian Theory

There are many versions of libertarian theory, but their characteristic doctrine is that coercion may only be used to prevent or punish physical harm, theft, and fraud, and to enforce contracts. Perhaps the most influential and systematic recent instance of Libertarianism is the theory presented by Robert Nozick in *Anarchy, State, and Utopia* [5]. In Nozick's theory of justice, as in libertarian theories generally, the right to private property is fundamental and determines both the legitimate role of the state and the most basic principles of individual conduct.

Nozick contends that individuals have a property right in their persons and in whatever 'holdings' they come to have through actions which conform to (1) "the principle of justice in [initial] acquisition" and (2) "the principle of justice in transfer" ([5], p. 151). The first principle specifies the ways in which an individual may come to own hitherto unowned things without violating anyone else's rights. Here Nozick largely follows John Locke's famous account of how one makes natural objects one's own by "mixing one's labor" with them or improving them through one's labor. Though Nozick does not actually formulate a principle of justice in (initial) acquisition, he does argue that whatever the appropriate formulation is it must include a 'Lockean Proviso,' which places a constraint on the holdings which one may acquire through one's labor. Nozick maintains that one may appropriate as much of an unowned item as one desires so long as (a) one's appropriation does not worsen the conditions of others in a special way, namely, by creating a situation in which others are "no longer...able to use freely [without exclusively appropriating] what [they]...previously could" or (b) one properly compensates those whose condition is worsened by one's appropriation in the way specified in (a) ([5], pp. 178–179). Nozick emphasizes that the Proviso only picks out one way in which one's appropriation may worsen the condition of others; it does not forbid appropriation or require compensation in cases in which one's appropriation of an unowned thing worsens another's condition merely by limiting his opportunities to appropriate (rather than merely use) that thing, i.e., to make it his property.

The second principle states that one may justly transfer one's legitimate holdings to another through sale, trade, gift or bequest and that one is entitled to whatever one receives in any of these ways, so long as the person from whom one receives it was entitled to that which he transferred to you. The right to property which Nozick advances is the right to exclusive control over anything one can get through initial appropriation (subject to the Lockean Proviso) or through voluntary exchanges with others entitled to what they transfer. Nozick concludes that a distribtuion is just if and only if it arose from another just distribution by legitimate means. The principle of justice in initial acquisition specifies the legitimate 'first moves,' while the principle of justice in transfers specifies the legitimate ways of moving from one distribution to another: "Whatever arises from a just situation by just steps is itself just" ([5], p. 151).

Since not all existing holdings arose through the 'just steps' specified by the principles of justice in acquisition and transfer, there will be a need for a *principle of rectification* of past injustices. Though Nozick does not attempt to formulate such a principle he thinks that it might well require significant redistribution of holdings.

Apart from the case of rectifying past violations of the principles of acquisition and transfer, however, Nozick's theory is strikingly anti-redistributive. Nozick contends that attempts to force anyone to contribute any part of his legitimate holdings to the welfare of others is a violation of that person's property rights, whether it is undertaken by private individuals or the state. On this view, coercively backed taxation to raise funds for welfare programs of any kind is literally theft. Thus, a large proportion of the activities now engaged in by the government involve gross injustices.

After stating his theory of rights, Nozick tries to show that the state is legitimate so long as it limits its activities to the enforcement of these rights and eschews

redistributive functions. To do this he employs an 'invisible hand explanation,' which purports to show how the minimal state could arise as an unintended consequence of a series of voluntary transactions which violate no one's rights. The phrase 'invisible hand explanation' is chosen to stress that the process by which the minimal state could emerge fits Adam Smith's famous account of how individuals freely pursuing their own private ends in the market collectively produce benefits which are not the aim of anyone.

The process by which the minimal state could arise without violating anyone's rights is said to include four main steps ([5], pp. 10–25).[5] First, individuals in a 'state of nature' in which (Libertarian) moral principles are generally respected would form a plurality of 'protective agencies' to enforce their libertarian rights, since individual efforts at enforcement would be inefficient and liable to abuse. Second, through competition for clients, a 'dominant protective agency' would eventually emerge in given geographical area. Third, such an agency would eventually become a 'minimal state' by asserting a claim of monopoly over protective services in order to prevent less reliable efforts at enforcement which might endanger its clients: it would forbid 'independents' (those who refused to purchase its services) from seeking other forms of enforcement. Fourth, again assuming that correct moral principles are generally followed, those belonging to the dominant protective agency would compensate the 'independents,' presumably by providing them with free or partially subsidized protection services. With the exception of taxing its clients to provide compensation for the independents, the minimal state would act only to protect persons against physical injury, theft, fraud, and violations of contracts.

It is striking that Nozick does not attempt to provide any systematic *justification* for the Lockean rights principles he advocates. In this respect he departs radically from Rawls. Instead, Nozick assumes the correctness of the Lockean principles and then, on the basis of that assumption, argues that the minimal state and only the minimal stated is compatible with the rights those principles specify.

He does, however, offer some arguments against the more-than-minimal state which purport to be independent of that particular theory of property rights which he assumes. These arguments may provide indirect support for his principles insofar as they are designed to make alternative principles, such as Rawls's, unattractive. Perhaps most important of these is an argument designed to show that any principle of justice which demands a certain distributive end state or pattern of holdings will require frequent and gross disruptions of individuals' holdings for the sake of maintaining that end state or pattern. Nozick supports this general conclusion by a vivid example. He asks us to suppose that there is some distribution of holdings 'D$_1$' which is required by some end-state or patterned theory of justice and that 'D$_1$' is achieved at time 'T.' Now suppose that Wilt Chamberlain, the renowned basketball player, signs a contract stipulating that he is to receive twenty-five cents from the price of each ticket to the home games in which he performs, and suppose that he nets $250,000, from this arrangement. We now have a new distribution 'D$_2$'. Is 'D$_2$' unjust? Notice that by hypothesis those who paid the price of admission were entitled to control over the resources they held in 'D$_1$' (as were Chamberlain and the team's owners). The new distribution arose through *voluntary exchanges of legitimate holdings*, so it is difficult to see how it could be unjust, even if it does diverge from 'D$_1$.' From this and like examples, Nozick concludes that attempts to maintain any end-state or patterned distributive principle would require continuous interference in peoples' lives ([5], pp. 161–163).

As in the cases of Utilitarianism and Rawls's theory, Nozick and libertarians generally do not limit morality to justice. Thus, Nozick and others emphasize that a libertarian theory of individual rights is to be supplemented by a libertarian theory of virtues which recognizes that not all moral principles are suitable objects of enforcement and that moral life includes more than the nonviolation of rights. Libertarians invoke the distinction between justice and charity to reply to those who complain that a Lockean theory of property rights legitimizes crushing poverty for millions. They stress that while justice demands that we not be *forced* to contribute to the well-being of others, charity requires that we help even those who have no *right* to our aid.[6]

IMPLICATIONS FOR HEALTH CARE

Now that we have a grasp of the main ideas of three major theories of justice, we can explore briefly some of their implications for health care. To do this we may confront the theories with four questions:

1. Is there a right to health care? (If so, what is its basis and what is its content?)

2. How, in order of priority, is health care related to other goods, or how are health care needs re-

lated to other needs? (If there is a right to health care, how is it related to other rights?)

3. How, in order of priority, are various forms of health care related to one another?

4. What can we conclude about the justice or injustice of the current health care system?

In some cases, as we shall see, the theories will provide opposing answers to the same question; in others, the theories may be unhelpfully silent.

We have already seen that the Utilitarian position on rights in general is complex. If by a right we mean a right in the strict sense, i.e., a claim which takes precedence over mere appeals to utility at all levels, including the most basic institutional level, then Utilitarianism denies the existence of rights in general, including the right to health care. If, on the other hand, we mean by right a claim that takes precedence over mere appeals to utility at the level of particular actions or at some institutional level short of the most basic, but which is justified ultimately by appeal to the utility of the total set of institutions, then Utilitarianism does not exclude, and indeed may even require rights, including a right to health care. Whether or not the total institutional array which maximizes utility will include a right to health care will depend upon a wealth of *empirical facts* not deducible from the principle of utility itself. The nature and complexity of the relevant facts can best be appreciated by considering briefly the bearing of Utilitarianism on questions (2) and (3). A utilitarian system of (derivative) rights will pick out certain goods as those which make an especially large contribution to the maximization of utility. It is reasonable to assume, on the basis of empirical data, that health care, or at least certain forms of health care, is among them. Consider, for example, prenatal care, broadly conceived as including genetic screening and counseling (at least for special risk groups), prenatal nutritional care and medical examinations for expectant mothers, medical care during delivery, and basic pediatric services in the crucial months after birth. If empirical research indicates (1) that a system of institutional arrangements which maximizes utility would include such services and (2) that such services can best be assured if they are accorded the status of a right, with all that this implies, including the use of coercive sanctions where necessary, then according to Utilitarianism there is such a (derivative) right. The strength and content of this right relative to other (derivative) rights will be determined by the utility of health care as compared with other kinds of goods.

It is crucial to note that, for the utilitarian, empirical research must determine not only whether certain health care services are to be provided as a matter of right, but also whether the right in question is to be an equal right enjoyed by all persons. No commitment to equality of rights is included in the utilitarian principle itself, nor is there any commitment to equal distribution of any kind. Utilitarianism is egalitarian only in the sense that in calculating what will maximize utility each person's welfare is to be included.

Utilitarian arguments, sometimes based on empirical data, have been advanced to show that providing health care free of charge as a matter of right would encourage wasteful use of scarce and costly resources because the individual would have no incentive to restrain his 'consumption' of health care. The cumulative result, it is said, would be quite disutilitarian: a breakdown of the health care system or a disastrous curtailment of other basic services to cover the spiraling costs of health care. In contrast (proponents of this argument continue) a *market* in health care encourages 'consumers' to use resources wisely because the costs of the services an individual receives are borne by that individual.

On the other side of the utilitarian ledger, empirical evidence may be marshalled to show that the benefits of a right to health care outweigh the costs, including the costs of possible over-use, and that a market in health care would not maximize utility because those who need health care the most may not be able to afford it.

Similarly, even if there is a utilitarian justification for a right to health care, empirical evidence must again be presented to show that it should be an equal right. For it is certainly conceivable that, under certain circumstances at least, utility could be maximized by providing extensive health care only for some groups, perhaps even a minority, rather than for all persons.

Utilitarians who advocate a right to health care often argue that this right, like other basic rights, should be equal, on the basis of the assumption of diminishing marginal utility. The idea, roughly, is that with respect to many goods, including health care, there is a finite upper bound to the satisfaction a person can gain from being provided with additional amounts of the goods in question. Hence, if in general we are all subject to the phenomenon of diminishing marginal utility in the case of health care and if the threshold of diminishing marginal utility is in general sufficiently low, then there are sound utilitarian reasons for distributing health care equally.

Finally, it should be clear that for the utilitarian the issue of priorities within health care, as well as that of priorities between health care and other goods, must again be settled by empirical research. If, as seems likely, utility maximization requires more resources for prevention and health maintenance rather than for curative intervention after pathology has already developed, then this will be reflected in the content of the utilitarian right to health care. If, as many writers have contended, the current emphasis in the U.S. on high technology intervention produces less utility than would a system which stresses prevention and health maintenance (for example through stricter control of pollution and other environmental determinants of disease), then the utilitarian may conclude that the current system is unjust in this respect. Empirical data would also be needed to ascertain whether more social resources should be devoted to high- or low-technology intervention: for example, neonatal intensive care units versus 'well-baby clinics.' These examples are intended merely to illustrate the breadth and complexity of the empirical research needed to apply Utilitarianism to crucial issues in health care.

Libertarian theories such as Nozick's rely much less heavily upon empirical premises for answers to questions (1)–(4). Since the libertarian is interested only in preventing violations of libertarian rights, and since the latter are rights against certain sorts of interferences rather than rights to be provided with anything, the question of what will maximize utility is irrelevant. Further, any effort to implement any right to health care whatsoever is an injustice, according to the libertarian.

There are only two points at which empirical data are relevant for Nozick. First, whether or not any current case of appropriation of hitherto unheld things satisfies the Lockean Proviso is a matter of fact to be ascertained by empirical methods. Second, empirical historical research is needed to determine what sort of redistribution for the sake of rectifying past injustices is necessary. If, for example, physicians' higher incomes are due in part to government policies which violate libertarian rights, then rectificatory redistribution may be required. And indeed libertarians have argued that two basic features of the current health care system do involve gross violations of libertarian rights. First, compulsory taxation to provide equipment, hospital facilities, research funds, and educational subsidies for medical personnel is literally theft. Second, some argue that government enforced occupational licensing laws which prohibit all but the established forms of medical practice violate the right to freedom of contract (3).

Those who raise this second objection also usually argue that the function of such laws is to secure a monopoly for the medical establishment while sharply limiting the supply of doctors so as to keep medical fees artificially high. Whether or not such arguments are sound it is important to note that Libertarianism is not to be confused with Conservatism. A theory which would institute a free market in medical services, abolish government subsidies, and reduce government regulation of medical practice to the prevention of injury and fraud and the enforcement of contracts has radical implications for changing the current system.

Libertarianism offers straightforward answers to questions (2) and (3). Even if it can be shown that health care in general, and certain forms of health care more than others, are especially important for the happiness or even the freedom of most persons, this fact is quite irrelevant from the perspective of a libertarian theory of justice, though it is no doubt significant for the libertarian concerned with charity or other virtues which exceed the requirements of justice. Nozick and other libertarians recognize that a free market in medical services may in fact produce severe inequalities and that there is no assurance that all or even most will be able to afford adequate medical care. Though the humane libertarian will find this condition unfortunate and will aid those in need and encourage others to do likewise voluntarily, he remains adamant that no one has a right to health care and that hence none may rightly be forced to aid another.

According to Rawls, the most basic questions about health care are not to be decided either by consideration of utility or by market processes. Instead they are to be settled ultimately by appeal to those principles of justice which would be chosen in the original position. As we shall see, however, the implications of Rawls's principles for health care are far from clear.[7]

No principle explicitly specifying a right to health care is included among Rawls's principles of justice. Further, since those principles are intended to regulate the basic structure of society as a whole, they are not themselves intended to guide the decisions individuals make in particular health care situations, nor are they themselves to be applied directly to health care institutions. We are not to assume that either individual physicians or administrators of particular policies or programs are to attempt to allocate health care so as to maximize the prospects of the worse off. In Rawls's theory, as in Utilitarianism, the rightness or wrongness of

particular actions or policies depends ultimately upon the nature of the entire institutional structure within which they exist. Hence, Rawls's theory can provide us with fruitful answers at the micro level only if its implications at the macro level are adequately developed.

If Rawls's theory includes a right to health care, it must be a right which is in some way derivative upon the basic rights laid down by the Principle of Greatest Equal Liberty, the Principle of Equality of Fair Opportunity, and the Difference Principle. And if there is to be such a derivative right to health care, then health care must either be among the primary goods covered by the three principles or it must be importantly connected with some of those goods. Now at least some forms of health care (such as broad services for prevention and health maintenance, including mental health) seem to share the earmarks of Rawlsian primary goods: they facilitate the effective pursuit of ends in general and may also enhance our ability to criticize and revise our conceptions of the good. Nonetheless, Rawls does not explicitly list health care among the social primary goods included under the three principles. However, he does include wealth under the Difference Principle and defines it so broadly that it might be thought to include access to health care services. In "Fairness to Goodness" Rawls defines wealth as virtually any legally exchangeable social asset; this would cover health care 'vouchers' if they could be cashed or exchanged for other goods ([7], p. 540).

Let us suppose that health care is either itself a primary good covered by the Difference Principle or that health care may be purchased with income or some other form of wealth which is included under the Difference Principle. In the former case, depending upon various empirical conditions, it might turn out that the best way to insure that the basic structure satisfies the Difference Principle is to establish a state-enforced right to health care. But whether maximizing the prospects of the worst off will require such a right and what the content of the right will be will depend upon what weight is to be assigned to health care relative to other primary goods included under the Difference Principle. Similarly, a weighting must also be assigned if we are to determine whether the share of wealth one receives under the Difference Principle would be sufficient both for health care needs and for other ends. Unfortunatley, though Rawls acknowledges that a weighted index of primary goods is needed if we are to be able to determine what would maximize the prospects of the worst off, he offers no account of how the weighting is to be achieved.

The problem is especially acute in the case of health care, because some forms of health care are so costly that an unrestrained commitment to them would undercut any serious commitment to providing other important goods. Thus, it appears that until we have some solution to the weighting problem Rawls's theory can shed only a limited light upon the question of priority relations between health care and other goods and among various forms of health care. Rawls's conception of primary goods may explain what distinguishes health care from those things that are not primary goods, but this is clearly not sufficient.

Perhaps because he is aware of the exorbitant demands which certain health care needs may place upon social resources, Rawls stipulates that the parties in the original position are to choose principles of justice on the assumption that their needs fall within the 'normal range' ([9], pp. 9–10). His ideal may be that the satisfaction of extremely costly special needs for health care may not be a matter of justice but rather of *charity*. If some reasonable way of drawing the line between 'normal' needs which fall within the gambit of principles of justice and 'special' needs which are the proper object of the virtue of charity could be developed, then this would be a step towards solving the priority problems mentioned above.

It has been suggested that the Principle of Equality of Fair Opportunity, rather than the Difference Principle, might provide the basis for a Rawlsian right to health care ([2], pp. 16–18). While I cannot accord this proposal the consideration it deserves here, I wish to point out that there are four difficulties which make it problematic. First, priority problems still remain. For now we are faced with the task of assigning a weight to health care relative to those other factors (such as education) which are also determinants of opportunity. Further, since the Principle of Equality of Fair Opportunity is lexically prior to the Difference Principle, we must again face the prospect that commitment to the former principle might swallow up social resources needed for providing important goods included under the latter.

Second, because it refers only to opportunities for occupying social *positions* and *offices*, rather than to opportunities in general, the Principle of Equality of Fair Opportunity might be thought too narrow to provide an adequate foundation for a right to health care. Rawls might respond either by defining 'position' rather broadly or by arguing that opportunities for attaining positions and offices are related to opportunities in gen-

eral in such a way that equality in the former insures equality in the latter.

Third, and more importantly, Rawls's Principle of Equality of Fair Opportunity takes 'abilities' and 'skills' as given, requiring only that persons with equal or similar abilities and skills are to have equal prospects of attaining social positions and offices. Yet clearly inequalities in health care can produce severe inequalities in abilities and skills. For example, poor nutrition and medical care during gestation can result in mental retardation, and many health problems hinder the development of skills and abilities. Hence it might be argued that if the Principle of Opportunity is to provide an adequate basis for a right to health care it must be reformulated to capture the crucial influence of health care or the lack of it upon individual development.

Each of the theories of justice under consideration offers a theoretical basis for answering some basic questions concerning justice in health care. We have seen, however, that none of them provides unambiguous answers to all of the questions and that each depends for its application upon a wealth of empirical premises, many of which may not now be available. Each theory does at least rule out some answers and each supplies us with a perspective from which to pursue issues which we cannot ignore. Nonetheless, almost all of the work in developing an account of justice in health care remains to be done.[8]

NOTES

1 In this essay I shall be concerned for the most part with utilitarianism at the institutional level, and I shall proceed on the assumption that a set of institutions which maximizes utility will include rules which bar other direct applications of the principle of utility itself. Consequently, I will mainly be concerned with Rule Utilitarianism, rather than Act Utilitarianism (the latter being the view that the rightness or wrongness of a given act depends solely upon whether it maximizes utility). For an original and interesting attempt to show that Act Utilitarianism is compatible with social norms that bar direct appeals to utility, see [10].

2 Rawls sometimes refers to the "Principle of Equality of Fair Opportunity" and sometimes to the "Principle of Fair Equality of Opportunity." For convenience I will stay with the former label.

3 The phrase "worst off" refers to those who are worst off with respect to prospects of the social primary goods regulated by the Difference Principle.

4 For a detailed elaboration of this point, see [1].

5 For a fundamental objection to Nozick's invisible hand explanation, see [11].

6 P. Singer [12], expanding an argument developed earlier by R. Titmuss, argues that the existence of markets for certain goods may in fact undermine the motivation for charity.

7 See [2].

8 I would like to thank Earl Shelp and William Hanson for their very helpful comments on an earlier draft of this paper.

REFERENCES

1 Buchanan, A. "Revisability and Rational Choice." *Canadian Journal of Philosophy* 5:395–408, 1975.

2 Daniels, N. "Rights to Health Care and Distributive Justice: Programmatic Worries." *Journal of Medicine and Philosophy* 4:174–191, 1979.

3 Friedman, M. *Capitalism and Freedom.* Chicago: University of Chicago Press, 1962, pp. 137–160.

4 Kant, I. *Foundations of the Metaphysics of Morals* (transl. by L. W. Beck), New York: Bobbs-Merrill, 1959, Part III.

5 Nozick, R. *Anarchy, State and Utopia.* New York: Basic Books, 1974.

6 Rawls, J. *A Theory of Justice.* Cambridge, Mass.: Harvard University Press, 1971.

7 Rawls, J. "Fairness to Goodness." *Philosophical Review* 84:536–554, 1975.

8 Rawls, J. "Reply to Alexander and Musgrave." *Quarterly Journal of Economics* 88:633–655, November 1974.

9 Rawls, J. "Responsibility for Ends." Stanford University, Unpublished Lecture, 1979.

10 Sartorius, R. *Individual Conduct and Social Norms.* Encino, Calif.: Dickenson Publishing, 1975.

11 Sartorius, R. "The Limits of Libertarianism." In *Liberty and the Rule of Law*, edited by R. L. Cunningham, 87–131. College Station, Texas: Texas A and M University Press, 1979.

12 Singer, P. "Rights and the Market." In *Justice and Economic Distribution*, edited by J. Arthur and W. Shaw, pp. 207–221. Englewood Cliffs, N.J.: Prentice-Hall, 1978.

Autonomy, Equality and a Just Health Care System
Kai Nielsen

Kai Nielsen is professor and chair of the department of philosophy at the University of Calgary and an editor of the *Canadian Journal of Philosophy.* He is the author of *Equality and Liberty: A Defense of Radical Egalitarianism* (1985) and *Marxism and the Moral Point of View: Morality, Ideology, and Historical Materialism* (1988).

Acording to Nielsen, justice requires social institutions that work on the premise of moral equality—the life of everyone matters and matters equally. Beginning with this premise and an analysis of basic needs, Nielsen argues that individuals have a moral right to have their health-care needs met. Furthermore, on his account, a commitment to egalitarianism is incompatible with a two- or three-tier system of medical care. Moral equality requires the open and free provision of medical treatment of the same extent and quality to everyone in society. In his view, a system intended to achieve this end would have to take medicine out of the private sector altogether and place both the ownership and control of medicine in the public sector.

Reprinted with permission of the publisher from *The International Journal of Applied Philosophy*, vol. 4 (Spring 1989), pp. 39–44.

I

Autonomy and equality are both fundamental values in our firmament of values, and they are frequently thought to be in conflict. Indeed the standard liberal view is that we must make difficult and often morally ambiguous trade-offs between them.[1] I shall argue that this common view is mistaken and that autonomy cannot be widespread or secure in a society which is not egalitarian: where, that is, equality is not also a very fundamental value which has an operative role within the society.[2] I shall further argue that, given human needs and a commitment to an autonomy respecting egalitarianism, a very different health care system would come into being than that which exists at present in the United States.

I shall first turn to a discussion of autonomy and equality and then, in terms of those conceptions, to a conception of justice. In modernizing societies of Western Europe, a perfectly just society will be a society of equals and in such societies there will be a belief held across the political spectrum in what has been called *moral* equality. That is to say, when viewed with the impartiality required by morality, the life of everyone matters and matters equally.[3] Individuals will, of course, and rightly so, have their local attachments but they will acknowledge that justice requires that the social institutions of the society should be such that they work on the premise that the life of everyone matters and matters equally. Some privileged elite or other group cannot be given special treatment simply because they are that group. Moreover, for there to be a society of equals there must be a rough equality of condition in the society. Power must be sufficiently equally shared for it to be securely the case that no group or class or gender can dominate others through the social structures either by means of their frequently thoroughly unacknowledged latent functions or more explicitly and manifestly by institutional arrangements sanctioned by law or custom. Roughly equal material resources or power are not things which are desirable in themselves, but they are essential instrumentalities for the very possibility of equal well-being and for as many people as possible having as thorough and as complete a control over their own lives as is compatible with this being true for everyone alike. Liberty cannot flourish without something approaching this equality of condition, and people without autonomous lives will surely live impoverished lives. These are mere commonplaces. In fine, a commitment to achieving equality of condition, far from undermining

liberty and autonomy, is essential for their extensive flourishing.

If we genuinely believe in moral equality, we will want to see come into existence a world in which all people capable of self-direction have, and have as nearly as is feasible equally, control over their own lives and can, as far as the institutional arrangements for it obtaining are concerned, all live flourishing lives where their needs and desires as individuals are met as fully as possible and as fully and extensively as is compatible with that possibility being open to everyone alike. The thing is to provide institutional arrangements that are conducive to that.

People, we need to remind ourselves, plainly have different capacities and sensibilities. However, even in the extreme case of people for whom little in the way of human flourishing is possible, their needs and desires, as far as possible, should still also be satisfied in the way I have just described. Everyone in this respect at least has equal moral standing. No preference or pride of place should be given to those capable, in varying degrees, of rational self-direction. The more rational, or, for that matter, the more loveable, among us should not be given preference. No one should. Our needs should determine what is to be done.

People committed to achieving and sustaining a society of equals will seek to bring into stable existence conditions such that it would be possible for everyone, if they were personally capable of it, to enjoy an equally worthwhile and satisfying life or at least a life in which, for all of them, their needs, starting with and giving priority to their more urgent needs, were met and met as equally and as fully as possible, even where their needs are not entirely the same needs. This, at least, is the heuristic, though we might, to gain something more nearly feasible, have to scale down talk of meeting needs to providing conditions propitious for the equal satisfaction for everyone of their *basic* needs. Believers in equality want to see a world in which everyone, as far as this is possible, have equal whole life prospects. This requires an equal consideration of their needs and interests and a refusal to just override anyone's interests: to just regard anyone's interests as something which comes to naught, which can simply be set aside as expendable. Minimally, an egalitarian must believe that taking the moral point of view requires that each person's good is afforded equal consideration. Moreover, this is not just a bit of egalitarian ideology but is a deeply embedded considered judgment in modern Western culture capable of being put into wide reflective equilibrium.[4]

II

What is a need, how do we identify needs and what are our really basic needs, needs that are presumptively universal? Do these basic needs in most circumstances at least trump our other needs and our reflective considered preferences?

Let us start this examination by asking if we can come up with a list of universal needs correctly ascribable to all human beings in all cultures. In doing this we should, as David Braybrooke has, distinguish *adventitious* and *course-of-life* needs.[5] Moreover, it is the latter that it is essential to focus on. Adventitious needs, like the need for a really good fly rod or computer, come and go with particular projects. Course-of-life needs, such as the need for exercise, sleep or food, are such that every human being may be expected to have them all at least at some stage of life.

Still, we need to step back a bit and ask: how do we determine what is a need, course-of-life need or otherwise? We need a relational formula to spot needs. We say, where we are speaking of needs, B needs x in order to y, as in Janet needs milk or some other form of calcium in order to protect her bone structure. With course-of-life needs the relation comes out platitudinously as in 'People need food and water in order to live' or 'People need exercise in order to function normally or well'. This, in the very identification of the need, refers to human flourishing or to human well-being, thereby giving to understand that they are basic needs. Perhaps it is better to say instead that this is to specify in part what it is for something to be a basic need. Be that as it may, there are these basic needs we *must* have to live well. If this is really so, then, where they are things we as individuals can have without jeopardy to others, no further question arises, or can arise, about the desirability of satisfying them. They are just things that in such circumstances ought to be met in our lives if they can. The satisfying of such needs is an unequivocally good thing. The questions 'Does Janet need to live?' and 'Does Sven need to function well?' are at best otiose.

In this context David Braybrooke has quite properly remarked that being "essential to living or to functioning normally may be taken as a criterion for being a basic need. Questions about whether needs are genuine, or well-founded, come to an end of the line when the needs have been connected with life or health."[6] Certainly to flourish we must have these things and in some instances they must be met at least to a certain extent

even to survive. This being so, we can quite properly call them basic needs. Where these needs do not clash or the satisfying of them by one person does not conflict with the satisfying of the equally basic needs of another no question about justifying the meeting of them arises.

By linking the identification of needs with what we must have to function well and linking course-of-life and basic needs with what all people, or at least almost all people, must have to function well, a list of basic needs can readily be set out. I shall give such a list, though surely the list is incomplete. However, what will be added is the same sort of thing similarly identified. First there are needs connected closely to our physical functioning, namely the need for food and water, the need for excretion, for exercise, for rest (including sleep), for a life supporting relation to the environment, and the need for whatever is indispensable to preserve the body intact. Similarly there are basic needs connected with our function as social beings. We have needs for companionship, education, social acceptance and recognition, for sexual activity, freedom from harassment, freedom from domination, for some meaningful work, for recreation and relaxation and the like.[7]

The list, as I remarked initially, is surely incomplete. But it does catch many of the basic things which are in fact necessary for us to live or to function well. Now an autonomy respecting egalitarian society with an interest in the well-being of its citizens—something moral beings could hardly be without—would (trivially) be a society of equals, and as a society of equals it would be committed to (a) *moral* equality and (b) an equality of *condition* which would, under conditions of moderate abundance, in turn expect the equality of condition to be rough and to be principally understood (cashed in) in terms of providing the conditions (as far as that is possible) for meeting the needs (including most centrally the basic needs) of everyone and meeting them equally, as far as either of these things is feasible.

III

What kind of health care system would such an autonomy respecting egalitarian society have under conditions of moderate abundance such as we find in Canada and the United States?

The following are health care needs which are also basic needs: being healthy and having conditions treated which impede one's functioning well or which adversely affect one's well-being or cause suffering. These are plainly things we need. Where societies have the economic and technical capacity to do so, as these societies plainly do, without undermining other equally urgent or more urgent needs, these health needs, as basic needs, must be met, and the right to have such medical care is a right for everyone in the society regardless of her capacity to pay. This just follows from a commitment to *moral* equality and to an equality of condition. Where we have the belief, a belief which is very basic in nonfascistic modernizing societies, that each person's good is to be given equal consideration, it is hard not to go in that way, given a plausible conception of needs and reasonable list of needs based on that conception.[8] If there is the need for some particular regime of care and the society has the resources to meet that need, without undermining structures protecting other at least equally urgent needs, then, *ceteris paribus*, the society, if it is a decent society, must do so. The commitment to more equality—the commitment to the belief that the life of each person matters and matters equally—entails, given a few plausible empirical premises, that each person's health needs will be the object of an equal regard. Each has an equal claim, *prima facie*, to have her needs satisfied where this is possible. That does not, of course, mean that people should all be treated alike in the sense of their all getting the same thing. Not everyone needs flu shots, braces, a dialysis machine, a psychiatrist, or a triple bypass. What should be equal is that each person's health needs should be the object of equal societal concern since each person's good should be given equal consideration.[9] This does not mean that equal energy should be directed to Hans's rash as to Frank's cancer. Here one person's need for a cure is much greater than the other, and the greater need clearly takes precedence. Both should be met where possible, but where they both cannot then the greater need has pride of place. But what should not count in the treatment of Hans and Frank is that Hans is wealthy or prestigious or creative and Frank is not. Everyone should have their health needs met where possible. Moreover, where the need is the same, they should have (where possible), and where other at least equally urgent needs are not thereby undermined, the same quality treatment. No differentiation should be made between them on the basis of their ability to pay or on the basis of their being (one more so than the other) important people. There should, in short, where this is possible, be open and free medical treatment of the same quality and extent available to everyone in the society. And no two- or three-tier system should be allowed to obtain, and treatment should only vary (subject to the above qualification) on the basis of variable needs and unavoidable differences in different places in supply and personnel, e.g., differences between town and country. Furthermore, these latter differences should be remedied where technically and economically feasible. The underlying aim should be to meet the health care needs of everyone and meet them, in the sense explicated, equally: everybody's needs here should be met as fully as possible; different treatment is only justified where the need is different or where both needs cannot be met. Special treatment for one person rather than another is only justified where, as I remarked, both needs cannot be met or cannot as adequately be met. Constrained by ought implies can; where these circumstances obtain, priority should be given to the greater need that can feasibly be met. A moral system or a social policy, plainly, cannot be reasonably asked to do the impossible. But my account does not ask that.

To have such a health care system would, I think, involve taking medicine out of the private sector altogether including, of course, out of private entrepreneurship where the governing rationale has to be profit and where supply and demand rules the roost. Instead there must be a health care system firmly in the public sector (publicly owned and controlled) where the rationale of the system is to meet as efficiently and as fully as possible the health care needs of everyone in the society in question. The health care system should not be viewed as a business anymore than a university should be viewed as a business—compare a university and a large hospital—but as a set of institutions and practices designed to meet urgent human needs.

I do not mean that we should ignore costs or efficiency. The state-run railroad system in Switzerland, to argue by analogy, is very efficient. The state cannot, of course, ignore costs in running it. But the aim is not to make a profit. The aim is to produce the most rapid, safe, efficient and comfortable service meeting travellers' needs within the parameters of the overall socio-economic priorities of the state and the society. Moreover, since the state in question is a democracy, if its citizens do not like the policies of the government here (or elsewhere) they can replace it with a government with different priorities and policies. Indeed the option is there (probably never to be exercised) to shift the railroad into the private sector.

Governments, understandably, worry with aging populations about mounting health care costs. This is slightly ludicrous in the United States, given its military and space exploration budgets, but is also a reality in Canada and even in Iceland where there is no military or space budget at all. There should, of course, be concern about containing health costs, but this can be done effectively with a state-run system. Modern societies need systems of socialized medicine, something that obtains in almost all civilized modernizing societies. The United States and South Africa are, I believe, the only exceptions. But, as is evident from my own country (Canada), socialized health care systems often need altering, and their costs need monitoring. As a cost-cutting and as an efficiency measure that would at the same time improve health care, doctors, like university professors and government bureaucrats, should be put on salaries and they should work in medical units. They should, I hasten to add, have good salaries but salaries all the same; the last vestiges of petty entrepreneurship should be taken from the medical profession. This measure would save the state-run health care system a considerable amount of money, would improve the quality of medical care with greater cooperation and consultation resulting from economies of scale and a more extensive division of labor with larger and better equipped medical units. (There would also be less duplication of equipment.) The overall quality of care would also improve with a better balance between health care in the country and in the large cities, with doctors being systematically and rationally deployed throughout the society. In such a system doctors, no more than university professors or state bureaucrats, could not just set up a practice anywhere. They would no more be free to do this than university professors or state bureaucrats. In the altered system there would be no cultural space for it. Placing doctors on salary, though not at a piece work rate, would also result in its being the case that the financial need to see as many patients as possible as quickly as possible would be removed. This would plainly enhance the quality of medical care. It would also be the case that a different sort of person would go into the medical profession. People would go into it more frequently because they were actually interested in medicine and less frequently because this is a rather good way (though hardly the best way) of building a stock portfolio.

There should also be a rethinking of the respective roles of nurses (in all their variety), paramedics and doctors. Much more of the routine work done in medicine—taking the trout fly out of my ear for example—can be done by nurses or paramedics. Doctors, with their more extensive training, could be freed up for other more demanding tasks worthy of their expertise. This would require somewhat different training for all of these different medical personnel and a rethinking of the authority structure in the health care system. But doing this in a reasonable way would improve the teamwork in hospitals, make morale all around a lot better, improve medical treatment and save a very considerable amount of money. (It is no secret that the relations between doctors and nurses are not good.) Finally, a far greater emphasis should be placed on preventative medicine than is done now. This, if really extensively done, utilizing the considerable educational and fiscal powers of the state, would result in very considerable health care savings and a very much healthier and perhaps even happier population. (Whether with the states we actually have we are likely to get anything like that is—to understate it—questionable. I wouldn't hold my breath in the United States. Still, Finland and Sweden are very different places from the United States and South Africa.)

IV

It is moves of this *general* sort that an egalitarian and autonomy loving society under conditions of moderate scarcity should implement. (I say 'general sort' for I am more likely to be wrong about some of the specifics than about the general thrust of my argument.) It would, if in place, limit the freedom of some people, including some doctors and some patients, to do what they want to do. That is obvious enough. But any society, any society at all, as long as it had norms (legal and otherwise) will limit freedom in some way.[10] There is no living in society without some limitation on the freedom to do some things. Indeed a society without norms and thus without any limitation on freedom is a contradiction in terms. Such a mass of people wouldn't be a society. They, without norms, would just be a mass of people. (If these are 'grammatical remarks,' make the most of them.) In our societies I am not free to go for a spin in your car without your permission, to practice law or medicine without a license, to marry your wife while she is still your wife and the like. Many restrictions on our liberties, because they are so common, so widely accepted and thought by most of us to be so reasonable, hardly *seem* like restrictions on our liberty. But they are all the same. No doubt some members of the medical profession would feel quite reined in if the measures I propose were adopted. (These measures are not part of conventional wisdom.) But the restrictions on the freedom of the medical profession and on patients I am proposing would make for both a greater liberty all around, everything considered, and, as well, for greater well-being in the society. Sometimes we have to restrict certain liberties in order to enhance the overall system of liberty. Not speaking out of turn in parliamentary debate is a familiar example. Many people who now have a rather limited access to medical treatment would come to have it and have it in a more adequate way with such a socialized system in place. Often we have to choose between a greater or lesser liberty in a society, and, at least under conditions of abundance, the answer almost always should be 'Choose the greater liberty'. If we really prize human autonomy, if, that is, we want a world in which as many people as possible have as full as is possible control over their own lives, then we will be egalitarians. Our very egalitarianism will commit us to something like the health care system I described, but so will the realization that, without reasonable health on the part of the population, autonomy can hardly flourish or be very extensive. Without the kind of equitability and increased coverage in health care that goes with a properly administered socialized medicine, the number of healthy people will be far less than could otherwise feasibly be the case. With that being the case, autonomy and well-being as well will be neither as extensive nor so thorough as it could otherwise be. Autonomy, like everything else, has its material conditions. And to will the end is to will the necessary means to the end.

To take—to sum up—what since the Enlightenment has come to be seen as the moral point of view, and to take morality seriously, is to take it as axiomatic that each person's good be given equal consideration.[11] I have argued that (a) where that is accepted, and (b) where we are tolerably clear about the facts (including facts about human needs), and (c) where we live under conditions of moderate abundance, a health care system bearing at least a family resemblance to the one I have gestured at will be put in place. It is a health care system befitting an autonomy respecting democracy committed to the democratic and egalitarian belief that the life of everyone matters and matters equally.

NOTES

1 Isaiah Berlin, "On the Pursuit of the Ideal," *The New York Review of Books* XXXV (March 1987), pp. 11–18. See also his "Equality" in his *Concepts and Categories* (Oxford, England: Oxford University Press, 1980), pp. 81–102. I have criticized that latter paper in my "Formulating Egalitarianism: Animadversions on Berlin," *Philosophia* 13:3–4 (October 1983), pp. 299–315.

2 For three defenses of such a view see Kai Nielsen, *Equality and Liberty* (Totowa, New Jersey: Rowman and Allanheld, 1985), Richard Norman, *Free and Equal* (Oxford, England: Oxford University Press, 1987), and John Baker, *Arguing for Equality* (London: Verso Press, 1987).

3 Will Kymlicka, "Rawls on Teleology and Deontology," *Philosophy and Public Affairs* 17:3 (Summer 1988), pp. 173–190 and John Rawls, "The Priority of Right and Ideas of the Good," *Philosophy and Public Affairs* 17:4 (Fall 1988), pp. 251–276.

4 Kai Nielsen, "Searching for an Emancipatory Perspective: Wide Reflective Equilibrium and the Hermeneutical Circle" in Evan Simpson (ed.), *Anti-Foundationalism and Practical Reasoning* (Edmonton, Alberta: Academic Printing and Publishing, 1987), pp. 143–164 and Kai Nielsen, "In Defense of Wide Reflective Equilibrium" in Douglas Odegard (ed.) *Ethics and Justification* (Edmonton, Alberta: Academic Printing and Publishing, 1988), pp. 19–37.

5 David Braybrooke, *Meeting Needs* (Princeton, New Jersey: Princeton University Press, 1987), p. 29.

6 *Ibid.*, p. 31.

7 *Ibid.*, p. 37.

8 Will Kymlicka, *op cit.*, p. 190.

9 *Ibid.*

10 Ralf Dahrendorf, *Essays in the Theory of Society* (Stanford, California: Stanford University Press, 1968), pp. 151–78 and G. A. Cohen, "The Structure of Proletarian Unfreedom," *Philosophy and Public Affairs* 12 (1983), pp. 2–33.

11 Will Kymlicka, *op cit.*, p. 190.

An Ethical Framework for Access to Health Care
President's Commission for the Study of Ethical Problems in Medicine and Biomedical and Behavioral Research

A descriptive account of the President's Commission is found on page 92.

The Commission maintains that society, understood as the collective U.S. community, has an *obligation* to ensure that every member of the society is able to secure an adequate level of health care without being subject to excessive burdens. It bases this obligation on the special nature of health care, which it sees as both promoting personal well-being and broadening a person's range of opportunities. In developing its position, the Commission raises and responds to several important questions, including the following: (1) What should be the role of government in ensuring that society's obligation is met? (2) What constitutes an adequate level of health care?

Most Americans believe that because health care is special, access to it raises special ethical concerns. In part, this is because good health is by definition important to well-being. Health care can relieve pain and suffering, restore functioning, and prevent death; it can enhance good health and improve an individual's opportunity to pursue a life plan; and it can provide valuable information about a person's overall health. Beyond its practical importance, the involvement of health care with the most significant and awesome events of life—birth, illness, and death—adds a symbolic aspect to health care: it is special because it signifies not only mutual empathy and caring but the mysterious aspects of curing and healing.

Furthermore, while people have some ability—through choice of life-style and through preventive measures—to influence their health status, many health problems are beyond their control and are therefore undeserved. Besides the burdens of genetics, environment, and chance, individuals become ill because of things they do or fail to do—but it is often difficult for an individual to choose to do otherwise or even to know with enough specificity and confidence what he or she ought to do to remain healthy. Finally, the incidence and severity of ill health is distributed very unevenly among people. Basic needs for housing and food are predictable, but even the most hardworking and prudent

person may suddenly be faced with overwhelming needs for health care. Together, these considerations lend weight to the belief that health care is different from most other goods and services. In a society concerned not only with fairness and equality of opportunity but also with the redemptive powers of science, there is a felt obligation to ensure that some level of health services is available to all....

THE SPECIAL IMPORTANCE OF HEALTH CARE

Although the importance of health care may, at first blush, appear obvious, this assumption is often based on instinct rather than reasoning. Yet it is possible to step back and examine those properties of health care that lead to the ethical conclusion that it ought to be distributed equitably.

Well-Being

Ethical concern about the distribution of health care derives from the special importance of health care in promoting personal well-being by preventing or relieving pain, suffering, and disability and by avoiding loss of life. The fundamental importance of the latter is obvious; pain and suffering are also experiences that people have strong desires to avoid, both because of the intrinsic quality of the experience and because of their effects on the capacity to pursue and achieve other goals and

Reprinted from President's Commission for the Study of Ethical Problems in Medicine and Biomedical and Behavioral Research, *Securing Access to Health Care*, Volume One (1983), pp. 11–12, 16–21, 22–23, 31–33, 34–38.

purposes. Similarly, untreated disability can prevent people from leading rewarding and fully active lives.

Health, insofar as it is the absence of pain, suffering, or serious disability, is what has been called a primary good, that is, there is no need to know what a particular person's other ends, preferences, and values are in order to know that health is good for that individual. It generally helps people carry out their life plans, whatever they may happen to be. This is not to say that everyone defines good health in the same way or assigns the same weight or importance to different aspects of being healthy, or to health in comparison with the other goods of life. Yet though people may differ over each of these matters, their disagreement takes place within a framework of basic agreement on the importance of health. Likewise, people differ in their beliefs about the value of health and medical care and their use of it as a means of achieving good health, as well as in their attitudes toward the various benefits and risks of different treatments.

Opportunity

Health care can also broaden a person's range of opportunities, that is, the array of life plans that is reasonable to pursue within the conditions obtaining in society. In the United States equality of opportunity is a widely accepted value that is reflected throughout public policy. The effects that meeting (or failing to meet) people's health needs have on the distribution of opportunity in a society become apparent if diseases are thought of as adverse departures from a normal level of functioning. In this view, health care is that which people need to maintain or restore normal functioning or to compensate for inability to function normally. Health is thus comparable in importance to education in determining the opportunities available to people to pursue different life plans.

Information

The special importance of health care stems in part from its ability to relieve worry and to enable patients to adjust to their situation by supplying reliable information about their health. Most people do not understand the true nature of a health problem when it first develops. Health professionals can then perform the worthwhile function of informing people about their conditions and about the expected prognosis with or without various treatments. Though information sometimes creates concern, often it reassures patients either by ruling out a feared disease or by revealing the self-limiting nature of a condition and, thus, the lack of need for further treatment. Although health care in many situations may thus not be necessary for good physical health, a great deal of relief from unnecessary concern—and even avoidance of pointless or potentially harmful steps—is achieved by health care in the form of expert information provided to worried patients. Even when a prognosis is unfavorable and health professionals have little treatment to offer, accurate information can help patients plan how to cope with their situation.

The Interpersonal Significance of Illness, Birth, and Death

It is no accident that religious organizations have played a major role in the care of the sick and dying and in the process of birth. Since all human beings are vulnerable to disease and all die, health care has a special interpersonal significance: it expresses and nurtures bonds of empathy and compassion. The depth of a society's concern about health care can be seen as a measure of its sense of solidarity in the face of suffering and death. Moreover, health care takes on special meaning because of its role in the beginning of a human being's life as well as the end. In spite of all the advances in the scientific understanding of birth, disease, and death, these profound and universal experiences remain shared mysteries that touch the spiritual side of human nature. For these reasons a society's commitment to health care reflects some of its most basic attitudes about what it is to be a member of the human community.

THE CONCEPT OF EQUITABLE ACCESS TO HEALTH CARE

The special nature of health care helps to explain why it ought to be accessible, in a fair fashion, to all. But if this ethical conclusion is to provide a basis for evaluating current patterns of access to health care and proposed health policies, the meaning of fairness or equity in this context must be clarified. The concept of equitable access needs definition in its two main aspects: the level of care that ought to be available to all and the extent to which burdens can be imposed on those who obtain these services.

Access to What?

"Equitable access" could be interpreted in a number of ways: equality of access, access to whatever an individual needs or would benefit from, or access to an adequate level of care.

Equity as Equality   It has been suggested that equity is achieved either when everyone is assured of receiving an equal quantity of health care dollars or when people enjoy equal health. The most common characterization of equity as equality, however, is as providing everyone with the same level of health care. In this view, it follows that if a given level of care is available to one individual it must be available to all. If the initial standard is set high, by reference to the highest level of care presently received, an enormous drain would result on the resources needed to provide other goods. Alternatively, if the standard is set low in order to avoid an excessive use of resources, some beneficial services would have to be withheld from people who wished to purchase them. In other words, no one would be allowed access to more services or services of higher quality than those available to everyone else, even if he or she were willing to pay for those services from his or her personal resources.

As long as significant inequalities in income and wealth persist, inequalities in the use of health care can be expected beyond those created by differences in need. Given people with the same pattern of preferences and equal health care needs, those with greater financial resources will purchase more health care. Conversely, given equal financial resources, the different patterns of health care preferences that typically exist in any population will result in a different use of health services by people with equal health care needs. Trying to prevent such inequalities would require interfering with people's liberty to use their income to purchase an important good like health care while leaving them free to use it for frivolous or inessential ends. Prohibiting people with higher incomes or stronger preferences for health care from purchasing more care than everyone else gets would not be feasible, and would probably result in a black market for health care.

Equity as Access Solely According to Benefit or Need

Interpreting equitable access to mean that everyone must receive all health care that is of any benefit to them also has unacceptable implications. Unless health is the only good or resources are unlimited, it would be irrational for a society—as for an individual—to make a commitment to provide whatever health care might be beneficial regardless of cost. Although health care is of special importance, it is surely not all that is important to people. Pushed to an extreme, this criterion might swallow up all of society's resources, since there is virtually no end to the funds that could be devoted to possibly beneficial care for diseases and disabilities and to their prevention.

Equitable access to health care must take into account not only the benefits of care but also the cost in comparison with other goods and services to which those resources might be allocated. Society will reasonably devote some resources to health care but reserve most resources for other goals. This, in turn, will mean that some health services (even of a lifesaving sort) will not be developed or employed because they would produce too few benefits in relation to their costs and to the other ways the resources for them might be used.

It might be argued that the notion of "need" provides a way to limit access to only that care that confers especially important benefits. In this view, equity as access according to need would place less severe demands on social resources than equity according to benefit would. There are, however, difficulties with the notion of need in this context. On the one hand, medical need is often not narrowly defined but refers to any condition for which medical treatment might be effective. Thus, "equity as access according to need" collapses into "access according to whatever is of benefit."

On the other hand, "need" could be even more expansive in scope than "benefit." Philosophical and economic writings do not provide any clear distinction between "needs" and "wants" or "preferences." Since the term means different things to different people, "access according to need" could become "access to any health service a person wants." Conversely, need could be interpreted very narrowly to encompass only a very minimal level of services—for example, those "necessary to prevent death."

Equity as an Adequate Level of Health Care   Although neither "everything needed" nor "everything beneficial" nor "everything that anyone else is getting" are defensible ways of understanding equitable access, the special nature of health care dictates that everyone have access to *some* level of care: enough care to achieve sufficient welfare, opportunity, information, and evidence of interpersonal concern to facilitate a reasonably full and satisfying life. That level can be termed "an adequate level of health care." The difficulty of sharpening this amorphous notion into a workable foundation for health policy is a major problem in the United States today. This concept is not new; it is implicit in the public debate over health policy and has manifested itself in the history of public policy in this country. In this chapter, the Commission attempts to demonstrate the value of the concept, to clarify its content, and to apply it to the problems facing health policymakers.

Understanding equitable access to health care to mean that everyone should be able to secure an adequate level of care has several strengths. Because an adequate level of care may be less than "all beneficial care" and because it does not require that all needs be satisfied, it acknowledges the need for setting priorities within health care and signals a clear recognition that society's resources are limited and that there are other goods besides health. Thus, interpreting equity as access to adequate care does not generate an open-ended obligation. One of the chief dangers of interpretations of equity that require virtually unlimited resources for health care is that they encourage the view that equitable access is an impossible ideal. Defining equity as an adequate level of care for all avoids an impossible commitment of resources without falling into the opposite error of abandoning the enterprise of seeking to ensure that health care is in fact available for everyone.

In addition, since providing an adequate level of care is a limited moral requirement, this definition also avoids the unacceptable restriction on individual liberty entailed by the view that equity requires equality. Provided that an adequate level is available to all, those who prefer to use their resources to obtain care that exceeds that level do not offend any ethical principle in doing so. Finally, the concept of adequacy, as the Commission understands it, is society-relative. The content of adequate care will depend upon the overall resources available in a given society, and can take into account a consensus of expectations about what is adequate in a particular society at a particular time in its historical development. This permits the definition of adequacy to be altered as societal resources and expectations change.

With What Burdens?

It is not enough to focus on the care that individuals receive; attention must be paid to the burdens they must bear in order to obtain it—waiting and travel time, the cost and availability of transport, the financial cost of the care itself. Equity requires not only that adequate care

be available to all, but also that these burdens not be excessive.

If individuals must travel unreasonably long distances, wait for unreasonably long hours, or spend most of their financial resources to obtain care, some will be deterred from obtaining adequate care, with adverse effects on their health and well-being. Others may bear the burdens, but only at the expense of their ability to meet other important needs. If one of the main reasons for providing adequate care is that health care increases welfare and opportunity, then a system that required large numbers of individuals to forego food, shelter, or educational advancement in order to obtain care would be self-defeating and irrational.

The concept of acceptable burdens in obtaining care, as opposed to excessive ones, parallels in some respects the concept of adequacy. Just as equity does not require equal access, neither must the burdens of obtaining adequate care be equal for all persons. What is crucial is that the variations in burdens fall within an acceptable range. As in determining an adequate level of care, there is no simple formula for ascertaining when the burdens of obtaining care fall within such a range. Yet some guidelines can be formulated. To illustrate, since a given financial outlay represents a greater sacrifice to a poor person than to a rich person, "excessive" must be understood in relation to income. Obviously everyone cannot live the same distance from a health care facility, and some individuals choose to locate in remote and sparsely populated areas. Concern about an inequitable burden would be appropriate, however, when identifiable groups must travel a great distance or long time to receive care—though people may appropriately be expected to travel farther to get specialized care, for example, than to obtain primary or emergency care....

A SOCIETAL OBLIGATION

Society has a moral obligation to ensure that everyone has access to adequate care without being subject to excessive burdens. In speaking of a societal obligation the Commission makes reference to society in the broadest sense—the collective American community. The community is made up of individuals, who are in turn members of many other, overlapping groups, both public and private: local, state, regional, and national units; professional and workplace organizations; religious, educational, and charitable organizations; and family, kinship, and ethnic groups. All these entities play a role in discharging societal obligations.

The Commission believes it is important to distinguish between society, in this inclusive sense, and government as one institution among others in society. Thus the recognition of a collective or societal obligation does not imply that government should be the only or even the primary institution involved in the complex enterprise of making health care available. It is the Commission's view that the societal obligation to ensure equitable access for everyone may best be fulfilled in this country by a pluralistic approach that relies upon the coordinated contributions of actions by both the private and public sectors.

Securing equitable access is a societal rather than a merely private or individual responsibility for several reasons. First, while health is of special importance for human beings, health care—especially scientific health care—is a social product requiring the skills and efforts of many individuals; it is not something that individuals can provide for themselves solely through their own efforts. Second, because the need for health care is both unevenly distributed among persons and highly unpredictable and because the cost of securing care may be great, few individuals could secure adequate care without relying on some social mechanism for sharing the costs. Third, if persons generally deserved their health conditions or if the need for health care were fully within the individual's control, the fact that some lack adequate care would not be viewed as an inequity. But differences in health status, and hence differences in health care needs, are largely undeserved because they are, for the most part, not within the individual's control....

WHO SHOULD ENSURE THAT SOCIETY'S OBLIGATION IS MET?

The Limitations of Relying upon the Government
Although the Commission recognizes the necessity of government involvement in ensuring equity of access, it believes that such activity must be carefully crafted and implemented in order to achieve its intended purpose. Public concern about the inability of the market and of private charity to secure access to health care for all has led to extensive government involvement in the financing and delivery of health care. This involvement has come about largely as a result of ad hoc responses to specific problems; the result has been a patch-work of public initiatives at the local, state, and Federal level. These efforts have done much to make health care more widely available to all citizens, but...they have not achieved equity of access.

To a large extent, this is the result of a lack of consensus about the nature of the goal and the proper role of government in pursuing it. But to some degree, it may also be the product of the nature of government activity. In some instances, government programs (of all types, not just health-related) have not been designed well enough to achieve the purposes intended or have been subverted to serve purposes explicitly not intended.

In the case of health care, it is extremely difficult to devise public strategies that, on the one hand, do not encourage the misuse of health services and, on the other hand, are not so restrictive as to unnecessarily or arbitrarily limit available care. There is a growing concern, for example, that government assistance in the form of tax exemptions for the purchase of employment-related health insurance has led to the overuse of many services of only very marginal benefit. Similarly, government programs that pay for health care directly (such as Medicaid) have been subject to fraud and abuse by both beneficiaries and providers. Alternatively, efforts to avoid misuse and abuse have at times caused local, state, and Federal programs to suffer from excessive bureaucracy, red tape, inflexibility, and unreasonable interference in individual choice. Also, as with private charity, government programs have not always avoided the unfortunate effects on the human spirit of "discretionary benevolence," especially in those programs requiring income or means tests.

It is also possible that as the government role in health care increases, the private sector's role will decrease in unforeseen and undesired ways. For example, government efforts to ensure access to nursing home care might lead to a lessening of support from family, friends, and other private sources for people who could be cared for in their homes. Although these kinds of problems do not inevitably accompany governmental involvement, they do occur and their presence provides evidence of the need for thoughtful and careful structuring of any government enterprise.

A Right to Health Care?

Often the issue of equitable access to health care is framed in the language of rights. Some who view health care from the perspective of distributive justice argue that the considerations discussed in this chapter show not only that society has a moral obligation to provide equitable access, but also that every individual has a moral right to such access. The Commission has chosen not to develop the case for achieving equitable access through the assertion of a right to health care. Instead it has sought to frame the issues in terms of the special nature of health care and of society's moral obligation to achieve equity, without taking a position on whether the term "obligation" should be read as entailing a moral right. The Commission reaches this conclusion for several reasons: first, such a right is not legally or Constitutionally recognized at the present time; second, it is not a logical corollary of an ethical obligation of the type the Commission has enunciated; and third, it is not necessary as a foundation for appropriate governmental actions to secure adequate health care for all.

Legal Rights   Neither the Supreme Court nor any appellate court has found a constitutional right to health or to health care. However, most Federal statutes and many state statutes that fund or regulate health care have been interpreted to provide statutory rights in the form of entitlements for the intended beneficiaries of the program or for members of the group protected by the regulatory authority. As a consequence, a host of legal decisions have developed significant legal protections for program beneficiaries. These protections have prevented Federal and state agencies and private providers from withholding authorized benefits and services. They have required agencies and providers to deliver health care to eligible individuals—the poor, elderly, handicapped, children, and others....

Moral Obligations and Rights   The relationship between the concept of a moral right and that of a moral obligation is complex. To say that a person has a moral right to something is always to say that it is that person's due, that is, he or she is morally entitled to it. In contrast, the term "obligation" is used in two different senses. All moral rights imply corresponding obligations, but, depending on the sense of the term that is being used, moral obligations may or may not imply corresponding rights. In the broad sense, to say that society has a moral obligation to do something is to say that it ought morally to do that thing and that failure to do it makes society liable to serious moral criticism. This does not, however, mean that there is a corresponding right. For example, a person may have a moral obligation to help those in need, even though the needy cannot, strictly speaking, demand that person's aid as something they are due.

The government's responsibility for seeing that the obligation to achieve equity is met is independent of the existence of a corresponding moral right to health care. There are many forms of government involvement, such as enforcement of traffic rules or taxation to support national defense, to protect the environment, or to promote biomedical research, that do not presuppose corresponding moral rights but that are nonetheless legitimate and almost universally recognized as such. In a democracy, at least, the people may assign to government the responsibility for seeing that important collective obligations are met, provided that doing so does not violate important moral rights.

As long as the debate over the ethical assessment of patterns of access to health care is carried on simply by the assertion and refutation of a "right to health care," the debate will be incapable of guiding policy. At the very least, the nature of the right must be made clear and competing accounts of it compared and evaluated. Moreover, if claims of rights are to guide policy they must be supported by sound ethical reasoning and the connections between various rights must be systematically developed, especially where rights are potentially in conflict with one another. At present, however, there is a great deal of dispute among competing theories of rights, with most theories being so abstract and inadequately developed that their implications for health care are not obvious. Rather than attempt to adjudicate among competing theories of rights, the Commission has chosen to concentrate on what it believes to be the more important part of the question: what is the nature of the societal obligation, which exists whether or not people can claim a corresponding right to health care, and how should this societal obligation be fulfilled?

MEETING THE SOCIETAL OBLIGATION

How Much Care Is Enough?

Before the concept of an adequate level of care can be used as a tool to evaluate patterns of access and efforts to improve equity, it must be fleshed out. Since there is no objective formula for doing this, reasonable people can disagree about whether particular patterns and policies meet the demands of adequacy. The Commission does not attempt to spell out in detail what adequate care should include. Rather it frames the terms in which those who discuss or critique health care issues can consider ethics as well as economics, medical science, and other dimensions.

Characteristics of Adequacy First, the Commission considers it clear that health care can only be judged adequate in relation to an individual's health condition. To begin with a list of techniques or procedures, for example, is not sensible: A CT scan for an accident victim with a serious head injury might be the best way to make a diagnosis essential for the appropriate treatment of that patient; a CT scan for a person with headaches might not be considered essential for adequate care. To focus only on the technique, therefore, rather than on the individual's health and the impact the procedure will have on that individual's welfare and opportunity, would lead to inappropriate policy.

Disagreement will arise about whether the care of some health conditions falls within the demands of adequacy. Most people will agree, however, that some conditions should not be included in the societal obligation to ensure access to adequate care. A relatively uncontroversial example would be changing the shape of a functioning, normal nose or retarding the normal effects of aging (through cosmetic surgery). By the same token, there are some conditions, such as pregnancy, for which care would be regarded as an important component of adequacy. In determining adequacy, it is important to consider how people's welfare, opportunities, and requirements for information and interpersonal caring are affected by their health condition.

Any assessment of adequacy must consider also the types, amounts, and quality of care necessary to respond to each health condition. It is important to emphasize that these questions are implicitly comparative: the standard of adequacy for a condition must reflect the fact that resources used for it will not be available to respond to other conditions. Consequently, the level of care deemed adequate should reflect a reasoned judgment not only about the impact of the condition on the welfare and opportunity of the individual but also about the efficacy and the cost of the care itself in relation to other conditions and the efficacy and cost of the care that is available for them. Since individual cases differ so much, the health care professional and patient must be flexible. Thus adequacy, even in relation to a particular health condition, generally refers to a range of options.

The Relationship of Costs and Benefits The level of care that is available will be determined by the level of resources devoted to producing it. Such allocation should reflect the benefits and costs of the care provided. It should be emphasized that these "benefits," as well as their "costs," should be interpreted broadly, and not re-

stricted only to effects easily quantifiable in monetary terms. Personal benefits include improvements in individuals' functioning and in their quality of life, and the reassurance from worry and the provision of information that are a product of health care. Broader social benefits should be included as well, such as strengthening the sense of community and the belief that no one in serious need of health care will be left without it. Similarly, costs are not merely the funds spent for a treatment but include other less tangible and quantifiable adverse consequences, such as diverting funds away from other socially desirable endeavors including education, welfare, and other social services.

There is no objectively correct value that these various costs and benefits have or that can be discovered by the tools of cost/benefit analysis. Still, such an analysis, as a recent report of the Office of Technology Assessment noted, "can be very helpful to decisionmakers because the process of analysis gives structure to the problem, allows an open consideration of all relevant effects of a decision, and forces the explicit treatment of key assumptions."[1] But the valuation of the various effects of alternative treatments for different conditions rests on people's values and goals, about which individuals will reasonably disagree. In a democracy, the appropriate values to be assigned to the consequences of policies must ultimately be determined by people expressing their values through social and political processes as well as in the marketplace.

Approximating Adequacy The intention of the Commission is to provide a frame of reference for policymakers, not to resolve these complex questions. Nevertheless, it is possible to raise some of the specific issues that should be considered in determining what constitutes adequate care. It is important, for example, to gather accurate information about and compare the costs and effects, both favorable and unfavorable, of various treatment or management options. The options that better serve the goals that make health care of special importance should be assigned a higher value. As already noted, the assessment of costs must take two factors into account: the cost of a proposed option in relation to alternative forms of care that would achieve the same goal of enhancing the welfare and opportunities of the patient, and the cost of each proposed option in terms of foregone opportunities to apply the same resources to social goals other than that of ensuring equitable access.

Furthermore, a reasonable specification of adequate care must reflect an assessment of the relative importance of many different characteristics of a given form of care for a particular condition. Sometimes the problem is posed as: What *amounts* of care and what *quality* of care? Such a formulation reduces a complex problem to only two dimensions, implying that all care can readily be ranked as better or worse. Because two alternative forms of care may vary along a number of dimensions, there may be no consensus among reasonable and informed individuals about which form is of higher overall quality. It is worth bearing in mind that adequacy does not mean the highest possible level of quality or strictly equal quality any more than it requires equal amounts of care; of course, adequacy does require that everyone receive care that meets standards of sound medical practice.

Any combination of arrangements for achieving adequacy will presumably include some health care deliv-ery settings that mainly serve certain groups, such as the poor or those covered by public programs. The fact that patients receive care in different settings or from differ-ent providers does not itself show that some are receiv-ing inadequate care. The Commission believes that there is no moral objection to such a system so long as all re-ceive care that is adequate in amount and quality and all patients are treated with concern and respect....

NOTE

1 Office of Technology Assessment, U.S. Congress, THE IMPLICATIONS OF COST-EFFECTIVENESS ANALYSIS OF MEDICAL TECHNOLOGY, SUMMARY, U.S. Govern-ment Printing Office, Washington (1980) at 8.

Macroallocation and the Problem of Rationing

Meeting Needs and Rationing Care
Daniel Callahan

A biographical sketch of Daniel Callahan is found on page 445.

Callahan identifies two overriding but apparently contradictory needs of the health-care system in the United States: the need to provide an adequate minimal level of care for all and the need to find a permanent and effective way to control the constant escalation of health-care costs. He maintains that if both these needs are to be met, we must recognize the necessity for rationing. Callahan distinguishes between hard and soft rationing. Soft rationing is "the casual and unsystematic way in which, under the market system, some people get things that others do not." Hard rationing occurs when "choices are openly specified, and then a specific still open decision is made to choose one possible health good rather than another." Callahan con-demns soft rationing, which is the dominant form of rationing in our society, because it is often unfair. He prefers hard rationing because it is much more subject to debate and broadly considered moral judgment. Callahan argues that the standard, traditional excuses for not deal-ing directly with questions of rationing and setting limits have failed. He discusses the demo-graphic, technological, political, and moral forces that, on his view, render an expansive sys-tem of health care inevitable unless there is a fundamental change in our thinking about health care. Callahan concludes by advancing three propositions for public debate: (1) We must rec-ognize that we cannot hope to meet all individual needs and expectations in the area of human health. (2) We should shift the focus of national attention from individual to social need. (3) We will have to set limits in many directions, and we will have to be prepared to create the kind of psychological expectations necessary to do that.

Reprinted with permission of the publisher (American Society of Law and Medicine) from *Law, Medicine, and Health Care*, vol. 16 (Winter 1988), pp. 261–266.

I think it is fair to say that there have been two overriding needs of the health care system in the United States for the past couple of decades. One of them is to provide an adequate minimal level of care for all, especially for the underinsured and for those who could be faced by catastrophic health care costs. That need points to an expansion of health care expenditures and to the creation of new programs and strategies. The second need is that of finding a permanent and effective way of controlling the constant escalation of health care costs, and of the proportion of health care costs in our overall economy. That need points to restraint and limitations, not constant expansion.

We are left, then, with two apparently contradictory needs, each pointing to a major problem, but each standing, it would seem, directly in the path of the other. To look at the matter from another perspective, let me suggest the following two propositions: We should not further expand entitlement programs until we have found some way to set limits to the growth of the system; and we should not set limits on the system until we have found some way of meeting unmet needs. How in the world can we combine such disparate needs, as well as such contradictory goals? I believe the answer to that question lies in recognizing the necessity for rationing, for a fresh and more circumscribed understanding of the nature of the health care system, and for a guaranteed level of care for all. That possibility lies in creating a system that begins turning inward upon itself rather than continuing to expand outward; and that process of turning inward will provide the possible key to setting an acceptable set of boundaries to the health care system. The most important point at the outset, however, is to recognize the need quite openly to ration health care.

Let me make some necessary distinctions about the use of the word "rationing." There is a standard distinction made between allocation and rationing. Allocation is often taken to refer to the relative weight and role to be given health in the distribution of resources across a variety of social areas, including education, defense, housing, and so on. Rationing, by contrast, involves making distinctions within a particular category, in this case health, deciding which needs are comparatively more or less important and should be dealt with first. To those distinctions, I would add a distinction between "soft" and "hard" rationing. By soft rationing I mean the casual and unsystematic way in which, under the market system, some people get things that others do not. There are no conscious choices made about rationing but the combination of interest group pressures and market forces means that some will have things that others do not have. Soft rationing might also be understood to include the use of covert or tacit methods of making decisions; things simply happen without public debate, but manipulations nonetheless are going on which make a difference in who gets what. Hard rationing, by contrast, would occur in those situations where choices are openly specified, and then a specific, still open decision is made to choose one possible health good rather than another.

In our own American situation, soft rationing is the most common reality. It is very rare—as in Oregon in 1987—that an open decision is made to provide one good rather than another (i.e., prenatal care rather than organ transplantation for Medicaid beneficiaries). Soft rationing is usually preferred because it is less conspicuous, and thus less politically volatile. Soft rationing by means of bureaucratic manipulation seems, moreover, to be significantly on the rise. The increasing difficulty of people gaining Medicare or other forms of entitlements which are their right because of bureaucratic impediments put in their way is a good example of this. The discharge of patients from hospitals who are not medically ready to leave could also be seen as an instance of soft rationing.

Soft rationing is often unfair, and we need to limit it significantly. It is not publicly open and accountable, depends on decisions made by a few, and does not open up the possibility of alternative choices being made. There is no doubt that in many ways hard rationing is more painful, because more obvious and open; but it is also likely to be much more subject to debate and broadly considered moral judgment.

One might well ask why there is any need to discuss rationing, or even to have any serious discussion about the allocation of resources. The most obvious reason is that expenditures on health care in this country now exceed $500 billion, that they have been increasing at a rate far in excess of the general pace of inflation, and that they show no signs of leveling off in the near future. At the same time, there are between 35 and 40 million people who are uninsured, and the number who are uninsured—or not sufficiently insured—continues to rise. For those faced with catastrophic illnesses, or the need for long-term care, the problems are obvious, dramatically and painfully so.

Behind those statistics lies the well-recognized fact that fewer and fewer individuals are able to pay for high technology medicine out of their own pocket, and that some significant forms of social support and entitlements are necessary, whether through employer insurance plans or public entitlement programs. At the same time, the increase in life expectancy and the increased incremental cost of adding further healthy life to the years we already have adds to our problems. That the most significant remaining set of lethal diseases—cancer, heart disease, and stroke—are chronic diseases rather than acute means that the cost of their control is very high both individually and collectively. The question before us now as a nation is whether the cost of our collective care, not just our individual care, may run beyond our social resources. I believe that is the situation.

Until a few years ago, it was possible to deny the existence of a real problem altogether. It was widely believed that a successful program of cost-containment would effectively deal with the economic stress upon the system. The most common phrase was that of "cutting the fat," and any number of studies appeared to show that significant savings could be made by greater efficiency, savings in the vicinity of $40–60 billion a year. It was assumed that there was no deep issue but simply a problem of manipulating the system better, providing in particular the necessary incentives and disincentives to bring about more efficient health care delivery.

It is beginning to become obvious, however, that cost containment has failed as a general movement. That movement has been going on in this country since at least 1970, with the beginning of the Nixon administration, and has yet to show any significant success. Just about every reform method introduced within the past decade or so to bring down costs, or to contain costs, has failed. Increased competition was thought by the Reagan Administration to be one method of doing that, but it has become evident that competition among providers increases costs rather than decreases them. It was also believed that a greater control by corporations over the way they purchased health care would make a great difference. In 1988, despite those efforts, health care costs for corporations increased anywhere from 20–70 percent. The DRG system, introduced in the early 1980s to control hospital costs, has been a relative success so far as the cost of in-patient care is concerned. What it has also done, however, is simply to push many patients out of hospitals sooner and into either out-patient care or nursing home settings. Total costs have remained about the same; they have just been pushed from one place to another. Other methods of cost containment—HMOs, for instance—have not been noticeably successful either.

One mistake that has been made with all of these methods has been to assume that they could be effective without requiring severe restrictions, not unlike rationing: a required change in physician and patient standards, for example, and all of the severity associated

with difficult choices. In addition, under the assumption that the problem is simply one of efficiency, there has been an evasion of the nasty reality that effective control of costs requires a significant institutional control of behavior. There has, finally, been a great confusion between the possibility of controlling costs and the probability of doing so; optimistic prospects for the former have distracted attention from the latter, where optimism is less justified.

Another reason for denying the necessity of severe rationing and the setting of limits has been the belief that it makes no difference if the percentage of the gross national product devoted to health care rises. So what if we go from 11 percent—the present figure—to 14 or 15 percent, or even 20 percent? An answer is that such a rise means that money must be transferred from other sources of our social life and expenditures, and that will be done without adequate discussion of whether it is a good or wise change. Moreover, there are at least some prominent economists who have argued that a constant increase in expenditures for health care does not represent a good national investment. It represents essentially consumption investment rather than the kind that creates new wealth.

Another diversionary argument is that we live in a society that is wasteful, both in private and public consumption. The Department of Defense spends well over $300 billion a year, and much of that is notoriously wasted, lining the pockets of the defense industry. Why should we pick on health care needs when that goes on? The obvious answer is that we have a political system that allows people, through their elected president and representatives, to choose defense as a way of allocating resources. While there is indeed much waste in the Department of Defense, the simple fact of the matter is that in 1980 the United States elected a President whose plank was to increase defense expenditures and to lower spending on domestic welfare programs. There is no reason to believe that, in 1988 or shortly thereafter, the American people are prepared for any significant decrease in defense expenditures; and in any event they have a right to make those choices under our system. That money is wasted on cosmetics and other trivia is no less true, but it should be evident that people desire to spend money on things other than health in this country; and, again, they have a right to do so. We may deplore these choices—and I am prepared to deplore them—but they are real, a part of life in a democratic society.

There is a last illusion to be shattered. There has been a long-standing assumption that the public is seriously enough concerned about health care needs to spend much more on them, and particularly to spend more tax money. Any number of surveys over the years seem to have indicated just that. More recent surveys indicate, however, that while people are enthused about providing health care for all, for supporting catastrophic health care costs, for improving long-term care, and for a lengthy shopping list of other health care needs, there is actually a significant limitation on their willingness to pay the additional costs. Here the American people seem to be caught in a situation of utter contradiction: they say they want more, but they do not seem to be willing to pay more of their tax money to get it. Legislators well recognize this, and it helps to explain why they have been reluctant to vote more money for health care needs, however popular it might seem such expenditures would be.

All of this is simply to say that the traditional, and standard, excuses for not dealing directly with questions of rationing and setting limits have now failed. There are few reasons to be optimistic that greater efficiency is going to be the answer, or that people are going to be willing to pay significantly higher taxes, or that it would be wise to casually let investment in health care grow as a proportion of our gross national product. Put another way: the time for rationalization is over and we must take seriously the problem of rationing.

We still must ask, however, just why we have a problem, and it is important here to set aside a number of the reasons most commonly believed. Among those reasons are, most notably, a widespread public belief that the high fees of doctors represent the major problem. But doctors' fees represent about 20 percent of health care expenditures in this country, and it has been estimated that, at best, a significant reduction in physicians' fees would bring about no more than a 4 or 5 percent drop in costs. Even if that could happen, there is now a severe shortage of nurses, and the necessity of increasing their pay would be more than likely to offset any gains from a reduction in physicians' fees. There is also a growing shortage of medical technicians, and they will also require higher salaries if they are to be retained once they have been added to the health care work force.

There is no doubt that malpractice worries lead physicians to overdiagnose, and to overtreat, and sometimes to employ useless treatment. But there is no evidence to suggest that a significant relief of worry on the part of physicians would make a genuinely dramatic difference in health care costs, though it would no doubt help. And of course there is waste in the system, and a reduction of that waste could greatly help as well. But when one is looking at health care costs that are increasing at an annual rate two or three times that of inflation, one must be very wary of any belief that some specific set of reforms is going to make a decisive difference.

The unfortunate reality behind the increase in costs is simply that some important structural features drive up costs, not one of which is going to yield itself to any simple solution. The aging of the population has to have a high place among those features, not so much because people are getting older as such, but because there is a steady intensification of care—more technology more intensively applied—with older patients. Technological development, with its constant emphasis on change and improvement, and its constant desire for increased profits, is also a significant reason for increased costs. The drive to find improved ways of delivering care, and the reliance upon technological means to do that, are powerful and central parts of our health care system. To the reality of demographic change and constant technological development must be added the broad range of interest group demands that are part of the system as well: there are the demands of health care workers, of medical suppliers and technology producers, of the various groups looking for cures to assorted diseases, and of the large number of other people who have a stake in the delivery of health care. Those interest groups are for the most part intent simply on getting *more* and *more*, and it is in the very nature of the interest groups system that they do not coordinate their efforts, much less give way to each other to allow the setting of national priorities.

The most important source of increased costs, however, underlying all of the others, is that of public demand. Public demand might simply be understood as the powerful desire of people to have more and better health care. Not only is demand very powerful, but we have expanded the scope of health care—which now encompasses mental health and substance abuse—and at the same time we have seen a constant expansion of what counts as a "need" and of the acceptability of moving desires into the category of needs. We have developed almost unlimited expectations about good health, and at the same time those expectations have continued to run ahead of whatever the actual state of health is. There is good evidence that people now feel no healthier or better off than they did some decades ago, despite the fact that they are indeed healthier and that more of their earlier expressed needs are being met. But the very nature of public demand, stimulated by technological development, is such that more is always wanted.

Behind that desire for more lie some fundamental American values. We typically put freedom of choice higher than justice on our scale of political values. Our health care system has been one which seems to believe that the patient should have as many free choices as possible, and that physicians and other health care workers should have as much freedom as possible in providing that care. Any restraints, either on patients or providers, are considered a fundamental insult to our values, and they have rarely been accepted without a great deal of muttering and a sense of betrayal. When a desire for maximal freedom is combined with interest group politics one has a set of values that is expansive of its very nature. To that emphasis more recently has been added a focus on "quality" health care. It is assumed that, somehow, we are to meet everyone's needs, do so in an efficient way, and yet provide constantly improved "quality." All of that is combined with very strong resistance to government control, to any very formal evaluation and assessment of "quality," and even to specifying a very clear definition of the term.

When one looks at the dynamic behind the American health care system, then, one sees a powerful set of forces, both structural, and political. The combination of demographic, technological, and political and moral forces is such that an expansive system is and remains inevitable.

In trying to think about this dynamic, I find it helpful to categorize the problems we face in our health care system at three levels. The first might be termed the "technical" level. I refer to the various institutions, mechanisms, and systems already in place to deliver health care. The second level might be termed the "entitlement" level. Here we make decisions about who is entitled to what kind of care at government expense, who should pay for it out of their own pocket, and what is a fair way of allocating resources. The third level I think of as that of our "way of life." By that I mean the combination of our political values, our understanding of health and its place in our individual and national life, and our understanding of illness, decline, and death.

In trying to devise a strategy for our health care problems, it is useful to look at the way we have dealt with those three levels. Almost all of the serious efforts in health care reform have taken place at the first level, the technical. It is at that level that we have put in place cost containment programs and mechanisms of incentives and disincentives to control provider behavior. We have also set up various delivery experiments, such as HMOs and competitive strategies, and have worked to deal with various financing mechanisms. This is the level at which politicians and administrators feel most comfortable. It is the level of incremental change, of political negotiation, and of the avoidance of deep, disturbing

moral questions, questions that begin to touch on some fundamental American political and social values. The problem, of course, is that we have failed very badly in dealing with the problem at that level. What we have tried to do is tinker ourselves into good shape at the technical level, and that tinkering has been a notable failure so far.

There have also been efforts made to manipulate the second level, that of entitlements. We have seen changes in the various formulas for Medicare entitlements, with shifts in the amount of money required out of pocket, and various changes in conditions for receiving Medicare support. The same has been true of Medicaid, and over the years it has become obvious that a diminishing proportion of people who live below the poverty line have in fact been eligible at the state level to receive support for their health care needs. Because of the concern about growing health care costs, and probably because of perceptions that public tolerance for increased taxes is not very great, there have been very few efforts to expand entitlement programs. Those few efforts have been primarily attempts to modify, tinker with, and manipulate the present programs.

Modifications solely at the technical and the entitlement levels are insufficient. The forces facing the system are far too great to be dealt with significantly at those levels alone; something more is needed. Our ultimate problem really lies with our way of life. Unless we get ourselves straight at that level we cannot solve the problems at the other levels. We will not be able to work out the large entitlement issues, much less find a way at the technical level to manipulate the system into good shape. Any ultimate solution will involve all three levels, but it is becoming increasingly clear that the crucial and determining level is that of the third level.

At that level we must change public opinion and expectations about what we can afford and what we need in the way of health care. We must scale down our aspirations for good health and for high quality care. We must learn to manage and severely control our technological expectations and desires. We must learn to live within our economic means, and to do that we must learn to change our way of life.

But how are we to bring about a change at so deep, and difficult, a level as that of our entire "way of life"? I can offer no simple way of achieving that, but would simply note that—under public pressure, and in the presence of strong public debate—we have been able over a period of decades to make deep changes in American values on other crucial issues in the recent past. Think of the change in values on civil rights, feminism, and environmental issues, for example, over the past 20 to 30 years. There is no reason in principle we cannot do that now with health care. We will have to accept some significant changes in the way we think about health care, about its place in our private lives and its place in our societal, communal lives.

Let me propose some propositions for debate. They are of increasing severity in the demands they might place upon us, but they are necessary for consideration if we are to make progress here.

The first proposition is that we cannot hope to meet all individual needs and expectations in the area of human health. Our thirst for a longer, and healthier, and happier life has become an unlimited one; we cannot slake that thirst. The human body forces limits upon us, and thus it will always be the case that our expectations will outrun real possibilities. We must recognize that final limitation, and be willing to settle for less than we now want. We must recognize also that much of what we construe as desperate individual need is very much a function of our sense of technological possibility and the malleability of the world.

Need, in short, is a function of the way we construct our social and individual world, and not something in the very nature of things. I do not believe it even possible conceptually to specify what individual "need" means anymore. It is too much a function of the state of available technology and what people think they require in order to be happy—and that is something that changes all the time. Moreover, we cannot talk in any clear way about a "right to health care," since that requires a notion of need upon which it can be based, and of the place of health in human life, neither of which we have, or are likely to have in the near future.

A second proposition is that we should shift the focus of national attention from individual to social need. The great emphasis on health care in this country has been to focus upon the meeting of individual needs. We can, however, more fundamentally and perhaps successfully ask what we need as a community. At what point does bad health begin to interfere with our collective sense of well-being and with our national prosperity? My own belief is that we already have a significantly decent level of health in this country. Increasing our average life expectancy from 75 to 85 or more will not add significantly to our national welfare or to our collective happiness. There is no good evidence that a longer life as such makes for a stronger nation or society, or that further investments in increasing our general level of health will do more than improve health for individuals, as distinguished from creating a stronger society or commu-

nity. This is certainly not to deny the needs of some underserved groups—the poor, minorities, and a large number of the elderly and disabled. Their special needs should certainly be met. One could indeed make a strong argument that it is the meeting of the needs of the underserved that should take the priority, not the improvement of general health in this country. Some groups are not able to make their full contribution to the society because of poor health. Those groups should be enabled to come up to a common standard.

The third proposition is that we will have to set limits in many directions, and we will have to be prepared to create the kind of psychological expectations necessary to do that. In Setting Limits[1] I have argued that we will probably have eventually to use age as a standard to set limits on health care entitlements for the elderly. Care for the elderly is the open, endless frontier of medicine, and there will always be needs to be met and new possibilities of improved health to be explored. Given the impossibility of solving the problem of the elderly by trying endlessly to deal with ever-changing, everescalating individual need, we will not be able to allocate resources to the elderly on that basis any more than we can successfully do so at other levels. We must then consider the possibility of trying to close off the frontier of aging by using age itself as a standard for the denial of some forms of care, at least under public entitlement programs.

At the same time, we will have to set limits on the provision of some kinds of expensive care for every other age group as well. This means, for example, coming to accept the necessity of high levels of success rates as a justification for public entitlements in the care of newborn infants, of middle-aged persons, or of people suffering from rare and unusual diseases. We simply cannot pursue an endless improvement of efficacious outcomes while trying to deal with every possible condition that affects human health.

Even though we will have to set limits on trying to meet many individual needs, we can also modify the impact of that kind of policy by trying to spend money more wisely on all those areas of life that do yield a health payoff along with other gains as well. We know that good housing, education, and income are themselves a source of good health, and thus it makes considerable sense to look at those fundamental needs of society that take care of a number of human wants while at the same time resulting in a good health dividend.

What I am suggesting is that we should now have a national debate at the third level, about the place of health in our way of life. We are not going to be able to have all the good health we want, or that science can bring us. We are not as individuals going to be able to have everything we need to flourish. We should adopt a communal standard for the provision of health, or at least to give that kind of a standard priority over our individual needs. We are going to have to limit the choice of patients and providers. We are going to have to find a way to give priority to the unmet needs of the underserved at the expense of trying to improve overall quality. We are going to have to accept the reality that we cannot pay for everything we want.

Let me return to my original proposition. There is certainly a reasonable demand to provide some minimal level of guaranteed care for all, just as there is a reasonable demand to set economic limits to the health care system. To meet those demands we should stop hoping and dreaming for bureaucratic miracles that will control our costs, or some theory of justice that will enable us, with perfect equity, to meet all individual health care needs. We should instead be willing to look to our communal needs in establishing a minimal guaranteed level for all, and at the same time be prepared to set firm upper limits to what we provide. That way we might have a system that is not inherently expansive, but one which, though it may shorten and limit our lives to less than what is theoretically or scientifically possible, may provide a more coherent, rounded system. It would be a system that provides some level of guaranteed care for all, but does not promise either to bankrupt the nation or to give health a higher priority in human life than it should have. We cannot, and should not, have the former unless we are prepared to embrace the latter.

NOTE

[1] Daniel Callahan, *Setting Limits: Medical Goals in an Aging Society* (New York: Simon and Schuster, 1987).

Age-Based Rationing

Ensuring Care, Respect, and Fairness for the Elderly
James F. Childress

A biographical sketch of James F. Childress is found on page 401.

Childress grants that in principle, under ideal conditions, some age-based rationing of health care can be compatible with the demands of justice and the overall demands of morality. However, he advances several cautionary observations. First, in our less-than-ideal world, attempts to apply some ideal theory often produce new injustices and aggravate existing injustices. Second, using age as a criterion in limiting health-care provision in our society at this time could have negative symbolic significance—the abandonment and exclusion of the elderly from communal care. Third, since our health-care policies are often shaped by our sociocultural metaphors, the dominant medical metaphor of warfare results in an inability to visualize alternative priorities in allocating health-care resources, especially for the elderly. Childress concludes by suggesting that attention to the metaphor of *nursing* might enable us to avoid some of the negative implications of the warfare metaphor and thereby enable us to envision alternative priorities.

Perhaps in the nineteenth century it was still plausible to say with Robert Browning:

Reprinted with permission of the author and the publisher from *Hastings Center Report*, vol. 14 (October 1984), pp. 27–31.

Grow old along with me
The best is yet to be
The last of life for which the first was made.

That sentiment does not ring true in the last part of the twentieth century, in part because of both the successes and the failures of medicine and health care. It is impossible to deal with the distribution and allocation of health care apart from those successes and failures. As a case study, consider the debates about the treatment of end-stage renal failure in Britain, where age is used as a criterion for admission to and exclusion from dialysis.

AGE AND DIALYSIS: THE BRITISH CASE

The British exclude many patients with end-stage renal failure, such as diabetics, who would be treated in many other countries. But, contrary to many popular analyses, "There are no special British rules about which patients with end-stage renal failure may or may not be treated. Nevertheless, limited facilities for treatment have made it necessary for British physicians to practice selection to a degree which seems strange, even barbaric, to ... colleagues in other civilized countries."[1] In one study, physicians in twenty-five renal units were given the clinical and social details of forty patients and were asked to select thirty for treatment. Several discrepancies emerged: only one-third of the patients would have been treated in all twenty-five units, and no single patient would have been rejected by all units. One patient who would have been rejected by nineteen of the twenty-five centers was sixty years old and had poor home facilities and marital status. Fifteen of the nineteen centers that would have rejected him gave his age as one reason. Although some centers also mentioned his social conditions, only a few appealed to accompanying or underlying disease. Even more striking was a sixty-eight-year-old patient who would have been rejected by twelve of the twenty-five centers: age was the only reason given.

In the United Kingdom, patients over sixty-five are five times less likely to receive dialysis than in Europe.[2] In general, local physicians reduce the need for dialysis centers to reject applicants by serving as "gatekeepers" to the system. But the society's allocation of funds maintains the scarcity; it has been estimated that an additional fifty million pounds a year would be required to treat the approximately two thousand people who need but do not receive dialysis in Britain.[3] (The British system with its commitment to equal access to health care has used age as a criterion for admission to dialysis, while the United States with a half-hearted commitment to a decent minimum has extended dialysis—and dialysis alone—to almost all who need it, rejecting any criterion of age and perhaps even treating patients who do not benefit.) Is age a morally relevant criterion for admission to or rejection from dialysis?

THE CRITERION OF AGE

The use of the age criterion is clearly a form of discrimination, but it is often important to make "discriminating" judgments, and discrimination is not always unjust or unjustified. The question is whether age discrimination in the allocation and distribution of health care is unjust and unjustified. There are several possibilities: discrimination might be (1) just and justified; (2) unjust but justified; (3) just but unjustified; or (4) unjust and unjustified. These distinctions presuppose that justice is central in moral assessments but that it does not exhaust such assessments. Thus, justice and justification may vary independently, even though, of course, the justice or injustice of a policy will figure prominently in its overall justification.

In all moral assessments it is important to treat similar cases in a similar way as a reflection of the principle of formal justice or universalizability. Then the fundamental question of material or substantive justice is: which similarities and which dissimilarities are morally relevant? The major argument against using some properties such as race or sex or IQ for the distribution of such goods as health care is that it is *unfair* to "treat people differently in ways that profoundly affect their lives because of differences for which they have no responsibility."[4] The standard of fairness or fair opportunity indicates why racism and sexism are unjust and unjustified, and it also excludes the distribution of health care according to race or sex. Ageism, like racism and sexism, involves a set of beliefs, attitudes, and practices that unjustly and unjustifiably discriminate against a group. We have no responsibility for our aging; if we live long enough, we will age. On at least one level, then, ageism is comparable to racism and sexism and should be rejected for similar reasons, which also appear to exclude the use of age as a criterion for the distribution of medical care.

But matters are more complex. Age is frequently introduced not as a standard in and of itself, but as a shorthand expression for several characteristics that may be morally relevant. For example, age sometimes may be a way to suggest that underlying medical problems may make a treatment such as dialysis optional rather than medically indicated. But this suggestion is unfair to elderly individuals who do not have other medical problems that might make a particular treatment less successful. It is also a form of disrespect, insult, and indignity—a violation of the principle of respect for persons—not to pay attention to the characteristics of individuals who may not fit the generalizations about their age cohort.

Regarding both fairness and respect, it is important to stress that the aged are not homogeneous; they constitute a heterogeneous group, similar in age but dissimilar in most other respects.

THE STAGES OF LIFE

Is there a way around these moral issues? One way, which has emerged in some traditional societies, is poignantly depicted in Jack London's short story, "The Law of Life."[5] An elderly, failing man is left to die in the snow with a small pile of wood as his tribe breaks camp. Reliving his memories and anxious about his impending death, he "did not complain": "It was the way of life, and it was just. He had been born close to the earth, close to the earth he had lived, and the law thereof was not new to him." He accepts his abandonment without complaint because this law of life is also embodied in his tribe. He had abandoned his father one winter just as his son, the chief of the tribe, now abandons him (not, I might add, without appropriate rituals and gestures of concern). Abandonment to death was expected because each person benefited from this arrangement over his or her lifetime. As the "law of life," this duty to die was accepted as just and fair.

In the best philosophical analysis of age discrimination in health care, Norman Daniels notes one important difference between age discrimination and sex or race discrimination: although we do not (usually) change race or sex, we do become old. "Young birth cohorts age and are transformed into older age-groups."[6] Thus, he suggests, we should not consider issues of the distribution of health care according to age merely from a synchronic perspective, a time-slice, in which there is competition between age-cohorts. We also need to take a diachronic perspective: "From the perspective of institutions operating over time, the age criterion operates within a life and not between lives." The health care system has to treat people through various stages of their life, including aging. From this perspective, Daniels suggests that we view the question of discrimination according to age in the distribution of health care as one of *prudence* of actual or hypothetical persons: what distribution of health care would they want throughout their lives? People might rationally choose to participate in a lifetime health care package that would concentrate certain lifesaving technologies in their earlier years in order to increase their chances of reaching a normal lifespan. They thus would accept age as a criterion for distribution and withhold certain technologies from the elderly.

While this system obviously resembles the British case, the differences are important, and Daniels's proposal may not fit nonideal circumstances of the kind that have to be considered in health policies in both Britain and the United States. For example, rapidly developing technologies may make it very difficult to achieve equity and stability in a health care system. Conflicts between age-cohorts may become very divisive when several life-sustaining technologies, such as dialysis and transplantation, become available and are distributed to young people even though such technologies were not available to older people when they were young. In principle, rationing some health care by age can be just and justified. But unless conditions similar to Daniels's ideal scheme can be met, it is not clear that rationing by age can be publicly justified and accepted as just and fair. In Britain several factors mitigate the controversy (which does, however, exist) about the use of an age criterion in the distribution of dialysis. Rationing, particularly through queuing, has been accepted in part because of "the acceptance of scarcity as a general feature of British society and affection for the National Health Service."[7]

In addition, age is not an *official* criterion, and professional nondisclosure and perhaps even deception reduce potential friction: "For example, an internist confronted with a patient beyond the prevailing, if unofficial, age at which one's chances of receiving dialysis become slight is likely to tell the patient and family that nothing of medical benefit can be done and that he or she will simply make the patient as comfortable as possible."[8]

It is thus not clear whether the age criterion is publicly justifiable in Britain. Nevertheless, several schemes of allocation and distribution, including some appeals to the criterion of age, may be consistent with both prudence and justice and may be left to public democratic processes, at least within limits. Public discourse within those processes will in part concern the basis and scope of a political-legal right to health care.

A RIGHT TO HEALTH CARE

There are two common moral arguments for a political-legal right to health care (or for a societal obligation to provide health care), and these arguments encompass the elderly as well as all other people in a society. One argument rests on beneficence, care, or compassion; the other on justice or fairness. Both usually focus on the nature of health needs as largely the result of an impersonal, natural lottery and thus as largely undeserved. Such undeserved needs—the outcomes of chance—may be construed as *unfortunate* or as also *unfair*. If these needs are merely unfortunate (and not also unfair), they may be the object of beneficence, care or compassion; if they are also unfair, they become the object of justice.[9] I will not discuss the controversial argument from fairness in order to concentrate on beneficence, which is closely connected with the theme of community.

One version of the argument from beneficence holds that through establishing a political-legal right to health care, the society expresses, symbolizes, and conveys certain values, such as care and compassion for the victims of the natural lottery. There is an important distinction between realizing a goal and expressing a value, and this argument concentrates on the expressive significance of a political-legal right to health care. This theme echoes in *Securing Access to Health Care*, the report of the President's Commission:

> Since human beings are vulnerable to disease and all die, health care has a special interpersonal significance: it expresses and nurtures bonds of empathy and compassion. The depth of a society's concern about health care can be seen as a measure of its sense of solidarity in the face of suffering and death....a society's commitment to health care reflects some of its most basic attitudes about what it means to be a member of the human community.[10]

If this theme is sound, the use of an age criterion in the provision of health care in our society at this time could itself have negative symbolic significance: abandonment and exclusion from communal care. Nevertheless, it is morally possible to set certain limits on the provision of health care; its scope need not be unlimited. And denial of some life-sustaining technologies does not necessarily constitute abandonment and denial of communal care. But some methods to determine the content, scope, and limits of a political-legal right to health care may at least covertly violate strictures against age discrimination.

Obviously the moral basis of a political-legal right to health care will affect the way we determine its content, scope, and limits. The specification of a political-legal right to health care must be consistent with and guided by moral considerations, including the ones that support it. But these issues are somewhat independent. How can the society determine the content, scope, and limits of a political-legal right to health care? What would constitute an adequate level of care or a decent minimum of care? Negatively, there is no societal obligation to offer health care that has no reasonable chance of benefiting patients, and there is no obligation to provide health care if its costs outweigh its benefits.

But the methods we use for determining reasonable chance of benefit and the ratio of benefits and costs may themselves discriminate against the elderly. For example, the techniques of cost-benefit analysis and cost-effectiveness analysis tend to be biased against the elderly. In cost-benefit analysis, figures are assigned to benefits, such as prolonged life, by considering (a) discounted future earnings or human capital, or (b) willingness to pay (revealed preferences or disclosed preferences). From either standpoint, the figures are skewed against the elderly, whose discounted future earnings are obviously below others in the society and who may be less willing to pay to sustain life for various reasons. Even in cost-effectiveness analysis, which is generally less objectionable because the benefits are not reduced to common measurements such as dollars, problems emerge once we move beyond the number of lives saved to "quality adjusted life years."[11]

In general, when it is difficult to resolve disputes about substantive standards, such as adequacy of health care or a decent minimum of health care, there is a tendency to revert to procedures. This tendency is understandable and warranted if the procedures themselves are morally acceptable. Thus, the President's Commission rightly concludes: "It is reasonable for a society to turn to fair, democratic procedures to make a choice among just alternatives. Given the great imprecision in the notion of adequate health care, however, it is especially important that the procedures used to define that level be—and be perceived to be—fair."[12]

SOCIOCULTURAL METAPHORS

Our health care policies are often shaped by our sociocultural images and metaphors. Metaphors involve "seeing as." In each use of metaphor, we see something as something else; we experience or understand one thing through another. For example, we see X as Y, human beings as wolves, love as a journey, and argument as warfare. In their exciting book, *Metaphors We Live By*, George Lakoff and Mark Johnson argue that our metaphors (often subconsciously) shape how we think, what we experience, and what we do.[13] Take their example: argument as warfare. We develop *strategies* of argument, *contend* with one another, *attack* positions as *indefensible*, and so on. Imagine how different our interactions would be if we viewed argument as a collaborative work of art through which people seek the truth. It is clear from this example that metaphors both highlight and hide, as Lakoff and Johnson note. For example, the metaphor of argument as warfare highlights the conflict involved in argument, but it hides the cooperation and collaboration that are also indispensable.

The metaphor of warfare is also prominent in health care, especially in medicine, where it largely (but not completely) shapes our conception of what we do. The language that follows is drawn from conversations and from the literature: The physician as the captain leads the battle against disease, orders a battery of tests, develops a plan of attack, calls on the armamentarium or arsenal of medicine, directs allied health personnel, treats aggressively, and expects compliance. Good patients are those who fight vigorously and refuse to give up. Victory is sought and defeat is feared. Sometimes there is even hope for a "magic bullet" or a "silver bullet." Only professionals who stand on the firing line or in the trenches can really appreciate the moral problems of medicine. As medicine wages war against germs that invade the body and threaten its defenses, so the society itself may also declare war on cancer under the leadership of its chief medical officer—the Surgeon General. Articles and books may even herald the "Medical-Industrial Complex: Our National Defense."[14]

The military metaphor clearly structures much, though by no means all, of our conception of health care, and it both illuminates and distorts health care. Because its positive implications are widely recognized, I only want to identify some of its negative implications, especially for the allocation of resources that affect the elderly in need of health care. It is no accident, for example, that two major terms for allocation and distribution of health care under conditions of scarcity emerged from, or have been decisively shaped by, military experiences: triage and rationing. As Richard Rettig and Kathleen Lohr note,

> Earlier, policymakers spoke of the general problem of allocating scarce medical resources, a formulation that implied hard but generally manageable choices of a largely pragmatic nature. Now the discussion increasingly is of rationing scarce medical resources, a harsher term that connotes emergency—even war-time—circumstances requiring some societal triage mechanism.[15]

The first negative implication of the military metaphor is that the society's health care budget tends to be converted into a *defense budget* to prepare for and to conduct warfare against disease, trauma, and death. As a consequence, the society may put more resources into health care than it could justify, especially under a different metaphor, in relation to other social goods.

Second, the military metaphor also implies patterns of allocation within health care by assigning priority to *critical care* over prevention and chronic care. It tends to view health in negative rather than positive terms, as the absence of disease rather than a positive state of affairs, and concentrates on critical interventions to cure disease. It tends to neglect care when cure is impossible. Recently Lawrence Pray noted that he originally tried to conquer his diabetes, but after futile and counterproductive struggles and battles, he came to see his diabetes not as an "enemy" to be "conquered," but as a "teacher."[16]

A third point is closely connected: the military metaphor may direct attention to certain diseases rather than others for research and treatment. In particular, it tends to assign priority to *killer diseases* rather than disabling diseases. As Franz Ingelfinger once noted, if we concentrated research and treatment more on disabling diseases, such as arthritis, than on killer diseases, then national health expenditures would reflect the same values that individuals affirm: "It is more important to live a certain way than to die a certain way."[17] Anne Somers has suggested that the stroke is "a metaphor for the most difficult problems and challenges of geriatric medicine."[18] Although strokes are not, of course, limited to the elderly, they are more common among the elderly. Each year in the United States there are between 500,000 and 600,000 victims of stroke, 80 to 90 percent of them surviving their initial catastrophe, often with paralysis and aphasia, which have a terrible impact on both the victim and the family. Approximately 2.5 million victims of stroke are alive today, 90 percent of them with varying degrees of incapacity and misery. Even though it has been called the single most costly disease in the United States, stroke received only $18 million in research expenditures in 1979 in contrast to cancer, which received $937 million, and heart disease, which received $340 million. A major reason for this pattern of allocation is that after the first acute phase, the stroke victim does not fit into the prevalent model of health care, which emphasizes the specialist who uses various technological weapons.

A fourth implication of the military metaphor—medicine as warfare—is its emphasis on *technological intervention* and on particular technologies, such as intensive care units, over other technologies such as prostheses. It downplays less technological modes of care.

A fifth implication is *overtreatment*, particularly of terminally ill patients, because death is the ultimate enemy even if disease is the immediate foe. It is difficult for physicians and families under the spell of this metaphor to let a patient die. "Heroic" actions befit the military effort that must be undertaken against the ultimate enemy. As Paul Ramsey notes, "A culture that defines death as always a disaster [I would add enemy] will be one that is tempted to resolve these (allocation) questions in terms of triage-disaster medicine [I would add military-triage medicine]."[19]

I do not propose that we abandon the military metaphor—it illuminates and directs much of health care in morally significant ways. But its negative implications can be avoided in part if we supplement it with other metaphors. The military metaphor tends to assign priority to health care (especially medical care) over other goods and, within health care, to critical interventions over prevention and chronic care, killer over disabling diseases, technological interventions over care, and heroic treatment of dying patients. One of the most promising supplementary metaphors is *nursing*, which some have even proposed as a paradigm of future health care. This metaphor is not adequate by itself just as the military metaphor (or any other metaphor, such as business) is not adequate by itself, but it could direct the society to alternative priorities in the allocation of resources for and within health care, particularly for the elderly....

REFERENCES

1 A. J. Wing, "Why Don't the British Treat More Patients with Kidney Failure?" *British Medical Journal* 287 (October 22, 1983), 1157.

2 V. Parsons and P. Lock, "Triage and the Patient with Renal Failure," *Journal of Medical Ethics* 6 (1980), 173–76.

3 Wing, p. 1158.

4 William Frankena, "Some Beliefs about Justice," The Lindley Lecture, University of Kansas (March 2, 1966), p. 10.

5 Jack London, "The Law of Life," *The Unabridged Jack London*, edited by Lawrence Teacher and Richard E. Nicholls (Philadelphia: Running Press, 1981), pp. 279–84.

6 Norman Daniels, "Am I My Parents' Keeper?" in *Securing Access to Health Care* by the President's Commission for the Study of Ethical Problems in Medicine and Biomedical and Behavioral Research, Vol. 2 (Washington, D.C.: US Government Printing Office, March, 1983), Appendix K, pp. 265–91.

7 William B. Schwartz and Henry J. Aaron, "Rationing Hospital Care: Lessons from Britain," *New England Journal of Medicine* 310 (January 5, 1984), 56.

8 *Ibid*, p. 54.

9 See H. Tristram Engelhardt, Jr., "Health Care Allocations: Responses to the Unjust, the Unfortunate, and the Undesirable," in Earl E. Shelp, Jr., ed., *Justice and Health Care*, Philosophy and Medicine, vol. 8 (Boston, Mass.: Reidel, 1981), pp. 121–37; Engelhardt, "Shattuck Lecture—Allocating Scarce Medical Resources and the Availability of Organ Transplantation," *New England Journal of Medicine* 311 (July 5, 1984), 66–71.

10 President's Commission for the Study of Ethical Problems in Medicine and Biomedical and Behavioral Research, *Securing Access to Health Care*, Vol 1: Report (Washington, D.C.: US Government Printing Office, March 1983), p. 17.

11 Jerry Avorn, "Benefit and Cost Analysis in Geriatric Care: Turning Age Discrimination into Health Policy," *New England Journal of Medicine* 310 (May 17, 1984), 1294–1301.

12 President's Commission, *Securing Access to Health Care*, Vol 1: Report, p. 42.

13 George Lakoff and Mark Johnson, *Metaphors We Live By* (Chicago: University of Chicago Press, 1980).

14 For military metaphors in health care, see Virginia Warren, "A Powerful Metaphor: Medicine as War" (unpublished paper); Samuel Vaisrub, *Medicine's Metaphors: Messages and Menaces* (Oradell, N.J.: Medical Economics Company, 1977), chap. 1; and Susan Sontag, *Illness as Metaphor* (New York: Vintage Books, 1979).

15 Richard Rettig and Kathleen Lohr, "Ethical Dimensions of Allocating Scarce Resources in Medicine: A Cross-National Case Study of End-Stage Renal Disease," unpublished manuscript (1981).

16 Lawrence Pray, *Journey of a Diabetic* (New York: Simon & Schuster, 1983), and "How Diabetes Became My Teacher," *Washington Post*, July 31, 1983.

17 Franz Ingelfinger, Editorial, *New England Journal of Medicine* 287 (December 7, 1982), 1198–99.

18 Anne R. Somers, "The 'Geriatric Imperative' and Growing Economic Constraints," *Journal of Medical Education* 55 (February 1980); 89–98, from which the figures in the remainder of this paragraph have been drawn.

19 Paul Ramsey, *The Patient as Person* (New Haven: Yale University Press, 1970).

Aging and the Ends of Medicine
Daniel Callahan

A biographical sketch of Daniel Callahan is found on page 445.

Callahan maintains that since health-care resources are scarce, elderly individuals who have lived a natural life span should be offered care that relieves suffering but should be denied expensive life-prolonging technologies. In arguing for his position, Callahan stresses the need to reexamine questions about aging and the proper ends of medicine as well as the concept of a natural life span. He concludes that medicine should have two goals as it confronts aging: (1) averting premature death, that is, death prior to the completion of a natural life span and (2) the relief of suffering, rather than the extension of life, after that natural span has been completed.

In October of 1986, Dr. Thomas Starzl of the Presbyterian-University Hospital in Pittsburgh successfully transplanted a liver into a 76-year-old woman. The typical cost of such an operation is over $200,000. He thereby accelerated the extension to the elderly of the most expensive and most demanding form of high-technology medicine. Not long after that, Congress brought organ transplantation under Medicare coverage, thus guaranteeing an even greater extension of this form of life-saving care to older age groups.

This is, on the face of it, the kind of medical progress we have long grown to hail, a triumph of medical technology and a new-found benefit to be provided by an established entitlement program. But now an oddity. At the same time those events were taking place, a parallel government campaign for cost containment was under way, with a special targeting of health care to the aged under the Medicare program.

It was not hard to understand why. In 1980, the 11% of the population over age 65 consumed some 29% of the total American health care expenditures of $219.4 billion. By 1986, the percentage of consumption by the elderly had increased to 31% and total expenditures to $450 billion. Medicare costs are projected to rise from $75 billion in 1986 to $114 billion in the year 2000, and in real not inflated dollars.

There is every incentive for politicians, for those who care for the aged, and for those of us on the way to becoming old to avert our eyes from figures of that kind.

Reprinted with permission of the author and the publisher from *Annals of the New York Academy of Sciences*, vol. 530 (June 15, 1988), pp. 125–132.

We have tried as a society to see if we can simply muddle our way through. That, however, is no longer sufficient. The time has come, I am convinced, for a full and open reconsideration of our future direction. We can not for much longer continue on our present course. Even if we could find a way to radically increase the proportion of our health care dollar going to the elderly, it is not clear that that would be a good social investment.

Is it sensible, in the face of a rapidly increasing burden of health care costs for the elderly, to press forward with new and expensive ways of extending their lives? Is it possible to even hope to control costs while, simultaneously, supporting the innovative research that generates ever-new ways to spend money? These are now unavoidable questions. Medicare costs rise at an extraordinary pace, fueled by an ever-increasing number and proportion of the elderly. The fastest-growing age group in the United States are those over the age of 85, increasing at a rate of about 10% every two years. By the year 2040, it has been projected that the elderly will represent 21% of the population and consume 45% of all health care expenditures. Could costs of that magnitude be borne?

Yet even as this intimidating trend reveals itself, anyone who works closely with the elderly recognizes that the present Medicare and Medicaid programs are grossly inadequate in meeting the real and full needs of the elderly. They fail, most notably, in providing decent long-term care and medical care that does not constitute a heavy out-of-pocket drain. Members of minority groups, and single or widowed women, are particularly disadvantaged. How will it be possible, then, to keep pace with the growing number of elderly in even providing present levels of care, much less in ridding the system of its present inadequacies and inequities—and, at the same time, furiously adding expensive new technologies?

The straight answer is that it will not be possible to do all of those things and that, worse still, it may be harmful to even try. It may be harmful because of the economic burdens it will impose on younger age groups, and because of the skewing of national social priorities too heavily toward health care that it is coming to require. But it may also be harmful because it suggests to both the young and the old that the key to a happy old age is good health care. That may not be true.

It is not pleasant to raise possibilities of that kind. The struggle against what Dr. Robert Butler aptly and brilliantly called "ageism" in 1968 has been a difficult one. It has meant trying to persuade the public that not all the elderly are sick and senile. It has meant trying to convince Congress and state legislatures to provide more help for the old. It has meant trying to educate the elderly themselves to look upon their old age as a time of new, open possibilities. That campaign has met with only partial success. Despite great progress, the elderly are still subject to discrimination and stereotyping. The struggle against ageism is hardly over.

Three major concerns have, nonetheless, surfaced over the past few years. They are symptoms that a new era has arrived. The first is that an increasingly large share of health care is going to the elderly in comparison with benefits for children. The federal government, for instance, spends six times as much on health care for those over 65 as for those under 18. As the demographer Samuel Preston observed in a provocative 1984 presidential address to the Population Association of America:

> There is surely something to be said for a system in which things get better as we pass through life rather than worse. The great leveling off of age curves of psychological distress, suicide and income in the past two decades might simply reflect the fact that we have decided in some fundamental sense that we don't want to face futures that become continually bleaker. But let's be clear that the transfers from the working-age population to the elderly are also transfers away from children, since the working ages bear far more responsibility for childrearing than do the elderly.[1]

Preston's address had an immediate impact. The mainline aging advocacy groups responded with pained indignation, accusing Preston of fomenting a war be-

tween the generations. But led by Dave Durenberger, Republican Senator from Minnesota, it also stimulated the formation of Americans for Generational Equity (AGE), an organization created to promote debate on the burden to future generations, but particularly the Baby Boom generation, of "our major social insurance programs."[2] These two developments signalled the outburst of a struggle over what has come to be called "Intergenerational equity" that is only now gaining momentum.

The second concern is that the elderly dying consume a disproportionate share of health care costs. Stanford economist Victor Fuchs has noted:

> At present, the United States spends about 1 percent of the gross national product on health care for elderly persons who are in their last year of life.... One of the biggest challenges facing policy makers for the rest of this century will be how to strike an appropriate balance between care of the [elderly] dying and health services for the rest of the population.[3]

The third concern is summed up in an observation by Jerome L. Avorn, M.D., of the Harvard Medical School:

> With the exception of the birth-control pill, each of the medical-technology interventions developed since the 1950s has its most widespread impact on people who are past their fifties—the further past their fifties, the greater the impact.[4]

Many of these interventions were not intended for the elderly. Kidney dialysis, for example, was originally developed for those between the age of 15 and 45. Now some 30% of its recipients are over 65.

These three concerns have not gone unchallenged. They have, on the contrary, been strongly resisted, as has the more general assertion that some form of rationing of health care for the elderly might become necessary. To the charge that the elderly receive a disproportionate share of resources, the response has been that what helps the elderly helps every other age group. It both relieves the young of the burden of care for elderly parents they would otherwise have to bear and, since they too will eventually become old, promises them similar care when they come to need it. There is no guarantee, moreover, that any cutback in health care for the elderly would result in a transfer of the savings directly to the young. Our system is not that rational or that organized. And why, others ask, should we contemplate restricting care for the elderly when we wastefully spend hundreds of millions of dollars on an inflated defense budget?

The charge that the elderly dying receive a large share of funds hardly proves that it is an unjust or unreasonable amount. They are, after all, the most in need. As some important studies have shown, moreover, it is exceedingly difficult to know that someone is dying; the most expensive patients, it turns out, are those who are expected to live but who actually die. That most new technologies benefit the old more than the young is perfectly sensible: most of the killer diseases of the young have now been conquered.

These are reasonable responses. It would no doubt be possible to ignore the symptoms that the raising of such concerns represents, and to put off for at least a few more years any full confrontation with the overpowering tide of elderly now on the way. There is little incentive for politicians to think about, much less talk about, limits of any kind on health care for the aged; it is a politically hazardous topic. Perhaps also, as Dean Guido Calabresi of the Yale Law School and his colleague Philip Bobbitt observed in their thoughtful 1978 book *Tragic Choices*, when we are forced to make painful allocation choices, "Evasion, disguise, temporizing...[and] averting our eyes enables us to save some lives even when we will not save all."[5]

Yet however slight the incentives to take on this highly troubling issue, I believe it is inevitable that we must. Already rationing of health care under Medicare is a fact of life, though rarely labeled as such. The requirement that Medicare recipients pay the first $500 of the costs of hospital care, that there is a cutoff of reimbursement of care beyond 60 days, and a failure to cover long-term care, are nothing other than allocation and cost-saving devices. As sensitive as it is to the votes of the elderly, the Reagan administration only grudgingly agreed to support catastrophic health care costs of the elderly (a benefit that will not, in any event, help many of the aged). It is bound to be far more resistant to long-term care coverage, as will any administration.

But there are other reasons than economics to think about health care for the elderly. The coming economic crisis provides a much-needed opportunity to ask some deeper questions. Just what is it that we want medicine to do for us as we age? Earlier cultures believed that aging should be accepted, and that it should be in part a time of preparation for death. Our culture seems increasingly to reject that view, preferring instead, it often

seems, to think of aging as hardly more than another disease, to be fought and rejected. Which view is correct? To ask that question is only to note that disturbing puzzles about the ends of medicine and the ends of aging lie behind the more immediate financing worries. Without some kind of answer to them, there is no hope of finding a reasonable, and possibly even a humane, solution to the growing problem of health care for the elderly.

Let me put my own view directly. The future goal of medicine in the care of the aged should be that of improving the quality of their life, not in seeking ways to extend that life. In its longstanding ambition to forestall death, medicine has in the care of the aged reached its last frontier. That is hardly because death is absent elsewhere—children and young adults obviously still die of maladies that are open to potential cure—but because the largest number of deaths (some 70%) now occur among those over the age of 65, with the highest proportion in those over 85. If death is ever to be humbled, that is where the essentially endless work remains to be done. But however tempting that challenge, medicine should now restrain its ambition at that frontier. To do otherwise will, I believe, be to court harm to the needs of other age groups and to the old themselves.

Yet to ask medicine to restrain itself in the face of aging and death is to ask more than it, or the public that sustains it, is likely to find agreeable. Only a fresh understanding of the ends and meaning of aging, encompassing two conditions, are likely to make that a plausible stance. The first is that we—both young and old—need to understand that it is possible to live out a meaningful old age that is limited in time, one that does not require a compulsive effort to turn to medicine for more life to make it bearable. The second condition is that, as a culture, we need a more supportive context for aging and death, one that cherishes and respects the elderly while at the same time recognizing that their primary orientation should be to the young and the generations to come, not to their own age group. It will be no less necessary to recognize that in the passing of the generations lies the constant reinvigoration of biological life.

Neither of these conditions will be easy to realize. Our culture has, for one thing, worked hard to redefine old age as a time of liberation, not decline. The terms "modern maturity" or "prime time" have, after all, come to connote a time of travel, new ventures in education and self-discovery, the ever-accessible tennis court or golf course, and delightfully periodic but gratefully brief visits from well-behaved grandchildren.

This is, to be sure, an idealized picture. Its attraction lies not in its literal truth but as a widely-accepted utopian reference point. It projects the vision of an old age to which more and more believe they can aspire and which its proponents think an affluent country can afford if it so chooses. That it requires a medicine that is singleminded in its aggressiveness against the infirmities of old age is of a piece with its hopes. But as we have come to discover, the costs of that kind of war are prohibitive. No matter how much is spent the ultimate problem will still remain: people age and die. Worse still, by pretending that old age can be turned into a kind of endless middle age, we rob it of meaning and significance for the elderly themselves. It is a way of saying that old age can be acceptable only to the extent that it can mimic the vitality of the younger years.

There is a plausible alternative: that of a fresh vision of what it means to live a decently long and adequate life, what might be called a natural life span. Earlier generations accepted the idea that there was a natural life span—the biblical norm of three score years and ten captures that notion (even though, in fact, that was a much longer life span than was then typically the case). It is an idea well worth reconsidering, and would provide us with a meaningful and realizable goal. Modern medicine and biology have done much, however, to wean us away from that kind of thinking. They have insinuated the belief that the average life span is not a natural fact at all, but instead one that is strictly dependent upon the state of medical knowledge and skill. And there is much to that belief as a statistical fact: the average life expectancy continues to increase, with no end in sight.

But that is not what I think we ought to mean by a natural life span. We need a notion of a full life that is based on some deeper understanding of human need and sensible possibility, not the latest state of medical technology or medical possibility. We should instead think of a natural life span as the achievement of a life long enough to accomplish for the most part those opportunities that life typically affords people and which we ordinarily take to be the prime benefits of enjoying a life at all—that of loving and living, of raising a family, of finding and carrying out work that is satisfying, of reading and thinking, and of cherishing our friends and families.

If we envisioned a natural life span that way, then we could begin to intensify the devising of ways to get people to that stage of life, and to work to make certain they do so in good health and social dignity. People will

differ on what they might count as a natural life span; determining its appropriate range for social policy purposes would need extended thought and debate. My own view is that it can now be achieved by the late 70s or early 80s.

That many of the elderly discover new interests and new facets of themselves late in life—my mother took up painting in her seventies and was selling her paintings up until her death at 86—does not mean that we should necessarily encourage a kind of medicine that would make that the norm. Nor does it mean that we should base social and welfare policy on possibilities of that kind. A more reasonable approach is to ask how medicine can help most people live out a decently long life, and how that life can be enhanced along the way.

A longer life does not guarantee a better life—there is no inherent connection between the two. No matter how long medicine enabled people to live, death at any time—at age 90, or 100, or 110—would frustrate some possibility, some as-yet-unrealized goal. There is sadness in that realization, but not tragedy. An easily preventable death of a young child is an outrage. The death from an incurable disease of someone in the prime of young adulthood is a tragedy. But death at an old age, after a long and full life, is simply sad, a part of life itself.

As it confronts aging, medicine should have as its specific goal that of averting premature death, understood as death prior to a natural life span, and the relief of suffering thereafter. It should pursue those goals in order that the elderly can finish out their years with as little needless pain as possible, and with as much vigor as can be generated in contributing to the welfare of younger age groups and to the community of which they are a part. Above all, the elderly need to have a sense of the meaning and significance of their stage in life, one that is not dependent for its human value on economic productivity or physical vigor.

What would a medicine oriented toward the relief of suffering rather than the deliberate extension of life be like? We do not yet have a clear and ready answer to that question, so long-standing, central, and persistent has been the struggle against death as part of the self-conception of medicine. But the Hospice movement is providing us with much helpful evidence. It knows how to distinguish between the relief of suffering and the extension of life. A greater control by the elderly over their dying—and particularly a more readily respected and enforceable right to deny aggressive life-extending treatment—is a long-sought, minimally necessary goal.

What does this have to do with the rising cost of health care for the elderly? Everything. The indefinite extension of life combined with a never-satisfied improvement in the health of the elderly is a recipe for monomania and limitless spending. It fails to put health in its proper place as only one among many human goods. It fails to accept aging and death as part of the human condition. It fails to present to younger generations a model of wise stewardship.

How might we devise a plan to limit health care for the aged under public entitlement programs that is fair, humane, and sensitive to their special requirements and dignity? Let me suggest three principles to undergird a quest for limits. First, government has a duty, based on our collective social obligations to each other, to help people live out a natural life span, but not actively to help medically extend life beyond that point. Second, government is obliged to develop under its research subsidies, and pay for, under its entitlement programs, only that kind and degree of life-extending technology necessary for medicine to achieve and serve the end of a natural life span. The question is not whether a technology is available that can save the life of someone who has lived out a natural life span, but whether there is an obligation for society to provide them with that technology. I think not. Third, beyond the point of natural life span, government should provide only the means necessary for the relief of suffering, not life-extending technology. By proposing that we use age as a specific criterion for the limitation of life-extending health care, I am challenging one of the most revered norms of contemporary geriatrics: that medical need and not age should be the standard of care. Yet the use of age as a principle for the allocation of resources can be perfectly valid, both a necessary and legitimate basis for providing health care to the elderly. There is not likely to be any better or less arbitrary criterion for the limiting of resources in the face of the open-ended possibilities of medical advancement in therapy for the aged.

Medical "need," in particular, can no longer work as an allocation principle. It is too elastic a concept, too much a function of the state of medical art. A person of 100 dying from congestive heart failure "needs" a heart transplant no less than someone who is 30. Are we to treat both needs as equal? That is not economically feasible or, I would argue, a sensible way to allocate scarce resources. But it would be required by a strict need-based standard.

Age is also a legitimate basis for allocation because it is a meaningful and universal category. It can be understood at the level of common sense. It is concrete enough to be employed for policy purposes. It can also, most importantly, be of value to the aged themselves if combined with an ideal of old age that focuses on its quality rather than its indefinite extension.

I have become impressed with the philosophy underlying the British health care system and the way it meets the needs of the old and the chronically ill. It has, to begin with, a tacit allocation policy. It emphasizes improving the quality of life through primary care medicine and well-subsidized home care and institutional programs for the elderly rather than through life-extending acute care medicine. The well-known difficulty in getting dialysis after 55 is matched by like restrictions on access to open heart surgery, intensive care units, and other forms of expensive technology. An undergirding skepticism toward technology makes that a viable option. That attitude, together with a powerful drive for equity, "explains," as two commentators have noted, "why most British put a higher value on primary care for the population as a whole than on an abundance of sophisticated technology for the few who may benefit from it."[6]

That the British spend a significantly smaller proportion of their GNP (6.2%) on health care than Americans (10.8%) for an almost identical outcome in health status is itself a good advertisement for its priorities. Life expectancies are, for men, 70.0 years in the U.S. and 70.4 years in Great Britain; and, for women, 77.8 in the U.S. and 76.7 in Great Britain. There is, of course, a great difference in the ethos of the U.S. and Britain, and our individualism and love of technology stand in the way of a quick shift of priorities.

Yet our present American expectations about aging and death, it turns out, may not be all that reassuring. How many of us are really so certain that high-technology American medicine promises us all that much better an aging and death, even if some features appear improved and the process begins later than in earlier times? Between the widespread fear of death in an impersonal ICU, cozened about machines and invaded by tubes, on the one hand, or wasting away in the back ward of a nursing home, on the other, not many of us seem comforted.

Once we have reflected on those fears, it is not impossible that most people could be persuaded that a different, more limited set of expectations for health care could be made tolerable. That would be all the more possible if there was a greater assurance than at present that one could live out a full life span, that one's chronic illnesses would be better supported, and that long-term care and home care would be given a more powerful societal backing than is now the case. Though they would face a denial of life-extending medical care beyond a certain age, the old would not necessarily fear their aging anymore than they now do. They would, on the contrary, know that a better balance had been struck between making our later years as good as possible rather than simply trying to add more years.

This direction would not immediately bring down the costs of care of the elderly; it would add new costs. But it would set in place the beginning of a new understanding of old age, one that would admit of eventual stabilization and limits. The time has come to admit we can not go on much longer on the present course of open-ended health care for the elderly. Neither confident assertions about American affluence, nor tinkering with entitlement provisions and cost-containment strategies will work for more than a few more years. It is time for the dream that old age can be an infinite and open frontier to end, and for the unflagging, but self-deceptive, optimism that we can do anything we want with our economic system to be put aside.

The elderly will not be served by a belief that only a lack of resources, or better financing mechanisms, or political power, stand between them and the limitations of their bodies. The good of younger age groups will not be served by inspiring in them a desire to live to an old age that will simply extend the vitality of youth indefinitely, as if old age is nothing but a sign that medicine has failed in its mission. The future of our society will not be served by allowing expenditures on health care for the elderly endlessly and uncontrollably to escalate, fueled by a false altruism that thinks anything less is to deny the elderly their dignity. Nor will it be served by that pervasive kind of self-serving that urges the young to support such a crusade because they will eventually benefit from it also.

We require instead an understanding of the process of aging and death that looks to our obligation to the young and to the future, that recognizes the necessity of limits and the acceptance of decline and death, and that

values the old for their age and not for their continuing youthful vitality. In the name of accepting the elderly and repudiating discrimination against them, we have mainly succeeded in pretending that, with enough will and money, the unpleasant part of old age can be abolished. In the name of medical progress we have carried out a relentless war against death and decline, failing to ask in any probing way if that will give us a better society for all age groups.

The proper question is not whether we are succeeding in giving a longer life to the aged. It is whether we are making of old age a decent and honorable time of life. Neither a longer lifetime nor more life-extending technology are the way to that goal. The elderly themselves ask for greater financial security, for as much self-determination and independence as possible, for a decent quality of life and not just more life, and for a respected place in society.

The best way to achieve those goals is not simply to say more money and better programs are needed, however much they have their important place. We would do better to begin with a sense of limits, of the meaning of the human life cycle, and of the necessary coming and going of the generations. From that kind of starting point, we could devise a new understanding of old age.

REFERENCES

1 Preston, S. H. 1984. Children and the elderly: divergent paths for America's dependents. Demography 21: 491–495.
2 Americans for Generational Equity. Case Statement. May 1986.
3 Fuchs, V. R. 1984. Though much is taken: reflections on aging, health, and medical care. Milbank Mem. Fund Q. 62: 464–465.
4 Avorn, J. L. 1986. Medicine, health, and the geriatric transformation. Daedalus 115: 211–225.
5 Calabresi, G. & P. Bobbitt. 1978. Tragic Choices. W. W. Norton. New York, NY.
6 Miller, F. H. & G. A. H. Miller. 1986. The painful prescription: a procrustean perspective. N. Engl. J. Med. 314: 1385.

Spare the Old, Save the Young
Amitai Etzioni

Amitai Etzioni, a sociologist, is visiting professor at the Harvard Business School. He is the author of *Genetic Fix: The Next Technological Revolution* (1975), *Capital Corruption: The New Attack on American Democracy* (1984) and *The Moral Dimension: Toward a New Economics* (1988).

Etzioni rejects age-based rationing of health care and criticizes Callahan's position. On his view, such rationing would encourage intergenerational conflict. Furthermore, he argues, adopting Callahan's recommendations would start us on a slippery slope leading to growing restrictions on health care for other groups. Etzioni also suggests several ways in which funds required to avoid age-based health-care rationing might be raised.

In the coming years, Daniel Callahan's call to ration health care for the elderly, put forth in his book *Setting Limits*, is likely to have a growing appeal. Practically all economic observers expect the United States to go through a difficult time as it attempts to work its way out of its domestic (budgetary) and international (trade) deficits. Practically every serious analyst realizes that such an endeavor will initially entail slower growth, if not an outright cut in our standard of living, in order to release resources to these priorities. When the national economic "pie" grows more slowly, let alone contracts, the fight over how to divide it up intensifies. The elderly make an especially inviting target because they have been taking a growing slice of the resources (at least those dedicated to health care) and are expected to take even more in the future. Old people are widely held to be "nonproductive" and to constitute a growing "burden" on an ever-smaller proportion of society that is young and working. Also, the elderly are viewed as politically well-organized and powerful; hence "their" programs, especially Social Security and Medicare, have largely escaped the Reagan attempts to scale back social expenditures, while those aimed at other groups—especially the young, but even more so future generations—have been generally curtailed. There are now some signs that a backlash may be forming.

If a war between the generations, like that between the races and between the genders, does break out, his-

torians may accord former Governor Richard Lamm of Colorado the dubious honor of having fired the opening shot in his statement that the elderly ill have "got a duty to die and get out of the way." Phillip Longman, in his book *Born to Pay*, sounded an early alarm. However, the historians may well say, it was left to Daniel Callahan, a social philosopher and ethicist, to provide a detailed rationale and blueprint for limiting the care to the elderly, explicitly in order to free resources for the young [see Daniel Callahan, "Limiting Health Care for the Old," *The Nation*, August 15/22, 1987]. Callahan's thesis deserves close examination because he attempts to deal with the numerous objections his approach raises. If his thesis does not hold, the champions of limiting funds available to the old may have a long wait before they will find a new set of arguments on their behalf.

In order to free up economic resources for the young, Callahan offers the older generation a deal: Trade quantity for quality; the elderly should not be given life-*extending* services but better years while alive. Instead of the relentless attempt to push death to an older age, Callahan would stop all development of life-extending technologies and prohibit the use of ones at hand for those who outlive their "natural" life span, say, the age of 75. At the same time, the old would be granted more palliative medicine (e.g., pain killers) and more nursing-home and home-health care, to make their natural years more comfortable.

Callahan's call to break an existing ethical taboo and replace it with another raises the problem known among ethicists and sociologists as the "slippery slope." Once the precept that one should do "all one can" to avert death is given up, and attempts are made to fix a specific age for a full life, why stop there? If, for instance, the American economy experiences hard times in the 1990s, should the "maximum" age be reduced to 72, 65—or lower? And should the care for other so-called unproductive groups be cut off, even if they are even younger? Should countries that are economically worse off than the United States set their limit, say, at 55?

This is not an idle thought, because the idea of limiting the care the elderly receive in itself represents a partial slide down such a slope. Originally, Callahan, the Hastings Center (which he directs) and other think tanks played an important role in redefining the concept of death. Death used to be seen by the public at large as occurring when the lungs stopped functioning and, above all, the heart stopped beating. In numerous old movies and novels, those attending the dying would hold a mirror to their faces to see if it fogged over, or put an ear to their chests to see if the heart had stopped. However, high technology made these criteria obsolete by mechanically ventilating people and keeping their hearts pumping. Hastings et al. led the way to provide a new technological definition of death: brain death. Increasingly this has been accepted, both in the medical community and by the public at large, as the point of demise, the point at which care should stop even if it means turning off life-extending machines, because people who are brain dead do not regain consciousness. At the same time, most doctors and a majority of the public as well continue strongly to oppose terminating care to people who are conscious, even if there is little prospect for recovery, despite considerable debate about certain special cases.

Callahan now suggests turning off life-extending technology for all those above a certain age, even if they could recover their full human capacity if treated. It is instructive to look at the list of technologies he would withhold: mechanical ventilation, artificial resuscitation, antibiotics and artificial nutrition and hydration. Note that while several of these are used to maintain brain-dead bodies, they are also used for individuals who are temporarily incapacitated but able to recover fully; indeed, they are used to save young lives, say, after a car accident. But there is no way to stop the development of such new technologies and the improvement of existing ones without depriving the young of benefit as well. (Antibiotics are on the list because of an imminent "high cost" technological advance—administering them with a

pump implanted in the body, which makes their introduction more reliable and better distributes dosages.)

One may say that this is Callahan's particular list; other lists may well be drawn. But any of them would start us down the slope, because the savings that are achieved by turning off the machines that keep brain-dead people alive are minimal compared with those that would result from the measures sought by the people calling for new equity between the generations. And any significant foray into deliberately withholding medical care for those who can recover does raise the question, Once society has embarked on such a slope, where will it stop?

Those opposed to Callahan, Lamm and the other advocates of limiting care to the old, but who also favor extending the frontier of life, must answer the question, Where will the resources come from? One answer is found in the realization that defining people as old at the age of 65 is obsolescent. That age limit was set generations ago, before changes in life styles and medicines much extended not only life but also the number and quality of productive years. One might recognize that many of the "elderly" can contribute to society not merely by providing love, companionship and wisdom to the young but also by continuing to work, in the traditional sense of the term. Indeed, many already work in the underground economy because of the large penalty—a cut in Social Security benefits—exacted from them if they hold a job "on the books."

Allowing elderly people to retain their Social Security benefits while working, typically part-time, would immediately raise significant tax revenues, dramatically change the much-feared dependency-to-dependent ratio, provide a much-needed source of child-care workers and increase contributions to Social Security (under the assumption that anybody who will continue to work will continue to contribute to the program). There is also evidence that people who continue to have meaningful work will live longer and healthier lives, without requiring more health care, because psychic well-being in our society is so deeply associated with meaningful work. Other policy changes, such as deferring retirement, modifying Social Security benefits by a small, gradual stretching out of the age of full-benefit entitlement, plus some other shifts under way, could be used readily to gain more resources. Such changes might be justified prima facie because as we extend life and its quality, the payouts to the old may also be stretched out.

Beyond the question of whether to cut care or stretch out Social Security payouts, policies that seek to promote intergenerational equity must be assessed as to how they deal with another matter of equity: that between the poor and the rich. A policy that would stop Federal support for certain kinds of care, as Callahan and others propose, would halt treatment for the aged, poor, the near-poor and even the less-well-off segment of the middle class (although for the latter at a later point), while the rich would continue to buy all the care they wished to. Callahan's suggestion that a consensus of doctors would stop certain kinds of care for all elderly people is quite impractical; for it to work, most if not all doctors would have to agree to participate. Even if this somehow happened, the rich would buy their services overseas either by going there or by importing the services. There is little enough we can do to significantly enhance economic equality. Do we want to exacerbate the inequalities that already exist by completely eliminating access to major categories of health care services for those who cannot afford to pay for them?

In addition to concern about slipping down the slope of less (and less) care, the *way* the limitations are to be introduced raises a serious question. The advocates of changing the intergenerational allocation of resources favor rationing health care for the elderly but nothing else. This is a major intellectual weakness of their argument. There are other major targets to consider within health care, as well as other areas, which seem, at least by some criteria, much more inviting than terminating care to those above a certain age. Within the medical sector, for example, why not stop all interventions for which there is no hard evidence that they are beneficial? Say, public financing of psychotherapy and coronary bypass operations? Why not take the $2 billion or so from plastic surgery dedicated to face lifts, reducing behinds and the like? Or require that all burials be done by low-cost cremations rather than using high-cost coffins?

Once we extend our reach beyond medical care to health care, if we cannot stop people from blowing $25 billion per year on cigarettes and convince them to use the money to serve the young, shouldn't we at least cut out public subsidies to tobacco growers before we save funds by denying antibiotics to old people? And there is the matter of profits. The high-technology medicine Callahan targets for savings is actually a minor cause of the increase in health care costs for the elderly or for anyone—about 4 percent. A major factor is the very high standard of living American doctors have, compared to those of many other nations. Indeed, many doctors tell interviewers that they love their work and would do it

for half their current income as long as the incomes of their fellow practitioners were also cut. Another important area of saving is the exorbitant profits made by the nondoctor owners of dialysis units and nursing homes. If we dare ask how many years of life are enough, should we not also be able to ask how much profit is "enough"? This profit, by the way, is largely set not by the market but by public policy.

Last but not least, as the United States enters a time of economic constraints, should we draw new lines of conflict or should we focus on matters that sustain our societal fabric? During the 1960s numerous groups gained in political consciousness and actively sought to address injustices done to them. The result has been some redress and an increase in the level of societal stress (witness the deeply troubled relationships between the genders). But these conflicts occurred in an affluent society and redressed deeply felt grievances. Are the young like blacks and women, except that they have not yet discovered their oppressors—a group whose consciousness should be raised, so it will rally and gain its due share?

The answer is in the eye of the beholder. There are no objective criteria that can be used here the way they can be used between the races or between the genders. While women and minorities have the same rights to the same jobs at the same pay as white males, the needs of the young and the aged are so different that no simple criteria of equity come to mind. Thus, no one would argue that the teen-agers and those above 75 have the same need for schooling or nursing homes.

At the same time, it is easy to see that those who try to mobilize the young—led by a new Washington research group, Americans for Generational Equity (AGE), formed to fight for the needs of the younger generation—offer many arguments that do not hold. For instance, they often argue that today's young, age 35 or less, will pay for old people's Social Security, but by the time that they come of age they will not be able to collect, because Social Security will be bankrupt. However, this argument is based on extremely farfetched assumptions about the future. In effect, Social Security is now and for the foreseeable future overprovided, and its surplus is used to reduce deficits caused by other expenditures, such as Star Wars, in what is still an integrated budget. And, if Social Security runs into the red again somewhere after the year 2020, relatively small adjustments in premiums and payouts would restore it to financial health.

Above all, it is a dubious sociological achievement to foment conflict between the generations, because, unlike the minorities and the white majority, or men and women, many millions of Americans are neither young nor old but of intermediate ages. We should not avoid issues just because we face stressing times in an already strained society; but maybe we should declare a moratorium on raising new conflicts until more compelling arguments can be found in their favor, and more evidence that this particular line of divisiveness is called for.

Age-Based Allocation: Discrimination or Justice?
Robert M. Veatch

A biographical sketch of Robert M. Veatch is found on page 55.

Veatch discusses and criticizes two kinds of arguments given in defense of age-based rationing (which he calls "allocation"): arguments from utility and arguments from justice. He rejects arguments based on utility that would ground rationing either on considerations of social usefulness or on statistical predictions of the medical usefulness of interventions. However, he accepts the possibility of establishing fair and reasonable social policies that use age as a basis for excluding the elderly from some types of medical care.

It is widely reported that in Britain patients over the age of 65 are excluded from hemodialysis. In fact, this is not official policy, but one study reported that 80% of United Kingdom dialysis centers excluded patients over 65. Whether official or not, the idea is horrifying to many Americans. Although health care resources are limited, excluding patients solely on the basis of age sounds wrong.

Americans may not be free of age-based allocation, however. The Diagnosis Related Group (DRG) system has many groups defined not just by illness but by age, typically beginning at age 70; patients with the same ailments but of different ages generate different reimbursements. Medicare funding of heart transplants is likely to include an upper age limit. Already, liver transplants are authorized on the basis of age.

Congress's Office of Technology Assessment was so concerned that it commissioned a study of the social and

ethical problems of distributing life-sustaining technologies, including the role of age in setting limits. Two kinds of arguments are given defending age-based limits: utility and justice.

The argument of utility bases cut-offs on the judgment that elderly people are no longer useful members of society. Dialyzing persons over age 65 takes resources away from younger, more useful members of the society—those who could lead productive lives. If that is their basis, defenders of age-based limits are in for considerable argument.

In the first place, it is just not true that persons over 65 are necessarily less useful. Some are still working efficiently in important jobs. Calculations would also have to include more subtle values: role models, loving care givers, and compassionate grandparents, for example. More fundamentally, most people find the idea of allocating resources on the basis of usefulness simply repulsive. Scholars, such as Jerry Avorn, James Childress, and Harry Moody, have all challenged the ethics of allocating resources to younger persons on this basis.

At this point, defenders shift to medical usefulness. Medical risks make heart transplants contraindicated above age 55. Age is only a marker for success, not blatant age discrimination per se. That sounds more accept-able but still raises questions. We cannot simply identify a specific age as a clear indicator that an intervention will or will not work. Age is, at best, statistically related to success.

Even if age is a predictor of success, there are still problems. Society is increasingly skeptical of using social indicators in allocating resources. For some medical interventions, men statistically do better than women, the rich better than the poor, or whites better than blacks. It seems wrong to use these sociological facts to eliminate those interventions for groups doing worse statistically. Medical usefulness based on a statistical prediction of usefulness is only a social criterion in disguise; it is not based on any evidence of success in the individual. If we reject the argument that only the social groups that do statistically better are entitled to treatment, wouldn't we reject age as a social criterion for allocating resources?

The defense of age as a predictor of usefulness is a difficult one. Many doubt that the health care system should simply do as much good as possible, independent of how benefits are distributed.

The other basis for using age focuses more on fairness and justice. At least three different examples of this kind of reasoning have appeared recently.

REASONABLE LIMITS

Daniel Callahan, Director of The Hastings Center, argues in his book *Setting Limits*... that the goal of medicine should be "to help people live out a natural life span and, after that, not actively to help extend life." Beyond that point, only care necessary to relieve suffering is appropriate. He appeals to the reasonable limits of the life span, not a calculation of usefulness, medical or social.

Norman Daniels, a professor of philosophy at Tufts University, argues that age-based allocation is fundamentally different from allocation based on sex or race or other social categories. He asks us to imagine ourselves trying to decide what portion of our resources we would want to allocate to health care at different stages of our personal life cycles. He suggests that the reasonable thing to do would be to provide enough care to have fair opportunities at each age range. Daniels proposes that we would rationally want health insurance that would give us opportunities for normal functioning at all stages in the life cycle. This would mean different care for persons of different ages that is not based on their useful-ness as persons or on the effectiveness of interventions for their age group.

According to Daniels, justice requires that a society adopt insurance schemes that provide such age-specific opportunities. Both Callahan and Daniels end up with moral defenses of age-based limits that are grounded more in what is just or fair than what is efficient or useful.

A third attempt to establish age-based limits in justice starts with the premise that people should be given health care necessary for them to have a chance for opportunities for equality. The key ethical issue, however, then becomes one of deciding how people can be treated equally. There are two ways to treat people equally. We could assess the medical needs at a moment in time. Two people of different ages suffering from equally life-threatening end-stage renal disease (ESRD) could, from the "moment-in-time" perspective, be said to have equal need. On the other hand, people could be entitled to the health care needed to give them equal opportunities over their lifetimes. From the "over-a-lifetime" perspective, an elderly and a young person suffering equally serious kidney problems are not at all comparable. The elderly person has had a lifetime of opportunity. By contrast, the younger person in ESRD has much greater need in order to have a lifetime of opportunities. Treating them equally from this lifetime perspective means that the young person deserves priority.

But if justice requires priority for younger persons, on what grounds could the elderly qualify for any medical care at all? On what grounds could they get pain relief and the basics of nursing care? It seems obvious that ethics requires giving the elderly at least these basics of care. Using the moment-in-time perspective for such basics and possibly for relatively safe, simple, and sure remedies for acute illness seems necessary. The two different ways of interpreting equality may be appropriate for different kinds of care.

DISCRIMINATION?

There are important differences among these perspectives. Callahan's scheme draws a sharp division between those who have completed the major stages of the life cycle and those who have not. He provides no basis for distinguishing between those who have recently reached this point and those who have long since reached it. Likewise, he seems to provide no basis for assigning age-based priority between an 18-year-old and someone nearing the end of the life cycle (say, someone in his late sixties). Daniels's approach recognizes different ranges of normal opportunity at different life stages and could easily account for different allocations to the 18- and 68-year-olds. The over-a-lifetime view recognizes gradations of claims over the entire life cycle, thus avoiding Callahan's unrealistically sharp chasm between those who have completed their life cycle and those who have not and Daniels's separation of claims into different age groups.

AGE-BASED LIMITS

None of these approaches accepts any age-based limits for relief of suffering or the basics of medical care. Most important, none would ground age-based allocations on either social usefulness or on statistical predictions of the medical usefulness of interventions.

Ethical discussion of limiting health care is no longer taboo. People are realizing that resources are limited and that some criteria are needed for allocating health care—based not on social utility, but on fairness. Age, at first, looks like it is just another social discrimination. More careful examination seems to be taking us in an unexpected direction. Some are beginning to conclude that if we are reasonable and fair about planning what we would like for ourselves when we are elderly, some interventions would be excluded. Deciding whether we can establish fair social policies that exclude on the basis of age is a crucial ethical project for the next decade.

Microallocation Decisions

The Allocation of Exotic Medical Lifesaving Therapy
Nicholas P. Rescher

Nicholas P. Rescher is professor of philosophy at the University of Pittsburgh. Among his many books are *Distributive Justice: A Constructive Critique of the Utilitarian Theory of Distribution* (1966), *Welfare: The Social Issues in Philosophical Perspective* (1972), *Unselfishness: The Role of the Vicarious Affects in Moral Philosophy* (1975), *Dialectics: A Controversy Oriented Approach to the Theory of Knowledge* (1977), and *Empirical Inquiry* (1982). Rescher's published articles include "Ethical Issues Regarding the Delivery of Health-Care Services."

Rescher focuses on *microallocation* decisions regarding scarce medical lifesaving therapies. He attempts to set forth the criteria that should govern the selection process when the decisions made determine who will be given and who will be denied the opportunity to survive. Rescher advocates a two-tiered, cluster-of-criteria system. He suggests one set of criteria that should be used to determine who will be placed in the pool of applicants from which some will be chosen to receive treatment. The main criterion here seems to be the "prospect of success factor." Rescher then proposes a second set of criteria that should be used to select individuals from the first pool. In presenting this second set of criteria, Rescher appeals to both utility and justice. He concludes by arguing that if there are no really significant disparities within the pool of candidates selected by this two-step process, a random selection process should be used in making the final decisions.

Reprinted with permission of the author and the publisher from *Ethics*, vol. 79, no. 3 (April 1969), pp. 173–86. Copyright © 1969 by The University of Chicago.

I THE PROBLEM

Technological progress has in recent years transformed the limits of the possible in medical therapy. However, the elevated state of sophistication of modern medical technology has brought the economists' classic problem of scarcity in its wake as an unfortunate side product. The enormously sophisticated and complex equipment and the highly trained teams of experts requisite for its utilization are scarce resources in relation to potential demand. The administrators of the great medical institutions that preside over these scarce resources thus come to be faced increasingly with the awesome choice: *Whose life to save?*

A (somewhat hypothetical) paradigm example of this problem may be sketched within the following set of definitive assumptions: We suppose that persons in some particular medically morbid condition are "mortally afflicted": It is virtually certain that they will die within a short time period (say ninety days). We assume that some very complex course of treatment (e.g., a heart transplant) represents a substantial probability of life prolongation for persons in this mortally afflicted condition. We assume that the facilities available in terms of human resources, mechanical instrumentalities, and requisite materials (e.g., hearts in the case of a heart transplant) make it possible to give a certain treatment—this "exotic (medical) lifesaving therapy," or ELT for short—to a certain, relatively small number of people. And finally we assume that a substantially greater pool of people in the mortally afflicted condition is at hand. The problem then may be formulated as follows: How is one to select within the pool of afflicted patients the ones to be given the ELT treatment in question: how to select those "whose lives are to be saved"? Faced with many candidates for an ELT process that can be made available to only a few, doctors and medical administrators confront the decision of who is to be given a chance at survival and who is, in effect, to be condemned to die.

As has already been implied, the "heroic" variety of spare-part surgery can pretty well be assimilated to this paradigm. One can foresee the time when heart transplantation, for example, will have become pretty much a routine medical procedure, albeit on a very limited basis, since a cardiac surgeon with the technical competence to transplant hearts can operate at best a rather small number of times each week and the elaborate facilities for such operations will most probably exist on a modest scale. Moreover, in "spare-part" surgery there is always

the problem of availability of the "spare parts" themselves. A report in one British newspaper gives the following picture: "Of the 150,000 who die of heart disease each year [in the U.K.], Mr. Donald Longmore, research surgeon at the National Heart Hospital [in London] estimates that 22,000 might be eligible for heart surgery. Another 30,000 would need heart and lung transplants. But there are probably only between 7,000 and 14,000 potential donors a year."[1] Envisaging this situation in which at the very most something like one in four heart-malfunction victims can be saved, we clearly confront a problem in ELT allocation.

A perhaps even more drastic case in point is afforded by long-term haemodialysis, an ongoing process by which a complex device—an "artificial kidney machine"—is used periodically in cases of chronic renal failure to substitute for a non-functional kidney in "cleaning" potential poisons from the blood. Only a few major institutions have chronic haemodialysis units, whose complex operation is an extremely expensive proposition. For the present and the foreseeable future the situation is that "the number of places available for chronic haemodialysis is hopelessly inadequate."[2]

The traditional medical ethos has insulated the physician against facing the very existence of this problem. When swearing the Hippocratic Oath, he commits himself to work for the benefit of the sick in "whatsoever house I enter."[3] In taking this stance, the physician substantially renounces the explicit choice of saving certain lives rather than others. Of course, doctors have always in fact had to face such choices on the battlefield or in times of disaster, but there the issue had to be resolved hurriedly, under pressure, and in circumstances in which the very nature of the case effectively precluded calm deliberation by the decision maker as well as criticism by others. In sharp contrast, however, cases of the type we have postulated in the present discussion arise predictably, and represent choices to be made deliberately and "in cold blood."

It is, to begin with, appropriate to remark that this problem is not fundamentally a medical problem. For when there are sufficiently many afflicted candidates for ELT then—so we may assume—there will also be more than enough for whom the purely medical grounds for ELT allocation are decisively strong in any individual case, and just about equally strong throughout the group. But in this circumstance a selection of some afflicted patients over and against others cannot *ex hypothesi* be made on the basis of purely medical considerations.

The selection problem, as we have said, is in substantial measure not a medical one. It is a problem *for* medical men, which must somehow be solved by them, but that does not make it a medical issue—any more than the problem of hospital building is a medical issue. As a problem it belongs to the category of philosophical problems—specifically a problem of moral philosophy or ethics. Structurally, it bears a substantial kinship with those issues in this field that revolve about the notorious whom-to-save-on-the-lifeboat and whom-to-throw-to-the-wolves-pursuing-the-sled questions. But whereas questions of this just-indicated sort are artificial, hypothetical, and far-fetched, the ELT issue poses a *genuine* policy question for the responsible administrators in medical institutions, indeed a question that threatens to become commonplace in the foreseeable future.

Now what the medical administrator needs to have, and what the philosopher is presumably *ex officio* in a position to help in providing, is a body of *rational guidelines* for making choices in these literally life-or-death situations. This is an issue in which many interested parties have a substantial stake, including the responsible decision maker who wants to satisfy his conscience that he is acting in a reasonable way. Moreover, the family and associates of the man who is turned away—to say nothing of the man himself—have the right to an acceptable explanation. And indeed even the general public wants to know that what is being done is fitting and proper. All of these interested parties are entitled to insist that a reasonable code of operating principles provides a defensible rationale for making the life-and-death choices involved in ELT.

II   THE TWO TYPES OF CRITERIA

Two distinguishable types of criteria are bound up in the issue of making ELT choices. We shall call these *Criteria of Inclusion* and *Criteria of Comparison*, respectively. The distinction at issue here requires some explanation. We can think of the selection as being made by a two-stage process: (1) the selection from among all possible candidates (by a suitable screening process) of a group to be taken under serious consideration as candidates for therapy, and then (2) the actual singling out, within this group, of the particular individuals to whom therapy is to be given. Thus the first process narrows down the range of comparative choice by eliminating *en bloc* whole categories of potential candidates. The second process

calls for a more refined, case-by-case comparison of those candidates that remain. By means of the first set of criteria one forms a selection group; by means of the second set, an actual selection is made within this group.

Thus what we shall call a "selection system" for the choice of patients to receive therapy of the ELT type will consist of criteria of these two kinds. Such a system will be acceptable only when the reasonableness of its component criteria can be established.

III   ESSENTIAL FEATURES OF AN ACCEPTABLE ELT SELECTION SYSTEM

To qualify as reasonable, an ELT selection must meet two important "regulative" requirements: it must be *simple* enough to be readily intelligible, and it must be *plausible*, that is, patently reasonable in a way that can be apprehended easily and without involving ramified subtleties. Those medical administrators responsible for ELT choices must follow a modus operandi that virtually all the people involved can readily understand to be acceptable (at a reasonable level of generality, at any rate). Appearances are critically important here. It is not enough that the choice be made in a *justifiable* way; it must be possible for people—*plain* people—to "see" (i.e., understand without elaborate teaching or indoctrination) that *it is justified*, insofar as any mode of procedure can be justified in cases of this sort.

One "constitutive" requirement is obviously an essential feature of a reasonable selection system: all of its component criteria—those of inclusion and those of comparison alike—must be reasonable in the sense of being *rationally defensible*. The ramifications of this requirement call for detailed consideration. But one of its aspects should be noted without further ado: it must be *fair*—it must treat relevantly like cases alike, leaving no room for "influence" or favoritism, etc.

IV   THE BASIC SCREENING STAGE: CRITERIA OF INCLUSION (AND EXCLUSION)

Three sorts of considerations are prominent among the plausible criteria of inclusion/exclusion at the basic screening stage: the constituency factor, the progress-of-science factor, and the prospect-of-success factor.

A The Constituency Factor

It is a "fact of life" that ELT can be available only in the institutional setting of a hospital or medical institute or the like. Such institutions generally have normal clientele boundaries. A veterans' hospital will not concern itself primarily with treating nonveterans, a children's hospital cannot be expected to accommodate the "senior citizen," an army hospital can regard college professors as outside its sphere. Sometimes the boundaries are geographic—a state hospital may admit only residents of a certain state. (There are, of course, indefensible constituency principles—say race or religion, party membership, or ability to pay; and there are cases of borderline legitimacy, e.g., sex.[4]) A medical institution is justified in considering for ELT only persons within its own constituency, provided this constituency is constituted upon a defensible basis. Thus the haemodialysis selection committee in Seattle "agreed to consider only those applicants who were residents of the state of Washington.... They justified this stand on the grounds that since the basic research...had been done at...a state-supported institution—the people whose taxes had paid for the research should be its first beneficiaries."[5]

While thus insisting that constituency considerations represent a valid and legitimate factor in ELT selection, I do feel there is much to be said for minimizing their role in life-or-death cases. Indeed a refusal to recognize them at all is a significant part of medical tradition, going back to the very oath of Hippocrates. They represent a departure from the ideal arising with the institutionalization of medicine, moving it away from its original status as an art practiced by an individual practitioner.

B The Progress-of-Science Factor

The needs of medical research can provide a second valid principle of inclusion. The research interests of the medical staff in relation to the specific nature of the cases at issue is a significant consideration. It may be important for the progress of medical science—and thus of potential benefit to many persons in the future—to determine how effective the ELT at issue is with diabetics or persons over sixty or with a negative RH factor. Considerations of this sort represent another type of legitimate factor in ELT selection.

A very definitely *borderline* case under this head would revolve around the question of a patient's willing-ness to pay, not in monetary terms, but in offering himself as an experimental subject, say by contracting to return at designated times for a series of tests substantially unrelated to his own health, but yielding data of importance to medical knowledge in general.

C The Prospect-of-Success Factor

It may be that while the ELT at issue is not without *some* effectiveness in general, it has been established to be highly effective only with patients in certain specific categories (e.g., females under forty of a specific blood type). This difference in effectiveness—in the absolute or in the probability of success—is (we assume) so marked as to constitute virtually a difference in kind rather than in degree. In this case, it would be perfectly legitimate to adopt the general rule of making the ELT at issue available only or primarily to persons in this substantial-promise-of-success category. (It is on grounds of this sort that young children and persons over fifty are generally ruled out as candidates for haemodialysis.)

We have maintained that the three factors of constituency, progress of science, and prospect of success represent legitimate criteria of inclusion for ELT selection. But it remains to examine the considerations which legitimate them. The legitimating factors are in the final analysis practical or pragmatic in nature. From the practical angle, it is advantageous—indeed to some extent necessary—that the arrangements governing medical institutions should embody certain constituency principles. It makes good pragmatic and utilitarian sense that progress-of-science considerations should be operative here. And, finally, the practical aspect is reinforced by a whole host of other considerations—including moral ones—in supporting the prospect-of-success criterion. The workings of each of these factors are of course conditioned by the ever-present element of limited availability. They are operative only in this context, that is, prospect of success is a legitimate consideration at all only because we are dealing with a situation of scarcity.

V THE FINAL SELECTION STAGE: CRITERIA OF SELECTION

Five sorts of elements must, as we see it, figure primarily among the plausible criteria of selection that are to be brought to bear in further screening the group constituted after application of the criteria of inclusion: the relative-likelihood-of-success factor, the life-expectancy factor, the family role factor, the potential-contributions factor, and the services-rendered factor. The first two represent the *biomedical* aspect, the second three the *social* aspect.

A The Relative-Likelihood-of-Success Factor

It is clear that the relative likelihood of success is a legitimate and appropriate factor in making a selection within the group of qualified patients that are to receive ELT. This is obviously one of the considerations that must count very significantly in a reasonable selection procedure.

The present criterion is of course closely related to item C of the preceding section. There we were concerned with prospect-of-success considerations categorically and *en bloc*. Here at present they come into play in a particularized case-by-case comparison among individuals. If the therapy at issue is not a once-and-for-all proposition and requires ongoing treatment, cognate considerations must be brought in. Thus, for example, in the case of a chronic ELT procedure such as haemodialysis it would clearly make sense to give priority to patients with a potentially reversible condition (who would thus need treatment for only a fraction of their remaining lives).

B The Life-Expectancy Factor

Even if the ELT is "successful" in the patient's case he may, considering his age and/or other aspects of his general medical condition, look forward to only a very short probable future life. This is obviously another factor that must be taken into account.

C The Family Role Factor

A person's life is a thing of importance not only to himself but to others—friends, associates, neighbors, colleagues, etc. But his (or her) relationship to his immediate family is a thing of unique intimacy and significance. The nature of his relationship to his wife, children, and parents, and the issue of their financial and psychological dependence upon him, are obviously matters that deserve to be given weight in the ELT selection process. Other things being anything like equal, the mother of minor children must take priority over the middle-aged bachelor.

D The Potential Future-Contributions Factor (Prospective Service)

In "choosing to save" one life rather than another, "the society," through the mediation of the particular medical institution in question—which should certainly look upon itself as a trustee for the social interest—is clearly warranted in considering the likely pattern of future *services to be rendered* by the patient (adequate recovery assumed), considering his age, talent, training, and past record of performance. In its allocations of ELT, society "invests" a scarce resource in one person as against another and is thus entitled to look to the probable prospective "return" on its investment.

It may well be that a thoroughly egalitarian society is reluctant to put someone's social contribution into the scale in situations of the sort at issue. One popular article states that "the most difficult standard would be the candidate's value to society," and goes on to quote someone who said: "You can't just pick a brilliant painter over a laborer. The average citizen would be quickly eliminated."[6] But what if it were not a brilliant painter but a brilliant surgeon or medical researcher that was at issue? One wonders if the author of the *obiter dictum* that one "can't just pick" would still feel equally sure of his ground. In any case, the fact that the standard is difficult to apply is certainly no reason for not attempting to apply it. The problem of ELT selection is inevitably burdened with difficult standards.

Some might feel that in assessing a patient's value to society one should ask not only who if permitted to continue living can make the greatest contribution to society in some creative or constructive way, but also who by dying would leave behind the greatest burden on society in assuming the discharge of their residual responsibilities.[7] Certainly the philosophical utilitarian would give equal weight to both these considerations. Just here is where I would part ways with orthodox utilitarianism. For—though this is not the place to do so—I should be prepared to argue that a civilized society has an obligation to promote the furtherance of positive achievements in cultural and related areas even if this means the assumption of certain added burdens.[8]

E   The Past Services-Rendered Factor
(Retrospective Service)

A person's services to another person or group have always been taken to constitute a valid basis for a claim
upon this person or group—of course a moral and not
necessarily a legal claim. Society's obligation for the recognition and reward of services rendered—an obligation
whose discharge is also very possibly conducive to self-
interest in the long run—is thus another factor to be
taken into account. This should be viewed as a morally
necessary correlative of the previously considered factor
of *prospective* service. It would be morally indefensible of
society in effect to say: "Never mind about services you
rendered yesterday—it is only the services to be rendered tomorrow that will count with us today." We live
in very future-oriented times, constantly preoccupied in
a distinctly utilitarian way with future satisfactions. And
this disinclines us to give much recognition to past services. But parity considerations of the sort just adduced
indicate that such recognition should be given *on grounds
of equity*. No doubt a justification for giving weight to
services rendered can also be attempted along utilitarian
lines. ("The reward of past services rendered spurs people on to greater future efforts and is thus socially advantageous in the long-run future.") In saying that past
services should be counted "on grounds of equity"—
rather than "on grounds of utility"—I take the view that
even if this utilitarian defense could somehow be shown
to be fallacious, I should still be prepared to maintain
the propriety of taking services rendered into account.
The position does not rest on a utilitarian basis and so
would not collapse with the removal of such a basis.[9]

As we have said, these five factors fall into three
groups: the biomedical factors A and B, the familial factor C, and the social factors D and E. With items A and
B the need for a detailed analysis of the medical considerations comes to the fore. The age of the patient, his
medical history, his physical and psychological condition, his specific disease, etc., will all need to be taken
into exact account. These biomedical factors represent
technical issues: they call for the physicians' expert judgment and the medical statisticians' hard data. And they
are ethically uncontroversial factors—their legitimacy
and appropriateness are evident from the very nature of
the case.

Greater problems arise with the familial and social
factors. They involve intangibles that are difficult to
judge. How is one to develop subcriteria for weighing

the relative social contributions of (say) an architect or a
librarian or a mother of young children? And they involve highly problematic issues. (For example, should
good moral character be rated a plus and bad a minus in
judging services rendered?) And there is something
strikingly unpleasant in grappling with issues of this sort
for people brought up in times greatly inclined towards
maxims of the type "Judge not!" and "Live and let
live!" All the same, in the situation that concerns us here
such distasteful problems must be faced, since a failure
to choose to save some is tantamount to sentencing all.
Unpleasant choices are intrinsic to the problem of ELT
selection; they are of the very essence of the matter.[10]

But is reference to all these factors indeed inevitable? The justification for taking account of the medical
factors is pretty obvious. But why should the social aspect of services rendered and to be rendered be taken
into account at all? The answer is that they must be
taken into account not from the *medical* but from the *ethical* point of view. Despite disagreement on many fundamental issues, moral philosophers of the present day
are pretty well in consensus that the justification of human actions is to be sought largely and primarily—if not
exclusively—in the principles of utility and of justice.[11]
But utility requires reference of services to be rendered
and justice calls for a recognition of services that have
been rendered. Moral considerations would thus demand recognition of these two factors. (This, of course,
still leaves open the question of whether the point of
view provides a valid basis of action: Why base one's actions upon moral principles?—or, to put it bluntly—
Why be moral? The present paper is, however, hardly
the place to grapple with so fundamental an issue, which
has been canvassed in the literature of philosophical ethics since Plato.)

VI   MORE THAN MEDICAL ISSUES
ARE INVOLVED

An active controversy has of late sprung up in medical
circles over the question of whether non-physician laymen should be given a role in ELT selection (in the specific context of chronic haemodialysis). One physician
writes: "I think that the assessment of the candidates
should be made by a senior doctor on the [dialysis] unit,
but I am sure that it would be helpful to him—both in
sharing responsibility and in avoiding personal pressure—if a small unnamed group of people [presumably

including laymen] officially made the final decision. I visualize the doctor bringing the data to the group, explaining the points in relation to each case, and obtaining their approval of his order of priority.[12]

Essentially this procedure of a selection committee of laymen has for some years been in use in one of the most publicized chronic dialysis units, that of the Swedish Hospital of Seattle, Washington.[13] Many physicians are apparently reluctant to see the choice of allocation of medical therapy pass out of strictly medical hands. Thus in a recent symposium on the "Selection of Patients for Haemodialysis,"[14] Dr. Ralph Shakman writes: "Who is to implement the selection? In my opinion it must ultimately be the responsibility of the consultants in charge of the renal units...I can see no reason for delegating this responsibility to lay persons. Surely the latter would be better employed if they could be persuaded to devote their time and energy to raise more and more money for us to spend on our patients."[15] Other contributors to this symposium strike much the same note. Dr. F. M. Parsons writes: "In an attempt to overcome... difficulties in selection some have advocated introducing certain specified lay people into the discussions. Is it wise? I doubt whether a committee of this type can adjudicate as satisfactorily as two medical colleagues, particularly as successful therapy involves close cooperation between doctor and patient."[16] And Dr. M. A. Wilson writes in the same symposium: "The suggestion has been made that lay panels should select individuals for dialysis from among a group who are medically suitable. Though this would relieve the doctor-in-charge of a heavy load of responsibility, it would place the burden on those who have no personal knowledge and have to base their judgments on medical or social reports. I do not believe this would result in better decisions for the group or improve the doctor-patient relationship in individual cases."[17]

But no amount of flag waving about the doctor's facing up to his responsibility—or prostrations before the idol of the doctor-patient relationship and reluctance to admit laymen into the sacred precincts of the conference chambers of medical consultations—can obscure the essential fact that ELT selection is not a wholly medical problem. When there are more than enough places in an ELT program to accommodate all who need it, then it will clearly be a medical question to decide who does have the need and which among these would successfully respond. But when an admitted gross insufficiency of places exists, when there are ten or fifty or one hundred highly eligible candidates for each place in the

program, then it is unrealistic to take the view that purely medical criteria can furnish a sufficient basis for selection. The question of ELT selection becomes serious as a phenomenon of scale—because, as more candidates present themselves, strictly medical factors are increasingly less adequate as a selection criterion precisely because by numerical category-crowding there will be more and more cases whose "status is much the same" so far as purely medical considerations go.

The ELT selection problem clearly poses issues that transcend the medical sphere because—in the nature of the case—many residual issues remain to be dealt with once *all* of the medical questions have been faced. Because of this there is good reason why laymen as well as physicians should be involved in the selection process. Once the medical considerations have been brought to bear, fundamental social issues remain to be resolved. The instrumentalities of ELT have been created through the social investment of scarce resources, and the interests of the society deserve to play a role in their utilization. As representatives of their social interests, lay opinions should function to complement and supplement medical views once the proper arena of medical considerations is left behind.[18] Those physicians who have urged the presence of lay members on selection panels can, from this point of view, be recognized as having seen the issue in proper perspective.

One physician has argued against lay representation on selection panels for haemodialysis as follows: "If the doctor advises dialysis and the lay panel refuses, the patient will regard this as a death sentence passed by an anonymous court from which he has no right of appeal."[19] But this drawback is not specific to the use of a lay panel. Rather, it is a feature inherent in every selection procedure, regardless of whether the selection is done by the head doctor of the unit, by a panel of physicians, etc. No matter who does the selecting among patients recommended for dialysis, the feelings of the patient who has been rejected (and knows it) can be expected to be much the same, provided that he recognizes the actual nature of the choice (and is not deceived by the possibly convenient but ultimately poisonous fiction that because the selection was made by physicians it was made entirely on medical grounds).

In summary, then, the question of ELT selection would appear to be one that is in its very nature heavily laden with issues of medical research, practice, and administration. But it will not be a question that can be resolved on solely medical grounds. Strictly social issues of justice and utility will invariably arise in this area—questions going outside the medical area in whose resolution medical laymen can and should play a substantial role.

VII   THE INHERENT IMPERFECTION (NON-OPTIMALITY) OF ANY SELECTION SYSTEM

Our discussion to this point of the design of a selection system for ELT has left a gap that is a very fundamental and serious omission. We have argued that five factors must be taken into substantial and explicit account:

A. *Relative likelihood of success.*—Is the chance of the treatment's being "successful" to be rated as high, good, average, etc.?[20]

B. *Expectancy of future life.*—Assuming the "success" of the treatment, how much longer does the patient stand a good chance (75 per cent or better) of living—considering his age and general condition?

C. *Family role.*—To what extent does the patient have responsibilities to others in his immediate family?

D. *Social contributions rendered.*—Are the patient's past services to his society outstanding, substantial, average, etc.?

E. *Social contributions to be rendered.*—Considering his age, talents, training, and past record of performance, is there a substantial probability that the patient will—*adequate recovery being assumed*—render in the future services to his society that can be characterized as outstanding, substantial, average, etc.?

This list is clearly insufficient for the construction of a reasonable selection system, since that would require not only *that these factors be taken into account* (somehow or other), but—going beyond this—would specify *a specific set of procedures for taking account of them.* The specific procedures that would constitute such a system would have to take account of the interrelationship of these factors (e.g., B and E), and to set out exact guidelines as to the relevant weight that is to be given to each of them. This is something our discussion has not as yet considered.

In fact, I should want to maintain that there is no such thing here as a single rationally superior selection system. The position of affairs seems to me to be something like this: (1) It is necessary (for reasons already canvassed) to *have* a system, and to have a system that is rationally defensible, and (2) to be rationally defensible, this system must take the factors A–E into substantial and explicit account. But (3) the exact manner in which a rationally defensible system takes account of these factors cannot be fixed in any one specific way on the basis of general considerations. Any of the variety of ways that give A–E "their due" will be acceptable and viable. One cannot hope to find within this range of workable systems some one that is *optimal* in relation to the alternatives. There is no one system that does "the (uniquely) best"—only a variety of systems that do "as well as one can expect to do" in cases of this sort.

The situation is structurally very much akin to that of rules of partition of an estate among the relations of a decedent. It is important *that there be* such rules. And it is reasonable that spouse, children, parents, siblings, etc., be taken account of in these rules. But the question of the exact method of division—say that when the decedent has neither living spouse nor living children then his estate is to be divided, dividing 60 per cent between parents, 40 per cent between siblings versus dividing 90 per cent between parents, 10 per cent between siblings—cannot be settled on the basis of any general abstract considerations of reasonableness. Within broad limits, a *variety* of resolutions are all perfectly acceptable—so that no one procedure can justifiably be regarded as "the (uniquely) best" because it is superior to all others.[21]

VIII   A POSSIBLE BASIS FOR A REASONABLE SELECTION SYSTEM

Having said that there is no such thing as the *optimal* selection system for ELT, I want now to sketch out the broad features of what I would regard as *one acceptable* system.

The basis for the system would be a point rating. The scoring here at issue would give roughly equal weight to the medical considerations (A and B) in comparison with the extramedical considerations (C = family role, D = services rendered, and E = services to be rendered), also giving roughly equal weight to the three items involved here (C, D, and E). The result of such a scoring procedure would provide the essential *starting point* of our ELT selection mechanism. I deliberately say "starting point" because it seems to me that one should not follow the results of this scoring in an *automatic* way. I would propose that the actual selection should only be guided but not actually be dictated by this scoring procedure, along lines now to be explained.

IX THE DESIRABILITY OF INTRODUCING AN ELEMENT OF CHANCE

The detailed procedure I would propose—not of course as optimal (for reasons we have seen), but as eminently acceptable—would combine the scoring procedure just discussed with an element of chance. The resulting selection system would function as follows:

1. First the criteria of inclusion of Section IV above would be applied to constitute a *first phase selection group*—which (we shall suppose) is substantially larger than the number *n* of persons who can actually be accommodated with ELT.

2. Next the criteria of selection of Section V are brought to bear via a scoring procedure of the type described in Section VIII. On this basis a *second phase selection group* is constituted which is only *somewhat* larger—say by a third or a half—than the critical number *n* at issue.

3. If this second phase selection group is relatively homogeneous as regards rating by the scoring procedure—that is, if there are no really major disparities within this group (as would be likely if the initial group was significantly larger than *n*)—then the final selection is made by *random* selection of *n* persons from within this group.

This introduction of the element of chance—in what could be dramatized as a "lottery of life and death"—must be justified. The fact is that such a procedure would bring with it three substantial advantages.

First as we have argued above (in Section VII), any acceptable selection system is inherently non-optimal. The introduction of the element of chance prevents the results that life-and-death choices are made by the automatic application of an admittedly imperfect selection method.

Second, a recourse to chance would doubtless make matters easier for the rejected patient and those who

have a specific interest in him. It would surely be quite hard for them to accept his exclusion by relatively mechanical application of objective criteria in whose implementation subjective judgment is involved. But the circumstances of life have conditioned us to accept the workings of chance and to tolerate the element of luck (good or bad): human life is an inherently contingent process. Nobody, after all, has an absolute right to ELT—but most of us would feel that we have "every bit as much right" to it as anyone else in significantly similar circumstances. The introduction of the element of chance assures a like handling of like cases over the widest possible area that seems reasonable in the circumstances.

Third (and perhaps least), such a recourse to random selection does much to relieve the administrators of the selection system of the awesome burden of ultimate and absolute responsibility.

These three considerations would seem to build up a substantial case for introducing the element of chance into the mechanism of the system for ELT selection in a way limited and circumscribed by other weightier considerations, along some such lines as those set forth above.[22]

It should be recognized that this injection of *man-made* chance supplements the element of *natural* chance that is present inevitably and in any case (apart from the role of chance in singling out certain persons as victims for the affliction at issue). As F. M. Parsons has observed: "any vacancies [in an ELT program—specifically haemodialysis] will be filled immediately by the first suitable patients, even though their claims for therapy may subsequently prove less than those of other patients refused later."[23] Life is a chancy business and even the most rational of human arrangements can cover this over to a very limited extent at best.[24]

NOTES

1 Christine Doyle, "Spare-Part Heart Surgeons Worried by Their Success," *Observer*, May 12, 1968.

2 J. D. N. Nabarro, "Selection of Patients for Haemodialysis," *British Medical Journal* (March 11, 1967), p. 623. Although several thousand patients die in the U.K. each year from renal failure—there are about thirty new cases per million of population—only 10 per cent of these can for the foreseeable future be accommodated with chronic haemodialysis. Kidney transplantation—itself a very

tricky procedure—cannot make a more than minor contribution here. As this article goes to press, I learn that patients can be maintained in home dialysis at an operating cost about half that of maintaining them in a hospital dialysis unit (roughly an $8,000 minimum). In the United States, around 7,000 patients with terminal uremia who could benefit from haemodialysis evolve yearly. As of mid-1968, some 1,000 of these can be accommodated in existing hospital units. By June 1967, a world-wide total of some 120 patients were in treatment by home dialysis. (Data from a forthcoming paper, "Home Dialysis," by C. M. Conty and H. V. Murdaugh. See also R. A. Baillod *et al.*, "Overnight Haemodialysis in the Home," *Proceedings of the European Dialysis and Transplant Association*, VI [1965], 99 ff.).

3 For the Hippocratic Oath see *Hippocrates: Works* (Loeb ed.; London, 1959), I, p. 298.

4 Another example of borderline legitimacy is posed by an endowment "with strings attached," e.g., "In accepting this legacy the hospital agrees to admit and provide all needed treatment for any direct descendant of myself, its founder."

5 Shana Alexander, "They Decide Who Lives, Who Dies," *Life*, LIII (November 9, 1962), 102–25 (see p. 107).

6 Lawrence Lader, "Who Has the Right To Live?" *Good Housekeeping* (January 1968), p. 144.

7 This approach could thus be continued to embrace the previous factor, that of family role, the preceding item (C).

8 Moreover a doctrinaire utilitarian would presumably be willing to withdraw a continuing mode of ELT such as haemodialysis from a patient to make room for a more promising candidate who came to view at a later stage and who could not otherwise be accommodated. I should be unwilling to adopt this course, partly on grounds of utility (with a view to the demoralization of insecurity), partly on the non-utilitarian ground that a "moral commitment" has been made and must be honored.

9 Of course the difficult question remains of the relative weight that should be given to prospective and retrospective service in cases where these factors conflict. There is a good reason to treat them on a par.

10 This in the symposium on "Selection of Patients for Haemodialysis," *British Medical Journal* (March 11, 1967), pp. 622–24. F. M. Parsons writes: "But other forms of selecting patients [distinct from first come, first served] are suspect in my view if they imply

evaluation of man by man. What criteria could be used? Who could justify a claim that the life of a mayor would be more valuable than that of the humblest citizen of his borough? Whatever we may think as individuals none of us is indispensable." But having just set out this hard-line view he immediately backs away from it: "On the other hand, to assume that there was little to choose between Alexander Fleming and Adolf Hitler...would be nonsense, and we should be naive if we were to pretend that we could not be influenced by their achievements and characters if we had to choose between the two of them. Whether we like it or not we cannot escape the fact that this kind of selection for long-term haemodialysis will be required until very large sums of money become available for equipment and services [so that *everyone* who needs treatment can be accommodated]."

11 The relative fundamentality of these principles is, however, a substantially disputed issue.

12 J. D. N. Nabarro, *op. cit.*, p. 622.

13 See Shana Alexander, *op. cit.*

14 *British Medical Journal* (March 11, 1967), pp. 622–24.

15 *Ibid.*, p. 624. Another contributor writes in the same symposium, "The selection of the few [to receive haemodialysis] is proving very difficult—a true 'Doctor's Dilemma'—for almost everybody would agree that this must be a medical decision, preferably reached by consultation among colleagues" (Dr. F. M. Parsons, *ibid.*, p. 623).

16 "Selection of Patients for Haemodialysis," *op. cit.* (n. 10 above), p. 623.

17 Dr. Wilson's article concludes with the perplexing suggestion—wildly beside the point given the structure of the situation at issue—that "the final decision will be made by the patient." But this contention is only marginally more ludicrous than Parsons' contention that in selecting patients for haemodialysis "gainful employment in a well chosen occupation is necessary to achieve the best results" since "only the minority wish to live on charity" (*ibid.*).

18 To say this is of course not to deny that such questions of applied medical ethics will invariably involve a host of medical considerations—it is only to insist that extramedical considerations will also invariably be at issue.

19 M. A. Wilson, "Selection of Patients for Haemodialysis," *op. cit.*, p. 624.

20 In the case of an ongoing treatment involving complex procedure and dietary and other mode-of-life re-

strictions—and chronic haemodialysis definitely falls into this category—the patient's psychological make-up, his willpower to "stick with it" in the face of substantial discouragements—will obviously also be a substantial factor here. The man who gives up, takes not his life alone, but (figuratively speaking) also that of the person he replaced in the treatment schedule.

21 To say that acceptable solutions can range over broad limits is *not* to say that there are no limits at all. It is an obviously intriguing and fundamental problem to raise the question of the factors that set these limits. This complex issue cannot be dealt with adequately here. Suffice it to say that considerations regarding precedent and people's expectations, factors of social utility, and matters of fairness and sense of justice all come into play.

22 One writer has mooted the suggestion that: "Perhaps the right thing to do, difficult as it may be to accept, is to select [for haemodialysis] from among the medically and psychologically qualified patients on a strictly random basis" (S. Gorovitz, "Ethics and the Allocation of Medical Resources," *Medical Research Engineering*, V [1966], p. 7). Outright random selection would, however, seem indefensible because of its refusal to give weight to considerations which, un-

der the circumstances, *deserve* to be given weight. The proposed procedure of superimposing a certain degree of randomness upon the rational-choice criteria would seem to combine the advantages of the two without importing the worst defects of either.

23 "Selection of Patients for Haemodialysis," *op. cit.*, p. 623. The question of whether a patient for chronic treatment should ever be terminated from the program (say if he contracts cancer) poses a variety of difficult ethical problems with which we need not at present concern ourselves. But it does seem plausible to take the (somewhat anti-utilitarian) view that a patient should not be terminated simply because a "better qualified" patient comes along later on. It would seem that a quasi-contractual relationship has been created through established expectations and reciprocal understandings, and that the situation is in this regard akin to that of the man who, having undertaken to sell his house to one buyer, cannot afterward unilaterally undo this arrangement to sell it to a higher bidder who "needs it worse" (thus maximizing the over-all utility).

24 I acknowledge with thanks the help of Miss Hazel Johnson, Reference Librarian at the University of Pittsburgh Library, in connection with the works cited.

The Prostitute, the Playboy, and the Poet: Rationing Schemes for Organ Transplantation
George J. Annas

A biographical sketch of George J. Annas is found on page 137.

Annas examines and compares the respective merits of four major approaches to the microallocation of scarce medical resources: (1) the market approach, (2) the committee-selection process, (3) the lottery approach, and (4) the customary approach. He maintains that the last approach, although apparently relying exclusively on medical criteria, contains many hidden social-worth criteria. Annas condemns the use of social-worth criteria as inconsistent with important value commitments. He advocates a combination of approaches in the interest of fairness and equality as well as efficiency and concludes that a "first come, first served" policy would be preferable as long as it allowed those in imminent danger of death to "jump the queue."

From *American Journal of Public Health*, vol. 75 (1985), pp. 187–189. Copyright © 1985, George J. Annas. Reprinted with permission.

In the public debate about the availability of heart and liver transplants, the issue of rationing on a massive scale has been credibly raised for the first time in United States medical care. In an era of scarce resources, the eventual arrival of such a discussion was, of course, inevitable.[1] Unless we decide to ban heart and liver transplantation, or make them available to everyone, some rationing scheme must be used to choose among potential transplant candidates. The debate has existed throughout the history of medical ethics. Traditionally it has been stated as a choice between saving one of two patients, both of whom require the immediate assistance of the only available physician to survive.

National attention was focused on decisions regarding the rationing of kidney dialysis machines when they were first used on a limited basis in the late 1960s. As one commentator described the debate within the medical profession:

> Shall machines or organs go to the sickest, or to the ones with most promise of recovery; on a first-come, first-served basis; to the most "valuable" patient (based on wealth, education, position, what?); to the one with the most dependents; to women and children first; to those who can pay; to whom? Or should lots be cast, impersonally and uncritically?[2]

In Seattle, Washington, an anonymous screening committee was set up to pick who among competing candidates would receive the life-saving technology. One lay member of the screening committe is quoted as saying:

> The choices were hard...I remember voting against a young woman who was a known prostitute. I found I couldn't vote for her, rather than another candidate, a young wife and mother. I also voted against a young man who, until he learned he had renal failure, had been a ne'er do-well, a real playboy. He promised he would reform his character, go back to school, and so on, if only he were selected for treatment. But I felt I'd lived long enough to know that a person like that won't really do what he was promising at the time.[3]

When the biases and selection criteria of the committee were made public, there was a general negative reaction against this type of arbitrary device. Two experts reacted to the "numbing accounts of how close to the surface lie the prejudices and mindless cliches that pollute the committee's deliberations," by concluding that the committee was "measuring persons in accordance with its own middle-class values." The committee

process, they noted, ruled out "creative nonconformists" and made the Pacific Northwest "no place for a Henry David Thoreau with bad kidneys."[4]

To avoid having to make such explicit, arbitrary, "social worth" determinations, the Congress, in 1972, enacted legislation that provided federal funds for virtually all kidney dialysis and kidney transplantation procedures in the United States.[5] This decision, however, simply served to postpone the time when identical decisions will have to be made about candidates for heart and liver transplantation in a society that does not provide sufficient financial and medical resources to provide all "suitable" candidates with the operation.

There are four major approaches to rationing scarce medical resources: the market approach; the selection committee approach; the lottery approach; and the "customary" approach.[1]

THE MARKET APPROACH

The market approach would provide an organ to everyone who could pay for it with their own funds or private insurance. It puts a very high value on individual rights, and a very low value on equality and fairness. It has properly been criticized on a number of bases, including that the transplant technologies have been developed and are supported with public funds, that medical resources used for transplantation will not be available for higher priority care, and that financial success alone is an insufficient justification for demanding a medical procedure. Most telling is its complete lack of concern for fairness and equity.[6]

A "bake sale" or charity approach that requires the less financially fortunate to make public appeals for funding is demeaning to the individuals involved, and to society as a whole. Rationing by financial ability says we do not believe in equality, but believe that a price can and should be placed on human life and that it should be paid by the individual whose life is at stake. Neither belief is tolerable in a society in which income is inequitably distributed.

THE COMMITTEE SELECTION PROCESS

The Seattle Selection Committee is a model of the committee process. Ethics Committees set up in some hospitals to decide whether or not certain handicapped newborn infants should be given medical care may represent another.[7] These committees have developed because it was seen as unworkable or unwise to explicitly set forth the criteria on which selection decisions would be made. But only two results are possible, as Professor Guido Calabresi has pointed out: either a pattern of decision-making will develop or it will not. If a pattern does develop (e.g., in Seattle, the imposition of middle-class values), then it can be articulated and those decision "rules" codified and used directly, without resort to the committee. If a pattern does not develop, the committee is vulnerable to the charge that it is acting arbitrarily, or dishonestly, and therefore cannot be permitted to continue to make such important decisions.[1]

In the end, public designation of a committee to make selection decisions on vague criteria will fail because it too closely involves the state and all members of society in explicitly preferring specific individuals over others, and in devaluing the interests those others have in living. It thus directly undermines, as surely as the market system does, society's view of equality and the value of human life.

THE LOTTERY APPROACH

The lottery approach is the ultimate equalizer which puts equality ahead of every other value. This makes it extremely attractive, since all comers have an equal chance at selection regardless of race, color, creed, or financial status. On the other hand, it offends our notions of efficiency and fairness since it makes *no* distinctions among such things as the strength of the desires of the candidates, their potential survival, and their quality of life. In this sense it is a mindless method of trying to solve society's dilemma which is caused by its unwillingness or inability to spend enough resources to make a lottery unnecessary. By making this macro spending decision evident to all, it also undermines society's view of the pricelessness of human life. A first-come, first-served system is a type of natural lottery since referral to a transplant program is generally random in time. Nonetheless, higher income groups have quicker access to referral networks and thus have an inherent advantage over the poor in a strict first-come, first-served system.[8, 9]

THE CUSTOMARY APPROACH

Society has traditionally attempted to avoid explicitly recognizing that we are making a choice not to save individual lives because it is too expensive to do so. As long as such decisions are not explicitly acknowledged, they can be tolerated by society. For example, until recently there was said to be a general understanding among general practitioners in Britain that individuals over age 55 suffering from end-stage kidney disease not be referred for dialysis or transplant. In 1984, however, this unwritten practice became highly publicized, with figures that showed a rate of new cases of end-stage kidney disease treated in Britain at 40 per million (versus the US figure of 80 per million) resulting in 1500–3000 "unnecessary deaths" annually.[10] This has, predictably, led to movements to enlarge the National Health Service budget to expand dialysis services to meet this need, a more socially acceptable solution than permitting the now publicly recognized situation to continue.

In the US, the customary approach permits individual physicians to select their patients on the basis of medical criteria or clinical suitability. This, however, contains much hidden social worth criteria. For example, one criterion, common in the transplant literature, requires an individual to have sufficient family support for successful aftercare. This discriminates against individuals without families and those who have become alienated from their families. The criterion may be relevant, but it is hardly medical.

Similar observations can be made about medical criteria that include IQ, mental illness, criminal records, employment, indigency, alcoholism, drug addiction, or geographical location. Age is perhaps more difficult, since it may be impressionistically related to outcome. But it is not medically logical to assume that an individual who is 49 years old is necessarily a better medical candidate for a transplant than one who is 50 years old. Unless specific examination of the characteristics of older persons that make them less desirable candidates is undertaken, such a cut off is arbitrary, and thus devalues the lives of older citizens. The same can be said of blanket exclusions of alcoholics and drug addicts.

In short, the customary approach has one great advantage for society and one great disadvantage: it gives us the illusion that we do not have to make choices; but the cost is mass deception, and when this deception is uncovered, we must deal with it either by universal entitlement or by choosing another method of patient selection.

A COMBINATION OF APPROACHES

A socially acceptable approach must be fair, efficient, and reflective of important social values. The most important values at stake in organ transplantation are fairness itself, equity in the sense of equality, and the value of life. To promote efficiency, it is important that no one receive a transplant unless they want one and are likely to obtain significant benefit from it in the sense of years of life at a reasonable level of functioning.

Accordingly, it is appropriate for there to be an initial screening process that is based *exclusively* on medical criteria designed to measure the probability of a successful transplant, i.e., one in which the patient survives for at least a number of years and is rehabilitated. There is room in medical criteria for social worth judgments, but there is probably no way to avoid this completely. For example, it has been noted that "in many respects social and medical criteria are inextricably intertwined" and that therefore medical criteria might "exclude the poor and disadvantaged because health and socioeconomic status are highly interdependent."[11] Roger Evans gives an example. In the End Stage Renal Disease Program, "those of lower socioeconomic status are likely to have multiple comorbid health conditions such as diabetes, hepatitis, and hypertension" making them both less desirable candidates and more expensive to treat.[11]

To prevent the gulf between the haves and have nots from widening, we must make every reasonable attempt to develop medical criteria that are objective and independent of social worth categories. One minimal way to approach this is to require that medical screening be reviewed and approved by an ethics committee with significant public representation, filed with a public agency, and made readily available to the public for comment. In the event that more than one hospital in a state or region is offering a particular transplant service, it would be most fair and efficient for the individual hospitals to perform the initial medical screening themselves (based on the uniform, objective criteria), but to have all subsequent nonmedical selection done by a method approved by a single selection committee composed of representatives of all hospitals engaged in a particular transplant procedure, as well as significant representation of the public at large.

As this implies, after the medical screening is performed, there may be more acceptable candidates in the "pool" than there are organs or surgical teams to go around. Selection among waiting candidates will then be necessary. This situation occurs now in kidney transplantation, but since the organ matching is much more sophisticated than in hearts and livers (permitting much more precise matching of organ and recipient), and since dialysis permits individuals to wait almost indefinitely for an organ without risking death, the situations are not close enough to permit use of the same matching criteria. On the other hand, to the extent that organs are specifically tissue- and size-matched and fairly distributed to the best matched candidate, the organ distribution system itself will resemble a natural lottery.

When a pool of acceptable candidates is developed, a decision about who gets the next available, suitable organ must be made. We must choose between using a conscious, value-laden, social worth selection criterion (including a committee to make the actual choice), or some type of random device. In view of the unacceptability and arbitrariness of social worth criteria being applied, implicitly or explicitly, by committee, this method is neither viable nor proper. On the other hand, strict adherence to a lottery might create a situation where an individual who has only a one-in-four chance of living five years with a transplant (but who could survive another six months without one) would get an organ before an individual who could survive as long or longer, but who will die within days or hours if he or she is not immediately transplanted. Accordingly, the most reasonable approach seems to be to allocate organs on a first-come, first-served basis to members of the pool but permit individuals to "jump" the queue if the second level selection committee believes they are in immediate danger of death (but still have a reasonable prospect for long-term survival with a transplant) and the person who would otherwise get the organ can survive long enough to be reasonably assured that he or she will be able to get another organ.

The first-come, first-served method of basic selection (after a medical screen) seems the preferred method because it most closely approximates the randomness of a straight lottery without the obviousness of making equity the only promoted value. Some unfairness is introduced by the fact that the more wealthy and medically astute will likely get into the pool first, and thus be ahead in line, but this advantage should decrease sharply as public awareness of the system grows. The possibility of unfairness is also inherent in permitting individuals to jump the queue, but some flexibility needs to be retained in the system to permit it to respond to reasonable contingencies.

We will have to face the fact that should the resources devoted to organ transplantation be limited (as they are now and are likely to be in the future), at some point it is likely that significant numbers of individuals will die in the pool waiting for a transplant. Three things can be done to avoid this: 1) medical criteria can be made stricter, perhaps by adding a more rigorous notion of "quality" of life to longevity and prospects for rehabilitation; 2) resources devoted to transplantation and organ procurement can be increased; or 3) individuals can be persuaded not to attempt to join the pool.

Of these three options, only the third has the promise of both conserving resources and promoting autonomy. While most persons medically eligible for a transplant would probably want one, some would not—at least if they understood all that was involved, including the need for a lifetime commitment to daily immunosuppression medications, and periodic medical monitoring for rejection symptoms. Accordingly, it makes public policy sense to publicize the risks and side effects of transplantation, and to require careful explanations of the procedure be given to prospective patients *before* they undergo medical screening. It is likely that by the time patients come to the transplant center they have made up their minds and would do almost anything to get the transplant. Nonetheless, if there are patients who, when confronted with all the facts, would voluntarily elect not to proceed, we enhance both their own freedom and the efficiency and cost-effectiveness of the transplantation system by screening them out as early as possible.

CONCLUSION

Choices among patients that seem to condemn some to death and give others an opportunity to survive will always be tragic. Society has developed a number of mechanisms to make such decisions more acceptable by camouflaging them. In an era of scarce resources and conscious cost containment, such mechanisms will become public, and they will be usable only if they are fair and efficient. If they are not so perceived, we will shift from one mechanism to another in an effort to continue the illusion that tragic choices really don't have to be made, and that we can simultaneously move toward equity of access, quality of services, and cost containment without any challenges to our values. Along with the prostitute, the playboy, and the poet, we all need to be involved in the development of an access model to extreme and expensive medical technologies with which we can live.

NOTES

1 Calabresi G, Bobbitt P: *Tragic Choices*. New York: Norton, 1978.

2 Fletcher J: Our shameful waste of human tissue. *In: Cutler* DR (ed): The Religious Situation. Boston: Beacon Press, 1969; 223–252.

3 Quoted in Fox R, Swazey J: *The Courage to Fail.* Chicago: Univ of Chicago Press, 1974; 232.

4 Sanders & Dukeminier: Medical advance and legal lag: hemodialysis and kidney transplantation. UCLA L Rev 1968; 15:357.

5 Rettig RA: The policy debate on patient care financing for victims of end stage renal disease. Law & Contemporary Problems 1976; 40:196.

6 President's Commission for the Study of Ethical Problems in Medicine and Biomedical and Behavioral Research: *Securing Access to Health Care.* US Govt Printing Office, 1983; 25.

7 Annas GJ: Ethics committees on neonatal care: substantive protection or procedural diversion? Am J Public Health 1984; 74:843–845.

8 Bayer R: Justice and health care in an era of cost containment: allocating scarce medical resources. Soc Responsibility 1984; 9:37–52.

9 Annas GJ: Allocation of artificial hearts in the year 2002: *Minerva v National Health Agency.* Am J Law Med 1977; 3:59–76.

10 Commentary: UK's poor record in treatment of renal failure. Lancet July 7, 1984; 53.

11 Evans R: Health care technology and the inevitability of resource allocation and rationing decisions, Part II. JAMA 1983; 249:2208, 2217.

Voluntary Risks to Health: The Ethical Issues
Robert M. Veatch

A biographical sketch of Robert M. Veatch is found on page 55.

Veatch explores some of the empirical, conceptual, and ethical issues raised by the correlation between life-styles and health. He first addresses a question whose answer embodies both empirical and conceptual considerations: "Are health risks voluntary?" In response, Veatch presents four conceptual approaches, or models: (1) the voluntary model, (2) the medical model, (3) the psychological model, and (4) the social structural model. Citing the limitations of each of these models, Veatch argues for the adoption of a multicausal model. He then distinguishes between responsibility and culpability and explores some of the pro and con arguments regarding the just treatment of individuals who squander their opportunity for good health. Veatch defends the view that if individuals have equal opportunities to be healthy, it is just to treat those who waste their opportunities by engaging in voluntary high-risk behavior differently from those who do not. Policies adopted in keeping with such differential treatment might include taxes on cigarettes or special insurance plans for those on an unhealthy diet.

In an earlier era, one's health was thought to be determined by the gods or by fate. The individual had little responsibility for personal health. In terms of the personal responsibility for health and disease, the modern medical model has required little change in this view. One of the primary elements of the medical model was the belief that people were exempt from responsibility for their condition.[1] If one had good health in old age, from the vantage point of the belief system of the medical model, one would say he had been blessed with good health. Disease was the result of mysterious, uncontrollable microorganisms or the random process of genetic fate.

A few years ago we developed a case study[2] involving a purely hypothetical proposal that smokers should be required to pay for the costs of their extra health care required over and above that of nonsmokers. The scheme involved taxing tobacco at a rate calculated to add to the nation's budget an amount equal to the marginal health cost of smoking.

Recently a number of proposals have been put forth that imply that individuals are in some sense personally responsible for the state of their health. The town of Alexandria, Va., refuses to hire smokers as fire fighters, in part because smokers increase the cost of health and dis-

Reprinted with permission of the author and the publisher from *Journal of the American Medical Association*, vol. 243 (January 4, 1980), pp. 50–55.

ability insurance (*The New York Times*, Dec. 18, 1977, p. 28). Oral Roberts University insists that students meet weight requirements to attend school. Claiming that the school was concerned about the whole person, the school dean said that the school was just as concerned about the students' physical growth as their intellectual and spiritual growth (*The New York Times*, Oct. 9, 1977, p. 77). Behaviors as highly diverse as smoking, skiing, playing professional football, compulsive eating, omitting exercise, exposing oneself excessively to the sun, skipping needed immunizations, automobile racing, and mountain climbing all can be viewed as having a substantial voluntary component. Health care needed as a result of any voluntary behavior might generate very different claims on a health care system from care conceptualized as growing out of some other causal nexus. Keith Reemtsma, M.D., chairman of the Department of Surgery at Columbia University's College of Physicians and Surgeons, has called for "a more rational approach to improving national health," involving "a reward/punishment system based on individual choices." Persons who smoked cigarettes, drank whiskey, drove cars, and owned guns would be taxed for the medical consequences of their choices (*The New York Times*, Oct. 14, 1976, p. 37). That individuals should be personally responsible for their health is a new theme, implying a new model for health care and perhaps for funding of health care.[3–6]

Some data correlating life-style to health status are being generated. They seem to support the conceptual shift toward a model that sees the individual as more personally responsible for his health status. The data of Belloc and Breslow[7-9] make those of us who lead the slovenly life-style very uncomfortable. As Morison[3] has pointed out, John Wesley and his puritan brothers of the covenant may not have been far from wrong after all. Belloc and Breslow identify seven empirical correlates of good health: eating moderately, eating regularly, eating breakfast, no cigarette smoking, moderate or no use of alcohol, at least moderate exercise, and seven to eight hours of sleep nightly. They all seem to be well within human control, far less mysterious than the viruses and genes that exceed the comprehension of the average citizen. The authors found that the average physical health of persons aged 70 years who reported all of the preceding good health practices was about the same as persons aged 35 to 44 years who reported fewer than three.

We have just begun to realize the policy implications and the ethical impact of the conceptual shift that begins viewing health[7] status as, in part, a result of voluntary risk taking in personal behavior and life-style choices. If individuals are responsible to some degree for their health and their need for health resources, why should they not also be responsible for the costs involved? If national health insurance is on the horizon, it will be even more questionable that individuals should have such health care paid for out of the same money pool generated by society to pay for other kinds of health care. Even with existing insurance plans, is it equitable that all persons contributing to the insurance money pool pay the extra costs of those who voluntarily run the risk of increasing their need for medical services?

The most obvious policy proposals—banning from the health care system risky behaviors and persons who have medical needs resulting from such risks—turns out to be the least plausible.[10, 11] For one thing, it is going to be extremely difficult to establish precisely the cause of the lung tumor at the time the patient is standing at the hospital door. Those who have carcinoma of the lung possibly from smoking or from unknown causes should not be excluded.

Even if the voluntary component of the cause could be determined, it is unlikely that our society could or would choose to implement a policy of barring the doors. While we have demonstrated a capacity to risk statistical lives or to risk the lives of citizens with certain socioeconomic characteristics, it is unlikely that we would be prepared to follow an overall policy of refusing medical service to those who voluntarily brought on their own conditions. We fought a similar battle over social security and concluded that—in part for reasons of the stress placed on family members and on society as a whole—individuals would not be permitted to take the risk of staying outside the social security system.

A number of policy options are more plausible. Additional health fees on health-risk behavior calculated to reimburse the health care system would redistribute the burden of the cost of such care to those who have chosen to engage in it. Separating health insurance pools for persons who engage in health-risk behavior and requiring them to pay out of pocket the marginal cost of their health care is another alternative. In some cases the economic cost is not the critical factor, it may be scarce personnel or equipment. Some behaviors might have to be banned to free the best neurosurgeons or orthopedic specialists for those who need their services for reasons other than for injuries suffered from the motorcycle accident or skiing tumble. Of course, all of these policy options require not only judgments about whether these behaviors are truly voluntary, but also ethical judgments about the rights and responsibilities of the individual and the other, more social components of the society.

There are several ethical principles that could lead us to be concerned about these apparently voluntary behaviors and even lead us to justify decisions to change our social policy about paying for or providing health care needed as a result of such behavior. The most obvious, the most traditional, medical ethical basis for concern is that the welfare of the individual is at stake. The Hippocratic tradition is committed to having the physician do what he thinks will benefit the patient. If one were developing an insurance policy or a mode of approaching the individual patient for private practice, paternalistic concern about the medical welfare of the patient might lead to a conclusion that, for the good of the patient, this behavior ought to be prevented or deferred. The paternalistic Hippocratic ethic, however, is suspect in circles outside the medical profession and is even coming under attack from within the physician community itself.[12] The Hippocratic ethic leaves no room for the principle of self-determination—a principle at the core of liberal Western thought. The freedom of choice to smoke, ski, and even race automobiles may well justify avoiding more coercive policies regarding these behaviors—assuming that it is the individual's own welfare that is at stake. The hyperindividualistic ethics of Hippocratism also leaves no room for concern for the welfare of others or the distribution of burdens within the society. A totally different rationale for concern is being put forward, however. Some, such as Tom Beauchamp,[13] have argued that we have a right to be concerned about such behaviors because of their social costs. He leaves unanswered the question of why it would be considered fair or just to regulate these voluntary behaviors when and only when their total social costs exceed the total social benefits of the behavior. This is a question we must explore.

Clearly, the argument is a complex one requiring many empirical, conceptual, and ethical judgments. Those judgments will have to be made regardless of whether we decide to continue the present policy or adopt one of the proposed alternatives. At this point, we need a thorough statement of the kinds of questions that must be addressed and the types of judgments that must be made.

ARE HEALTH RISKS VOLUNTARY?

The first question, addressed to those advocating policy shifts based on the notion that persons are in some sense responsible for their own health, melds the conceptual and empirical issues. Are health risks voluntary? Several models are competing for the conceptual attention of those working in the field.

The Voluntary Model

The model that considers the individual as personally responsible for his health has a great deal going for it. The empirical correlations of life-style choices with health status are impressive. The view of humans as personally responsible for their destiny is attractive to those of us within modern Western society. Its appeal extends beyond the view of the human as subject to the forces of fate and even the medical model, which as late as the 1950s saw disease as an attack on the individual coming from outside the person and outside his control.

The Medical Model

Of course, that it is attractive cannot justify opting for the voluntarist model if it flies in the face of the empirical reality. The theory of external and uncontrollable causation is central to the medical model.[14] It is still probably the case that organic causal chains almost totally outside human control account now and then for a

disease. But the medical model has been under such an onslaught of reality testing in the last decade that it can hardly provide a credible alternative to the voluntarist model. Even for those conditions that undeniably have an organic causal component, the luxury of human innocence is no longer a plausible defense against human accountability. The more we learn about disease and health and their causal chains, the more we have the possibility of intervening to change those chains of causation. Since the days of the movement for public health, sanitation, and control of contagion, there has been a rational basis for human responsibility. Even for those conditions that do not yet lend themselves to such direct voluntary control, the chronic diseases and even genetic diseases, there exists the possibility of purposeful, rational decisions that have an indirect impact on the risk. Choices can be made to minimize our exposure to potential carcinogens and risk factors for cardiovascular disease. Parents now have a variety of potential choices to minimize genetic disease risk and even eliminate it in certain cases. We may not be far from the day when we can say that all health problems can be viewed as someone's fault—if not our own fault for poor sanitary practices and life-style choices, then the fault of our parents for avoiding carrier status diagnosis, amniocentesis, and selective abortion; the fault of industries that pollute our environment; or the fault of the National Institutes of Health for failing to make the scientific breakthroughs to understand the causal chain so that we could intervene. Although there remains a streak of plausibility in the medical model as an account of disease and health, it is fading rapidly and may soon remain only as a fossil-like trace in our model of health.

The Psychological Model

While the medical model seems to offer at best a limited counter to the policy options rooted in the voluntarist model, other theories of determinism may be more plausible. Any policy to control health care services that are viewed as necessitated by voluntary choices to risk one's health is based on the judgment that the behavior is indeed voluntary. The primary argument countering policies to tax or control smoking to be fair in distributing the burdens for treating smokers' health problems is that the smoker is not really responsible for his medical problems. The argument is not normally based on organic or genetic theories of determinism, but on more psychological theories. The smoker's personality and even the initial pattern of smoking are developed at such an early point in life that they could be viewed as beyond voluntary control. If the smoker's behavior is the result of toilet training rather than rational decision making, then to blame the smoker for the toilet training seems odd.

Many of the other presumably voluntary risks to health might also be seen as psychologically determined and therefore not truly voluntary. Compulsive eating, the sedentary life-style, and the choice of a high-stress life pattern may all be psychologically determined.

Football playing is a medically risky behavior. For the professional, the choice seems to be made consciously and voluntarily. But the choice to participate in high school and even grade school competitive leagues may not really be the voluntary choice of the student. Then, if reward systems are generated from these early choices, certainly college level football could be the result. The continuum from partially nonvoluntary choices of the youngster to the career choice of the professional athlete may have a heavy psychological overlay after all.

If so-called voluntary health risks are really psychologically determined, then the ethical and policy implications collapse. But it must seriously be questioned whether the model of psychological determinism is a much more plausible monocausal explanation of these behaviors than the medical model. Choosing to be a professional football player, or even to continue smoking, simply cannot be viewed as determined and beyond personal choice because of demonstrated irresistible psychological forces. The fact that so many people have stopped smoking or drinking or even playing professional sports reveals that such choices are fundamentally different from monocausally determined behaviors. Although state of mind may be a component in all disease, it seems that an attempt to will away pneumonia or a carcinoma of the pancreas is much less likely to be decisively influential than using the will to control the behaviors that are now being grouped as voluntary.

The Social Structural Model

Perhaps the most plausible competition to the voluntarist model comes not from a theory of organic or even psychological determinism, but from a social structural model. The correlations of disease, mortality, and even so-called voluntary health-risk behavior with socioeconomic class are impressive. Recent data from Great Britain and from the Medicaid system in the United States[15] reveal that these correlations persist even with elaborate schemes that attempt to make health care more equitably available to all social classes. In Great Britain, for instance, it has recently been revealed that differences in death rates by social class continue, with inequalities essentially undiminished, since the advent of the National Health Service. Continuing to press the voluntarist model of personal responsibility for health risk in the face of a social structural model of the patterns of health and disease could be nothing more than blaming the victim,[16–19] avoiding the reality of the true causes of disease, and escaping proper social responsibility for changing the underlying social inequalities of the society and its modes of production.

This is a powerful counter to the voluntarist thesis. Even if it is shown that health and disease are governed by behaviors and risk factors subject to human control, it does not follow that the individual should bear the sole or even primary responsibility for bringing about the changes necessary to produce better health. If it is the case that for virtually every disease, those who are the poorest, those who are in the lowest socioeconomic classes, are at the greatest risk,[20–22] then there is a piously evasive quality to proposals that insist on individuals changing their life-styles to improve their positions and their health potential. The smoker may not be forced into his behavior so much by toilet training as by the social forces of the workplace or the society. The professional football player may be forced into that role by the work alternatives available to him, especially if he is a victim of racial, economic, and educational inequities.

If one had to make a forced choice between the voluntarist model and the social structural model, the choice would be difficult. The knowledge that some socially deprived persons have pulled themselves up by their bootstraps is cited as evidence for the voluntarist model, but the overwhelming power of the social system to hold most individuals in their social place cannot be ignored.

A Multicausal Model and Its Implications

The only reasonable alternative is to adopt a multicausal model; one that has a place for organic, psychological, and social theories of causation, as well as voluntarist elements, in an account of the cause of a disease or health pattern. One of the great conceptual issues confronting persons working in this area will be whether it is logically or psychologically possible to maintain simultaneously voluntarist and deterministic theories. In other areas of competing causal theories, such as theories of crime, drug addiction, and occupational achievement, we have not been very successful in maintaining the two types of explanation simultaneously. I am not convinced that it is impossible. A theory of criminal behavior that simultaneously lets the individual view criminal behavior as voluntary while the society views it as socially or psychologically determined has provocative and attractive implications. In the end it may be no more illogical or implausible than a reductionistic, monocausal theory.

The problem parallels one of the classic problems of philosophy and theology: How is it that there can be freedom of the will while at the same time the world is orderly and predictable? In more theological language, how can humans be free to choose good and evil while at the same time affirming that they are dependent on divine grace and that there is a transcendent order to the world? The tension is apparent in the Biblical authors, the Pelagian controversy of the fourth century, Arminius's struggle with the Calvinists, and contemporary secular arguments over free will. The conclusion that freedom of choice is a pseudo-problem, that it is compatible with predictability in the social order, may be the most plausible of the alternative, seemingly paradoxical answers.

The same conclusions may be reached regarding voluntary health risks. It would be a serious problem if a voluntarist theory led to abandoning any sense of social structural responsibility for health patterns. On the other hand, it seems clear that there are disease and health differentials even within socioeconomic classes and that some element of voluntary choice of life-style remains that leads to illness, even for the elite of the capitalist society and even for the members of the classless society. The voluntarist model seems at least to apply to differentials in behavior within socioeconomic classes or within groups similarly situated. Admitting the possibility of a theory of causation that includes a voluntary element may so distract the society from attention to the social and economic components in the causal nexus that the move would become counterproductive. On the other hand, important values are affirmed in the view that the human is in some sense responsible for his own medical destiny, that he is not merely the receptacle for external forces. These values are important in countering the trend toward the professionalization of medical decisions and the reduction of the individual to a passive object to be manipulated. They are so important that some risk may well be necessary. This is one of the core

problems in any discussion of the ethics of the voluntary health-risk perspecitve. One of the most difficult research questions posed by the voluntary health-risk theme is teasing out the implications of the theme for a theory of the causation of health patterns.

RESPONSIBILITY AND CULPABILITY

Even in cases where we conclude that the voluntarist model may be relevant—where voluntary choices are at least a minor component of the pattern of health—it is still unclear what to make of the voluntarist conclusion. If we say that a person is responsible for his health, it still does not follow that the person is culpable for the harm that comes from voluntary choices. It may be that society still would want to bear the burden of providing health care needed to patch up a person who has voluntarily taken a health risk.

To take an extreme example, a member of a community may choose to become a professional fire fighter. Certainly this is a health-risking choice. Presumably it could be a relatively voluntary one. Still it does not follow that the person is culpable for the harms done to his health. Responsible, yes, but culpable, no.

To decide in favor of any policy incorporating the so-called presumption that health risks are voluntary, it will be necessary to decide not only that the risk is voluntary, but also that it is not worthy of public subsidy. Fire fighting, an occupation undertaken in the public interest, probably would be worthy of subsidy. It seems that very few such activities, however, are so evaluated. Professional automobile racing, for instance, hardly seems socially ennobling, even if it does provide entertainment and diversion. A more plausible course would be requiring auto racers to purchase a license for a fee equal to their predicted extra health costs.

But what about the health risks of casual automobile driving for business or personal reasons? There are currently marginal health costs that are not built into the insurance system, e.g., risks from automobile exhaust pollution, from stress, and from the discouraging of exercise. It seems as though, in principle, there would be nothing wrong with recovering the economic part of those costs, if it could be done. A health tax on gasoline, for instance, might be sensible as a progressive way of funding a national health service. The evidence for the direct causal links and the exact costs will be hard, probably impossible, to discover. That difficulty, however, may not be decisive, provided there is general agreement that there are some costs, that the behavior is not socially ennobling, and that the funds are obtained more or less equitably in any case. It would certainly be no worse than some other luxury tax.

THE ARGUMENTS FROM JUSTICE

The core of the argument over policies deriving from the voluntary health-risks thesis is the argument over what is fair or just. Regardless of whether individuals have a general right to health care, or whether justice in general requires the social provision of health services, it seems as though what justice requires for a risk voluntarily assumed is quite different from what it might require in the more usual medical need.

Two responses have been offered to the problem of justice in providing health care for medical needs resulting from voluntarily assumed risks. One by Dan Beauchamp[19, 23] and others resolves the problem by attacking the category of voluntary risk. He implies that so-called voluntary behaviors are, in reality, the result of social and cultural forces. Since voluntary behavior is a null set, the special implications of meritorious or blameworthy behavior for a theory of justice are of no importance. Beauchamp begins forcefully with a somewhat egalitarian theory of social justice, which leads to a moral right to health for all citizens. There is no need to amend that theory to account for fairness of the claims of citizens who bring on their need for health care through their voluntary choices, because there are no voluntary choices.

It seems reasonable to concede to Dan Beauchamp that the medical model has been overly individualistic, that socioeconomic and cultural forces play a much greater role in the causal nexus of health problems than is normally assumed. Indeed, they probably play the dominant role. But the total elimination of voluntarism from our understanding of human behavior is quite implausible. Injuries to the socioeconomic elite while mountain climbing or waterskiing are not reasonably seen as primarily the result of social structural determinism. If there remains a residuum of the voluntary theory, then one of justice for health care will have to take that into account.

A second approach is that of Tom Beauchamp,[13] who goes further than Dan Beauchamp. He attacks the principle of justice itself. Dan Beauchamp seems to hold that justice or fairness requires us to distribute resources according to need. Since needs are not the result of voluntary choices, a subsidiary consideration of whether the need results from foolish, voluntary behavior is unnecessary. Tom Beauchamp, on the other hand, rejects the idea that needs per se have a claim on us as a society. He seems to accept the idea that at least occasionally behaviors may be voluntary. He questions whether need alone provides a plausible basis for deciding what is fair in cases where the individual has voluntarily risked his health and is subsequently in need of medical services. He offers a utilitarian alternative, claiming that the crucial dimension is the total social costs of the behaviors. He argues:

> Hazardous personal behaviors should be restricted if, and only if: (1) the behavior creates risks of harm to persons other than those who engage in such activities, and (2) a cost-benefit analysis reveals that the social investment in controlling such behaviors would produce a net increase in social utility, rather than a net decrease.

The implication is that any social advantage to the society that can come from controlling these behaviors would justify intervention, regardless of how the benefits and burdens of the policy are distributed.

A totally independent, nonpaternalistic argument is based much more in the principle of justice. This approach examines not only the impact of disease, but also questions of fairness. It is asked, is it fair that society as a whole should bear the burden of providing medical care needed only because of voluntarily taken risks to one's health? From this point of view, even if the net benefit of letting the behavior continue exceeded the benefits of prohibiting it, the behavior justifiably might be prohibited, or at least controlled, on nonpaternalistic grounds. Consider the case, for instance, where the benefits accrue overwhelmingly to persons who do engage in the behavior and the costs to those who do not. If the need for medical care is the result of the voluntary choice to engage in the behavior, then those arguing from the standpoint of equity or fairness might conclude that the behavior should still be controlled even though it produces a net benefit in aggregate.

Both Beauchamps downplay a secondary dimension of the argument over the principle of justice. Even those who accept the egalitarian formula ought to concede that all an individual is entitled to is an equal opportunity for a chance to be as healthy, insofar as possible, as other people.[24] Since those who are voluntarily risking their health (assuming for the moment that the behavior really is voluntary) do have an opportunity to be healthy, it is not the egalitarian dimensions of the principle of justice that are relevant to the voluntary health-risks question. It is the question of what is just treatment of those who have had opportunity and have not taken advantage of it. The question is one of what to do with persons who have not made use of their chance. Even the most egalitarian theories of justice—of which I consider myself to be a proponent—must at times deal with the secondary question of what to do in cases where individuals voluntarily have chosen to use their opportunities unequally. Unless there is no such thing as voluntary health-risk behavior, as Dan Beauchamp implies, this must remain a problem for the more egalitarian theories of justice.

In principle I see nothing wrong with the conclusion, which even an egalitarian would hold, that those who have not used fairly their opportunities receive inequalities of outcome. I emphasize that this is an argument in principle. It would not apply to persons who are truly not equal in their opportunity because of their social or psychological conditions. It would not apply to those who are forced into their health-risky behavior because of social oppression or stress in the mode of production.

From this application of a subsidiary component of the principle of justice, I reach the conclusion that it is fair, that it is just, if persons in need of health services resulting from true, voluntary risks are treated differently from those in need of the same services for other reasons. In fact, it would be unfair if the two groups were treated equally.

For most cases this would justify only the funding of the needed health care separately in cases where the need results from voluntary behavior. In extreme circumstances, however, where the resources needed are scarce and cannot be supplemented with more funds (e.g., when it is the skill that is scarce), then actual prohibition of the behavior may be the only plausible option, if one is arguing from this kind of principle of justice.

This essentially egalitarian principle, which says that like cases should be treated alike, leaves us with one final problem under the rubric of justice. If all voluntary risks ought to be treated alike, what do we make of the fact that only certain of the behaviors are monitorable? Is it unfair to place a health tax on smoking, automobile racing, skiing at organized resorts with ski lifts, and other organized activities that one can monitor, while letting slip by failing to exercise, mountain climbing, skiing on the hill on one's farm, and other behaviors that

cannot be monitored? In a sense it may be. The problem is perhaps like the unfairness of being able to treat the respiratory problems of pneumonia, but not those of trisomy E syndrome or other incurable diseases. There may be some essential unfairness in life. This may appear in the inequities of policy proposals to control or tax monitorable behavior, but not behavior that cannot be monitored. Actually some ingenuity may generate ways to tax what seems untaxable—taxing gasoline for the health risks of automobiles, taxing mountain climbing equipment (assuming it is not an ennobling activity), or creating special insurance pools for persons who eat a bad diet. The devices probably would be crude and not necessarily in exact proportion to the risks involved. Some people engaged in equally risky behaviors probably would not be treated equally. That may be a necessary implication of the crudeness of any public policy mechanism. Whether the inequities of not being able to treat equally people taking comparable risks constitute such a serious problem that it would be better to abandon entirely the principle of equality of opportunity for health is the policy question that will have to be resolved.

COST-SAVING HEALTH-RISK BEHAVIORS

Another argument is mounted against the application of the principle of equity to voluntarily health-risking behaviors. What ought to be done with behaviors that are health risky, but that end up either not costing society or actually saving society's scarce resources? This question will separate clearly those who argue for intervention on paternalistic grounds from those who argue on utilitarian grounds or on the basis of the principle of justice. What ought to be done about a behavior that would risk a person's health, but risk it in such a way that he would die rapidly and cheaply at about retirement age? If the concern is from the unfair burden that these behaviors generate on the rest of society, and, if the society is required to bear the costs and to use scarce resources, then a health-risk behavior that did not involve such social costs would surely be exempt from any social policy oriented to controlling such unfair behavior. In fact, if social utility were the only concern, then this particular type of risky behavior ought to be encouraged. Since our social policy is one that ought to incorporate many ethical concerns, it seems unlikely that we would want to encourage these behaviors even if such encouragement were cost-effective. This, indeed, shows the weakness of approaches that focus only on aggregate costs and benefits.

REVULSION AGAINST THE RATIONAL, CALCULATING LIFE

There is one final, last-ditch argument against adoption of a health policy that incorporates an equitable handling of voluntary health risks. Some would argue that, although the behavior might be voluntary and supplying health care to meet the resulting needs unfair to the rest of the society, the alternative would be even worse. Such a policy might require the conversion of many decisions in life from spontaneous expressions based on long tradition and life-style patterns to cold, rational, calculating decisions based on health and economic elements.

It is not clear to me that that would be the result. Placing a health fee on a package of cigarettes or on a ski-lift ticket may not make those decisions any more rational calculations than they are now. The current warning on tobacco has not had much of an impact. Even if rational decision making were the outcome, however, I am not sure that it would be wrong to elevate such health-risking decisions to a level of consciousness in which one had to think about what one was doing. At least it seems that as a side effect of a policy that would permit health resources to be paid for and used more equitably, this would not be an overwhelming or decisive counterargument.

CONCLUSION

The health policy decisions that must be made in an era in which a multicausal theory is the only plausible one are going to be much harder than the ones made in the simpler era of the medical model—but then, those were harder than some of the ones that had to be made in the era where health was in the hands of the gods. Several serious questions remain to be answered. These are both empirical and normative. They may constitute a research agenda for pursuing the question of ethics and health policy for an era when some risks to health may be seen, at least by some people, as voluntary.

REFERENCES

1 Parsons, T., *The Social System*. New York, The Free Press, 1951, p. 437.

2 Steinfels, P., Veatch, R. M., Who should pay for smokers' medical care? *Hastings Cent. Rep.* 4:8–10, 1974.

3 Morison, R. S., Rights and responsibilities: Redressing the uneasy balance. *Hastings Cent. Rep.* 4:1–4, 1974.

4 Vayda, E., Keeping people well: A new approach to medicine. *Hum. Nature* 1:64–71, 1978.

5 Somers, A. R., Hayden, M. C., Rights and responsibilities in prevention. *Health Educ.* 9:37–39, 1978.

6 Kass, L., Regarding the end of medicine and the pursuit of health. *Public Interest* 40:11–42, 1975.

7 Belloc, N. B., Breslow, L., Relationship of physical status health and health practices. *Prev. Med.* 1:409–421, 1972.

8 Belloc, N. B., Relationship of health practices and mortality. *Prev. Med.* 2:68–81, 1973.

9 Breslow, L., Prospects for improving health through reducing risk factors. *Prev. Med.* 7:449–458, 1978.

10 Wikler, D., Coercive measures in health promotion: Can they be justified? *Health Educ. Monogr.* 6:223–241, 1978.

11 Wikler, D., Persuasion and coercion for health: Ethical issues in government efforts to change life-styles. *Milbank Mem. Fund Q.* 56:303–338, 1978.

12 Veatch, R. M., The Hippocratic ethic: Consequentialism, individualism and paternalism, in Smith, D. H., Bernstein, L. M. (eds.), *No Rush to Judgment: Essays on Medical Ethics*. Bloomington, Ind., The Poynter Center, Indiana University, 1978, pp. 238–264.

13 Beauchamp, T., The regulation of hazards and hazardous behaviors. *Health Educ. Monogr.* 6:242–257, 1978.

14 Veatch, R. M., The medical model: Its nature and problems. *Hastings Cent. Rep.* 1:59–76, 1973.

15 Morris, J. N., Social inequalities undiminished. *Lancet* 1:87–90, 1979.

16 Ryan, W., *Blaming the Victim*. New York, Vintage Books, 1971.

17 Crawford, R., Sickness as sin. *Health Policy Advisory Center Bull.* 80:10–16, 1978.

18 Crawford, R., You are dangerous to your health. *Social Policy* 8:11–20, 1978.

19 Beauchamp, D. E., Public health as social justice. *Inquiry* 13:3–14, 1976.

20 Syme, L., Berkman, I., Social class, susceptibility and sickness. *Am. J. Epidemiol.* 104:1–8, 1976.

21 Conover, P. W., Social class and chronic illness. *Int. J. Health Serv.* 3:357–368, 1973.

22 *Health of the Disadvantaged: Chart Book*, publication (HRA) 77-628. Hyattsville, Md., U.S. Dept. of

Health, Education, and Welfare, Public Health Service, Health Resources Administration, 1977.

23 Beauchamp, D. E., Alcoholism as blaming the alcoholic. *Int. J. Addict.* 11:41–52, 1976.

24 Veatch, R. M., What is a "just" health care delivery? in Branson, R., Veatch, R. M. (eds.), *Ethics and Health Policy.* Cambridge, Mass., Ballinger Publishing Co., 1976, pp. 127–153.

ANNOTATED BIBLIOGRAPHY: CHAPTER 10

Blackstone, William R.: "On Health Care as a Legal Right: An Exploration of Legal and Moral Grounds," *Georgia Law Review* 10 (1976), pp. 391–418. Blackstone examines a number of legal and moral positions that can be used to argue for or against some kind of right to health care. He argues in favor of a public, socialized, or nationalized health system.

Callahan, Daniel: *Setting Limits: Medical Goals in an Aging Society* (New York: Simon and Schuster, 1987). This is a much expanded version of the reasoning Callahan advances in the two articles in this chapter.

Caplan, Arthur L.: "Beg, Borrow, or Steal: The Ethics of Solid Organ Procurement." In Deborah Mathieu, ed., *Organ Substitution Technology: Ethical, Legal and Public Policy Issues* (Boulder, Colo.: Westview Press, 1988), pp. 59–68. Caplan reviews the history of the evolution of the field of solid organ transplantation and of the related evolution of social policies regarding organ procurement. He notes that the "required request approach" is becoming the policy of choice in most areas in the United States.

Childress, James F.: "Priorities in the Allocation of Health Care Resources," *Soundings* 62 (Fall 1979), pp. 258–269. Childress focuses on macroallocation decisions that require choices between (1) health care and other social goods and (2) prevention and crisis or rescue medicine.

————: "Who Shall Live When Not All Can Live?" *Soundings* 53 (Winter 1970), pp. 339–355. Childress advocates a two-stage selection process for making decisions about the microallocation of scarce resources. The first step involves the use of medical criteria to establish a pool of medically acceptable candidates. The second step is a random selection proces.

Daniels, Norman: "Am I My Parents' Keeper?" In *Securing Access to Health Care* by the President's Commission for the Study of Ethical Problems in Medicine and Biomedical and Behavioral Research, Vol. 2 (Washington, D.C.: U.S. Government Printing Office, March 1983), Appendix K, pp. 265–291. In his excellent philosophical analysis, Daniels argues that we should not view the problem of age-based rationing as one of intergenerational conflict. He suggests that we should view it as a problem of individual prudence.

————: "Health-Care Needs and Distributive Justice," *Philosophy and Public Affairs* 10 (1981), pp. 146–179. Daniels defends the following claim: If an acceptable theory of justice includes a principle providing for fair equality of opportunity, then health-care institutions should be among those governed by the principle of fair equality of opportunity. His article includes an account of basic needs in general and health-care needs in particular. He identifies basic needs, including health-care needs, with those important to maintaining normal species functioning and sees such normal functioning as an important determinant of the range of opportunity open to an individual.

Fried, Charles: "Equality and Rights in Medical Care," *Hastings Center Report* 6 (February 1976), pp. 29–34. Fried argues that a right to health care does not imply a right to equal access. He does, however, argue that it is profoundly wrong not to afford a decent standard of care to all our citizens.

Fuchs, Victor R.: *The Health Economy* (Cambridge, Mass.: Harvard University Press, 1986). Fuchs provides a framework for thinking about the issues of cost, efficiency, access, and quality in regard to health care.

Guttmann, Amy: "For and against Equal Access to Health Care," *Milbank Memorial Fund Quarterly/Health and Society* 59 (Fall 1981), pp. 542–560. Guttmann rejects both the free-market approach and the decent-minimum approach to the provision of health care. Drawing on the values of self-respect, equal relief from pain, and equality of opportunity, she argues for equal access to health care as a moral ideal.

Hiatt, Howard H.: *America's Health in the Balance: Choice or Chance* (New York: Harper & Row, 1987). Hiatt discusses the economic, social, and medical factors that contribute to the strengths and weaknesses of health care in the United States. He compares our system of health care with the British and Canadian systems and recommends some policies intended to lead to a more effective and equitable system of care.

Journal of Medicine and Philosophy 13 (February 1988). The theme of this special issue is "Justice between Generations and Health Care for the Elderly." Of particular note is Theodore R. Marmor's "Reflections on Medicare." Marmor provides both a historical and a political overview of Medicare's development and a discussion of some of the problems faced by Medicare in respect to equitable resource allocation.

Stern, Lawrence: "Opportunity and Health Care: Criticisms and Suggestions," *The Journal of Medicine and Philosophy* 8 (1983), pp. 339–361. Stern criticizes Norman Daniels's proposal that health care should be distributed on the basis of fair equality of opportunity. He then advances his own position on health care and justice and argues for a health-voucher system that will provide roughly equal access to health care for all classes.

Veatch, Robert M.: *The Foundations of Justice: Why the Retarded and the Rest of Us Have Claims to Equality* (New York: Oxford University Press, 1986). Veatch examines current conceptions of justice, equality, and social responsibility as he discusses the question of how to fairly allocate limited resources, especially to people with inexhaustible needs and very little capacity for improvement.

Wikler, Daniel I.: "Persuasion and Coercion for Health," *Milbank Memorial Fund Quarterly/ Health and Society* 56 (Summer 1978), pp. 303–335. Wikler examines two of the central arguments invoked in discussions of the government's role in promoting health-preserving personal behavior: the argument from paternalism and the fair-distribution-of-burdens argument.

APPENDIX

Case Studies

This appendix contains a set of case studies for analysis and discussion. Most of the cases are essentially records of actual situations. Others, however, are only loosely based on actual happenings, and a few have been constructed simply for their perceived pedagogical value. Most of the cases are developed only up to a crucial "decision point," but some are supplemented by information about what happened after a decision was actually made. In assessing a decision that was actually made in a given case, it is important to focus on the information available to the decision maker prior to the decision and not be overly influenced by the element of hindsight. Case studies of the type presented here may pose another problem. Individuals involved in analyzing such cases often feel that it would be desirable to have more factual details, especially clinical ones. This recurrent desire reflects the well-based axiom that good decision making must be based on "good facts." However, a perceived lack of factual detail should not be allowed to paralyze analysis and discussion. If the proper decision in a certain case is thought to be dependent on information not provided in the case description, and if it is reasonable to believe that the desired information would or could be available to those confronted with the decision, a discussion of the case can include an examination of the precise way in which the desired information is relevant to the decision.

Two final points are worth noting. First, the last paragraph of each case study identifies some questions raised by the case. These questions are not the only ones worthy of consideration, but they can be used to facilitate analysis and discussion. Second, the title of each case study is followed by a number or numbers within brackets. These numbers refer to the various chapters in this book. Thus the chapter or chapters most directly relevant to each case are identified.

CASE 1

A Patient's Role in Determining Therapy [2]

Andrew W. is a 56-year-old male who has contracted colon cancer. He is an intelligent man who has considerable research skills. The cancer is in its early stages, and Andrew W. could benefit from the proper chemotherapy. Andrew W. has read that the National Institutes of Health has developed a test to determine the sensitivity of cancer cells to the combinations of chemotherapy. This test (while still somewhat experimental) has proven effective to the point that NIH is offering it as a service to physicians around the country. Andrew W. talks to his physician, Dr. M., about sending a sample of his cancer cells to NIH to determine the most effective form of chemotherapy. Dr. M. is upset by the suggestion and says that treatment determination is the prerogative of the physician and that he knows what is effective for the treatment of colon cancer. He tells Andrew W. that, if he wants the NIH test, he will have to find another oncologist. Andrew W. goes to another physician, undergoes the test, and has the chemotherapy indicated by the test. Three years later Andrew W. is still disease free.

(1) Was Andrew W. within his rights in asking for or even demanding the test? (2) Did Dr. M. act ethically toward Andrew W.? Did Dr. M. act in the best interests of his patient?

CASE 2

A Physician's Abandonment of a Patient [2]

Todd Z. is a 75-year-old male who has been diagnosed as having lung cancer with brain metastases. His physician of thirty years, Dr. S., is seriously concerned that, if told of his diagnosis, Todd Z. will go into a deep depression and spend the remainder of his life in that state. Dr. S. keeps the information from Todd Z. and orders Todd Z.'s wife and three sons not to tell Todd Z. of the diagnosis. He tells them that he wants to keep Todd Z. in the hospital for a couple of weeks for brain radiation and promises to make up some excuse for the treatment. After the treatment is concluded, the family can take him home to die. Dr. S. promises that he will visit Todd Z. at his home every week and care for him until he dies because he has been very fond of Todd Z. and lives nearby. Todd Z. becomes increasingly persistent with his questions about his physical condition. By the third week the family breaks down and tells him about the diagnosis. Todd Z. does go into the predictable depression, but it is not as severe as Dr. S. had feared. Dr. S. is angered by the fact that the family had disobeyed his orders. He releases Todd Z. from the hospital and does not keep his promise to visit him at home. He never visits Todd Z. during the six-month period from Todd Z.'s departure from the hospital to the day of his death. During that six-month period Dr. S. is very uncooperative. When the family contacts him to discuss the medication program, he is very curt with them, and when they ask him about a particular condition that is developing, he asserts that they will have to bring Todd Z. to the office or to the hospital. He even refuses to talk with Todd Z. on the telephone.

(1) Did Dr. S. break his fiduciary relationship with the patient and abandon him? (2) Is it appropriate for a physician to set conditions such as deception for full involvement in caring for a patient?

CASE 3

Withholding Information about Risks [2]

Marcia W. is a 40-year-old female with multiple myeloma, who upon diagnosis shows great interest in having all the information that is necessary to make a decision about further treatment. Dr. C. tells her that the response rates to chemotherapy with this disease are very good and that recent research has shown that 50 percent of patients can hope for long-term survival rates, which are tantamount to cure. The other 50 percent of patients die within a year or two. What Dr. C. neglects to tell her is that preliminary studies are showing that in twenty years, 10 percent of the 50 percent who survive contract a form of leukemia that is highly resistant to treatment. When her treatment is discussed in a staff meeting, Dr. C. says that he did not want to tell Marcia W. about the 10 percent because he was afraid that it might unduly alarm her and cause her not to take treatment, thereby spoiling her chances for long-term survival. Moreover, he states (a) that the research is not conclusive enough to suit him and (b) that 10 percent is such a low figure that he is not morally required to communicate the risk. After all, he suggests, one cannot inform a patient of *every* risk.

(1) Did Marcia W. have a right to the information about the possible risk of leukemia? (2) Is this 10 percent chance of contracting leukemia significant for her decision making? (3) Will this information harm her by making it impossible for her to make an autonomous decision? (4) Is the low 10 percent figure counterbalanced by the seriousness of the consequences?

CASE 4
Voluntary Sterilization and a Young Unmarried Man [2]

Gregory X., who is 25 years old, unmarried, and childless, wants a vasectomy. (Vasectomy is a sterilization procedure that is considered irreversible, although research is being done to make it reversible.) He comes to Dr. H., a urologist in a clinic in a large city hospital, because he cannot afford the surgery elsewhere. He tells Dr. H. that he has decided, after several years of thought, never to be a parent. The vasectomy will now ensure that and make it unnecessary for any woman he loves to run the various risks associated with the available means of contraception. Dr. H. has doubts about performing the surgery on a young, unmarried man. He asks Gregory X. to consider the feelings of a possible future wife who will not have any say about the sterilization decision. Gregory X. insists on the surgery.

(1) Should Dr. H. accede to Gregory X.'s request despite his reservations, since Gregory X. cannot afford the vasectomy otherwise? (2) Is there anything morally problematic about Gregory X.'s request?

CASE 5
The Dentist and Patient Autonomy [2]

A 36-year-old man, Patrick M., contacts the office of an endodontist. (Endodontics is a specialized field of dentistry.) Patrick M. wants to arrange for a procedure commonly called a "root canal" to be performed on each of his teeth. A root canal is a common (somewhat involved) procedure used as an alternative to extracting a diseased tooth. It consists of removing the damaged or diseased blood vessels and nerves contained within the tooth. The tooth is thus "devital" but functions normally. If this procedure is not done on a diseased tooth or if the tooth is not extracted, infection will very likely develop in the necrotic tissue and spread into the jaw bone and surrounding tissues.

The endodontist is startled by the idea of performing a root canal on all of Patrick M.'s teeth. Further discussion makes Patrick M.'s motivation clear. He is a fervent survivalist, dedicated to planning for every contingency in the expectation that some conflagration is about to destroy society. Patrick M. is attempting to ensure—by having all of his teeth desensitized—that he will never suffer a toothache. Although the endodontist cannot escape a sense of amusement over what he considers a bizarre situation, Patrick M. seems fully prepared both to undergo a difficult set of procedures and to pay what will be a huge overall bill. Still, the endodontist feels that it would be unethical to remove healthy tissue. He feels that he is being asked to perform a procedure that is not indicated by the existing conditions and may never be indicated, judging by the excellent overall health of the teeth.

(1) Is there any significant difference between the dentist-patient relationship and the physician-patient relationship? (2) Should the endodontist accede to Patrick M.'s desires?

CASE 6
The Nurse and Informed Consent [2, 3]

Michael G., who is dying of leukemia, is in a hospital where he is receiving chemotherapy. A registered nurse involved in his care, Nurse L., learns that he has never received information about alternative natural therapies. She gives Michael G. the information and discusses the advantages and disadvantages of the various alternatives. After extensive reflection and consultation with his family, Michael G. decides to leave the hospital and to make arrangements to try one of the alternative therapies. He informs the attending oncologist of his decision. When the oncologist learns about the source of Michael G.'s information, he charges Nurse L. with unprofessional conduct and asks that her nursing license be revoked. Nurse L. argues that the patient has the right to know about the alternatives and that a failure to inform him vitiates his "informed consent" to the chemotherapy.

(1) Was Nurse L. acting in a morally correct way when she gave Michael G. the information? (2) Should the physician in charge have the final word about the information a patient should receive? (3) If Michael G. did not know about the alternative therapies, was his assent to the chemotherapy *informed* consent?

CASE 7

The Office Nurse and Informed Consent [2, 3]

Joan R. is going through menopause. Her physician, Dr. W., wants her to begin estrogen therapy. After talking with the physician, Joan R. agrees to the therapy. She stops at the nurse's desk in Dr. W.'s office to pick up her prescription. In the course of the conversation, Nurse M. realizes that Dr. W. has not informed Joan R. that other options are available to her and that there is wide disagreement about which option is preferable. Instead of taking only estrogen, Joan R. could choose to take estrogen together with a progestin, or she could choose to take no hormones at all. Each of these options is thought to carry different potential benefits and risks.

(1) Should Nurse M. provide Joan R. with that information? (2) Should Nurse M. suggest to Joan R. that she initiate an additional discussion with Dr. W. in order to obtain more information? (3) If Nurse M. approaches the problem from the perspective of the rights model of advocacy, what would she do? If she approaches it from the perspective of the existential advocacy model, what would she do? Would the proper resolution of this case be different if the patient were in a hospital and Nurse M. were directly involved in her care?

CASE 8

A Nurse's Obligations and a Patient's Living Will [2, 3]

George G., who is 70 years old and has no family, has a history of coronary disease and myocardial infarctions. He is also suffering from a large and advanced carcinoma of the stomach. George G. tells Nurse C. that he has given his physician, Dr. E., a copy of a living will, which requests that no heroic measures be taken to prolong his life. After a further myocardial collapse occurs, Nurse C. learns that Dr. E.'s orders had called for maximum therapeutic efforts in the event of such a collapse, including resuscitation, if necessary. The patient is resuscitated, and his life continues. George G. expresses a desire to die, but his condition has deteriorated to such an extent that his competence to make decisions on his own behalf is questionable. If the existence of his living will were known, his present expressions of a desire not to be subjected to further therapy would be given more credence. There is no explicit hospital policy regarding living wills; such matters are left to the physician's discretion.

(1) Does Nurse C. have an obligation to inform other hospital personnel about George G.'s living will? (2) Does Nurse C. have an obligation to defend George G.'s interests even if this means challenging Dr. E.'s course of treatment? (3) Has Dr. E. violated George G.'s rights?

CASE 9

An HIV-Infected Surgeon and a Duty to Disclose [2, 3]

Dr. M., a surgeon, has learned that he has been infected with the human immunodeficiency virus (HIV). Studies have shown that a surgeon will cut a glove while performing surgery in about one out of four cases and will sustain a significant skin cut in about one out of every forty cases. Given the fact that during surgery a surgeon is in significant contact with a patient's organs and blood as well as the fact that HIV can be transmitted through the blood, there is at least some risk that a patient being operated on by Dr. M. will be infected.

(1) Does Dr. M. have an obligation to refrain from performing surgery? (2) If not, does Dr. M. have an obligation to inform those on whom he plans to operate that he is infected with the virus? (3) Suppose the position were reversed and a patient, Dorothea L., is the one infected. Is Dorothea L. obligated to inform Dr. M. of her infection?

CASE 10

Who Communicates with the Patient? [2, 3]

Thomas P. is a 56-year-old male with head and neck cancer. After radical surgery, which left him quite disfigured, he was apparently disease free. However, the disease reoccurred two years later, and the tumor grew in such a way that it eventually closed off his trachea. He agreed to a tracheotomy to allow him to breathe, but due to complications in surgery he became respirator dependent. His daughter, and only relative, Wanda G., asked the physician in charge, Dr. Z., to extubate Thomas P., that is, remove him from the respirator. Dr. Z. agreed that it might be appropriate to extubate Thomas P. but stated that Thomas P. should be consulted during his conscious periods. Wanda G. agreed that this was the proper procedure and told Dr. Z. to ask her father as quickly as possible. Dr. Z. protested, saying that he had no intention of asking the father. Since the extubation was the daughter's idea, the physician asserted, she should discuss the matter with her father. Wanda G., already grieving because of her father's long illness and impending death, said that she could not discuss the matter with her father. She subsequently asked the nurse taking care of her father to discuss the extubation with him. The nurse refused, saying that it was not her job.

(1) Who has the primary responsibility to discuss this decision with the patient? (2) If the person who has primary responsibility refuses to act on that responsibility, how should the patient's best interests be protected?

CASE 11

Alzheimer's Disease, Memory Continuity, and Autonomy [2, 3]

Thomas P. is a 78-year-old male who has cancer, with a primary site in the lung and metastases to the bone. It has been determined that nothing genuinely therapeutic can be done for the lung disease. Now he faces a decision as to whether he should have radiation to the bones to reduce the possibility of fractures. The radiation proposed has already been used once in the course of the disease, and it made the patient very ill for about six weeks. There is every reason to believe that the same morbidity will occur this time. Thomas P. must now decide if he wants to undergo a similar treatment, with its accompanying side effects, for the bone metastases. He is cared for at home by his wife, and he has five children who have genuine loving concern for him.

Thomas P.'s situation is complicated by the fact that he has Alzheimer's disease. His memory does not always serve him well. He remembers the side effects of the previous radiation, and he seems to be well acquainted with the disease process. However, he does not always remember what his physician tells him and then is forced to make decisions based on incomplete or unrecalled information. Furthermore, he cannot always remember what he has consented to and what he has not consented to. His locutions sometimes take the form of "Did I agree to that?" He sometimes seems to be persuaded by whomever he is discussing the matter with at the time. This ambivalence, together with the lapses in memory continuity, raises questions about his competence in making decisions.

(1) Is Thomas P. sufficiently autonomous to make his own decisions? (2) How seriously should his health-care professionals consult with him about his mode of treatment? To what extent should the family be involved?

CASE 12

Hospitals, Surgeons, and Economic Incentives [2, 3]

A large, for-profit hospital chain (RASA) offers to share the profits generated by the use of its operating rooms with the staff surgeons who use them. Dr. G. is one of these surgeons. Thus she benefits financially in two ways when she operates on a patient in a RASA hospital—she is paid for the operation and she receives a share of the hospital's profits. There are other, equally equipped hospitals in the community whose facilities Dr. G. could use.

(1)Is Dr. G. acting in a morally acceptable way by referring her patients to a RASA hospital? (2) is RASA's profit-sharing policy morally acceptable? (3) Does RASA's policy work to the detriment of the patient?

CASE 13

A Randomized Clinical Trial and a Physician's Responsibility to a Patient [2, 4]

Dr. L. has agreed to include his patients in a RCT designed to test a new drug whose purpose is to treat and cure a disease that is about 70 percent fatal. One of the participants in the trial, Bruce W., has been a patient of Dr. L.'s for eleven years. There are a total of thirty participants in the RCT. Twelve are given placebos. The other eighteen are given the new drug. None of the patients are told which treatment they are receiving, although all know that they are taking part in a randomized clinical trial. After eight of the twelve patients on placebos and five of those receiving the new drug die, Dr. L. is asked by Bruce W. whether he is one of the placebo recipients and whether there is any good reason to think that the new drug is effective. Dr. L. knows that Bruce W. is a placebo recipient and that the data so far support the view that the experimental drug may be effective and prevent death. Dr. L. and the other physicians involved in the trial are unwilling to end the experiment because of their concern about the validity of the study if it is terminated too soon.

(1) Should the experiment be ended and the remaining patients put on the new therapy immediately? (2) Should Dr. L. lie to Bruce W., if necessary, in order to continue the experiment? (3) Does Dr. L. have an obligation to his patient, Bruce W., which should take precedence over his concern with establishing the validity of the results of the RCT?

CASE 14

Enrolling Ineligible Patients in a Clinical Trial [2, 4]

Participation in the clinical trial of a drug intended to benefit cancer patients is contingent on the fulfillment of certain requirements. These include having only a certain type of cancer, having at least an eight-week life expectancy, having normal kidney, liver, and heart functioning, and having the ability to perform everyday functions. The validity of the trial depends on the enforcement of these requirements. The trial is being conducted by colleagues of Dr. T. who have asked him to enroll eligible patients in the trial, with the latters' consent, of course. Dr. Y., who is Dr. T.'s patient, has exhausted the therapies available for his form of cancer. Dr. Y hears about the clinical trial. Although he knows that he cannot meet the requirements for participation, he tells Dr. T. that he wants to be enrolled and asks that Dr. T. fudge the data, if necessary, since otherwise he has no chance for survival.

(1) Should Dr. T. fudge the data to give Dr. Y. one last chance? (2) Since Dr. Y is also a physician and understands that his participation will compromise the validity of the trial, is his insistence on participation incompatible with his professional commitment?

CASE 15

A Teenager's Consent to Participate in Research [4]

One hundred high school sophomores are asked to participate in an experimental trial of a new soap intended to prevent acne or at least to mitigate its severity. In the planned randomized clinical trial, half the students will receive the new soap while the other half will be given a facsimile without the ingredients thought to be effective against acne. No risks to the students are anticipated. The students are given consent forms to take home for their parents' signature. Lisa H.'s parents refuse to consent on Lisa's behalf although Lisa wants to participate in the project.

(1) Should Lisa's consent override her parents' refusal? (2) Would the answer be different if a similar situation occurred involving children whose ages ranged from 7 to 9?

CASE 16

Liberty and the Elderly Patient [2, 3, 5]

Ronald X. is 71 years old. A widower, he lives alone in an apartment but he receives some assistance from a cleaning woman and a friendly neighbor. Ronald X. is presently in a hospital because of a broken leg, but he is ready to be discharged. Ronald X. also suffers from arteriosclerosis, however, a condition which results in his experiencing periods of confusion during which he sometimes wanders purposelessly around the city, running some risks to himself. Ronald X.'s children do not want him to return to his home. They believe that he needs the supervised care provided in a nursing home. Ronald X., when not in a confused state, repeatedly expresses his awareness of the problems he faces stemming from his arteriosclerosis and of the resultant risks he runs. Nonetheless, he would rather run those risks than be confined to institutional care. The medical professionals and Ronald X.'s children decide that he will not be discharged from the hospital until an appropriate nursing home is found. At that time, he will be sent to the nursing home. When Ronald X. insists on being discharged from the hospital, the medical professionals sedate him to a level sufficient to gain his compliance.

(1) Are the health professionals and Ronald X.'s children making an unjustified leap from his occasional risk-running behavior to the conclusion that he lacks sufficient competence to determine the shape of his own life? (2) Is this paternalistic limitation on Ronald X.'s liberty morally obligatory? Morally permissible? Morally reprehensible?

CASE 17

Privacy and Monitoring Systems in a Mental Institution [3, 5]

The new superintendent of the Meller Valley Mental Institute, Dr. R., has decided to install television monitoring devices in all the patients' rooms as well as in the hallways and visiting rooms of the Institute. His primary purposes are to make it easier to locate personnel when they are needed in a hurry and to help the staff, which is short-handed, keep an eye on the doings of patients, a small number of whom are prone to violence. Patients know about the surveillance, but visitors are not informed. Some of the members of Dr. R.'s staff object, arguing that the system is a gross violation of the privacy of both patients and visitors.

(1) Is Dr. R. morally justified in establishing the monitoring system? (2) Are patients' and visitors' rights being violated?

CASE 18

Autonomy and Mental Illness [5]

Humphrey W., a 40-year-old businessman, is committed to a mental hospital at the instigation of his wife and without his consent after repeated manic episodes in public and a suicide attempt. During some of his manic episodes he has thrown money around on street corners, harangued passers-by, raged aganst his fellow employees, and boasted of nonexistent business deals to his boss. After commitment, Humphrey W. refuses tranquilizing medication, which psychiatrists consider necessary to control his "manic flights" and strengthen his own control over his behavior.

(1) Would it be morally correct for the psychiatrists to give him the tranquilizers (e.g., by means of a syringe) against his expressed dissent? (2) Was it morally correct to commit him to the institution without his consent?

CASE 19

A Schizophrenic Son's Refusal of Therapy [5]

William T., who is 22 years old, has a troubled history. He has been diagnosed as suffering from chronic undifferentiated schizophrenia. He has been expelled from several schools due to his severely disruptive conduct and a continuing serious deterioration in his school performance. William T. has been a multiple drug abuser, he has threatened various members of his family, and his behavior has sometimes been catatonic. He has persistently refused to take any medication and has rejected all other forms of treatment. Now William T. is in a state hospital after being charged with attempted armed robbery, assault, and battery. He continues to reject all treatment. William T.'s father, Joseph T., who has been appointed his temporary guardian, wants to consent to the administration of medication to William T. The father thinks that William T. may pose a danger to others if he is discharged without treatment and thereby poses a threat of harm both to himself and others. Joseph T. maintains that he is acting in the best interests of his son, who is incompetent to decide what is best for himself.

(1) Should parents in such cases be allowed to make treatment decisions that go against the expressed wishes of their children? (2) Is William T.'s autonomy sufficiently diminished so that his father's actions on his behalf are an example of weak rather than strong paternalism? (3) Is forcing medication on patients inconsistent with respecting them as persons?

CASE 20

Sterilization and the Mentally Retarded [5]

The parents of a 19 year old, Mindy G., who has Down's syndrome and an I.Q. in the upper 30s range, ask her physician to implant a drug-delivery system that will serve as a relatively long-term contraceptive. The parents argue that the prevention of pregnancy will serve Mindy's long-term interests, since if she becomes pregnant she will neither understand her condition nor be able to care for the baby on her own. Furthermore, they are concerned about what will happen to Mindy after they die. They would like to see her settled in a group home for retarded adults and working in a sheltered workshop. They argue that continuous and dependable contraception is a prerequisite for these kinds of changes in her life.

(1) Putting aside any legal complications, would it be morally correct for the physician to implant the contraceptive device? (2) Is it plausible to see such long-term contraception as serving Mindy's long-term interests and, perhaps, as even maximizing her freedom? (3) Would surgical sterilization (tubal ligation), which would permanently prevent pregnancy, be a preferable option given Mindy G.'s parents' concern with her well-being after their death?

CASE 21

Refusal of Life-Sustaining Treatment by a Minor [2, 6]

Charlie R. is an 11-year-old boy who suffers from lymphoma with a prognosis of six months to live. The oncologist has indicated that the condition is terminal and that aggressive chemotherapy can be done, but its results would be at best a three-month to six-month extension of his life. Charlie is also compromised by a neurological disease that he has had for several years. The neurological disease will eventually make it impossible for him to walk, talk, use his hands effectively, or control his excretory functions. Already his speech is slurred, and he cannot hold a pencil. Even without the lymphoma, the prognosis for him because of the neurological disease is death by age 18 at the latest. Charlie has been raised in a strong religious environment, and his belief in God has been an important comforting factor in the course of his disease. He has accepted his disease and his impending death after having the facts fully explained to him. He has said that he is ready to "go to God," and he does not want the chemotherapy. His father has consulted with his local parish priest, who says that the Catholic Church requires that in such cases chemotherapy be used because it is seen as therapeutic and not as merely prolonging the dying process. As a result of this consultation the father decides to override Charlie's decision and agrees to the chemotherapy.

(1) Is chemotherapy genuinely therapeutic in this case? (2) Should minors of Charlie's age be permitted to participate in decisions of this magnitude? (3) Whose decision, the father's or the child's, should be decisive?

CASE 22

Depression and Autonomy [2, 6]

John Q. is a 56-year-old male with a wife and two grown children. He has just suffered his third heart attack in five years, and his cardiologist, Dr. Y., has told him that he must have bypass surgery if he is going to live. Dr. Y. has also told him that because of the already existent damage to the heart muscles he will be a semi-invalid for the rest of his life even with the surgery. John Q. had been an active businessman until his first attack, and he has resentfully had to cut back on his activity since that attack. Now the possibility of extensive surgery and living as a semi-invalid is too much for him to bear. He goes into a depressed state and refuses the surgery, saying that he is "tired of being sick" and that life holds no meaning for him any longer. He is adamant about not having the surgery. The family asks for a psychiatric consultation, and Dr. Y. supports the idea because he believes that the psychiatrist might be able to talk John Q. into the surgery. The psychiatrist says the depression obviously indicates that John Q. is incapable of making a rational judgment and that the family and Dr. Y. should make the decision and ignore the patient's wishes.

(1) Does depression after hearing "bad news" automatically indicate that a patient is incompetent to make decisions regarding treatment? (2) Is it the consulting psychiatrist's role to try to talk the patient into doing what the attending physician wants to do? (3) How can the family serve the best interests of the patient in this situation?

CASE 23

Suicide and Pain Control [2, 6]

Beverly S., a 67-year-old female, is suffering the terminal stages of breast cancer with metastases to the bone. The bone pain has become a major problem in the management of her disease. She is cared for at home by her husband, a daughter, and a nurse from a home health service. She has been troubled so much by the pain that she talks frequently of suicide. She has even made three suicide attempts. After the third attempt, which was almost successful, a health-care counselor was called. In the ensuing discussions, it is determined that Beverly S.'s physician is probably not paying sufficient attention to her pain medication needs. When it is suggested that she might want to change to another physician in the area who is well known for her ability to control pain in cancer patients, Beverly S. replies that she does not want to offend her current physician. Eventually, she agrees to contact the other physician, who begins to care for her immediately. She dies, relatively pain free, about six weeks later.

(1) Was intervention in Beverly S.'s suicide attempts appropriate? (2) Should health-care counselors encourage patients to explore alternatives with other physicians, or will such encouragement tend to undermine the trust patients have in their physicians? Are patient trust and loyalty to the physician important elements in fostering the patient's well-being?

CASE 24

Physician Disagreement Regarding a Patient's Wishes [2, 6]

John H., a 59-year-old male, has been diagnosed as having cancer, the primary site of which is the pancreas. His condition is rapidly deteriorating. John H. has requested that he not be resuscitated if he should go into cardiac arrest. He has also stated that he wishes no further treatment. Dr. W., who is John H.'s personal physician, and Dr. R., the oncologist in the case, agree that he should not be resuscitated, and "Do not resuscitate" is written on his chart. However, when John H. begins to experience severe internal bleeding, he asks his physicians if they can do something. Dr. W. does not want to take measures to stop the bleeding, in keeping with John H.'s request for no further treatment. Dr. R. sees the request "to do something" as taking precedence over the earlier request for no additional treatment. If they do not act quickly to stop the internal bleeding, John H. will die as a result of blood loss.

(1) When the personal physician and the attending specialist disagree, who should decide the course of treatment? (2) When a patient who is in a great deal of pain, weak, and close to death makes a request that seems at odds with a decision he made when he may have been more fully autonomous, which request should guide those caring for him?

CASE 25

Honoring the Living Will [2, 6, 7]

Esther K., a 65-year-old woman with a long history of diabetes, has been diagnosed as having pancreatic cancer. At the time of diagnosis, she refused all aggressive therapies and later wrote a "living will," in which she stated clearly that she did not want any "extraordinary means" used to prolong her life. She specified the "extraordinary means" as chemotherapy, respirators, or resuscitation efforts. Three months after diagnosis, Esther K. was admitted to the hospital in a confused state with discoloration on her foot and some evidence of necrotic tissue on the top of her foot. Observation over the next couple of days revealed that the necrosis had spread, and the surgeon, Dr. P., diagnosed gangrene. Dr. P. wanted to remove the foot before the gangrene spread. Esther K. was still somewhat confused but nonetheless agreed to the surgery. The family was very upset with Dr. P. for suggesting the surgery and for considering her competent to give consent. The family thinks that in the spirit of the "living will" she would not want the surgery, which would fall into the class of "extraordinary means." Furthermore, the family thinks that Esther K. is too confused to give reflective consent, and this may be borne out by the fact that the patient whispered to the nurse that she consented only because she was afraid Dr. P. would no longer take care of her and might order her out of the hospital.

(1) How specific must a "living will" be in order for it to be morally decisive? (2) Is there a danger of assuming that a consent is valid merely because it coincides with what the physician wishes to do? (3) What weight should be given to the family's judgment in this case?

CASE 26

Discriminating among Life-Sustaining Therapies [2, 6, 7]

Shirley W. is a 26-year-old female, unmarried with no dependents. She has reached the end stage of leukemia, has accepted her impending death, and has told her physician that she wishes to have no heroic measures used to preserve her life, although she also wishes to be kept comfortable. Her physician, Dr. Q., wants to honor her request but is concerned with her rapidly falling platelet count. The lower the platelet count, the greater the chance of hemorrhage. The physician does not know whether to interpret possible platelet transfusions as "heroic measures." On the one hand, a hemorrhage would cause Shirley W. to die soon, and a transfusion would extend the dying process. On the other hand, if the hemorrhage occurred in the mouth, the death would be very uncomfortable because the patient would choke. If the latter were allowed to happen, Dr. Q.'s promise to keep the patient comfortable would be broken.

Not knowing quite how to proceed, Dr. Q. consults with the staff and as a result offers the patient the following mode of treatment. If a hemorrhage were to occur in the mouth, the patient would be given platelets as a comfort-producing measure. Thus the platelets would be seen as serving a palliative function in keeping with the patient's desire to be kept comfortable and would not be seen as a heroic measure whose primary function is to prolong life. However, if the hemorrhage were to occur in some other part of the body, the priorities would be reversed, the platelets would be seen as heroic measures, and they would not be given. Shirley W. agreed to this approach and died two days later as the result of a cerebral hemorrhage.

(1) Is the concept of "heroic measures" a useful one for purposes of ethical analysis? If so, how should one determine "heroic measures" in general? (2) Did Dr. Q handle this situation in an appropriate manner?

CASE 27

Refusing Life-Sustaining Treatment [6, 7]

Rita M., a 78-year-old female, has suffered from chronic obstructive pulmonary disease for about twenty years. She comes to the hospital in crisis about once a year and spends some time on a respirator. Currently, she is a resident of a nursing home where there is decent care for residents but little in the way of diversionary activity. Rita M. says that she is bored there most of the time. She seems decently attached to her son, but he cannot visit her frequently because he lives some distance from the nursing home. Another crisis occurs, and she is admitted to the hospital. This crisis, however, is worse than usual, and Rita M. is told that she will have to remain on a respirator for the rest of her life. The attending physician, Dr. E., informs her that a tracheotomy can make the respirator dependency more comfortable and that she can then return to the nursing home to live out the rest of her life. After several days, Rita M. informs Dr. E. that she does not want to have the tracheotomy and that she wants to be removed from the respirator and allowed to die. Dr. E., who is concerned about this decision, develops the following options in consultation with the house staff who accompany him on rounds: (1) the patient could have the tracheotomy and return to the nursing home; (2) the patient could be removed from the respirator, and nature would then take its course; (3) the patient could be removed from the respirator and receive morphine injections to alleviate pain when it occurred; or (4) the patient could receive a morphine injection prior to removal from the respirator and subsequent injections as needed. Dr. E. presented these options to Rita M., who chose the fourth one. She was subsequently given the injection and extubated. She died twenty hours later.

(1) Is this a case of suicide? Is this a case of euthanasia? (2) Was Rita M.'s refusal of treatment based on her assessment of what constitutes an acceptable quality of life?

CASE 28

Is Nutrition Expendable? [6, 7]

Mildred D., a 78-year-old woman, suffers from diabetes, which has been controlled largely by diet. She has a history of heart disease and has suffered two heart attacks. She has now had a stroke, which has rendered her semicomatose and paralyzed. She must be fed through an NG tube, and the sustenance that she receives in this way is the only thing that keeps her going. Mildred D. has previously indicated to her family that in such a circumstance she would not want to be resuscitated. Her condition is slowly deteriorating, but it looks as though the dying process will be a long one. It seems that she will never return from the twilight zone in which she now resides. Angiography indicates that a substantial portion of the brain has been destroyed by the stroke. Her three children want to stop the tube feedings, but the physician objects that it is unethical to "starve" a patient so that she will die sooner.

(1) Is it morally legitimate to withhold nutrition in this case? (2) Does the family have the right to make such a decision for the patient? (3) Should the refusal of resuscitation be considered an indicator that the patient would also refuse nutrition?

CASE 29

Neonatal Care and the Problem of Uncertainty [7]

Bobbie C. is now six months old. He was born prematurely with a birth weight of 800 grams and had multiple problems from the beginning. Bobbie developed Hyaline Membrane disease due to his undeveloped lungs and the need for a respirator. He also developed rickets. A CAT scan revealed some calcium deposits in the brain that might or might not compromise his mental functions. Within the first month, Bobbie developed thrombocytopenia (low platelet count), for which he was given transfusions. He now suffers from a depression of his immunological system, the cause of which may be AIDS contracted through the blood transfusions. He shows little interest in eating, and all attempts to bottle feed him have failed after a couple of days. His health-care costs are being supported by Medicaid, and they are estimated to be in the neighborhood of $550,000 for his six months of hospitalization. Now the health-care staff and the attending physician are considering the possibility of a bone marrow transplant to deal with the thrombocytopenia and the immunosuppression. The chances of success in an infant this small are minimal, and the procedure is largely experimental in infants having this condition. If the transplant is successful, it will only alleviate one of his many problems.

(1) In view of the many uncertainties in this case, what is the proper treatment decision? (2) Should society be expected to shoulder such an expense for an infant who is so physiologically and, perhaps, mentally compromised? (3) Do the parents have a right to reject further aggressive therapies?

CASE 30

Anencephalic Newborns, Organ Donation, and Social Policy [7]

It is estimated that 2000 to 3000 babies are born in the United States each year with anencephaly, the total or almost total absence of the cerebral hemispheres. Many of these infants are stillborn; the prognosis for those born alive is that they will live for only a few hours, days, or weeks. Although the organ systems of some anencephalic infants are underdeveloped, there are many cases in which organs (e.g., a heart or kidneys) could be transplanted to other infants whose lives might thereby be saved. Some parents of anencephalic infants would undoubtedly consent to organ donation as a way of creating some redeeming value out of a tragic situation. Still, numerous reservations have been expressed about the idea of transplanting the organs of anencephalic infants, and at present there is no legal mechanism through which organ donation can be accomplished.

(1) Is it disrespectful, unfair, or otherwise immoral to transplant the organs of an anencephalic infant? (2) Should we adopt a social policy that would permit (with parental consent) harvesting the organs of an anencephalic infant? (3) If an anencephalic infant is stillborn, would it be justifiable to attempt resuscitation purely for the purpose of keeping organs intact until they can be harvested? (4) If it is justifiable to harvest the organs of an anencephalic infant, would it be justifiable to harvest the organs of someone in a persistent vegetative state?

CASE 31

A Brain-Dead Mother Gives Birth [7, 8]

Rosa J. suffered a fatal seizure while she was twenty-three weeks pregnant. After the seizure, Rosa J. was hooked to life-support systems but was declared brain-dead the next day. She was kept on life-support systems for nine weeks, however, until she gave birth to a healthy baby girl by cesarean section. During this time the physicians used steroids to help the lungs of the fetus to mature and monitored fetal growth with ultrasound examinations. Rosa J. was fed intravenously and given antibiotics for infections when necessary. After the birth, the woman's life-support systems were disconnected. The baby was given an excellent chance to survive, although she weighed only three pounds. From the time of the seizure, all decisions about Rosa J. and the fetus she was carrying were made by physicians in consultation with Rosa J.'s family.

(1) Should Rosa J. have been kept on life-support systems for nine weeks after being declared brain-dead simply in order to give the child she was carrying a better chance to survive? (2) Was Rosa J. being used merely as a means to others' ends? (3) Is someone who is brain-dead a "person" and, therefore, on a Kantian account an individual who cannot be used merely as a means to others' ends?

CASE 32

RU 486 and Social Policy [8]

RU 486, a drug developed in France, functions to terminate early pregnancy. In most cases, when the drug is taken in repeated oral doses within ten days of a missed menstrual period, menses is induced and pregnancy is terminated. There are some minor side effects (e.g., heavier bleeding, nausea, and fatigue) but no apparent long-term bad effects. Worries about safety aside, RU 486 has been warmly endorsed by right-to-choose forces. If the drug were to become legally available in the United States, it would largely "privatize" abortion decisions. However, right-to-life forces are bitterly opposed to the legal availability of RU 486. They refer to the drug as a "human pesticide" and denounce its employment as "chemical warfare on the unborn."

(1) If concerns about safety can be adequately addressed, should RU 486 be legally available in the United States? Would any restrictions be appropriate? (2) Would easy access to RU 486 provide a disincentive to responsible birth control and/or encourage uncritical, automatic decisions to abort?

CASE 33

Maternal PKU and Fetal Welfare [8]

Martha J., a 23-year-old female, was born with PKU (phenylketonuria), an enzyme deficiency that prevents the metabolization of phenylalanine. Children born with PKU are ordinarily placed on a special low-phenylalanine diet for at least the first five years of their life. Although the diet is necessary to prevent severe retardation, it is very burdensome, not only because normal foods are very limited but also because the main source of protein is a bad-tasting "medical food." Since Martha J. was placed on this special diet in her childhood, she does not suffer from retardation.

Martha J. is four-months pregnant. Although her inability to metabolize phenylalanine is no longer a problem for her own well-being, there is a problem for the fetus she is carrying. Unless Martha J. maintains the same low-phenylalanine diet throughout the course of her pregnancy, her fetus is at grave risk for severe retardation, microcephaly, congenital heart disease, and other disorders. Martha J.'s religious beliefs have motivated her to decide against abortion. Nevertheless, she is ambivalent about her pregnancy, because she is unmarried and depressed by the breakdown of her relationship with the child's father. She is also finding it very difficult to adhere to the same dietary restrictions that she found so oppressive in her childhood. Dr. R., the obstetrician who is caring for Martha J., has repeatedly emphasized the importance of adhering to the prescribed diet, but Martha J. acknowledges that she has been inconstant in doing so.

(1) Should Dr. R. encourage Martha J. to reconsider the possibility of abortion? (2) If Martha J. is resolved to carry her fetus to term, how should Dr. R. deal with the fact that she is not maintaining the prescribed diet? (3) If all else fails, should Dr. R. seek a court order that would place Martha J. in a supervised setting where dietary restrictions could be enforced?

CASE 34

Prenatal Diagnosis and Sex Selection [8, 9]

A 32-year-old woman, Lisa B., comes to the prenatal diagnostic center of a major hospital. She is intent on arranging for chorionic villi sampling (CVS) in order to determine the sex of the fetus she is carrying. A genetic counselor explains to her that the Center has an established policy against making prenatal diagnosis (whether CVS or amniocentesis) available for purposes of sex selection. The genetic counselor, in defending the policy, tells her that there is a collective sense at the Center that abortion purely on grounds of sex selection is both morally and socially problematic.

Lisa B. proceeds to explain her situation. She and her husband already have three children, all of whom are girls. They want very much to have a male child but, for economic reasons, are determined to have no more than one more child. Indeed, if they had a boy among their three children, they would not even consider having a fourth. They feel so strongly about this fourth child being a boy that if they cannot gain assurance that it is a male they will elect abortion. Lisa B. insists that it is unfair for the Center to deny her access to prenatal diagnosis.

(1) Should the Center consider this case an exceptional one and make CVS available? (2) Would the Center be well advised to develop a different policy regarding the availability of prenatal diagnosis for purposes of sex selection?

CASE 35

Sickle-Cell Disease and a Question of Paternity [9]

Harry B. is a 1-year-old black male who has been admitted to the hospital in extreme distress and pain. Hematology has discovered that Harry is suffering from sickle-cell crisis. Harry is the first child born in this marriage. Sickle-cell disease is genetic in origin and is passed on in an autosomal recessive pattern of inheritance. This means that for the child to be born with the disease, both parents must either have the disease or be carriers (with a recessive trait). The offspring cannot inherit the disease from one carrier parent, although the child of such a parent might be a carrier. The hospital initiates treatment for Harry, a treatment he will have to undergo every time he goes into crisis. At the physicians' suggestion, the parents undergo a screening blood test to determine their carrier status. The results from the laboratory indicate that the mother is a carrier of the sickle-cell trait but that her husband is not. This means it is virtually certain the husband cannot be Harry's father, although Harry was born after the couple had been married about two years.
(1) Was it necessary for the hospital to run the screening tests on the parents? Did the screening tests assist in the treatment of the child? (2) Should the results of the tests be communicated to the parents, thereby jeopardizing their young marriage?

CASE 36

Children at Risk for Huntington's Chorea [9]

Marcia C. is a 38-year-old female who has just been diagnosed with Huntington's chorea, an autosomal dominant genetic disease whose symptoms first emerge (ordinarily) sometime between the ages of 30 and 50. Because her father was a victim of Huntington's chorea, Marcia C. had known since she was a teenager that she was at 50 percent risk for the disease. But now her worst fears have been confirmed. Like her father before her, she can expect an extended period of progressive physical and mental deterioration leading inevitably to death in ten to fifteen years. Although Marcia C. is deeply distressed, and experiences bouts of depression, her mental capacities appear to be essentially uncompromised at the present time.
One of Marcia C.'s principal concerns is the well-being of her children, a girl 10 years old and a boy 8 years old. If Marcia C. had not inherited the disease from her father, her own children would not have been at risk, but now it is clear that each of her children is at 50 percent risk for the disease. A genetic counselor has told Marcia C. and her husband that it is very likely that a reliable presymptomatic test for Huntington's chorea will soon be available. Thus it would be possible to determine if Marcia C.'s children have inherited the disease. Neither Marcia C. nor her husband regret the fact that they had decided to have children, but Marcia C. feels that she has a special obligation to decide with her husband (before her mental powers become too badly compromised) what is best for her children. Should the children be tested when the presymptomatic test becomes available? If so, should they be informed of the results? Or perhaps the testing should be postponed, thus allowing the children to decide for themselves when they are grown whether or not to have the testing done. When the genetic counselor is asked what should be done, the counselor responds that it is for Marcia C. and her husband to decide.

(1) What course of action is in the best interests of Marcia C.'s children? (2) Should the genetic counselor have adopted a more "directive" approach in this case?

CASE 37

A Feminist Sperm Bank [9]

The Oakland (California) Feminist Women's Health Center is a sperm bank that was founded in order to make AID (artificial insemination by donor) available in a manner that is consistent with feminist ideals. Although genetic and medical screening is provided, the keynote of the Center's operation is the fact that no *social* screening of applicants is done. Lesbians and unmarried women are expressly invited, along with more traditional candidates for AID, to make use of the Center's services. In addition, neither standards of economics nor standards of intelligence are employed to exclude applicants, and racial matching is not done.

(1) Is the operational philosophy of this sperm bank morally sound? (2) Should a sperm bank be held accountable to society for a social screening of its applicants for AID? If so, what factors would be sufficient to disqualify an applicant?

CASE 38

Patient Responsibility [2, 10]

Brian B., a 57-year-old male, has been a patient of Dr. L.'s for thirty years. Every time he has come to Dr. L. for assistance, Dr. L. has inquired about his smoking habits and has repeatedly advised him to curtail his smoking. Despite repeated warnings, Brian B. has continued his heavy smoking, even after developing signs of emphysema in his early fifties. Now at age 57, Brian B. has developed lung cancer. He is very angry because the cancer was not detected earlier so that effective treatment could have been given, and he blames Dr. L. Now he has become very passive in the treatment decisions for the cancer. He first tells Dr. L. to decide whether to initiate treatment. When the physician refuses to make the decision, Brian B. tells his wife and two children to make the decision. The family does not know what to do as Brian B. sinks more and more into a depressed state.

(1) What is Brian B.'s responsibility for contracting the cancer? (2) What is Brian B.'s responsibility for his depressed state? (3) Can Brian B. morally surrender his role in the decision-making process leading to treatment?

CASE 39

Justice, Mental Retardation, and Public Policy [5, 10]

State representative Amanda S. has introduced a state bill that calls for the establishment of community-based homes for the care and education of the mentally retarded. The bill would provide one home for every fifteen persons presently institutionalized in five state institutions for the mentally retarded. The present annual cost of maintaining the five institutions is 90 million dollars. Providing the new kind of care for the present institutionalized population of 8,000 is expected to cost about $112 million annually.

Amanda S. argues that the mentally retarded who are presently in the five state institutions live in antiquated buildings lacking basic human necessities and amenities. Many of them are unclothed, spending their days huddled in dark, drab rooms, supervised by an overworked staff, many of whom have no professional training. She contends that justice requires that the mentally retarded be taken out of such subhuman surroundings and given at least a minimal chance for a "normal" life.

A physician, Dr. M., testifying before the House of Representatives, argues that the money required to make the change could be used more efficiently to provide health care for three groups: normal or more nearly normal children, pregnant women, and individuals potentially engaged in productive labor. He argues that a great deal of mental retardation can be eliminated through prenatal diagnosis, which would cost about $400 per case for Down's syndrome, compared to the suggested $14,000 needed for each mentally retarded individual annually in the proposed facilities and $11,250 in the present facilities. Even if some of those presently institutionalized might be gainfully employed if they were in the proposed high-quality community homes, the savings from spending the funds on detection rather than on more expensive forms of institutionalized care are enormous.

(1) Should the proposed bill be enacted into law? (2) Do the mentally retarded have a "right" to lead a life as "normal" as possible given their limitations?

CASE 40

Justice, Kidney Dialysis, and a Mentally Retarded Boy [5, 6, 7, 10]

Joey C. is a 13-year-old retarded boy living in a state-supported home for the mentally retarded. He has no relatives. Joey is suffering from uremic poisoning. Ordinarily someone in Joey's condition would be treated by dialysis three times a week. If Joey does not receive dialysis treatments, he will die. Joey is examined by four kidney experts, all of whom decide against dialysis. They give two reasons for their decision. (1) Joey will not understand the need for the therapy; he will consider the needles and the frequent confinements to the machine as torture, and, as a result, he will be unmanageable. (2) The state institution cannot provide Joey with the necessary hygienic and dietary care required for dialysis. The physicians conclude that the alternative to adopt for Joey is a slow, easy death.

Several employees of the institution protest and argue that Joey should not simply be allowed to die but should be given dialysis treatments. They offer the following reasons: (1) Retardation should not be a criterion for dialysis. (2) Any form of therapy can be perceived as a form of torture by a patient, depending on how the health professionals in charge handle the patient. (3) Other retarded children on dialysis have often been model patients. In fact, retarded young adults are sometimes perceived as overly compliant, meticulously following orders about their care.

(1) When a child has no parents or close relatives and is not competent to understand what is at issue in a life or death decision, who should make the decision for the child? Physicians? The courts? A guardian appointed by the courts? (2) Is severe mental retardation a morally relevant criterion when decisions are made about the use of expensive medical resources?

CASE 41

Determining the Quality of Life [6, 7, 10]

George K. is a 25-year-old male who is unmarried and has no dependents. Medicaid supports him in his health-care needs, which are considerable since he suffers from muscular dystrophy. George K. is totally paralyzed and therefore confined to bed. In addition to being quadriplegic, he cannot speak, and he is respirator dependent through a tracheotomy. Ordinarily he resides in a nursing home, but periodically he must be brought to the intensive care unit of a local hospital for crisis care related to the respirator dependency. He has a girl friend who visits him occasionally as well as a mother who visits him regularly. George K. communicates through smiles and raising and lowering his eyebrows. He seems to enjoy watching television and is a great fan of the Dallas Cowboys and the Detroit Tigers.

(1) What assessment should be made of George K.'s quality of life? (2) Should discussions be initiated with George K. about withholding treatment in the case of future crises? (3) Can society afford to support, for long periods of time, individuals who constitute such a drain on health-care resources?

CASE 42

Justice and Abortion Funding [8, 10]

Sara G. is a 35-year-old mother of four children whose husband deserted her about a month after she became pregnant with her fifth child. The age of her four children ranges from 1 year old to 6 years old. She knows nothing about her husband's whereabouts and is currently being supported by welfare payments including Aid to Dependent Children (ADC). Sara G. is less than three months pregnant and wants an abortion. Her reasons are as follows. (1) She does not have the skills to get a job whose earnings will even come close to the welfare payments she receives. If she has to pay for child care from whatever meager wages she could earn, the money left could not support her family at even the subsistence level. So, at least until the children are older, she will be dependent on welfare and ADC. The sums she receives are barely adequate to take care of her present family. Adding another member would mean even further deprivation for her present family. (2) Her welfare caseworker has agreed that when the four children are a bit older, Sara G. will go into a job-training program that will enable her to get a job paying enough to get the family off public assistance and to give her children a better start in life. Sara G. has undergone a battery of psychological tests to help determine what kind of work she should be capable of doing with the right education and training. The social worker and psychological counselor are both confident that Sara G. can do the work necessary to make a good living for herself and her family. Having another child would only postpone the time when Sara G. will be self-supporting, and in the meantime her family would be living at a very inadequate level.

Because Sara G. is on welfare, she must get an authorization from the social work agency for any medical procedure that is not necessitated by an emergency. In cases involving abortion, the final decision is made by a social worker.

(1) Should the social worker authorize the abortion? (2) What moral justification could be advanced to support an authorization? A refusal to authorize the abortion? (3) What social policy should be adopted to deal with such cases?

CASE 43

Justice, Age, and Personal Responsibility [10]

The intensive care unit (ICU) at a local hospital has one available bed. Two patients are in immediate and desperate need of ICU care. The first is Jeffrey O., who is 71 years old and has been severely injured in an automobile accident. Jeffrey O. was in good physical shape prior to the accident and does not suffer from any debilitating condition. However, his present condition is extremely critical due to the accident. The second patient is Donald R., a 22-year-old drug addict whose present equally critical condition is the result of drug use.

(1) Which of the two should receive the ICU bed? (2) Would the answer be different if Donald R. were 71 years old and Jeffrey O. were 22? (3) Suppose Donald R. were not a drug addict but a previously healthy 22 year old severely injured in an automobile accident. And suppose that Jeffrey O. had been admitted to the hospital about an hour before Donald R., but the decision about putting each of them in the ICU is being made at the same time. Who should get the bed?

CASE 44

Justice, Health Care, and Poverty [10]

Amanda R. is 25 years old. Although she holds both a full-time and a part-time job, she has a very low income and does not have any health-care insurance. At the same time, Amanda R.'s income is just high enough to prevent her from qualifying for any government-funded health care such as that provided by Medicaid. While experiencing severe chest pain and difficulty in breathing, Amanda R. goes to the emergency room of a local for-profit hospital. Before she receives any care, clerical personnel in the hospital determine her financial status and the fact that she is uninsured. By the time she is examined, Amanda R.'s chest pains stop, and her breathing difficulties disappear. A medical staff member gives her a cursory examination, which does not include an electrocardiogram, and sends her home, suggesting that she go to her own physician the next day for a more thorough examination. That same night while sleeping, Amanda suffers a massive coronary and dies.

(1) If the medical staff member's decision not to give Amanda R. a more thorough examination and not to admit her for further observation was based on her lack of health-care insurance, can that decision be morally justified? (2) Suppose that Amanda R.'s symptoms had not eased while she was in the emergency room and that the medical staff had decided that Amanda R. did need hospital admittance, observation, and testing. But suppose that instead of admitting her to their hospital, they had sent her by ambulance to a community (not-for-profit) hospital and she had died en route. Would their behavior have been morally acceptable?

CASE 45

Justice, Financial Incentives, and Organ Donations [10]

Many patients who currently undergo dialysis because of end-stage renal disease could dispense with the machines and live a relatively normal life if they were to receive a kidney transplant. However, the supply of cadaver kidneys is severely limited. To meet the need, a member of the U.S. Congress introduces a bill that would provide a tax incentive for "gifts of life." Any individual who donates an organ such as a heart, liver, or kidney, would gain the following financial benefits: (1) a $30,000 deduction on his or her last taxable year and (2) a $30,000 exclusion from estate taxes. In order to qualify for these benefits, the individual's organ would have to be in a condition suitable for transplantation and removed from the cadaver for the purposes of transplantation. If the source of the organ is a dependent, the same tax incentives would be granted to the parents. Since renal dialysis is extremely costly for the United States government, the projected savings are enormous. In addition, those patients who received a transplant could lead a more satisfactory life because they would no longer need dialysis three times a week.

(1) Will the financial incentive affect families' decisions to donate organs in the case of both children and adults who have not expressed any desire to make such a donation? If yes, is this a good reason not to enact the bill into law? (2) Is there something morally questionable about offering significant cash benefits for consent to organ donation? Since poorer individuals with no estate to leave and much lower tax bills would not have the same opportunities to gain financially from organ donation, is the proposed bill unjust?